Gastrointestinal and Hepatic Infections

CHRISTINA SURAWICZ, M.D.
Associate Professor of Medicine
University of Washington
Seattle, Washington
Chief, Gastroenterology,
Harborview Medical Center
Seattle, Washington

ROBERT L. OWEN, M.D.
Professor of Medicine,
Epidemiology and Biostatistics
University of California
San Francisco, California
Chief, Environmental Health and Consultant
in Gastrointestinal Infectious Diseases
Veterans Affairs Medical Center
San Francisco, California

Gastrointestinal and Hepatic Infections

W.B. SAUNDERS COMPANY
A Division of Harcourt Brace & Company

Philadelphia London Toronto Montreal Sydney Tokyo

W.B. SAUNDERS COMPANY
A Division of
Harcourt Brace & Company

The Curtis Center
Independence Square West
Philadelphia, Pennsylvania 19106

Library of Congress Cataloging-in-Publication Data

Gastrointestinal and hepatic infections / [edited by] Christina Surawicz, Robert Owen.—1st ed.

p.   cm.

ISBN 0–7216–4062–1

1. Gastrointestinal system—Infections.   2. Liver—Infections.   3. Biliary tract—Infections.   I. Surawicz, Christina.   II. Owen, Robert.

[DNLM: 1. Gastrointestinal Diseases—diagnosis.
2. Gastrointestinal Diseases—therapy.   3. Infection Control.   4. Liver Diseases—diagnosis.   5. Liver Diseases—therapy.   WI 100 G25825 1995]

RC840.I53G37   1995

616.3′3—dc20
DNLM/DLC   93–15671

Gastrointestinal and Hepatic Infections   ISBN 0–7216–4062–1

Printed in the United States of America.

Last digit is the print number: 9   8   7   6   5   4   3   2   1

I wish to dedicate my efforts in preparing this book to
Roger A. Feldman and Eugene J. Gangarosa,
who awakened my interest
in the epidemiology and clinical consequences of intestinal infectious diseases;
Lloyd L. Brandborg,
who introduced me to
the fascinating and varied morphology and manifestations of intestinal parasites;
Nathaniel F. Pierce,
who encouraged me to
explore basic pathophysiologic mechanisms during our collaborative investigations of *Vibrio cholerae;*
and Richard Wayne La Blue,
a naturalist, inveterate traveler, and patient,
who sacrificed his personal comfort and,
at times, dignity, to help my colleagues and me in our initial understanding
of microsporida as human intestinal pathogens.

ROBERT L. OWEN, M.D.

For Borys and Frida
for their love and support,
and for Jim, Jesse, Joe, and Daniel
with my love,

CHRISTINA SURAWICZ, M.D.

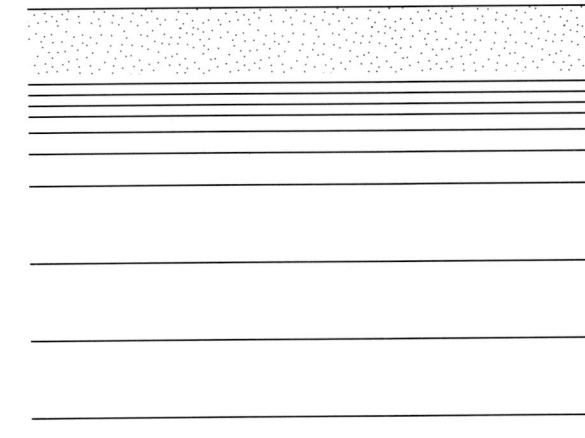

Contributors

PAUL H. BAEHR, M.D.
Senior Fellow, University of Washington and Fred Hutchinson Cancer Research Center, Seattle, Washington; Attending Staff, Fred Hutchinson Cancer Research Center, University of Washington Medical Center, Harborview Medical Center, Pacific Medical Center, Seattle VA Hospital, and Providence Medical Center, Seattle, Washington
Infections of the Esophagus

ROBERT C. BOLLINGER, M.D., M.P.H.
Assistant Professor, Division of Infectious Diseases, Department of Medicine, Johns Hopkins Medical School and Department of International Health, Johns Hopkins School of Hygiene and Public Health, Baltimore, Maryland; Attending Staff, Johns Hopkins Hospital, Baltimore, Maryland
Approach to Gastrointestinal Infection in Immunosuppressed Patients

RALPH T. BRYAN, M.D.
Medical Epidemiologist, National Center for Infectious Diseases, Centers for Disease Control and Prevention, Atlanta, Georgia; Clinical Assistant Professor of Medicine, Emory University School of Medicine, Atlanta, Georgia
Parasitic Infections of the Liver and Biliary Tree

MARCIA IRENE F. CANTO, M.D.
Instructor, Case Western Reserve University, Cleveland, Ohio
Bacterial Infections of the Liver and Biliary System

JOHN H. CROSS, Ph.D.
Professor, Tropical Public Health, Department of Preventive Medicine and Biometrics, Uniformed Services University of the Health Sciences, Bethesda, Maryland
Parasites of the Small Intestine

ANNA MAE DIEHL, M.D.
Associate Professor of Medicine, Johns Hopkins University School of Medicine, Baltimore, Maryland; Gastroenterology Division, Johns Hopkins Hospital, Baltimore, Maryland
Bacterial Infections of the Liver and Biliary System

HERBERT L. DuPONT, M.D.
Mary W. Kelsey Professor of the Medical Sciences, The University of Texas–Houston Medical School (Department of Internal Medicine) and School of Public Health (Center for Infectious Diseases), Houston, Texas; Attending Physician, Hermann Hospital, Methodist Hospital, and M.D. Anderson Cancer Center, Houston, Texas
Traveler's Diarrhea and Foodborne Diseases

CECILIA FENOGLIO-PREISER, M.D.
Mackenzie Professor of Pathology and
Laboratory Medicine, University of Cincinnati
College of Medicine, Cincinnati, Ohio;
Director of Pathology and Laboratory
Medicine, University of Cincinnati Medical
Center, Cincinnati, Ohio
Laboratory Performance in the Diagnosis of Gastro-
intestinal Infections

SCOTT L. FRIEDMAN, M.D.
Associate Professor of Medicine, UCSF School
of Medicine, San Francisco, California;
Attending Physician and Director,
Gastrointestinal Clinic, San Francisco General
Hospital, San Francisco, California
Hepatobiliary Infections in AIDS

J. GORDON FRIERSON, M.D.
Clinical Professor, Department of
Epidemiology and Biostatistics and Department
of Medicine, University of California Medical
Center, San Francisco, California; Medical
Staff, Summit Medical Center, Oakland,
California

ROBERT M. GENTA, M.D., D.T.M.&H.
Associate Professor of Pathology, Medicine, and
Immunology and Microbiology, Baylor College
of Medicine, Houston, Texas; Chief, Anatomic
Pathology, Ben Taub General Hospital; Staff
Pathologist, VA Medical Center; Staff
Pathologist, The Methodist Hospital, Houston,
Texas
Infectious Gastritis

MAE F. GO, M.D.
Assistant Professor, Department of Medicine,
Baylor College of Medicine, Houston, Texas;
Staff Physician; Houston VA Medical Center,
Houston, Texas
Infectious Gastritis

RICHARD W. GOODGAME, M.D.
Associate Professor of Medicine, Baylor College
of Medicine, Houston, Texas; Chief of
Endoscopy, Ben Taub General Hospital,
Houston, Texas
Infectious Gastritis

DAVID Y. GRAHAM, M.D.
Professor of Medicine and Molecular Virology,
Baylor College of Medicine, Houston, Texas;
Chief, Digestive Disease, VA Medical Center,

Houston, Texas; Chief, Gastroenterology
Section, Baylor College of Medicine, Houston,
Texas
Infectious Gastritis

JANE S. GREATOREX, F.I.M.L.S.
Research Technician, Department of Medicine,
Addenbrookes Hospital, Cambridge, England
Evaluation of Diarrhea, Including Molecular Diag-
nostic Methods and Interpretation of Diagnostic Tests

MELVIN B. HEYMAN, M.D., M.P.H.
Associate Professor of Pediatrics and Chief,
Pediatric Gastroenterology and Nutrition,
University of California, San Francisco,
California
Diarrhea in Infants and Children

EDWARD N. JANOFF, M.D.
Associate Professor of Medicine, Infectious
Disease Division, Veterans Affairs Medical
Center, University of Minnesota, Minneapolis,
Minnesota; Attending Staff, Veterans Affairs
Medical Center, University of Minnesota,
Minneapolis, Minnesota
Diarrheal Disease with Viral Enteric Infections in Im-
munocompromised Patients

ABIODUN O. JOHNSON, M.D., F.R.C.P.
Professor of Pediatrics, School of Medicine,
Meharry Medical College, Nashville, Tennessee
Diarrhea in Infants and Children

ALBERT Z. KAPIKIAN, M.D.
Head, Epidemiology Section, Laboratory of
Infectious Diseases, National Institute of
Allergy and Infectious Diseases, National
Institutes of Health, Bethesda, Maryland
Viral Gastroenteritis

NANCY B. KIVIAT, M.D.
Professor, Department of Pathology, University
of Washington, Seattle, Washington
Anal Papillomavirus Infections

RAYMOND S. KOFF, M.D.
Professor of Medicine, University of
Massachusetts Medical School, Worcester,
Massachusetts; Chairman, Department of
Medicine, MetroWest Medical Center,
Framingham, Massachusetts
Diagnosis of Viral Hepatitis

JANE M. KUYPERS, PH.D.
Director, DNA Probe Laboratory, Department of Pathology, University of Washington, Seattle, Washington
Anal Papillomavirus Infections

MYRON M. LEVINE, M.D., D.T.P.H.
Professor and Director, Center for Vaccine Development, University of Maryland School of Medicine, Baltimore, Maryland
The Treatment of Acute Diarrhea

JUDY F. LEW, M.D.
Assistant Clinical Professor of Pediatrics, Georgetown University Medical Center, Washington, D.C.
Gastrointestinal Infections in the Elderly

GEORGE B. McDONALD, M.D.
Professor of Medicine, University of Washington School of Medicine, and Member, Fred Hutchinson Cancer Research Center, Seattle, Washington; Attending Staff, Fred Hutchinson Cancer Research Center, University of Washington Medical Center, Harborview Medical Center, Pacific Medical Center, Veterans Affairs Medical Center, Providence Medical Center, and Swedish Medical Center, Seattle, Washington
Infections of the Esophagus

LYNNE McFARLAND, M.S., PH.D.
Research Assistant Professor, Department of Medicinal Chemistry, School of Pharmacy, University of Washington, Seattle, Washington
Clostridium difficile–Associated Disease

JOHN G. McHUTCHISON, M.D.
Assistant Professor of Medicine, University of California, San Diego, California; Attending Staff, Scripps Clinic and Research Foundation, La Jolla, California
Spontaneous Bacterial Peritonitis

MARCO K. MICHELSON, M.D.
Assistant Professor of Medicine, SUNY at Stony Brook School of Medicine, Stony Brook, New York; Director, AIDS Program, Nassau County Medical Center, East Meadow, New York
Parasitic Infections of the Liver and Biliary Tree

KAREN MIDTHUN, M.D.
Adjunct Assistant Professor, Johns Hopkins University School of Hygiene and Public Health, Department of International Health, Baltimore, Maryland
Viral Gastroenteritis

ROBERT L. OWEN, M.D.
Professor of Medicine, Epidemiology and Biostatistics, University of California, San Francisco, California; Chief, Environmental Health and Consultant in Gastrointestinal Infectious Diseases, Veterans Affairs Medical Center, San Francisco, California
Gastrointestinal Infections in the Elderly

THOMAS C. QUINN, M.D., M.Sc.
Professor of Medicine, Johns Hopkins University School of Medicine, Baltimore, Maryland; Professor of Medicine, Johns Hopkins University Hospital, Baltimore, Maryland
Approach to Gastrointestinal Infection in Immunosuppressed Patients

BRUCE A. RUNYON, M.D.
Professor of Medicine, University of Louisville, Louisville, Kentucky; Medical Director—Liver Transplantation and Director—Liver Service, University of Louisville Medical Center, Louisville, Kentucky
Spontaneous Bacterial Peritonitis

STEPHEN SAVARINO, M.D., M.P.H.
Assistant Professor, Department of Pediatrics, Uniformed Services University of the Health Sciences, Bethesda, Maryland
The Treatment of Acute Diarrhea

JOHN D. SNYDER, M.D.
Associate Professor of Pediatrics, UCSF School of Medicine, San Francisco, California
Diarrhea in Infants and Children

JACK D. SOBEL, M.D.
Professor of Medicine, Wayne State University School of Medicine, Detroit, Michigan; Chief, Section of Infectious Diseases, Harper Hospital, and Chief, Section of Infectious Diseases, Hutzel Hospital, Detroit, Michigan
Fungal Infections of the Gastrointestinal Tract

PAUL E. STEELE, M.D.
Assistant Professor of Pathology and Laboratory Medicine, University of Cincinnati College of Medicine, Cincinnati, Ohio; Associate Director, Diagnostic Immunology, University of Cincinnati Medical Center, Cincinnati, Ohio
Laboratory Performance in the Diagnosis of Gastrointestinal Infections

CHRISTINA M. SURAWICZ, M.D.
Associate Professor of Medicine, University of Washington, Seattle, Washington; Chief, Gastroenterology, Harborview Medical Center, Seattle, Washington
Colorectal Spirochetosis

PHILLIP I. TARR, M.D.
Assistant Professor, University of Washington School of Medicine, Seattle, Washington; Attending Physician, Children's Hospital and Medical Center, Seattle, Washington
Approach to the Patient with Acute Bloody Diarrhea

GRACE M. THORNE, Ph.D.
Assistant Professor of Pediatrics, Harvard Medical School, Boston, Massachusetts; Director, Rapid Diagnostics Program, Children's Hospital, Boston, Massachusetts
Evaluation of Diarrhea, Including Molecular Diagnostic Methods and Interpretation of Diagnostic Tests

JOSÉ A. VAZQUEZ, M.D.
Assistant Professor of Medicine, Wayne State University School of Medicine, Detroit, Michigan
Fungal Infections of the Gastrointestinal Tract

RICHARD A. WILLSON, M.D.
Associate Professor of Medicine, University of Washington, Seattle, Washington; Chief, Hepatology Section, Harborview Medical Center, Seattle, Washington
Treatment of Chronic Viral Hepatitis

LOWELL S. YOUNG, M.D.
Clinical Professor of Medicine, University of California, San Francisco, California; Director, Kuzell Institute for Arthritis and Infectious Diseases, Medical Research Institute, California Pacific Medical Center, San Francisco, California; Chief, Division of Infectious Diseases, California Pacific Medical Center, San Francisco, California
Gastrointestinal Mycobacterial Disease

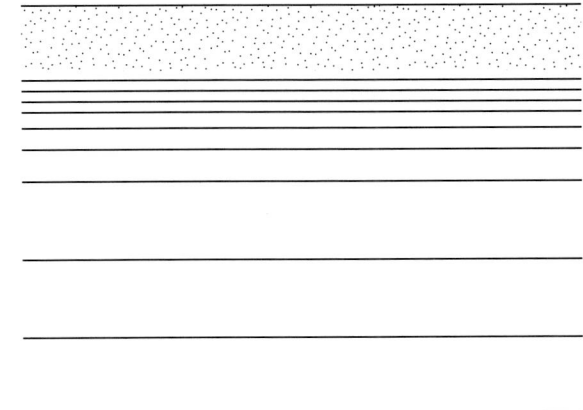

Preface

The manifestations of gastrointestinal and hepatic infections are varied, and infections are increasingly frequent. In the last 10 years, we have recognized new organisms that cause intestinal and hepatic disease in both immunocompetent and immunosuppressed individuals. Prominent examples include *Escherichia coli* O157:H7 infection, parasites such as Microsporida that appear to be major causes of diarrhea in persons with AIDS, and bacillary angiomatosis, also seen with HIV infection. With the occurrence of an ever-increasing population of immunosuppressed individuals, more frequent travel and migration, and population pressures on water treatment and sewer systems, gastrointestinal infections are increasingly common and more varied.

We saw the need for a book on gastrointestinal and hepatic infections that would delineate infectious organisms throughout the gastrointestinal tract and liver organized by clinical syndromes rather than by organisms. This is not an encyclopedic book, yet it is meant to be inclusive and authoritative.

A major challenge in a multiauthored book is to reduce redundancies. We have chosen not to eliminate all overlaps, however, because it is important to make each chapter coherent without reference to other chapters.

Although the book was designed with general internists and gastroenterologists in mind, we believe that it will be of interest to all clinicians faced with diagnosing and managing intestinal or hepatic infections.

CHRISTINA M. SURAWICZ, M.D.
ROBERT L. OWEN, M.D.

Contents

Part 4
Hepatobiliary Disorders

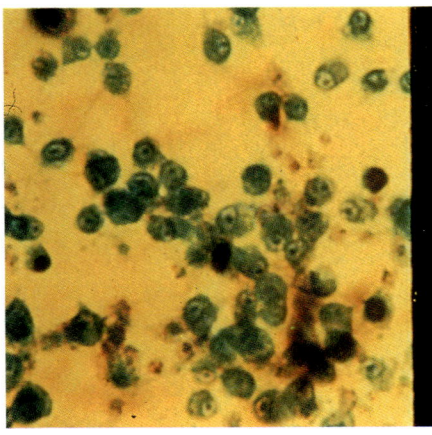

FIGURE 6–1.
Cytopathic effect of cytotoxin from *Clostridium difficile* on tissue culture monolayers. *A*, A monolayer with *C. difficile* cytotoxin and rounded fibroblastic cells; *B*, monolayer with no cytotoxin. SOURCE: Courtesy of Dr Robert Fekety. Dept Infectious Diseases, University of Michigan, Ann Arbor.

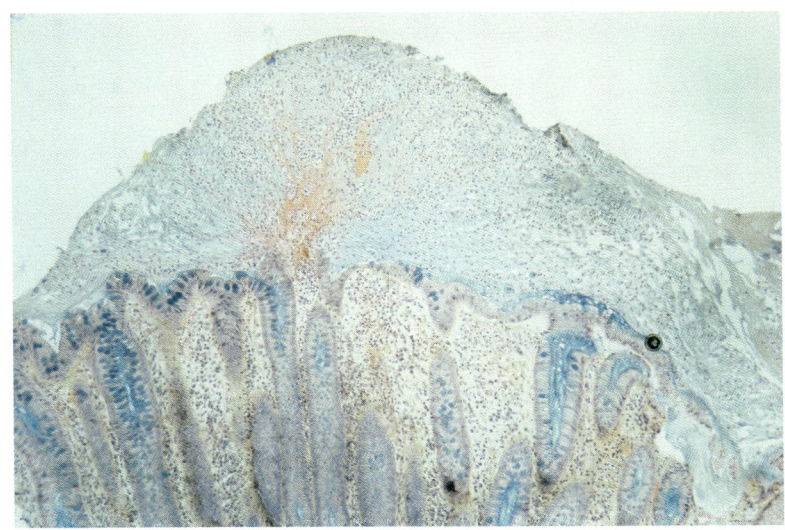

FIGURE 6–3.
Histologic appearance of pseudomembrane. SOURCE: Courtesy of Dr Christina Surawicz. Dept of Medicine, University of Washington, Seattle.

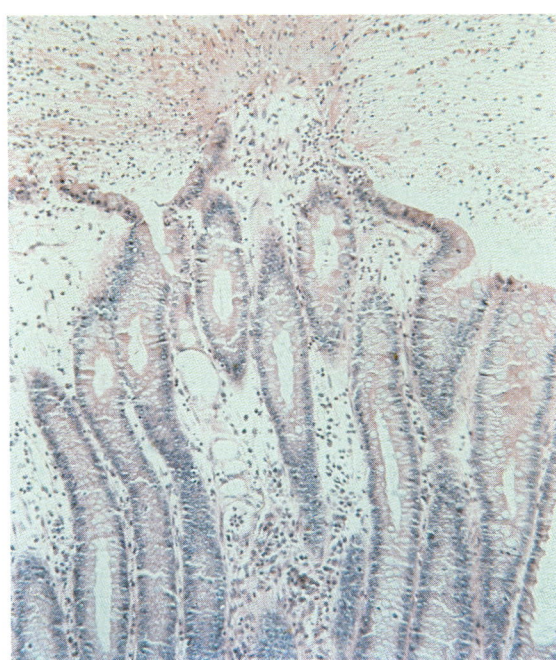

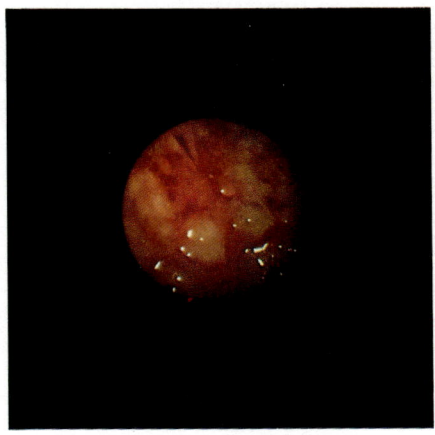

FIGURE 6–2.
Summitlike lesion noted in a patient with *C. difficile* colitis. SOURCE: Courtesy of Dr Christina Surawicz. Dept of Medicine, University of Washington, Seattle.

FIGURE 6–4.
Gross appearance of pseudomembrane in a patient with *C. difficile*–associated pseudomembranous colitis. SOURCE: Courtesy of Dr Christina Surawicz. Dept of Medicine, University of Washington, Seattle.

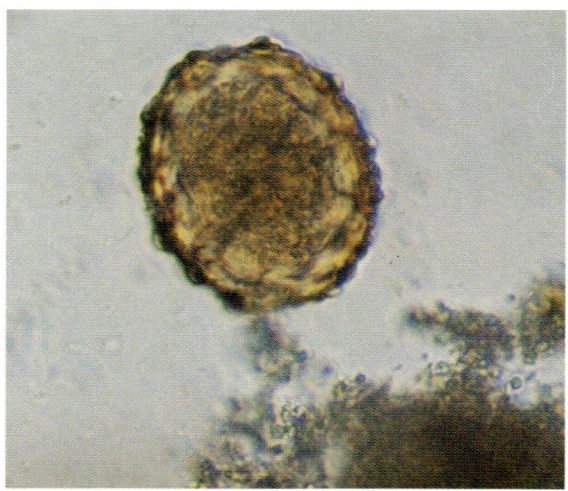

FIGURE 7–1.
Regular fertilized egg of *Ascaris lumbricoides* (55–75 × 35–50 μm).

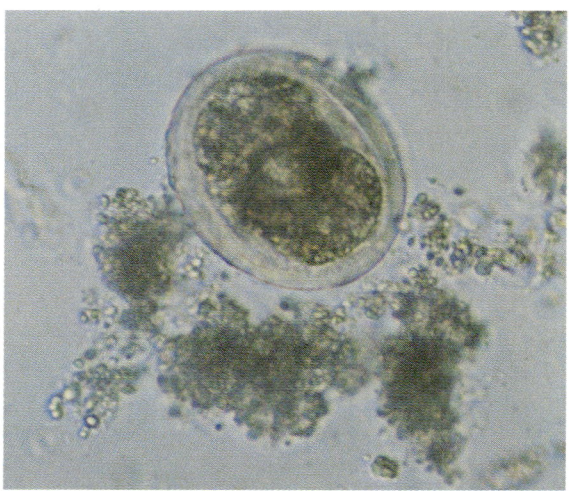

FIGURE 7–2.
Decorticated egg of *Ascaris lumbricoides* (30–40 μm).

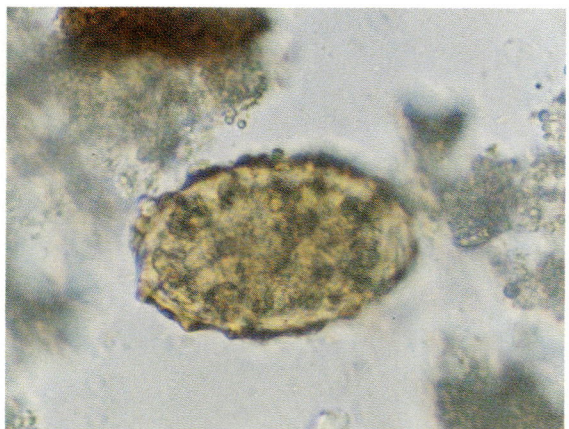

FIGURE 7–3.
Unfertilized egg of *Ascaris lumbricoides* (85 × 45 μm).

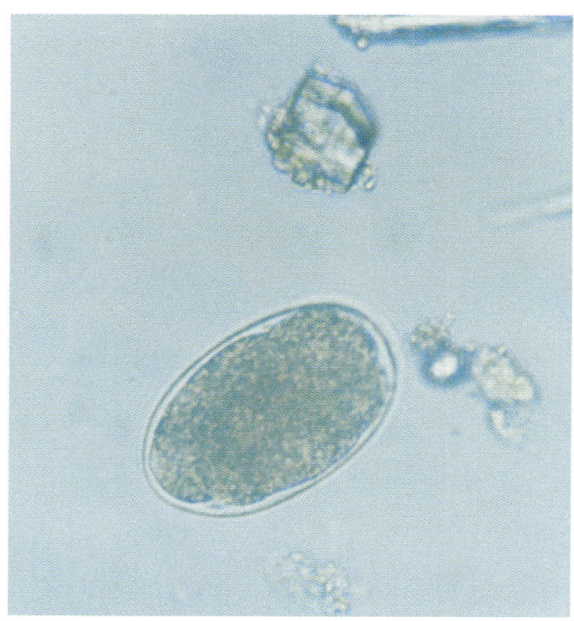

FIGURE 7–4.
Hookworm egg (65 × 40 μm).

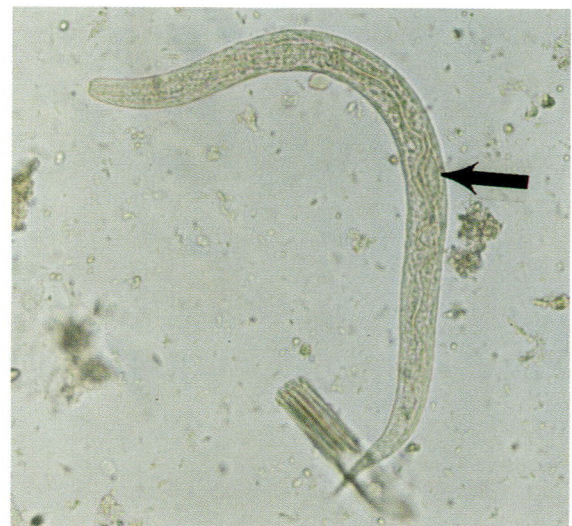

FIGURE 7–5.
Rhabditiform larvae of *Strongyloides stercoralis* (250 × 15 μm); note small buccal capsule and large genital primordium *(arrow).*

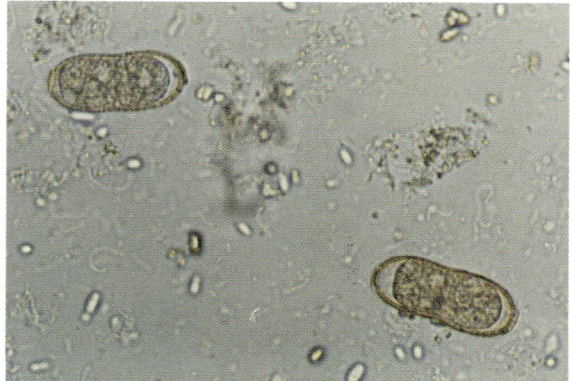

FIGURE 7–7.
Egg of *Capillaria philippinensis* (36–45 × 21 μm); note flattened bipolar plugs.

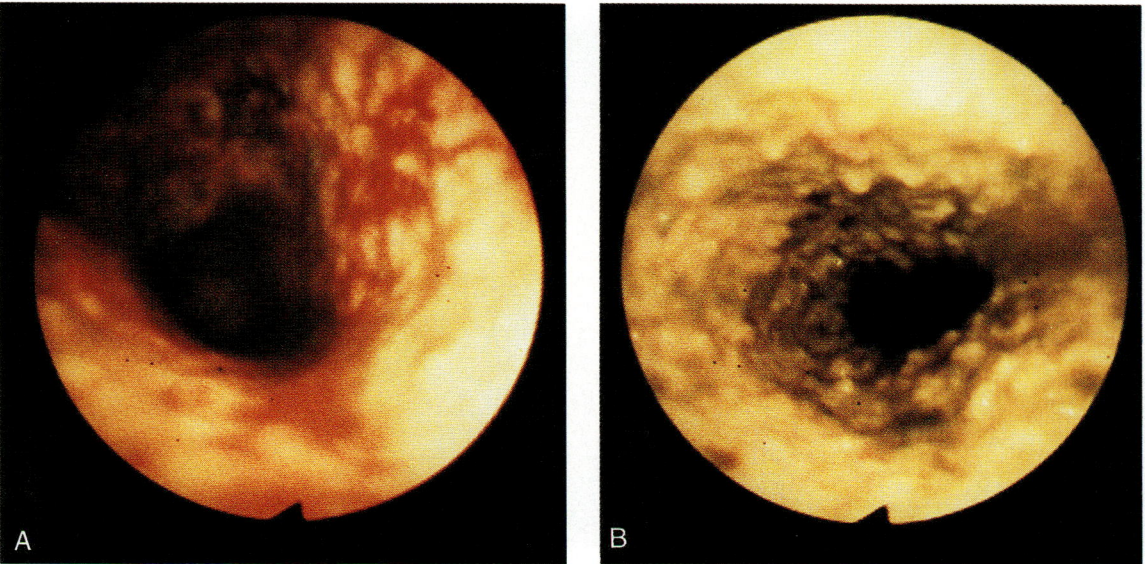

FIGURE 9–2.
A, intense congestion, erythema, and white exudative plaques, which have become confluent in *B*. SOURCE: Kennedy MJ. Regulation of *Candida albicans* populations in the gastrointestinal tract: Mechanisms and significance in GI and systemic candidiasis. Curr Top Med Mycol. 1989;3:315–402.

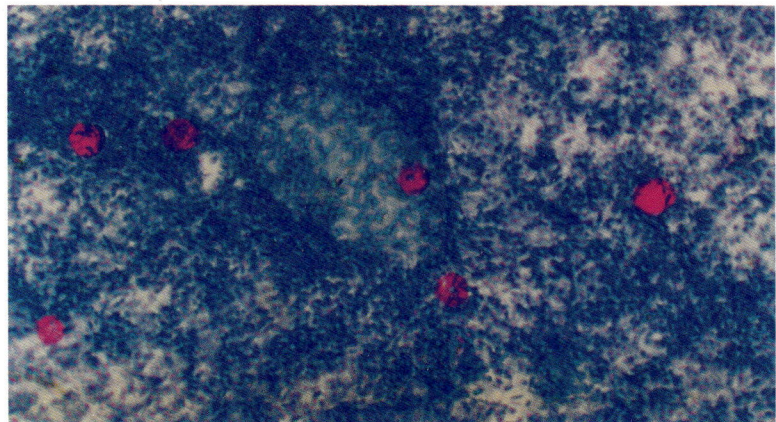

FIGURE 10–8.
Stool sample stained with modified acid-fast method, showing the cryptosporidial oocysts stained in red. SOURCE: Courtesy of John H. Cross, PhD. Dept Preventive Medicine and Biometrics, Uniformed Services University of the Health Sciences, Bethesda MD.

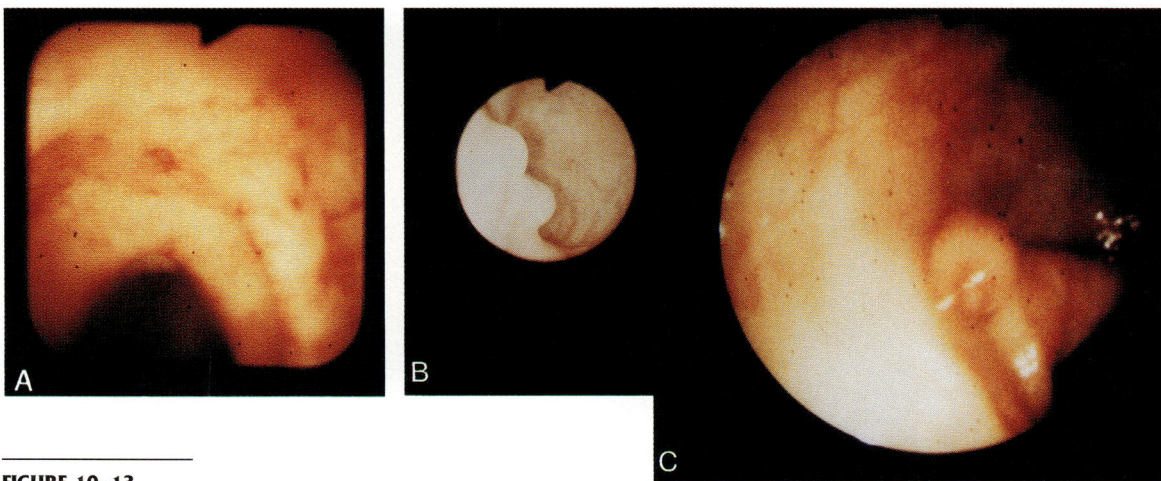

FIGURE 10–13.
Manson's schistosomiasis as seen through the sigmoidoscope. *A*, Scattered hyperemia and petechial hemorrhages in the colon. *B*, Schistosomal rectal varices. *C*, Schistosomal colonic polyp. These patients were all examined in Saudi Arabia. SOURCE: Courtesy of Dr AE Mohamed, Riyadh Armed Forces Hospital, Riyadh, Saudi Arabia.

FIGURE 16–1.

Microscopic appearance of bacillary peliosis hepatis. Photomicrograph of liver biopsy specimen revealing dilated peliotic spaces containing red blood cells. Dark clusters within the stroma or adjacent to vascular lakes are clumps of bacteria. (hematoxylin and eosin, ×500) SOURCE: Courtesy of Dr Linda Ferrell.

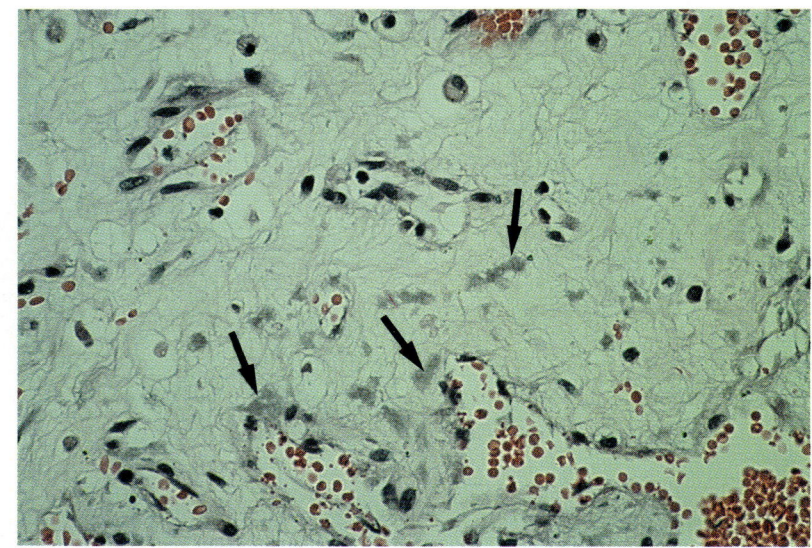

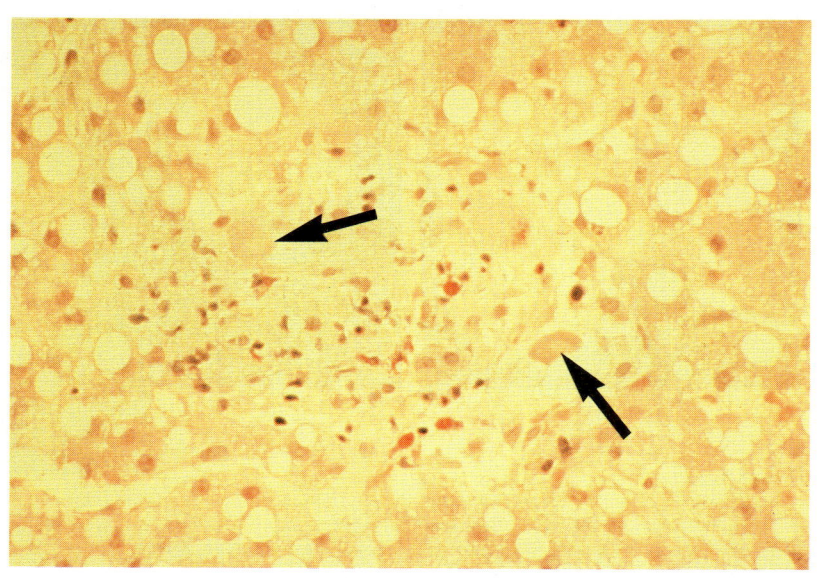

FIGURE 16–2.

Hepatic granuloma in AIDS. Liver biopsy from a patient with AIDS demonstrating a granuloma, without associated microorganisms. Granulomata are frequently identified as a nonspecific finding in patients with AIDS. (hematoxylin and eosin, ×325) SOURCE: Courtesy of Dr Linda Ferrell.

FIGURE 16–3.

Hepatic cytomegalovirus infection. Liver biopsy specimen demonstrating giant cell formation with "owl's eye" appearance, fatty change, and mononuclear infiltration, all typical of hepatic CMV disease. (hematoxylin and eosin, ×250) SOURCE: Courtesy of Dr Linda Ferrell.

Gastrointestinal and Hepatic Infections

The Esophagus

1

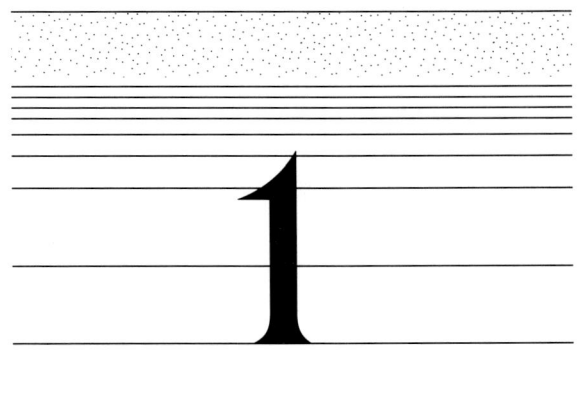

Infections of the Esophagus

PAUL H. BAEHR, M.D.
GEORGE B. McDONALD, M.D.

Infections of the esophagus have become a cause of considerable morbidity over the past decade owing to an increase in the number of individuals with altered immune defenses as a result of human immunodeficiency virus (HIV) infection, organ transplantation, and aggressive chemotherapy for malignant disease. The widespread use of fiberoptic endoscopy has also led to the documentation of opportunistic infections of the esophagus in persons with alcoholism, diabetes, malignancy, and congenital immunodeficiency syndromes. Only rarely do otherwise normal hosts develop candidal or herpes simplex virus (HSV) esophagitis. When organisms or agents other than *Candida* or HSV are found in esophageal lesions, there is almost always an underlying defect in cell-mediated immunity.

CLINICAL SIGNS AND SYMPTOMS

The presenting signs and symptoms of the five most common infectious causes of esophagitis have been compiled from 57 journal articles (Table 1–1). This information provides a framework for discussion and offers a guide for the clinician in determining an approach toward a correct diagnosis.

Difficult or Painful Swallowing

Dysphagia, or difficulty in swallowing, and odynophagia, pain on swallowing, are the most common presenting symptoms of infectious esophagitis (see Table 1–1). These symptoms were reported in 59 to 95% of patients with documented esophageal infection. In some patients, pain is brought on by swallowing liquids or solids, but in others the pain is a constant cervical or retrosternal discomfort that worsens with swallowing. An absence of pain cannot be used as evidence against infection, since up to 40% of patients with proven infections have no pain referable to the esophagus (see Table 1–1).

Although in many cases infection is the direct cause of painful esophageal ulcerations, acid-pepsin reflux onto infected, ulcerated mucosa also causes symptoms. Reflux of gastric contents occurs frequently throughout the day, and although normal individuals readily clear acid from the esophagus through salivary neutralization and peristalsis,[1] patients with an inflamed esophagus fail to clear acid efficiently.[2, 3] It is our impression that persistent acid-pepsin reflux plays an important role in the constant retrosternal pain, painful swallowing, and large size of infectious ulcers. This impression is sup-

3

TABLE 1–1. PRESENTING SIGNS AND SYMPTOMS OF PATIENTS WITH ESOPHAGEAL INFECTION

SIGNS AND SYMPTOMS	CANDIDA n = 177	HSV n = 48	CMV n = 69	TB n = 81	HIV n = 41
Difficult or painful swallowing	111 (63%)	38 (79%)	41 (59%)	52 (64%)	39 (95%)
Abdominal pain	8 (5%)	1 (2%)	13 (19%)	1 (1%)	2 (5%)
Nausea or vomiting	9 (5%)	7 (15%)	29 (42%)	1 (1%)	1 (2%)
Oral lesions	66 (37%)	14 (29%)	—	5 (6%)	11 (27%)
Gastrointestinal bleeding	4 (2%)	8 (17%)	7 (10%)	3 (4%)	6 (15%)
Weight loss	2 (1%)	1 (2%)	17 (25%)	28 (35%)	11 (27%)
Diarrhea	—	1 (2%)	14 (20%)	—	8 (20%)
Fever	3 (2%)	2 (4%)	14 (20%)	16 (20%)	5 (12%)
Rash	2 (1%)	—	—	—	20 (49%)
Sore throat	5 (3%)	—	—	—	16 (39%)
Cough	—	—	—	18 (22%)	—
Asymptomatic	41 (23%)	—	—	—	—
References	5,8–12, 16, 25, 32, 33, 46, 48, 49, 63, 75, 92	5, 13, 33, 51, 115, 117, 118, 119, 121, 125	4, 5, 17, 31, 33, 145, 161	18, 22, 23, 244, 245, 248, 257, 259, 260	14, 19, 24, 26–28, 76, 204–206

KEY: CMV = cytomegalovirus, HIV = human immunodeficiency virus–associated idiopathic esophageal ulcers, HSV = herpes simplex virus, TB = *Mycobacterium tuberculosis*.
SOURCE: Data are compiled from clinical information contained in 57 published articles.

ported by an improvement in the symptoms of patients with cytomegalovirus (CMV) esophagitis after the initiation of antireflux and acid-suppressive therapy and by the exacerbation of symptoms when these patients ingest acidic fruit juices.[4]

Abdominal Pain

Abdominal pain was reported in 2 to 19% of patients with documented esophageal infection (see Table 1–1). Abdominal pain in association with esophageal infection may be referred from distal esophageal ulcers, or it may indicate a concurrent intra-abdominal visceral involvement. For example, CMV esophagitis is frequently accompanied by evidence of CMV infection in the stomach and intestine,[4, 5] while *Candida* esophagitis in a granulocytopenic patient may be accompanied by abdominal pain from splenic, renal, or hepatic fungal abscesses. Likewise, by the time HIV-infected patients develop opportunistic esophageal infections, several coexisting infectious causes of abdominal pain may be present.[6]

Nausea and Vomiting

Nausea and vomiting were present in 1 to 42% of patients with documented esophageal infection (see Table 1–1). Cytomegalovirus esophagitis frequently presents with nausea, vomiting, and anorexia in transplant patients,[5, 7–9] many of whom lack symptoms that direct attention to the esophagus. Often CMV esophagitis is not an isolated finding, and evidence of productive CMV infection can usually be found elsewhere.[4, 5] Among anorexic patients with AIDS, the actual prevalence of CMV esophagitis is not known because endoscopy, which would document its presence, is typically reserved for those patients with esophageal symptoms. Herpes simplex virus esophagitis occasionally presents with nausea and vomiting in the absence of esophageal symptoms or the typical oral-labial lesions (see Table 1–1).[5, 7] Other causes of infectious esophagitis are rarely associated with nausea and vomiting.

Oral Lesions

Oral lesions were present in 27 to 37% of patients with documented fungal, herpetic, and HIV-related esophagitis (see Table 1–1). Because both esophageal and oropharyngeal mucosa are lined with squamous epithelium, it is not surprising that they are subject to similar mucosal infections. Oral candidiasis, known as thrush, is very common among immunocompromised patients, especially those with AIDS. Among articles that specifically reported the presence or absence of oral thrush accompanying *Candida* esophagitis, oral thrush was present in approximately 75% of cases. Prospective studies have found that 71 to 100% of patients with AIDS who present with both oral thrush and painful swallowing have endoscopic evidence of esophageal candidiasis.[10-12] The presence of oral thrush does not preclude esophageal infection with organisms other than *Candida*, nor does the absence of oral thrush exclude *Candida* esophagitis. Oral thrush serves as a marker for immunodeficiency, and the presence of both oral thrush and esophageal symptoms is a strong predictor for an underlying esophageal infection. To illustrate, thrush was the oral lesion reported in 7 of the 14 patients with HSV esophagitis[13] and in 2 of 10 patients with HIV ulcers of the esophagus (see Table 1–1).[14] Herpetic oropharyngeal lesions were associated with HSV esophagitis in 14 (29%) of the 48 cases listed in Table 1–1. Herpes simplex virus esophagitis in noncompromised patients is probably underreported because endoscopy is not often warranted when symptoms are self-limited and characteristic HSV nasolabial lesions are present. Skin rash, sore throat, and discrete oral mucosal lesions were frequently reported in HIV-associated esophagitis (see Table 1–1). In addition to the aphthous lesions of a primary HIV infection, oral "hairy" leukoplakia due to Epstein-Barr virus (EBV) is associated with HIV infection and usually presents after clinically observable AIDS has developed.[15]

Gastrointestinal Bleeding

Gastrointestinal bleeding was present in 2 to 17% of patients with documented esophageal infection (see Table 1–1). Gross gastrointestinal bleeding in infectious esophagitis is uncommon in patients whose platelet counts and coagulation parameters are normal. Certain groups of patients are at high risk for bleeding from otherwise superficial lesions in the esophagus because of abnormal hemostasis. These groups of patients include those who are receiving chemotherapy for malignancy, those with marrow failure, those in the preengraftment phase after marrow transplantation, and those with hepatic failure. Severely immunocompromised patients suffer the most significant bleeding, probably because they have deeper lesions that involve the submucosa. Among severely immunocompromised patients, both fungi and viruses have been implicated as direct causes of massive bleeding,[9, 16, 17] but bleeding appears to be more frequent with HSV and CMV than with candidal infection. Aortoenteric fistulae and other rare vascular catastrophes have been ascribed to esophageal fistulae, erosions, or abscesses caused by tuberculosis, HIV ulcers, and syphilis.[18-20]

To establish a diagnosis of esophageal infection in the presence of bleeding presents a dilemma. One is hesitant to perform a biopsy on a bleeding lesion, especially in the esophagus, where there is a risk of perforating an already deep ulcer, yet a diagnosis is necessary so that appropriate therapy can be instituted. If HSV infection is suspected, the edges of ulcers can often be brushed without aggravating the bleeding. Another approach is to sample lesions remote from the bleeding site, including the stomach and duodenum, especially if CMV infection is under consideration. Oropharyngeal culture may occasionally be useful for diagnosis of either HSV or CMV excretion, which, combined with the endoscopic appearance, may be sufficient to determine therapy.[5, 7] Alternatively, after hemostatic abnormalities have been corrected by the transfusion of platelets or fresh plasma, endoscopy can be repeated.

Weight Loss

Weight loss in a patient with esophageal infection may be a result of severe debilitation caused by a wasting systemic illness such as metastatic cancer or, alternatively, it may be due to an esophageal infection that is the primary pathologic process. Weight loss was reported in 25% of patients with esophageal infection secondary to CMV infection, in 35% of those with mycobacterial infection, and in 22% of those with HIV-associated esophagitis (see Table 1–1). Each of these three infections involves the esophagus as part of a more widespread systemic infection. In the posttransplant patient, protracted nausea, vomiting, and anorexia caused by CMV infection limit oral caloric intake. Frequently these patients must be supported with parenteral nutrition to prevent wasting, since these symptoms are slow to respond to antiviral therapy.[4, 7] By contrast, weight loss is seldom reported with *Candida* or HSV esophagitis.

Diarrhea

Diarrhea was a reported symptom in 20% of patients with CMV and HIV esophagitis and was virtually unreported among patients with candidal, HSV, or mycobacterial disease (see Table 1–1). As CMV infection is rarely limited to the esophagus, the association of diarrhea and CMV esophagitis is expected, given the widespread nature of this infection. Diarrhea among HIV-infected individuals presumably reflects the high incidence of enteric infection by CMV and other pathogens suffered by this population.[21]

Fever

Fever accompanying esophageal symptoms is more common in patients with CMV and mycobacterial infections than in those who have HSV, candidal, or HIV-associated idiopathic esophageal ulcerations (see Table 1–1). As patients suffering from CMV enteritis are immunocompromised, fever in these patients may be secondary to CMV or other opportunistic pathogens. Likewise, fever in an HIV-infected individual may be secondary to HIV as well as to other pathogens. In patients with mycobacterial esophagitis, fever is a manifestation of either the mycobacterial infection itself or complications of mycobacterial infection, such as mediastinal abscesses secondary to esophageal perforation or bacterial pneumonitis secondary to bronchotracheal-esophageal fistulae.[22, 23]

Rash

A skin rash is reported at the time of presentation in approximately one half of the patients diagnosed with HIV-associated esophageal lesions. This rash is predominantly a maculopapular truncal eruption and often correlates temporally with HIV seroconversion. A rash was not reported in the CMV, HSV, or mycobacterial case reports that we reviewed, and only very rarely in *Candida* cases (see Table 1–1). The development of a truncal skin rash in conjunction with esophageal symptoms should significantly raise the clinician's suspicion of HIV infection involving the esophagus. This diagnosis may be erroneously excluded on the basis of a negative response to HIV antibody testing, since esophageal symptoms may precede HIV seroconversion.[24] If risk factors for HIV infection are present and the patient presents with rash, fever, and malaise in addition to esophageal symptoms, the diagnosis of HIV esophagitis secondary to acute HIV infection must be included in the differential diagnosis.

Cough

Among 56 published studies of infectious esophagitis, coughing was reported exclusively in cases of mycobacterial infections (see Table 1–1). The majority of case reports of mycobacterial esophagitis involved the esophagus through direct extension of a mediastinal or pulmonary nidus of infection. Although cough in some cases indicated a primarily pulmonic process, coughing paroxysms upon swallowing led typically to a diagnosis of tracheoesophageal fistula or high-grade esophageal obstruction.[22, 23]

Asymptomatic

Asymptomatic candidal esophagitis is reported in the AIDS literature as well as population-based studies.[10, 12, 25] In our review of published studies, 23% of patients diagnosed with esophageal candidiasis were asymptomatic. As the majority of these cases were chance discoveries, the actual prevalence of *Candida* esophagitis is not known. The endoscopic findings in asymptomatic patients are typically small, scattered adherent plaques, with confirmation of *Candida* by positive brush cytology or culture.

RISK FACTORS

The major risk factors for esophageal infection are defective immune surveillance, altered microbial flora, and abnormal esophageal function (Table 1–2). These risk factors are not mutually exclusive, and patients who have multiple risk factors are likely to have more severe disease. On occasion apparently normal individuals develop esophageal infections with certain organisms.

Defective Immune Surveillance

Human Immunodeficiency Virus Infection

Human immunodeficiency virus infection is currently the most significant risk factor for the development of esophageal infections. Although HIV appears to be an esophageal pathogen,[24–28] it is best known as a cause of lymphocyte deficiency leading to secondary opportunistic infections. Esophageal lesions at the time of acute HIV infection and seroconversion have been attributed both to primary HIV infection of the esophagus and to opportunistic *Candida* infection secondary to a transient decrease in lymphocytes.[29, 30] Esophageal disease later in the course of HIV infection occurs most often with *Candida albicans* and herpesviruses. The risk of candidal or viral esophagitis relates directly to the severity of immunodeficiency.[31] This correlation is supported by the hierarchal pattern of mucosal

TABLE 1–2. RISK FACTORS FOR DEVELOPMENT OF ESOPHAGEAL INFECTIONS

RISK FACTOR	ORGANISMS THAT CAUSE ESOPHAGEAL INFECTION	
	FREQUENT CAUSES	INFREQUENT CAUSES
Defective Immune Surveillance		
Primary HIV infection	*Candida*, HIV	
AIDS	*Candida*, CMV, HSV, HIV	*Mycobacterium tuberculosis, Aspergillus*, EBV, *Mycobacterium avium-intracellulare, Histoplasma, Cryptosporidium*, papovavirus, *Pneumocystis carinii*
Leukemia, lymphoma	*Candida*, HSV, CMV	VZV
Chemotherapy	*Candida*, HSV, CMV	Oropharyngeal flora
Congenital defects	*Candida*	—
Corticosteroid therapy	*Candida*	HSV, CMV
Immunosuppressive drugs	*Candida*	HSV, CMV
Solid organ transplantation	*Candida*, HSV, CMV	—
Bone marrow transplantation	*Candida*, HSV, CMV	VZV, oropharyngeal flora
Diabetes mellitus	*Candida*	—
Malnutrition	*Candida*	—
Older age	*Candida*	—
Altered Microbial Flora		
Antibiotic therapy	*Candida*	
Prolonged antifungal therapy		Non-*albicans Candida* species, *Aspergillus* species
Prolonged antiviral therapy		Resistant HSV, CMV
Hypochlorhydria (H₂-receptor antagonists, omeprazole, gastric surgery, AIDS gastrophathy)	*Candida*	—
Abnormal Esophageal Structure and Function		
Motility disorders (systemic sclerosis, achalasia)	*Candida*	—
Obstruction	*Candida*	—
Diverticulosis	*Candida*	—
Mucosal ulceration	*Candida*	Oropharyngeal flora
Exposure to an Infecting Organism		
Recurrent herpes infections (normal host)	HSV	—
Chagas's disease (endemic areas)	*Trypanosoma cruzi*	—
Papillomatosis	—	Human papillomavirus
Tuberculosis	—	*M. tuberculosis*
Histoplasmosis	—	*H. capsulatum*
Syphilis	—	*T. pallidum*

KEY: AIDS = acquired immunodeficiency syndrome, CMV = cytomegalovirus, EBV = Epstein-Barr virus, HIV = human immunodeficiency virus–associated idiopathic esophageal ulcers, HSV = herpes simplex virus, VZV = varicella-zoster virus.

candidal infection in HIV-positive women, in whom oropharyngeal infection occurred when CD4 lymphocytes were moderately decreased, and esophageal infection occurred when CD4 lymphocyte counts were very low.[32] The most severely immunocompromised AIDS patients may have concurrent opportunistic infections with *Candida*, HSV, and CMV.[33] *Mycobacterium tuberculosis, Mycobacterium avium-intracellulare* complex (MAC), *Pneumocystis carinii, Cryptosporidium, Aspergillus, Histoplasma*, and EBV are less common esophageal pathogens in patients with AIDS.

Hematologic Malignancy and the Sequelae of Chemotherapy

The prevalence of esophageal infections secondary to impaired immune surveillance and low granulocyte counts is high among patients with cancer, particularly those with hematologic malignancies. In two prospective endoscopic series totaling 3725 patients, *C. albicans* esophagitis was associated with an underlying malignancy in 20 of 80 patients.[25, 34] Another review of 15 patients with adult T-cell leukemia found 4 patients (27%) with esophageal candidiasis at the time of endoscopy.[35] Although *C. albicans* is the most frequently recovered opportunistic pathogen among patients with hematologic malignancy, this finding may be due to an underdiagnosis of viruses in these patients.[36]

Chemotherapy for the treatment of malignancy predisposes the patient to infectious esophagitis via two pathways. Aggressive chemotherapeutic protocols often cause profound and prolonged leukopenia. The absence of functional granulocytes results in impaired defense against dissemination of bacteria and fungi. Chemotherapy may also result in loss of normal esophageal mucosal integrity through its effect on rapidly dividing germinal epithelial layers. Thus, chemotherapy interferes with both normal immune surveillance and mechanical barriers to infection. Empirical antibacterial and antifungal therapy during intensive chemotherapy has reduced, but not eliminated, the incidence of bacterial sepsis and disseminated fungal infection.

Congenital Defects

Although many of the congenital immunodeficiency syndromes result in intestinal infection, esophageal involvement is not common, except in those patients with chronic mucocutaneous candidiasis.[37] In this disease there is defective chemotaxis of neutrophils and monocytes, which leads to chronic *Candida* infections of the skin and mucous membranes, including the esophagus.

Immunosuppressive Drug Therapy

Corticosteroids are known to suppress both lymphocyte and granulocyte function.[38] Their use is associated with the development of infectious esophagitis. Suppression of lymphocyte function predisposes the patient to mucosal infection, primarily with *Candida*, and granulocyte dysfunction may permit deep mucosal invasion and disseminated fungal or bacterial infection. In addition to risks of disseminated infection, high-dose parenteral steroid use can lead to bleeding from deep esophageal *Candida* ulcers.[16] Aerosolized beclomethasone, a topical inhaled corticosteroid used by asthmatics, has also been associated with *Candida* esophagitis in an otherwise healthy adult.[39] Long-term, high-dose corticosteroid use may lead to infection with HSV and CMV, but they are less common than *Candida*.

Treatment of autoimmune disorders with cytotoxic agents such as cyclophosphamide, azathioprine, chlorambucil, and methotrexate can compromise cellular immunity by suppressing the leukocyte count and interfering with monocyte-macrophage interaction. *Candida* is again the most likely infective cause of esophagitis, but because leukocyte counts are seldom allowed to fall below set levels, severe infections are uncommon.

Transplantation

Among 292 solid organ transplant recipients who had nonspecific upper intestinal symptoms,

the incidence of infectious esophagitis was approximately 6%.[8, 9, 40, 41] In the first few weeks following transplant surgery, *C. albicans* is the most common cause of infectious esophagitis, probably as a result of a combination of factors, including immune deficiency from surgical trauma and therapy with perioperative antibiotics, H_2 receptor antagonists, and immunosuppressive drugs given to prevent graft rejection. Candidal esophagitis is encountered more frequently following renal transplantation than following liver or heart transplantation.[8] This discrepancy is likely to be related to the concurrent risk factor of diabetes mellitus in the renal transplant patient population.[9] Cytomegaloviral and HSV esophagitis typically present several weeks after transplantation as a result either of primary viral infection from transfused blood products or the transplanted organ or of the reactivation of a virus that was latent during immunosuppressive drug therapy. The widespread routine use of antifungal and antiviral prophylaxis following solid organ transplantation has significantly reduced morbidity from opportunistic pathogens.[42, 43]

Marrow transplantation differs from solid organ transplantation in several respects: Most patients have an underlying malignant disease; the high-dose cytoreductive therapy given prior to marrow infusion causes profound immunosuppression until the new marrow becomes functional; and an immune disorder, graft-versus-host disease, may affect recipients of allogeneic marrow. Each of these is an independent risk factor for the development of opportunistic fungal, viral, and bacterial esophagitis.[5] The most common causes of infectious esophagitis in bone marrow transplantation patients are *C. albicans*, HSV, and CMV.[5] Such infections were once common in these patients but recently have almost disappeared because of effective prophylaxis against these organisms. Bacterial esophagitis has been reported in granulocytopenic marrow transplant patients, often in conjunction with *Candida*, CMV, or HSV.[5, 44] Non-*albicans* series of *Candida*, other fungi, varicella zostervirus (VZV), and herpesviruses resistant to acyclovir and ganciclovir may also be seen in these patients.

Other Medical Disorders

Patients with diabetes mellitus are at an increased risk for *Candida* esophagitis, particularly those patients who are persistently hyperglycemic, since granulocyte dysfunction has been related to glycemia.[45] Sporadic cases of candidiasis are found in most busy endoscopic practices that include diabetics. In a large series of 224 renal transplant patients, of whom 144 were diabetic, all 5 cases of esophageal candidiasis occurred among diabetic patients.[9] Candidal esophagitis was also demonstrated endoscopically in 3 of 20 patients (15%) with nausea and vomiting initially thought to be secondary to diabetic gastroparesis.[46] Alcoholism has been implicated as a risk factor for esophageal candidiasis.[47] Aging has also been suggested as a risk factor for esophageal infection. In a series of 224 consecutive upper endoscopies, 39 cases of Candida esophagitis were diagnosed, among which were 3 patients who had no recognized predisposing illness or medication. A common feature of these 3 patients was their advanced age, their mean age being 82 years.[34] Herpesvirus infections of the esophagus are uncommon in both diabetic and aged patients unless additional immunosuppressive factors are present.

Altered Microbial Flora

Antimicrobial Therapy

Altered microbial flora is a risk factor for mucosal Candida infections. Low levels of C. albicans are present in normal oral flora. Institution of antibiotics alters the normal competitive balance among the various bacterial and fungal species. In this setting, overgrowth of C. albicans can occur and can progress to infectious esophagitis, especially in the presence of other risk factors for infectious esophagitis. Prolonged antifungal therapy in immunocompromised patients with recurrent oropharyngeal or esophageal candidiasis increases the risk for colonization by Candida species other than C. albicans, and other opportunistic fungi such as the Aspergillus species,[48] as well as the risk for development of resistant C. albicans strains.[49] Similarly, prolonged antiviral maintenance therapy among AIDS patients and bone marrow transplant recipients is associated with the emergence of strains of HSV and CMV resistant to acyclovir and ganciclovir.[50–56]

Hypochlorhydria

Since gastric acidity is an important factor in the defense of the upper intestinal tract, it is not surprising that suppression of acid secretion leads to overgrowth of bacteria and fungi in the upper gut. Hypochlorhydria secondary to the use of H_2 receptor antagonists or omeprazole or to gastric surgery or AIDS gastropathy is in each instance associated with an increased risk for Candida esophagitis.[25, 57]

Abnormal Esophageal Structure and Function

Lack of normal esophageal motility predisposes a patient to colonization and epithelial infection with Candida. This is most clearly seen in patients with progressive systemic sclerosis (PSS), among whom esophageal dysmotility is present in 75 to 85%.[58] The esophageal manifestations of PSS include impaired peristalsis, gastroesophageal reflux, erosive esophagitis, and esophageal stricture. Candidal esophagitis was diagnosed in approximately 35% of 193 dyspeptic PSS patients from 3 series of studies.[47, 59, 60] In most cases of PSS, Candida esophagitis is not associated with painful swallowing or other symptoms typical of acute candidal esophagitis, but rather is a secondary finding in patients undergoing upper endoscopy for nonspecific symptoms. When PSS patients who were not receiving potent antacid therapy for reflux symptoms were compared with those who were, the incidence of fungal esophagitis increased from 44% (21 of 48 patients) to 89% (16 of 18 patients).[47] This implies that the suppression of gastric acid secretion increases the incidence of Candida esophagitis by removing the acid barrier to fungal colonization. Candidal infection in an aperistaltic esophagus is difficult to eradicate; recurrence rates after discontinuation of antifungal therapy approach 100%.[47] Stasis and dysmotility also accompany achalasia, esophageal diverticula, esophageal pseudodiverticula, and obstructing tumors. Each of these conditions is associated with an increased risk for superficial Candida esophagitis through interference with the normal housekeeping function of esophageal peristalsis.[61] Oral bacterial flora can also be cultured from esophageal mucosal ulcerations and necrotic areas of esophageal tumors, but they are seldom a cause of specific symptoms.

Exposure to an Infecting Organism

Normal hosts occasionally develop esophageal infection with Candida or HSV. In addition, in certain geographic regions other organisms have been reported to affect the esophagi of normal hosts. Trypanosoma cruzi, the South American parasite responsible for Chagas's disease, progressively destroys ganglion cells throughout the body, producing esophageal manifestations similar to those of achalasia as well as heart, intestinal, and gallbladder dysfunction. *M. tuberculosis* infection infrequently involves the esophagus via direct extension of mediastinal lymphangitic foci, although primary *M. tuberculosis* infection of the esophagus has been reported. *Histoplasma capsulatum* is a fungus that on rare occasions has caused esophagitis through direct extension from the mediastinum. Syphilis secondary to *Treponema pallidum* has been reported to involve the esophagus directly.[20] These organisms are discussed later in this review.

FUNGAL INFECTIONS

Fungal infections of the esophagus are predominantly caused by *C. albicans,* a yeast that is part of the normal human oral flora.[62, 63] Other *Candida* species such as *C. tropicalis, C. glabrata, C. parapsilosis,* and *C. krusei* are occasionally pathogenic in patients who have received chronic antifungal therapy to which these fungi are resistant.[64] Predisposing factors for fungal esophagitis include colonization with *Candida* species, altered microbial flora, T lymphocyte deficiency, impaired granulocyte function, dysmotility, and achlorhydria. Impaired cellular immunity, from HIV infection of lymphocytes, for example, predisposes the patient to localized fungal infection, though generally not to disseminated fungal infection. The normal defense against systemic fungal infection depends on the opsonization of fungal forms by antibodies and complement, which permits their recognition and destruction by granulocytes and macrophages.[62] Thus, the loss of functioning granulocytes predisposes patients to disseminated fungal infection via impaired phagocytosis.[63–66] Patients with AIDS may become granulocytopenic secondary to infection (e.g., MAI) or drug toxicity (e.g., zidovudine [formerly AZT] or ganciclovir). Patients not infected with HIV may become granulocytopenic because of marrow failure, leukemia, cytotoxic therapy, bone marrow transplantation, or adverse medication reactions.

Candida Species

Mycology

Candida species are yeasts that grow as round to oval eukaryotic cells and reproduce asexually by budding.[62] They grow well on common culture media and appear as creamy colonies in 48 to 72 hours. Additional morphologic features include pseudohyphae, which are linear arrangements of buds, or blastoconidia, and occasionally true septate hyphae, which form under stress of 5 to 10% CO_2 or low oxygen tension, as in infected host tissues. *Candida albicans* is the most common human fungal pathogen. Identification of *C. albicans* in cultured specimens is rapid and simple, since of the medically important yeasts, only *C. albicans* forms a germ tube after 2 to 4 hours of incubation in fetal bovine serum at 37°C.[62]

In patients at risk for candidiasis, candidal colonization is the first pathologic stage, followed by epithelial infection, then deeper invasion. *Candida albicans* is more adept at colonizing mucosal surfaces than are other *Candida* species because of its fibrillar peptidomannan components that adhere to fibronectin on the host cell.[62] A population-based study of candidal colonization of the esophagus in healthy ambulatory Danish adults found a prevalence of approximately 20%.[67] *Candida albicans* invades locally into squamous mucosa, with advancing pseudohyphae and hyphae, where fungal proteases are thought to play a role.[62, 68] In patients capable of an immune response, an associated acute inflammation usually limits *Candida* penetration at the epithelium. Although *C. albicans* is adept at colonization, *C. tropicalis* is reported to be a more virulent organism in granulocytopenic patients because it invades more deeply and more frequently involves the entire alimentary tract.[68]

Clinical Presentation

Candidal esophagitis is frequently asymptomatic, especially when patients are immunologically intact and have only scattered adherent plaques in their esophagus. Of the 177 cases of documented *Candida* esophagitis compiled in Table 1–1, 23% were asymptomatic. In a prospective study of 3501 patients undergoing upper endoscopy, 41 patients with *Candida* esophagitis were diagnosed, of whom 27 (67%) were asymptomatic.[25] In a prospective study of 57 AIDS patients, 25 cases of candidal esophagitis were diagnosed, of whom 10 (40%) were asymptomatic.[10] Because asymptomatic patients are seldom subjected to endoscopy, the prevalence of fungal esophagitis among patients with minor abnormalities of motility and immunity is underreported. As asymptomatic *Candida* esophagitis does not necessarily progress and is likely to recur after therapy, clinicians should not feel compelled to treat all cases. Risk factors for esophageal infection, such as corticosteroid therapy or hyperglycemia, should be considered and modified when possible. By contrast, patients with more advanced abnormalities of immune function are usually symptomatic, with painful or difficult swallowing as the initial manifestation of *Candida* esophagitis. The presence of oral thrush is often an indicator of the pathologic esophageal process, though documented candidal esophagitis occurs in the absence of thrush in approximately 15% of cases.[12, 39, 69–73]

Transient *Candida* esophagitis presenting with difficult, painful swallowing has been associated with acute HIV infection, also known as HIV seroconversion syndrome.[71, 74, 75] These patients do not have persistent immunodeficiency but rather develop a transient decrease in CD4$^+$ cell counts, lymphocyte hyporesponsiveness, and mucosal ulceration from HIV.[24, 26, 76–79]

Diagnosis

CLINICAL DATA

In the AIDS patient, a diagnosis of *Candida* esophagitis can often be derived from a careful history and physical examination. In consecutive upper endoscopies in 57 hospitalized patients with AIDS, the prevalence of oral candidiasis and esophageal candidiasis was 62% and 48%, respectively.[10] In this series of studies the presence of both esophageal symptoms and oral candidiasis had a positive predictive value for esophageal candidiasis of 100%, and the absence both of symptoms and of oral candidiasis had a negative predictive value of 96%. In a similar study of 10 hospitalized AIDS patients with oral candidiasis, esophageal candidiasis was found by cytology in all patients, but 3 of the patients were asymptomatic.[12] Of 66 AIDS patients with esophageal symptoms who were evaluated for oral and esophageal candidiasis, thrush was present in 20 of 28 patients (71%) who had documented *Candida* esophagitis. Thrush was also seen, however, in 8 of 38 symptomatic patients (21%) who did not have esophageal candidiasis. Thus, in this series of studies of patients with AIDS, the presence of both esophageal symptoms and oral candidiasis had a positive predictive value for esophageal candidiasis of only 71%.[11]

The magnitude of the AIDS epidemic has imposed practical considerations on the diagnostic evaluation and management of HIV-infected subjects. In centers evaluating hundreds of HIV-infected patients, the demand to perform fiberoptic esophagoscopy on AIDS patients presenting with esophageal symptoms is overwhelming.[72] This has prompted a modified approach

in caring for these patients. If a patient is in a high risk group for *Candida* infection, such as AIDS, and presents with painful or difficult swallowing, *Candida* esophagitis should be suspected. If physical examination reveals oral candidiasis, many physicians would treat empirically with systemic antifungal medications, reserving further diagnostic studies for patients in whom a second esophageal pathogen is more likely (see Table 1–1) and for patients who fail to respond to empirical therapy.

Unfortunately, in immunocompromised patients, the law of parsimony of diagnosis does not always apply, particularly if the degree of immunocompromise is profound. The presence of esophageal infection with multiple organisms has been frequently reported in both transplant and AIDS patients.[7, 11, 33, 48] When a patient with oral thrush and esophageal symptoms also complains of persistent nausea and vomiting, abdominal pain, intestinal bleeding, fever, cough, or diarrhea, *Candida* is not likely to be the only infecting organism (see Table 1–1) and further diagnostic studies are indicated.

RADIOLOGY

Of available radiographic studies, the air-contrast esophagogram is preferred in the assessment of esophageal mucosal disease. This technique demonstrates subtle mucosal features not seen on single-contrast examinations. Obtaining an air-contrast esophagogram requires patient cooperation and may be uncomfortable for patients with severe esophageal symptoms.

Candidal esophagitis classically appears on an esophageal radiograph as discrete plaquelike lesions. These lesions tend to orient longitudinally and to display irregular linear filling defects. The margins of the lesions may have distinct borders formed by trapped barium.[80] Other patients may have upper to midesophageal tiny nodular lesions that have a granular appearance similar to lesions seen in the distal esophagus in reflux esophagitis.[81] In severe *Candida* esophagitis, coalescing plaques and pseudomembranes may produce a grossly irregular, or shaggy pattern (Fig. 1–1).[82]

Unfortunately, many patients with *Candida* esophagitis do not have typical lesions on esophagogram. The esophagogram may appear normal or, alternatively, have nonspecific abnormalities such as stricture, ulceration, tumorlike masses, polyps, mucosal bridging, and fistula formation.[25, 80, 82, 83] A coexisting viral infection is likely to be missed. Radiographic studies are most useful to assess motility, to exclude mechanical obstruction, to evaluate for the pres-

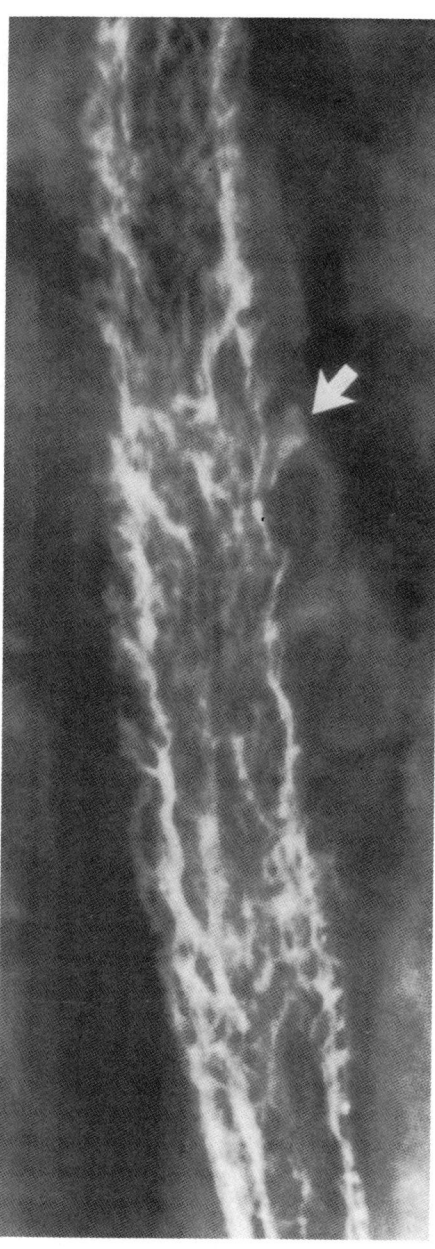

FIGURE 1–1.
A double-contrast esophagogram demonstrating severe candidal esophagitis in a patient with AIDS. Note the grossly irregular, or shaggy, contour produced by coalescing plaques and pseudomembranes (arrow). A deep ulcer is also present. SOURCE: Levine MS. Radiology of the esophagus: A pattern approach. Radiology. 1991;179(1):2.

ence of perforation or fistula, and to assist in diagnosis when fiberoptic esophagoscopy is unavailable or contraindicated. Radiologic contrast studies of the esophagus are not usually necessary if endoscopy is planned independently of the radiologic findings.

BLIND ESOPHAGEAL BRUSHING

Blind brush cytology is a technique of sampling esophageal material without recourse to the technical skill, equipment, time, and personnel required by endoscopy. The technique uses a perorally or transnasally placed sheathed brush to sample the esophageal lining. The brush is sheathed to minimize nasopharyngeal and oropharyngeal contamination during passage into and removal from the esophagus. After the instrument has been placed in the esophagus, the brush is exposed, moved to and fro, resheathed, and then removed. Blind transnasal cytology had a sensitivity of 87.5% and a specificity of 100% when compared with endoscopically directed cytology in 24 patients with esophageal candidiasis.[73] Oral thrush was present in all patients with documented esophageal candidiasis. A second study with perorally placed brush cytology was diagnostic in 27 of 28 endoscopically documented cases (sensitivity 96%), but with false positive findings in 5 of 38 symptomatic patients without *Candida* esophagitis (specificity 87%).[80] These two studies demonstrate that blind brush cytology is more sensitive and more specific than the presence of oral thrush in predicting esophageal candidiasis in AIDS patients. The disadvantages of blind esophageal brushings are the inability to inspect the extent and severity of disease, the inability to direct the sampling brush, and the inability to obtain tissue biopsies for histologic examination.

ENDOSCOPY

Endoscopy with brushings and biopsy is currently the gold-standard technique for definitive diagnosis of esophageal infections because its sensitivity and specificity are superior to those of radiography in the diagnosis of *Candida* esophagitis (Fig. 1–2). At endoscopy the severity of fungal esophagitis can be assessed and categorized as follows: grade 1, few raised white plaques up to 2 mm in size, but no ulceration; grade 2, multiple raised white plaques greater than 2 mm in size, but no ulceration; grade 3, confluent, linear, and nodular elevated plaques with ulceration; grade 4, findings of grade 3 with narrowing of the lumen.[84] The gross appearance of the mucosa at endoscopy may be misleading, however, since not all white exudative lesions are fungal, and for this reason recovery of specimens is essential. Similar white exudative lesions can be seen with HSV or CMV infection, bacterial esophagitis, pill esophagitis, and sucralfate ingestion. Swallowed bits of adherent material containing fungi can also be

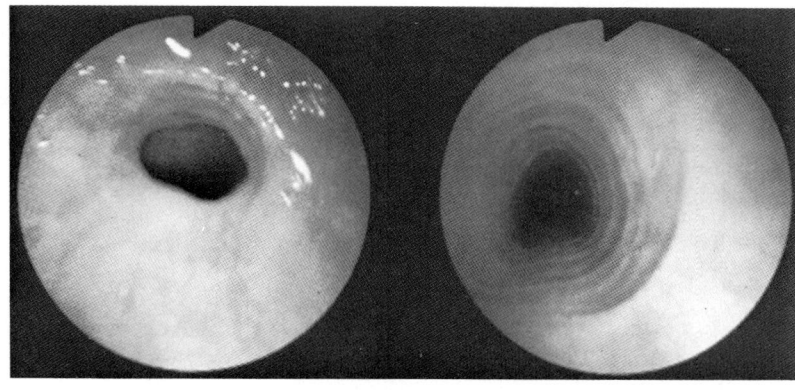

FIGURE 1–2.
Two endoscopic photographs of severe candidal esophagitis in patients with AIDS. Note the underlying erythema and linear exudates typical of this infection. SOURCE: Silverstein FE, Tytgat GNJ. Atlas of Gastrointestinal Endoscopy. 2nd ed. New York: Gower Medical Publishing; 1991: 3.21.

seen in the esophagus of patients with oral thrush or poorly cleaned dentures, but these wash off the epithelial surface of the esophagus and do not indicate fungal esophagitis. Candidal plaques in the esophagus cannot be washed away; when they are brushed, there is usually bleeding at the site of attachment.

Not all patients with candidal esophagitis have white exudates. For example, an inflammatory stricture with no hint of fungal etiology may prove to have invasive fungal elements on brushing or biopsy. It is essential at endoscopy to perform biopsies and brushings—platelet count and coagulation parameters permitting—to confirm the presence of infection and to avoid misdiagnoses. Specimens obtained by sheathed brush should be smeared onto slides for fungal and bacterial stains and shaken into transport medium for viral cultures.

HISTOLOGY

Biopsies should be placed in fixative for histologic examination, using routine H&E staining and specific stains for fungi and bacteria, including mycobacteria, if indicated. Budding yeast cells, hyphae, and pseudohyphae are best seen by silver stain, periodic acid–Schiff (PAS) stain, or Gram stain and are diagnostic of *Candida* infection.[62, 85, 86] Morphology is best preserved by fixing tissue in Bouin's, Hollande's, or B5, but buffered formalin fixation is better for immunohistology and in situ hybridization methods to identify viruses in tissue sections. Pathologists should be alerted to the history and endoscopic findings, since not every stain in the histologic repertoire needs to be applied to every specimen.

CULTURE

We do not routinely culture esophageal specimens for fungi or bacteria, since cultures do not differentiate reliably among normal flora, colonization, and infection. If an unusual infection such as *Aspergillus* infection, tuberculosis, or bacterial esophagitis is suspected on clinical or endoscopic grounds, however, cultures can be useful, particularly if sensitivity to antimicrobial drugs is available from these cultures. Most *Candida* species grow well on enriched bacteriologic media, blood agar, and Sabouraud's medium.[62] The primary feature that differentiates *C. albicans* from other *Candida* species is the development of a sproutlike hypha, termed a germ tube, within 2 to 3 hours of incubation in serum at 37°C.[62, 85] Viral culture of both brushings and biopsies is the most accurate method of diagnosis of herpesvirus esophagitis and should be routine when viral esophagitis is in the differential diagnosis, even when *Candida* esophagitis is obvious.

Drug Therapy for *Candida* Esophagitis

Mucosal fungal infections may be treated by nonabsorbable topical agents, systemically absorbed oral medications, or parenterally administered drugs (Table 1–3). Appropriate treatment is determined by the severity of fungal infection and the degree to which immune defenses are compromised.

PATIENT STRATIFICATION FOR THE TREATMENT OF CANDIDAL ESOPHAGITIS

No or Minimal Lymphocyte Defects and Normal Granulocytes. Most general medical patients, such as patients on chronic prednisone therapy, diabetics, and the elderly, who are found to have *Candida* esophagitis have minimal defects in lymphocyte and granulocyte function. Clotrimazole troches or tablets are tolerated well and are effective for these patients when taken at regular intervals since they act topically. Oral fluconazole is more convenient, with its

TABLE 1–3. TREATMENT OF CANDIDAL ESOPHAGITIS

DRUGS AVAILABLE	NO OR MINIMAL LYMPHOCYTE DEFECTS AND NORMAL GRANULOCYTES	DECREASED LYMPHOCYTE FUNCTION BUT NORMAL GRANULOCYTES	DECREASED LYMPHOCYTE AND GRANULOCYTE FUNCTION
Oral Nonabsorbable			
Nystatin suspension (1 million u/ml)	1–3 million U qid	N/A	N/A
Amphotericin B lozenge (10 mg) or suspension (100 mg/ml)*	1–2 lozenges or 1 ml suspension qid	N/A	N/A
Miconazole oral gel (25 mg/ml)	10 ml qid	N/A	N/A
Clotrimazole troches (10 mg)	*10-mg troche dissolved in mouth 5 times daily*	N/A	N/A
Clotrimazole vaginal tablets (100 mg)	100-mg tablet dissolved in mouth tid	100-mg tablet dissolved in mouth 3–5 times daily	N/A
Oral Absorbable			
Ketoconazole tablets (200 mg)	200 mg once daily	400–800 mg once daily	400–800 mg once daily
Fluconazole capsules (50 or 100 mg)	*50 mg once daily*	*100 mg once daily*	100–200 mg once daily
Flucytosine capsules (250 or 500 mg)†	N/A	N/A	50–150 mg/kg/d at 6 h intervals
Intravenous			
Amphotericin B for IV use (5 mg/ml)	N/A	0.3 mg/kg/d	*0.5 mg/kg/d*
Miconazole for IV use (10 mg/ml)	N/A	N/A	600–1800 mg q 8 h
Fluconazole for IV use (2 mg/ml)‡	100 mg once daily	100 mg once daily	100–200 mg once daily

NOTE: Italic type indicates therapy of choice.
*Not available in the USA.
†Not for use as a single agent. (See text for discussion on the use of this drug.)
‡When oral route is not available.

once-daily dosing, but may cause adverse reactions because it is absorbed systemically. Oral nystatin is an inexpensive and usually effective nonabsorbable drug, though most patients find it unpalatable. Duration of therapy with these agents is usually 7 to 10 days, or until resolution of Candida-related symptoms. It may not be possible to eradicate Candida in patients who have anatomic or motility defects that lead to colonization, or in those whose mild immune defects persist. A lower dosage of an oral nonabsorbable drug taken chronically may be useful in controlling candidal colonization, particularly if recurrent symptomatic infections are bothersome.

Decreased Lymphocyte Function but Normal Granulocytes. Patients who have defects in lymphocyte function but normal granulocytes are exemplified by patients with AIDS. The treatment of choice in this population is oral fluconazole, which can be taken in once daily dosing (see Table 1–3). In randomized controlled trials in patients with AIDS, fluconazole was superior to standard-dose ketoconazole.[87] Ketoconazole is effective in higher dosages (400–800 mg/d), however, since the higher dosages compensate

for the hypochlorhydria of AIDS gastropathy.[57, 88] Clotrimazole tablets (100 mg) dissolved in the mouth have been reported to be effective as well.[69] Intravenous fluconazole and low-dose amphotericin (0.3 mg/kg/d) are available for initiating therapy in patients who are unable to swallow capsules. Duration of therapy is usually 10 to 14 days, but many centers continue antifungal therapy in full doses for 1 to 2 weeks after resolution of symptoms. As the lymphocyte defect in AIDS is persistent, prophylactic antifungal therapy may be needed to prevent recurrent symptomatic esophagitis. The oral nonabsorbable drugs listed in Table 1–3 limit the degree of colonization. The major complications of chronic imidazole therapy are emergence of resistant organisms and adverse systemic reactions.[89–91]

Decreased Granulocyte Function. Patients with granulocytopenia who have Candida esophagitis must be treated aggressively because they are at risk for disseminated fungal disease. The patients at highest risk are cancer patients who have received high-dose chemotherapy regimens, marrow transplant patients, and patients with AIDS whose granulocyte counts have fallen, usually as a result of drug therapy with AZT or ganciclovir. Oral nonabsorbable drugs are inappropriate in this setting. The drug of choice is intravenous amphotericin B at 0.5 mg/kg/d, particularly when the patient is febrile or has clinical evidence of *Candida* infection of the liver, spleen, kidneys, or bloodstream. New liposomal and lipid dispersion forms of amphotericin B that aim at reducing toxicity without losing efficacy are under investigation. Intravenous fluconazole is available as an alternative parenteral drug, but it has not displaced amphotericin B as the drug of choice for severe fungal infections. Oral fluconazole or ketoconazole should be reserved for patients who have had a good response to intravenous antifungal therapy or for those with mild esophageal candidiasis despite their granulocytopenia. Duration of therapy is usually 10 to 14 days for uncomplicated esophageal candidiasis and longer if bloodstream infection or visceral involvement has been documented. Attention should also be given to correction of any reversible predisposing factors, for example, discontinuation of corticosteroids or antibiotics and restoration of granulocyte counts with colony-stimulating factors. If the granulocyte counts remain low, prophylactic therapy with oral nonabsorbable drugs or fluconazole is usually indicated.

ANTIFUNGAL FORMULARY FOR THE TREATMENT OF CANDIDAL ESOPHAGITIS

Topical Agents. Topical antifungal agents are in wide use primarily because of the safety of their administration. As the drugs are not systemically absorbed, little risk of adverse effects arises. Nystatin is a topical polyene antifungal drug that binds to sterols in fungal cytoplasmic membranes, causing disruption and cell death.[62] Although nystatin solution is not so effective in the treatment of established esophageal candidiasis as are systemically absorbed or parenterally administered antifungal agents, it is frequently used for oral candidiasis prophylaxis during intensive chemotherapy, in radiation therapy, in organ transplantation, and in AIDS. The efficacy of topical nystatin therapy is directly related to the dosage and interval of administration. For example, renal transplant patients who developed *Candida* esophagitis despite low-dose nystatin prophylaxis responded well to higher dose therapy of 400,000 units swished and swallowed 6 times a day.[8]

Amphotericin B is also a polyene antifungal drug that is insoluble in water and poorly absorbed from the gastrointestinal tract. It has been used for topical prophylaxis and treatment of fungal infections in Japan and Europe. Oral amphotericin has demonstrated some utility in the treatment of *Candida* esophagitis. Thirteen of nineteen patients with esophageal candidiasis treated with amphotericin B syrup had an effective clinical response to oral amphotericin.[25] Oral amphotericin B was found to be ineffective therapy, however, for fungal esophagitis in renal transplant patients.[9]

Oral miconazole is a nonabsorbable fungistatic imidazole that limits ergosterol synthesis, thereby altering fungal cytoplasmic membrane integrity. Twelve Haitian AIDS patients with endoscopically documented moderate to severe *Candida* esophagitis were randomized to treatment with either oral miconazole or ketoconazole.[92] The 6 patients treated with 50 mg of miconazole gel 4 times a day had complete symptomatic response within 3 to 5 days, and repeat endoscopy after completion of the ten-day course showed normal esophageal mucosa in all 6 patients.

Clotrimazole is also a nonabsorbable imidazole antimicrobial drug. Successful treatment of *Candida* esophagitis in non-AIDS patients with 10 mg buccal troches of clotrimazole has been reported.[93] Twenty-five AIDS patients with moderately severe *Candida* esophagitis were treated with 100 mg vaginal tablets of clotrimazole dissolved in the mouth 3 times a day for 7 days.[69] There was complete clearing of symptoms with normal mucosa on repeat endoscopy in all patients.

Systemic Oral Agents. Absorbable imidazole derivatives such as ketoconazole and fluconazole have become the mainstay of therapy for mild to moderate esophageal candidiasis. They are more effective than nonsystemically absorbed drugs and are favored over parenteral amphotericin B owing to ease of administration and lower toxicity. Imidazole drugs inhibit the biosynthesis of ergosterol, thereby causing changes in the permeability of the fungal cell membrane.[62, 94]

Ketoconazole, the first absorbable imidazole, is widely used for the treatment of superficial *Candida* species infection. The usual dosage of ketoconazole is 200 mg daily, and it is effective in non-AIDS patients. In AIDS patients, a starting dose of 400 mg daily is recommended but dosages of up to 800 mg daily may be required for effective therapy.[12] Ketoconazole is best absorbed at a low pH, and hypochlorhydria secondary to AIDS gastropathy or acid suppressive therapy may contribute to the poor response in AIDS patients with *Candida* esophagitis.[57] It is not available as a parenteral agent, and it penetrates poorly into cerebrospinal fluid (CSF), limiting its use in fungal cerebritis or meningitis. Ketoconazole affects hepatic cytochrome P-450 enzymes and alters metabolism of several drugs, among them cyclosporine, warfarin, isoniazid, and rifampin.[62] Adverse effects of ketoconazole therapy include nausea, especially with high doses, hepatotoxicity, and adrenal insufficiency.[94]

Fluconazole is a water-soluble triazole with several advantages over ketoconazole. It is more water-soluble, has a larger volume of distribution, and has a longer half-life, and its absorption is not affected by hypochlorhydria. It is available in both oral and parenteral forms. Fluconazole has excellent penetration into the CSF. A randomized, double-blind trial of fluconazole (100 mg/d) versus ketoconazole (200 mg/d) for documented *Candida* esophagitis found that resolution of both symptoms and endoscopic findings was more frequent with fluconazole.[87] Single-dose therapy with fluconazole (400 mg) has been reported as curative for esophageal candidiasis in AIDS patients,[95] but immunodeficiency persists and recurrence of candidal infection is common in these patients. A double-blind placebo-controlled trial of maintenance therapy in 14 AIDS patients after clinical cure of oropharyngeal and esophageal candidiasis found that all placebo recipients relapsed within 6 weeks, but 7 of 9 (78%) receiving weekly fluconazole (150 mg) were maintained free from recurrent disease.[70] Side effects appear to cause fewer problems with fluconazole than with ketoconazole, though it, too, interferes with metabolism of other medications. Fluconazole is cleared by the kidneys, and dosage should be adjusted for renal insufficiency. Emergence of *Candida* resistance to ketoconazole and fluconazole has become a problem in the long-term management of immunocompromised patients.[49, 96] Isolates may be resistant to several imidazole derivatives and may demonstrate in vitro resistance to other classes of antifungal agents.[89, 91, 97] Compromised patients on long-term fungal prophylaxis are also at increased risk for infection with noncandidal fungi resistant to the usual oral medications such as *Aspergillus* species.[48]

Flucytosine (5-fluorocytosine, 50–150 mg/kg/d in divided doses every 6 h) is an orally absorbed analog of cytosine that, when converted by the fungus into 5-fluorouracil, becomes incorporated into RNA (ribonucleic acid), disrupting protein synthesis.[62, 94] It is active against most clinically important yeasts, and is absorbed well in CSF. Its use is limited by rapid development of resistance when used as single-agent therapy.

It can be used as single-agent therapy in uncomplicated lower urinary tract infections, but it is used primarily in combination with parenteral amphotericin B in the treatment of life-threatening disseminated fungal infections.[62] It is not indicated for uncomplicated esophageal candidiasis. A principal toxicity of flucytosine is reversible bone marrow suppression. Other toxicities include liver damage and gastrointestinal disturbance.[94] Serum levels should be monitored frequently and maintained between 50 and 100 μg/ml to avoid excessive myelosuppression. Since the drug is cleared by the kidneys, dosage should be adjusted for patients with renal insufficiency.

Parenteral Agents. Amphotericin B, a polyene that disrupts fungal cytoplasmic membrane integrity, is the antifungal therapy of choice for patients with life-threatening disseminated fungal infections.[62, 94] Almost all fungi are susceptible to this drug. Despite its severe toxicities, it is also the drug of choice for granulocytopenic patients with *Candida* esophagitis because these patients are at a high risk for developing systemic fungal infection.[87] The drug is first administered with a test dose of 1 mg, and if no severe adverse reaction, such as anaphylaxis, occurs, the dosage can be incrementally increased to 0.5 mg/kg/d by slow intravenous infusion. For disseminated *Candida* infections, a cumulative dose of 1.5 to 2.0 g should be given during a period of 6 to 12 weeks. In the absence of disseminated infection, treatment of *Candida* esophagitis in a granulocytopenic patient with a shorter, seven- to ten-day, course of amphotericin B at 0.5 mg/kg/d is usually effective. Amphotericin B is also appropriate therapy for treatment of *Candida* esophagitis among nongranulocytopenic patients who fail to respond to systemic imidazole therapy. These patients are at low risk for disseminated fungal infection and a lower dose regimen of amphotericin B at 0.3 mg/kg/d for 7 to 10 days is recommended to reduce dose-related adverse effects. Premedication with acetaminophen, antihistamines, and hydrocortisone can reduce side effects during infusion. Adverse reactions to amphotericin B include fever, chills, headache, dyspnea, delirium, hypotension, hypertension, hypokalemia, and anemia. Nephrotoxicity is found in virtually all patients receiving a course of the drug, and renal function must be followed closely with dosages adjusted accordingly.[62] Amphotericin B penetrates CSF poorly and should be used in conjunction with other agents such as flucytosine for treatment of meningitis or cerebritis. Although this combination is synergistic in some instances, the dosage of amphotericin B should not be lowered.[94] Such patients must be monitored for bone marrow toxicity from flucytosine and nephrotoxicity from amphotericin B. Simultaneous use of imidazole drugs and amphotericin B should be avoided because of potential antagonism between the two drugs.[68, 98]

Miconazole, a first-generation imidazole, also has severe toxicity when administered parenterally, and it has largely been supplanted by newer imidazole drugs. It is given in dosages of 600 to 1200 mg intravenously 3 times daily. Side effects include fever, chills, arrhythmias, phlebitis, hyponatremia, anemia, thrombocytosis, and hyperlipidemia.[62]

Fluconazole is available in an intravenous formulation. Dosage is equivalent to that of the oral formulation, since the oral drug's bioavailability approaches 100%. This route of administration is appropriate when the patient is unable to swallow or is unable to keep medications down secondary to intractable vomiting.

Prevention of Candidal Esophagitis

Patients whose immune defects cannot be reversed are at high risk for recurrent fungal infection. Antifungal prophylaxis is appropriate for many of these individuals. One must strike a balance, however, between clinical effectiveness and adverse side effects, including development of resistant strains and drug toxicity.[90] It has become clear that it is nearly impossible to eradicate fungi completely from the intestinal tract, but control of the number of fungi may be enough to prevent epithelial infection. Among patients with AIDS, 150 mg of fluconazole given orally each week was effective in reducing the risk of a recurrence of oropharyngeal infection.[70] Oral amphotericin B (10 or 50 mg/d) reduced the incidence of esophageal candidiasis among patients with hematologic disorders who were in intensive care units.[99, 100] In a double-blind randomized trial among bone marrow transplant recipients, fluconazole (400 mg/d) prophylaxis reduced the incidence of both systemic and superficial fungal infections.[101]

Complications and Outcome

After therapy with antifungal drugs, patients generally recover with no persistent sequelae. Patients who present with severe fungal esophagitis complicated by fistula formation, perforation, or stricture may, however, still have these anatomic defects after successful antifungal therapy. Patients with chronic mucocutaneous candidiasis frequently develop esophageal strictures.[102] Granulocytopenic patients with severe esophagitis may succumb from disseminated fungal infection, and those who survive may suffer chronic renal insufficiency or renal failure from cumulative amphotericin B toxicity.

Aspergillus Species

Mycology

Aspergillus species are ubiquitous, rapidly growing molds. The most important of these species in human infections are A. fumigatus and A. flavus.[94] Aspergilli can be differentiated from Candida organisms by their morphology. They have septate hyphae that are 2–4 μm wide, are dichotomously branched at 45 degrees, and have smooth parallel walls. On a culture plate, aspergilli appear as white, yellow, or green colonies. Characteristic conidiophores, if present, aid in the microscopic identification of Aspergillus species.

Clinical Presentation

Aspergillus is primarily a pulmonary pathogen, infecting patients with preexisting pulmonary disease, particularly bullous disease, via sequential colonization and growth, followed by invasion. Invasiveness is promoted by factors that suppress granulocyte function, such as high-dose corticosteroid therapy in patients with obstructive airway disease. In profoundly immunocompromised hosts, Aspergillus infection behaves aggressively, infecting the sinuses, lungs, and adjacent organs by direct extension across tissue planes.[94] Aspergillar infection in severely compromised cancer and AIDS patients may cause deep mucosal lesions in the esophagus, with progression to tracheoesophageal fistula formation.[48, 103] Patients with Aspergillus esophagitis typically present with symptoms of painful or difficult swallowing. Weight loss and concurrent mucosal candidiasis are also frequently present.[103] Aspergillosis should be considered in patients whose condition presents like Candida esophagitis but fails to respond to first-line antifungal therapy. An illustrative case is a patient with AIDS and a history of Candida esophagitis.[48] While on fluconazole maintenance therapy the patient developed a recrudescence of dysphagia, weight loss, and oral thrush. Endoscopy documented erythematous and friable esophageal mucosa with abundant white exudates consistent with candidiasis. Brushings and biopsies revealed both Candida and Aspergillus. Treatment with intravenous amphotericin B (total dose 500 mg) completely resolved both symptoms and endoscopic findings in this case.

Diagnosis

Endoscopic brushings and biopsies are essential for an accurate diagnosis of *Aspergillus* esophagitis. No specific diagnostic features for esophageal aspergillosis are revealed by esophageal radiography or by endoscopy. Blind brushings alone are of limited utility because *Aspergillus* is a common laboratory contaminant and occasionally a colonizing fungus. Endoscopically directed brushings and biopsies are more specific for the diagnosis of *Aspergillus* infection. Silver stain or PAS stain demonstrates the dichotomously branched septate hyphae of aspergilli and occasionally shows the characteristic conidiophores as well. A presumptive histologic diagnosis of aspergillosis should be confirmed by fungal culture, since in the absence of characteristic conidial features on tissue section, the identification of *Aspergillus* is tenuous.

Drug Therapy for Aspergillar Esophagitis

Treatment of *Aspergillus* esophagitis is with intravenous amphotericin B, since *Aspergillus* organism are resistant to the commonly used imidazoles, ketoconazole and fluconazole. Itraconazole, a new absorbable imidazole derivative, is active against *Aspergillus* organisms and may prove useful in the treatment of mucosal *Aspergillus* infections.[94] Meanwhile, amphotericin B remains the drug of choice. Adverse systemic side effects and nephrotoxicity are the major limiting factors in the use of amphotericin B. Studies are in progress to assess whether delivery of amphotericin B as a colloidal suspension or liposomal preparation reduces toxicity while maintaining therapeutic efficacy.[104]

Histoplasma Species

Mycology

Histoplasma capsulatum infection is the most common respiratory mycosis in the United States.[105] The principal endemic areas are the central United States and some scattered tropical, subtropical, and temperate zones of the world.[105] The fungus exists in soil in its mycelial phase but converts to yeast phase at the body temperature of mammalian hosts. The mycelial form consists of septate branching hyphae, bearing either macroconidia or microconidia at lateral and terminal positions. The primary infection is via inhalation of the infectious conidia, which are of appropriate size to reach the alveoli, where the organism infects the reticuloendothelial system (RES). There *Histoplasma* assumes the yeast form, which is ovoid (1.5–2.0 μm × 3.0–3.5 μm) and reproduces via budding. Growth is almost entirely within the phagocytic macrophages of infected tissues.[105] Generally, most infections are mild and self-limited. Occasionally, patients develop progressive pulmonary and lymphatic disease.[62] Disseminated histoplasmosis is a rare and potentially fatal development that is considered to be due to a defect in host immunity.[105] The esophagus is not known to be colonized or primarily infected by *Histoplasma*, but rather is involved via direct extension from the lungs and mediastinum or from hematogenous spread.[106, 107]

Clinical Presentation

Systemic symptoms of acute *Histoplasma* infection are nonspecific and include fever, headache, chills, cough, and aching chest pain. Dysphagia secondary to extrinsic compression of the esophagus by mediastinal lymph nodes or secondary to progressive mediastinal fibrosis is the most common presenting symptom of esophageal involvement. Less common presenting symptoms include bleeding and esophago-bronchial fistula formation.[108, 109]

Diagnosis

Physical findings are meager in histoplasmosis. Occasionally, hepatosplenomegaly is present, particularly in children. The examiner may note cachexia. Positive complement fixation serology for yeast phase antigens is suggestive of an acute or recent *Histoplasma* infection.[105] Chest radiographs in pulmonary histoplasmosis may reveal mediastinal adenopathy, pulmonary nodules, calcified nodes, and infiltrates, and an esophagogram may demonstrate extrinsic compression in the region of the right paratracheal or middle mediastinal lymph nodes. Endoscopy is unlikely to provide a diagnosis because the epithelium is not generally involved. Any mucosal lesions should, however, be brushed and a biopsy performed, with specimens submitted for analysis by silver stain and acid-fast stain as well as by routine preparations. Samples should also be sent for fungal and mycobacterial cultures. Bronchoscopy, mediastinoscopy, or thoracotomy may be required to obtain a tissue diagnosis. Silver stain reveals *H. capsulatum* in oval budding yeast forms, and H&E stain may show caseating granulomata.

Drug Therapy for Histoplasma Esophagitis

Esophageal complications from histoplasmosis have been treated traditionally with surgery. Clearly, patients with esophageal perforation or fistulization, related sepsis, or severe symptoms are more suited to surgical intervention. A subset of patients with extrinsic esophageal compression and mild symptoms without sepsis warrant more conservative therapy. Amphotericin B has been the mainstay of histoplasmosis therapy and was effective in resolving a tracheoesophageal fistula secondary to histoplasmosis. Ketoconazole and other new imidazoles are also active against *Histoplasma* and may replace amphotericin B in some clinical settings.[63]

VIRAL INFECTIONS

Herpes Simplex Virus

Virology

Herpes simplex virus is a member of the herpesvirus family, which comprise large, enveloped, double-stranded DNA viruses. The two distinct types of HSV—HSV I and HSV II—each have numerous strains. The HSV I type is the predominant cause of nasolabial, oropharyngeal, and esophageal infection, while HSV II primarily causes genital and perianal herpes. Herpes simplex virus causes an initial acute infection followed by latency. Sites of HSV I latency include the trigeminal nerve root ganglion and the autonomic ganglion of the superior cervical and vagus nerves.[110] During latency, viral DNA is in a circular form within the nerve cell nucleus, and transcription occurs in only a small portion of the viral genome.[111] Reactivation of HSV, with viral DNA replication, transcription, translation, encapsulation, and shedding, is dependent on host-virus interaction. In healthy individuals, reactivation episodes are milder than the initial infection owing to partial immunity. Immunocompromised patients suffer more frequent and more severe episodes of reactivation. Endogenous reactivation is much more common than exogenous reinfection.[112]

Herpes simplex virus infection is found worldwide, and humans are the only known reservoir of HSV. Herpesvirus is transmitted by direct contact with infected secretions. Primary HSV gingivostomatitis is a common self-limited illness of three- to five-year-old children.[111] Reactivation may occur without symptoms, and HSV has been isolated from saliva in 5 to 8% of asymptomatic children and 1 to 2% of adults.[111]

During primary infection, HSV preferentially invades squamous epithelium of skin and mucosa. Cell destruction, viral replication, and the host inflammatory response produce the characteristic painful vesicles with erythematous bases.[112] Vesicles become pustular and coalesce to form larger ulcers. Virus can be isolated from these vesicles and squamous epithelial cells at the edge of the ulcerations.[111] Although primary infection may occur, HSV esophagitis most often results from reactivation of latent HSV in the distribution of the vagus nerve.[110, 113] The advent of acyclovir prophylaxis has significantly reduced HSV reactivation among groups at risk. If host response to HSV infection is compromised, primary infection or reactivation may be severe and may progress to viremia, with visceral dissemination to liver, lungs, central nervous system (CNS), and in rare instances, the gut.[112]

Clinical Presentation

Herpes simplex virus esophagitis is a self-limited illness in the normal host, but in the compromised host HSV infection can be severe and prolonged. Patients typically present with an acute onset of severely painful and difficult swallowing (see Table 1–1). Constant retrosternal pain may be present as well as nausea, vomiting, and hematemesis. One series of studies reported that persistent nausea and vomiting were the primary symptoms of HSV esophagitis in marrow transplant patients.[7] Labial and oropharyngeal epithelia should be inspected carefully for lesions, since a fourth of reported HSV esophagitis patients had evidence of either HSV or *Candida* infection at these sites (see Table 1–1). Intestinal bleeding from HSV esophagitis can be a presenting sign, especially if platelet counts are low. Because HSV infection is usually confined to squamous epithelium, even in compromised hosts, systemic and intra-abdominal symptoms are uncommon, which is not the case with other infectious agents that cause esophagitis (see Table 1–1).

Diagnosis

CLINICAL DATA

A careful history and physical examination can provide a diagnosis of HSV esophagitis. A previously healthy, immunocompetent patient having a history of recurrent coldsores and presenting with nasolabial herpetic lesions concurrent with the onset of esophageal symptoms is likely to have HSV esophagitis. Further diagnostic evaluation is warranted when symptoms are atypical, the onset of esophageal symptoms does not correlate with visible lesions, oral thrush is present, undiagnosed immunodeficiency is suspected, or the patient is in severe distress.

RADIOLOGY

A double-contrast esophagogram can make the diagnosis of HSV esophagitis. Typical findings include discrete, superficial stellate ulcers in the midesophagus and otherwise normal-appearing mucosa (Fig. 1–3).[14, 114] Advanced HSV esophagitis may show plaques, cobblestoning, or a shaggy ulcerative appearance indistinguishable from that of *Candida* esophagitis.[115] Alternatively, radiographic examination of the esophagus may be normal, depending on the severity of mucosal involvement.[116] Radiographs seldom identify the vesicular stage of HSV esophagitis. *Candida* co-infection is frequently present in immunosuppressed hosts, making accurate radiographic diagnosis difficult. As often as not, radiographic findings are nonspecific in HSV esophagitis, and endoscopy is necessary to provide the diagnosis.[13]

ENDOSCOPY

Endoscopic appearance of HSV esophagitis depends on the amount of time the infection has been present. Rounded 1- to 3-mm vesicles are the earliest lesions, seen predominantly in the mid- to distal esophagus. The tip of vesicles may have a reticulated appearance just before the epithelium in this area is sloughed to produce small, 1- to 2-mm ulcers. Vesicles are fragile and rarely seen at the time of endoscopy. Characteristic sharply demarcated ulcers with raised margins and yellow-gray bases are formed after each vesicle sloughs most of its HSV-infected squamous cells (Fig. 1–4). These "punched-out" ulcers may have surrounding erythema, but the uninvolved mucosa is otherwise normal. If the infection progresses, ulcers begin to coalesce, and inflammatory exudates grossly resembling those of *Candida* esophagitis may develop.[115, 117–119] Confluent ulceration with denudement of the esophagus is found in severe HSV infection. These cases are difficult for the endoscopist because the area of ulceration can occupy the entire esophagus, leaving no squamous mucosal edge to provide perspective. As HSV preferentially infects squamous epithelium, margins of esophageal ulcers and islands of squamous epithelium must undergo biopsy and be brushed thoroughly to confirm the diagnosis of HSV esophagitis (Fig. 1–5). Biopsies of the ulcer base are inadequate to diagnose

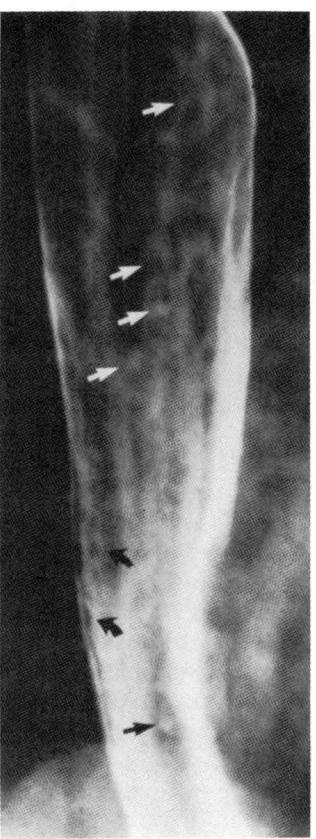

FIGURE 1–3.
A case of confirmed HSV esophagitis diagnosed on double-contrast esophagogram. Note the discrete, widely separated ulcers in the middle and distal esophagus, some of which have radiolucent halos of edematous mucosa (arrows). SOURCE: Levine MS, Loevner LA, Saul SH, et al. Herpes esophagitis: Sensitivity of double-contrast esophagography. Am J Roentgenol. 1988;151:59.

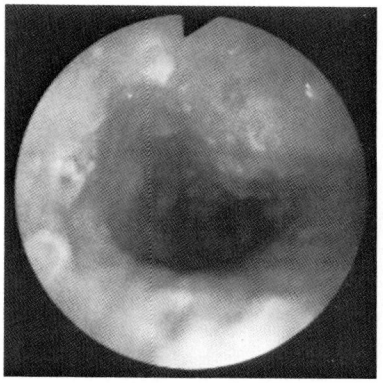

FIGURE 1–4.
Endoscopic photograph of HSV esophagitis showing sharply demarcated multiple ulcers with exudative bases. SOURCE: Silverstein FE, Tytgat GNJ. Atlas of Gastrointestinal Endoscopy. 2nd ed. New York: Gower Medical Publishing; 1991:3.19.

HSV infection. Brushings and biopsy samples should be submitted for cytology, routine histology, histochemical stains, and viral culture. Brushed material should be smeared on glass slides, some of which are then fixed in Papanicolaou's fixative, whereas others are air-dried. If low platelet counts preclude biopsy, analysis of brushings of the edges of ulcers is often sufficient to diagnose HSV infection. Biopsy specimens should be fixed in buffered formalin and B5 fixative, if available. Picric acid solutions (Bouin's, Hollande's) should not be used alone as a fixative because viral antigens are not preserved well for immunostaining.

HISTOLOGY

The pathologist should be notified that herpesviruses are being considered so that appropriate immunohistologic stains are used in the event that cytology and routine stains prove nondiagnostic. Diagnostic changes of HSV infection include multinucleated giant cells, ballooning degeneration, "ground glass" intranuclear Cowdry type A inclusion bodies, and margination of chromatin. Unlike CMV infection, herpetic infection demonstrates no cytoplasmic inclusion bodies. One blind study suggests that aggregates of macrophages are characteristic of the inflammatory response in ulcerative herpetic esophagitis when compared with nonherpetic ulcerative lesions (including *Candida* and bacteria).[120] Immunohistologic stains using monoclonal antibodies to HSV antigens may show infected cells that have no morphologic changes. The combination of directed brushings and biopsies improves the sensitivity of endoscopic diagnosis.[121] In contrast to CMV ulceration, an HSV ulcer rarely invades below the epithelial layer, and biopsies of the ulcer base are generally nondiagnostic. Thus, in a denuded esophagus, histologic diagnosis of HSV may be difficult.

CULTURE

Brushed material and biopsy specimens should be submitted in viral transport media for later culture. Viral culture is more sensitive than microscopic examination for diagnosis of HSV infection.[122] Herpes simplex virus grows readily in diploid fibroblast or rabbit kidney cells. Cytopathic changes are usually evident 24 to 96 hours after inoculation.[111] Alternatively, HSV can be identified rapidly by immunohistochemical staining of a centrifuged culture suspension by shell vial culture technique after 24 to 36 hours.[123] Although highly sensitive and specific, viral culture methods are dependent on viability of the cell cultures; a report of toxic indicates that nonspecific cellular damage has occurred and that no diagnostic viral culture results are forthcoming.

Drug Therapy for HSV Esophagitis

Herpes simplex virus esophagitis in the immunocompetent patient typically requires only simple supportive care, such as analgesics and possibly topical anesthetics.[114] On occasion, intravenous hydration may be necessary for patients unable to maintain adequate fluid intake secondary to painful swallowing. Symptoms should resolve completely within several days, though reepithelialization of mucosa may take longer. A double-blind, randomized, placebo-controlled trial of high-dose oral acyclovir in the treatment of 174 nonimmunocompromised patients with recurrent labial HSV found that initiation of drug within 1 hour of the first sign or symptom hastened time to lesion resolution by 27% and time to pain resolution by 36%.[124] It is reasonable to assume that acyclovir therapy immediately after onset of esophageal symptoms would be effective in hastening recovery from HSV esophagitis, but unfortunately the diagnosis of HSV esophagitis is rarely established so

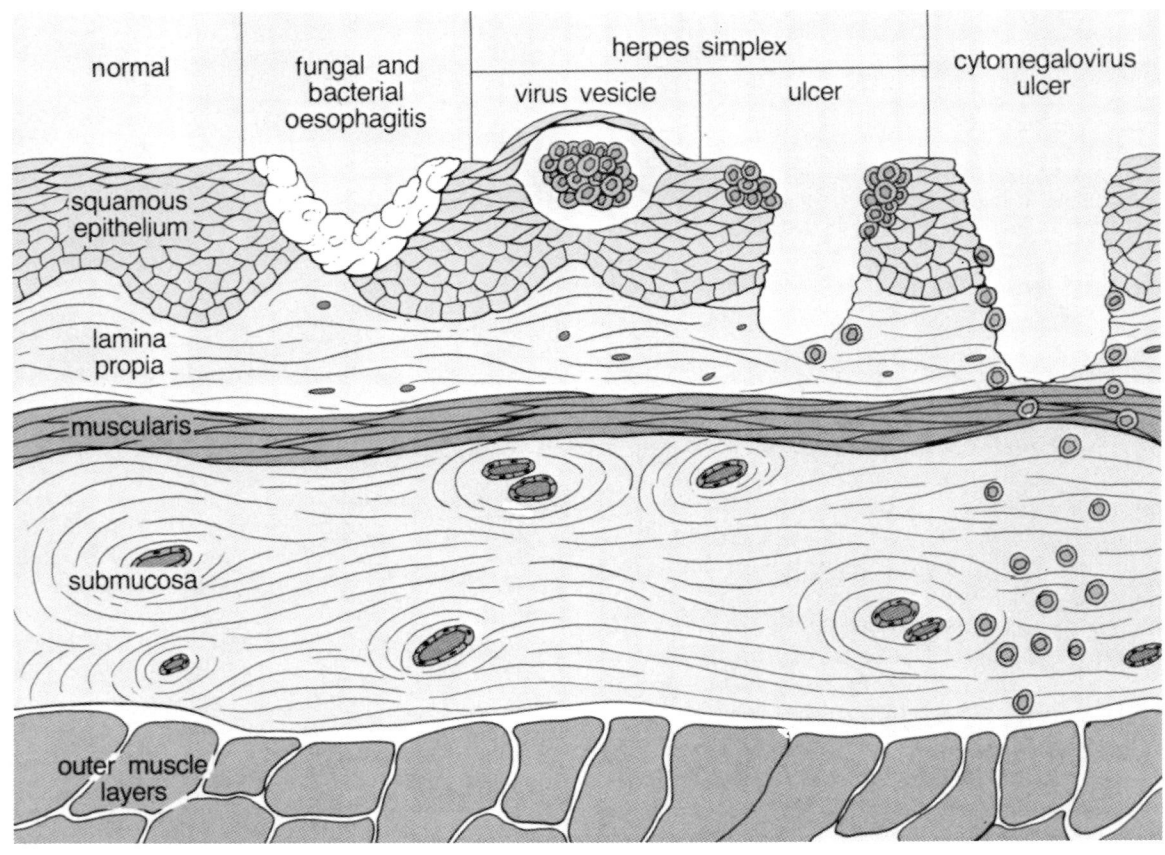

FIGURE 1–5.
Guide for diagnostic endoscopic biopsy. Note HSV tropism for the squamous epithelium and CMV tropism for subepithelial esophageal tissues. For accurate diagnosis in an ulcerated esophagus, biopsies must be obtained from ulcer margins to detect HSV and from the ulcer base to detect CMV. SOURCE: Silverstein FE, Tytgat GNJ. Atlas of Gastrointestinal Endoscopy. 2nd ed. New York: Gower Medical Publishing; 1991:3.23.

quickly. Since symptoms usually persist for only a few days, any clinical utility in treating immunocompetent patients with high-dose oral acyclovir is unlikely. Such spontaneous healing of HSV esophagitis is not always the case in a compromised host, in whom HSV infection may persist until treated or until adequate immune function returns. Complications of progressive HSV esophagitis include bleeding, HSV pneumonia, and superinfection of the injured esophagus.[113, 125] Antiviral therapy has proved to be effective in both prophylaxis and treatment of HSV esophagitis among immunocompromised patients.

Acyclovir, the mainstay of HSV infection treatment, is a nucleoside analog that is phosphorylated by viral and cellular thymidine kinase to a triphosphate form. This molecule is a potent inhibitor of viral DNA polymerase.[126] Acyclovir does not eradicate the virus, but it is effective in reducing the severity of primary HSV infections and in suppressing reactivation. Therapy for es-

tablished HSV esophagitis is with 250 mg/m^2 of parenteral acyclovir every 8 hours for 7 to 10 days (see Table 1–4). Acyclovir is generally tolerated well. Adverse reactions include gastrointestinal disturbances and headaches with oral acyclovir, crystalline nephropathy with high-dosage intravenous (IV) acyclovir, and encephalopathy with either acyclovir form.[127]

Strains of HSV resistant to acyclovir have emerged via mutations in viral DNA polymerase and thymidine kinase.[50, 51] Although most reported strains of acyclovir-resistant HSV have attenuated virulence, progression of clinical disease in immunocompromised patients has been reported.[51, 52] Foscarnet (trisodium phosphonoformate), a pyrophosphate derivative that inhibits viral DNA polymerase at the pyrophosphate binding site, is effective in treating most strains of acyclovir-resistant HSV, although isolates resistant to both foscarnet and acyclovir have been reported.[51, 128–132] Foscarnet is administered as a 60-mg/kg slow intravenous infusion every 8

TABLE 1–4. PREVENTION AND TREATMENT OF HERPES SIMPLEX VIRUS (HSV) ESOPHAGITIS

DRUGS AVAILABLE	PREVENTION OF ACTIVE HSV INFECTION (FOR PATIENTS AT RISK)	TREATMENT OF ESTABLISHED HSV INFECTION
Acyclovir capsules (200 mg)	200–400 mg po 4–5 times daily or 800 mg bid	200–400 mg po 5 times daily
Acyclovir for IV use (500 mg/10 ml vial, admixed to final conc. <7 mg/ml)	250 mg/m² IV q 12 h	250 mg/m² IV q 8 h
Foscarnet for IV use (12 gm/500 ml)*	N/A	60 mg/kg IV q 8 h for 2 wk, then 90–120 mg/kg daily for 2 wk

*For treatment of HSV resistant to acyclovir.

hours for 2 weeks, often followed by maintenance therapy with 90–120 mg/kg daily for an additional 2 weeks. It is more expensive and less well tolerated than acyclovir. Toxicities of foscarnet therapy are significant and include renal insufficiency and electrolyte imbalances such as hypocalcemia.[53, 133]

Vidarabine (adenine arabinoside) is a purine analog that preferentially inhibits herpes group viral polymerases.[126] It reduces the mortality from herpes encephalitis, neonatal HSV infection, and HSV infection in immunocompromised patients. A randomized comparison of foscarnet versus vidarabine in AIDS patients who had acyclovir-resistant mucocutaneous herpetic lesions found that foscarnet had superior efficacy and less toxicity than vidarabine.[129] In high dosages, vidarabine's use is limited by bone marrow toxicity and neurologic abnormalities.[126, 132] Bone marrow toxicity limits the clinical utility of vidarabine because the drug can weaken an already impaired immune system.

Prevention of HSV Esophagitis

Herpes simplex virus prophylaxis is indicated for immunosuppressed patients who are at risk for reactivation of HSV infection. These cases include HSV seropositive transplant recipients and AIDS patients with recurrent herpetic infections. Acyclovir prophylactic therapy in HSV-seropositive patients has almost eliminated HSV esophagitis among solid organ and bone marrow transplant recipients.[134–136] Table 1–4 gives recommended dosing schedules for HSV prophylaxis in immunocompromised patients with either oral or intravenous acyclovir.

Complications and Outcome

Among immunocompetent individuals, the initial episode of HSV esophagitis is self-limited, and if reactivation occurs, the episodes are generally mild, with no long-term complications. Among immunocompromised hosts, however, reactivation of HSV infection may follow a more harmful course. Complications of severe, unresponsive, or untreated HSV esophagitis include mucosal necrosis, mucosal superinfection, hemorrhage, strictures, HSV pneumonia, tracheoesophageal fistula formation, and disseminated HSV infection (Fig. 1–6). A case of esophageal perforation associated with HSV infection has been reported.[137] In patients with prolonged immunodeficiency, HSV prophylaxis with acyclovir reduces recurrence, though virulent strains of resistant HSV have developed in some patients on long-term prophylaxis.

Cytomegalovirus

Virology

Cytomegalovirus is a ubiquitous herpesvirus that, subject to geographic variation, results in positive serology in roughly 80% of the world's adult population.[111] Primary CMV infection has two epidemiologic peaks, in preschool children and young adults. Studies using the method of in situ hybridization demonstrate that CMV DNA can be found in a talent form in most of the organs of the body.[138] Latent infection of leukocytes is responsible for the high incidence of transmission of CMV infection by blood product transfusions from CMV-seropositive blood donors into CMV-seronegative recipients.[139]

Both humoral and cellular immune responses are important in controlling CMV infections. Seropositive patients with prolonged deficiency of cellular immunity are at high risk for reactivation of latent CMV infection in spite of high levels of circulating antibody to CMV.[111] Primary CMV infections in immunosuppressed patients tend to be more severe than in immunocompetent hosts. Systemic CMV infection can suppress hemopoiesis, resulting in marrow hypoplasia[140–143] and an increased risk for additional infections.[144]

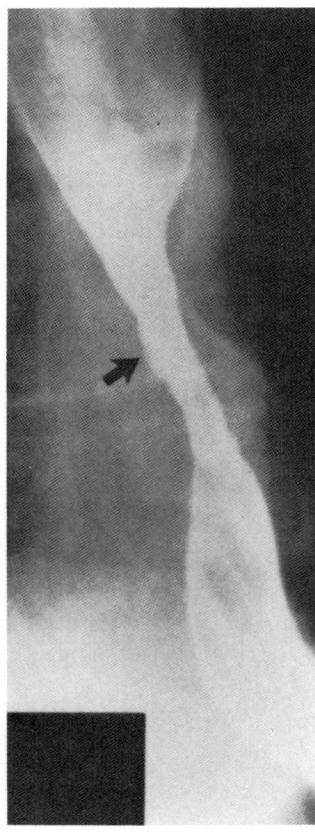

FIGURE 1–6.
An esophagogram from a case of severe HSV esophagitis and ulceration that was complicated by the development of a midesophageal stricture as the herpetic lesions healed. SOURCE: Levine MS, Loevner LA, Saul SH, et al. Herpes esophagitis: Sensitivity of double-contrast esophagography. Am J Roentgenol. 1988;151:61.

Clinical Presentation

Cytomegalovirus esophagitis differs in its clinical presentation from other viral and fungal infections. Onset of symptoms is typically more gradual than with HSV esophagitis. Painful, difficult swallowing and retrosternal pain are less common, but nausea, vomiting, fever, epigastric pain, diarrhea, and weight loss are more prominent symptoms (see Table 1–1),[4, 5, 145] reflecting the fact that CMV infection is systemic and involves multiple organs in addition to the esophagus. The esophagus may, however, be the first site at which CMV infection is clinically manifest.[4] CMV esophagitis may coexist with both HSV and candidal infection in transplant recipients and patients with AIDS.[5, 33] In recent cases of coexisting *Candida* and CMV esophagitis among patients with AIDS, pain and dysphagia ceased after treatment with antifungal drugs, suggesting that CMV lesions were not the cause of dysphagia.[81]

Diagnosis

RADIOLOGY

Double-contrast barium radiographs of CMV esophagitis may demonstrate discrete small su-

perficial ulcerative lesions indistinguishable from those of HSV esophagitis, but in other patients the esophagogram may appear normal or have one or more large flat elongate ulcers.[14] These ovoid or elongated ulcers may extend for several centimeters or more (Fig. 1–7). On occasion, a radiolucent rim of edematous mucosa is apparent. Since HSV esophageal ulcers are rarely as long as several centimeters, the presence of one or more giant ulcers is suggestive of CMV esophagitis in patients with AIDS, although HIV-related idiopathic esophageal ulcers may also be several centimeters in length.[14]

ENDOSCOPY

The diagnosis of CMV esophagitis is usually dependent on endoscopic biopsies because neither clinical assessment nor radiology is sufficiently accurate to commit a patient to antiviral therapy. Cytomegalovirus infection of the esophagus is typically most prominent in the mid- to distal esophagus, with a characteristic early appearance of superficial erosions with geographic, serpiginous, nonraised borders (Fig. 1–8).[116, 146] As the infection progresses, shallow ulcerations can extend for 10 to 15 cm in length. In contrast to HSV ulcers, complete

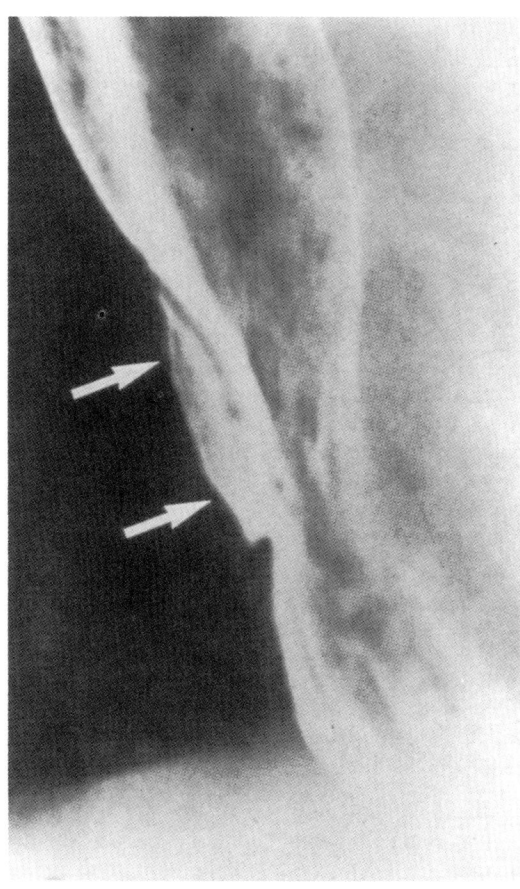

FIGURE 1–7.
A single-contrast esophagogram demonstrating a large, flat CMV ulcer (arrows) in a patient with AIDS. Endoscopic biopsy and cultures are required for a definitive diagnosis. SOURCE: Levine MS. Radiology of the esophagus: A pattern approach. Radiology. 1991;179(1):5.

denudation of the esophagus is unusual with CMV infection. Although shallow ulcers are typical, deep ulcerations with raised margins have also been reported.[116] Since CMV-infected fibroblasts and endothelial cells are found in the base of esophageal ulcers but never in squamous epithelium, multiple biopsies should be taken from the center of the ulcer crater.[5, 146] Biopsies containing only squamous epithelium are not evaluable for CMV, and superficial brushings for cytology do little to increase the diagnostic yield for CMV infection. Biopsy specimens should be placed into buffered formalin and B5 fixatives as well as viral transport media. As CMV is capable of infecting both epithelial and lamina propria cells of the stomach and intestines, biopsies of abnormal mucosa in these areas should also be sent for histologic study and culture for patients at risk for CMV infection.

HISTOLOGY

Characteristic histologic features of CMV infection are large cells in the subepithelial layer, with amphophilic intranuclear inclusions, a halo surrounding the nucleus, and, unlike HSV and VZV, multiple small cytoplasmic inclusions (Fig. 1–9). Immunohistochemical staining for early, intermediate, and late antigens and in situ hybridization for CMV DNA can confirm the diagnosis of CMV infection when infected cells are neither megaloid nor inclusion-bearing.[147] The sensitivity of histologic and immunohistologic methods, however, is only about half that of viral culture methods.[148] For this reason, we suggest that the biopsy specimen that is best targeted in the ulcer base be sent for viral culture. This is usually the first biopsy taken, since a bloody endoscopic field may hinder accurate placement of the forceps. On occasion, biopsy specimens document concurrent HSV, fungal, or bacterial esophagitis.[33]

CULTURE

Cytomegalovirus can be isolated in human diploid fibroblast cultures. Such cultures are very sensitive but are of limited clinical utility

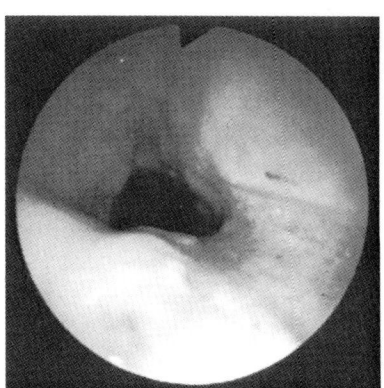

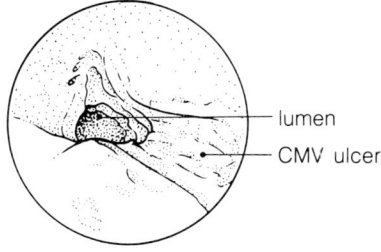

lumen
CMV ulcer

FIGURE 1–8.
Endoscopic photograph of a large CMV ulcer of the esophagus in a patient with AIDS. Biopsies should be taken from the base of this lesion to confirm CMV infection. SOURCE: Silverstein FE, Tytgat GNJ. Atlas of Gastrointestinal Endoscopy. 2nd ed. New York: Gower Medical Publishing; 1991:3.22.

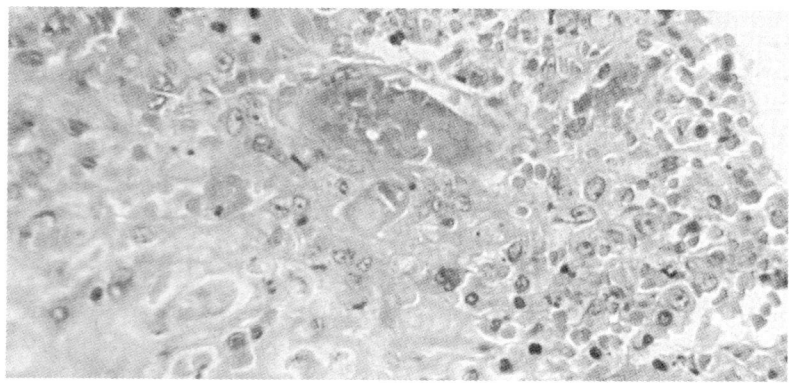

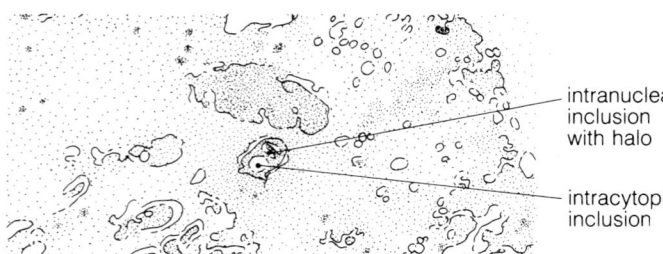

intranuclear
inclusion
with halo

intracytoplasmic
inclusion

FIGURE 1–9.
The typical cellular changes associated with CMV infection. The indicated cell has an intranuclear inclusion with surrounding halo and multiple cytoplasmic inclusions. SOURCE: Silverstein FE, Tytgat GNJ. Atlas of Gastrointestinal Endoscopy. 2nd ed. New York: Gower Medical Publishing; 1991:3.22.

because cytopathic changes may take 3 to 14 days to develop.[111] By contrast, newer techniques using immunologic staining of centrifugation cultures can provide a diagnosis of CMV infection in only 1 to 2 days.[127] A report of toxic on viral culture means that nonspecific tissue culture damage has occurred and that no results will be forthcoming.

Drug Therapy for CMV Esophagitis

Ganciclovir and foscarnet are both effective antiviral drugs in the treatment of CMV infection (Table 1–5).[149, 150] The two drugs have different mechanisms of action and differing adverse effects. Ganciclovir, or dehydroxyphenylglycol (DHPG), is an acyclovir analog that

TABLE 1–5. PREVENTION AND TREATMENT OF CYTOMEGALOVIRUS (CMV) ESOPHAGITIS

	PREVENTION OF CMV DISEASE (FOR PATIENTS AT RISK)	TREATMENT OF ESTABLISHED CMV DISEASE
Drugs Available		
Acyclovir for IV use (500 mg/10ml vial, admixed to final concentration of <7 mg/ml)*	For seropositive patients‡ or recipients of organs from seropositive donors: 500 mg/m² IV 9 8 h	N/A
Ganciclovir for IV use (500 mg/10ml vial, admixed to final concentration of <10 mg/ml)†	For seropositive patients‡ or recipients of organs from seropositive donors: 5 mg/kg IV q 12 h for 5 d then once daily as maintenance therapy	5 mg/kg IV q 12 h for 2 wk, then once daily for 2 wk
Foscarnet for IV use (12 g/500ml)	N/A	60 mg/kg IV q 8 h for 2 wk, then 90–120 mg/kg daily for 2 wk
Epidemiologic Methods	For seronegative patients: Transfusion of CMV seronegative blood products Organ transplants from CMV seronegative donors Leukofiltration of CMV seropositive blood products	N/A

*Adjust dose for renal function.
†Use of oral ganciclovir formulations are under study.
‡Marrow transplant patients; trials of prophylactic ganciclovir for HIV-infected patients have not been completed.

inhibits the DNA polymerase of human herpesviruses, including CMV. Ganciclovir, administered 5 mg/kg intravenously every 12 hours for 2 weeks, was effective in clearing CMV from esophageal ulcers when compared with a placebo, although patient symptoms and endoscopic findings were not significantly different after 2 weeks of therapy.[4] Several uncontrolled studies of ganciclovir therapy in both organ transplant recipients and AIDS patients report clinical improvement in intestinal symptoms in CMV infection.[149, 150–155] As recurrence of CMV infection is common after 2 weeks of therapy with ganciclovir, full-dose therapy should be administered for 2 weeks and followed by maintenance therapy for several additional weeks or until immunosuppression resolves. AIDS patients often remain on indefinite maintenance therapy for recurrent CMV infection. Adverse effects of ganciclovir therapy include bone marrow toxicity. Myelosuppression may be severe when ganciclovir is administered concurrently with zidovudine.[156] Dosage must be adjusted for renal insufficiency.[157] Long-term therapy with ganciclovir has seen an emergence of ganciclovir-resistant strains of CMV.[54–56, 158]

The use of foscarnet has increased among patients with CMV disease who have failed to respond to ganciclovir or have insufficient bone marrow reserve to tolerate the neutropenic side effect of ganciclovir.[145, 159] Fifteen of 18 cases (83%) of CMV esophagitis in AIDS patients underwent rapid resolution of symptoms following treatment with foscarnet.[159] Relapse occurred in 3 of the 15 cases. A group of 5 AIDS patients with CMV esophagitis unresponsive to ganciclovir all had resolution of symptoms with foscarnet.[158] Foscarnet has proved to be valuable in CMV-infected organ transplant patients as well.[55, 149] Typically, patients are treated with foscarnet for 2 to 3 weeks, followed by maintenance therapy for several weeks or until immune reconstitution. Treatment with foscarnet has seen the emergence of foscarnet-resistant strains of CMV.[160] A case of successful simultaneous treatment with combined ganciclovir and foscarnet for CMV retinitis refractory to either agent alone has been reported.[161] Adverse effects of foscarnet therapy include renal insufficiency and electrolyte disturbances, particularly low-ionized calcium.[158, 162] Dosage should be adjusted for renal function.[163] Patients must be well-hydrated and monitored for iatrogenic complications.

Prevention of CMV Infection

Screening of all blood products for CMV antibodies has decreased significantly the morbidity and mortality from primary CMV infection among CMV-seronegative organ transplant recipients who received CMV-seronegative donor organs. Organ transplant recipients who are either CMV-seropositive or who receive organs from CMV-seropositive donors should receive antiviral prophylaxis (see Table 1–5). Prophylaxis with both acyclovir and ganciclovir has been studied. Their disparate efficacies and adverse effects influence their usefulness. In the case of CMV infection, ganciclovir is the more efficacious agent, but its use is hampered by bone marrow suppression, and although acyclovir is significantly less effective, it has a more acceptable side effect profile. Oral acyclovir has proved partially effective in suppressing productive CMV infection in both renal and hepatic transplant recipients.[164, 165] In CMV seropositive bone marrow transplant recipients, prophylaxis with acyclovir provides partial protection until successful engraftment and rising leukocyte counts allow therapy with ganciclovir.[166] In the marrow transplant patient, ganciclovir treatment of early CMV infection (i.e., excretion of virus) has proved highly effective in preventing symptomatic CMV disease.[149, 167] Many patients, however, develop CMV infection and clinical disease simultaneously. Recent randomized trials have demonstrated that prophylactic ganciclovir following solid organ transplantation or bone marrow transplantation is highly effective in preventing both infection and disease.[43, 165, 168]

Because blood bank supplies of seronegative blood products are limited, several studies have examined the concept that elimination of CMV-bearing leukocytes from blood product transfusions might lower the risk of transmitting CMV.[169] This is particularly relevant for solid organ transplant recipients and patients who undergo open heart surgery, for whom transfusion requirements can be large. Several methods are effective in achieving leukocyte depletion. Centrifugation alone reduced the risk of CMV transmission in open heart surgery patients despite removing only 60% of the leukocytes present in each unit of blood.[170] Centrifugation and subsequent saline washing remove 89% of leukocytes from units of red cells, and some investigators have found a reduced risk for CMV transmission.[171] Studies of frozen, deglycerolized blood products show little, if any, risk for transmission of CMV.[172, 173] In-line filtration of red cells and platelets at the time of transfusion appears to be a very effective and practical technique for leukocyte depletion. Among 32 bone marrow transplant patients who received on average 20 units of red cells and 130 units of platelets from a donor pool with CMV seroprevalence of 50%, none developed CMV disease, and only 1 patient developed a positive surveillance culture for CMV.[174]

Complications and Outcome

Lesions resulting from esophageal CMV infection can be a source of persistent nausea, anorexia, and intestinal bleeding even after the virus has been effectively eliminated from tissue. Large esophageal ulcers require months to re-epithelialize under the best of circumstances and may take longer if there is acid-pepsin reflux or superinfection with fungi and bacteria. While severe immunosuppression persists the risk of reactivation of CMV and reinfection is high. Stricture formation may occur, although perforation is rare after CMV esophagitis.[175]

Varicella-Zoster Virus

Virology

Varicella-zoster virus is a double-stranded DNA virus morphologically identical to HSV. The lesions of VZV infection are similar to those of HSV as well. Primary VZV infection in children causes the characteristic generalized pruritic vesicular eruptions of chickenpox. Primary VZV infection among immunocompromised children is frequently severe, with visceral dissemination in 20 to 30% and a mortality rate of 7 to 30%.[111] The lung is the major target of viscerally disseminated VZV, followed by brain and liver. Symptomatic esophageal involvement with chickenpox is uncommon, although oropharyngeal lesions are common in normal children. The esophagus is rarely involved in cases of herpes zoster, or reactivation of latent VZV.

Clinical Presentation

As VZV esophagitis is a rare manifestation of VZV infection, no typical presentation is known.[5, 176-179] Case reports have almost all been of either severely immunocompromised or very ill patients. Symptoms of VZV esophagitis are similar to those of HSV esophagitis, including painful or difficult swallowing. Key to the diagnosis of VZV esophagitis is the finding of concurrent dermatologic VZV lesions in all reported cases.

Diagnosis

CLINICAL DATA

Primary VZV infection (chickenpox) or secondary VZV infection (herpes zoster) can al-most always be diagnosed clinically based on the characteristic evolving appearance and distribution of dermatologic lesions. Rarely, HSV infection in an immunocompromised patient can masquerade as VZV, producing a varicelliform or zosteriform eruption distinguishable only by culture or immunostaining of fluid from fresh vesicles.[111] Consequently, though esophageal VZV infection may be suspected on clinical grounds, endoscopy is warranted to confirm the diagnosis and to exclude other causes of esophageal symptoms such as concurrent infections, pill esophagitis, or reflux esophagitis.

ENDOSCOPY

Varicella-zoster virus esophagitis can have an endoscopic appearance indistinguishable from that of HSV, with occasional vesicles, discrete ulcerative lesions, and confluence of ulcerations. The lesions can progress to form necrotizing esophagitis in severely immunosuppressed patients.[176, 179] Esophageal lesions should be biopsied and brushed thoroughly for culture, histology, and cytology.

HISTOLOGY

Epithelial VZV lesion histology is characterized by edema, ballooning degeneration, and vesicles lined by multinucleated giant cells that contain intranuclear eosinophilic inclusion bodies.[112, 180] Immunohistochemical staining using monoclonal antibodies to VZV antigens is helpful in the confirmation of clinically suspected VZV infection.[112]

CULTURE

Varicella-zoster virus is more difficult to isolate in tissue culture than is HSV. It grows best in fresh human embryo lung fibroblast culture, although other tissues such as human foreskin fibroblasts or melanoma cells are sometimes used.[180] Cytopathic changes are similar to those in HSV but are not present until after 3 to 10 days.[112] Consequently, routine culture techniques are of limited clinical utility.

Drug Therapy for VZV Esophagitis

Acyclovir and vidarabine (adenine arabinoside) are effective agents in the treatment of VZV infections.[181, 182] A multicenter controlled trial of acyclovir for chickenpox in normal children found a reduction in duration and severity of disease compared with children taking placebo.[183] Among immunocompromised children with primary VZV infection, acyclovir and vidarabine were equally effective in shortening the time to complete crusting of all lesions.[184] Relapses of VZV infection have occurred in immunocompromised children following short-course therapy with acyclovir for 5 days, suggesting that longer courses of acyclovir may be necessary in these patients.[185] Varicella-zoster infection developed in 14 (21%) of 67 pediatric liver transplant patients on maintenance immunosuppression.[186] Despite treatment with intravenous acyclovir, 2 of these patients died of VZV-related complications.

Adult AIDS patients may develop recurrent VZV eruptions, requiring prolonged oral acyclovir therapy. Emergence of acyclovir resistance has become a problem in these patients. The reported mechanism of acyclovir resistance in VZV strains is thymidine kinase deficiency.[187, 188] This is also the mechanism of resistance for some strains of HSV.[50, 51] Foscarnet appears to be a viable alternative therapy for treatment of acyclovir-resistant VZV infection among AIDS patients.[190, 191]

Prevention of VZV Infection

Varicella-zoster immune globulin (VZIG) prophylaxis of varicella is recommended for susceptible patients with an immunocompromising illness or those who are within 96 hours of exposure to VZV.[191] Prophylaxis with VZIG against primary infection should not be delayed because immune globulin is ineffective during clinical VZV infection. Vaccination with a live attenuated VZV virus has been used in both healthy and immunocompromised children, demonstrating safety and efficacy in the prevention of chickenpox.[192, 193] Prophylaxis against VZV reactivation with intravenous, then oral, acyclovir in bone marrow transplant patients has significantly reduced clinical VZV infection during the first 6 months posttransplant.[133]

Complications and Outcome

Necrotizing esophagitis has been reported in patients with severe immunodeficiency and disseminated VZV infection.[175, 178] The esophageal component may be relatively minor in comparison with other manifestations of disseminated VZV infection in these patients, such as varicella encephalitis, pneumonitis, and fulminant hepatitis. Little is known of the long-term sequelae of VZV esophagitis, but necrotic lesions may lead to perforation and esophageal stricture.

Epstein-Barr Virus

Virology

Epstein-Barr virus is a double-stranded DNA virus of the herpesvirus family that is present worldwide and is the cause of heterophile antibody–positive infectious mononucleosis. Epstein-Barr virus is also implicated, through DNA hybridization studies, in African Burkitt's lymphoma and nasopharyngeal carcinoma[111, 112] as well as lymphoproliferative syndromes, lymphomas, and oral hairy leukoplakia among immunocompromised subjects.[194] Oral hairy leukoplakia is a white, raised mucosal lesion typically found on the lateral tongue margin of patients with AIDS.

Clinical Presentation

Reports of esophageal manifestations of EBV in healthy subjects are rare. In infectious mononucleosis, a sore throat is a nearly universal complaint. As a diagnosis of EBV is often clinically apparent, further investigation of throat pain with endoscopy is generally not warranted. Odynophagia and hematemesis have, however, been reported in an otherwise healthy patient with infectious mononucleosis.[195] In this case, esophageal ulceration was attributed to EBV, as no other etiology was apparent. Similarly, immunodeficient patients with HIV infection have presented with esophageal symptoms of dysphagia, pain, sore throat, and weight loss that were eventually attributed to EBV.[196]

Diagnosis

ENDOSCOPY

Endoscopy of one immunocompetent patient with acute EBV infection revealed multiple 3 to 5 mm esophageal ulcerations with erythematous rims and gray gelatinous bases.[195] Histologic studies were nondiagnostic, and cultures for CMV and HSV were negative. In this case, the diagnosis of EBV esophagitis was presumptive, based on serology. Epstein-Barr viral infection of the esophagus was diagnosed in 5 of 18 AIDS patients with discrete esophageal ulcerations.[197] The diagnosis of EBV infection was based on in situ DNA hybridization in 3 cases and on histologic changes in 2 cases. These esophageal EBV ulcers were different from typical HSV ulcers in that they were deep, often linear and located in the midesophagus.

HISTOLOGY

A diagnosis of EBV infection can be confirmed by DNA hybridization studies of tissue biopsies using Southern blot or in situ techniques.[197] In situ DNA hybridization did demonstrate EBV DNA in squamous epithelial cells of esophageal biopsy specimens from 3 to 5 patients with esophageal ulcers and 0 among control AIDS patients. Of interest, the histologic features of EBV-infected esophageal mucosa are identical to those of oral hairy leukoplakia in AIDS patients (epithelial hyperplasia, parakeratosis, koilocytosis), suggesting that the lesions in the esophagus are variants of oral hairy leukoplakia.[15, 196]

CULTURE

Human umbilical cord B lymphocytes are favored as indicator cells for EBV isolation because of their susceptibility to infection. Lymphoid tissues and leukocytes from seronegative adults are not useful for cultivation of EBV because of suppressive interference from T cells. Virus-positive cultures show clusters of large proliferating lymphoblastoid cells. Identification is via indirect immunofluorescence assay for EBV antigen.[198]

Drug Therapy for Epstein-Barr Virus Infection

Treatment of infectious mononucleosis is supportive, and full recovery is the rule in almost all otherwise healthy individuals. Oral hairy leukoplakia lesions have been effectively cleared with oral acyclovir in patients with AIDS.[200] As EBV has been demonstrated both in oral hairy leukoplakia lesions and in histologically identical esophageal ulcers, acyclovir would be reasonable therapy for treatment of these esophageal lesions.[15, 196] The response of oral hairy leukoplakia to oral acyclovir is dependent on continuing presence of the drug; when acyclovir is withdrawn, oral hairy leukoplakia recurs.[200, 201] Therefore, successful treatment of symptomatic esophageal EBV lesions may require long-term maintenance acyclovir therapy.

Complications and Outcome

Long-term sequelae of EBV esophageal infection are unknown, but since few patients with AIDS suffer significant complications of oral hairy leukoplakia, significant complications of the histologically identical esophageal lesions are also unlikely. Some increased risk for malignant transformation of EBV-infected esophageal tissues is possible, given the association between EBV and nasopharyngeal carcinoma.

Human Immunodeficiency Virus

Virology

Human immunodeficiency virus type I is a 100-nm diameter single-stranded diploid RNA retrovirus that preferentially infects CD4 surface antigen-presenting lymphocytes.[202] Upon entering host cells, viral RNA is transcribed by viral reverse-transcriptase into double-stranded DNA. The virally encoded DNA then enters the nucleus and is integrated into the host cell DNA. HIV genome and viral particles have been demonstrated in esophageal ulcerations in the absence of other identifiable pathogens.[24, 26]

Clinical Presentation

Painful esophageal mucosal ulcerations can develop during acute HIV seroconversion syndrome.[24, 26, 27] This syndrome is a 2-week long, flulike illness experienced by many HIV-infected patients approximately 2 to 3 weeks after HIV exposure. Characteristics include a macular erythematous eruption, fever, chills, and malaise.[26, 27, 203] Symptoms of a sore throat, severe odynophagia, dysphagia, and weight loss may precede HIV seroconversion and lead to a diagnosis of ulcerative esophagitis. The presence of HIV I P24 antigen in serum or the cultures of blood and biopsy tissues has confirmed HIV infection in these seronegative patients.[24, 27] Other HIV-infected patients developed esophageal ulcers well after developing positive HIV serology or clinically overt AIDS.[14, 19, 76, 204, 205] These patients also present with acute onset of painful, difficult swallowing as the most common symptom. Concurrent clinical findings often include weight loss, painful oropharyngeal lesions, oral thrush, diarrhea, and gastrointestinal bleeding (see Table 1–1).

Diagnosis

RADIOLOGY

Radiographic findings in HIV-related esophagitis are varied. Several case reports describe single giant ulcers up to 4.5 cm in length, with smooth, irregular, or undermining margins (Fig. 1–10).[14, 28, 204] Other findings have included multiple discrete ulcerations.[14] The majority of radiographic lesions are located in the middle to distal esophagus.

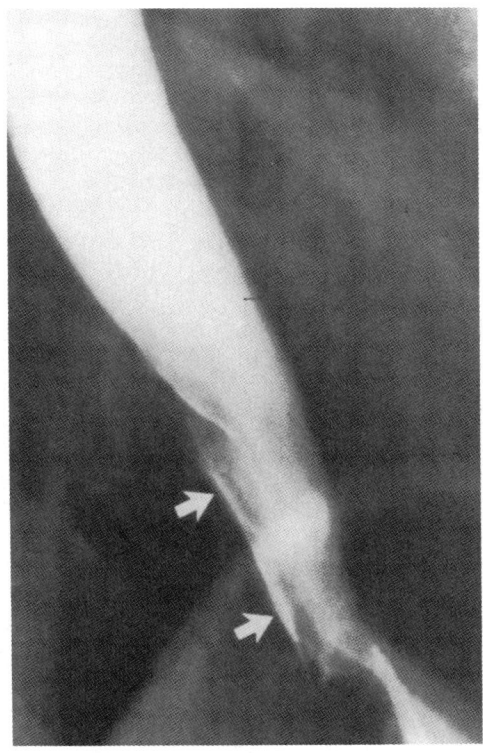

FIGURE 1–10.
Single-contrast esophagogram showing a giant HIV-related ulcer (arrows) in the distal esophagus of a patient with AIDS. Endoscopic biopsies, brushings, and cultures did not detect an identifiable pathogen. Note the similar radiographic appearance of the large CMV ulcer demonstrated in Figure 2–7. SOURCE: Levine MS, Loercher G, Katzka DA, et al. Giant, human immunodeficiency virus–related ulcers in the esophagus. Radiology. 1991;180:325.

ENDOSCOPY

At endoscopy the esophageal ulcers described in acute HIV seroconversion illness are multiple, superficial, and small.[24, 26, 27] Both small shallow aphthoid lesions and large deep ulcers have been described in patients who are HIV seropositive, both without and with AIDS (Fig. 1–11).[14, 28, 76, 206] In these cases, endoscopic biopsies, cytology, and cultures have been nondiagnostic for any of the usual opportunistic viral or fungal organisms associated with AIDS. The number and location of biopsies are not often reported explicitly, and CMV, HSV, and possibly EBV can be missed in endoscopic biopsy specimens for the reasons outlined earlier.

HISTOLOGY

Electron micrographs from margins of some small shallow ulcers have demonstrated viral particles with the morphologic characteristics of

retroviruses,[26] and in situ hybridization has documented HIV RNA in lymphocytes and mononuclear cells from these idiopathic esophageal ulcers in patients with AIDS.[24, 28] Analysis utilizing the polymerase chain reaction (PCR) has also demonstrated HIV genome in 12 of 14 tissue specimens (86%) obtained from HIV-associated idiopathic esophageal ulcers.[207] Of note, PCR detected the HIV genome in the same high percentage of tissue samples from AIDS patients with CMV ulcers of the esophagus.[207] This suggests that while HIV can be repeatedly demonstrated in esophageal lesions of HIV-infected patients, HIV may not be playing a direct causal role in every esophageal ulcer.

CULTURE

Routine viral cultures of these idiopathic esophageal ulcers do not grow HIV; specialized monocyte-macrophage culture systems are required to support growth. Tissue biopsies from one patient who developed idiopathic esophageal ulcers during HIV seroconversion syndrome did grow HIV virus in monocyte-macrophage cell cultures.[24] This supports the data from electron microscopy, in situ hybridization,

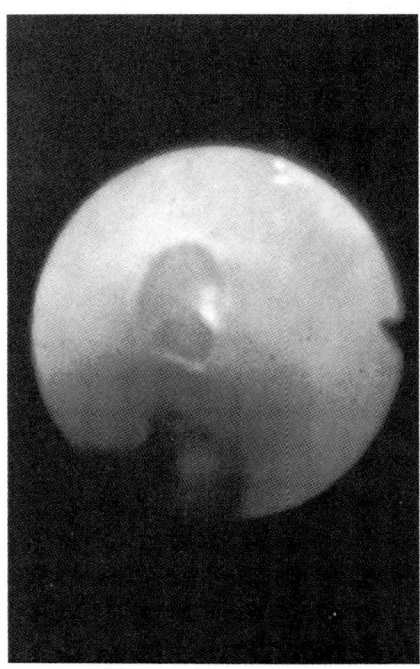

FIGURE 1–11.
Endoscopic photograph of a solitary esophageal ulcer in an HIV-infected patient. The ulcer is approximately 1 cm long with a sharply demarcated margin. Surrounding mucosa appears normal. SOURCE: Rabeneck L, Popovic M, Gartner S, et al. Acute HIV infection presenting with painful swallowing and esophageal ulcers. JAMA. 1990;263(17):2320. American Medical Association.

and PCR assay documenting the presence of HIV in tissue from the idiopathic esophageal lesions of HIV-infected individuals.

Drug Therapy for HIV-Associated Esophagitis

Idiopathic esophageal ulcers associated with HIV fail to respond to empirical antiviral or antifungal therapies.[76] Systemic steroid therapy has been temporally associated with ulcer healing in some patients.[28, 76] Caution must be advised, however, since systemic steroid therapy can lead to serious complications in an already immunocompromised host. A thorough search, including endoscopic biopsies, for treatable infectious causes must be undertaken prior to contemplating corticosteroid therapy. Local therapy with a slurry of sulcralfate (1 g) and dexamethasone (0.5 mg) orally 4 times daily may be a viable alternative, since 4 patients with AIDS and giant esophageal ulcers were clinically improved with this therapy.[205] Similarly, intralesional injection of corticosteroids has provided relief in some patients. Thalidomide, which has immunomodulatory activity, has also been reported to be useful but is not generally available.[208, 209]

Complications and Outcome

Although esophageal symptoms seem to improve with corticosteroid therapy, repeat endoscopy in several reports has shown variable healing. Persistent esophageal symptoms and anorexia may result from these chronic giant ulcers, and HIV ulcers may ultimately become complicated by superinfection or hemorrhage.[19]

Papillomavirus

Virology

Human papillomaviruses (HPV) are small (55 nm) unenveloped double-stranded DNA viruses that cause hyperplastic, verrucous, and papillomatous lesions in squamous epithelium of immunocompetent subjects.[111, 202] Typical sites of HPV infection include the female genital tract, skin, trachea, and larynx, but HPV infection in the esophagus is an unusual finding, and the lesions are rarely symptomatic.[210–217] Transmission of the virus is primarily through close personal contact, sexual contact, or, less frequently, vertical transmission from mother to child.[218] Infection with HPV has been implicated as a factor in the development of some squamous cell carcinomas, especially those of the cervix.[219]

Clinical Presentation

Most esophageal infections with HPV are asymptomatic, given the evidence that HPV has been found in large numbers of patients with esophageal carcinoma but in fewer than 10 patients who presented with dysphagia. Two cases of symptomatic HPV esophageal lesions have been reported. Summaries of these cases are presented here. In one previously healthy 35-year-old man who presented with dysphagia, a barium radiograph showed a bulky, irregularly shaped, broad-based polypoid lesion and several smaller lesions in the midesophagus at the level of the carina. Upper gastrointestinal endoscopy revealed multiple white, verrucous lesions of various sizes and shapes in the midesophagus at 30 cm from the lips. Histologic examination and DNA analysis confirmed the presence of HPV infection. Attempted laser ablation of the symptomatic lesions was unsatisfactory, as was heater probe application. Direct injection with sclerosant produced only minor shrinkage. Finally, removal of the majority of the papillomas with an electrocautery snare was successful in resolving symptoms and endoscopic lesions. After 1 year the patient was still asymptomatic.[220]

Another healthy 27-year-old man with a remote history of hand warts presented with epigastric pain and dysphagia. Esophagoscopy revealed multiple papillomas in the most distal part of the esophagus, protruding into the cardia. Biopsies showed viral and mildly dysplastic changes limited to the epithelium. After 5 months, he had lost 15 kg in weight and required parenteral feeding. Repeat esophagoscopy found the distal esophageal lumen almost obliterated by papillomatous lesions. Multiple attempts at laser fulguration were ineffective. The lesions did improve initially with interferon-α subcutaneous injections, then recurred despite dosage escalation and topical interferon-α jelly. By 1 year after onset of symptoms, he was unable to swallow his saliva. Pulmonary symptoms ensued, and endobronchial papillomas were diagnosed. Treatment with intralesional injections of interferon-α was ineffective. Resection via thoracotomy was attempted but unsuccessful, and therapy with bleomycin, followed by VP-16, was futile. The patient later died of sudden cardiovascular collapse.[221]

Diagnosis

ENDOSCOPY

Appearance at endoscopy is varied. Human papillomavirus lesions in the esophagus may appear as erythematous areas, white plaques, nodules, exuberant frondlike lesions, or even ulcerations (Fig. 1–12).[220, 222, 223] These lesions are most frequently found in the middle to distal esophagus and may become so large as to protrude into the cardia of the stomach.[221] The gross appearance of such large lesions can be mistaken for malignancy, and small lesions may be mistaken for glycogenic acanthosis.[116] Diagnosis in this setting requires endoscopic biopsies for histology and hybridization studies.

HISTOLOGY

The primary histologic feature associated with HPV infection of squamous epithelium is koilocytosis. Other characteristic cytologic atypia include giant cells, cytoplasmic vacuolization, multinucleate cells, nuclear hyperchromasia, and disturbances in maturation. Immunohistochemical evaluation utilizing polyclonal HPV antisera may confirm a diagnosis of HPV infection, but in one series this technique was less sensitive than routine histology.[222, 223]

MOLECULAR BIOLOGY

Human papillomavirus can be detected in biopsy specimens through techniques of PCR and in situ hybridization for HPV DNA sequences. The PCR technique utilizes oligonucleotide primers of highly conserved regions of the HPV genome, which through cycled incubation of biopsy extracts amplifies complementary HPV DNA sequences to levels detectable by HPV hybridization probes.[224] In situ hybridization is a technique for the detection of specific nucleotide sequences within material mounted on a microscope slide. To detect HPV within squamous epithelial cells, probes complementary to highly conserved regions of HPV DNA are constructed and labeled. If HPV DNA is present within a cell, under appropriate conditions the labeled probes hybridize to the complementary sequences in situ. Through immunocytochemical reactions the hybridized probe can then be visualized, using fluorescent or light microscopy.

Therapy for Papillomaviral Esophageal Lesions

Treatment of esophageal papillomas is seldom indicated, because the lesions are typically incidental findings. As most common skin and orogenital papillomas regress spontaneously,[218] esophageal papillomas are likely to behave similarly. Persistent or symptomatic skin warts are typically treated with topical agents such as podophyllin and 5-fluorouracil, cryotherapy, or surgical resection.[218] Interferon-α has been used for both intralesional injection and systemic treatment of skin warts and has produced significant improvement.[218] Experience in the treatment of esophageal papillomas with these means is limited. Local resection of large symptomatic esophageal lesions with snare electrocautery was effective in the case described earlier, but local destruction of these lesions with a heater probe or laser ablation appears to be less effective. Case reports also include treatment of symptomatic esophageal lesions with systemic interferon-α, bleomycin, and VP-16, with varying results.[218, 221, 225]

Complications and Outcome

As malignant transformation of genital HPV lesions is believed to be a cause of cervical carcinoma, a similar causative role for HPV infection in the development of squamous cell carcinoma of the esophagus has been suggested. The incidence of esophageal carcinoma is remarkably high in particular regions of China, Iran, South Africa, and Alaska, prompting investigation in these geographic regions. Although early epidemiologic studies in China, Iran, and South

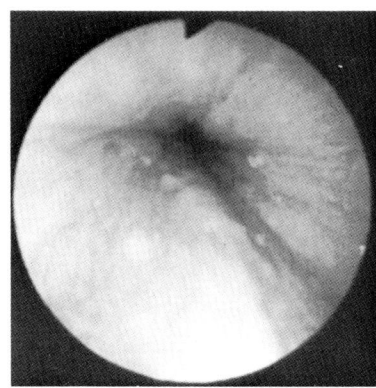

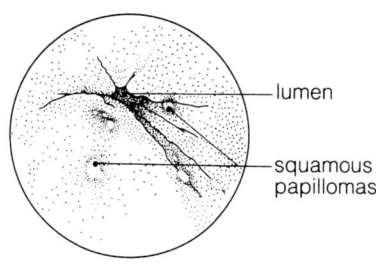

FIGURE 1–12.
Endoscopic photograph of several small squamous papillomas in the distal esophagus. SOURCE: Silverstein FE, Tytgat GNJ. Atlas of Gastrointestinal Endoscopy. 2nd ed. New York: Gower Medical Publishing; 1991: 3.2.

lumen

squamous papillomas

Africa focused on vitamins (A, B, and C), minerals, nitrosamines in moldy foodstuffs, alcohol, and tobacco in the search for esophageal cancer risk factors,[226–228] more recent studies from these regions have supported a role for HPV in the multifactorial genesis of esophageal cancer. In Linxian, China, tissues from 51 patients with invasive squamous cell carcinoma were analyzed histologically and by in situ DNA hybridization; histologic changes consistent with HPV infection in and adjacent to malignant tissue were found in 25 cases (49%) and evidence for HPV DNA by in situ hybridization in 22 cases (43%).[229, 230] Studies in South Africa using PCR found HPV DNA in 10 of 14 (71%) patients with esophageal carcinoma.[231] In native Alaskans of North America, a population among whom the prevalence of anogenital HPV infection is high,[232] HPV DNA was detected by PCR in 10 of 22 (45%) esophageal squamous cell carcinoma specimens.[233]

Studies from other geographic regions have not supported a role for HPV in the development of esophageal squamous cell carcinoma. In the continental United States, where tobacco and alcohol abuse are associated with the development of esophageal carcinoma,[228] HPV DNA was not detected by PCR in any of 13 esophageal squamous cell carcinoma specimens.[234] Similarly, in Hong Kong, where the prevalence of anogenital HPV infection is low relative to that of most Western countries,[235] DNA hybridization studies of specimens from 37 cases of esophageal squamous cell carcinoma found no evidence for HPV DNA.[236]

This geographic disparity supports a multifactorial etiology for squamous cell carcinoma of the esophagus. It appears likely that HPV infection is one of several cofactors contributing to but not necessary for the development of esophageal malignancy.

Poliovirus

Dysphagia has been described in postpolio syndromes. Acute bulbar poliomyelitis results in abnormal neuromuscular control of swallowing, leading to transfer dysphagia.[237, 238]

BACTERIAL INFECTION

Bacteria from the Normal Oropharyngeal Flora

Microbiology

Of the reported cases of bacterial esophagitis, the most common infecting organisms are found in the normal oral flora. These include *Staphylococcus aureus*, *Staphylococcus epidermidis*, *Streptococcus viridans*, *Bacillus* species, and *Klebsiella* species. Previously, bacteria found in esophageal ulcers were often believed to represent colonization by commensal organisms. Subsequent investigations have reported that in settings of immunodeficiency, invasive bacterial esophagitis occurs in as much as 11 to 16% of infectious esophagitis cases.[5, 44] Many cases represent secondary infection of epithelium injured by acid-pepsin reflux and by other organisms.

Granulocytopenia secondary to hematologic malignancy, intensive chemotherapy, or bone marrow transplantation is the most significant risk factor for bacterial esophagitis,[5, 240] although there have been reports of bacterial esophagitis among apparently immunocompetent subjects.[239, 240] Although HIV infection combined with poorly controlled diabetes was associated with bacterial esophagitis in one case,[241] the prevalence of bacterial esophagitis in the AIDS population is less than in oncology patients, owing to relative sparing of granulocyte function.

Clinical Presentation

Symptoms associated with bacterial esophagitis include painful difficult swallowing and retrosternal pain.[44, 241] Fever was reported in only a minority of cases.[44]

Diagnosis

ENDOSCOPY

Fiberoptic esophagoscopy with brushings and biopsies is the procedure of choice in the diagnostic workup of esophageal symptoms in the granulocytopenic patient. Gross endoscopic findings in bacterial esophagitis are nonspecific and may include middle to distal esophageal friability, plaques, pseudomembranes, and ulcerations.[44, 241] Ulceration and pseudomembrane formation serve as a marker of the severity of bacterial esophagitis, and these were present in 2 of 4 patients with concurrent bacteremia and in only 1 of 19 without.[44]

HISTOLOGY

The histologic appearance of bacterial esophagitis includes sheets or masses of confluent bacteria in the lamina propria that are best seen by examining tissue sections stained with a Gram stain under an oil-immersion lens. Several bacterial species are usually present, supporting the polymicrobial nature of these infections. Biopsy materials stained only with H&E are unsatisfactory. Severe ulceration and pseudomembranes of necrotic material may be present. As these patients are granulocytopenic, often no significant inflammatory reaction accompanies the infection. In fact, an inverse relationship between the number of bacteria and the intensity of inflammatory reaction has been described.[44]

CULTURE

Bacterial cultures of endoscopic biopsies are not routinely performed in most endoscopy suites owing to the infrequency of invasive bacterial esophagitis and the unavoidable bacterial contamination of the endoscope secondary to passage through the oral cavity. If the clinical suspicion for bacterial esophagitis is high, then cultures of tissue biopsies for anaerobic as well as aerobic bacteria can identify organisms seen on histologic stains of tissues from the corresponding site and can provide sensitivity information to guide antimicrobial therapy. As bacterial esophagitis was associated with bacteremia in 4 of 23 reported cases (17%),[44] cultures of esophageal biopsies may confirm the esophagus as the source of bacteremia.

Drug Therapy for Bacterial Esophagitis

Acute onset of painful or difficult swallowing in the setting of granulocytopenia is suggestive of infectious esophagitis, and prompt diagnostic endoscopy should be considered. Pending results from biopsies, broad-spectrum antibiotic coverage against oral flora should be initiated. For odontogenic soft tissue infections in a compromised host, treatment with a broad-spectrum β-lactam antibiotic such as piperacillin, cefoxitin, ticarcillin/clavulanate, or imipenem/cilastatin is recommended, generally in combination with an aminoglycoside.[242] Clinical response and culture results can then be used to tailor subsequent antimicrobial therapy. Appropriate antimicrobial coverage should be continued until adequate granulocyte function recovers.

Complications and Outcome

The most significant complication of bacterial esophageal infection is sepsis. The risk of bacteremia correlates with the severity of esophagitis. Esophageal perforation and fistula formation are not prominent features, since these are generally features of a more indolent infection.

The outcome of bacterial esophagitis is generally favorable, provided appropriate antibiotic coverage and other supportive measures are instituted promptly and granulocyte dysfunction is reversible.

Mycobacterium tuberculosis

Microbiology

Mycobacterium tuberculosis is a slow-growing rod-shaped organism that is strongly acid fast on histologic staining and pathogenic in normal humans.[243] Infection is transmitted by inhalation of aerosolized droplet nuclei containing the organism, although the infection can also be transmitted through the intestinal tract or a skin lesion. Primary infection is usually handled well by the normal host, in whom *M. tuberculosis* organisms are phagocytized and destroyed by macrophages. In regional lymph nodes, the infected macrophages stimulate cell-mediated immunity and chemotaxis of activated macrophages and fibroblasts to form a granuloma. Central necrosis within the inflammatory granuloma provides the nearly pathognomonic histologic appearance of a caseating granuloma. Some bacilli in granulomas may survive and be a source of reactivation of *M. tuberculosis* infection, should immune surveillance lapse, months to years later. Reactivation of latent infection is responsible for the increased incidence of mycobacterial esophageal infections among immunocompromised subjects, especially those with AIDS. The diagnosis of *M. tuberculosis* esophageal infection can be difficult in this population because these patients are often coinfected by candidal and viral organisms.

Clinical Presentation

Presenting signs and symptoms of dysphagia, weight loss, fever, chest pain, and cough support the diagnosis of esophageal tuberculosis (see Table 2-1). Although the AIDS epidemic has increased the frequency of esophageal tuberculosis in developed countries, the majority of case reports are of immunocompetent patients from geographic regions with a high prevalence of *M. tuberculosis* infection. Presenting symptoms depend on the extent of esophageal involvement and the severity of the extraesophageal infection. Symptoms from extrinsic esophageal compression by mediastinal lymphadenopathy range from mild to severe dysphagia. Alternatively, mediastinal or hilar nodes can erode directly into the esophagus, causing bleeding, esophageal perforation with mediastinitis, or formation of fistulae between the tracheobronchial tree and the esophagus, resulting in bacterial pneumonitis.[23, 244] Coughing after swallowing is a common presenting symptom among patients with tubercular tracheoesophageal fistulae.[23, 244]

Reports of primary tuberculous infection limited to the esophagus are rare, reflecting the hostile esophageal environment of peristalsis, stratified squamous epithelia, protective mucus, and salivary secretions. A few cases of mycobacterial esophagitis with no apparent pulmonary, hilar, or mediastinal disease have, however, been described.[245, 248]

Diagnosis

RADIOGRAPHY

Radiographic findings in esophageal tuberculosis may be striking. An esophagogram may demonstrate intramural pseudodiverticulosis,[18, 249, 250] extrinsic compression or displacement of the midesophagus by mediastinal lymph nodes,[244, 249, 250] and sinus tracts extending into the mediastinum (Fig. 1–13).[249, 251–254] Fistulae may be

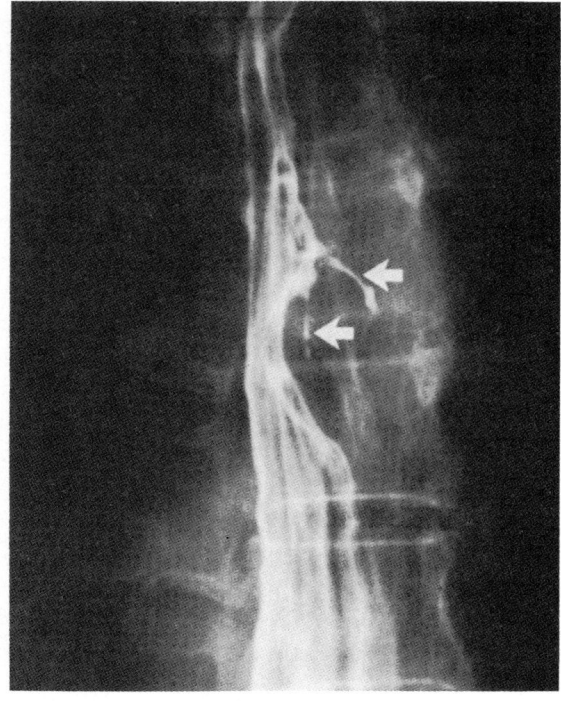

FIGURE 1–13.
Esophagogram documenting extrinsic compression of the esophagus and two sinus tracts in a patient with esophageal tuberculosis (arrows). SOURCE: Eng J, Sabanathan S. Tuberculosis of the esophagus. Dig Dis Sci. 1991:36(4):537.

obvious between the esophagus and the tracheobronchial tree or even between segments of the esophagus, resulting in a "double-barrel" esophagus.[244, 252, 254] Filling defects suggestive of esophageal neoplasms have also been reported.[255, 256] Computed tomography (CT) scan may help to demonstrate mediastinal adenopathy, esophageal involvement, and extraesophageal air (Fig. 1–14).[23, 245, 251, 254]

ENDOSCOPY

Although a diagnosis of esophageal tuberculosis may be suggested by radiographic findings, endoscopy is often necessary for confirmation. At endoscopy, the majority of tuberculous lesions appear as distinct shallow ulcers, having a necrotic base[245, 257] and ranging in size from small mucosal defects to large linear ulcerations.[245] Probing a necrotic ulcer base may reveal a fistulous tract.[245] Endoscopic features of other cases include heaped-up mucosal lesions mimicking neoplasms or extrinsic compression of the esophageal lumen with no mucosal lesions.[255, 256, 258, 259] Mucosal lesions should be thoroughly biopsied and specimens sent for acid-fast stain and mycobacterial culture, in addition to routine histologic studies. If the patient is immunocompromised, the possibility of concurrent infections should be investigated with viral culture and with stains for viruses, fungi, and bacteria.

BRONCHOSCOPY, MEDIASTINOSCOPY, SURGERY

In some cases, radiographs and esophagoscopy are nondiagnostic, and bronchoscopy or mediastinoscopy may be necessary to confirm involvement of the esophagus by tuberculous lymphadenopathy.[22] Bronchoscopy has been diagnostic in cases of bronchoesophageal fistulae, revealing acid-fast bacteria in bronchoalveolar lavage specimens and noncaseating granulomas on biopsy.[249] One advantage of mediastinoscopy and mediastinotomy over endoscopy is the ability to obtain larger pieces of tissue for histology and culture.[244] Thoracotomy has also been employed in the diagnosis and treatment of esophageal lesions, perforations, and fistulae secondary to *M. tuberculosis*.[23, 256, 260]

HISTOLOGY

Diagnostic biopsies may demonstrate acute and chronic inflammation, caseating granulomas, and acid-fast staining bacilli.[18, 245, 249, 259] Smears of sputum samples from patients with tracheoesophageal fistulae are also useful in detecting acid-fast bacilli.[244]

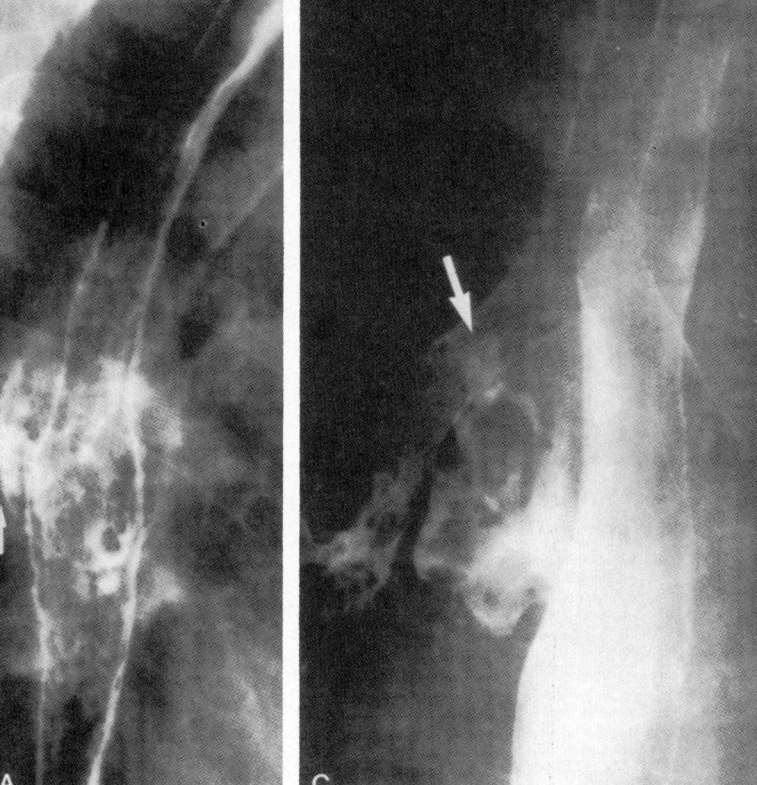

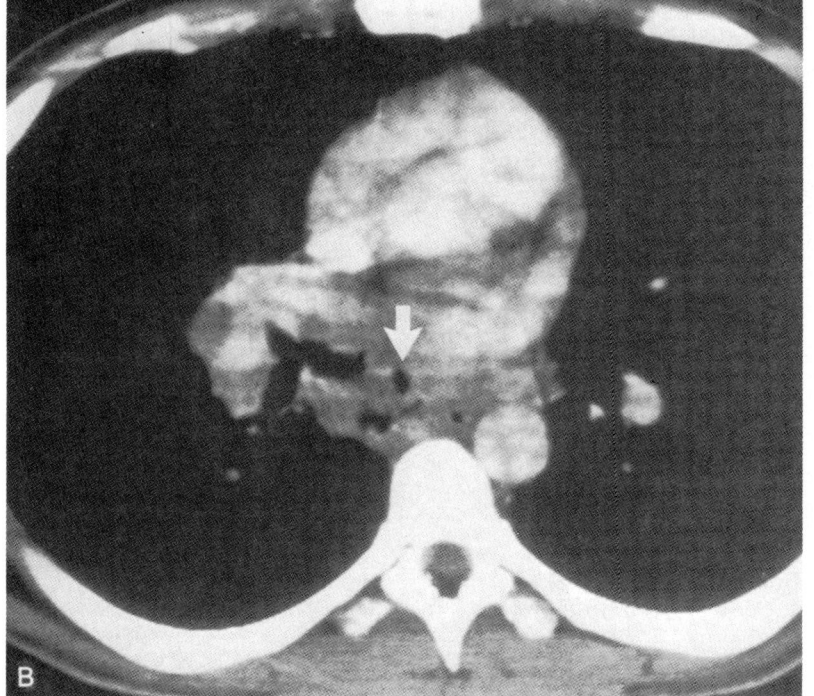

FIGURE 1–14.
Two esophagograms and chest CT scan from a patient with esophageal tuberculosis. *A,* The first esophagogram demonstrates diffuse mucosal irregularity and a large periesophageal fluid collection in the subcarinal region. *B,* The chest CT scan demonstrates extensive mediastinal lymphadenopathy, with scattered air pockets among subcarinal nodes, suggesting communication between the mediastinum and the esophageal lumen. At a later date the patient developed a cough when swallowing. *C,* A later esophagogram showed an esophagomediastinobronchial fistula. SOURCE: de Silva R, Stoopack PM, Raufman JP. Esophageal fistulas associated with mycobacterial infection in patients at risk for AIDS. Radiology. 1990;175: 451.

CULTURE

Endoscopic biopsy specimens should be cultured for *Mycobacterium* species. Cultures are of no short-term clinical utility, since *M. tuberculosis* is slow-growing on complex media and colonies may take 3 to 6 weeks to appear.[243] They are useful, however, when histology is nondiagnostic, and they are a useful guide to therapy because some isolates may be resistant to conventional therapy.[257]

Therapy for Mycobacterial Esophagitis

The immunocompetent patient generally responds well to standard antituberculous therapy, although surgery may be required for repair of perforations and fistulae.[22, 23, 244, 245, 259] Emergence of drug-resistant strains of *M. tuberculosis* has raised concerns as to the future management of tuberculous infection. Among cases of esophageal tuberculosis, however, none was due to a resistant strain.

Complications and Outcome

As a group, HIV-infected patients have a poorer response to drug therapy than do immunocompetent patients. None of 5 AIDS patients with tuberculous fistulae demonstrated resolution of fistulous tracts with drug therapy.[22, 254] The major cause for treatment failure in tuberculosis is poor compliance of patients with lengthy, multiple drug regimens.[261] One elderly patient died of hemorrhage from an aortic aneurysmal esophageal tuberculous fistula 1 month after initiation of antituberculous drug therapy.[18] Surgical intervention is appropriate in cases of hemorrhage, obstruction, and perforation.[250, 259, 260]

Mycobacterium avium-intracellulare

Mycobacterium avium-intracellulare complex is a group of opportunistic mycobacteria rarely reported in humans prior to the AIDS epidemic, but it is one of the most common opportunistic pathogens reported in advanced AIDS. In these patients, MAC is widely disseminated, response to therapy is marginal, and prognosis is very poor.[243] Although MAC is frequently isolated from the duodenum and small bowel in patients with AIDS, esophageal involvement is unusual.[33] Clinical presentation of MAC esophagitis can include fever, chills, dyspnea, weight loss, and difficult painful swallowing.[254] Radiographic studies in 1 case demonstrated a large esopha-

goesophageal fistula on esophagogram and retrosternal adenopathy on CT scan.[254] Subsequent endoscopy found esophageal ulcerations, and biopsy material eventually grew MAC.

Helicobacter pylori

Helicobacter pylori has been found in the esophagus of patients with gastric *H. pylori*,[262, 263] but is never present in the absence of gastric *H. pylori* infection.[264] Investigators have found no association between *H. pylori* and esophagitis, esophageal ulceration, or Barrett's esophagus.[263–267] The presence of *H. pylori* in the normal esophagus or in Barrett's epithelium probably represents commensalism or contamination, not esophageal infection.[262, 263]

Treponema pallidum

Treponema pallidum is the causative organism of syphilis, a disease that is still prominent in some geographic regions. Earlier literature described gummata, diffuse ulceration, and strictures of the esophagus in tertiary syphilis.[268, 269] The diagnosis should be considered a possibility in a patient with an inflammatory esophageal stricture and evidence of tertiary lues elsewhere. Histology shows perivascular lymphocytic infiltration; specific immunostaining should be done if this diagnosis is a possibility. A rare case of rupture of a syphilitic aortic aneurysm into the esophagus has been reported.[20]

Corynebacterium diphtheriae

Diphtheria is a disease caused by the potent toxin of *Corynebacterium diphtheriae* and is marked by severe mucosal inflammation with fibrinous exudative membranes of the pharynx, throat, nose, and, occasionally, the tracheobronchial tree. Diphtheria may also involve the esophagus through extension of inflammatory membranes from the oropharynx.

Clostridium tetani

Tetanus is a disease marked by painful tonic muscular contractions caused by the neurotropic toxin of *Clostridium tetani* acting on the CNS. Dysphagia may rarely be the presenting symptom.[270–272]

TABLE 1–6. NONINFECTIOUS INFLAMMATORY CONDITIONS OF THE ESOPHAGUS: SYMPTOMS AND ENDOSCOPIC APPEARANCE MAY MIMIC AN INFECTION

ACID-PEPSIN DISEASE	**CHEMICAL, THERMAL, OR**
Reflux esophagitis	**TRAUMATIC INJURY**
Barrett's ulcer	Pill esophagitis
ONCOLOGIC THERAPY	Caustic ingestion (alkali or acid)
Cytotoxic drug	Scalding liquid
Acute radiation esophagitis	Foreign body
Chronic radiation esophagitis	Sclerotherapy injection
DERMATOLOGIC DISEASE	**OTHER INFLAMMATORY DISEASE**
Dystrophic epidermolysis bullosa	Aphthous stomatitis
Pemphigus vulgaris	Behçet's disease
Bullous pemphigoid	Crohn's disease
Benign mucous membrane	Sarcoidosis
pemphigoid	Chronic graft-versus-host disease
Lichen planus	Chronic granulomatous disease
Toxic epidermal necrolysis	
(Stevens–Johnson syndrome)	

PARASITIC INFECTION

Trypanosoma cruzi

Trypanosoma cruzi is a parasite endemic to South America that causes Chagas's disease through progressive destruction of ganglion cells throughout the body. Esophageal manifestations of chronic Chagas's disease are similar to those of achalasia and present 10 to 30 years after the acute infection. Symptoms include dysphagia and regurgitation. Diagnosis of chagasic esophagus depends on finding other involved organs and on serologic tests. Manometric study of the body of the chagasic esophagus reveals findings identical to those of achalasia, but lower esophageal sphincter pressure is below normal with Chagas's disease.[273] A chagasic esophagus may be responsive to nitrate therapy.[274] Symptoms may also abate after balloon dilation of the gastroesophageal junction.[275] Ultimately, patients may undergo myectomy at the esophagogastric junction or esophagectomy for advanced disease.[276] Chronic stasis secondary to chagasic megaesophagus leads to esophageal mucosal alterations such as hyperplasia and malignancy.[277]

Pneumocystis carinii

Disseminated *Pneumocystis carinii* infection, including esophageal invasion, has been reported in an AIDS patient.[278] The patient had a history of recurrent pneumocystic pneumonia and presented with dysphagia. Endoscopy revealed a diffuse white esophageal exudate containing pneumocystic cysts with focal superficial ulceration. Postmortem examination revealed dissemination to multiple organs.

Cryptosporidium

Cryptosporidium is a protozoan parasite known to infect birds and domesticated animals and more recently identified as a common cause of acute self-limited diarrhea in humans. It is an opportunistic pathogen in the compromised host, especially patients with AIDS.[21] Esophageal involvement has been reported in 2 patients who had widely disseminated cryptosporidiosis.[279, 280] Marked dysphagia, frequent vomiting, and voluminous diarrhea were reported.[280]

NONINFECTIOUS CONDITIONS OF THE ESOPHAGUS THAT MIMIC INFECTION

Table 1–6 lists noninfectious conditions that should be considered in the differential diagnosis of patients with inflammatory lesions of the esophagus.[281] Of these conditions, peptic esophagitis, ulceration, and stricture formation are the most common causes of esophageal pain and dysphagia in the general population. Also common are chemical, thermal, and traumatic esophageal injuries, the causes of which either are immediately apparent (e.g., caustic ingestion, scalding) or can be derived from a careful medical history (e.g., pill esophagitis, sclerotherapy ulceration). Among patients with cancer, symptomatic esophageal injury, such as mucosal ulceration and sloughing, can develop after treatment with cytotoxic drugs and radiation therapy. Over time, chronic radiation esophagitis may result from progressive arteriolar obliterative changes, leading to bleeding, ulceration, and stricture formation. Dermatologic diseases can also involve the esophagus, occasionally leading to desquamation, webs, and strictures.[282] Primary treatment of these diseases typically includes immunosuppressive drugs, particularly corticosteroids. When esophageal symptoms appear, endoscopy is often indicated to exclude infection and to dilate esophageal webs and strictures mechanically. Chronic graft-versus-host disease, an immunologic reaction against host tissues by donor lymphoid cells following allogeneic bone marrow transplantation, involves multiple systems and results in esophageal symptoms secondary to progressive fibrosis. Several other inflammatory conditions of the esophagus also result in esophageal symptoms that mimic infection. The clinician must consider risk factors for esophageal infection in each of these conditions, such as immunodeficiency and altered mucosal integrity, and exclude infection when appropriate.

REFERENCES

1. Orlando RC. Reflux esophagitis. In: Yamada T, Alpers DH, Owyang C, et al. Textbook of Gastroenterology. Philadelphia: JB Lippincott; 1991;55:1123–1147.
2. Biancani P, Barwick K, Selling J, et al. Effects of acute experimental esophagitis on mechanical properties of the lower esophageal sphincter. Gastroenterology. 1984;87:8–16.
3. Eastwood GI, Castell DO, Higgs RH. Experimental esophagitis in cats impairs lower esophageal sphincter pressure. Gastroenterology. 1975;69:146–151.
4. Reed EC, Wolford JL, Kopecky KJ, et al. Ganciclovir for the treatment of cytomegalovirus gastroenteritis in bone marrow transplant patients: A randomized, placebo-controlled trial. Ann Intern Med. 1990;112:505–510.
5. McDonald GB, Sharma P, Hackman RC, et al. Esophageal infections in immunosuppressed patients after marrow transplantation. Gastroenterology. 1985;88:1111–1117.
6. Kotler DP. Gastrointestinal complications of the acquired immunodeficiency syndrome. In: Yamada T, Alpers DH, Owyang C, et al. Textbook of Gastroenterology. Philadelphia: Lippincott; 1991;103:2086–2103.
7. Spencer GD, Hackman RC, McDonald GB, et al. A prospective study of unexplained nausea and vomiting after marrow transplantation. Transplantation. 1986;42:602–607.
8. Alexander JA, Brouillette DE, Chien MC, et al. Infectious esophagitis following liver and renal transplantation. Dig Dis Sci. 1988;33:1121–1126.
9. Frick T, Fryd DS, Goodale RL, et al. Incidence and treatment of Candida esophagitis in patients undergoing renal transplantation: Data from the Minnesota prospective randomized trial of cyclosporine versus antilymphocyte globulin-azathioprine. Am J Surg. 1988;155:311–313.
10. Porro GB, Parente F, Cernushi M. The diagnosis of esophageal candidiasis in patients with acquired immune deficiency syndrome: Is endoscopy always necessary? Am J Gastroenterol. 1989;84:143–146.
11. Bonacini M, Laine L, Gal AA, et al. Prospective evaluation of blind brushings in the esophagus for Candida esophagitis in patients with human immunodeficiency virus infection. Am J Gastroenterol. 1990;85:385–389.
12. Tavitian A, Raufman JP, Rosenthal LE. Oral candidiasis as a marker for esophageal candidiasis in acquired immunodeficiency syndrome. Ann Intern Med. 1986;104:54–55.
13. Levine MS, Loevner LA, Saul SH, et al. Herpes esophagitis: Sensitivity of double-contrast esophagography. Am J Roentgentol. 1988;151:57–62.
14. Levine MS, Loercher G, Katzka DA, et al. Giant, human immunodeficiency virus–related ulcers in the esophagus. Radiology. 1991;180:323–326.
15. Greenspan JS, Greenspan D, Lennette ET, et al. Replication of Epstein-Barr virus within the epithelial cells of oral "hairy" leukoplakia, an AIDS associated lesion. N Engl J Med. 1985;313:1564–1571.
16. Kaplan D, Warren J. Massive gastrointestinal hemorrhage due to Candida esophagitis. Am J Gastroenterol. 1988;83:463–464.
17. Mayeux GP, Smith JW. Massive esophageal bleeding from cytomegalovirus esophagitis. Am J Gastroenterol. 1990;85:626.
18. Catinella FP, Kittle CF. Tuberculous esophagitis with aortic aneurysm fistula. Ann Thorac Surg. 1988;45:87–88.
19. Pedro-Botet J, Miralles R, Sauleda J, et al. Idiopathic ulcer of the esophagus in the AIDS syndrome: A potential life-threatening complication. Gastrointest Endosc. 1989;35:470–475.
20. Zagrebin VM, Fomin SD. A rare case of rupture of a syphilitic aneurysm into the esophagus. Ter Arkh. 1988;60:70–71.
21. Smith PD, Quinn TC, Strober W, et al. Gastrointestinal infections in AIDS. Ann Intern Med. 1992;116:63–77.
22. Allen CM, Craze J, Grundy A. Tuberculosis broncho-oesophageal fistula in the acquired immunodeficiency syndrome. Clin Radiol. 1991;43:60–62.
23. Raghu G, Dillard D. Esophagobronchial fistula and mediastinal tuberculosis. Ann Thorac Surg. 1990;50:647–649.
24. Rabeneck L, Popovic M, Gartner S, et al. Acute HIV infection presenting with painful swallowing and esophageal ulcers. JAMA. 1990;263:2318–2322.
25. Naito Y, Yoshikawa T, Oyamada H, et al. Esophageal candidiasis. Gastroenterol Jpn. 1988;23:363–370.
26. Rabeneck L, Boyko WJ, McLean DM, et al. Unusual esophageal ulcers containing enveloped viruslike particles in homosexual men. Gastroenterology. 1986;90:1882–1889.
27. Bartelsman JF, Lange JM, van Leeuwen R, et al. Acute primary HIV-esophagitis. Endoscopy. 1990;22:184–185.
28. Kotler DP, Wilson CS, Haroutiounian G, et al. Detection of human immunodeficiency virus-1 by 35S-RNA in situ hybridization in solitary esophageal ulcers in two patients with the acquired immune deficiency syndrome. Am J Gastroenterol. 1989;84:313–317.
29. Clotet B, Romeau J, Casals A, et al. Spontaneous resolution of Candida esophagitis in a seroconverting patient for HIV antibodies. Am J Gastroenterol. 1988;83:1433–1434.
30. Decker CF, Tiernan R, Paparello SF. Esophageal candidiasis associated with acute infection due to human immunodeficiency virus. Clin Infect Dis. 1992;14:791–797.
31. Wilcox CM, Diehl DL, Cello JP, et al. Cytomegalovirus esophagitis in patients with AIDS: A clinical, endoscopic, and pathologic correlation. Ann Intern Med. 1990;113:589–593.
32. Imam N, Carpenter CCJ, Mayer KH, et al. Hierarchical pattern of mucosal Candida infections in MIV-seropositive women. Am J Med. 1990;89:142–146.

33. Connolly GM, Hawkins D, Harcourt-Webster JN, et al. Oesophageal symptoms, their causes, treatment, and prognosis in patients with the acquired immunodeficiency syndrome. Gut. 1989;30:1033–1039.

34. Vermeersch B, Rysselaere M, Dekeyser K, et al. Fungal colonization of the esophagus. Am J Gastroenterol. 1989;84:1079–1083.

35. Obata S, Matsuzaki H, Nishimura H, et al. Gastroduodenal complications in patients with adult T-cell leukemia. Jpn J Clin Oncol. 1988;18:335–342.

36. Meunier F. Infections in patients with acute leukemia and lymphoma. In: Mandell GL, Douglas RG, Bennett JE, eds. Principles and Practices of Infectious Diseases. 3rd ed. New York: Churchill Livingstone; 1990; 287:2265–2275.

37. Ammann AJ, Hong R. Disorders of the T cell system. In: Stiehm ER, ed. Immunologic Disorders in Infants and Children. Philadelphia: WB Saunders, 1989;286.

38. Katz P, Fauci AS. Immunosuppressives and immunoadjuvants. In: Samter M, Talmage DW, Frank MM, et al., eds. Immunological Diseases, 4th ed. Boston: Little, Brown; 1988;675.

39. Kesten S, Hyland RH, Pruzanski WR, et al. Esophageal candidiasis associated with beclomethasone dipropionate aerosol therapy. Drug Intell Clin Pharm. 1988;22:568–569.

40. Brouilette DE, Alexander J, Yoo YK, et al. T-cell populations in liver and renal transplant recipients with infectious esophagitis. Dig Dis Sci. 1989;34:92–96.

41. Johnson R, Peitzman AB, Webster MW, et al. Upper gastrointestinal endoscopy after cardiac transplantation. Surgery. 1988;103:300–306.

42. Stratta RJ, Shaeffer MS, Markin RS, et al. Cytomegalovirus infection and disease after liver transplantation: An overview. Dig Dis Sci. 1992;37:673–688.

43. Merigan TC, Renlund DG, Keay S, et al. A controlled trial of ganciclovir to prevent cytomegalovirus disease after heart transplant. N Engl J Med. 1992;326:1182–1186.

44. Walsh TJ, Belitos NJ, Hamilton SR. Bacterial esophagitis in immunocompromised patients. Arch Intern Med. 1986;146:1345–1348.

45. Handwerger BS. The immunology of diabetes mellitus. In: Samter M, Talmage DW, Frank MD, eds. Immunological Diseases, 4th ed. Boston: Little, Brown; 1988:1765.

46. Parkman HP, Schwartz SS. Esophagitis and gastroduodenal disorders associated with diabetic gastroparesis. Arch Intern Med. 1987;147:1477–1480.

47. Hendel L, Svejgaard E, Walsoe I, et al. Esophageal candidosis in progressive systemic sclerosis: Occurrence, significance, and treatment with fluconazole. Scand J Gastroenterol. 1988;23:1182–1186.

48. Bluhm CS, Backerstaff CA, Holt S. Refractory esophageal candidiasis in acquired immune deficiency syndrome (AIDS). Am J Gastroenterol. 1990;85:479–480.

49. Kitchen VS, Savage M, Harris JRW. Candida albicans resistance in AIDS. J Infect. 1991;22:204–205.

50. Collins P, Larder BA, Oliver NM, et al. Characterization of a DNA polymerase mutant of herpes simplex virus from a severely immunocompromised patient receiving acyclovir. J Gen Virol. 1989;70:375–378.

51. Sacks SL, Wanklin RJ, Reece DE, et al. Progressive esophagitis from acyclovir-resistant herpes simplex: Clinical roles for DNA polymerase mutants and viral heterogeneity? Ann Intern Med. 1989;111:893–899.

52. Ljungman P, Ellis MN, Hackman RC, et al. Acyclovir-resistant herpes simplex virus causing pneumonia after marrow transplantation. J Infect Dis. 1990;162:244–248.

53. Jacobson MA, Gambertoglio JG, Aweeka FT, et al. Foscarnet-induced hypocalcemia and effects of foscarnet on calcium metabolism. J Clin Endocrinol Metab. 1991;72:1130–1135.

54. Dieterich D, Dicker M, Tepper R. Foscarnet treatment of cytomegalovirus gastrointestinal infections in HIV patients who have failed ganciclovir. Gastroenterology. 1991;100:A575.

55. Drobyski WR, Knox KK, Carrigan DR, Ash RC. Foscarnet therapy of ganciclovir-resistant cytomegalovirus in marrow transplantation. Transplantation. 1991;52:155–157.

56. Drew WL, Miner RC, Busch DF, et al. Prevalence of resistence in patients receiving ganciclovir for serious cytomegalovirus infection. J Infect Dis. 1991;163:716–719.

57. Lake-Bakaar G, Tom W, Lake-Bakaar D, et al. Gastropathy and ketoconazole malabsorption in the acquired immunodeficiency syndrome (AIDS). Ann Intern Med. 1988;109:471–478.

58. Richter JE. Motility disorders of the esophagus. In: Yamada T, Alpers DH, Owyang C, et al. Textbook of Gastroenterology. Philadelphia: JB Lippincott; 1991; 54:1083–1122.

59. Zamost BJ, Hirshberg J, Ippoliti AF, et al. Esophagitis in scleroderma: Prevalence and risk factors. Gastroenterology. 1987;92:421–428.

60. Geirssom AJ, Akesson A, Gustafson, et al. Cineradiography identifies esophageal candidiasis in progressive systemic sclerosis. Clin Exp Rheumatol. 1989;7:43–46.

61. Bhatia V, Kochhar R, Talwar P, et al. Association of Candida with carcinoma of esophagus. Indian Gastroenterol. 1989;8:171–172.

62. Ryan KJ. Candida and other opportunistic fungi. In: Sherris JC, ed. Medical Microbiology. New York: Elsevier; 1990;47:651–660.

63. Francis P, Walsh TJ. Current approaches to the management of fungal infections in cancer patients: Part 1. Oncology. 1992;6:81–100.

64. Tom W, Aaron JS. Esophageal ulcers caused by Torulopsis glabrata in a patient with acquired immune deficiency syndrome. Am J Gastroenterol. 1987;82:766–768.

65. Meunier F. Fungal infection in the compromised host. In: Rubin RH, Young LS, eds. Clinical Approach to Infection in the Compromised Host. 2nd ed. New York: Plenum, 1988;8:193–220.

66. Niedt GW, Schinella RA. Acquired immunodeficiency syndrome: Clinicopathologic study of 56 autopsies. Arch Pathol Lab Med. 1986;105:145.

67. Andersen LI, Frederiksen H-J, Appleyard M. Prevalence of esophageal Candida colonization in a Danish population, with special reference to esophageal symptoms, benign esophageal disorders, and pulmonary disease. J Infect Dis 1992;165:389–392.

68. Walsh TJ, Pizzo PA. Nosocomial fungal infections. Annu Rev Microbiol. 1988;42:517.

69. Lalor E, Rabeneck L. Esophageal candidiasis in AIDS: Successful therapy with clotrimazole vaginal tablets taken by mouth. Dig Dis Sci. 1991;36:279–281.

70. Leen CLS, Dunbar EM, Ellis ME, et al. Once-weekly fluconazole to prevent recurrence of oropharyngeal candidiasis in patients with AIDS and AIDS-related complex: A double-blind placebo-controlled study. J Infect. 1990;21:55–60.

71. Pena HM, Martinez-Lopez MA, Arnalich F, et al. Esophageal candidiasis associated with acute infection due to human immunodeficiency virus: Case report and review. Rev Infect Dis. 1991;13:872–875.

72. Raufman JP. Esophagoscopy in acquired immune deficiency syndrome. Gastroenterology. 1987;92:838.

73. Rosario MT, Raso CL, Comer GM, et al. Transnasal

brush cytology for the diagnosis of *Candida* esophagitis in the acquired immunodeficiency syndrome. Gastrointest Endosc. 1998;35:102–103.

74. Clotet B, Casals A, Reverter J, et al. *Candida* esophagitis in patients infected by human immune deficiency virus: Treatment and prognostic significance. Am J Gastroenterol. 1988;83:1008.

75. Pedersen C, Gerstoft J, Lindhardt BO, et al. *Candida* esophagitis associated with acute human immunodeficiency virus infection. J Infect Dis. 1987;156:529–530.

76. Bach MC, Valenti AJ, Howell DA, et al. Odynophagia from aphthous ulcers of the pharynx and esophagus in the acquired immunodeficiency (AIDS). Ann Intern Med. 1988;109:338–339.

77. Cooper DA, MacLean P, Finlayson R, et al. Acute AIDS retrovirus infection: Definition of a clinical illness associated with seroconversion. Lancet. 1985;1:537–540.

78. Kessler HA, Blaauw B, Spear J, et al. Diagnosis of human immunodeficiency virus infection in seronegative homosexuals presenting with an acute viral syndrome. JAMA. 1987;258:1196–1199.

79. Cooper DA, Tindall B, Wilson EJ, et al. Characterization of T lymphocyte responses during primary infection with human immunodeficiency virus. J Infect Dis. 1988;157:889–896.

80. Bonacini M, Young T, Laine L. The causes of esophageal symptoms in human immunodeficiency virus infection: A prospective study of 110 patients. Arch Intern Med. 1991;151:1567–1572.

81. Laine L, Bonacini M, Sattler F, et al. Cytomegalovirus (CMV) and *Candida* esophagitis (CE) in patients with AIDS. Gastroenterology. 1991;100:A591. Abstract.

82. Levine MS, Rubesin SE, Ott DJ. Update on esophageal radiology. Am J Roentgenol. 1990;155:933.

83. Levine MS. Radiology of the esophagus: A pattern approach. Radiology. 1991;179:1–7.

84. Kodsi BE, Wickremesinghe PC, Kozinn PJ, et al. *Candida* esophagitis: A prospective study of 27 cases. Gastroenterology. 1976;71:715–719.

85. Warren NG, Shadomy HJ. Yeasts of medical importance. In: Balows A, Hauser WJ Jr, Herrmann KL, et al., eds. Manual of Clinical Microbiology. 5th ed. Washington, DC. American Society for Microbiology, 1991;63:617–629.

86. Walsh TJ, Merz WG. Pathologic features in the human alimentary tract associated with invasiveness of *Candida tropicalis*. Am J Clin Pathol. 1986;85:498–502.

87. Laine L, Conteas C, Islam MZ, et al. A prospective, randomized, double-blind trial of fluconazole vs. ketoconazole for *Candida* esophagitis. Gastroenterology. In press.

88. Tavitian A, Raufman JP, Rosenthal LE, et al. Ketoconazole-resistant *Candida* esophagitis in patients with acquired immunodeficiency syndrome. Gastroenterology. 1986;90:443.

89. Wingard JR, Merz WG, Rinaldi MG, et al. Increase in *Candida krusei* infection among patients with bone marrow transplantation and neutropenia treated prophylactically with fluconazole. N Engl J Med. 1991;325:1274–1277.

90. Parente F, Cernuschi M, Rizzardini G, et al. Opportunistic infections of the esophagus not responding to oral systemic antifungals in patients with AIDS: Their frequency and treatment. Am J Gastroenterol. 1991;86:1729–1734.

91. Morace G, Manzara S, Dettori G. In vitro susceptibility of 119 yeast isolates to fluconazole, 5-fluorocytosine, amphotericin B, and ketoconazole. Chemotherapy. 1991;37:23–31.

92. Deschamps MH, Pape JW, Verdier RI, et al. Treatment of *Candida* esophagitis in AIDS patients. Am J Gastroenterol. 1988;83:20–21.

93. Ginsberg CH, Braden GL, Tauber AI, et al. Oral clotrimazole in the treatment of esophageal candidiasis. Am J Med. 1981;71:891–895.

94. Francis P, Walsh TJ. Approaches to management of fungal infections in cancer patients: Part 2. Oncology. 1992;6:133–148.

95. Chave JP, Franciolo P, Hirschel B, et al. Single-dose therapy for esophageal candidiasis with fluconazole. AIDS. 1990;4:1034–1037.

96. Warnock DW, Burke J, Cope NJ, et al. Fluconazole resistance in *Candida glabrata*. Lancet. 1988;2:1310.

97. Parente F, Trogi L, Cernushi M, et al. Is oral antifungal prophylaxis effective in preventing symptomatic relapses of esophageal candidiasis in patients with AIDS? Part 2. Gastroenterology. 1992;102:A677. Abstract.

98. Medoff G. Controversial areas in antifungal chemotherapy: Short course and combination therapy with amphotericin B. Rev Infect Dis. 1987;9:403.

99. Oh H, Hiruma K, Hirasawa A, et al. Effects of amphotericin B for prophylaxis of fungal infection in hematologic disorders. Exp Hematol. 1989;17:728.

100. Leon A, Toubas D, Renard P, et al. Diagnosis and prevention of candidiasis in intensive care patients. Agressologie. 1990;31:514.

101. Goodman JL, Winston DJ, Greenfield RA, et al. A controlled trial of fluconazole to prevent fungal infections in patients undergoing bone marrow transplantation. N Engl J Med. 1992;326:845–851.

102. Rohrman CA, Kidd R. Chronic mucocutaneous candidiasis: Radiologic abnormalities in the esophagus. Am J Radiol. 1978;130:473–477.

103. Obrecht WF, Richter JE, Olympio GA, et al. Tracheoesophageal fistula: A serious complication of infectious esophagitis. Gastroenterology. 1984;87:1174.

104. Lasic DD. Mixed micelles in drug delivery. Nature. 1992;355:279–280.

105. Loyd JE, desPrez RM, Goodwin RA Jr. *Histoplasma capsulatum*. In: Mandell GL, Douglas RG, Bennett JE, eds. Principles and Practices of Infectious Diseases. 3rd ed. New York: Churchill Livingstone; 1990;242:1989–1999.

106. Lee JH, Newman DA, Welsh JD. Disseminated histoplasmosis presenting with esophageal symptomatology. Dig Dis. 1977;22:831–834.

107. Goodwin RA, Nickell JA, desPrez RM. Mediastinal fibrosis complicating healed primary histoplasmosis and tuberculosis. Medicine (Baltimore). 1972;51:227–246.

108. Forsmark CE, Wilcox CM, Darragh TM, et al. Disseminated histoplasmosis in AIDS: An unusual case of esophageal involvement and gastrointestinal bleeding. Gastrointest Endos. 1990;36:604.

109. Coss KC, Wheat LJ, Conces DJ, et al. Esophageal fistula complicating mediastinal histoplasmosis: Response to amphotericin B. Am J Med. 1987;83:343–346.

110. Warren KG, Brown SM, Wroblewska Z, et al. Isolation of latent herpes simplex virus from the superior cervical and vagus ganglions of human beings. N Engl J Med. 1978;298:1068–1070.

111. Corey L. Herpesviruses. In: Sherris J, ed. Medical Microbiology. 2nd ed. New York: Elsevier; 1990;37:559–575.

112. Hirsch MS. Herpes group virus infections in the compromised host. In: Rubin RH, Young LS, eds. Clinical approach to infection in the compromised host. 2nd ed. New York: Plenum; 1988;13:347–366.

113. Nash G, Ross JS. Herpetic esophagitis: A common cause of esophageal ulceration. Hum Pathol. 1974;5:339–345.

114. Shortsleeve MJ, Levine MS. Herpes esophagitis in otherwise healthy patients: Clinical and radiographic findings. Radiology. 1992;182:859–861.

115. Ginaldi S, Burgert W, Paulk T. Herpes esophagitis in

immunocompetent patients. Am Fam Physician. 1987;36:160–164.

116. Silverstein FE, Tytgat GNJ. Atlas of gastrointestinal endoscopy. 2nd ed. New York; Gower Medical Publishing; 1991;2.1–3.22.

117. Jenkins D, Wick ACB. Herpes simplex esophagitis in a renal transplant patient: The need for antiviral therapy. Am J Gastroenterol. 1988;83:331–332.

118. Watts SJ, Alexander LC, Fawcett K, et al. Herpes simplex esophagitis in a renal transplant patient treated with cyclosporin A: A case report. Am J Gastroenterol. 1986;81:185–188.

119. Byard RW, Champion MC, Orizaga M. Variability in the clinical presentation and endoscopic findings of herpetic esophagitis. Endoscopy. 1987;19:153–155.

120. Greenson JK, Beschorner WE, Boitnott JK, et al. Prominent mononuclear cell infiltrate is characteristic of herpes esophagitis. Hum Pathol. 1991;22:541–549.

121. Cardillo MR, Forte F. Brush cytology in the diagnosis of herpetic esophagitis: A case report. Endoscopy. 1988;20:156–157.

122. McBane RD, Gross JB Jr. Herpes esophagitis: Clinical syndrome, endoscopic appearance, and diagnosis in 23 patients. Gastrointest Endosc. 1991;37:600–603.

123. Gleaves CA, Reed EC, Hackman RC, et al. Rapid diagnosis of invasive cytomegalovirus infection by examination of tissue specimens in centrifugation culture. Am J Clin Pathol. 1987;88:354.

124. Spruance SL, Stewart JC, Rowe NH, et al. Treatment of recurrent herpes simplex labialis with oral acyclovir. J Infect Dis. 1990;161:185–190.

125. Agha FP, Horchang HL, Nostrandt TT. Herpetic esophagitis: A diagnostic challenge in immunocompromised patients. Am J Gastroenterol. 1986;81:246–253.

126. Sherris JC, Plorde JJ. Antimicrobics and chemotherapy of bacterial and viral infections. In: Sherris JC, ed. Medical Microbiology. 2nd ed. New York: Elsevier; 1990;13:197–232.

127. Eck P, Silver S, Clark E. Acute renal failure and coma after a high dose of acyclovir. N Engl J Med. 1991;325:1178–1179.

128. Dolin R. Antiviral chemotherapy and prophylaxis. Science. 1985;227:1296–1303.

129. Safrin S, Crumpacker C, Chatis P, et al. A controlled trial comparing foscarnet with vidarabine for acyclovir-resistant mucocutaneous herpes simplex in the acquired immunodeficiency syndrome. N Engl J Med. 1991;325:551–555.

130. Birch CJ, Tachedjian G, Doherty RR, et al. Altered sensitivity to antiviral drugs of herpes simplex virus isolates from a patient with the acquired immunodeficiency syndrome. J Infect Dis. 1990;162:731–734.

131. Sall RK, Kauffman CL, Levy CS. Successful treatment of progressive acyclovir-resistant herpes simplex virus using intravenous foscarnet in a patient with the acquired immunodeficiency syndrome. Arch Dermatol. 1989;125:1548–1550.

132. Safrin S, Assaykeen T, Follansbee S, et al. Foscarnet therapy for acyclovir-resistant mucocutaneous herpes simplex virus infection in 26 AIDS patients: Preliminary data. J Infect Dis. 1990;161:1078–1084.

133. Minor JR, Baltz JK. Foscarnet sodium. DICP. 1991;25:41–47.

134. Selby PJ, Powles RL, Easton D, et al. The prophylactic role of intravenous and long-term oral acyclovir after allogeneic bone marrow transplantation. Br J Cancer. 1989;59:434–438.

135. Redding SW, Montgomery MT. Acyclovir for oral herpes simplex virus infection in patients with bone marrow transplants. Oral Surg Oral Med Oral Pathol. 1989;67:680–683.

136. Tang IY, Maddux MS, Veremis SA, et al. Low-dose oral acyclovir for prevention of herpes simplex virus infection during OKT3 therapy. Transplant Proc. 1989;21:1758–1760.

137. Cronstedt JL, Bouchama A, Hainau B, et al. Spontaneous esophageal perforation in herpes simplex esophagitis. Am J Gastroenterol. 1992;87:124–127.

138. Myerson D, Hackman RC, Nelson JA, et al. Widespread presence of histologically occult cytomegalovirus. Hum Pathol. 1984;15:430–439.

139. Adler SP. Transfusion-associated cytomegalovirus infections. Rev Infect Dis. 1983;5:977–993.

140. Preiksaitis JK, Janowska-Wieczorek A. Persistence of cytomegalovirus in human long-term bone marrow culture: Relationship to hemopoiesis. J Med Virol. 1991;35:76–84.

141. Reddehase MJ. Bone marrow dysfunction in irradiated, cytomegalovirus-infected mice. Transplant Proc. 1991;23:10–11.

142. Duncombe AS, Grundy JE, Prentice HG, Brenner MK. IL2 activated killer cells may contribute to cytomegalovirus induced marrow hypoplasia after bone marrow transplantation. Bone Marrow Transplant. 1991;7:81–87.

143. Sing GK, Ruscetti FW. Preferential suppression of myelopoiesis in normal human bone marrow cells after in vitro challenge with human cytomegalovirus. Blood. 1990;75:1965–1973.

144. Rook AH. Interactions of cytomegalovirus with the human immune system. Rev Infect Dis. 1988;10(suppl 3):S460–S467.

145. Weber JN, Thom W, Barrison I, et al. Cytomegalovirus colitis and oesophageal ulceration in the context of AIDS: Clinical manifestations and preliminary report of treatment with foscarnet. Gut. 1987;28:482–487.

146. Wilcox CD, Theise ND, Rotterdam H, Dieterich D. Cytomegalovirus esophagitis in AIDS: Diagnosis by endoscopic biopsy. Am J Gastroenterol. 1991;86:1123–1126.

147. Schwartz DA, Wilcox CM. Atypical cytomegalovirus inclusions in gastrointestinal biopsy specimens from patients with the acquired immunodeficiency syndrome: diagnostic role of in situ nucleic acid hybridization. Hum Pathol. 1992;23:1019–1026.

148. Hackman RC, Wolford JL, Gleaves GA, et al. Recognition and rapid diagnosis of upper gastrointestinal cytomegalovirus infection in marrow transplant recipients: A comparison of seven virologic methods. Transplantation. In press.

149. Meyers JD. Prevention and treatment of cytomegalovirus infections. Annu Rev Med. 1991;42:179–187.

150. Jacobson MA. Ganciclovir therapy for opportunistic cytomegalovirus disease in AIDS. AIDS Clin Rev. 1990;149–163.

151. Mayoral JL, Loeffler CM, Fasola CG, et al. Diagnosis and treatment of cytomegalovirus disease in transplant patients based on gastrointestinal tract manifestations. Arch Surg. 1991;126:202–206.

152. Stratta RJ, Shaefer MS, Markin RS, et al. Clinical patterns of cytomegalovirus disease after liver transplantation. Arch Surg. 1989;124:1443–1449.

153. Thomson MH, Jeffries DJ. Ganciclovir therapy in iatrogenically immunosuppressed patients with cytomegalovirus disease. J Antimicrob Chemother. 1989;23:61–70.

154. Grossi P, Revello MG, Minolo L, et al. Three year experience with human cytomegalovirus infections in heart transplant recipients. J Heart Transplant. 1990;9:712.

155. Dunn DL, Mayoral JL, Gillingham KJ, et al. Treatment of invasive cytomegalovirus disease in solid organ transplant patients with ganciclovir. Transplantation. 1991;51:98–106.

156. Hochster H, Dieterich D, Bozzette S, et al. Toxicity of combined ganciclovir and zidovudine for cytomegalovirus disease associated with AIDS: An AIDS clinical trials group study. Ann Intern Med. 1990;113:111–117.

157. Swan SK, Munar MY, Wigger MA, et al. Pharmacokinetics of ganciclovir in a patient undergoing hemodialysis. Am J Kidney Dis. 1991;17:69–72.

158. Jacobson MA, Drew WL, Feinberg J, et al. Foscarnet therapy for ganciclovir-resistant cytomegalovirus retinitis in patients with AIDS. J Infect Dis. 1991;163:1348–1351.

159. Nelson MR, Connolly GM, Hawkins DA, et al. Foscarnet in the treatment of cytomegalovirus infection of the esophagus and colon in patients with the acquired immune deficiency syndrome. Am J Gastroenterol. 1991;86:876–881.

160. Knox K, Drobyski W, Carrigan D. Cytomegalovirus isolate resistant to ganciclovir and foscarnet from a marrow transplant recipient. Lancet. 1991;337:1292–1293.

161. Nelson MR, Barter G, Hawkins D, et al. Simultaneous treatment of cytomegalovirus retinitis with ganciclovir and foscarnet. Lancet. 1991;338:250.

162. Deray G, Katlama C, Dohin E. Prevention of foscarnet nephrotoxicity. Ann Intern Med. 1990;113:332.

163. Aweeka F, Gamgertoglio J, Mills J, et al. Pharmacokinetics of intermittently administered intravenous foscarnet in the treatment of acquired immunodeficiency syndrome patients with serious cytomegalovirus retinitis. Antimicrob Agents Chemother. 1989;33:742–745.

164. Balfour HH, Chace BA, Stapleton JT, et al. A randomized, placebo-controlled trial of oral acyclovir for the prevention of cytomegalovirus disease in recipients of renal allografts. N Engl J Med. 1989;320:1381–1387.

165. Stratta RJ, Shaefer MS, Cushing KA, et al. Successful prophylaxis of cytomegalovirus disease after primary CMV exposure in liver transplant recipients. Transplantation. 1991;51:90–97.

166. Meyers JD, Reed EC, Shepp DH, et al. Acyclovir for prevention of cytomegalovirus infection and disease after allogeneic marrow transplantation. N Engl J Med. 1988;318:70–75.

167. Goodrich JM, Mori M, Gleaves CA, et al. Early treatment with ganciclovir to prevent cytomegalovirus disease after allogeneic bone marrow transplantation. N Engl J Med. 1991;325:1601–1607.

168. Schmidt GM, Horak DA, Niland JC, et al. A randomized, controlled trial of prophylactic ganciclovir for cytomegalovirus pulmonary infection in recipients of allogeneic bone marrow transplants. The City of Hope—Stanford—Syntex CMV Study Group. N Engl J Med. 1991;324:1005–1011.

169. Sayers MH, Anderson KC, Goodnough LT, et al. Reducing the risk for transfusion-transmitted cytomegalovirus infection. Ann Intern Med. 1992;116:55–62.

170. Lang DJ, Ebert PA, Rodgers BM, et al. Reduction on postperfusion cytomegalovirus infections following the use of leukocyte depleted blood. Transfusion. 1977;17:391–395.

171. Luban NL, Williams AE, McDonald MG, et al. Low incidence of cytomegalovirus infection in neonates transfused with washed red blood cells. Am J Dis Child. 1987;141:416–419.

172. Tolkoff-Rubin NA, Rubin RH, Keller EE, et al. Cytomegalovirus infection in dialysis patients and personnel. Ann Intern Med. 1978;89:625–628.

173. Verdonck LF, de Graan-Hentzen YC, Dekker AW, et al. Cytomegalovirus seronegative platelets and leukocyte-poor red blood cells from random donors can prevent primary cytomegalovirus infection after bone marrow transplantation. Bone Marrow Transplant. 1987;2:73–78.

174. Bowden RA, Sayers MH, Cays M, et al. The role of blood product filtration in the prevention of transfusion associated cytomegalovirus (CMV) infection after marrow transplant. Transfusion. 1989;29:57S. Abstract.

175. Goodgame RW, Ross PG, Kim H, et al. Esophageal stricture after cytomegalovirus ulcer therapy with ganciclovir. J Clin Gastroenterol. 1991;13:678–681.

176. Gill RA, Gebhard RL, Dozeman RL, et al. Shingles esophagitis: Endoscopic diagnosis in two patients. Gastrointest Endosc. 1984;30:26.

177. Buss DH, Scharyi M. Herpes virus infection of the esophagus and other visceral organs in adults: Incidence and clinical significance. Am J Med. 1979;77:44.

178. Rosen P, Hadju S. Visceral herpesvirus infections in patients with cancer. Am J Clin Pathol. 1971;56:459.

179. Sherman RA, Silva J, Gandour-Edwards R. Fatal varicella in an adult: Case report and review of the gastrointestinal complications of chickenpox. Rev Infect Dis. 1991;13:424.

180. Gelb LD. Varicella-zoster virus. In: Fields BN, Knipe DM, et al., eds. Virology. 2nd ed. New York: Raven Press; 1990;71:2011–2054.

181. Whitley RJ, Soong SJ, Dolin R, et al. Early vidarabine therapy to control the complications of herpes zoster in the immunosuppressed: NIAID Collaborative Antiviral Study. N Engl J Med. 1982;307:971–975.

182. Shepp DH, Dandliker PS, Meyers JD. Treatment of varicella-zoster virus infection in severely immunocompromised patients: A randomized comparison of acyclovir and vidarabine. N Engl J Med. 1986;314:208–214.

183. Dunkle LM, Arvin AM, Whitley RJ, et al. A controlled trial of acyclovir for chickenpox in normal children. N Engl J Med. 1991;325:1539–1544.

184. Kunitomi T, Akazai A, Ikeda M, et al. Comparison of acyclovir and vidarabine in immunocompromised children with varicella-zoster virus infection. Acta Paediatrica Jpn. 1989;31:702–705.

185. Meszner Z, Gyarmati E, Nyerges G, et al. Early relapses of varicella-zoster virus infection in immunocompromised children treated with acyclovir. Acta Paediatrica Hung. 1990;30:263–270.

186. McGregor RS, Zitelli BJ, Urbach AH, et al. Varicella in pediatric orthotopic liver transplant recipients. Pediatrics. 1989;83:256–261.

187. Linnemann CC Jr, Biron KK, Hoppenjamns WG, et al. Emergence of acyclovir resistant varicella-zoster virus in an AIDS patient on prolonged acyclovir therapy. AIDS. 1990;4:577–579.

188. Jacobson MA, Berger TG, Fikrig S, et al. Acyclovir resistant varicella-zoster virus infection after chronic oral acyclovir therapy in patients with the acquired immunodeficiency syndrome (AIDS). Ann Intern Med. 1990;112:187–191.

189. Safrin S, Berger TG, Gilson I, et al. Foscarnet therapy in five patients with AIDS and acyclovir-resistant varicella-zoster virus infection. Ann Intern Med. 1991;115:19–21.

190. Smith KJ, Kahlter DC, Davis C, et al. Acyclovir-resistant varicella-zoster responsive to foscarnet. Arch Dermatol. 1991;127:1069–1071. Letter.

191. Varicella-zoster immune globulin for the prevention of chickenpox: Recommendation of the Immunization Practices Advisory Committee (ACIP). MMWR. 1984;33:84–100.

192. Weibel RE, Neff BJ, Kuter BJK, et al. Live attenuated varicella virus vaccine-efficacy in healthy children. N Engl J Med. 1984;310:1409–1415.

193. Gershon A, Steinberg S, Gelb L, et al. Liver attenuated varicella vaccine: Efficacy for children with leukemia in remission. JAMA. 1984;255:355–362.

194. Eversole LR, Stone CE, Beckman AM. Detection of EBV and HPV DNA sequences in oral "hairy" leukoplakia by in situ hybridization. J Med Virol. 1988;26:271–277.

195. Tilbe KS, Lloyd DA. A case of viral esophagitis. J Clin Gastroenterol. 1886;8:494–495.

196. Kitchen VS, Helbert M, Francis ND, et al. Epstein-Barr virus associated oesophageal ulcers in AIDS. Gut. 1990; 31:1223–1225.

197. Miller G. Epstein-Barr virus: Biology, pathology, and medical aspects. In: Fields BN, Knipe DM, et al., eds. Virology. 2nd ed. New York: Raven Press; 1990; 68:1921–1958.

198. Lennett ET. Epstein-Barr virus. In: Balows A, Hausler WJ Jr, Herrmann KL, et al., eds. Manual of Medical Microbiology. 5th ed. Washington: American Society for Microbiology; 1991;78:847–852.

199. Friedman-Kein AE. Viral origin of hairy leukoplakia. Lancet. 1986;2:694.

200. Samaranayake LP, Pindborg JJ. Hairy leukoplakia. Br Med J. 1989;298:270–271.

201. Resnik L, Herbst JS, Ablashi DV, et al. Regression of oral hairy leukoplakia after orally administered acyclovir therapy. JAMA. 1988;259:384–388.

202. Murphy FA, Kingsbury DW. Virus taxonomy. In: Fields BN, Knipe DM, et al., eds. Virology. 2nd ed. New York: Raven Press; 1990;2:9–35.

203. Gaines H, vonSydow M, Pehrson PO, et al. Clinical picture of primary HIV-infection presenting as a glandular-fever-like illness. Br Med J. 1988;297:1363.

204. Kumar A, Posner G, Colby S, et al. Giant esophageal ulcers in AIDS-related complex. Gastrointest Endosc. 1988;34:153–154.

205. Sokol-Anderson ML, Prelutsky DJ, Westblom TU. Giant esophageal aphthous ulcers in AIDS patients: Treatment with low-dose corticosteroids. AIDS. 1991;5:1537–1538.

206. Dretler RH, Rausher DB. Giant esophageal ulcer healed with steroid therapy in an AIDS patient. Rev Infect Dis. 1989;11:768–769.

207. Wilcox CM, Schwartz DA, Coffield LM, et al. Evaluation of idiopathic esophageal ulcers (IEU) for human immunodeficiency virus (HIV) by polymerase chain reaction (PCR): Is HIV an esophageal pathogen? Part 2. Gastroenterology. 1992;102:A712.

208. Georgehiou PR, Kemp RJ. HIV-associated oesophageal ulcers treated with thalidomide. Med J Aust. 1990;152:382–383.

209. Bernardo P, Arrizabalaga J, Iribarren JA, Garde C. Effectiveness of thalidomide in nonspecific esophageal ulcer in patients with acquired immunodeficiency syndrome. Med Clin (Barc). 1990;94:638–639.

210. Lombardi JP, Tang D, Myhre OA. Squamous cell papilloma of the esophagus: A case report and review of the literature. Int Surg. 1980;65:459–461.

211. Franzin G, Musola R, Qambomi G, et al. Squamous papilloma of the esophagus. Gastrointest Endosc. 1983;29:104–106.

212. Jadvan P, Pitman ER. Squamous papilloma of esophagus. Dig Dis Sci. 1984;29:317–320.

213. de Borges RJ, Acevedo F, Miralles E, et al. Squamous papilloma of the esophagus diagnosed by cytology: Report of a case with concurrent occult epidermoid carcinoma. Acta Cytol. 1986;30:487–490.

214. Syrjanen KJ. Histological changes identical to those of condylomatous lesions found in esophageal squamous cell carcinomas. Arch Geswelstforsch. 1982;52:283–292.

215. Weitzner S, Hendel W. Squamous papilloma of the esophagus: Case report and review of the literature. Am J Gastroenterol. 1968;50:391–396.

216. Zeabart LE, Fabian J, Nord HG. Squamous papilloma of the esophagus: Report of three cases. Gastrointest Endosc. 1979;25:18–20.

217. Colina F, Solis JA, Munoz MT. Squamous papilloma of the esophagus: A report of three cases and review of literature. Am J Gastroenterol. 1980;74:410–414.

218. Shah KV, Howley PM. Papillomaviruses. In: Fields BN, Knipe DM, et al. Virology. 2nd ed. New York: Raven Press; 1990;59:1651–1676.

219. zur Hausen H. Minireview: Human papillomavirus in the pathogenesis of anogenital cancer. Virology. 1991;184:9–13.

220. Janson JA, Baille J, Pollack M. Endoscopic removal of esophageal condylomata acuminatum containing human papilloma virus. Gastrointest Endosc. 1991; 37:367–369.

221. Hording M, Hording U, Daugaard S, et al. Human papilloma varus type 11 in a fatal case of esophageal and bronchial papillomatosis. Scand J Infect Dis. 1989;21:229–231.

222. Winkler B, Capo V, Reumann W, et al. Human papillomavirus infection of the esophagus: A clinicopathologic study with demonstration of papillomavirus antigen by the immunoperoxidase technique. Cancer. 1985;55:149–155.

223. Schechter M, Pannain VLN, de Oliveira V. Papovavirus-associated esophageal ulceration in a patient with AIDS. AIDS. 1991;5:238.

224. van de Brule AJC, Claas AJC, du Maine HCJ, et al. Use of anti-contamination primers in the polymerase chain reaction for the detection of human papillomavirus genotypes in cervical scrapes and biopsies. J Med Virol. 1989;29:20–27.

225. Leventhal BG, Kashima HK, Mounts P, et al. Long-term response of recurrent respiratory papillomatosis to treatment with lymphoblastoid interferon alfa-n1. N Engl J Med. 1991;325:613–617.

226. Yang CS. Research on esophageal cancer in China: A review. Cancer Res. 1980;40:2633–2644.

227. Joint Iran/IARC Study Group. Oesophageal cancer studies in the Caspian littoral of Iran: Results of population studies, a prodrome. J Natl Cancer Inst. 1977;59:1127–1138.

228. Wynder EL, Bross IJ. A study of etiologic factors in cancer of the esophagus. Cancer. 1961;14:389–411.

229. Chang F, Shen Q, Zhou J, et al. Detection of human papillomavirus DNA in cytologic specimens derived from esophageal precancer lesions and cancer. Scand J Gastroenterol. 1990;25:383–388.

230. Chang F, Syrjanen S, Shen Q, et al. Human papillomavirus (HPV) DNA in esophageal precancer lesions and squamous cell carcinomas from China. Int J Cancer. 1990;45:21–25.

231. Williamson AL, Jaskiesicz K, Gunning A. The detection of human papillomavirus in oesophageal lesions. Anticancer Res. 1991;11:263–265.

232. Davidson M, Parkinson A, Schloss M, et al. Prevalence of cervical infections with human papillomavirus in Alaska native women. Interscience Conference on Antimicrobial Agents and Chemotherapy, Atlanta, GA, October 1990.

233. Miller BA, Davidson M, Myerson D, et al. Human papillomavirus (HPV) DNA in esophageal carcinoma from Alaska natives. Submitted for publication, Int J Cancer.

234. Kiyabu MT, Shibata D, Arnheim N, et al. Detection of human papillomavirus in formalin-fixed, invasive squamous carcinoma using the polymerase chain reaction. Am J Surg Pathol. 1989;13:221–224.

235. Collins RJ, Ngan HYS, Hsu C, et al. Proceedings of the Thirty-Fourth Annual Scientific Meeting of the Royal College of Pathologists of Australia, 1989. Abstract.

236. Loke SL, Ma L, Wong M, et al. Human papillomavirus in oesophageal squamous cell carcinoma. J Clin Pathol. 1990;43:909–912.

237. Coelho CA, Ferrante R. Dysphagia in postpolio sequelae: Report of three cases. Arch Phys Med Rehabil. 1988;69:634–636.

238. Buchholz D. Dysphagia in post-polio patients. Birth Defects. 1987;23:55–62.

239. McManus JPA, Webb JN. A yeast-like infection of the esophagus caused by *Lactobacillus acidophilus*. Gastroenterology. 1975;68:583–586.

240. Howlett SA. Acute streptococcal esophagitis. Gastrointest Endosc. 1979;25:150–151.

241. Ezzell JH, Bremer J, Adamec TA. Bacterial esophagitis: An often forgotten cause of odynophagia. Am J Gastroenterol. 1990;85:296–298.

242. Chow AW. Infections of the oral cavity, neck, and head. In: Mandell GL, Douglas RG, Bennett JE, eds. Principles and practices of infectious diseases. 3rd ed. New York: Churchill Livingstone; 1990;49:516–529.

243. Sherris JC, Plodre JJ. Mycobacteria. In: Sherris JC, ed. Medical Microbiology. 2nd ed. New York: Elsevier; 1990;27:443–462.

244. McNamara M, Williams CE, Brown TS, et al. Tuberculosis affecting the oesophagus. Clin Radiol. 1987;38:419–422.

245. Gordon AH, Marshall JB. Esophageal tuberculosis: Definitive diagnosis by endoscopy. Am J Gastroenterol. 1990;85:174–177.

246. Dow C. Esophageal tuberculosis: Four cases. Gut. 1981;22:234–236.

247. Fahmy AR, Guindi R, Farid A. Tuberculosis of the oesophagus. Thorax. 1969;24:254–256.

248. Al-Idrissi HY, Satti MB, Al-Quirain A, et al. Granulomatous esophagitis: A case of tuberculosis limited to the oesophagus. Ann Trop Med Parasitol. 1987;81:129–133.

249. Eng J, Sbaratnam S. Tuberculosis of the esophagus. Dig Dis Sci. 1991;36:536–540.

250. Sinha SN, Tesar P, Seta W, et al. Primary oesophageal tuberculosis. Br J Clin Pract. 1988;42:391–394.

251. Rosario MT, Raso CL, Comer GM. Esophageal tuberculosis. Dig Dis Sci. 1989;34:1281–1284.

252. Ramakantan R, Shah P. Tuberculous fistulas of the pharynx and esophagus. Gastrointest Radiol. 1990;15:145–147.

253. Goodman P, Pinero SS, Rance RM, et al. Mycobacterial esophagitis in AIDS. Gastrointest Radiol. 1989;14:103–105.

254. de Silva R, Stoopack PM, Raufman JP. Esophageal fistulas associated with mycobacterial infection in patients at risk for AIDS. Radiology. 1990;175:449–453.

255. Damtew B, Frengley D, Wolinski E, et al. Esophageal tuberculosis: Mimicry of gastrointestinal malignancy. Rev Infect Dis. 1987;9:140–146.

256. Bárcena R, Erdozain JC, Lopez–San Roman A, et al. Tuberculous mediastinal adenopathy mimicking esophageal leiomyoma. Endoscopy. 1990;22:57–58.

257. Pina Cabral JE, Toste M, Correia Leitao M, et al. Endoscopic diagnosis of esophageal tuberculosis. Am J Gastroenterol. 1990;85:1431–1432.

258. Tornieporth N, Lorenz R, Gain T, et al. An unusual case of active tuberculosis of the oesophagus in an adult. Endoscopy. 1991;23:294–296.

259. Newman RM, Fleshner PR, Lajam FE, et al. Esophageal tuberculosis: A rare presentation with hematemesis. Am J Gastroenterol. 1991;86:751–755.

260. Adkins MS, Raccuia JS, Acinapura AJ. Esophageal perforation in a patient with acquired immunodeficiency syndrome. Ann Thorac Surg. 1990;50:299–300.

261. van Scoy RE, Wilkowske CJ. Antituberculous agents. Mayo Clin Proc. 1992;67:179–187.

262. Coelho LGV, Payne A, Karim QN, et al. *Campylobacter pylori* in esophagus, antrum, and duodenum: A histological and microbiological study. Dig Dis Sci. 1989;34:445–448.

263. Walker SJ, Birch PJ, Stewart M, et al. Patterns of colonization of *Campylobacter pylori* in the oesophagus, stomach, and duodenum. Gut. 1989;30:1334–1338.

264. Paull G, Yardley JH. Gastric and esophageal *Campylobacter pylori* in patients with Barrett's esophagus. Gastroenterology. 1988;95:216–218.

265. Shallcross TM, Wyatt JI, Rathbone BJ, et al. Non-steroidal anti-inflammatory drugs, hiatus hernia, and *Helicobacter pylori*, in patients with oesophageal ulceration. Br J Rheumatol. 1990;29:288–290.

266. Cheng EH, Bermanski P, Silversmith M, et al. Prevalence of *Campylobacter pylori* in esophagitis, gastritis, and duodenal disease. Arch Intern Med. 1989;149:1373–1375.

267. Houck JA, Lucas JG. Absence of campylobacter-like organisms in Barrett's esophagus. Arch Pathol Lab Med. 1989;113:470–472.

268. Hudson TR, Head JR. Syphilis of the esophagus. J Thorac Surg. 1950;20:216.

269. Stone J, Friedberg SA. Obstructive syphilitic esophagitis. JAMA. 1961;177:711.

270. Lathrop DL, Griebel M, Horner J. Dysphagia in tetanus: Evaluation and outcome. Dysphagia. 1989;4:173–175.

271. Kasanzew M, Brown B, Dawes P. Tetanus presenting as dysphagia. J Laryngol Otol. 1989;103:229–230.

272. Scholz DG, Olson JM, Thurber DL, et al. Tetanus: An uncommon cause of dysphagia. Mayo Clinic Proc. 1989;64:335–338.

273. Dantas RO, Godoy RA, de Oliveira RB, et al. Lower esophageal sphincter pressure in Chagas's disease. Dig Dis Sci. 1990;35:508–512.

274. Rezende FJ, de Oliveira RB, Dantas RO, et al. The effect of isosorbide dinitrate on esophageal emptying in chagasic megaesophagus. Arq Gastroenterol. 1990;27:115–119.

275. Esper FE, Muneiro V, dos Santos EP, et al. Dilation of the cardia in treating dysphagia in patients with chagasic megaesophagus. Arq Gastroenterol. 1988;25:69–74.

276. Pinotti HW, Felix VN, Zilberstein B, Cecconello I. Surgical complications of Chagas' disease: Megaesophagus, achalasia of the pylorus, and cholelithiasis. World J Surg. 1991;15:198–204.

277. Zucoloto S, de Rezende JM. Mucosal alterations in human chronic chagasic esophagopathy. Digestion. 1990;47:138–142.

278. Grimes MM, LaPook JD, Bar MH, et al. Disseminated *Pneumocystis carinii* in a patient with acquired immunodeficiency syndrome. Hum Pathol. 1987;18:307–308.

279. Ditrich O, Palkovic L, Sterba J, et al. The first finding of *Cryptosporidium baileyi* in man. Parasitol Res. 1991;77:44–47.

280. Kazlow PG, Shah K, Benkov KJ, et al. Esophageal cryptosporidiosis in a child with acquired immune deficiency syndrome. Gastroenterology. 1986;91:1301–1303.

281. McDonald GB. Esophageal diseases caused by infection, systemic illness, and trauma. In: Sleisenger MH, Fordtran JS, eds. Gastrointestinal Disease: Pathophysiology, Diagnosis, Management. 5th ed. Philadelphia: WB Saunders; 1993; 427–441.

282. Walton S, Bennet JR. Skin and gullet. Gut. 1991;32:694–697.

The Stomach

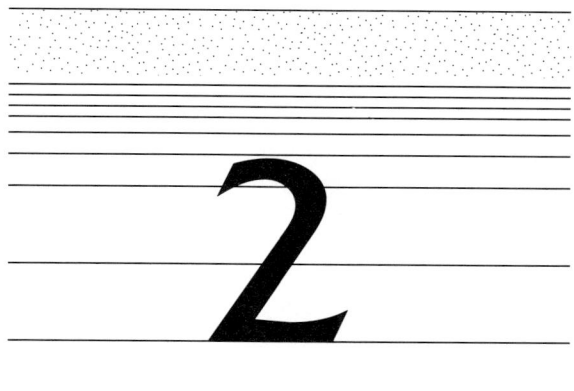

2

Infectious Gastritis

RICHARD W. GOODGAME, M.D.
ROBERT M. GENTA, M.D., D.T.M. & H.
MAE F. GO, M.D.
DAVID Y. GRAHAM, M.D.

WHAT IS GASTRITIS?

Gastritis is a term that conveys different meanings to different people. Pathologists view gastritis as an inflammatory process that involves the gastric mucosa. Endoscopists often associate the term with mucosal erythema or erosions. To many clinicians and lay persons the term gastritis evokes a wide spectrum of poorly defined upper abdominal signs and symptoms. Efforts to correlate the endoscopic findings with the histopathologic characteristics of the gastric mucosa have been unsuccessful.[1] Furthermore, neither the endoscopic nor the histopathologic features of the stomach show a consistent association with the clinical manifestations. In addition, histologic gastritis is present in a large segment of the normal asymptomatic population. This lack of correlation between clinical, endoscopic, and histopathologic findings probably accounts for the disorder that still pervades the classification of gastritis.[2]

Another crucial reason for difficulties in classifying gastritis is that the gastric mucosa reacts to injury with a relatively limited spectrum of responses. For example, polymorphonuclear or mononuclear inflammatory cells may gather with various degrees of density in different locations of the lamina propria; or they may infiltrate and destroy the epithelium; or, after they destroy the epithelium, it may regenerate in an imperfect fashion, losing some of its elements or acquiring the characteristics of other epithelium and thus adapting to a changed environment. These are, in essence, the features of acute and chronic gastritis, of atrophy, and of intestinal metaplasia. This scarcity of histopathologic findings and their lack of etiologic specificity account for the fact that most gastritides were, in the past, labeled idiopathic and that they gave rise to frequent speculation about dietary, toxic, immunologic, or infectious causes.

Until recently, infective gastritides included only a very small portion of the gastric diseases seen by clinicians and an even smaller portion of the histologic specimens examined by pathologists. Phlegmonous gastritis, caused by a variety of common bacteria, was, and remains, exceedingly rare. Syphilitic gastritis, probably common in the prepenicillin era, has become a medical curiosity. Tuberculosis of the stomach was occasionally reported, mostly in patients from developing or Eastern European countries.[3, 4] Although a variety of pathogenic and saprophytic fungi may colonize preexisting lesions of the stomach, such as peptic ulcers and ulcerated neoplasms, they are almost never a primary cause of gastritis. Cytomegalovirus (CMV) and herpesvirus infections of the stomach were also uncommon. A few cases of parasitic gastritis have been reported during the course of disseminated strongyloidiasis,[5] and several cases of gastric perforation were reported in association with anisakiasis.[6] Overall, until the early 1980s, microorganisms were rarely searched for and even more rarely identified in the evaluation of gastritis.

Two events in the 1980s produced a dramatic change in this state of affairs. First was the discovery that the majority of cases of chronic gastritis are caused by *Helicobacter pylori*. Second, the pandemic of the acquired immunodeficiency syndrome (AIDS) plus the widespread use of immunosuppressive treatment in conjunction with organ transplants and cancer chemotherapy has increased the frequency of previously uncommon viral, fungal, and mycobacterial infection. Gastric infections are now the most prominent categories in the etiologic classification of gastritis.

A number of classification systems for gastritis have been proposed. The most recent is the Sydney system, which includes both histologic and endoscopic components.[7] The histologic component is divided into etiology (including pathogenic associations), topography, and morphology. Each division is important and may predict the spectrum of disease associated with the gastritis. The two most common causes of gastritis are an autoimmune process leading to pernicious anemia and infection with *H. pylori*. The more common infectious causes are given in Table 2–1. In this chapter we shall address

three types of infectious gastritis. *H. pylori* gastritis is discussed because of its widespread prevalence and its role in the causation of peptic ulcer disease and gastric carcinoma. Because the early stages of *H. pylori* and *Treponema pallidum* infections of the stomach may be deceptively similar and because of the increasing prevalence of syphilis in recent years, we also have included a discussion of syphilitic gastritis. Cytomegalovirus was chosen for discussion because it is the most common cause of opportunistic gastritis seen in immunosuppressed patients.

Acute Gastritis

The distinction between acute and chronic gastritis has greatly suffered from the pathologists' tendency to use the term acute as synonymous with neutrophilic infiltration, and the term chronic as synonymous with mononuclear infiltration. Although this general principle of pathology is often correct, when used in descriptions of the gastrointestinal mucosa it may be seriously misleading. For example, ulcerative colitis is a process that may last for decades, yet much of the inflammatory infiltrate in the colonic mucosa consists of polymorphonuclear cells. Similarly, as discussed later, neutrophils are an essential part of the inflammatory response to lifelong infection with *H. pylori*. The presence of neutrophils on a background of mononuclear inflammation may be better defined as active inflammation, a term that conveys the image of a dynamic process without suggesting artificial chronologic constraints.

Acute gastritis, as a clinical syndrome accompanied by a histopathologic picture of acute inflammation, has long been recognized. Osler's 1925 textbook devoted a section to acute gastritis, for which the synonyms gastritis, acute gastric catarrh, and acute dyspepsia were given.[8] Attacks were described as lasting from 1 to 3 days, occasionally longer. The symptoms of acute gastritis were described as an uncomfortable feeling in the abdomen, headache, depression, nausea, eructation, and vomiting, which usually gave relief. The abdomen was described as often somewhat distended and tender in the epigastric area. All three infections discussed in this chapter can have a clinical presentation that fits this description. Examination of the vomitus showed, as a rule, absence of hydrochloric acid, a feature of acute *H. pylori* and syphilitic gastritis. Osler's textbook referred to Beaumont's study of St. Martin, which ''showed in acute catarrh that the mucous membrane is

TABLE 2–1. FREQUENT CAUSES OF INFECTIVE GASTRITIS

BACTERIAL
Helicobacter sp, especially *H. pylori*
Treponema pallidum
Mouth bacteria (phlegmonous gastritis)
Mycobacterium tuberculosis
VIRAL
Cytomegalovirus
Herpes simplex
FUNGAL
Candida albicans
PARASITIC
Strongyloides stercoralis
Anisakis spp

reddened and swollen, less gastric juice is secreted, and mucus covers the surface. Slight hemorrhages or even small erosions may occur. The submucosa may be somewhat edematous. Microscopically, the changes are chiefly noticeable in the mucous and peptic cells, which are swollen and more granular, and in an infiltration of the intertubular tissues by leucocytes."[8] Even recently, similar descriptions have been written characterizing acute *H. pylori* gastritis.

Sugimachi and coworkers proposed a classification of acute gastritis based on the findings of upper gastrointestinal series and endoscopy.[9] They studied patients presenting to their outpatient departments with sudden onset of epigastric pain, nausea, and vomiting; over a 13-year period, 160 patients with acute findings, mainly in the antrum, were seen. The mean age of the patients was 38 years. These investigators classified the cases into 3 types: edematous (44%), hemorrhagic (34%), and ulcerous (22%). Nausea and anorexia were more frequent in the hemorrhagic and ulcerous types (80–90%) than in the edematous type. Vomiting was rare with the edematous type (3%), but frequent with the hemorrhagic (65%) and ulcerous (91%) types. The duration of symptoms was related to the endoscopic severity, averaging 5.9 days for the edematous type, 7.1 days for the hemorrhagic, and 10.5 days for the ulcerative type. The duration of symptoms of the ulcerative type was statistically longer than that of the edematous type. Histologic examination showed only mucosal edema in the edematous type, necrosis with neutrophils in the hemorrhagic type, and more severe necrosis in the ulcerative type. We suspect that the hemorrhagic and ulcerous types were part of the spectrum of the same disease and, in our opinion, most likely indicate acute *H. pylori* infection. Both the clinical presentations and the endoscopic findings are, however, compatible with the much less common syphilitic and CMV gastritis.

The temporal imprecision of the term acute gastritis is well illustrated by the three infections discussed in this chapter. Acute *H. pylori* gastritis occurs a few days after oral inoculation in a previously uninfected host. Acute syphilitic gastritis occurs in the secondary phase of syphilis, days to weeks after the primary cutaneous or mucous membrane inoculation. Acute CMV gastritis is most often the result of reactivation of a latent infection that may have been present for many years prior to the onset of gastric injury. All three of these infectious agents need to be considered when approaching a patient with acute upper intestinal symptoms and endoscopic abnormalities suggestive of active mucosal injury.

Chronic Gastritis

If the concept of acute gastritis was unclear because of the misuse of the terms acute and chronic in describing inflammatory infiltrates and chronology, the histologic definition of chronic gastritis is even further plagued by two additional problems. One is that the lamina propria of the normal stomach contains a generous population of mononuclear cells, the spectrum of which still awaits rigorous definition. Therefore, some pathologists call normal what others call chronic inflammation, and no immediately applicable way to regulate these subjective interpretations is apparent. The other problem is that some forms of gastric injury that histopathologically do not satisfy the criteria for inflammation have traditionally been called gastritis. One example is reactive (or chemical, or bile reflux) gastritis, which is characterized by hyperplasia of the foveolar cells and absence of an abnormal inflammatory infiltrate. Another example is gastric atrophy. Should this condition still be considered gastritis, even in the absence of inflammation, only because it is believed to be part of the spectrum of chronic gastritis? Because infectious chronic gastritis is essentially synonymous with *H. pylori* infection, we shall discuss further these and other issues pertinent to chronic gastritis under that heading. Chronic gummatous syphilis may cause confusion histologically, but clinically the suspicion is of malignancy and not gastritis. Gastric CMV infection can be protracted, and the patient can relapse, but symptoms, mucosal lesions, and histologic findings remain the same and could never be confused with those of the chronic gastritis produced by *H. pylori* infection.

SYPHILITIC GASTRITIS

Gastric syphilis is the infection of the stomach by *T. pallidum*. Involvement of the digestive tract in syphilis, which may occur during the secondary or the tertiary stage, is rarely detected because it responds promptly to penicillin treatment. Symptomatic gastritis is estimated to occur in less than 1% of the patients with secondary or tertiary syphilis.[10] Syphilitic gastritis is diagnosed when three criteria are met: Gastric mucosal lesions are present; serologic evidence of active syphilis or histologic demonstration of

T. pallidum in the stomach exists; and other causes of gastritis have been ruled out.

Epidemiology

The incidence of syphilis in the United States declined steadily from 1943 to 1977, when it started to increase, and it reached 103,437 reported cases in 1988.[11] The epidemic of the late 1980s and the '90s affects primarily black and Hispanic heterosexual men and women, largely in urban areas. The peak incidence occurs in those who are between the ages of 15 and 34 years.

Pathogenesis and Pathology

Syphilis is a chronic systemic infection that is usually transmitted by sexual contact. Following an incubation period averaging 3 weeks, a primary lesion appears at the portal of entry, usually the genital organs, and is often associated with regional lymphadenopathy. A secondary bacteremic stage is manifested by generalized mucocutaneous lesions and lymphadenopathy. This is followed by a latent period of subclinical infection that lasts many years. In approximately one third of untreated patients a tertiary stage eventually appears, characterized by various combinations of destructive mucocutaneous, musculoskeletal, or parenchymal lesions; cardiovascular involvement; and symptomatic central nervous system disease.[12] The basic pathogenetic mechanism of all stages of syphilis is the development of obliterative endarteritis, a process that starts with the invasion of perivascular lymphatics by spirochetes and is followed by perivascular infiltration by mononuclear cells, particularly plasma cells.[12] The obliteration of small arteries results in foci of ischemic necrosis, which, depending on their size, location, and the host's immune status, may cause a large ulcerating nodule (the primary chancre), small superficial erosions (the pustules of secondary syphilis), or large indolent liquefactive nodules walled by fibrous and inflammatory tissue (the gummata of tertiary syphilis).

The type of gastric lesions parallels the systemic behavior of the infection. In secondary syphilis, the disease is a disseminated one, with myriad ulcerating pustules on skin and mucosal surfaces. In the more indolent phase of tertiary syphilis, the lesions demonstrate a more proliferative appearance, with the slow development of discrete masses. Similarly, two types of lesions may occur in the stomach: the diffuse gastritis and its variants, typical of the secondary stage, and the widely infiltrating lesions or gastric masses that resemble carcinoma seen in patients with tertiary syphilis.

In acute syphilitic gastritis, the gross appearance of the stomach may be that of diffuse erosive gastritis, usually more severe in the antrum, or it may show multiple or single ulcers, occasionally with a serpiginous appearance.[10, 13, 14] In some cases, however, nonulcerated mucosal folds have been described.[15] Microscopically, in addition to mucosal erosion or ulceration, severe plasmacytic, mononuclear inflammation of the mucosa, described in milder cases as perivascular, may be seen.[16] Spirochetes are usually difficult to find but may be seen by using the silver impregnation stains of Levaditi or Dieterle[14] or by immunofluorescent microscopy.[17]

During the course of tertiary syphilis, gastric lesions clinically and radiographically similar to infiltrative gastric carcinoma have been identified.[18] The histopathologic diagnosis of these lesions is given as very severe chronic gastritis, fibrosis, and, occasionally, gummata. Because treponemes are not usually detectable in tertiary lesions, the causal association with syphilis is suggested only by response to several weeks of penicillin therapy.

Clinical Manifestations

Most patients with endoscopic evidence of gastric involvement during secondary syphilis are asymptomatic.[10] Patients with symptomatic syphilitic gastritis often have concurrent or recent cutaneous evidence of secondary syphilis. The typical patient presents with several weeks of epigastric pain and vomiting. The pain is exacerbated by eating and awakens the patient at night; marked weight loss is common. Gastric secretion is usually reduced and hypo- or achlorhydria is common.[19, 20]

The clinical presentation of patients with infiltrative or fungating gummatous lesions of tertiary syphilis is indistinguishable from that of patients with gastric malignancies. These syphilitic patients present with a history of epigastric discomfort that becomes progressively worse over a period of several years.[18, 20]

Diagnosis and Treatment

Syphilitic gastritis should be suspected in patients with secondary syphilis and concomitant upper gastrointestinal symptoms. Because treatment with penicillin for syphilis promptly relieves the symptoms of syphilitic gastritis, further investigation of the gastrointestinal complaints is warranted only if a rapid improvement does not occur. In patients with no clinical evidence of syphilis but an endoscopic appearance suggestive of acute erosive gastritis, the possibility of syphilis should be investigated by serology. Endoscopic biopsy to confirm suspected gastric syphilis requires consultation with the pathologist because certain tests, for example, immunofluorescence, need to be performed on unfixed frozen sections, whereas others, such as darkfield examinations, require fresh tissue. If syphilis is suspected only after a biopsy has already been performed, the pathologist should be informed of this possibility because without special silver stains and a painstaking search for *T. pallidum*, the biopsy may be interpreted as chronic gastritis or even as plasmacytic lymphoma.

Gastric involvement of the stomach in tertiary syphilis is difficult to diagnose, and many reported cases were suspected to be syphilis only after a stomach resected for infiltrating carcinoma revealed not carcinoma but chronic inflammation and fibrosis. Patients with a so-called leather-bottle radiographic appearance of the stomach should be tested for syphilis. If serology is positive for syphilis and biopsies fail to reveal malignant tumor, an 8-week course of penicillin may be indicated.

HELICOBACTER PYLORI GASTRITIS

Helicobacter pylori is a gram-negative, spiral bacterium that was not cultured until the mid-1980s.[21] Infection by *H. pylori* is predominantly antral but can be found anywhere gastric epithelium is present. It has a distinctive spiral shape that is easily identified in histologic specimens. Infection with this organism is now accepted as the most common cause of gastritis in humans. *Helicobacter pylori* gastritis is defined as the presence of the typical inflammatory changes in the gastric epithelium, combined with histologic or culture evidence of infection with this organism.

Epidemiology

The epidemiology of *H. pylori* is the epidemiology of gastritis, and previous demographic and disease associations with gastritis have now been documented to apply to *H. pylori*.[22] These include associations with age, low socioeconomic status, gastric ulcer, duodenal ulcer, and gastric cancer. Therefore, we discuss the epidemiology of *H. pylori* in conjuction with data concerning its link to ulcers and cancer.

In Western and westernizing societies, the prevalence of peptic ulcer and gastric cancer has changed. Duodenal ulcer disease appeared in the last century as a new disease, and its incidence has gradually diminished. Gastric cancer has also become steadily less common. These changes suggest that the epidemiology of *H. pylori*, or one or more important unknown cofactors, has also changed. Analysis of the mortality data for peptic ulcer available from a number of countries shows that the risk of mortality for peptic ulcer was highest for those born in the latter part of the 1800s. The higher risk was carried by this group throughout their lives, and the risk decreased steadily for each subsequent birth cohort.[23–25] We have elsewhere drawn attention to the analogy between the appearance of peptic ulcer disease and the appearance of paralytic poliomyelitis.[22, 26, 27] Infection with polio virus was almost universal in childhood but did not result in a recognizable disease. Improvements in sanitation and standards of living resulted in failure to become infected during infancy. Development of a polio infection as an older child or as an adult resulted in the appearance of a new disease, paralytic poliomyelitis. Duodenal ulcer disease was first recognized about the same time as paralytic poliomyelitis, and the groups most likely to be affected were the upper classes. We hypothesized that the age of the patient at the time of acquisition of the infection was a major factor in determining the *H. pylori* disease associations observed, and this hypothesis has been supported by further studies.

In developing countries, *H. pylori* infection is almost universal at an early age, and atrophic gastritis is common in young adults.[22] According to our age-at-acquisition hypothesis, *H. pylori* infection in early childhood usually results in atrophic gastritis and gastric atrophy, limiting the stomach's ability to make acid and preventing duodenal ulcer disease from appearing. Data from Peru have been consistent with this hypothesis, showing that in an area where childhood *H. pylori* infection was virtually universal, gastric ulcer and gastric cancer were common, but duodenal ulcer was rare.[28] This hypothesis is also consistent with the previous observations concerning the epidemiology of gastric cancer in Japanese who emmigrated from Japan to Hawaii.[29] Immigrants retained the high risk that they had acquired in childhood, but their children born in Hawaii, a low-risk environment, experienced a marked reduction in the risk of developing gastric carcinoma. It would appear unlikely that *H. pylori* alone is responsible for gastric cancer but rather that it provides the proper environment, for example, chronic gastritis and intestinal metaplasia. Numerous studies have shown that the risk of cancer can be further modified by factors that are unlikely to affect *H. pylori*, such as the ingestion of fruits and vegetables containing the antioxidant vitamin C.[30, 31] Important studies have shown that *H. pylori* infection may limit the transport of vitamin C into the gastric juice.[32] The role of this mechanism in limiting the protective effect of vitamin C is unknown.

Many investigators subscribe to the hypothesis that atrophic gastritis, in combination with as yet unidentified cofactors (candidates include nitrates and salt), is responsible for the observed frequency of gastric cancer in a population.[33, 34] These data are consistent worldwide. A strong association exists between *H. pylori* prevalence in a population and the intestinal type of gastric carcinoma.[22, 35–48] More importantly, gastric carcinoma is rare in populations in which *H. pylori* is infrequent.

The progression from atrophic gastritis to gastric cancer takes several decades, and any increase in the average age of acquisition of the infection decreases the incidence of gastric carcinoma in that population. Such postponement of onset allows the infected individuals to reach their natural life span before sufficient time has elapsed for gastric cancer to develop. As would be expected from this hypothesis, gastric cancer in the United States is most prevalent in populations with low socioeconomic status (i.e., high *H. pylori* prevalence at an early age), such as blacks and Hispanics.[35, 42, 43, 49–51]

A number of excellent indirect studies showing consistency between the frequency of *H. pylori* and the prevalence of gastric carcinoma in various populations have been published.[34–45] More recently, the results of three case-control studies have appeared confirming and extending the indirect associations between *H. pylori* and gastric cancer.[46–48] Overall, the relative risk attributable to *H. pylori* was relatively low, but this is probably a reflection of an age-at-acquisition bias within the study populations. Studies from Finland have shown that a very high relative risk for gastric cancer is related to gastric morphology, with the highest risk being experienced by those with severe pangastritis,[38] which is considered the end result of long-standing gastritis[52] and probably serves to negate any age-of-acquisition bias present in recent prospective studies.[46–48] Although these case-control studies show the expected significant association between gastric cancer and *H. pylori* infection, the role of *H. pylori* in the etiology of gastric cancer remains unclear.

Pathogenesis of *H. pylori* Gastritis

The steps and mediators in *H. pylori* infection and inflammation are unknown. The proportion of *H. pylori* ingestions that result in initial colonization is not known, nor is the proportion of early infections eradicated by the host known. The difficulty in transmitting infection to 2 subjects who ingested bacterial cultures[53, 54] suggests that infection follows ingestion, infrequently, or that the host can eradicate the bacteria (as occurred in Dr. Marshall's ingestion),[53] or that in vitro cultured strains lack important virulence factors.

The initial steps are probably ingestion, followed by penetration of the mucous layer, "swimming" through the mucous layer to the mucosa, leading to attachment, and multiplication (Table 2–2). The first reaction of the host is neutrophilic. This is an important phase of the infection and one in which the bacterium and any bacterial toxins are unfettered by a local secretory immunoglobulin A (S-IgA) response. The mediators of the neutrophilic reaction at this stage are unknown, but local or systemic antibody is unlikely to be involved because the reaction precedes their appearance. One feature that may be especially common during the acute phase is for *H. pylori* to invade between mucocytes.[55]

Polymorphonuclear neutrophil (PMN) cells are evident wherever *H. pylori* is present. Bacterial products such as endotoxin, peptidoglycans, and formylpeptides have been found in damaged tissue along with host products such as activated complement components. This process results in a vigorous local and systemic immune response. Little is known about the proportion of *H. pylori* infections that start as a

TABLE 2–2. POSTULATED STEPS IN *HELICOBACTER PYLORI* INFECTION

Ingestion of *H. pylori*
Movement into and through mucus layer
Attachment to mucosa
Bacterial multiplication
Invasion, tissue damage
Internalization
Active eradication attempt by host
   Neutrophilic response
   Chronic inflammatory cell response
   Humoral immune response
Control of infection and down regulation of immune
   response to the pattern of chronic disease

vigorous acute neutrophilic reaction or the proportion that starts slowly and insidiously. We have seen patients in whom the initial infection was a severe symptomatic infection with achlorhydria and the second infection, a year or more after eradication of the initial infection, was subclinical. It is likely that the local and systemic immune response to infection plays a significant role in the later stages of the infection. We have also followed a second individual without treatment and observed the transformation of the disease from an acute neutrophilic achlorhydria syndrome with innumerable *H. pylori* to a mild gastritis with few *H. pylori*.[56] Other data (David Y. Graham, unpublished data, 1992) confirm these observations. This is not unexpected; the host's response to infection is to attempt to eradicate it, and, failing that (e.g., the pathogen is successful), to contain it as much as possible.

The second phase of the infection includes continuation of acute inflammation but also infiltration with chronic inflammatory cells. Later, the acute inflammatory response seems to fade but never to resolve completely. The role of the local and systemic immune response both in controlling the infection and in neutralizing any *H. pylori* toxins has aroused considerable interest. Little or no information exists concerning the critical factors responsible for either the neutrophilic or the mononuclear inflammatory response. Among the factors that deserve study are the relationship between the histologic findings and bacterial density. Examination of histologic sections from patients infected with *H. pylori* suggests that bacterial density may be a determining factor and may be directly correlated with the intensity of the acute immune response.[57, 58]

Different *H. pylori* diseases may be related to the ability of the body to control either the number of *H. pylori* organisms present or their products. One can imagine that the events leading to control could reside with the host, with the organism, or with both. For example, we hypothesized that *H. pylori* gastritis may be localized to the antrum of patients with duodenal ulcer (antral predominant gastritis) because the preexisting high rate of acid secretion prevents effective colonization of the gastric body.[59] In other instances, differences in the virulence of the *H. pylori* strain may be responsible for the differences in ability to evade the host's immune response, leading to varying severity of inflammation.

Data suggest that differences in strain among *H. pylori* organisms may relate to the degree of inflammation and, indirectly, to poor control of the infection by the immune system.[60] Genetic studies using DNA and DNA hybridization techniques in solution had previously shown that *H. pylori* organisms obtained from subjects with asymptomatic gastritis were in a hybridization group different from that of strains obtained from patients with duodenal ulcer.[61] *Helicobacter pylori* infection is associated with a brisk humoral immune response, both locally and systemically. Antibodies are directed against a large number of *H. pylori* proteins, which is consistent with *H. pylori* being invasive and accessible to the immune system. One approach to the identification of specific strains or markers for virulence is to examine the target of IgA produced by antral mucosal biopsies and gastric mononuclear cell cultures.[60] A number of different proteins were recognized by Immunoblot. Such data should be interpreted with the caveat that the number and variety of antigens identified is dependent on the procedure used to separate antigens and identify antigen-antibody reactions. The resulting conclusions from such an experiment may greatly underestimate the number and variety of antigens actually recognized by the immune system. Nevertheless, the study just described provided the first clear indication of an association between a protein, or class of proteins, and the severity of the gastritis. One *H. pylori* protein, molecular weight 120,000 (120K), was associated with fairly severe gastritis, that is, PMN infiltration and epithelial surface degeneration, and with peptic ulcer disease. This finding suggests that differences in strain exist among *H. pylori* organisms and either that the 120K protein is involved in the process or that it is a marker for an *H. pylori* factor or *H. pylori*–host interaction that leads to relatively severe gastritis. The severe gastritis-associated mucosal immune response to the 120K protein is not carried over to the systemic immune response, in which a reaction to a 120K protein band (not necessarily the same protein, since a number of proteins may have the same or similar apparent molecular weight) does not predict the severity of the gastritis. Further studies are needed to clarify the role of these proteins and their association with various conditions.

Pathology of Acute *Helicobacter pylori* Gastritis

Although the endoscopic appearance of acute *H. pylori* gastritis may be very similar to that of syphilitic gastritis, the histologic features are quite different. Biopsy specimens obtained from areas seen endoscopically as erythematous

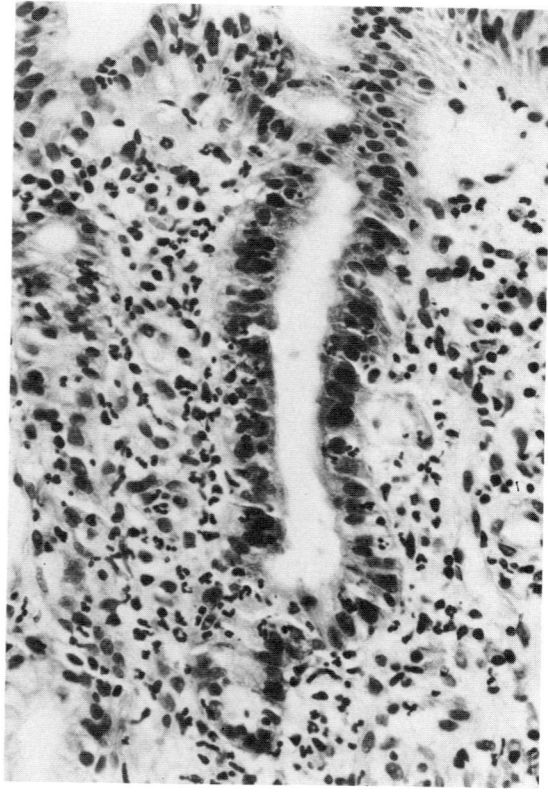

FIGURE 2–1.
Acute *H. pylori* infection: red patches, with prominent neutro-philic infiltrate of surface and glandular epithelium, a large num-ber of neutrophils in the lamina propria, and a nearly normal background of lymphocytes and plasma cells.

patches show preservation of the mucosal archi-tecture with extensive infiltration of both lam-ina propria and epithelial lining by numerous neutrophils. Lymphocytes and plasma cells, al-though present in larger numbers than in the normal gastric mucosa, appear as a background to the neutrophils without achieving particular prominence (Fig. 2–1). In these areas, small to moderate numbers of *H. pylori* may be visible, particularly on the surface of the foveolar epi-thelium. Specimens acquired from endoscopic white patches show aggregates of necrotic de-bris, fibrin, and neutrophils attached to eroded gastric epithelium, in some cases showing a dis-tinct resemblance to the erupting lesions seen in pseudomembranous colitis (Fig. 2–2). *H. py-lori* organisms are usually absent from these le-sions and from the immediately adjacent gastric mucosa.

The evolution of the untreated disease is

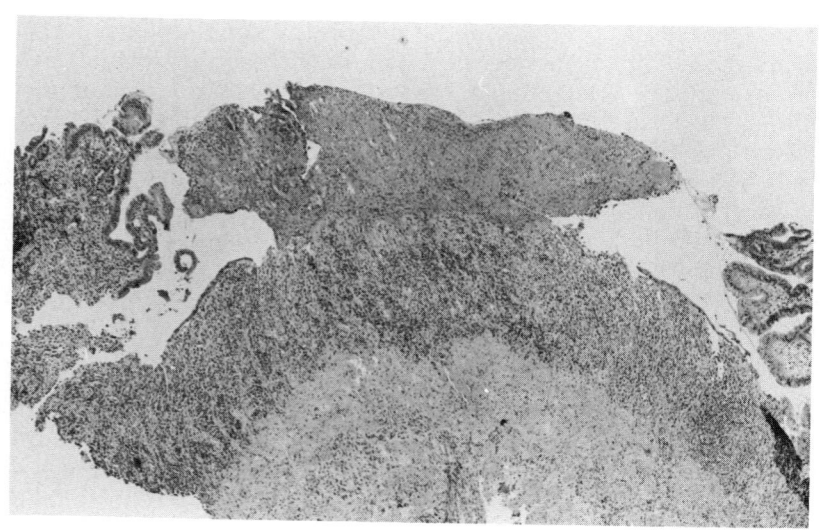

FIGURE 2–2.
A low-power photomicrograph of a white patch seen in acute *H. py-lori* infection. The gastric mucosa is virtually destroyed by a mixed in-filtrate of inflammatory cells. At-tached to the eroded mucosa may be seen a large aggregate of fibri-nopurulent material, reminiscent of the pseudomembranes seen in *C. difficile*–associated colitis.

known in only a few cases. The infiltrate becomes increasingly mononuclear, lymphoid aggregates develop, and larger numbers of *H. pylori* become visible as the histologic features merge with those of chronic gastritis.

Pathology of Chronic *Helicobacter pylori* Gastritis

The histopathology of chronic *H. pylori* infection includes the wide spectrum of histopathologic changes previously associated with chronic active gastritis. Because these changes usually vary considerably in antrum and corpus, we shall consider them separately.

The typical appearance of *H. pylori* chronic antral gastritis is depicted in Figure 2–3. The architecture of the mucosa is well preserved, with minor disarray of the pits caused by the lymphocytic and plasmacytic infiltrate occupying the lamina propria. Neutrophils, and usually a much smaller number of eosinophils, are mixed with the mononuclear infiltrate, but they are most prominent within the surface and foveolar epithelium, where they are seen individually or in tiny clusters. Small aggregates of neutrophils, usually without fibrin, can often be seen on the surface epithelium and within the pits and are termed pit abscesses. The antral mucous glands may be separated by the infiltrate in the lamina propria, but only by exception do they contain inflammatory cells within their epithelium and virtually never in the lumen. Organisms of *H. pylori* are located singly or in clusters along the surface and foveolar epithelium (Fig. 2–4A). They may appear to be entrapped within mucous strands, freely floating in the foveolar spaces, or adherent to the columnar cells. This apparent difference in location is probably due to the limitations of the bidimensional observation of a tridimensional structure rather than the actual distribution of the bacteria. Only rarely, however, perhaps once in 20 or 30 infected biopsy specimens examined, are isolated organisms seen in the lumen of mucous glands (Fig. 2–4B). This typical appearance can vary considerably, depending on the size and relative proportions of the different components of the inflammatory infiltrate. Intraepithelial neutrophils may be so rare that they are difficult to find, even when many organisms are present. Gross destruction of heavily infiltrated and dilated pits may be seen, and large numbers of PMN cells may be mixed with the background mononuclear infiltrate. Eosinophils may be prominent in some cases, for reasons that are not known.

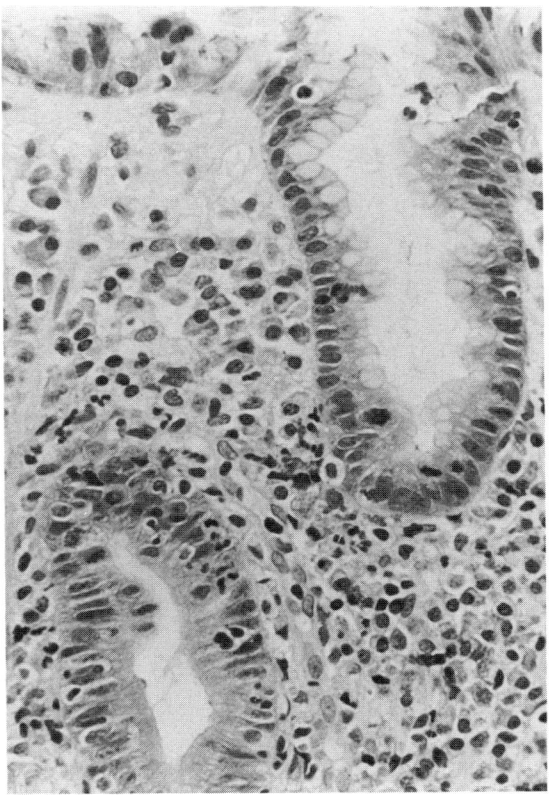

FIGURE 2–3.
This high-power photomicrograph of an antral biopsy specimen shows an increased number of plasma cells and lymphocytes in the lamina propria, a moderate number of polymorphonuclear cells that have infiltrated the foveolar and the surface epithelium, and aggregates of organisms within the pit on the right and on the mucosal surface.

The variation in the quantity of PMN cells may be pathogenetically important, but it is rarely a source of confusion in the interpretation of gastric biopsies, since the aphorism "if you see polys, look for *H. pylori*" is, or should be, well embedded in every pathologist's diagnostic algorithm. In contrast, the presence of an unusually dense mononuclear infiltrate, particularly if neutrophils are few and inconspicuous, may suggest an infiltrative, or even a proliferative, process, such as lymphoma. In such cases, as illustrated in Figure 2–5, compact aggregates of mononuclear cells expand the lamina propria and obfuscate the foveolar and glandular structures, giving the impression of atrophy. Furthermore, lymphocytes infiltrate into the epithelium and may damage its structures, in a manner considered typical of mucosa-associated lymphoid tissue lymphomas (MALTomas).[62] When closely observed, however, the lymphocytes have a mature benign appearance and, in their intraepithelial location, are surrounded by

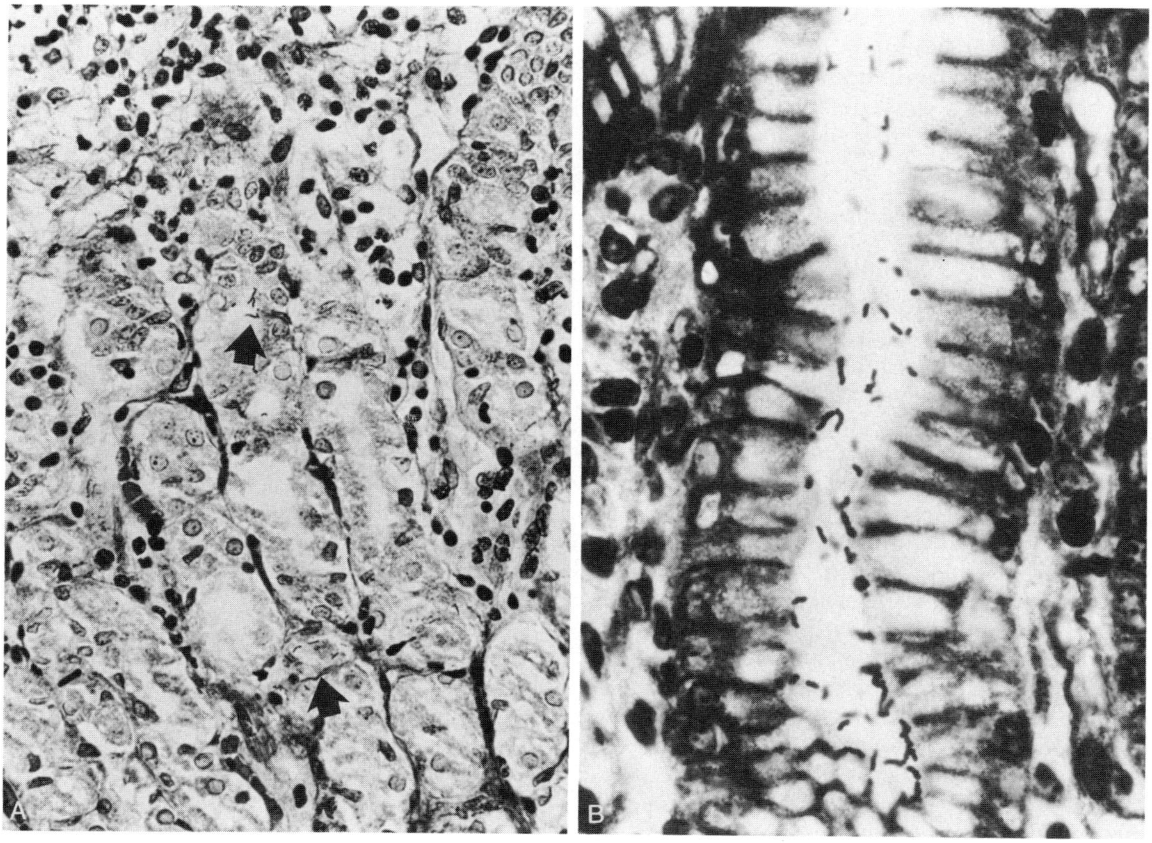

FIGURE 2–4.
A, The typical location of *H. pylori* is dramatized by this high-power photomicrograph of a Warthin-Starry silver stain. *B*, This medium-power photomicrograph shows *H. pylori* organisms *(arrows)* in an unusual location: deeply seated inside fundic glands.

a clear halo, considered to be the hallmark of benign inflammatory infiltrates.[62] In these cases, a careful search for *H. pylori* organisms is necessary because they tend to be rare. One must also bear in mind that finding *H. pylori* organisms does not exclude the possibility of a concurrent lymphoma; therefore, a close follow-up of suspect cases with extensive biopsy sampling after

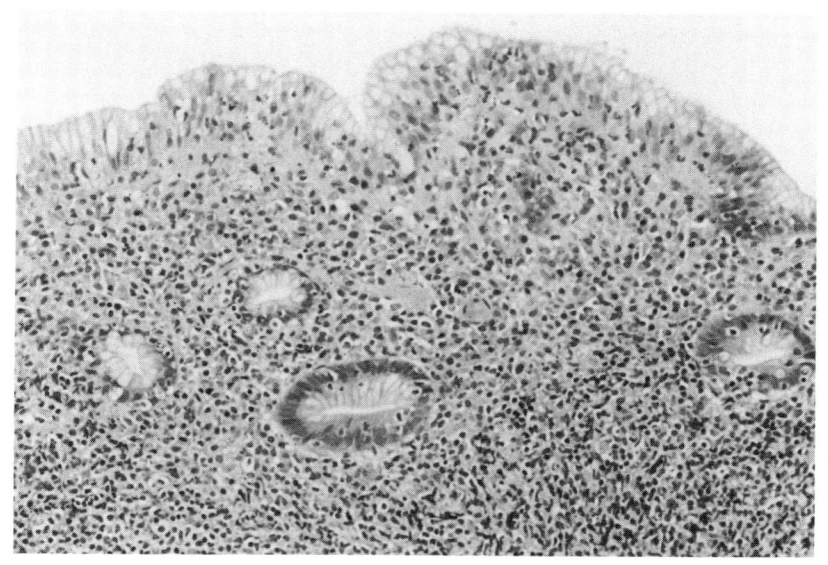

FIGURE 2–5.
The antral lamina propria of this patient with *H. pylori*–associated gastritis is virtually obliterated by a dense, predominantly lymphocytic infiltrate. After triple therapy, the mucosal architecture remained moderately distorted, but the inflammatory infiltrates resolved completely. A small number of *H. pylori* organisms were present but difficult to see.

attempting the eradication of the organisms is mandatory.

A less dramatic lymphocytic infiltrate may still be the most conspicuous response to *H. pylori* in some subjects. The resulting picture is what has been called lymphocytic gastritis, a recently described entity found to be associated with *H. pylori* infection in approximately half the cases.[63]

Irrespective of the relative prevalence of different inflammatory cell types, one feature that, in our experience, is present in virtually every *H. pylori*–infected antrum is the lymphoid aggregate with germinal center (LAGC) (Fig. 2–6). Long regarded as normal structures of the gastric mucosa (in the days when some degree of chronic gastritis was considered by many to be part of the normal aging process), LAGCs are being increasingly recognized as typical, if not pathognomonic, of *H. pylori* infection, both in adults[64] and in children.[65] By examining at least 5 biopsy specimens from more than 40 patients with documented *H. pylori* gastritis, we found LAGCs in all of them, whereas none of the specimens from the stomachs of 18 normal subjects that had negative serologic and histologic findings contained these structures.[66] We do not know yet whether LAGCs are the expression of a specific immune response to an organism, but studies are under way to address this issue.

The gastric corpus in *H. pylori*–infected stomachs may be entirely normal, with neither visible organisms nor inflammatory responses, even when the antrum shows evidence of severe infection. In adequately sampled cases, organisms are often detected on the surface epithelium and in the short foveolar spaces, but no inflammatory response seems to accompany the mucosal colonization. When inflammation is present, it often has the appearance of what was once known as superficial gastritis.[67] A bandlike infiltrate of mononuclear cells separates the slightly elongated pits from the subjacent oxyntic mucosa, and usually very small numbers of neutrophils populate the columnar epithelium (Fig. 2–7). Scattered eosinophils are frequently seen between the glandular spaces of the oxyntic mucosa, but bacteria are always absent from this location. Frequently LAGCs are found in the corporal mucosa, even in cases in which this area shows no other evidence of infection.

Usually, but not always, the overall inflammatory response is less intense in the corpus than in the antrum. Although uncommon, chronic active gastritis limited to the corpus may be seen. Surface epithelial damage that, in various degrees of intensity, almost invariably accompanies *H. pylori* infection occurs in both antrum and corpus. These cellular alterations, described in elegant detail by Chan and coworkers,[68] include flattening of the surface cells, formation of hyperplastic-looking cellular tufts, and other subtler changes. Such alterations are found even in areas not otherwise damaged by intraepithelial inflammatory cells, and they are believed to be a direct consequence of the presence of the adhering organisms.

Our understanding of the natural evolution of the histopathologic features of *H. pylori*–associated gastritis is limited by the dearth of prospective long-term cohort studies. Data obtained from cross-sectional studies in populations with high prevalence of *H. pylori* infection suggest that in a considerable percentage of patients the inflammation may eventually become exclusively mononuclear and may slowly vanish over a period of years, while at the same time the gastric glands decrease in number and the surface and foveolar epithelium undergo intestinal metaplasia. The sequence of these changes describes the hypothetical pathway from *H. pylori*–associated chronic active gastritis to atrophic

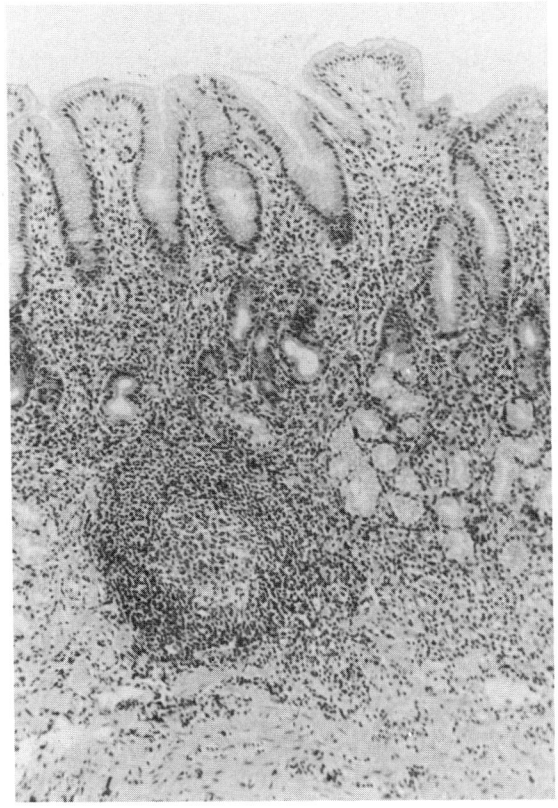

FIGURE 2–6.
A lymphoid aggregate with a germinal center located deep in the lamina propria of the antral mucosa. Such structures are strongly associated with *H. pylori* infection and persist for years after the successful eradication of the organisms.

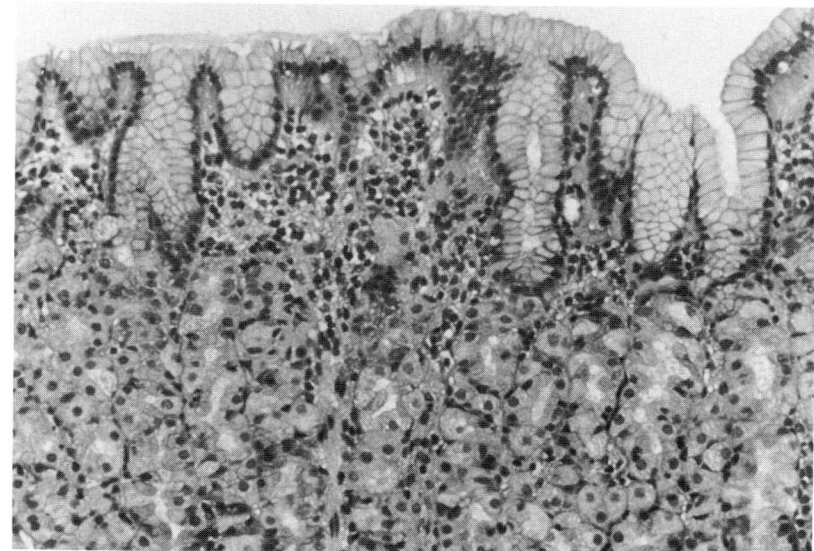

FIGURE 2–7.
Superficial gastritis in the fundic mucosa. Note the thin rim of mostly mononuclear cells that expand the subepithelial space. *H. pylori* with this histologic appearance may often be seen in the gastric corpus without any appreciable neutrophilic inflammation.

gastritis and eventually to gastric metaplasia and atrophy.

Successful eradication of *H. pylori* results in the rapid disappearance of neutrophils from the gastric mucosa, which can be seen as early as 2 or 3 days after the beginning of triple therapy.[69] Again, long-term studies of treated patients are rare. We have studied 15 subjects with histologically documented *H. pylori* infection for periods of 2 to 3 years after therapy by repeated endoscopies and extensive biopsy sampling. The rapid disappearance of neutrophils was accompanied in most subjects by an initial increase in eosinophils, but the degree of mononuclear inflammation decreased at a much slower pace, in some cases taking more than 1 year to return to normal. Lymphoid follicles with germinal centers did not completely disappear in any of the subjects within the time of the study.

Clinical Manifestations

Acute *Helicobacter pylori* Gastritis

The clinical presentation of acute gastritis due to *H. pylori* is similar to Osler's description quoted earlier. The proportion of patients that present with a recognizable symptomatic illness is unknown. At least 60% of iatrogenic *H. pylori* gastritis has been reported as symptomatic. Symptoms usually last 1 to 3 days, but we have seen patients with *H. pylori* presenting with symptoms lasting for several weeks, associated with marked weight loss. Hypochlorhydria or achlorhydria is common. Endoscopic abnormalities are seen mainly in the antrum and include erythema, subepithelial hemorrhage, and raised white plaques. The acute changes usually resolve spontaneously, and acid secretion returns to normal.

Chronic *Helicobacter pylori* Gastritis

An *H. pylori* infection and resultant chronic gastritis are almost universal in individuals living in or emigrating from developing countries and in those with duodenal or gastric ulcer disease. Unless complicated by ulcer disease, the gastric infection is asymptomatic. Most studies trying to link chronic *H. pylori* gastritis to the non-ulcer dyspepsia syndrome have failed to prove an association between the symptoms and the infection.[70–74]

Diagnosis

We now have an all but bewildering number of ways to diagnose *H. pylori* infection (Table 2–3).[75] Tests can be divided into invasive (requiring endoscopy or gastric intubation) and noninvasive types.

Serology

Because untreated *H. pylori* infection is essentially lifelong and because it is associated with a brisk systemic immune response, the presence of serum immunoglobulin G (IgG) antibody against *H. pylori* antigens provides a reliable method of detecting the presence of an infection. A number of serologic tests are now available commercially. The first-generation assays were based on total *H. pylori* surface antigens,

TABLE 2–3. TESTS IN USE TO DETECT
HELICOBACTER PYLORI INFECTION

NONINVASIVE (INDIRECT)
Urea breath tests
Antibody detection (serum, saliva, urine)
INVASIVE
Direct microscopy
Rapid urease tests (biopsy, brush)
Histology (special strains, immunohistochemical)
Culture
Endoscopic spray dye tests (phenol red and urea)
Gastric ammonium: urea ratio
Nucleic acid tests (polymerase chain reaction, restriction
    endonuclease profile)
Endoscopic spray techniques (phenol red, Congo red, red
    cabbage)

but the newer second-generation assays use specific purified antigens for greater sensitivity and specificity. Serologic tests are particularly useful for determining an existing infection or a previous exposure to *H. pylori*. A progressive decline in antibody titers can also be used to confirm eradication of an *H. pylori* infection.

Urea Breath Test

The fact that *H. pylori* organisms have an extremely high urease activity has allowed the development of urea breath tests based on either the radioactive carbon isotope ^{14}C or the stable ^{13}C. The principle of the urea breath test is that, in the presence of the enzyme urease, orally administered urea is hydrolyzed to CO_2 and ammonia. If the urea carbon is labeled with either ^{13}C or ^{14}C it can be detected in the breath as labeled CO_2. The *H. pylori* organism is the most common urease-containing gastric pathogen, and therefore a positive urea breath test can generally be equated with the presence of an *H. pylori* infection.[58, 76] The urea breath test has proved reliable, and almost any variant of the original test attains a specificity and sensitivity of more than 80%.[77]

Biopsy Urease Test

The simplest technique at endoscopy is a rapid biopsy urease test. Because of the patchy nature of the infection, 2 antral biopsy specimens should be taken: one near the pylorus and the other on the lesser curvature on the pyloric side of the angulus incisura. Biopsy specimens are placed into the test medium. The ingredients of biopsy urease test media are similar in the different tests: urea, a pH indicator, a buffer, and a bacteriostatic agent. The latter is added to make certain that only preformed enzyme is detected and to suppress extraneous urease-containing organisms that, if present, may contaminate and spoil the medium before use or, upon incubation, produce a false-positive result. The nature of the test media is relatively unimportant; results are best when one obtains large tissue specimens and places them into small volumes of indicator media. The sensitivity of rapid urease tests is between 70 and 90%, and the specificity exceeds 90%. The relatively expensive CLO (*Campylobacter*-like organism) test (Delta West Pty Ltd, Western Australia) is available commercially. Inexpensive biopsy urease tests can be easily made by any hospital laboratory. We suggest the recipe of Hazell and coworkers; each test costs a few pennies.[78] A biopsy specimen is added directly to 50 μl of test solution in a 0.5 dram vial. The solution contains 2 g of urea, 10 ml of 0.5% (w/v) phenol red, and 20 mg of sodium azide in 100 ml of 0.01 M sodium phosphate buffer, pH 6.5. The test is positive for *H. pylori* if the medium changes from orange to a definite pink.

Microscopic Examination of Biopsy Material

If, at the time of endoscopy, it is important to confirm whether *H. pylori* infection is present, one should use techniques that result in a permanent record and provide objective data concerning the presence of the bacteria and the status of the gastric mucosa. The simplest approach is histologic examination of mucosal biopsy specimens. Best results are obtained when at least two large biopsies, as outlined earlier, are obtained from the antrum. Formalin fixation is satisfactory.

A number of factors must be considered for optimal specimen evaluation.[75] Since *H. pylori* predominantly inhabits the mucous layer overlying the stomach and the area within the gastric pits, biopsies should be handled in such a manner as to minimize tissue distortion and to dislodge as little mucus as possible. Thus, methods that involve placing the fresh biopsy material on a supporting structure such as a piece of filter paper should be avoided. Although many of the biopsy specimen tend to curl owing to contraction of the smooth muscle of the muscularis mucosae, optimal orientation of the tissue at the time of paraffin embedding is easily achieved by a trained technician.

Various methods for identification of bacteria in tissue sections have been suggested, including the modified Giemsa, the Gimenez stain, and a number of Gram stains, including Brown-Brenn, Brown-Hopps, and half-Gram. Each of these varies in difficulty, cost, ease of interpretation, and differential staining of the tissue.

The choice of staining method should be based on the information sought. In a routine clinical setting, where one simply wishes to determine the presence of *H. pylori*, the H&E stain is often adequate, and one can usually find the organism on randomly oriented sections. The most important asset is an interested and cooperative pathologist.

Culture

Culture of *H. pylori* is generally unnecessary, and most hospital laboratories have a relatively low yield of positive cultures, even in patients known to be infected. Culture can easily add several hundred dollars to the cost of the procedure. If antibiotic sensitivity testing becomes useful to guide therapy, culture may become important; it is not so now. With present knowledge and therapies, culture is not recommended, except in the research setting. If the specimens are kept at 4°C, processing of tissue specimens for culture can be safely delayed more than 4 hours without an appreciable decrease in growth. A transport medium is recommended, especially if the microbiology laboratory is some distance from the endoscopy unit and a delay in transportation or processing is expected. Possible transport media include cystine-Brucella broth, normal saline, and glucose. In our experience, cysteine Brucella broth with 20% glycerol is a good choice because it is an excellent transport medium, and biopsy specimens can also be frozen in it (at −70°C), without loss of *H. pylori* viability, for more than a year. The organisms of *H. pylori* are closely associated with the gastric mucosa, and culture from tissue biopsies has a yield superior to that from gastric aspirates or brushings.

Since noninvasive tests are now available and allow one to readily diagnose the presence of *H. pylori*, patients need not undergo invasive procedures to obtain tissue simply for *H. pylori* detection.

Treatment

Most cases of acute *H. pylori* gastritis are self-limited. Chronic *H. pylori* gastritis is typically asymptomatic, and no therapy is needed. It has become evident that peptic ulcers can be cured by eradication of *H. pylori* infection,[79–84] and evidence suggests that eradication of *H. pylori* also prevents recurrence of ulcer complications in those who have previously experienced them.[85] Numerous trials have tested the susceptibility of *H. pylori* to various antimicrobial and antiulcer drugs.[86] It has become evident that *H. pylori* is susceptible to many drugs and is relatively easy to suppress, but it is extraordinarily difficult to eradicate.[86, 87] Initially, investigators did not fully realize that the gastric environment was a very hostile one for antimicrobial agents and that excellent results with in vitro antimicrobial sensitivity tests would not predict in vivo effectiveness. Among the reasons for this discrepancy are diminished antimicrobial activity on exposure to the acid conditions of the stomach, rapid development of acquired resistance, patient noncompliance, and the fact that adherent orgnisms have a susceptibility different from those that are not attached.[87, 88] Eradication rates reported with most antimicrobial monotherapies have been very low, leading to the development of triple therapies.[86] Triple-drug regimens have been relatively effective in eradicating *H. pylori*, and eradication rates above 90% have been achieved with combinations of bismuth salts plus two antimicrobial agents.[86, 89] Our current triple therapy is a 2-week course of tetracycline (500 mg) with meals and at bedtime, metronidazole (250 mg) with meals, and bismuth subsalicylate tablets, 2 with meals and at bedtime.[89] Metronidazole, or the similar tinidazole, is the most effective antimicrobial, other than bismuth, and the combination of bismuth and metronidazole forms the cornerstone of current successful therapies. Unfortunately, resistance to metronidazole develops rapidly, and populations in which metronidazole use is widespread have a high proportion of metronidazole-resistant *H. pylori*.[90] Eradication of *H. pylori* infection is defined as absence of infection 4 or more weeks after ending therapy. Table 2–4 shows methods for confirming eradication.

CYTOMEGALOVIRUS GASTRITIS

The criteria for a diagnosis of gastric CMV infection are an erosive or ulcerative process, usually occurring in the presence of immune deficiency; a mucosal biopsy that demonstrates CMV by the presence of cytomegalic cells, CMV antigen, or DNA, or by culture; and the exclusion of other explanations for the mucosal damage. This simple guideline is useful for diagnosis and clinical decision making, but CMV infection occurs in a variety of different settings and has a complicated and controversial pathogenesis.

Epidemiology and Pathology

Evidence of CMV infection is found in 40 to 100% of individuals in various populations. The

TABLE 2–4. BÖRSCH AND GRAHAM'S CRITERIA FOR ERADICATION OF *HELICOBACTER PYLORI*

Laboratory: Not to be done until 4 or more weeks after ending therapy.

INVASIVE

Failure to culture *H. pylori* from at least 2 gastric mucosal biopsies, at least taken from the antrum

Failure to visualize *H. pylori* on gastric mucosal biopsy specimens (at least antral) using sensitive special stains or, preferably, specific immunohistochemical techniques

Continued improvement in the histology of the gastric mucosa with a return to or toward normal and absence of polymorphonuclear infiltration

NONINVASIVE

Continued fall in titer of specific anti-*H. pylori* antibodies

Continued negative findings on urea breath tests

CLINICAL

Absence of duodenal or gastric ulcer recurrence

Risk of developing a duodenal or gastric ulcer less than that of a control population (for those who have not had duodenal or gastric ulcer)

SOURCE: Adapted from: Börsch GMA, Graham DY. *Helicobacter pylori.* In: Benjamin SB, Cullen MJ, eds. Handbook of Experimental Pharmacology: Pharmacology of Peptic Ulcer Disease. Berlin: Springer-Verlag; 1991;99:107–148.

prevalence correlates directly with socioeconomic status and sexual habits.[91] Most CMV infections are acquired during the perinatal period and infancy or through sexual contacts as an adult. Acute infections are frequently asymptomatic, but once the infection is acquired, the pattern is one of lifelong latency with the possibility of intermittent reactivation. The predominant site of viral latency is not known,[92–94] but lymphocytes, monocytes, and PMNs probably harbor latent virus.[93] Latency has been hypothesized to occur in endothelial cells of organs that may be at risk for injury during future reactivation,[94, 95] suggesting that CMV gastritis may occasionally be due to reactivation of locally latent virus.[96]

Reactivation of virus and the production of symptomatic disease are most commonly seen in patients with altered immunity due to immunosuppressive drugs, as in organ transplantation, or in patients with AIDS.[91, 92, 97] Reactivation is associated with adequate CMV antibody but defective cell-mediated immunity, specifically, reduced numbers of cytotoxic T lymphocytes and natural killer cells.[92, 98, 99] Cytomegalovirus disease in an immunodeficient host is associated with one of three possible situations: primary CMV infection in a previously seronegative host, reactivation of latent virus, or reinfection with a new strain of CMV.[100] In transplant patients, all three mechanisms have been documented to lead to CMV disease, and the frequency and severity of CMV disease (particularly studied in reference to pulmonary disease)

is related to the source of CMV. Reactivation is the most common source of infection, but new infection is symptomatic more often than is reactivation.[92] In renal transplant patients who developed CMV pneumonitis, the offending CMV was shown by restriction enzyme analysis of viral DNA to be a new CMV strain rather than the reactivation of a preexisting strain.[100] No comparable data regarding the influence of the source of CMV on gastrointestinal cytomegalovirus infection exist in the setting of transplantation.

Whether CMV in AIDS patients is more commonly due to reactivation or to reinfection is unknown; prior infection is virtually universal.[100] Although reinfection with new virus subtypes has been documented in AIDS patients, no data exist regarding the importance of reinfection with CMV in the production of any CMV syndrome in AIDS patients.[100] Although it is intriguing to postulate that the frequency of esophagogastric or rectal CMV disease in AIDS patients is due to homosexual practices of swallowing CMV-laden semen or engaging in receptive anal intercourse, CMV infections of the esophagus and colon are common in transplant patients without such high risk of direct gastrointestinal inoculation of CMV. The high frequency of CMV retinitis in AIDS patients also tends to diminish the importance of direct inoculation of new virus subtypes in the pathogenesis of CMV disease in AIDS. In both AIDS and organ transplantation, the frequency and severity of gastrointestinal CMV disease parallels closely the degree of cellular immune dysfunction, suggesting that the source or subtype of CMV is not so crucial as is specific anti-CMV cellular immune function.

The organ system involved with reactivation disease varies according to the clinical setting; pneumonitis is more common in bone marrow transplant patients, but retinitis and gastrointestinal disease are more common in AIDS patients.[91, 92, 94, 97, 100] The spectrums of gastrointestinal lesions are the same, despite the reasons for reactivation.[97, 101] The factors that make the intestine vulnerable to CMV injury are unknown. In at-risk clinical settings, CMV organisms are frequently found in salivary glands and saliva as well as in the kidney and urine. Significant disease in these organs due to CMV occurs rarely if at all,[100] suggesting that there must be local factors in the intestine that predispose to CMV-mediated injury compared with other tissues. The same could be hypothesized about other target organs such as retina, liver, and lungs.

Macroscopically at endoscopy, surgery, or autopsy, mucosal hemorrhage, erosion, and ulceration are the dominant findings in gastrointestinal CMV disease. Histologic identification of the cytomegalic cell provides unequivocal evidence of tissue infection.[102–104] Numerous gastrointestinal cell types have been found to be infected in active disease, most commonly vascular endothelial cells,[102, 104–107] but also fibroblasts, smooth muscle cells, and glandular epithelium.[101, 104–106, 108] Many more cells are apparently infected than those that appear cytomegalic.[104, 106, 107, 109]

The pathogenesis of intestinal lesions has recently been reviewed.[100] It is a complex process involving direct mucosal CMV infection, with inflammation and tissue necrosis,[98] and vascular endothelial involvement, with subsequent ischemic mucosal injury.[101, 105, 107, 108, 110–112] Surface epithelial cells are frequently infected at the edge of the ulcerations and in nearby uninflamed mucosa,[105–109, 113, 114] suggesting that vaculitis may be either a marker of severe infection or an important cause of injury but not necessarily the only or the predominant cause. Local immune suppression or autoimmune factors may also play a role in the pathogenesis of gastrointestinal CMV disease,[93, 100] but they do not appear to be so central to the pathogenesis as they are to bone marrow transplant CMV-induced pneumonia.[100]

A widely held but controversial opinion asserts that CMV in the gastrointestinal tract is frequently a nonpathogenic bystander or a secondary invader.[115–118] Cytomegalovirus is said to be found with increased frequency in areas of inflammation, not because it is causing the inflammation, but because it is present in inflammatory cells and has a propensity to infect rapidly growing tissues, especially endothelial cells in granulation tissue.[97, 104, 116, 119–121] In an individual clinical situation, the significance of finding cytomegalic cells is frequently difficult to determine, as, for example, cytomegalic cells in an area of inflammation that also contains *H. pylori* or in a gastric ulcer in a patient receiving corticosteroids. Several lines of evidence suggest, however, that CMV causes gastrointestinal disease: CMV is often found in the absence of other pathogens; severity of disease is related to the number of CMV infected cells; antiviral therapy ameliorates the lesion and alleviates the symptoms; and in situations of sustained immune dysfunction such as AIDS, virologic, histologic, and clinical relapse often follow discontinuation of anti-CMV chemotherapy.

Why do some patients at risk for gastrointestinal CMV infection get it and others with the same apparent risks do not? The answer is not known, but the risk of acquiring gastrointestinal CMV disease is probably related to factors such as quantity of latent virus, location of latent virus, subtype of latent virus, populations of specific T-cell subsets, reinfection, route of infection, cytotoxic drug administration, and concomitant disease.

Clinical Setting

Acquired Immunodeficiency Syndrome

Most patients with AIDS are also infected with CMV.[122–124] Both asymptomatic infection with CMV[122, 125] and gastrointestinal disease caused by CMV are common.[102, 106, 122, 123, 126–129] Important interactions between human immunodeficiency virus (HIV) and CMV have recently been reviewed.[130] Most AIDS patients eventually develop active CMV infection[123]; the frequency increases when cluster designation 4 (CD4) counts are below 100/mm³. Cytomegalovirus is the most frequently found serious infection in many postmortem series.[102, 128] The organs most frequently involved are the lungs, adrenals, and gastrointestinal tract. All parts of the intestine can be affected, either alone or in combination.[106, 122, 128] Experience suggests the following descending order of frequency: colon, esophagus, stomach, small bowel. Cytomegalovirus is the most common cause for emergency or elective abdominal surgery in AIDS patients.[127] Gastric involvement in AIDS is seldom reported, but it is a definite clinical entity.[104, 106, 131–138]

Organ and Bone Marrow Transplant Recipients

The majority, 60 to 70%, of kidney, liver, bone marrow, and heart transplant recipients acquire CMV infection in the first 6 months after transplantation, making it the most common infectious complication of the procedure.[92, 139, 140] At least half are symptomatic. The factors that predispose to CMV infection are positive serology in recipient or donor, use of seropositive blood products for seronegative recipients, use of antithymocyte globulin, additional immunosuppressive agents with cyclosporine, and graft-versus-host disease.[92, 141] After pneumonia, the gastrointestinal tract is the most common site of CMV disease, with a frequency of about 10% in all transplant patients.[142] Three clinical series have documented the high rate (30–50%) of asymptomatic and endoscopically normal CMV infections of the gastroduodenal mucosa during the first month after transplantation.[140, 143, 144] Symptomatic CMV disease after transplantation has been documented, however, in all parts of the gastrointestinal tract, including the stomach.[142, 145-149] Bleeding from multiple gastric erosions after transplantation has been described,[149] as have gastric ulcers presenting as epigastric pain and bleeding after bone marrow[148, 150] or cardiac transplantation.[146]

Cancer and Cancer Chemotherapy Patients

Case reports and postmortem series have documented severe CMV disease in this group of patients, most frequently in those with myelo- or lymphoproliferative disorders and in those treated with corticosteroids.[113, 114, 151-153] Gastrointestinal CMV is well described, with ulcerative lesions in all parts of the intestine.[114] Most CMV gastrointestinal lesions now seen in AIDS and transplant patients were described in these types of patients before the early 1970s.[151, 152] Gastric CMV ulcers have occasionally preceded the diagnosis of cancer,[154] but more commonly have complicated the course of established cancer with pain or bleeding.[153]

Steroid Therapy

Gastric, duodenal, and colon lesions thought to be due to CMV have been associated with steroid therapy.[113, 114, 151, 152, 155] In most cases, steroids were being given for cancer as noted earlier, but occasionally they were prescribed for rheumatic diseases[155] or asthma.[112] Several pathologists have even raised the question of whether steroid-induced peptic ulcer disease might be gastric or duodenal CMV disease.[114, 155, 156] Reading case series gives credence to this idea for many but not all patients.[113] We suggest that when patients receiving steroids undergo endoscopy, the endoscopist perform a biopsy on any ulcers and alert the pathologist to the possibility of CMV infection. Healing of these lesions can occur with the cessation of steroids.[155]

Elderly and Normal Subjects

In the absence of the risk factors listed earlier, a small number of patients over age 65 have been reported to have gastrointestinal CMV disease in the form of colitis,[157, 158] gastric ulcer,[118] or small bowel perforation.[113, 159] These patients had diagnostic histologic studies, but few have had extensive follow-up or detailed immunologic studies. Early clinical series suggested that CMV could cause gastrointestinal disease in patients without obvious immunosuppression.[118]

Most normal people without immunosuppression who have been reported to be infected with gastrointestinal CMV have become so in the setting of acute primary CMV infection acquired in the community,[160-164] through blood transfusion[156, 165] or through sexual contact.[166] Gastric CMV ulcer can complicate the postperfusion syndrome,[156] the condition of multiple trauma treated with blood transfusion,[156] or the heterophil-negative mononucleosis syndrome caused by acute CMV infection.[164, 165] Several authors have reported an acute, self-limited gastropathy in childhood associated with marked hypertrophy of gastric folds and protein-losing enteropathy associated with serologic, histologic, or culture evidence of CMV infection.[167-170]

Clinical Manifestations

Since most diagnostic evaluations are prompted by symptoms, the prevalence and natural history of asymptomatic CMV infection of the stomach are not known. Organ transplant recipients develop positive gastric and duodenal CMV histology and cultures without symptoms in the posttransplant period.[140, 143, 144] Symptomatic disease usually presents with epigastric pain, nausea, and vomiting and often with fever.[101, 133, 135, 145, 153-155, 161, 162] Complications of ulcer disease, including bleeding,[147-149, 152, 156, 171] gastric outlet obstruction,[137] and perforation,[101, 171] have also been documented as presenting complaints. Unusual presentations have included gastrocolic fistula,[171] recurrent stomal ulcer after gastrectomy with afferent limb obstruction,[118] a 4-cm submucosal antral mass,[138] and an acute self-limited gastropathy in childhood associated with protein-losing enteropathy.[167-170]

Diagnosis

Serology

Serologic surveys indicate a prevalence of infection in the general population high enough to render antibody assay useless in most clinical situations.[102, 172-173] Immunoglobulin M (IgM) anti-CMV can be positive for CMV in acute infections or in reactivation of chronic disease.[93, 102, 173] In acute CMV infection in a normal host, serology has occasionally added important information, documenting that the gastrointestinal disease appeared in the setting of acute infection.[160-163, 165, 166] Serology has been used to identify uninfected patients before organ transplants to match them with uninfected donors and blood products in order to reduce the likelihood of posttransplant CMV disease.[174] Otherwise, serology is of little use in the clinical evaluation of patients.

Blood, Urine, Stool, and Oropharyngeal Culture

A blood culture positive for CMV is frequently associated with active CMV infection and carries a poor prognosis in the absence of improving or restored immune function.[142, 172] A positive blood culture does not, however, prove that gastrointestinal signs or symptoms are due to CMV, and a negative culture certainly does not exclude active gastrointestinal CMV infection.[102, 172, 173] Urine culture is frequently intermittently positive for CMV in healthy adults and bears little relationship to the presence of disease.[102] Stool culture is reported to show positive findings in only one third of patients with documented CMV colitis[102] and the results of oropharyngeal cultures are positive in about 30% of patients with proven esophageal CMV. False-positive stool and oropharyngeal cultures for CMV also occur, so it is not a useful diagnostic test.[142, 175] Multiple positive results of cultures from distant sites suggest the diagnosis of active gastrointestinal CMV when the initial gastrointestinal biopsies are negative; but this is an inefficient diagnostic approach.

Radiology

Upper gastrointestinal contrast studies from patients who later had endoscopy, surgery, or postmortem pathology that showed definite CMV have been described.[131, 133, 154, 176–178] The radiologic findings can be dramatic but are always nonspecific, such as thick gastric folds, antral narrowing, or ulcers of varying size and number.[131, 133, 135, 153, 154, 163, 168, 177] One case of gastric CMV infection was first suspected on computed tomography (CT) scan, which showed a thickened antral wall.[134] An asymptomatic submucosal antral mass in an AIDS patient seen by CT was found at laparotomy to be due to CMV.[138] Several authors have reported an acute self-limited gastropathy in childhood associated with marked hypertrophy of gastric folds and protein-losing enteropathy,[167, 170] but this has also been reported with *H. pylori* infection. The sensitivity of radiologic studies is unknown but must be quite low compared with endoscopy biopsy.

Endoscopy

Endoscopy is frequently used to evaluate upper gastrointestinal symptoms and signs in patients at risk for gastric CMV infection. The mucosa can be normal and yet biopsies show cytomegalic cells.[144, 179] Ulcers in all parts of the stomach have been described, as has a spectrum of endoscopic abnormalities, including erythema, subepithelial hemorrhage, erosion, and ulceration.[101, 122, 132, 145, 147, 149, 153–156, 163, 164] The variation in these factors is so great that no endoscopic feature is pathognomonic for CMV disease. Therefore, accurate diagnosis always depends on results from endoscopic or surgical biopsies.

Light Microscopy

Routine histopathologic examination looking for cytomegalic cells is frequently considered the gold standard for documenting CMV gastrointestinal disease.[102, 104, 122, 126, 175, 180–182] A CMV infection produces a characteristic cytopathic effect: a large 25 to 35-μm cell that contains a large basophilic intranuclear inclusion, frequently surrounded by a clear halo, known as the owl's-eye effect, and occasionally associated with clusters of intracytoplasmic inclusions (Fig. 2–8). Numerous studies have demonstrated the specificity for CMV of cytomegalic cells in gastrointestinal biopsies. These cells are always associated with CMV antigen[105, 119, 175, 180] or CMV DNA or both.[102, 103, 109, 119] In some clear-cut cases of gastrointestinal disease due to CMV, however, cytomegalic cells are uncommon[109, 123, 126, 161, 175, 183] and require a great deal of time and effort to find.[102, 103, 106, 184] Identification of specific CMV changes is a function of the number of biopsies, the competence and diligence of the pathologist, and the tissue that is being evaluated.[184a] Numerous diagnostic techniques have been advocated to enhance sensitivity of diagnosis of CMV infection in endoscopic biopsy specimens, but none purports to be more specific than the histologic demonstration of the typical cytopathy.

Biopsy Culture

Because of the absence of any gold-standard method for determining whether gastrointestinal disease is caused by CMV, the sensitivity and specificity of culture of endoscopic biopsy specimens are not known. Although some studies have shown good agreement between histology and culture,[108, 185] culture can be positive for CMV in the absence of symptoms or endoscopic

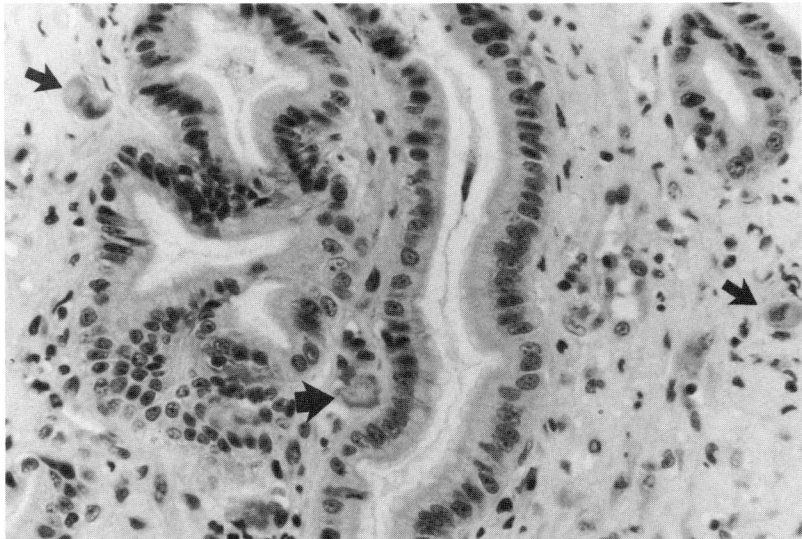

FIGURE 2–8.
A high-power view of the antrum of an HIV-infected patient. Numerous CMV inclusions are seen (arrows), but they have elicited a minimal inflammatory response. Frequently, prominent neutrophilic infiltration, granulation tissue, and ulceration may be seen in association with CMV infection.

lesions.[140, 143, 144, 173] Culture was found to be positive for CMV in only 50% of colonic and esophageal specimens showing cytomegalic cells in AIDS patients.[180, 182] Some investigators believe that culture of endoscopic specimens enhances sensitivity of diagnosis of CMV infection.[175, 183, 186] Some evidence supports the thesis that positive results of cultures do not correlate with gastrointestinal disease. In the one study that showed no effect of ganciclovir on gastrointestinal CMV disease, most patients were diagnosed based on a positive finding on biopsy culture.[187] Culture positivity rates in non-CMV lesions may be as high as 17% in at-risk AIDS patients.[182] We found that culture positivity, although low, was as frequent in endoscopic lesions as in normal mucosa.[184a] Culture of endoscopic biopsy specimens adds an expense that is not justified by any improvement in diagnostic accuracy over routine histopathology if sections are vigorously searched for cytomegalic cells.

For the greatest likelihood of recovering CMV in culture, freshly obtained forceps biopsies or brushings[186] should be placed immediately into refrigerated transport media on ice and processed as soon as possible without freezing or being allowed to remain at room temperature.[172] Commercially available transport media are adequate. They are balanced salt solutions (i.e., minimum essential medium—[MEM]) supplemented with protein, sugar, and antibiotics.[188] Multiple cultures and more tissue per culture are not better than a single culture. A big drawback to culture is the slow rate of CMV growth. Although heavy infections can produce positive results in 4 to 6 days, significant positive results of cultures are found up to 30 days after inoculation.[172] The new shell vial culture technology[173, 183] uses centrifugation to hasten viral entry, and positive findings may occur after 24 hours.

Immunohistochemistry and DNA Hybridization

In an effort to enhance the sensitivity and specificity of histopathology, two techniques have been compared with the histologic demonstration of cytomegalic cells in biopsy specimens: immunoperoxidase or immunofluorescence staining for CMV antigens using monoclonal antibodies (Fig. 2–9)[100, 101, 104, 124, 183, 184] and in situ DNA hybridization using a biotin-labeled probe.[101, 107, 182, 185] Most published series have not shown these assays to be more sensitive than routine histology. Two studies reported that immunoperoxidase stain was positive for CMV when routine histology failed to demonstrate cytomegalic cells.[104, 184] Comparable increased sensitivity was reported for in situ DNA hybridization.[185] None of these studies, however, reported how many biopsies of the lesions were examined before concluding that cytomegalic cells were absent. More extensive studies of these techniques must be performed before they can be recommended over the careful search of multiple biopsies for cytomegalic cells on routine histology.

Polymerase Chain Reaction

Polymerase chain reaction (PCR) has been used to identify CMV DNA in urine,[189] blood,[190] and tissue,[191] but its usefulness in gastrointes-

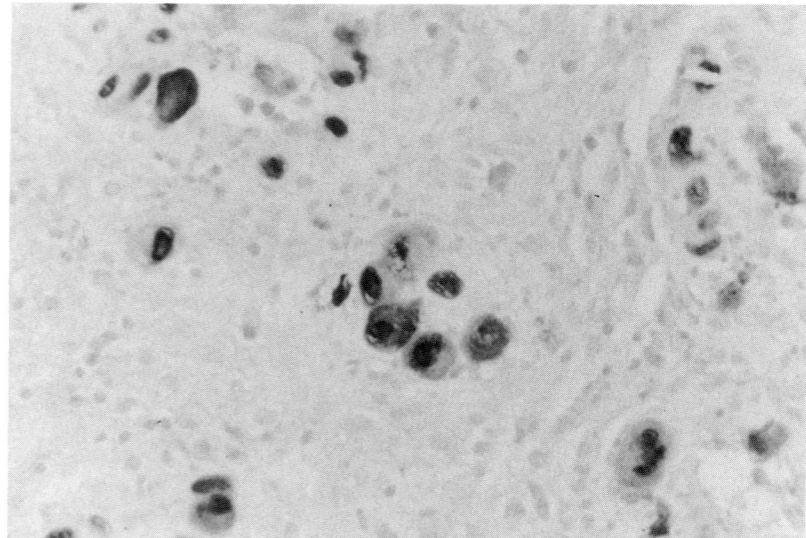

FIGURE 2–9.
Immunoperoxidase staining of CMV inclusions. Although it is not clear whether this technique reveals more inclusions than does a standard hematoxylin-eosin stain, the inclusions are undoubtedly easier to detect.

tinal biopsies has only recently been reported. In a small pilot study, PCR had the highest sensitivity for the diagnosis of active gastrointestinal CMV. The lack of any accepted gold-standard assay for CMV makes it difficult to substantiate this impression. The PCR method may emerge as a useful screening technique to exclude the diagnosis of CMV.

Treatment

Prevention of CMV disease in organ transplant recipients with blood product and donor organ screening, intravenous immunoglobulin, or high dosage of oral acyclovir is possible, but detailed discussion of the indications, risks, and benefits in various groups is beyond the scope of this chapter. Gastrointestinal CMV infection in immunologically normal hosts is frequently self-limited, and only supportive therapy is needed.[156, 160, 163–166] Similarly, some patients receiving corticosteroids, cancer chemotherapy, or drug therapy for posttransplant immune suppression may clear CMV infection without specific treatment if immunologic status improves.[144, 155] Good evidence suggests, however, that gastrointestinal disease in the setting of persistent immunodeficiency is a progressive disease with a high mortality[104, 120, 131, 135, 148, 181, 192] and one that frequently requires anti-CMV chemotherapy.

Ganciclovir is a nucleoside analog of thymidine that is structurally similar to acyclovir. It is a selective inhibitor of viral DNA polymerase, but its ability to be incorporated into human DNA increases its toxicity compared with that of acyclovir. Clinical experience suggests the efficacy of ganciclovir for gastric CMV infection, but it has not been studied extensively.[145, 181] Posttransplant patients with gastrointestinal (mostly gastric) CMV infection seemed to respond to ganciclovir.[145] Ganciclovir has been used in CMV esophageal ulcers[180] and in CMV colitis[192] in AIDS. Treatment of CMV colitis with ganciclovir in AIDS patients is associated with increased survival and improved quality of life.[193] Weight gain occurs with therapy, and progressive weight loss occurs without therapy. Ganciclovir must be given intravenously (IV) and is infused during 1 hour in the usual induction dose of 5 mg/kg twice daily for 3 weeks. The dosage must be reduced in a patient with renal impairment.[194] Since infection is suppressed but not eliminated, relapse is common. Repeat endoscopy after the 3-week induction period is useful to make a decision regarding response to therapy and to help assess relapse when it occurs. Relapse is treated with repeat induction if there was a good response originally, and then it is followed by maintenance of 5 mg/kg IV once daily. Even with maintenance therapy with anti-CMV drugs, CMV retinitis slowly progresses or recurs; similar observations have been made in gastrointestinal CMV infections. Resistance developed in 38% of 13 patients receiving ganciclovir for longer than 3 months but in no patient who had not been treated with the drug or had been treated for less than 3 months.[195] Since testing for ganciclovir resistance takes at least 6 weeks, the practical recommendation is to switch patients who are not responding to ganciclovir to foscarnet. The most frequent toxicities reported with ganciclovir are neutropenia, thrombocytopenia, rash, hypotension, nausea, vomiting, and headache.

Foscarnet (sodium phosphonoformate) is a nonnucleoside that competitively inhibits herpes DNA polymerase. The drug is virustatic and, unlike acyclovir and its analogs, it does not require thymidine kinase for activation; it is less potent in vitro than is acyclovir. It is active against all the most common herpesviruses (herpes simplex, CMV, Epstein-Barr, and varicella zoster) and against HIV. Unlike acyclovir and ganciclovir, it does not require phosphorylation to be activated; therefore it is usually effective when resistance to other drugs is a problem. Experience with gastric CMV is limited. Cytomegalovirus esophageal ulceration in 18 patients and colitis in 27 patients were treated with a continuous infusion of 200 mg/kg/d of foscarnet for 3 weeks.[196] Most patients responded in 7 to 14 days. All failures to alleviate esophageal disease were related to other disease or poor compliance. One colitis patient had absolute failure. The relapse was only about 20% during 6 months, and those patients responded to repeat treatment. Most toxicity and resistance studies have been done on patients with CMV retinitis, but certainly they are applicable to gastrointestinal patients. A randomized, placebo-controlled trial of foscarnet in 24 patients with CMV retinitis showed that retinitis progresses much less on foscarnet than on placebo.[197] The dosage was 60 mg/kg tid IV during a 3-week induction period. A higher maintenance dosage (90 mg/kg/d) was given than in previous studies (60 mg/kg/d). Side effects were mainly electrolyte abnormalities, with low magnesium, calcium, and phosphate in the majority of patients and increased creatinine in one third. Anemia is more common with foscarnet than with placebo, and transfusion requirements were significant. There were significant gastrointestinal side effects, including nausea, vomiting, diarrhea, and abdominal pain.

REFERENCES

1. Sausrbuch T, Schreiber MA, Schkusser P, Permanetter W. Endoscopy in the diagnosis of gastritis: Diagnostic value of endoscopic criteria in relation to histologic diagnosis. Endoscopy. 1984;16:101–104.
2. Rubin CE. Histological classification of gastritis: An iconoclastic view. Gastroenterology. 1992;102:360–361.
3. Mir-Madjlessi SH, Tavassolie H. Primary tuberculous granulomatous esophagogastro-duodenitis: A report of a case. J Trop Med Hyg. 1985;88:253–256.
4. Weissman D, Gumaste VV, Dave PB, Keh W. Bleeding from a tuberculous gastric ulcer. Am J Gastroenterol. 1990;85:742–744.
5. Genta RM, Caymmi-Gomes M. Pathology. In: Grove DA, ed. Strongyloidiasis, a major roundworm infection of man. London: Taylor & Francis; 1989:105–132.
6. Ikeda K, Kumashiro R, Kifune T. Nine cases of acute gastric anisakiasis. Gastrointest Endosc. 1989;35:304–305.
7. Price AB. The Sydney system: Histological division. J Gastroenterol Hepatol. 1991;6:209–222.
8. Osler W. Acute Gastritis. In: Disease of the Digestive System. McCrae T, ed. New York: D Appelton; 1925:474–476.
9. Sugimachi K, Inokuchi K, Kuwano H, Ooiwa T. Acute gastritis clinically classified in accordance with data from both upper GI series and endoscopy. Scand J Gastroenterol. 1984;19:31–37.
10. Manten HD, Harary AM. Chronic infections of the stomach. In: Berk JE, ed. Bockus Gastroenterology. 4th ed. Philadelphia: WB Saunders; 1985;2:1328–1342.
11. Rolfes RT, Nakashima AK. Epidemiology of primary and secondary syphilis in the U.S., 1981–1989. JAMA. 1990;264:1432–1437.
12. Tramont EC. *Treponema pallidum* (syphilis). In: Mandell GL, Douglas RG, Bennett JE, eds. Principle and Practice of Infectious Diseases. 3rd ed. New York: Churchill Livingstone; 1990:1794–1808.
13. Winters HA, Notar-Francesco V, Bromberg K, et al. Gastric syphilis: Five recent cases and a review of the literature. Ann Intern Med. 1992;116:314–319.
14. Besses C, Sans-Sabrafen J, Badia X. Ulceroinfiltrative syphilitic gastropathy: Silver stain diagnosis from biopsy specimen. Am J Gastroenterol. 1987;82:773–774.
15. Morin ME, Tan A. Diffuse enlargement of gastric folds as a manifestation of secondary syphilis. Am J Gastroenterol. 1980;74:170–172.
16. Bockus HL, Bank J. Upper gastro-intestinal disease associated with syphilis. JAMA. 1928;90:175–180.
17. Beckman JW, Schuman BM. Antral gastritis and ulceration in a patient with secondary syphilis. Gastrointest Endosc. 1986;32:355–356.
18. Madding GF, Baer LS, Kennedy PA. Gastric syphilis: A case report. Ann Surg. 1964;159:271–274.
19. Mitchell RD, Gonick HC, Grossman MI. Secretory and histologic changes after treatment of gastric syphilis. Gastroenterology. 1962;43:689–693.
20. Knight WA, Falk A. Tertiary gastric syphilis. Gastroenterology. 1947;9:17–27.
21. Marshall BJ, Royce H, Annear DI, et al. Original isolation of *Campylobacter pyloridis* for human gastric mucosa. Microbios Lett. 1984;25:83–88.
22. Graham DY. *Helicobacter pylori*: Its epidemiology and its role in duodenal ulcer disease. J Gastroenterol Hepatol. 1991;6:97–105.
23. Susser M. Period effects, generation effects and age effects in peptic ulcer mortality. J Chron Dis. 1982;35:29–40.
24. Sonnenberg A, Muller H. Cohort and period effects in peptic ulcer mortality from Japan. J Chron Dis. 1984;37:699–704.
25. Sonnenberg A. Occurrence of a cohort phenomenon in peptic ulcer mortality from Switzerland. Gastroenterology. 1984;86:398–401.
26. Graham DY, Adam E, Klein PD, et al. Epidemiology of *Campylobacter pylori*. Gastroenterol Clin Biol. 1989;13:84B–88B.
27. Graham DY. *Helicobacter pylori* in human populations: The present and predictions of the future based on the epidemiology of polio. In: Menge H, Gregor M, Tytgat GNJ, et al., eds. *Helicobacter pylori* 1990: Proceedings of the Second International Symposium on *Helicobacter pylori*. Berlin: Springer-Verlag; 1991:97–102.
28. Burstein M, Monge E, Leon-Baura R, et al. Low peptic ulcer and high gastric cancer prevalence in a develop-

ing country with a high prevalence of infection by *Helicobacter pylori.* J Clin Gastroenterol. 1991;13:154–156.

29. Haenszel W, Kurihara M, Segi M, Lee RKC. Stomach cancer among Japanese in Hawaii. J Natl Cancer Inst. 1972;49:969–988.

30. Fontham E, Zavala D, Correa P, et al. Diet and chronic atrophic gastritis: A case-control study. J Natl Cancer Inst. 1986;76:621–627.

31. Joossens JV, Geboers J. Diet and environment in the etiology of gastric cancer. In: Levin B, Riddell RH, eds. Frontiers in Gastrointestinal Cancer. New York: Elsevier; 1984:167–183.

32. Sobala GM, Crabtree JE, Dixon MG, et al. Acute *Helicobacter pylori* infection: Clinical features, local and systemic immune response, gastric mucosal histology, and gastric juice ascorbic acid concentrations. Gut. 1991;32:1415–1418.

33. Correa P. Clinical implications of recent developments in gastric cancer pathology and epidemiology. Semin Oncol. 1985;12:2–10.

34. Recavarren-Arce S, Leon-Barua R, Cok J, et al. *Helicobacter pylori* and progressive gastric pathology that predisposes to gastric cancer. Scand J Gastroenterol. 1991;26:51–57.

35. Correa P, Fox J, Fontham E, et al. *Helicobacter pylori* and gastric carcinoma: Serum antibody prevalence in populations with contrasting cancer risks. Cancer. 1990;66:2569–2574.

36. Cheng SCW, Sanderson CR, Waters TE, Goodwin CS. *Campylobacter pyloridis* in patients with gastric carcinoma. Med J Aust. 1987;147:202–203.

37. Loffeld RJLF, Willems I, Flendrig JA, Arends JW. *Helicobacter pylori* and gastric carcinoma. Histopathology. 1990;17:537–541.

38. Sipponen P, Kosunen TU, Valle J, et al. *Helicobacter pylori* infection and chronic gastritis in gastric cancer. J Clin Pathol. In press.

39. Feng Y-Y, Wang Y. *Campylobacter pylori* in patients with gastritis, peptic ulcer, and carcinoma of the stomach in Lanzhou, China. Lancet. 1988;1:1055–1056.

40. Sedgwick DM, Akoh JA, Macintyre IMC. Gastric cancer in Scotland: Changing epidemiology, unchanging workload. Br Med J. 1991;302:1305–1307.

41. Forman D, Sitas F, Newell DG, et al. Geographic association of *Helicobacter pylori* antibody prevalence and gastric cancer mortality in rural China. Int J Cancer. 1990;46:608–611.

42. Dehesa M, Dooly CP, Cohen H, et al. High prevalence of *Helicobacter pylori* infection and histologic gastritis in asymptomatic Hispanics. J Clin Microbiol. 1991; 29:1128–1131.

43. Fox JG, Correa P, Taylor NS, et al. *Campylobacter pylori*–associated gastritis and immune response in a population at increased risk of gastric carcinoma. Am J Gastroenterol. 1989;84:775–781.

44. Scott N, Lansdown M, Diament R, et al. *Helicobacter* gastritis and intestinal metaplasia in a gastric cancer family. Lancet. 1990;1:728.

45. Caruso ML, Fucci L. Histological identification of *Helicobacter pylori* in early and advanced gastric cancer. J Clin Gastroenterol. 1990;12:601–602.

46. Parsonnet J, Vandersteen D, Goates J, et al. *Helicobacter pylori* infection in intestinal- and diffuse-type gastric adenocarcinomas. J Natl Cancer Inst. 1991;83:640–643.

47. Forman D, Newell DG, Fullerton F, et al. Association between infection with *Helicobacter pylori* and risk of gastric cancer: Evidence from a prospective investigation. Br Med J. 1991;302:1302–1305.

48. Nomura A, Stemmermann GN, Chyou P-H, et al. *Helicobacter pylori* infection and gastric carcinoma among Japanese Americans in Hawaii. N Engl J Med. 1991;325:1132–1136.

49. Graham DY, Malaty HM, Evans DG, et al. Epidemiology of *Helicobacter pylori* in an asymptomatic population in the United States: Effect of age, race and socioeconomic status. Gastroenterology. 1991;100:1495–1501.

50. Fiedorek SC, Malaty HM, Evans DG, et al. Factors influencing the epidemiology of *Helicobacter pylori* infection in children. Pediatrics. 1991;87:578–582.

51. Malaty HM, Evans DG, Evans DJ Jr, Graham DY. *Helicobacter pylori* infection in Hispanics: Comparison with blacks and whites of similar age and socioeconomic class. Gastroenterology. 1992;103:813–816.

52. Siurala M, Sipponen P, Kekki M. Chronic gastritis: Dynamic and clinical aspects. Scand J Gastroenterol. 1985;20(suppl 109):69–76.

53. Marshall BJ, Armstrong JA, McGechie DB, Glancy RJ. Attempt to fulfil Koch's postulates for pyloric *Campylobacter.* Med J Aust. 1985;142:436–439.

54. Morris A, Nicholson G. Ingestion of *Campylobacter pyloridis* causes gastritis and raises fasting gastric pH. Am J Gastroenterol. 1987;82:192–199.

55. Graham DY. Pathogenic mechanisms leading to *Helicobacter pylori*–induced inflammation. Eur J Gastroenterol Hepatol. 1992;4:S9–S16.

56. Graham DY, Alpert LC, Smith JL, Yoshimura HH. Iatrogenic *Campylobacter pylori* infection is a cause of epidemic achlorhydria. Am J Gastroenterol. 1988;83:974–980.

57. Hessey SJ, Spencer J, Whatt JI, et al. Bacterial adhesion and disease activity in *Helicobacter* associated chronic gastritis. Gut. 1990;31:603–610.

58. Graham DY, Klein PD, Evans DJ, et al. *Campylobacter pyloridis* detected noninvasively by the ^{13}C-urea breath test. Lancet. 1987;1:1174–1177.

59. Graham DY. *Campylobacter pylori* and peptic ulcer disease. Gastroenterology. 1989;96(suppl):615–625.

60. Crabtree JE, Taylor JD, Wyatt JI, et al. Mucosal IgA recognition of *Helicobacter pylori* 120 kDa protein, peptic ulceration, and gastric pathology. Lancet. 1991;338:332–335.

61. Yoshimura HH, Evans DG, Graham DY. *H. pylori* strains from duodenal ulcer patients differ at the genomic level from those from patients with simple gastritis. Enferm Dig. 1990;78(suppl 1):22.

62. Zuckerberg LR, Ferry JA, Southern JF, Harris NL. Lymphoid infiltrates of the stomach: Evaluation of histologic criteria for the diagnosis of low-grade gastric lymphoma on endoscopic biopsy specimens. Am J Surg Pathol. 1990;14:1087–1099.

63. Dixon MF, Wyatt JI, Burke DA, Rathbone BJ. Lymphocytic gastritis: Relationship to *Campylobacter pylori* infection. J Pathol. 1988;154:125–132.

64. Stolte M, Eidt S. Lymphoid follicles in antral mucosa: Immune response to *Campylobacter pylori?* J Clin Pathol. 1989;42:1269–1271.

65. Rosh JR, Kurfist LA, Benkov KJ, et al. *Helicobacter pylori* and gastric lymphonodular hyperplasia in children. Am J Gastroenterol. 1992;87:135–139.

66. Genta RM, Hamner HW, Graham DY. Gastric lymphoid follicles in *Helicobacter pylori* infection: Frequency, distribution and response to triple therapy. Hum Pathol. 1993;24:575–582.

67. Correa P. Chronic gastritis: A clinico-pathological classification. Am J Gastroenterol. 1988;5:504–509.

68. Chan WY, Hui PK, Chan JKC, et al. Epithelial damage by *Helicobacter pylori* in gastric ulcers. Histopathology. 1991;19:47–53.

69. Alpert LC, Lew GM, Michaletz PA. Comparison of the extent and severity of *C. pylori* infection between duodenal ulcer patients and age-matched asymptomatic *C. pylori*–infected subjects. Gastroenterology. 1989; 96:A10.

70. McNulty CAM, Gearty JC, Crump B, et al. *Campylobacter pyloridis* and associated gastritis: Investigator blind, placebo controlled trial of bismuth salicylate and erythromycin ethylsuccinate. Br Med J. 1986;293:645–649.

71. Morgan D, Kraft W, Bender M, et al. Nitrofurans in the treatment of gastritis associated with *Campylobacter pylori*. Gastroenterology. 1988;95:1178–1184.

72. Loffeld RJLF, Potters HVJP, Stobberingh E, et al. *Campylobacter* associated gastritis in patients with non-ulcer dyspepsia: A double blind placebo controlled trial with colloidal bismuth subcitrate. Gut. 1989;30:1206–1212.

73. Strauss RM, Wang TC, Kelsey PB, et al. Association of *Helicobacter pylori* infection with dyspeptic symptoms in patients undergoing gastroduodenoscopy. Am J Med. 1990;89:464–469.

74. Kang JY, Tay HH, Wee A, et al. Effect of colloidal bismuth subcitrate on symptoms and gastric histology in non-ulcer dyspepsia: A double blind placebo controlled study. Gut. 1990;31:476–480.

75. Alpert LC, Graham DY, Evans DJ Jr, et al. Diagnostic possibilities for *Campylobacter pylori* infection. Eur J Gastroenterol Hepatol. 1989;1:17–26.

76. Klein PD, Graham DY. *Campylobacter pylori* detection by the ^{13}C-urea breath test. In: Rathbone B, Heatley V, eds. *Campylobacter pylori and Gastroduodenal Disease.* Oxford: Blackwell Scientific; 1989:94–106.

77. Graham DY, Klein PK. What you should know about the methods, problems, interpretations, and use of urea breath tests. Am J Gastroenterol. 1991;86:1118–1122.

78. Hazell SL, Borody TJ, Gal A, Lee A. *Campylobacter pyloridis* gastritis I: Detection of urease as a marker of bacterial colonization and gastritis. Am J Gastroenterol. 1987;82:292–296.

79. Coghlan JG, Gilligan D, Humphreys H, et al. *Campylobacter pylori* and recurrence of duodenal ulcers: A 12-month follow-up study. Lancet. 1987;2:1109–1111.

80. Lambert JR, Borromeo M, Korman MG, et al. Effect of colloidal bismuth (De-Nol) on healing and relapse of duodenal ulcers: Role of *Campylobacter pyloridis*. Gastroenterology. 1987;92:1489.

81. Marshall BJ, Goodwin CS, Warren JR, et al. Prospective double-blind trial of duodenal ulcer relapse after eradication of *Campylobacter pylori*. Lancet. 1988;2:1437–1442.

82. Rauws EAJ, Tytgat GNJ. Cure of duodenal ulcer associated with eradication of *Helicobacter pylori*. Lancet. 1990;335:1233–1235.

83. George LJ, Borody TJ, Andrews P, et al. Cure of duodenal ulcer after eradication of *Helicobacter pylori*. Med J Aust. 1990;153:145–149.

84. Graham DY, Lew GM, Klein PD, et al. Effect of treatment of *Helicobacter pylori* on the recurrence of gastric ulcers or duodenal ulcers: A randomized controlled study. Ann Intern Med. 1991;115:266–269.

85. Graham DY, Hepps KE, Ramirez FC, et al. Treatment of *H. pylori* reduces the rate of rebleeding in peptic ulcer disease. Scand J Gastroenterol. In press.

86. Börsch GMA, Graham DY. *Helicobacter pylori*. In: Benjamin SB, Collen MJ, eds. Handbook of Experimental Pharmacology: Pharmacology of Peptic Ulcer Disease. Berlin: Springer-Verlag; 1991;99:107–148.

87. Graham DY, Börsch GMA. The who's and when's of therapy for *Helicobacter pylori*. Am J Gastroenterol. 1990;85:1552–1555.

88. Megraud F, Trimoulet P, Lamouliatte H, Boyanova L. Bactericidal effect of amoxicillin on *H pylori* in an in vitro model using epithelial cells. Antimicrob Agents Chemother. 1991;35:869–872.

89. Graham DY, Lew GM, Malaty HM, et al. Factors influencing the eradication of *Helicobacter pylori* with triple therapy. Gastroenterology. 1992;102:493–496.

90. Glupczynski Y, Burette A. Drug therapy of *Helicobacter pylori* infection: Problems and pitfalls. Am J Gastroenterol. 1990;85:1545–1551.

91. Ho M. Epidemiology of cytomegalovirus infections. Rev Infect Dis. 1990;12(suppl 7):S701–S710.

92. Rubin R. Impact of cytomegalovirus on organ transplant recipients. Rev Infect Dis. 1990;12(suppl 7):S754–S766.

93. Merigan T, Resta S. Cytomegalovirus: Where have we been and where are we going? Rev Infect Dis. 1990;12(suppl 7):S693–S700.

94. Tyms A, Taylor D, Parkin J. Cytomegalovirus and the acquired immunodeficiency syndrome. J Antimicrob Chemother. 1989;23(suppl A):89–105.

95. Poland S, Costello P, Dekaban G, Rice G. Cytomegalovirus in the brain: In vitro infection of human brain-derived cells. J Infect Dis. 1990;162:1252–1262.

96. Roche J, Cheung K-S, Boldogh I, et al. Cytomegalovirus: Detection in human colonic and circulating mononuclear cells in association with gastrointestinal disease. Int J Cancer. 1981;27:659–667.

97. Griffiths P, Grundy J. The status of CMV as a human pathogen. Epidemiol Infect. 1988;100:1–15.

98. Pasternack M, Medearis D, Rubin R. Cell-mediated immunity in experimental cytomegalovirus infections: A perspective. Rev Infect Dis. 1990;12(suppl 7):S720–S726.

99. Jeffries D. The spectrum of cytomegalovirus infection and its management. J Antimicrob Chemother. 1989;23(suppl E):1–10.

100. Grundy J. Virologic and pathogenetic aspects of cytomegalovirus infection. Rev Infect Dis. 1990;12(suppl 7):S711–S719.

101. Iwasaki T. Alimentary tract lesions in cytomegalovirus infection. Acta Pathol Jpn. 1987;37:549–565.

102. Culpepper-Morgan J, Kotler D, Scholes J, Tierney A. Evaluation of diagnostic criteria for mucosal cytomegalovirus disease in the acquired immune deficiency syndrome. Am J Gastroenterol. 1987;82:1264–1270.

103. Robey S, Gage W, Kuhajda F. Comparison of immunoperoxidase and DNA in situ hybridization techniques in the diagnosis of cytomegalovirus colitis. Am J Clin Pathol. 1988;89:666–671.

104. Hinnart K, Rotterdam H, Bell E, Tapper M. Cytomegalovirus infection of the alimentary tract: A clincopathologic correlation. Am J Gastroenterol. 1986;81:944.

105. Foucar E, Mukai K, Foucar K, et al. Colonic ulceration in lethal cytomegalovirus infection. Am J Clin Pathol. 1981;76:788–801.

106. Francis N, Boylston A, Roberts A, et al. Cytomegalovirus infection in gastrointestinal tracts of patients infected with HIV-1 or AIDS. J Clin Pathol. 1989;42:1055–1064.

107. Roberts W, Sneddon J, Waldman J, Stephens R. Cytomegalovirus infection of gastrointestinal endothelium demonstrated by simultaneous nucleic acid hybridization and immunohistochemistry. Arch Pathol Lab Med. 1989;113:461–464.

108. Rene E, Marche C, Chevalier T, et al. Cytomegalovirus colitis in patients with acquired immunodeficiency syndrome. Dig Dis Sci. 1988;33:741–750.

109. Myerson D, Hackman R, Nelson J, et al. Widespread presence of histologically occult cytomegalovirus. Hum Pathol. 1984;15:430–439.

110. Goodman M, Porter O. Cytomegalovirus vasculitis with fatal colonic hemorrhage. Arch Pathol. 1973;96:281–284.

111. Meiselman M, Cello J, Margaretten W. Cytomegalovirus colitis: Report of the clinical endoscopic and pathologic findings in two patients with the acquired immunodeficiency syndrome. Gastroenterology. 1985;88:171–175.

112. Orloff JJ, Saito R, Lasky S, Dave H. Toxic megacolon in cytomegalovirus colitis. Am J Gastroenterol. 1989;84:794–797.

113. Henson D. Cytomegalovirus inclusion bodies in the gastrointestinal tract. Arch Pathol. 1972;93:477–482.

114. Rosen P, Hajdu S. Cytomegalovirus inclusion disease at autopsy of patients with cancer. Am J Clin Pathol. 1971;55:749–756.

115. Gangahar D, Liggett S, Casey J, et al. Two episodes of cytomegalovirus associated colon perforation after heart transplantation with successful result. J Heart Transplant. 1988;7:377–379.

116. Goodman Z, Boitnott J, Yardley J. Perforation of the colon associated with cytomegalovirus infection. Dig Dis Sci. 1979;24:376–380.

117. Rosen P, Armstrong D, Rice N. Gastrointestinal cytomegalovirus infection. Arch Intern Med. 1973;132:274–276.

118. Levine R, Warnker N, Johnson C. Cytomegalovirus inclusion disease in the gastrointestinal tract of adults. Ann Surg. 1964;159:37–48.

119. Eyre-Brook I, Dundas S. Incidence and clinical significance of colonic cytomegalovirus infection in idiopathic inflammatory bowel disease requiring colectomy. Gut. 1986;27:1419–1425.

120. Frank D, Raicht R. Intestinal perforation associated with cytomegalovirus infection in patients with acquired immunodeficiency syndrome. Am J Gastroenterol. 1984;79:201–204.

121. Vogel S. Enhanced susceptibility of proliferating endothelium to salivary gland virus under naturally occurring and experimental conditions. Am J Pathol. 1958;34:1069.

122. Jacobson M, Mills J. Serious cytomegalovirus disease in the acquired immunodeficiency syndrome (AIDS). Ann Intern Med. 1988;108:585–594.

123. Drew W. Cytomegalovirus infection in patients with AIDS. J Infect Dis. 1988;158:449–456.

124. Macher A, Reichert C, Straus S. Death in the AIDS patient: Role of cytomegalovirus. N Engl J Med. 1983;309:1454.

125. Blaser M, Cohn D. Opportunistic infections in patients with AIDS: Clues to the epidemiology of AIDS and to the relative virulence of pathogens. Rev Infect Dis. 1986;8:21–30.

126. Connolly G, Forbes A, Gazzard B. Investigation of seemingly pathogen-negative diarrhea in patients infected with HIV-1. Gut. 1990;31:886–889.

127. Wilson S, Robinson G, Williams R, et al. Acquired immune deficiency syndrome (AIDS): Indications for abdominal surgery, pathology and outcome. Ann Surg. 1989;210:428–434.

128. Guarda L, Luna M, Smith JJ, et al. Acquired immune deficiency syndrome: Postmortem findings. Am J Clin Pathol. 1984;81:549–557.

129. Reichert C, O'Leary T, Levens D, et al. Autopsy pathology in the acquired immune deficiency syndrome. Am J Pathol. 1983;12:357–382.

130. Schooley R. Cytomegalovirus in the setting of infection with human immunodeficiency virus. Rev Infect Dis. 1990;12(suppl 7):S811–S819.

131. Balthazar E, Megibow A, Hulnick D. Cytomegalovirus esophagitis and gastritis in AIDS. AJR Am J Roentgenol. 1985;144:1201–1204.

132. Knapp A, Horst D, Eliopoulos G, et al. Widespread cytomegalovirus gastroenterocolitis in a patient with acquired immunodeficiency syndrome. Gastroenterology. 1983;85:1399–1402.

133. Falcone S, Murphy B, Weinfeld A. Gastric manifestations of AIDS: Radiographic findings on upper gastrointestinal examination. Gastrointest Radiol. 1991;16:95–98.

134. Soulen M, Fishman E, Scatarige J, et al. Cryptosporidiosis of the gastric antrum: Detection using CT. Radiology. 1986;159:705–706.

135. Freedman P, Weiner B, Balthazar E. Cytomegalovirus esophagogastritis in a patient with acquired immunodeficiency syndrome. Am J Gastroenterol. 1985;80:434–437.

136. Goodgame R, Ross P, Kim H, et al. Esophageal stricture secondary to cytomegalovirus ulcer treated with ganciclovir. J Clin Gastroenterol. 1991;13:678–680.

137. Victoria M, Nangia B, Jindrak K. Cytomegalovirus pyloric obstruction in a child with acquired immunodeficiency syndrome. Pediatr Infect Dis J. 1985;4:550–552.

138. Elta G, Turnage R, Eckhauser F, et al. A submucosal antral mass caused by cytomegalovirus infection in a patient with acquired immunodeficiency syndrome. Am J Gastroenterol. 1986;81:714–717.

139. Dummer J. Cytomegalovirus infection after liver transplantation: Clinical manifestations and strategies for prevention. Rev Infect Dis. 1990;12(suppl 7):S767–S775.

140. Spencer G, Hackman R, McDonald G, et al. A prospective study of unexplained nausea and vomiting after marrow transplantation. Transplantation. 1986;42:602–607.

141. Meyers J, Flournoy N, Thomas E. Risk factors for cytomegalovirus infection after human marrow transplantation. J Infect Dis. 1986;153:478–488.

142. Meyers J, Ljungman P, Fisher L. Cytomegalovirus excretion as a predictor of cytomegalovirus disease after marrow transplantation: Importance of cytomegalovirus viremia. J Infect Dis. 1990;162:373–380.

143. Alexander J, Cuellar R, Fadden R, et al. Cytomegalovirus infection of the upper gastrointestinal tract before and after liver transplantation. Transplantation. 1988;46:378–382.

144. Franzin G, Muolo A, Griminelli T. Cytomegalovirus inclusions in the gastroduodenal mucosa of patients after renal transplantation. Gut. 1981;22:698.

145. Mayoral J, Loeffler C, Fasola C, et al. Diagnosis and treatment of cytomegalovirus disease in transplant patients based on gastrointestinal tract manifestations. Arch Surg. 1991;126:202–206.

146. Icenogle TB, Peterson E, Ray G, et al. DHPG effectively treats CMV infection in heart and heart-lung transplant patients: A preliminary report. J Heart Transpl. 1987;6:199–203.

147. Allen J, Silvis S, Sumner H, McClain C. Cytomegalovirus inclusion disease diagnosed endoscopically. Dig Dis Sci. 1981;26:133–135.

148. Strayer D, Phillips G, Barker K, et al. Gastric cytomegalovirus infection in bone marrow transplant patients: An indication of generalized disease. Cancer. 1981;48:1478–1483.

149. Diethelm A, Gore I, Ch'ien L, et al. Gastrointestinal hemorrhage secondary to CMV after renal transplantation. Am J Surg. 1976;131:370–374.

150. Minami H, Matsushita T, Sugihara T, et al. Cytomegalovirus-induced gastritis in a bone marrow transplant patient. Jpn J Med. 1990;29:433–435.

151. Rosen P. Cytomegalovirus infection in cancer patients. Pathol Annu. 1978;13:175–208.

152. Wong T, Warner N. Cytomegalic inclusion disease in adults: Report of 14 cases with review of literature. Arch Pathol. 1962;74:403–422.

153. Andrade J, Bambirra A, Lima F, et al. Gastric cytomegalic inclusion bodies diagnosed by histologic examination of endoscopic biosies in patients with gastric ulcer. Am J Clin Pathol. 1983;79:493–499.

154. Furukawa Y, Nakamura H, Sakamoto S, Miura Y. Cytomegalovirus gastritis as an initial manifestation of a

patient with adult T-cell leukemia. Acta Haematol (Basel) 1988;80:216–218.

155. Ayulo M, Aisner S, Margolis K, Moravec C. Cytomegalovirus-associated gastritis in a compromised host. JAMA. 1980;243:1364.

156. Campbell D, Piercy J, Shnitka T, et al. Cytomegalovirus associated gastric ulcer. Gastroenterology. 1977;72:533.

157. Spiegel J, Schwabe A. Disseminated cytomegalovirus infection with gastrointestinal involvement: The role of altered immunity in the elderly. Am J Gastroenterol. 1980;73:37–44.

158. Tamura H. Acute ulcerative colitis associated with cytomegalic inclusion virus. Arch Pathol Lab Med. 1973;96:164–167.

159. Nakoneczna J, Kay S. Fatal disseminated cytomegalic inclusion disease in an adult presenting with a lesion of the gastrointestinal tract. Am J Clin Pathol. 1967;47:124–128.

160. Surawitz C, Meyerson D. Self-limited cytomegalovirus colitis in immunocompetent individuals. Gastroenterology. 1988;94:194–199.

161. Diepersloot R, Kroes A, Visser W, et al. Acute ulcerative proctocolitis associated with primary cytomegalovirus infection. Arch Intern Med. 1990;150:1749–1751.

162. Cunningham M, Cantoni L, Humair L. Cytomegalovirus primoinfection in a patient with idiopathic proctitis. Am J Gastroenterol. 1986;81:586–588.

163. Garcia F, Garau J, Sierra M, Marco V. Cytomegalovirus mononucleosis–associated antral gastritis simulating malignancy. Arch Intern Med. 1987;147:787–788.

164. Spiller R, Lovell D, Silk D. Adult acquired cytomegalovirus infection with gastric and duodenal ulceration. Gut. 1988;29:1109–1111.

165. Villar L, Massanari R, Mitros F. Cytomegalovirus infection with acute erosive esophagitis. Am J Med. 1984;76:924–928.

166. Rabinowitz M, Bassan I, Robinson M. Sexually transmitted cytomegalovirus proctitis in a woman. Am J Gastroenterol. 1988;83:885–887.

167. Lachman R, Martin D, Vawter G. Thick gastric folds in childhood. AJR Am J Roentgenol. 1971;112:83–92.

168. Marks M, Lanza M, Kahlstrom E, et al. Pediatric hypertrophic gastropathy. AJR Am J Roentgenol. 1986; 147:1031–1034.

169. Leonidas J, Beatty E, Wenner H. Ménétrier's disease and cytomegalovirus infection in childhood. Am J Dis Child. 1973;126:806–808.

170. Stillman A, Sieber O, Manthei U, Pinnas J. Transient protein-losing enteropathy and enlarged gastric rugae in childhood. Am J Dis Child. 1981;135:29–33.

171. Agel N, Tanner P, Drury A, et al. Cytomegalovirus gastritis with perforation and gastrocolic fistula formation. Histopathology. 1991;18:165–168.

172. Drew W. Diagnosis of cytomegalovirus infection. Rev Infect Dis. 1988;10(suppl 3):S468–S476.

173. Chou S. Newer methods for the diagnosis of cytomegalovirus infection. Rev Infect Dis. 1990;12(suppl 7):S727–S736.

174. Meyers J. Prevention of cytomegalovirus infection after marrow transplantation. Rev Infect Dis. 1989;2(suppl 7):S1691–S1705.

175. McDonald G, Sharma P, Hackman R, et al. Esophageal infections in immunosuppressed patients after marrow transplantation. Gastroenterology. 1985;88:1111–1117.

176. Texador H, Honig C, Norsoph E, et al. Cytomegalovirus infection of the alimentary canal: Radiologic findings with pathologic correlation. Radiology. 1987;163:317–323.

177. Megibow A, Balthazar E, Hulnick D. Radiology of nonneoplastic gastrointestinal disorders in acquired immune deficiency syndrome. Semin Roentgenol. 1987;22:31–41.

178. Wall S, Ominsky S, Altman D, et al. Multifocal abnormalities of the gastrointestinal tract in AIDS. AJR Am J Roentgenol. 1986;146:1–5.

179. Franzin G, Novelli P, Fratten A. Histologic evidence of cytomegalovirus in the duodenal and gastric mucosa of patients with renal allograft. Endoscopy. 1980;12:117.

180. Wilcox C, Diehl D, Cello J, et al. Cytomegalovirus esophagitis in patients with AIDS: A clinical, endoscopic and pathologic correlation. Ann Intern Med. 1990;113:589–593.

181. Chachoua A, Dieterich D, Krasinski K, et al. 9-(1,3-dihydroxy-2-propoxymethyl) guanine (ganciclovir) in the treatment of cytomegalovirus gastrointestinal disease in the acquired immune deficiency syndrome. Ann Intern Med. 1987;107:133–137.

182. Clayton F, Klein E, Kotler D. Correlation of in situ hybridization with histology and viral culture in patients with acquired immunodeficiency syndrome with cytomegalovirus colitis. Arch Pathol Lab Med. 1989;113:1124–1126.

183. Gleaves C, Reed E, Hackman R, Meyers J. Rapid diagnosis of invasive cytomegalovirus infection by examination of tissue specimens in centrifugation culture. Am J Clin Pathol. 1987;88:354–358.

184. Theise N, Rotterdam H, Dieterich D. Cytomegalovirus esophagitis in AIDS: Diagnosis by endoscopic biopsy. Am J Gastroenterol. 1991;86:1123–1126.

184a. Goodgame RW, Genta RM, Estrada R, et al. Frequency of positive tests for cytomegalovirus in AIDS patients: Endoscopic lesions compared with normal mucosa. Am J Gastroenterol. 1993;88:338–343.

185. Robert W, Hammond S, Sneddon J, et al. In situ DNA hybridization for cytomegalovirus in colonoscopic biopsies. Arch Pathol Lab Med. 1988;112:1106–1109.

186. Bonacini M, Young T, Laine L. The causes of esophageal symptoms in human immunodeficiency virus infection: A prospective study of 110 patients. Arch Intern Med. 1991;151:1567–1572.

187. Reed E, Wolford J, Kopecky K, et al. Ganciclovir for the treatment of cytomegalovirus gastroenteritis in bone marrow transplant patients: A randomized, placebo-controlled trial. Ann Intern Med. 1990;112:505–510.

188. Schmidt NJ. Cell culture procedures for diagnostic virology. In: Schmidt NJ, Emmons RW, eds. Diagnostic Procedures for Viral, Rickettsial, and Chlamydial Infections. Washington: American Public Health Association; 1989:59–60.

189. Demmler G, Buffone G, Schimbor C, May R. Detection of cytomegalovirus in urine from newborns by using polymerase chain reaction DNA amplification. J Infect Dis. 1988;158:1177–1184.

190. Shibata D, Martin W, Appleman M, et al. Detection of cytomegalovirus DNA in peripheral blood of patients infected with human immunodeficiency virus. J Infect Dis. 1988;158:1185–1192.

191. Rogers B, Alpert L, Hine E, Buffone G. Analysis of DNA in fresh and fixed tissue by the polymerase chain reaction. Am J Pathol. 1990;136:541–548.

192. Kotler D, Teirney A, Altilio D, et al. Body mass repletion during ganciclovir treatment of cytomegalovirus infections in patients with acquired immunodeficiency syndrome. Arch Intern Med. 1989;149:901–905.

193. Kotler D. Cytomegalovirus colitis and wasting. J AIDS. 1991;4(suppl 1):S36–S41.

194. Drew W. Clinical use of ganciclovir for cytomegalovirus infection and the development of drug resistance. J AIDS. 1991;4(suppl 1):S42–S46.

195. Drew W, Miner R, Busch D, et al. Prevalence of resistance in patients receiving ganciclovir for serious cytomegalovirus infections. J Infect D. 1991;163:716–719.

196. Nelson M, Connolly G, Hawkins D, Gazzard B. Foscarnet in the treatment of cytomegalovirus infection of the esophagus and colon in patients with the acquired immune deficiency syndrome. Am J Gastroenterol. 1991;86:876–881.

197. Palestine A, Polis M, De Smet MD. A randomized, controlled trial of foscarnet in the treatment of cytomegalovirus retinitis in patients with AIDS. Ann Intern Med. 1991;115:665–673.

3

The Small Intestine and Colon

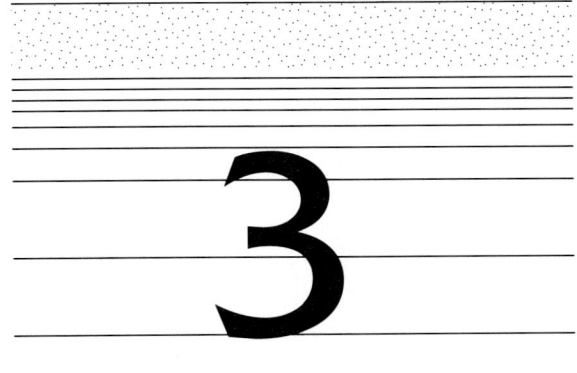

3

Viral Gastroenteritis

KAREN MIDTHUN, M.D.

ALBERT Z. KAPIKIAN, M.D.

Viral gastroenteritis is a common acute infectious disease characterized by vomiting or diarrhea or both. It is frequently a mild, self-limited illness of short duration but can lead to life-threatening dehydration, especially in infants and young children. The importance of this disease in a developed country was shown in the Cleveland Family Study, in which it accounted for 16% of 25,155 illnesses within a 10-year period.[1] The Centers for Disease Control (CDC) in Atlanta estimated that diarrheal illness in children younger than 5 years of age resulted in 209,000 hospitalizations and 517 deaths per year.[2] In the developing world, acute infectious diarrheal disease is one of the leading causes of morbidity and mortality. In a 1-year period from 1977 to 1978, an estimated 3 to 5 billion cases of diarrhea and 5 to 10 million diarrhea-related deaths occurred in Africa, Asia, and Latin America.[3]

Despite major discoveries in bacteriology and parasitology in the past century, the cause of most acute diarrheal illnesses remained elusive until electron microscopy (EM) led to the detection of several groups of previously unrecognized viruses, including Norwalk virus, rotavirus, fastidious adenovirus, calicivirus-like virus, and astrovirus.[4-7] Viruses that have an etiologic association with gastroenteritis are discussed in this chapter.

ROTAVIRUS

Description and Classification

Rotaviruses are classified as a genus in the family Reoviridae and are causal agents of diarrhea in humans and numerous animal species.[8] They are 70 nm in diameter, possess a distinctive double-layered capsid, and have 132 spoke-like capsomeres radiating from the inner capsid (Fig. 3–1).[9, 10] The virions have a density of 1.36 g per cm³ in cesium chloride and are antigenically distinct from the three reovirus serotypes. The genome consists of 11 segments of double-stranded ribonucleic acid (RNA) that encode at least six structural and four nonstructural proteins. Inner capsid polypeptides VP1, VP2, VP3, and VP6 are encoded by RNA segments 1, 2, 3, and 6, respectively. Outer capsid polypeptide VP4, which is present in the form of "spikes" protruding from the surface,[11] is encoded by segment 4, and outer capsid polypeptide VP7 by segments 7, 8, and 9. Rotaviruses possess three important antigenic specificities: group, subgroup, and serotype. The major inner capsid polypeptide, VP6, is the predominant bearer of the common group antigen that is shared by most human and animal strains and forms the basis for the classification of most strains as group A rotaviruses.[10] In most instances, VP6

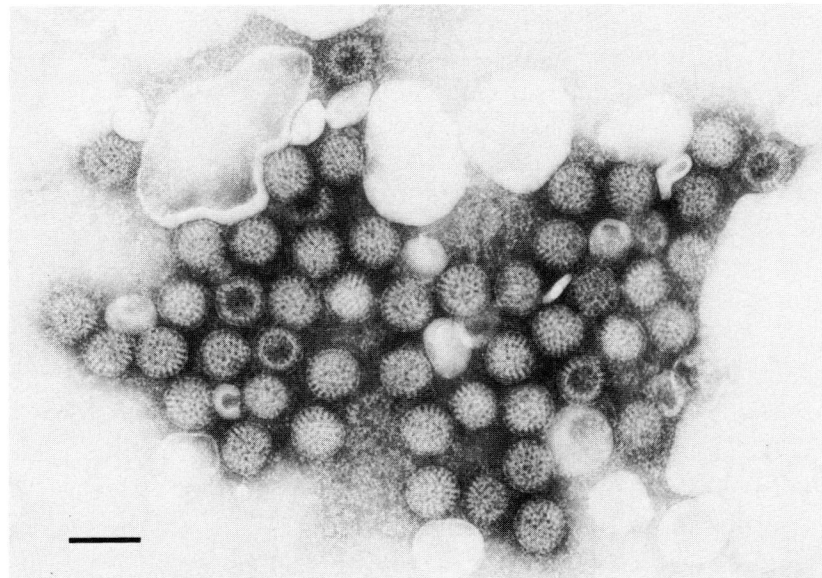

FIGURE 3–1.
Rotavirus particles, approximately 70 nm in diameter, observed by immune electron microscopy in a stool filtrate from a child admitted to the hospital with a diarrheal illness. The particles have a distinctive appearance highlighted by a double-shelled outer capsid. Occasional "empty" particles are seen. Scale bar indicates 100 nm. SOURCE: Kapikian AZ, Kim HW, Wyatt RG, et al. Human reovirus–like agent as the major pathogen associated with "winter" gastroenteritis in hospitalized infants and young children. N Engl J Med. 1976;294:965–972.

also carries one of two subgroup-specific antigens; monoclonal antibodies to these antigens can be used to divide most group A rotaviruses into subgroup I or II, although some isolates appear to carry both subgroup I and II specificities and a few do not belong to either subgroup.[12, 13] One of the two outer capsid polypeptides, VP4, is the hemagglutinin in certain rotaviruses and induces a neutralizing antibody that is associated with VP4 serotype specificity[14]; the cleavage of this protein enhances infectivity.[15] The major outer capsid polypeptide, VP7, induces large amounts of a neutralizing antibody that is responsible for the serotype classification currently in common use.[16] A serotyping scheme that takes into account both VP4 and VP7 specificities has been proposed.[14, 17] Indeed, in animal models, antibodies to both polypeptides are associated with protection against rotavirus illness.[18, 19]

Nine of 14 rotavirus serotypes, defined by VP7, have been recovered from humans, but only serotypes 1, 2, 3, and 4 appear to be of epidemiologic importance.[20–23] Each of the nine human rotavirus serotypes has a serotypically related animal strain.[16, 24–31] Initially, only animal rotaviruses could be cultivated in vitro. Subsequently, most human rotaviruses could be cultivated regularly after trypsin treatment and inoculation into roller tube cultures of monkey kidney cells.[32]

Several human and animal rotavirus strains that do not share the common group A antigen have been detected and classified into groups B through G according to their distinct group antigen. Although both group B and C rotavirus infections have occurred in humans, their distribution appears limited and they are not considered important causes of diarrhea in infants and young children.[33–35] The description of rotaviruses in this section is limited to group A strains unless specified otherwise.

Epidemiology

Rotavirus is the leading cause of severe diarrhea in infants and young children worldwide and is usually associated with sporadic and not epidemic gastroenteritis. In developed countries, rotavirus has been detected in 35 to 52% of infants and young children hospitalized with acute diarrhea (Fig. 3–2).[36–38] In the United States, the incidence of rotavirus diarrhea requiring hospitalization in the first and second years of life has been variously estimated to range from 3.68 and 2.22 per 1000, respectively,[39] to 11.1 and 5.8 per 1000, respectively.[40] Extrapolation from the study that reported the higher ranges suggested that 110,000 children are hospitalized each year in the United States with presumptive rotavirus diarrhea. In developing countries, rotaviruses are also the most frequently detected pathogen in children younger than 2 years with severe gastroenteritis, although bacterial agents play an important role as well.[41, 42] Rotaviruses cause significant morbidity and mortality in children younger than 5 years in the developing world, with an annual estimate of more than 125 million cases of rota-

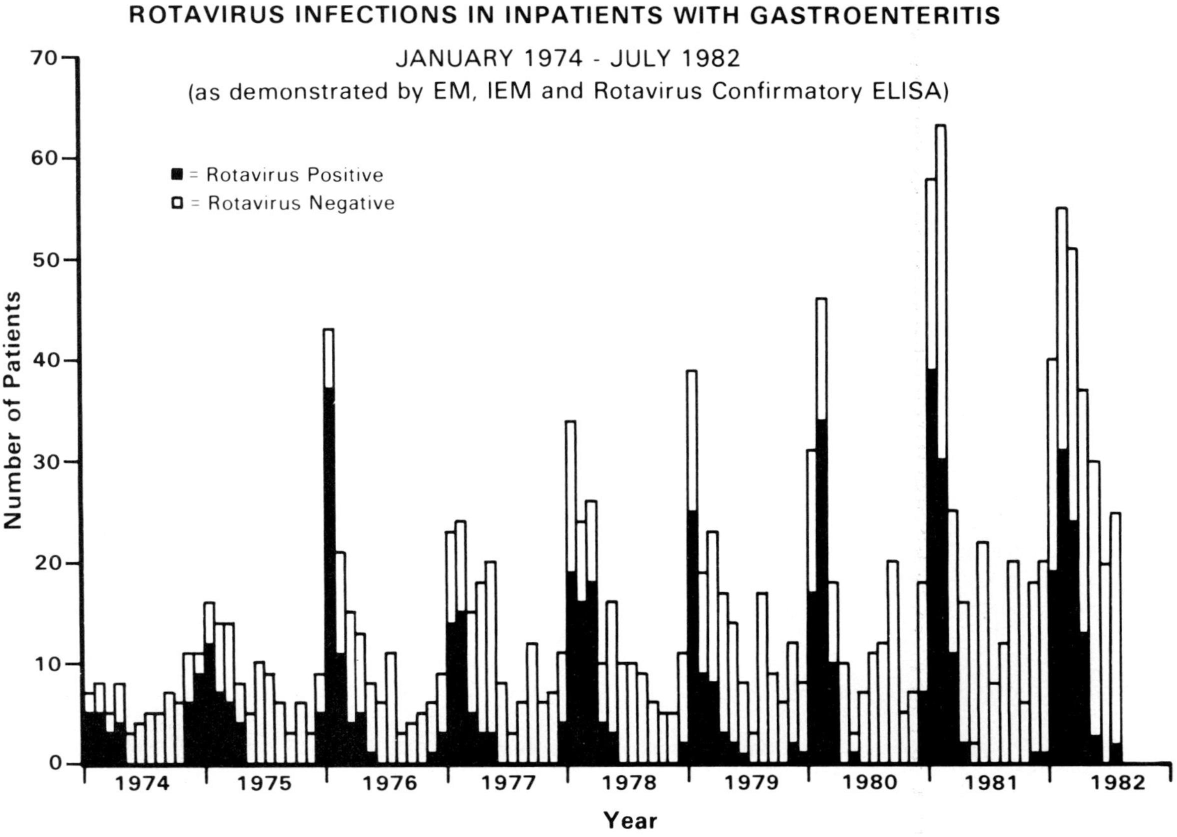

ROTAVIRUS INFECTIONS IN INPATIENTS WITH GASTROENTERITIS

FIGURE 3–2.
Seasonal distribution of rotavirus diarrhea among 1537 infants and young children hospitalized with gastroenteritis at Children's Hospital National Medical Center, Washington DC. KEY: ELISA = enzyme-linked immunosorbent assay, EM = electron microscopy, IEM = immune electron microscopy. SOURCE: Brandt CD, Kim HW, Rodriguez WJ, et al. Pediatric viral gastroenteritis during eight years of study. J Clin Microbiol. 1983;18:71–78.

virus diarrhea, of which 18 million are moderately severe or severe and 873,000 lead to death.[43] During longitudinal studies in a community setting in which all diarrheal episodes are monitored, the incidence of rotavirus diarrhea is lower than that of diarrhea caused by other pathogens but dehydration is more often associated with rotavirus than with other agents.

In temperate climates, most cases of rotavirus gastroenteritis occur during the colder months,[36, 44, 45] whereas in tropical countries, a seasonal pattern of illness is not usually observed.[46] Rotavirus diarrhea occurs most frequently in 6- to 36-month-old children, followed by infants younger than 6 months, although in a few studies, the younger group experienced the highest frequency.[45, 47] Infections have been reported frequently in newborn infants, but they are usually asymptomatic or associated with mild diarrhea.[48] The decreased susceptibility to serious rotavirus illness in this age group is unexplained. Rotavirus gastroenteritis occurs in-

frequently in adults, although subclinical infections are common.[49] Rotavirus infections have been observed in individuals with traveler's diarrhea but are not considered an important cause of this illness.[50]

The incubation period for rotavirus diarrhea is estimated to be less than 48 hours.[37] Rotaviruses are shed in large numbers in the feces and are transmitted by the fecal-oral route. The possibility of respiratory transmission has been considered because of the rapid acquisition of serum antibody in the first 3 years of life, regardless of hygienic conditions, and the failure to document fecal-oral spread in a few large outbreaks.[46, 51–53] Rotaviruses have been infrequently detected, however, in respiratory secretions.[54, 55] Animal-to-human transmission has not been documented under natural conditions, although the occasional similarity of human rotavirus isolates to animal strains has raised this possibility.[30, 56]

Nosocomial infections occur frequently in pediatric wards. In one study in the United States, 17% of 60 pediatric patients hospitalized for nondiarrheal disorders developed rotavirus diarrhea more than 72 hours after admission.[53] Asymptomatic nosocomial infections also occur commonly and have persisted in certain newborn nurseries for extended periods.[48, 57] Rotavirus gastroenteritis outbreaks have also occurred in nursing homes for the elderly.[58]

As noted earlier, rotavirus serotypes 1, 2, 3, and 4 are of epidemiologic importance. Although serotype 1 is detected most frequently, other serotypes may predominate during certain periods.[20-23] Of rotavirus groups other than group A, group B has been responsible for widespread outbreaks of gastroenteritis in adults in China and group C has been recovered occasionally from individuals with gastroenteritis in various countries.[33-35] Thus, with the exception of group B rotaviruses in China, the role of non–group A rotaviruses appears to be minor.

Pathology and Pathogenesis

In 1973, EM showed that viral particles were present in the enterocytes of duodenal mucosal biopsies from children with acute rotavirus diarrhea.[4] Histopathologic studies of such biopsy specimens revealed shortened and blunted villi with an intact mucosa, increased mononuclear cell infiltration of the lamina propria, and morphologically abnormal epithelial cells with a cuboidal appearance. The mucosal changes seen in association with the presence of rotavirus varied from mild to severe and tended to be patchy. Functional abnormalities included depressed disaccharidase levels (maltase, sucrase, lactase) in some patients with rotavirus infection.[4]

Greater understanding of the pathophysiology of rotavirus diarrhea has come from a series of studies in animals, particularly gnotobiotic colostrum-deprived calves infected with human rotaviruses.[59] In these studies, denuding of villi and flattening of epithelial cells were observed in the upper small intestine within half an hour after the onset of diarrhea, although viral antigen was not detected by immunofluorescence. At this time, the mucosa of the lower small intestine was intact, but swollen epithelial cells contained abundant viral antigens. The morphologic changes spread in a cephalocaudal direction and involved the lower small intestine after 7 hours of diarrhea. The changes were confined to the small intestine. Forty hours after onset of diarrhea, the intestine appeared relatively normal.

Studies of piglets infected with rotavirus have provided additional information on functional changes in intestinal epithelial cells.[60] Thymidine kinase and sucrase levels were measured in cells isolated from the tips of the villi of the small intestine. Within 72 hours of rotavirus infection, increased thymidine kinase and decreased sucrase levels were noted and the response of net sodium flux to glucose was abnormal (secretory). These changes presumably resulted from the transient replacement of mature, absorptive villus cells with immature crypt cells, which retained some of their secretory characteristics.

Immunity

The nature of the immune response to rotavirus infection is not well understood.[10, 61, 62] Studies of the natural history of disease and of volunteers challenged with wild-type human rotavirus suggest that serum antibody to rotavirus is associated with, but does not necessarily confer, protection from infection or disease.[63-68] Although reinfections are common, they are frequently asymptomatic in adults, who usually have detectable rotavirus antibody.[69] Likewise, children who had been infected as neonates had signficantly fewer episodes of severe rotavirus-associated diarrhea over the ensuing 3 years than did their previously uninfected counterparts, although the incidence of rotavirus infection was similar in the two groups.[48] Neonatal infections in general tend to be asymptomatic or associated only with mild diarrhea. Factors contributing to this phenomenon may include maternally acquired antibody, breast-feeding, host factors, and characteristics peculiar to neonatal rotavirus strains.[70-73]

The role of locally produced intestinal antibody in resistance to illness or infection has not been clearly established, but antibody administered via the alimentary tract to confer passive immunity has been shown to alter susceptibility to disease. In studies of newborn calves, lambs, and mice, the presence of colostrum- or serum-derived rotavirus antibody in the gut lumen at the time of challenge conferred protection against disease, whereas circulating serum antibody did not.[74-76] A recent study in gnotobiotic piglets has described a quantitative relationship between oral doses of virus-neutralizing antibody and protection from rotavirus infection or disease.[77] Passive protection has also been demonstrated in humans in various settings.[78-80] For example, in a study of low–birth-weight neonates, orally administered gamma globulin during the first week of life was associated with delayed viral excretion and milder illness when rotavirus infection occurred.[78]

Antibodies to a variety of rotavirus antigens develop during infection; neutralizing antibodies to both major neutralizing proteins, VP4 and VP7, have been shown to induce homotypic protection in animal studies.[9, 18, 19] Heterotypic immunity has been demonstrated, however, in several animal models.[81–83] The question of whether the serum neutralizing antibody response in infants after primary natural rotavirus infection is predominantly homotypic or also heterotypic needs further study because investigations have yielded variable results.[65, 84–88] Cell-mediated immunity appears to be involved in protection against rotavirus gastroenteritis in mice,[89, 90] but its importance in humans is unknown.

Clinical Findings and Diagnosis

Rotavirus infection may be asymptomatic or, alternatively, may cause diarrheal disease that ranges from mild to severe.[91–93] In a study reported in 1977, major findings associated with rotavirus diarrhea in a series of hospitalized children included vomiting, fever, and dehydration.[91] In this study, vomiting and dehydration were significantly more common in children with rotavirus diarrhea than in those with nonrotavirus diarrhea (96% vs 58% and 83% vs 40%, respectively). In the rotavirus group, the onset of vomiting frequently preceded that of diarrhea but the mean duration for vomiting was 2.6 days compared with 5 days for diarrhea; the average hospital stay was 4 days (range 2 to 14 days). The results of this study suggest that clinical laboratory findings may include elevations in blood urea nitrogen and urine specific gravity and a metabolic acidosis. Serum electrolytes and peripheral white blood cell counts are usually normal. Fecal leukocytes are occasionally found in cases of rotavirus diarrhea but are less common than in cases of diarrhea caused by bacterial pathogens.[91]

Rotavirus gastroenteritis is usually a self-limited disease when therapy for dehydration is given as needed. Diarrhea occasionally persists for longer than 14 days, often in association with lactose intolerance.[93, 94] Although severe life-threatening dehydration occurs in only a small percentage of children with rotavirus diarrhea, in developing countries it is nonetheless an important cause of mortality among children younger than 2 years. In Bangladesh, it was estimated that 42% of deaths from watery diarrhea

in this age group were due to rotavirus and that another 35% were caused by enterotoxigenic *Escherichia coli*.[42] Deaths from rotavirus diarrhea have also been documented in developed countries. In a 5-year study in Canada, 21 deaths in children 4 to 30 months of age were attributed to rotavirus. Rotavirus infection may also be especially severe or fatal in individuals immunosuppressed for bone marrow transplantation.[95] Likewise, children with severe combined immunodeficiency or malnutrition have developed persistent and severe disease.[96–99] Necrotizing enterocolitis and hemorrhagic gastroenteritis have also been associated with rotavirus infection in newborn and young infants.[100, 101]

Various conditions have been temporally associated with rotavirus infections, including Reye's syndrome, encephalitis, aseptic meningitis, benign convulsions, hemolytic-uremic syndrome, disseminated intravascular coagulation, sudden infant death syndrome, exanthem subitum, pneumonia, Kawasaki syndrome, and chronic diarrhea.[54, 55, 102–108] Because these clinical manifestations occur very infrequently in comparison with the incidence of rotavirus infection, the association appears to be temporal rather than causal.

Because clinical findings associated with rotavirus gastroenteritis are nonspecific, laboratory assays are essential to making the diagnosis. A variety of methods have been developed to detect rotavirus in feces. These methods include EM, enzyme immunoassay (EIA), latex agglutination, counterimmunoelectrophoresis, gel electrophoresis, reverse passive hemagglutination assay, dot hybridization, and polymerase chain reaction.[109–119] Although many tests for detection of group A rotaviruses are available commercially, the confirmatory EIA offers the most efficient and practical diagnostic method for large-scale epidemiologic surveys and clinical laboratories.[112, 119, 120] Electron microscopy is also highly efficient and specific and has the added advantage that it can detect both group A and non–group A rotaviruses. Enzyme immunoassays have been developed for the detection of human group B and group C rotaviruses, but the supply of reagents for these assays is limited to a few research settings.[121, 122] Although rotaviruses are almost always detected more frequently in infants and young children with diarrhea than in control subjects, subclinical infections have been observed with high frequency in certain settings.[49, 123] Therefore, the detection of rotavirus in the feces of an individual with diarrhea strongly suggests, but does not necessarily establish, an etiologic association.

The serotype and subgroup specificity of

group A rotavirus isolates can be determined by EIA and by solid-phase immune electron microscopy (SPIEM) using specialized reagents.[124–127] Many human rotaviruses can be amplified in cell cultures and then characterized further by a variety of tests, including neutralization assay and nucleotide sequence analysis.[16, 17, 72, 128, 129] The use of cell culture for the detection of rotavirus in stool specimens is impractical, however, and is somewhat less sensitive than other methods.

Rotavirus infection can also be diagnosed by serologic assays such as the complement fixation test, immune electron microscopy (IEM), and EIA.[10] The EIA can be adapted to measure levels of rotavirus-specific immunoglobulins G, M, and A (IgG, IgM, IgA) in serum, intestinal fluid, feces, and saliva.[130, 131] Neutralization assays in cell culture and epitope-blocking EIA using serotype-specific monoclonal antibodies are important techniques in defining serotype-specific serologic responses.[67, 132]

Therapy

Prevention or correction of dehydration and electrolyte imbalance is essential in the treatment of dehydrating gastroenteritis, regardless of its cause. The majority of infants and young children with mild to moderate dehydration can be treated with oral rehydration.[133–135] In cases of severe dehydration or failure of oral rehydration, intravenous fluids should be administered. The oral rehydration salts (ORS) solution recommended by the World Health Organization can be prepared by adding the following to 1 L of water: 3.5 g of sodium chloride, 1.5 g of potassium chloride, 2.9 g of trisodium citrate dihydrate (or 2.5 g of sodium bicarbonate), and 20 g of glucose.[136] The resulting solution contains 90 mmol/L of sodium, 20 mmol/L of potassium, 10 mmol/L of citrate (or 30 mmol/L of bicarbonate), and 111 mmol/L of glucose. Solutions that contain lower concentrations of sodium (50–75 mmol/L) or that are made with sucrose (40 g/L) instead of glucose have also shown good efficacy.[133, 136] In a recent study, rice-based ORS solution was associated with decreased stool output and greater absorption and retention of fluid and electrolytes compared with glucose-based ORS solution.[137] In oral rehydration therapy, the estimated fluid deficit is corrected with ORS solution within the first 6 to 8 hours. Subsequently, ORS solution and fluids such as breast milk or some other type of low-solute feeding are administered to replace losses from ongoing diarrhea and to furnish normal daily fluid requirements.

Chronic rotavirus infection in immunodeficient children has been treated successfully with human milk containing rotavirus antibodies. Treatment of normal children who have acute rotavirus diarrhea with colostrum or milk from cows immunized with human rotavirus was not, however, successful.[138] Antidiarrheal agents that alter motility of the gut are not indicated because they make it difficult to monitor continued fluid losses.[136] Oral bismuth subsalicylate used as an adjunct to rehydration therapy in infants and young children hospitalized with acute diarrhea was beneficial in mitigating clinical manifestations of illness.[139]

Prevention

Handwashing and decontamination of fomites are important measures in preventing nosocomial infections that are likely to be spread by person-to-person contact. The high incidence of rotavirus infections worldwide, regardless of hygienic conditions, underscores, however, the need for a rotavirus vaccine. Several live, attenuated oral vaccines have been evaluated in young infants. The protective efficacy of rotavirus vaccines of bovine (NCDV or WC3 strain, VP7 serotype 6) or simian (rhesus rotavirus, VP7 serotype 3) origin was highly variable, ranging from 0 to more than 80%.[140–147] A possible explanation for the variability is that monovalent vaccines do not elicit the production of heterotypic antibodies to each of the four epidemiologically important serotypes in young infants who have had no prior exposure to rotavirus. Thus, a quadrivalent vaccine composed of rhesus rotavirus (serotype 3) and human-rhesus rotavirus reassortant strains (serotypes 1, 2, and 4) is currently under evaluation.[148–150]

Other approaches to rotavirus vaccination include the use of human rotavirus strains that were isolated from neonates and may be naturally attenuated[148, 151] or that have been cold-adapted[152] as well as the use of subunit vaccines.[17, 153] Passive immunization with orally administered rotavirus antibodies is effective in preventing rotavirus illness in several animal models[75, 76] as well as in infants and young children.[79, 80, 154] Passive immunization is not practical, however, because it provides only short-lived protection.

NORWALK VIRUS GROUP AND HUMAN CALICIVIRUSES

Description and Classification

The Norwalk virus, a 27-nm particle, was first visualized by IEM in 1972. It is the prototype strain of a group of fastidious agents associated with outbreaks of acute nonbacterial gastroenteritis (Fig. 3–3).[6, 155, 156] Norwalk virus particles were found in a diarrheal stool filtrate of a volunteer who became ill after oral administration of a stool filtrate derived from a patient infected in an outbreak of acute epidemic diarrheal disease in Norwalk, OH.[157, 158] Most naturally and experimentally infected individuals developed a serologic response to the 27-nm particle visualized by IEM, providing evidence that the particle was the etiologic agent of Norwalk gastroenteritis.[6] The Norwalk virus has a single virion-associated protein with a molecular weight of 59,000 and a buoyant density in cesium chloride of 1.38 to 1.41 g per cm^3.[159, 160] The virus, which has not been cultivated in vitro, has been cloned and found to possess a single-stranded RNA genome of positive sense.[161, 162] Although the Norwalk virus does not have the classic surface morphology of most caliciviruses, it is similar to a calicivirus in its size, buoyant density, and single structural protein. Further evidence for classifying the Norwalk virus as a calicivirus was provided by a study in which 14 of 28 individuals infected with calicivirus developed a serologic response to Norwalk virus.[163] Other viruses that are morphologically similar to, but serologically distinct from, the Norwalk virus and have been associated with outbreaks of acute diarrheal disease include the Hawaii, Ditchling, and Snow Mountain agents.[156]

Human caliciviruses are 28- to 40-nm particles that have characteristically been detected in stools of pediatric patients with mild gastroenteritis.[164, 165] They have a buoyant density of 1.37 to 1.40 g per cm^3 in cesium chloride, a single-stranded RNA genome of positive sense, and a single structural protein with a molecular weight of 62,000.[166] They have cup-shaped indentations that form a six-pointed surface star with a central hollow when visualized by IEM.[167] Five distinct human calicivirus serotypes are recognized, but none has been successfully established in cell culture.[168] Antibody to calicivirus-like agents is rapidly acquired by 5 years of age,[169] suggesting that calicivirus infection is ubiquitous. Caliciviruses have been associated with outbreaks of gastroenteritis in infants and young children in an orphanage, a primary school, and day care centers.[170–175] Less frequently, caliciviruses have caused gastroenteritis outbreaks in adults, especially in the setting of nursing homes.[176, 177] A study in day care centers in the United States suggests that caliciviruses cause approximately 3% of diarrheal episodes.[173] Caliciviruses are infrequently associated with severe pediatric gastroenteritis; in studies conducted in the United States, Japan, and Ecuador, 0.3 to 1.6% of infants and young children hospitalized with diarrhea had calicivirus-like or other small, round viruses detected in their stools by EM.[36, 38, 178] With the development of an EIA for the detection of calicivirus

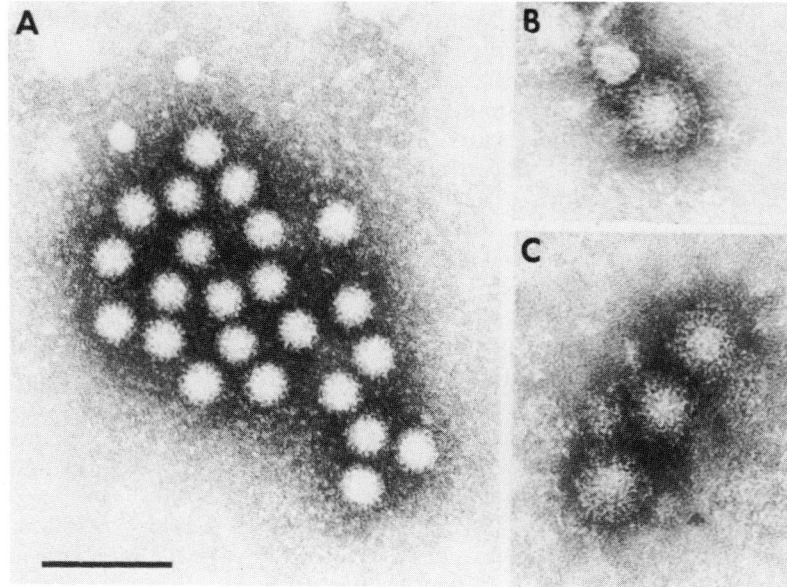

FIGURE 3–3.
Norwalk virus particles visualized by immune electron microscopy after incubation of a volunteer's prechallenge serum (*A*) and postchallenge serum (*B, C*) with Norwalk (8FIIa) stool filtrate. This volunteer developed gastroenteritis after challenge with a Norwalk stool filtrate. The quantity of antibody to Norwalk virus was rated 1 to 2 + in the prechallenge serum and 4 + in the postchallenge serum. The virus particles measure approximately 27 nm in diameter (scale bar = 100 nm applies to *A,B,* and *C*). SOURCE: Kapikian AZ, Feinstone SM, Purcell RH, et al. Detection and identification by immune electron microscopy of fastidious agents associated with respiratory illness, acute nonbacterial gastroenteritis, and hepatitis A. Perspect Virol. 1975;9:9–47.

antigen and antibody, a more thorough characterization of the epidemiology of human calicivirus infection should be possible.[179]

Other small, round viruses that are unrelated to the Norwalk group of viruses or to human caliciviruses have been detected in stools of patients with gastroenteritis, but their importance has not been established.[156] In this section, the Norwalk virus is discussed in detail as the prototype strain of the Norwalk group of agents.

Epidemiology

Norwalk virus is an important cause of acute epidemic gastroenteritis. In the original outbreak in an elementary school in Norwalk, OH, in 1968, the primary attack rate was 50% and the secondary attack rate among contacts of primary cases was approximately 32%.[157] In a survey by the CDC, 42% of 74 outbreaks of acute nonbacterial diarrheal disease that were studied serologically by radioimmunoassay (RIA) were associated with the Norwalk virus.[180] The outbreaks occurred year-round in recreational camps, cruise ships, community or family settings, and nursing homes and frequently could be attributed to a common contaminated source such as water or food. The outbreaks affected all age groups but tended to occur less frequently among infants and young children. In another study by the CDC, approximately 10% of 558 unselected outbreaks of gastroenteritis were thought to be associated with the Norwalk virus because of their clinical and epidemiologic characteristics.[181] The Snow Mountain agent, another member of the Norwalk virus group, has also been implicated in sharp outbreaks of gastroenteritis, but its overall importance has not yet been defined.[182-184]

Studies of serum antibody prevalence by RIA or immune adherence hemagglutination assay show that the Norwalk virus has a worldwide distribution.[185] In a study of the Washington, DC, area, acquisition of antibody to Norwalk virus occurred gradually during childhood and young adulthood, and by the age of 40 to 49 years, approximately 50% of individuals had detectable antibody.[52, 185] Pediatric populations in developing countries acquire antibodies to Norwalk more rapidly than do those in developed countries; for example, in Bangladesh, antibody prevalence increased from 7% in 2- to 7-month-old children to 100% in 4-year-old children.[64, 185] This study suggested that Norwalk infections might account for 1 to 2% of the episodes of mild gastroenteritis in young children in Bangladesh.[64] The Norwalk virus is not, however, an important causal agent of severe diarrheal disease in infants and young children since it is rarely found in the stools of children hospitalized with gastroenteritis.[36, 38, 178] Norwalk virus is occasionally associated with traveler's diarrhea.[186]

Norwalk virus is transmitted by the fecal-oral route, is highly infectious, and induces illness in approximately half of the volunteers studied after the oral administration of a bacteria-free stool filtrate containing the agent. The incubation period ranges from 10 to 51 hours, with a mean of 24 hours, and the illness usually lasts 12 to 60 hours.[180, 187]

Pathology and Pathogenesis

Biopsy specimens of stomach, proximal small intestine, and rectum obtained from volunteers inoculated with the Norwalk virus have been examined for histologic changes.[188, 189] Such changes were confined to the small intestine and included blunting of villi and mononuclear cell infiltration of the lamina propria; the mucosa remained intact. Selected brush border enzyme levels (alkaline phosphatase, sucrase, trehalase) were depressed during acute illness; adenylate cyclase levels were normal. Biopsy specimens obtained during the convalescent phase of illness were normal.

Immunity

Factors responsible for susceptibility to Norwalk virus infection are poorly understood. In volunteer studies, not only were preexisting serum and jejunal fluid antibodies not associated with protective immunity, but also individuals with high antibody levels were more likely to develop illness after initial challenge than were those with lower levels.[190-193] The potential for short-term immunity could be demonstrated in that volunteers who developed illness after challenge usually remained well if a rechallenge with the same inoculum occurred within a period of 6 months but not if it was delayed until 27 to 42 months after the original challenge.[192, 193] In contrast with volunteer studies, studies of natural infection in developing countries showed a correlation between the presence of serum antibody and the resistance to Norwalk virus infection.[64] Additional studies are needed to elucidate the mechanisms of short-term and long-term immunity to Norwalk virus.

Clinical Findings and Diagnosis

Norwalk gastroenteritis is characterized by the sudden onset of diarrhea or vomiting or both; fever, headache, abdominal cramps, and myalgias are common.[180] Vomiting has been observed more frequently than has diarrhea in children, whereas the reverse pattern has been observed in adults. The illnesses are usually mild and last 24 to 48 hours, although in rare instances severe dehydration requiring intravenous fluid replacement has occurred.[180] Definitive diagnosis of Norwalk gastroenteritis requires reagents that are not widely available and therefore is currently limited to research laboratories. Immune electron microscopy, RIA, and EIA have been used to detect Norwalk virus in stool specimens and to measure antibody responses in paired serum specimens.[6, 194–196] Similar assays have also been developed for the diagnosis of gastroenteritis caused by the Snow Mountain and Hawaii viruses.[196–198] The recent molecular cloning of the Norwalk genome may lead to the generation of reagents such as monoclonal antibodies and recombinant viral proteins that will greatly enhance the detection of virus particles and increases in serum antibody.[161, 162]

Therapy and Prevention

Norwalk disease is self-limited and of short duration. As with most diarrheal illnesses, oral fluid replacement is usually adequate, although intravenous rehydration may be required occasionally. Any discussion of prevention must await further studies of serotypes, immunity, and the importance of this group of viruses worldwide in acute diarrheal disease.

ASTROVIRUSES

Description and Classification

Astroviruses have been detected characteristically in stools of pediatric patients with mild gastroenteritis.[7, 155, 199, 200] They are approximately 28 nm in diameter and have a distinctive morphologic appearance under EM that is characterized by a smooth circular border, triangular surface hollows, and a five- or six-pointed surface star without a central hollow.[167] The stellate appearance may be present in about 10% of particles, and occasionally the typical morphologic features may be obscured by aggrega-

tion of the virus by antibody. The buoyant density reported for human astroviruses in cesium chloride ranges between 1.35 and 1.40 g per cm³.[201, 202] Astroviruses possess a positive-sense, single-stranded RNA genome,[202–204] but no consensus has yet been reached on the protein structure of the virus.[204] Although astroviruses share certain characteristics with both picornaviruses and caliciviruses, a final classification is not yet at hand. Five human astrovirus serotypes have been recognized; each has been cultivated successfully in cell cultures.[205]

Epidemiology

Human astroviruses have been observed worldwide in association with epidemic gastroenteritis and endemic childhood diarrhea.[7, 200, 202, 206–209] Their role in epidemic gastroenteritis appears to be minor, and their importance in childhood diarrhea is under study. Astroviruses appear to be more prevalent during the winter,[165, 210] and serotype 1 strains are detected most often.[202, 211] The acquisition of antibody to astrovirus occurs in early childhood, with over 70% of 5-year-old children having detectable antibody.[212] Astroviruses have been associated with outbreaks of diarrhea in newborn nurseries and pediatric wards[7, 199, 213, 214]; in community settings, affecting children and adults[201, 215]; and in nursing homes, affecting both patients and staff.[177, 216] Astroviruses have rarely been detected by EM examination of diarrheal stool specimens of infants and children hospitalized with gastroenteritis,[36, 38, 178] suggesting that astroviruses are not an important cause of severe gastroenteritis in this age group.

The recent development of an EIA using astrovirus-specific monoclonal antibodies has greatly enhanced the study of the epidemiology of astroviruses.[211] The EIA has been used to detect astroviruses in several recent studies of outpatient pediatric gastroenteritis. In one such study in Thailand, astroviruses were detected in 8.6% of children with gastroenteritis and 2% of children without gastroenteritis, whereas rotaviruses were detected in 19% of cases and 1% of controls, and enteric adenoviruses in 2.6% of cases and 0.5% of controls.[207] In a 2-year longitudinal study of 321 ambulatory children in Guatemala, astroviruses were detected in the specimens of 7.3% of the diarrhea episodes and in 2.4% of stool specimens obtained during diarrhea-free periods.[206] In both studies, astrovirus infection occurred most often in children younger than 1 year. A study conducted in day-care settings in the United States detected astrovirus in 4% of children with diarrhea and in fewer than 1% of controls.[208] Thus, astroviruses appear to be a relatively common cause of mild pediatric gastroenteritis.

Astroviruses are transmitted by the fecal-oral route. Two volunteer studies suggest that astrovirus is readily transmissible but of low pathogenicity in healthy adults.[217, 218] Only 1 of 17 adults (6%) and 1 of 19 adults (5%) in each study developed gastrointestinal illness characterized by vomiting and diarrhea, although serologic responses to astroviruses were detected in 10 of 16 (63%) and 9 of 19 (47%) volunteers who were tested. The illnesses in the 2 volunteers started 3 to 5 days after oral inoculation and lasted for 2 to 4 days.

Pathology and Pathogenesis

Astrovirus particles have been detected in biopsy specimens from the small intestine of 2 children hospitalized for the investigation of chronic gastrointestinal problems. Both children developed diarrhea in hospital, and astrovirus was detected by EM, within the epithelium in the lower part of the villus in one child and on the exposed surface epithelium of the other child, who had a "cow's milk–sensitive enteropathy."[219] Astrovirus was also found in the stool specimens obtained on the same day as the biopsy.[219] Although the pathogenesis of astrovirus infection in humans has not been studied further, the pathogenesis of ovine astrovirus infection in gnotobiotic lambs has been investigated. In these studies, astrovirus infected only the mature columnar epithelial cells covering the apical two thirds of the villi and the subepithelial macrophages of the small intestine. Virus particles were released when desquamated cells disintegrated in the gut lumen. Infected enterocytes were replaced by cuboidal cells from the crypts, and by 5 days after the onset of infection, the villi again appeared normal.[220, 221]

Immunity

Astrovirus infection early in life appears to provide long-lasting immunity because astrovirus gastroenteritis mainly affects infants and young children. Furthermore, healthy adult volunteers are relatively resistant to disease, and the presence of detectable antibody before inoculation is associated with resistance to infection.[217, 218]

Clinical Findings and Diagnosis

Two volunteer studies suggested that the incubation period for astrovirus gastroenteritis is 3 to 5 days, but a shorter incubation period of 24 to 36 hours was calculated from secondary transmission after an outbreak of astrovirus gastroenteritis in Japan.[201] Disease is characterized by diarrhea or vomiting or both; fever, abdominal pain, and dehydration may also occur.[201, 202, 206, 207, 216] The illness is usually of short duration, lasting 2 to 3 days in several outbreaks that affected 5- to 6-year-old children, adults, and the elderly.[177, 201, 216] In infants and children 3 years of age and younger, the median duration of disease has been 4 to 5 days,[206, 213] with a duration of as long as 35 days. Astrovirus gastroenteritis tends to be mild and self-limited and is rarely found in infants and children hospitalized with gastroenteritis.[36, 38, 178]

The diagnosis of astrovirus infection has been limited to the research setting, where EM, EIA, and immunofluorescence assay have been used to detect and to type astrovirus in stool specimens and to measure astrovirus antibodies in paired sera.[7, 202, 205, 211] The development of a broadly reactive astrovirus monoclonal antibody[211] has permitted the initiation of large epidemiologic studies to determine the role of astroviruses in gastroenteritis.

Therapy and Prevention

Astrovirus gastroenteritis is usually mild and of short duration and does not require specific therapy. As with any diarrheal disease, treatment includes oral rehydration and, if necessary, intravenous fluid administration. General hygienic measures such as handwashing and isolation strategies may be helpful in limiting person-to-person transmission in families, day care centers, and hospitals and other health care institutions. Further epidemiologic studies are needed to assess the overall importance of astrovirus and whether a vaccine might be a worthwhile objective.

ADENOVIRUS

Description and Classification

Enteric adenovirus is the second most common cause of viral diarrhea in infants and young children requiring hospitalization.[222, 223] Adenoviruses are 70 to 80 nm, double-stranded

DNA viruses that have icosahedral symmetry and a buoyant density of 1.34 g per cm^3 in cesium chloride. They are divided into six groups (A–F) and 47 serotypes.[224, 225] Enteric adenoviruses belong to group F and include serotypes 40 and 41.[226, 227] Although enteric adenoviruses have the same morphologic appearance by EM and the same group antigen as other adenoviruses, they differ in that they cannot be passaged serially in cell cultures such as human embryonic kidney and human diploid fibroblast cells that are routinely used for other adenovirus types.[228–230] The fastidious enteric types were able to be propagated in Graham 293 HEK, HeLa, HEp-2, Chang conjunctiva, and cynomolgus monkey kidney cells.[226, 227]

Epidemiology

Enteric adenovirus types 40 and 41 are second only to rotavirus in importance as causal agents of severe viral gastroenteritis in infants and children.[222, 223, 228, 231–233] They have a worldwide distribution, and acquisition of serum antibody occurs early in life and has been detected in approximately 50% of children by 4 to 5 years of age.[234, 235] Seasonal variation in enteric adenovirus infection has not usually been observed, although a summer decrease has been described.[223, 228, 231, 232, 236] Transmission presumably occurs only by the fecal-oral route because shedding of enteric adenovirus strains in the nasopharynx has not been demonstrated.[223]

In Sweden, almost 8% of acute diarrheal episodes in both hospitalized patients and outpatients combined were associated with enteric adenovirus, whereas 45% were associated with rotavirus. The median age for those infected with adenovirus type 40 or 41 was 12 months or 14 months, respectively.[233] In Korea, enteric adenovirus type 40 or 41 was detected in 9% of children hospitalized with diarrhea (mean age of 11 months) and in 2% of controls[232]; and in Italy, 8.3% of hospitalized infants and young children presumptively shed enteric adenovirus.[231] In a study of infants and young children hospitalized with diarrhea or other conditions in the United States, 4.1% of the group with diarrhea and 1% of the control group shed an adenovirus that was detectable by EM or IEM but not by tissue culture methods used to isolate nonenteric strains of adenoviruses; over 90% of such adenoviruses were identified as enteric adenoviruses by restriction endonuclease electrophoretic profile or by neutralization assay.[228] Children hospitalized with enteric adenovirus gastroenteritis ranged in age from 1 to 16 months, with a median age of 7 months. Rotaviruses were detected in 35% of a similar inpatient group hospitalized with diarrheal illness.[36]

In outpatient studies, enteric adenoviruses characteristically account for as much as 4% of acute diarrheal episodes.[207, 228, 237–239] They are also a common cause of pediatric gastroenteritis in day care settings.[208, 240]

Adenoviruses have occasionally been associated with fatal cases of gastroenteritis,[230, 241] and with intussusception.[242] Adenoviruses of unknown type were detected in 12 of 31 bone marrow transplant patients with gastroenteritis (39%) and were associated with 6 deaths (50%) in this group.[95] They have also been implicated as a cause of gastroenteritis in other immunosuppressed patients, of whom many had a fatal outcome.[95, 243, 244]

Clinical Findings and Diagnosis

Enteric adenovirus infections have an incubation period of 8 to 10 days, and illness is characterized by watery diarrhea with a mean duration of 9 days for serotype 40 and 12 days for serotype 41.[233] Prolonged diarrhea lasting 14 days or longer was observed in one third of children with type 40 infections. Vomiting, fever, and dehydration may occur and are usually mild.

Various techniques are available for the detection of adenovirus in stools. Diagnosis can be made by group-specific EIA, latex agglutination, or EM.[245–248] A serotype-specific EIA, IEM, or SPIEM can identify the enteric adenovirus types 40 and 41.[248–252] DNA restriction analysis and tissue culture neutralization are also useful in serotype identification.[226, 227, 253, 254] A commercially available EIA in which monoclonal antibodies to type 40 and 41 are used is available.[251] In a recent report, however, a variant of enteric adenovirus type 41 that was the most frequent cause of adenovirus gastroenteritis in a community could not be detected by the commercial kit.[255]

Therapy and Prevention

As with other diarrheal illnesses, the dehydration associated with adenovirus gastroenteritis should be treated with oral rehydration solutions or, if necessary, with parenteral rehydration. Basic hygienic measures should be practiced to limit transmission in hospital, clinical, and day care settings. Further study is needed to determine the need for a vaccine against enteric adenovirus.

REFERENCES

1. Dingle JH, Badger GF, Jordan WS. Illness in the Home: A Study of 25,000 Illnesses in a Group of Cleveland Families. Cleveland, OH: Case Western Reserve University Press; 1964:19.
2. Ho M-S, Glass RI, Pinsky PF, Anderson L. Rotavirus as a cause of diarrheal morbidity and mortality in the United States. J Infect Dis. 1988;158:1112–1116.
3. Walsh JA, Warren, KS. Selective primary health care: An interim strategy for disease control in developing countries. N Engl J Med. 1979;301:967–974.
4. Bishop RF, Davidson GP, Holmes IH, et al. Virus particles in epithelial cells of duodenal mucosa from children with acute gastroenteritis. Lancet. 1973;2:1281–1283.
5. Flewett TH, Bryden AS, Davies H. Diagnostic electron microscopy of faeces: I, The viral flora of the faeces as seen by electron microscopy. J Clin Pathol. 1974;27:603–608.
6. Kapikian AZ, Wyatt RG, Dolin R, et al. Visualization by immune electron microscopy of a 27-nm particle associated with acute infectious nonbacterial gastroenteritis. J Virol. 1972;10:1075–1081.
7. Madeley, CR, Cosgrove BP. Viruses in infantile gastroenteritis. Lancet. 1975;2:124.
8. Wyatt RG, Kalica AR, Mebus CA, et al. Reovirus-like agents (rotaviruses) associated with diarrheal illness in animals and man. In: Pollard M, ed. Perspectives in Virology. New York: Raven Press; 1978;10:121–145.
9. Estes MK. Rotaviruses and their replication. In: Fields BN, Knipe DM, Chanock RM, et al., eds. Virology. 2nd ed. New York: Raven Press; 1990:1329–1352.
10. Kapikian AZ, Chanock RM. Rotaviruses. In: Fields BN, Knipe DM, Chanock RM, et al., eds. Virology. 2nd ed. New York: Raven Press; 1990:1353–1404.
11. Prasad BV, Wang GJ, Clerx JPM, et al. Three-dimensional structure of rotavirus. J Mol Biol. 1988;199:269–275.
12. Browning GF, Chalmers RM, Fitzgerald TA, et al. Evidence for two serotype G3 subtypes among equine rotavirus. J Clin Microbiol. 1992;30:485–491.
13. Kalica AR, Greenberg HB, Wyatt RG, et al. Genes of human (strain Wa) and bovine (strain UK) rotaviruses that code for neutralization and subgroup antigens. Virology. 1981;112:385–390.
14. Hoshino Y, Sereno MM, Midthun K, et al. Independent segregation of two antigenic specificities (VP3 and VP7) involved in neutralization of rotavirus infectivity. Proc Natl Acad Sci U S A. 1985;82:8701–8704.
15. Kalica AR, Flores J, Greenberg HB. Identification of the rotaviral gene that codes for hemagglutination and protease-enhanced plaque formation. Virology. 1983;125:194–205.
16. Hoshino Y, Wyatt RG, Greenberg HB, et al. Serotypic similarity and diversity of rotaviruses of mammalian and avian origin as studied by plaque reduction neutralization. J Infect Dis. 1984;149:694–702.
17. Gorziglia M, Larralde G, Kapikian AZ, Chanock RM. Antigenic relationships among human rotaviruses as determined by outer capsid protein VP4. Proc Natl Acad Sci USA. 1989;159:753–757.
18. Hoshino Y, Saif LJ, Sereno MM, et al. Infection immunity of piglets to either VP3 or VP7 outer capsid protein confers resistance to challenge with a virulent rotavirus bearing the corresponding antigen. J Virol. 1988;62:744–748.
19. Offit PA, Clark HF, Blavat G, Greenberg HB. Reassortant rotaviruses containing structural proteins VP3 and VP7 from different parents induce antibodies protective against each parental serotype. J Virol. 1986;60:491–496.
20. Birch CJ, Heath RL, Gust ID. Use of serotype-specific monoclonal antibodies to study the epidemiology of rotavirus infection. J Med Virol. 1988;24:45–53.
21. Matson DO, Estes MK, Burns JW. Serotype variation of human group A rotaviruses in two regions in the USA. J Infect Dis. 1990;162:605–614.
22. Nakagomi O, Nakagomi T, Akatani K, et al. Relative frequency of rotavirus serotypes in Yamagata, Japan, over four consecutive rotavirus seasons. Res Virol. 1991;141:459–463.
23. Woods PA, Gentsch J, Gouvea V, et al. Distribution of serotypes of human rotavirus in different populations. J Clin Microbiol. 1992;30:781–785.
24. Hoshino Y, Kapikian AZ. Rotavirus antigens. Curr Top Microbiol Immunol. 1994;185:179–227.
25. Matsuno S, Hasegawa A, Mukoyama A, et al. A candidate for a new serotype of human rotavirus. J Virol. 1985;54:623–624.
26. Clark HF, Hoshino Y, Bell LM, et al. Rotavirus isolate W161 representing a presumptive new human serotype. J Clin Microbiol. 1987;25:1757–1762.
27. Urasawa S, Urasawa T, Wakasugi F, et al. Presumptive seventh serotype of human rotavirus. Arch Virol. 1990;113:279–282.
28. Browning GF, Chalmers RM, Fitzgerald TA, et al. Serological and genomic characterization of L338, a novel equine group G serotype. J Gen Virol. 1991;72:1059–1064.
29. Browning GF, Fitzgerald TA, Chalmers RM, et al. A novel group A rotavirus serotype: Serological and genomic characterization of equine isolate FI23. J Clin Microbiol. 1991;29:2043–2046.
30. Gerna G, Sarasini A, Parea M, et al. Isolation and characterization of two distinct human rotavirus strains with G6 specificity. J Clin Microbiol. 1992;30:9–16.
31. Beards G, Xu L, Ballard A, et al. A serotype 10 human rotavirus. J Clin Microbiol. 1992;30:1432–1435.
32. Urasawa T, Urasawa S, Taniguchi K. Sequential passages of human rotavirus in MA-104 cells. Microbiol Immunol. 1981;25:1025–1035.
33. Dai GZ, Sun M-S, Liu S-Q, et al. First report of an epidemic of diarrhea in human neonates involving the new rotavirus and biological characteristics of the epidemic strain (KMB/R85). J Med Virol. 1985;22:365–373.
34. Hung T. Rotavirus and adult diarrhea. Adv Virus Res. 1988;35:193–218.
35. Penaranda M, Cubitt WD, Sinarachatanant P, et al. Group C rotavirus infections in patients with diarrhea in Thailand, Nepal, and England. J Infect Dis. 1989;160:392–397.
36. Brandt CD, Kim HW, Rodriguez WJ, et al. Pediatric viral gastroenteritis during eight years of study. J Clin Microbiol. 1983;18:71–78.
37. Davidson GP, Bishop RF, Townley RR, et al. Importance of a new virus in acute sporadic enteritis in children. Lancet. 1975;1:242–245.
38. Konno T, Suzuki H, Katsushima N, et al. Influence of temperature and relative humidity on human rotavirus infection in Japan. J Infect Dis. 1983;147:125–128.
39. Rodriguez WJ, Kim HW, Brandt CD, et al. Rotavirus gastroenteritis in the Washington, DC area: Incidence of cases resulting in admission to the hospital. Am J Dis Child. 1980;134:777–779.

40. Matson DO, Estes MK. Impact of rotavirus infection at a large pediatric hospital. J Infect Dis. 1991;162:598–604.

41. Bingnan F, Unicomb L, Rahim Z, et al. Rotavirus-associated diarrhea in rural Bangladesh: Two-year study of incidence and serotype distribution. J Clin Microbiol. 1991;29:1359–1363.

42. Black RE, Merson MH, Mizanur Rahman ASM, et al. A 2-year study of bacterial, viral and parasitic agents associated with diarrhea in rural Bangladesh. J Infect Dis. 1980;142:660–664.

43. Institute of Medicine. Prospects for immunizing against rotavirus. In: New Vaccine Development, Establishing Priorities: Diseases of Importance in Developing Countries. Washington, DC: National Academy Press; 1986;12:308–318.

44. Brandt CD, Kim HW, Rodriguez WJ, et al. Gastroenteritis and human reovirus-like agent infection during the 1975–76 outbreak: An electron microscopic study. Clin Proc, Children's Hosp, Nat Med Center. 1977;33:21–26.

45. Kapikian AZ, Kim HW, Wyatt RG, et al. Human reovirus-like agent as the major pathogen associated with "winter" gastroenteritis in hospitalized infants and young children. N Engl J Med. 1976;294:965–972.

46. Cook SM, Glass RI, LeBaron CW, Ho M-S. Global seasonality of rotavirus infections. Bull WHO. 1990;68:171–177.

47. Birch CJ, Lewis FA, Kennett ML, et al. A study of prevalence of rotavirus infection in children with gastroenteritis admitted to an infectious diseases hospital. J Med Virol. 1977;1:69–77.

48. Bishop RF, Barnes GL, Cipriani E, et al. Clinical immunity after neonatal rotavirus infection: A prospective longitudinal study in young children. N Engl J Med. 1983;309:72–76.

49. Rodriguez, WJ, Kim HW, Brandt CD, et al. Longitudinal study of rotavirus infection and gastroenteritis in families served by a pediatric medical practice: Clinical and epidemiologic observations. Pediatr Infect Dis J. 1987;6:170–176.

50. Black RE. Epidemiology of travelers' diarrhea and relative importance of various pathogens. Rev Infect Dis. 1990;12:S73–S79.

51. Foster SO, Palmer EL, Gary GW Jr. Gastroenteritis due to rotavirus in an isolated Pacific island group: An epidemic of 3439 cases. J Infect Dis. 1980;141:32–39.

52. Kapikian AZ, Greenberg HB, Cline WL, et al. Prevalence of antibody to the Norwalk agent by a newly developed immune adherence hemagglutination assay. J Med Virol. 1978;2:281–294.

53. Ryder RW, McGowan JE, Hatch MH, et al. Reovirus-like agent as a cause of nosocomial diarrhea in infants. J Pediatr. 1977;90:698–702.

54. Santosham M, Yolken RH, Quiroz E, et al. Detection of rotavirus in respiratory secretions of children with pneumonia. J Pediatr. 1983;103:58.

55. Zhaori GT, Fu LT, Xu YH, et al. Detection of rotavirus antigen in tracheal aspirates of infants and children with pneumonia. Chin Med J. 1991;104:830–833.

56. Nakagomi O, Mochizuki M, Aboudy Y, et al. Hemagglutination by a human rotavirus isolate as evidence of transmission of animal rotavirus to humans. J Clin Microbiol. 1992;30:1011–1013.

57. Eiden JJ, Verleur DG, Vonderfecht SL, et al. Duration and pattern of asymptomatic rotavirus shedding by hospitalized children. Pediatr Infect Dis J. 1988;7:564–569.

58. Marrie TJ, Lee SHS, Faulkner RS, et al. Rotavirus infection in a geriatric population. Arch Intern Med. 1982;142:313–316.

59. Mebus CA, Wyatt RG, Kapikian AZ. Pathology of diarrhea in gnotobiotic calves induced by the human reovirus-like agent of infantile gastroenteritis. Vet Pathol. 1977;14:273–282.

60. Gall DG. Pathophysiology of viral diarrhea. In: Proceedings of 73rd Ross Conference on Pediatric Research: Etiology, pathology, and treatment of acute gastroenteritis, Ponte Vedra Beach, FL: March 20–22, 1977.

61. Bishop R, Lund J, Cipriani E, et al. Clinical, serological and intestinal immune responses to rotavirus infection of humans. Med Virol. 1990;9:85–109.

62. Matsui SM, Mackow ER, Greenberg HB. Molecular determinant of rotavirus neutralization and protection. Adv Virus Res. 1989;36:181–214.

63. Bernstein DI, Sander DS, Smith VE, et al. Protection from rotavirus reinfection: 2-year prospective study. J Infect Dis. 1991;164:277–283.

64. Black RE, Greenberg HB, Kapikian AZ, et al. Acquisition of serum antibody to Norwalk enteritis virus and rotavirus and relation to diarrhea in a longitudinal study of young children in rural Bangladesh. J Infect Dis. 1982;145:483–489.

65. Chiba S, Yokoyama T, Nakata S, et al. Protective effect of naturally acquired homotypic and heterotypic rotavirus antibodies. Lancet. 1986;2:417–421.

66. Clemens JD, Ward RL, Rao MR, et al. Seroepidemiologic evaluation of antibodies to rotavirus as correlates of risk of clinically significant rotavirus diarrhea in rural Bangladesh. J Infect Dis. 1992;165:161–165.

67. Kapikian AZ, Wyatt RG, Levine MM, et al. Oral administration of human rotavirus to volunteers: Induction of illness and correlates of resistance. J Infect Dis. 1983;147:95–106.

68. Ward RL, Bernstein DI, Shukla R, et al. Effects of antibody to rotavirus on protection of adults challenged with a human rotavirus. J Infect Dis. 1989;159:79–88.

69. Kim HW, Brandt CD, Kapikian AZ, et al. Human reovirus-like agent (HRVLA) infection: Occurrence in adult contacts of pediatric patients with gastroenteritis. JAMA. 1977;238:404–407.

70. Chrystie IL, Totterdell BM, Banatvala JE. Asymptomatic endemic rotavirus infection in the newborn. Lancet. 1978;1:1176–1178.

71. Flores J, Midthun K, Hoshino Y, et al. Conservation of the fourth gene among rotaviruses recovered from asymptomatic newborn infants and its possible role in attenuation. J Virol. 1986;60:972–979.

72. Gorziglia M, Green K, Nishikawa K, et al. Sequence of the fourth gene of human rotaviruses recovered from asymptomatic or symptomatic infections. J Virol. 1988;62:2978–2984.

73. Pichichero ME. Effect of breast feeding on oral rhesus rotavirus vaccine seroconversion: A meta-analysis. J Infect Dis. 1990;162:753–755.

74. Bridger JC, Woode GN. Neonatal calf diarrhea: Identification of a reovirus-like (rotavirus) agent in feces by immunofluorescence and immune electron microscopy. Br Vet J. 1975;131:528–535.

75. Offit PA, Clark HF. Protection against rotavirus-induced gastroenteritis in a murine model by passively acquired gastrointestinal but not circulating antibodies. J Virol. 1985;54:58–64.

76. Snodgrass DR, Wells PW. Rotavirus infection in lambs: Studies on passive protection. Arch Virol. 1976;52:201–205.

77. Shaller JP, Saif LJ, Cordle CT, et al. Prevention of human rotavirus-induced diarrhea in gnotobiotic piglets using bovine antibody. J Infect Dis. 1992;165:623–630.

78. Barnes GL, Doyle LW, Hewson PH, et al. A randomized trial of oral gamma globulin in low–birth-weight

infants infected with rotavirus. Lancet. 1982;1:1371–1373.

79. Davidson GP, Whyte PBD, Daniels E, et al. Passive immunization of children with bovine colostrum containing antibodies to human rotavirus. Lancet. 1989;2:709–712.

80. Ebina T, Sato A, Umezu K, et al. Prevention of rotavirus infection by oral administration of cow colostrum containing antihuman rotavirus antibody. Med Microbiol Immunol. 1985;174:177–185.

81. Bishop RF, Tzipori SR, Coulson BS, et al. Heterologous protection against rotavirus-induced disease in gnotobiotic piglets. J Clin Microbiol. 1986;24:1023–1028.

82. Wyatt RG, Mebus CA, Yolken RH, et al. Rotaviral immunity in gnotobiotic calves: Heterologous resistance to human virus induced by bovine virus. Science. 1975;203:548–550.

83. Zissis G, Lambert JP, Marbehant P, et al. Protection studies in colostrum-deprived piglets of a bovine rotavirus vaccine candidate using human rotavirus strains for challenge. J Infect Dis. 1983;148:1061–1068.

84. Brussow H, Werchau H, Lerner L, et al. Seroconversion patterns to four human rotavirus serotypes in hospitalized infants with acute rotavirus gastroenteritis. J Infect Dis. 1988;158:588–595.

85. Clark HF, Dolan K, Horton-Slight P, et al. Diverse serologic response to rotavirus infection of infants in a single epidemic. Pediatr Infect Dis. 1985;4:626–631.

86. Gerna G, Sarasini A, Torsellini M, et al. Group- and type-specific serologic response in infants and children with primary rotavirus infections and gastroenteritis caused by a strain of known serotype. J Infect Dis. 1990;161:1105–1111.

87. Puerto FI, Padilla-Noriega L, Zamoro-Chavez A, et al. Prevalent pattern of serotype-specific seroconversion in Mexican children infected with rotavirus. J Clin Microbiol. 1987;25:960–963.

88. Zheng B-J, Han S-X, Yan Y-K, et al. Development of neutralizing antibodies and group A common antibodies against natural infections with human rotavirus. J Clin Microbiol. 1988;26:1506–1512.

89. Dharakul T, Rott L, Greenberg HB. Recovery from chronic rotavirus infection in mice with severe combined immunodeficiency: Virus clearance mediated by adoptive transfer of immune CD8+ T lymphocytes. J Virol. 1990;64:4375–4382.

90. Offit PA, Dudzik KI. Rotavirus-specific cytotoxic T lymphocytes passively protect against gastroenteritis in suckling mice. J Virol. 1990;64:6325–6328.

91. Rodriguez WJ, Kim HW, Arrobio JO, et al. Clinical features of acute gastroenteritis associated with human reovirus-like agent in infants and young children. J Pediatr. 1977;91:188–193.

92. Shepherd RW, Truslow S, Walker-Smith JA, et al. Infantile gastroenteritis: A clinical study of reovirus-like agent infection. Lancet. 1975;2:1082–1084.

93. Tallet S, MacKenzie C, Middleton P, et al. Clinical, laboratory, and epidemiological features of a viral gastroenteritis in infants and children. Pediatrics. 1977;60:217–222.

94. Khoshoo V, Bhan MK, Jayashree S, et al. Rotavirus infection and persistent diarrhea in young children. Lancet. 1990;2:1314–1315.

95. Yolken RH, Bishop CA, Townsend TR, et al. Infectious gastroenteritis in bone-marrow transplant recipients. N Engl J Med. 1982;306:1009–1012.

96. Brown KH, Gilman RH, Gaffar A, et al. Infections associated with severe protein-calorie malnutrition in hospitalized infants and children. Nutr Res. 1981;1:33–46.

97. Dagan R, Bar-David Y, Sarov B, et al. Rotavirus diarrhea in Jewish and Bedouin children in the Negev region of Israel: Epidemiology, clinical aspects and possible role of malnutrition in severity of illness. Pediatr Infect Dis J. 1990;9:314–321.

98. Eiden J, Losonsky GA, Johnson J, Yolken RH. Rotavirus RNA variation during chronic infection of immunocompromised children. Pediatr Infect Dis. 1985;4:632–637.

99. Jarvis WR, Middleton PJ, Gelfand EW. Significance of viral infections in severe combined immunodeficiency disease. Pediatr Infect Dis. 1983;2:187–192.

100. Dearlove J, Latham P, Dearlove B, et al. Clinical range of neonatal rotavirus gastroenteritis. Br Med J. 1983;286:1473–1475.

101. Rotbart HA, Nelson WL, Glode MP, et al. Neonatal rotavirus-associated necrotizing enterocolitis: Case control study and prospective surveillance during an outbreak. J Pediatr. 1988;112:87–93.

102. Flewett TH. Clinical features of rotavirus infections. In: Tyrrell DAJ, Kapikian AZ, eds. Virus Infections of the Gastrointestinal Tract. New York: Marcel Dekker; 1982:125–145.

103. Matsuno S, Utagawa E, Sugiura A: Association of rotavirus infection with Kawasaki syndrome. J Infect Dis. 1983;148:177.

104. Saitoh Y, Matsuno S, Mukoyama A. Exanthem subitum and rotavirus. N Engl J Med 1981;304:845.

105. Salmi TT, Arstila P, Koivikko A. Central nervous system involvement in patients with rotavirus gastroenteritis. Scand J Infect Dis. 1978;10:29–31.

106. Ushijima H, Tajima T, Tagaya M, et al. Rotavirus and the central nervous system. Brain Dev. 1984;6:215.

107. Wong CJ, Price Z, Bruckner DA. Aseptic meningitis in an infant with rotavirus gastroenteritis. Pediatr Infect Dis. 1984;3:244–246.

108. Yolken RH, Murphy M. Sudden infant death syndrome associated with rotavirus infection. J Med Virol. 1982;10:291–296.

109. Bishop RF, Davidson GP, Holmes IH, et al. Detection of a new virus by electron microscopy of fecal extracts from children with acute gastroenteritis. Lancet. 1974;1:149–151.

110. Brandt CD, Kim HW, Rodriguez WJ, et al. Comparison of direct electron microscopy, immune electron microscopy, and rotavirus enzyme-linked immunosorbent assay for detection of gastroenteritis viruses in children. J Clin Microbiol. 1981;13:976–981.

111. Doern GV, Herrmann JE, Henderson P, et al. Detection of rotavirus with a new polyclonal antibody enzyme immunoassay (Rotazyme II) and a commercial latex agglutination test (Rotalex): Comparison with a monoclonal antibody enzyme immunoassay. J Clin Microbiol. 1986;23:226–229.

112. Flewett TH, Arias CF, Avendano LF, et al. Comparative evaluation of the WHO and DAKOPATTS enzyme-linked immunoassay kits for rotavirus detection. Bull WHO. 1989;67:369–374.

113. Flores J, Boeggeman E, Purcell RH, et al. A dot hybridization assay for detection of rotavirus. Lancet. 1983;1:555–558.

114. Hammond GW, Ahluwalia GS, Klisko B, et al. Human rotavirus detection by counterimmunoelectrophoresis versus enzyme immunoassay and electron microscopy after direct ultracentrifugation. J Clin Microbiol. 1984;19:439–441.

115. Herring AJ, Inglis NF, Ojeh CK, et al. Rapid diagnosis of rotavirus infection by direct detection of viral nucleic acid in silver-stained polyacrylamide gels. J Clin Microbiol. 1982;16:473–477.

116. Kapikian AZ, Kim HW, Wyatt RG, et al. Reovirus-like agent in stools: Association with infantile diarrhea and

development of serologic tests. Science. 1974; 185:1049–1053.

117. Sanekata T, Yoshida Y, Oda K. Detection of rotavirus from faeces by reversed passive hemagglutination method. J Clin Pathol. 1979;32:963.

118. Wilde J, Yolken R, Willoughby R, Eiden J. Improved detection of rotavirus shedding by polymerase chain reaction. Lancet. 1991;337:323–326.

119. Yolken RH, Wyatt RG, Kapikian AZ. ELISA for rotavirus. Lancet. 1977;2:819. Letter.

120. Kapikian AZ, Yolken RH, Greenberg HB, et al. Gastroenteritis viruses. In: Lennette EH, Schmidt NJ, eds. Diagnostic Procedures for Viral, Rickettsial, and Chlamydial Infections. Washington DC: American Public Health Association; 1979:927–995.

121. Fuji R, Kuzuya M, Hamano M, et al. Detection of human group C rotaviruses by an enzyme-linked immunosorbent assay using monoclonal antibodies. J Clin Microbiol. 1992;30:1307–1311.

122. Vonderfecht SL, Miskuff RL, Eiden JJ, et al. Enzyme immunoassay inhibition assay for detection of rat rotavirus-like agent in intestinal and fecal specimens obtained from diarrheic rats and humans. J Clin Microbiol. 1985;22:726–730.

123. Champosaur H, Questiaux E, Prevot J, et al. Rotavirus carriage, asymptomatic infection, and disease in the first two years of life: I, Virus shedding. J Infect Dis. 1984;149:667–674.

124. Gerna G, Passarani N, Battaglia M, et al. Rapid serotyping of human rotavirus strains by solid-phase immune electron microscopy. J Clin Microbiol. 1984;19:273–278.

125. Green KY, James HD Jr, Kapikian AZ. Evaluation of three panels of monoclonal antibodies for the identification of human rotavirus VP7 serotype by ELISA. Bull WHO. 1990;68:601–610.

126. Greenberg HB, McAuliffe V, Valdesuso J, et al. Serological analysis of the subgroup protein of rotavirus, using monoclonal antibodies. Infect Immun. 1983;39:91–99.

127. Taniguchi K, Urasawa T, Morita Y, et al. Direct serotyping of human rotavirus in stools using serotype 1-, 2-, 3-, and 4-specific monoclonal antibodies to VP7. J Infect Dis. 1987;155:1159–1166.

128. Green KY, Midthun K, Gorziglia M, et al. Comparison of amino acid sequences of the major neutralization protein of four human rotavirus serotypes. Virology. 1987;161:153–159.

129. Wyatt RG, James HD Jr, Pittman AL, et al. Direct isolation in cell culture of human rotaviruses and their characterization into four serotypes. J Clin Microbiol. 1983;18:310–317.

130. Grimwood K, Lund JCS, Coulson BS, et al. Comparison of serum and mucosal antibody responses following severe acute rotavirus gastroenteritis in young children. J Clin Microbiol. 1988;26:732–738.

131. Jayashree S, Bhan MK, Kumar R, et al. Serum and salivary antibodies as indicators of rotavirus infection in neonates. J Infect Dis. 1988;158:1117–1120.

132. Green KY, Taniguchi K, Mackow ER, Kapikian AZ. Homotypic and heterotypic epitope-specific antibody responses in adult and infant rotavirus vaccinees: Implications for vaccine development. J Infect Dis. 1990;161:667–679.

133. Sack DA, Chowdhury AMAK, Eusof A, et al. Oral rehydration in rotavirus diarrhea: A double blind comparison of sucrose with glucose electrolyte solution. Lancet. 1978;2:280–283.

134. Santosham M, Burns B, Nadkarni V, et al. Oral rehydration therapy for acute diarrhea in ambulatory children in the United States: A double-blind comparison of four different solutions. Pediatrics. 1985;76:159–166.

135. Santosham M, Daum RS, Dillman L, et al. Oral rehydration therapy of infantile diarrhea: A controlled study of well-nourished children hospitalized in the United States and Panama. N Engl J Med. 1982;306:1070–1076.

136. Avery ME, Snyder JD. Oral therapy for acute diarrhea: The underused simple solution. N Engl J Med. 1990;323:891–894.

137. Pizarro D, Posada G, Sandi L, Moran JR. Rice-based oral electrolyte solutions for the management of infantile diarrhea. N Engl J Med. 1991;324:517–521.

138. Hilpert H, Brussow H, Mietens C, et al. Use of bovine milk concentrate containing antibody to rotavirus to treat rotavirus gastroenteritis in infants. J Infect Dis. 1987;156:158–166.

139. Soriano-Brucher H, Avendano P, O'Ryan M, et al. Bismuth subsalicylate in the treatment of acute diarrhea in children. Pediatrics. 1991;87:18–27.

140. Bernstein DI, Smith VE, Sander DS, et al. Evaluation of WC3 rotavirus and correlates of protection in healthy infants. J Infect Dis. 1990;162:1055–1062.

141. Clark HF, Borian FE, Bell LM, et al. Protective effect of WC3 vaccine against rotavirus diarrhea in infants during a predominantly serotype 1 rotavirus season. J Infect Dis. 1988;158:570–587.

142. Flores J, Perez-Schael I, Gonzalez M, et al. Protection against severe rotavirus diarrhea by rhesus rotavirus vaccine in Venezuelan infants. Lancet. 1987;1:882–884.

143. Kapikian AZ, Flores J, Hoshino Y, et al. Rotavirus: The major etiologic agent of severe infantile diarrhea may be controlled by a "Jennerian" approach to vaccination. J Infect Dis. 1986;153:815–822.

144. Lanata CF, Black RE, del Aguila R, et al. Protection of Peruvian children against rotavirus diarrhea of specific serotypes by one, two, or three doses of the RIT 4237 attenuated bovine rotavirus vaccine. J Infect Dis. 1989;159:452–459.

145. Madore HP, Christy C, Pichichero M, et al. Field trial of rhesus rotavirus or human-rhesus rotavirus reassortant vaccine of VP7 serotype 3 or 1 specificity in infants. J Infect Dis. 1992;166:235–243.

146. Santosham M, Letson GW, Wolff M, et al. A field study of the safety and efficacy of two candidate rotavirus vaccines in a native American population. J Infect Dis. 1991;163:483–487.

147. Vesikari T, Isolauri E, D'Hondt E, et al. Protection of infants against rotavirus diarrhoea by RIT4237 attenuated bovine rotavirus strain vaccine. Lancet. 1984;1:977–981.

148. Flores J, Perez-Schael I, Blanco M, et al. Comparison of reactogenicity and antigenicity of M37 rotavirus vaccine and rhesus-rotavirus-based quadrivalent vaccine. Lancet. 1990;2:330–334.

149. Midthun K, Greenberg HB, Hoshino Y, et al. Reassortant rotaviruses as potential live rotavirus vaccine candidates. J Virol. 1985;53:949–954.

150. Midthun K, Hoshino Y, Kapikian AZ, Chanock RM. Single gene substitution rotavirus reassortants containing the major neutralization protein (VP7) of human rotavirus serotype 4. J Clin Microbiol. 1986;24:822–826.

151. Midthun K, Halsey NA, Jett-Goheen M, et al. Safety and immunogenicity of human rotavirus vaccine strains M37 in adults, children, and infants. J Infect Dis. 1991;164:792–796.

152. Matsuno S, Murakami S, Tagaki M, et al. Cold adaptation of human rotavirus. Virus Res. 1987;7:273–280.

153. Streckert H-J, Brussow H, Werchau H. A synthetic peptide corresponding to the cleavage region of VP3 from rotavirus SA11 induces neutralizing antibodies. J Virol. 1988;62:4265–4269.

154. Brussow H, Hilpert H, Walther I, et al. Bovine milk

immunoglobulins for passive immunity to infantile rotavirus gastroenteritis. J Clin Microbiol. 1987;25:982–
986.
155. Greenberg HB, Matsui SM. Astroviruses and caliciviruses: Emerging enteric pathogens. Infect Agents Dis—
Reviews, Issues and Commentary. 1992;1(2):71–91.
156. Kapikian AZ, Chanock RM. The Norwalk group of viruses. In: Fields BN, Knipe DM, Chanock RM, et al,
eds. Virology. 2nd ed. New York: Raven Press;
1990:671–693.
157. Adler I, Zickl R. Winter vomiting disease. J Infect Dis.
1969;119:668–673.
158. Dolin R, Blacklow NR, DuPont H, et al. Transmission
of acute infectious nonbacterial gastroenteritis to volunteers by oral administration of stool filtrates. J Infect
Dis. 1971;123:307–312.
159. Greenberg HB, Valdesuso J, Kalica AR, et al. Proteins
of Norwalk virus. J Virol. 1981;37:994–999.
160. Kapikian AZ, Gerin JL, Wyatt RG, et al. Density in
cesium chloride of the 27-nm "8FIIa" particle associated with acute infectious nonbacterial gastroenteritis:
Determination by ultracentrifugation and immune
electron microscopy. J Infect Dis. 1974;129:709–714.
161. Jiang X, Graham DY, Wang K, Estes MK. Norwalk virus
genome cloning and characterization. Science.
1990;250:1580–1583.
162. Matsui SM, Kim JP, Greenberg HB, et al. The isolation
and characterization of a Norwalk virus-specific DNA. J
Clin Invest. 1991;87:1456–1461.
163. Cubitt WD, Blacklow NR, Herrmann, JE, et al. Antigenic relationships between human caliciviruses and
Norwalk virus. J Infect Dis. 1987;156:806–814.
164. Madeley CR, Cosgrove BP. Caliciviruses in man. Lancet. 1976;1:199–200.
165. Monroe SS, Glass RI, Noah N, et al. Electron microscopic reporting of gastrointestinal viruses in the
United Kingdom, 1985–1987. J Med Virol.
1991;33:193–198.
166. Schaffer FL. Caliciviruses. In: Fraenkel-Conrat H, Wagner RR, eds. Comprehensive Virology. New York:
Plenum Press; 1979;14:249–284.
167. Madeley CR. Comparison of the features of astroviruses
and caliciviruses seen in samples of feces by electron
microscopy. J Infect Dis. 1979;139:519–523.
168. Cubitt WD. Human, small round structured viruses,
caliciviruses, and astroviruses. In: Farthing MJG, ed.
Baillière's Clinical Gastroenterology: Virus Infections
of the Gut and Liver. London: Baillière-Tindall;
1990;4:643–656.
169. Cubitt WD. Diagnosis, occurrence, and clinical significance of the human "candidate" caliciviruses. Prog
Med Virol. 1989;36:103–119.
170. Chiba S, Sakuma Y, Kogasaka R, et al. An outbreak of
gastroenteritis associated with calicivirus in an infant
home. J Med Virol. 1979;4:249–254.
171. Cubitt WD, McSwiggan DA, Moore W. Winter vomiting
disease caused by calicivirus. J Clin Pathol.
1979;32:786–793.
172. Grohmann G, Glass RI, Gold J, et al. Outbreak of human calicivirus gastroenteritis in a day-care center in
Sydney, Autralia. J Clin Microbiol. 1991;29:544–550.
173. Matson DO, Estes MK, Glass RI, et al. Human calicivi-
rus-associated diarrhea in children attending day care
centers. J Infect Dis. 1989;159:71–78.
174. Matson DO, Estes MK, Tanaka T, et al. Asymptomatic
human calicivirus infection in a day care center. Pediatr Infect Dis J. 1990;9:190–196.
175. McSwiggan DA, Cubitt D, Moore W. Calicivirus associated winter vomiting disease. Lancet. 1978;1:1215.
176. Cubitt WD, Pead PJ, Saeed AA. A new serotype of calicivirus associated with an outbreak of gastroenteritis in
a residential home for the elderly. J Clin Pathol.
1981;34:924–926.
177. Gray JJ, Wreghitt TG, Cubitt WD, Elliot PR. An outbreak of gastroenteritis in a home for the elderly associated with astrovirus type 1 and human calicivirus. J
Med Virol. 1987;23:377–381.
178. Suzuki H, Sato T, Kitaoka S, et al. Epidemiology of
rotavirus in Guayaquil, Ecuador. Am J Trop Med Hyg.
1986;35:372–375.
179. Nakata S, Estes MK, Chiba S. Detection of human calicivirus antigen and antibody by enzyme-linked immunosorbent assays. J Clin Microbiol. 1988;26:2001–2005.
180. Kaplan JE, Gary GW, Baron RC, et al. Epidemiology of
Norwalk gastroenteritis and the role of Norwalk virus
in outbreaks of acute nonbacterial gastroenteritis. Ann
Intern Med. 1982;96:756–761.
181. Kaplan JE, Feldman R, Campbell DS, et al. The frequency of a Norwalk-like pattern of illness in outbreaks
of acute gastroenteritis. Am J Public Health.
1982;72:1329–1332.
182. Brondum J, Spitalny KC, Vogt RL, et al. An outbreak
of gastroenteritis in Vermont attributed to Snow Mountain agent. J Infect Dis. 1985;152:834–837.
183. Guest C, Spitalny KC, Madore HP, et al. Food-borne
Snow Mountain agent gastroenteritis in a school cafe-
teria. Pediatrics. 1987;79:559–563.
184. Morens DM, Zweighaft RM, Vernon TM, et al. A waterborne outbreak of gastroenteritis with secondary person-to-person spread: Association with a viral agent.
Lancet. 1979;1:964–966.
185. Greenberg HB, Valdesuso J, Kapikian AZ, et al. Prevalence of antibody to the Norwalk virus in various countries. Infect Immun. 1979;26:270–273.
186. Johnson PC, Hoy J, Mathewson JJ, et al. Occurrence of
Norwalk virus infections among adults in Mexico. J
Infect Dis. 1990;162:389–393.
187. Blacklow NR, Dolin R, Fedson DS, et al. Acute infectious nonbacterial gastroenteritis: Etiology and pathogenesis. A combined clinical staff conference at the
Clinical Center of the National Institutes of Health.
Ann Intern Med. 1972;76:993–1008.
188. Agus SG, Dolin R, Wyatt RG, et al. Acute infectious
nonbacterial gastroenteritis: Intestinal histopathology.
Histologic and enzymatic alterations during illness produced by the Norwalk agent in man. Ann Intern Med.
1973;79:18–25.
189. Schreiber DS, Blacklow NR, Trier JS. The mucosal lesion of the proximal small intestine in acute infectious
nonbacterial gastroenteritis. N Engl J Med. 1973;
288:1318–1323.
190. Blacklow NR, Cukor G, Bedigian MK, et al. Immune
response and prevalence of antibody to Norwalk enteritis virus as determined by radioimmunoassay. J Clin
Microbiol. 1979;10:903–909.
191. Dolin R, Blacklow NR, DuPont H, et al. Biological
properties of Norwalk agent of acute infectious nonbacterial gastroenteritis. Proc Soc Exp Biol Med.
1972;140:578–583.
192. Johnson PC, Mathewson JJ, DuPont HL, Greenberg
HB. Multiple-challenge study of host susceptibility to
Norwalk gastroenteritis. J Infect Dis. 1990;161:18–21.
193. Parrino TA, Schreiber DS, Trier JS, et al. Clinical immunity in acute gastroenteritis caused by the Norwalk
agent. N Engl J Med. 1977;297:86–89.
194. Gary GW Jr, Kaplan JE, Stine SE, Anderson LJ. Detection of Norwalk virus antibodies and antigen with a
biotin-avidin immunoassay. J Clin Microbiol.
1985;22:274–278.
195. Greenberg HB, Wyatt RG, Valdesuso J, et al. Solid
phase microtiter radioimmunoassay for detection of
the Norwalk strain of acute nonbacterial epidemic gas-

troenteritis virus and its antibodies. J Med Virol. 1978;2:97–108.

196. Madore HP, Treanor JJ, Pray KA, Dolin R. Enzyme-linked immunosorbent assays for Snow Mountain and Norwalk agents of viral gastroenteritis. J Clin Microbiol. 1988;24:456–459.

197. Dolin R, Roessner KD, Treanor JJ, et al. Radioimmuno-assay for detection of the Snow Mountain agent of viral gastroenteritis. J Med Virol. 1986;19:11–18.

198. Treanor JJ, Madore HP, Dolin R. Development of an enzyme immunoassay for the Hawaii agent of viral gastroenteritis. J Virol Methods. 1988;22:207–214.

199. Appleton H, Higgins PG. Viruses and gastroenteritis in infants. Lancet. 1975;1:1297.

200. Madeley CR, Cosgrove BP. 28-nm particles in faeces in infantile gastroenteritis. Lancet. 1975;2:451–452.

201. Konno T, Suzuki H, Ishida N, et al. Astrovirus-associated epidemic gastroenteritis in Japan. J Med Virol. 1982;9:11–17.

202. Kurtz JB, Lee TW. Astrovirus: Human and animal. In: Bock G, Whelan J, eds. Novel Diarrhoea Viruses: Ciba Foundation Symposium 128. New York: John Wiley & Sons; 1987:92–107.

203. Matsui SM, Kim JP, Greenberg HB, et al. Identification and characterization of a human astrovirus-specific cDNA. Gastroenterology. 1991;100:A597.

204. Monroe SS, Stine SE, Gorelkin L, et al. Temporal synthesis of proteins and RNAs during human astrovirus infection in cultured cells. J Virol. 1991;65:641–648.

205. Kurtz JB, Lee TW. Human astrovirus serotypes. Lancet. 1984;2:1405.

206. Cruz JR, Bartlett AV, Herrmann JE, et al. Astrovirus-associated diarrhea among Guatemalan ambulatory rural children. J Clin Microbiol. 1992;30:1140–1144.

207. Herrmann JE, Taylor DN, Echeverria P, et al. Astroviruses as a cause of gastroenteritis in children. N Engl J Med. 1991;324:1757–1760.

208. Lew JF, Moe CL, Monroe SS, et al. Astrovirus and adenovirus associated with diarrhea in children in day care settings. J Infect Dis. 1991;164:673–678.

209. Moe CL, Allen JR, Monroe SS, et al. Detection of astrovirus in pediatric stool samples by immunoassay and RNA probe. J Clin Microbiol. 1991;29:2390–2395.

210. Lew JF, Glass RI, Petric M, et al. Six-year retrospective surveillance of gastroenteritis viruses identified at ten electron microscopy centers in the United States and Canada. Pediatr Infect Dis J. 1990;9:709–714.

211. Herrmann JE, Hudson RW, Perron-Henry DM, et al. Antigenic characterization of cell-cultivated astrovirus serotypes and development of astrovirus-specific monoclonal antibodies. J Infect Dis. 1988;158:182–185.

212. Kurtz J, Lee T. Astrovirus gastroenteritis: Age distribution of antibody. Med Microbiol Immunol. 1978; 166:227–230.

213. Esahli H, Breback K, Bennet R, et al. Astroviruses as a cause of nosocomial outbreaks of infant diarrhea. Pediatr Infect Dis J. 1991;10:511–515.

214. Kurtz JB, Lee TW, Pickering D. Astrovirus associated gastroenteritis in a children's ward. J Clin Path. 1977;30:948–952.

215. Yamashita T, Kobayashi S, Sakae K, et al. Isolation of cytopathic small round viruses with BS-C-1 cells from patients with gastroenteritis. J Infect Dis. 1991; 164:954–957.

216. Oshiro LS, Haley CE, Roberto RR, et al. A 27-nm virus isolated during an outbreak of acute infectious nonbacterial gastroenteritis in a convalescent hospital: A possible new serotype. J Infect Dis. 1981;143:791–795.

217. Kurtz JB, Lee TW, Craig JW, et al. Astrovirus infection in volunteers. J Med Virol. 1979;3:221–230.

218. Midthun K, Greenberg HB, Kurtz JB, et al. Characteri-

zation and seroepidemiology of a type 5 astrovirus associated with an outbreak of gastroenteritis in Marin County, California. J Clin Microbiol. 1993;31:955–962.

219. Phillips AD, Rice SJ, Walker-Smith JA. Astroviruses within human intestinal mucosa. Gut. 1982;23:A923–924.

220. Gray EW, Angus KW, Snodgrass DR. Ultrastructure of the small intestine in astrovirus-infected lambs. J Gen Virol. 1980;49:71–82.

221. Snodgrass DR, Angus KW, Gray EW, et al. Pathogenesis of diarrhea caused by astrovirus infections in lambs. Arch Virol. 1979;60:217–226.

222. Albert MJ. Enteric adenoviruses: Brief review. Arch Virol. 1986;88:1–17.

223. Uhnoo I, Svensson L, Wadell G. Enteric adenoviruses. In: Farthing MJG, ed. Baillière's Clinical Gastroenterology: Virus Infections of the Gut and Liver. London: Baillière-Tindall; 1990;4:627–642.

224. Hierholzer JC, Wigand R, Anderson LJ, et al. Adenoviruses from patients with AIDS: A plethora of serotypes and a description of five new serotypes of subgenus D (Types 43–47). J Infect Dis. 1988;158:804–813.

225. Horwitz MS. Adenoviruses. In: Fields BN, Knipe DM, Chanock RM, et al, eds. Virology. 2nd ed. New York: Raven Press; 1990:1723–1740.

226. de Jong JC, Wigand R, Kidd AH, et al. Candidate adenoviruses 40 and 41. J Med Virol. 1983;11:215–231.

227. Takiff HE, Straus SE, Garon CF. Propagation and in vitro studies of previously non-cultivable enteral adenoviruses in 293 cells. Lancet. 1981;2:832–834.

228. Brandt C, Kim HW, Rodriguez WJ, et al. Adenoviruses and pediatric gastroenteritis. J Infect Dis. 1985; 151:437–443.

229. Gary GW Jr, Hierholzer JC, Black RE. Characteristics of noncultivable adenoviruses associated with diarrhea in infants: A new subgroup of human adenoviruses. J Clin Microbiol. 1979;10:96–103.

230. Retter M, Middleton PJ, Tam JS, et al. Enteric adenoviruses: Detection, replication, and significance. J Clin Microbiol. 1979;10:574–578.

231. Cevinini R, Mazzaracchio R, Rumpianesi F, et al. Prevalence of enteric adenovirus from acute gastroenteritis: A five-year study. Eur J Epidemiol. 1987;3:147–150.

232. Kim K-H, Yang J-M, Joo S-I, et al. Importance of rotavirus and adenovirus types 40 and 41 in acute gastroenteritis in Korean children. J Clin Microbiol. 1990;28:2279–2284.

233. Uhnoo I, Wadell G, Svensson L, et al. Importance of enteric adenoviruses 40 and 41 in acute gastroenteritis in infants and young children. J Clin Microbiol. 1984;20:365–372.

234. Kidd AH, Banatvala JE, de Jong JC. Antibodies to fastidious faecal adenoviruses (species 40 and 41) in sera from children. J Med Virol. 1983;11:333–341.

235. Shinozaki T, Araki K, Ushijima H, Fujii R. Antibody response to enteric adenovirus types 40 and 41 in sera from people in various age groups. J Clin Microbiol. 1987;25:1679–1682.

236. Cruz JR, Caceres P, Cano F, et al. Adenovirus types 40 and 41 and rotaviruses associated with diarrhea in children from Guatemala. J Clin Microbiol. 1990;28:1780–1784.

237. Herrmann JE, Blacklow NR, Perron-Henry DM, et al. Incidence of enteric adenoviruses among children in Thailand and the significance of these viruses in gastroenteritis. J Clin Microbiol. 1988;26:1783–1786.

238. Kotloff KL, Losonsky GA, Morris JG, et al. Enteric adenovirus infection and childhood diarrhea: An epidemiologic study in three clinical settings. Pediatrics. 1989;84:219–225.

239. Leite JPG, Pereira HG, Azeredo RS, Schatzmayr HG.

Adenoviruses in faeces of children with acute gastroenteritis in Rio de Janeiro, Brazil. J Med Virol. 1985;15:203–209.

240. Paerregaard A, Hjelt K, Genner J, et al. Role of enteric adenoviruses in acute gastroenteritis in children attending day-care centers. Acta Paediatr Scand. 1990;79:370–371.

241. Whitelaw A, Davies H, Parry J. Electron microscopy of fatal adenovirus gastroenteritis. Lancet. 1977;1:361.

242. Gardner PS, Knox EG, Court SDM, et al. Virus infection and intussusception in childhood. Br Med J. 1962;2:697–700.

243. Krajden M, Brown M, Petrasek A, Middleton PJ. Clinical features of adenovirus enteritis: A review of 127 cases. Pediatr Infect Dis J. 1990;9:636–641.

244. Krilov LR, Rubin LG, Frogel M, et al. Disseminated adenovirus infection with hepatic necrosis in patients with human immunodeficiency virus infection and other immunodeficiency states. Rev Infect Dis. 1990;12:303–307.

245. August MJ, Warford AL. Evaluation of a commercial monoclonal antibody for detection of adenovirus antigen. J Clin Microbiol. 1987;25:2233–2235.

246. Brandt CD, Rodriguez WJ, Kim HW, et al. Rapid presumptive recognition of diarrhea-associated adenoviruses. J Clin Microbiol. 1984;20:1008–1009.

247. Grandien M, Patterson C-A, Svensson L, Uhnoo I. Latex agglutination test for adenovirus diagnosis in diarrheal disease. J Med Virol. 1987;23:311–316.

248. Johansson ME, Uhnoo I, Kidd AH. Direct identification of enteric adenovirus, a candidate new serotype, associated with infantile gastroenteritis. J Clin Microbiol. 1980;12:95–100.

249. Singh-Naz N, Rodriguez WJ, Kidd AH, Brandt CD. Monoclonal antibody enzyme-linked immunosorbent assay for specific identification and typing of subgroup F adenoviruses. J Clin Microbiol. 1988;26:297–300.

250. Svensson L, von Bonsdorff CH. Solid-phase immune electron microscopy (SPIEM) by use of protein A and its application for characterization of selected adenovirus serotypes. J Med Virol. 1982;10:242–253.

251. Wood DJ, Bijlsma K, de Jong JC, Tonkin C. Evaluation of a commercial monoclonal antibody-based enzyme immunoassay for detection of adenovirus types 40 and 41 in stool specimens. J Clin Microbiol. 1989;27:1155–1158.

252. Wood DJ, de Jong JC, Bijlsma K, et al. Development and evaluation of monoclonal antibody–based immune electron microscopy for diagnosis of adenovirus types 40 and 41. J Virol. Methods. 1989;25:241–250.

253. Brown NM. Laboratory identification of adenoviruses associated with gastroenteritis in Canada from 1983 to 1986. J Clin Microbiol. 1990;28:1525–1529.

254. Wadell G. Molecular epidemiology of human adenoviruses. Curr Top Microbiol Immunol. 1984;110:191–220.

255. Scott-Taylor T, Ahluwalia G, Klisko B, Hammond GW. Prevalent enteric adenovirus variant not detected by commercial monoclonal antibody enzyme immunoassay. J Clin Microbiol. 1990;28:2797–2801.

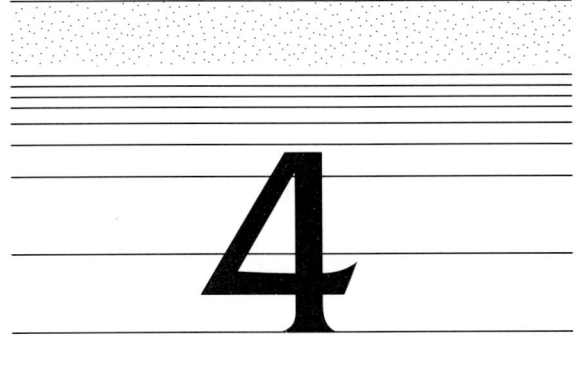

Diarrheal Disease with Viral Enteric Infections in Immunocompromised Patients

EDWARD N. JANOFF, M.D.

Diarrheal diseases affect many Americans once or twice a year. Typically, symptoms are mild and last only a few days. By contrast, in immunosuppressed patients, intestinal disease may be severe, prolonged, and even fatal. Increasing use of therapeutic immunosuppression in industrialized nations and the poorly controlled spread of human immunodeficiency virus (HIV) in both developed and developing countries expand the number of patients at risk. Chronic enteric disease in these patients may be associated with dehydration, malnutrition, fever, and abdominal pain. Chronic symptoms, particularly in persons afflicted with HIV infection, who are at high risk for this syndrome, may result in an inability to conduct routine daily activities and social interactions, to work, and ultimately to securely leave home. Viral infections, including those long recognized, those recently identified, and those yet to be appreciated, may figure prominently in the pathogenesis of these severe acute and chronic enteric syndromes.[1-3] The study of viral enteric pathogens has achieved clinical prominence and relevance owing to the convergence of advances in

diagnostic techniques, innovations in antiviral therapy, and an increasing population of profoundly immunosuppressed patients.

Symptomatic infections of mucosal surfaces, particularly of the lungs and gastrointestinal tract, are often the first clue that an immunodeficiency syndrome is present. Epithelial tissues exposed to the environment serve as the primary defensive barrier against infection. They act in concert with the host's immune system to limit microbial invasion and replication and subsequent disease. These observations highlight the importance of mucosa-associated lymphoid tissue (MALT)[4] and its interdependence with the systemic immune system in both immunocompetent and immunocompromised persons.[5]

Immunodeficiency may result from relatively uncommon primary intrinsic defects in immune development and regulation (Table 4–1).[6, 7] Compared with primary immunodeficiencies, however, secondary causes of immunosuppression have a much greater incidence and prevalence. Secondary immunodeficiency may result from malnutrition,[8-12] underlying diseases such

93

TABLE 4–1. RELATIONSHIP OF TYPES OF IMMUNOSUPPRESSION TO RISK AND TYPE OF VIRAL ENTERIC DISEASE

	IMMUNOSUPPRESSION		RELATIVE RISK OF ENTERIC VIRAL	
PATIENT GROUP	SOURCE	DURATION	INFECTION	VIRAL PATHOGENS
Primary Immunodeficiency				
Hypogammaglobulinemia	X-linked (Bruton's syndrome)	Prolonged	Low	Rotavirus (polio,* enteroviruses*, ECHO virus*)
	Transient in infancy	6–18 mo	Moderate	Rotavirus
	Common variable	Prolonged	Low	Rotavirus, ± CMV, (polio*)
	Selective IgA	Prolonged	None	
Severe combined immunodeficiency (SCID)		Prolonged	High	Rotavirus, adenovirus, picornavirus-like and parvovirus-like viruses, "mini-reo" virus, coxsackie virus A, calicivirus, astrovirus, small round viruses†
Severe T-cell defects	Cartilage hair hypoplasia	Prolonged	High (?)	Rotavirus, astrovirus, (polio*)
	DiGeorge syndrome	Prolonged	High (?)	Rotavirus
Phagocytic cell defects	Chronic granulomatous disease	Prolonged	None	
Secondary or Acquired Immunodeficiency				
Organ transplantation of kidney, liver, heart ± lung, bone marrow	Steroids, cyclosporine, azathioprine	Prolonged	High‡	CMV, adenovirus, HSV, rotavirus,§ coxsackievirus§
Cancer	Malignancy or chemotherapy	Transient	Moderate	CMV, adenovirus
Autoimmune disease, chronic obstructive lung disease (COPD)	Steroids	Prolonged or intermittent	Low to moderate	CMV, HSV
Viral infection	HIV	Prolonged	High	CMV, adenovirus, rotavirus
	Measles	Transient	High‖	Rotavirus
Selective neutropenia	Cyclic or drug-induced	Transient	None to low	
Splenectomy	Surgical or traumatic	Prolonged	None	

*May have increased incidence and rate of systemic manifestations, but not high incidence of enteric symptoms.
†Multiple enteric viruses may be identified simultaneously from children with SCID and chronic diarrhea.
‡Risk highest in months following transplantation.
§Reported primarily in pediatric bone marrow transplant recipients.
‖Primarily in developing countries, measles is associated with an increased risk of enteric symptoms, often in the presence of rotavirus infection.
KEY: CMV = cytomegalovirus, HSV = herpes simplex virus, IgA = immunoglobulin A.

as hematologic and solid malignancies, therapy of underlying diseases (such as cancer, autoimmune disease, chronic inflammatory diseases, and chronic obstructive lung disease), or transplantation of kidney, liver, heart, heart-lung, or allogeneic bone marrow. Acquired viral infections may also induce an immunodeficiency that is transient, as in infections with cytomegalovirus (CMV) and measles viruses,[13–17] or prolonged, as in HIV.[18]

Immune defects may involve a breach of the barrier function of skin and mucosal surfaces; decreased numbers or function of phagocytic cells, either polymorphonuclear cells or tissue macrophages; impaired humoral immunity, involving either antibodies or complement; or dysregulation of cell-mediated immunity, including CD4 + T lymphocytes, natural killer cells, cytotoxic T lymphocytes, and macrophages (Table 4–2). Most aspects of the immune response are affected by the activity of CD4 + T lymphocytes, commonly referred to as helper or inducer T cells.

Although selective defects of each component of the immune system are associated with an increased rate and severity of specific infections,[19] rates of viral enteric infections are higher in patients with cell-mediated defects[20–25] than they are in patients with humoral or phagocytic defects.[26–28] The highest rates of viral infection occur among patients with the most severe degrees of T-cell dysfunction[29–33] and among patients with prolonged immunodeficiency. A profound level of suppression of cell-

TABLE 4–2. FACTORS ASSOCIATED WITH THE INCIDENCE AND SEVERITY OF VIRAL ENTERIC INFECTIONS

FACTORS RELATED TO DEFECT IN IMMUNE SYSTEM OF HOST

Type of immune defect
  Barrier function: compromise of mucosal surfaces
  Humoral response: inadequacy of antibody or complement
  Phagocytic cells: insufficiency in number or function
  Cell-mediated immunity: dysregulation of natural killer cells, cytotoxic T cells, or macrophages*
Number of concomitant immune defects
Severity of immune defects
Duration of immune defects

FACTORS RELATED TO RELATION BETWEEN HOST AND INFECTIOUS ORGANISM

Pathogen-specific immunity of the host (prior exposure)
  Primary vs. reactivated infection
Prevalence of organism in environment (geographic, medical)
Biology of organism
  Tissue tropism, pathogenicity, latency

FACTORS RELATED TO THERAPY

Availability of sensitive and appropriate diagnostic tests
Availability of effective and acceptable therapy

*Most prominent immunologic risk factor for viral enteric disease.

mediated immunity is found among patients with primary T-cell defects, such as DiGeorge syndrome, cartilage hair hypoplasia,[34] and severe combined immunodeficiency (SCID)[29, 35]; those receiving organ transplantation,[30, 36] particularly allogeneic bone marrow transplantation[29, 30, 37]; and persons with the acquired immunodeficiency syndrome (AIDS).[5, 18] Each of these syndromes is associated with multiple immune defects of prolonged duration, including prominent cell-mediated immune dysfunction.

Factors that may affect the incidence, severity, and recognition of viral enteric infections in immunosuppressed populations are listed in Table 4–2. Prominent among these factors is the type of immune defect present. Patients with advanced HIV disease or SCID experience very high rates of viral enteric infections (see Table 4–1).[5, 35, 38] Recipients of organ and allogeneic bone marrow transplants are at significant risk of serious infections from such viruses as CMV, adenoviruses, and herpes simplex virus (HSV), but intestinal manifestations of infection are less frequent.[29, 30] Children with hypogammaglobulinemia may, however, be at increased risk of rotavirus infections, occasionally with prolonged symptomatic infections.[39, 40]

Other groups of immunodeficient patients are apparently at little or no increased risk of developing severe and prolonged viral enteric infections (see Table 4–1). Patients with defects of complement, with depletion or dysfunction of phagocytic cells, or with late-onset common variable immunodeficiency (CVI) do not develop enteric viral infections at particularly high rates.[27, 29, 30, 41–44] Neutropenic patients are at high risk for systemic fungal infections, such as candidemia, and for systemic, cutaneous, and enteric bacterial infections, such as typhlitis or neutropenic enterocolitis. Similarly, hypogammaglobulinemic patients may develop other chronic and often severe enteric infections with parasites such as *Giardia lamblia*,[40, 45, 46] or with bacteria such as *Campylobacter jejuni* or *Clostridium difficile*.[47] Some case reports describe serious systemic disease and prolonged excretion of enteroviruses, including coxsackieviruses, echoviruses, and polioviruses,[48] in children with X-linked agammaglobulinemia (XLA). Most viral infections, however, and particularly those causing enteric symptoms, are less common in patients with isolated complement, antibody, and phagocytic dysfunction than among patients with cell-mediated immunodeficiency, such as those with SCID or AIDS.

Unique biologic interactions with the host also determine the incidence and associated clinical spectrum of each virus. Enteroviruses, such as coxsackieviruses, may cause persistent invasive central nervous system infections in some immunodeficient subjects, but the virus shows little evidence of inducing intestinal pathologic conditions. By contrast, other viruses such as rotaviruses, CMV, and adenoviruses do induce pathologic effects in the gastrointestinal tract. Immunocompromised patients are particularly vulnerable to infections with CMV and adenoviruses because both viruses may be acquired early in life and establish latent infections that can reactivate.[29, 30] Patients infected with HIV are at high risk for reactivated CMV disease because their rates of prior exposure to the virus (>90%) usually exceed those in the general adult population (50–70%). Transplant patients are at risk for both secondary reactivated CMV infections and for primary infections after exposure through blood products of the transplanted organ.[49] Primary CMV infections are more common in children who receive transplants than in adults.[30] Immunocompromised children, particularly very young children with SCID, are less often infected with CMV. They are more likely to experience enteric infections with pathogens typical of childhood infection, such as rotaviruses, than are adults. Therefore, the biology of the virus, the tissue tropism of the organism, the host's exposure to a virus in the past or risk of exposure in the present based on age, behavior, and geography determine, in part, the risk of an immunocompromised patient for enteric viral disease.

The surge in numbers in the population susceptible to viral infection has been accompanied by the development of more sensitive diagnostic microbiologic techniques and the discovery of an extended range of viral enteric pathogens, which includes CMV, rotaviruses, adenoviruses, Norwalk and Norwalk-like agents, caliciviruses, astroviruses, coronaviruses, and picornavirus-like and parvovirus-like viruses (Table 4–3).[2, 3] The prevalence and manifestations of these viral infections are being defined in industrialized nations and in developing nations where technologic advances can be applied to local conditions. These advances and the introduction of potentially effective antiviral therapeutic regimens suggest that the management of serious viral infections, including those involving the gastrointestinal tract, will be an increasingly important component of basic research and clinical care.

INFECTIONS DEFINED BY TYPE OF IMMUNODEFICIENCY

Secondary or Acquired Immunodeficiency

Patients with acquired or secondary immunodeficiencies constitute the largest and most rapidly expanding group at risk of serious viral infections, including those involving the intestinal tract. As noted in Table 4–1, these patients may be at risk transiently or for prolonged periods, and their defects may involve cell-mediated immunity, reduction in neutrophil number or function, or splenic dysfunction. Selective acquired humoral immune deficiencies are unusual, but they may accompany the other defects listed. Patients with isolated neutropenia or phagocyte dysfunction, such as chronic granulomatous disease, are not at particular risk of

TABLE 4–3. POSSIBLE ENTERIC VIRAL PATHOGENS IN IMMUNOCOMPROMISED PERSONS

Cytomegalovirus
Rotavirus
Adenovirus
Herpes simplex virus
Enteroviruses
HIV
Other
Caliciviruses
Astroviruses
Picornavirus-like and parvovirus-like viruses

viral infections. Rates of viral infection are related, in part, to the duration and extent of immunosuppression. The highest rates of enteric viral infections occur in patients with advanced HIV disease and in some transplant patients, particularly those with graft-versus-host disease (GVHD).

Organ and Bone Marrow Transplantation

The majority of recipients of organ (kidney, heart, or heart and lung) and allogeneic bone marrow transplants develop clinically recognizable viral infections.[29, 30, 36, 37, 49–71] The specific viruses and the distribution and severity of clinical manifestations are dependent on a variety of factors, including those listed in Table 4–2. The majority of these infections become apparent within the first 4 months after transplantation.[19, 30, 68] Bone marrow transplant patients with GVHD are likely to experience serious infections with CMV and adenoviruses,[36, 66, 71] which compose the majority of important viral infections in children and adults. Children are also more susceptible to enteric rotavirus infections and experience a higher mortality rate with disseminated adenovirus infections than do older transplant patients.[29, 69] Children may also have lower rates of CMV disease owing to a lower prevalence of prior infection, and, therefore, of reactivation.[68] One study, however, describes a high rate of intestinal viral infections with serious sequelae, particularly from rotaviruses, in bone marrow transplant patients.[71]

Despite the overall frequency of systemic viral infections in transplant recipients, the frequency of intestinal manifestations, and specifically of virally induced diarrhea, is relatively low. Transplant patients, particularly those receiving allogeneic bone marrow, show high rates of intestinal symptoms and pathology. These findings are more likely to result from complications of chemotherapy, radiation, GVHD, bacterial enteritis, neutropenic enterocolitis (typhlitis), or C. difficile infection than from direct intestinal viral infection.[59] As noted, enteric CMV or adenovirus infection may coexist, and these infections occur more commonly with GVHD. Each of these syndromes may cause fever, abdominal pain, diarrhea, blood loss, bowel edema, and protein loss.

Lymphoproliferative disorders associated with Epstein-Barr virus infections and progressive intestinal lymphoid enlargement have also been described after bone marrow transplantation, severe GVHD, and treatment with anti–T-cell monoclonal antibodies.[36, 59] Each of these syndromes may be acute, life-threatening, and reversible, but each requires dramatically different therapy. Therefore, establishing a specific diagnosis of the origin of enteric symptoms in a patient with a recent transplant is critical for successful management of the infection.

Among pediatric bone marrow transplant patients, symptomatic viral enteric infections are also not usual. Wasserman and colleagues reported that among 95 children studied, infections with HSV were identified in 19 (20%), adenoviruses in 17 (18%), CMV in 17 (18%), and enteroviruses in 9 (9%). Intestinal symptoms are not described, even though adenoviruses were most often isolated from stool or rectal swab.[68] Case reports suggest that pediatric bone marrow transplant patients may also have serious illness with rotaviruses (group A and non–group A). As with CMV and adenovirus infections in these patients, the clinical, radiologic, and pathologic findings of rotavirus infections may be difficult to distinguish from those of GVHD.[69]

The incidence of CMV disease of the colon with diarrhea in organ and bone marrow transplant patients is relatively low.[72] Upper gastrointestinal disease (esophageal, gastric, and small bowel) is more frequently recognized and may result in ulceration, bleeding, or perforation.[56, 73, 74] In a prospective study that used well-defined endoscopic, histologic, and virologic entry criteria, invasive gastrointestinal CMV disease developed in 10 (10%) of 96 heart and 5 heart-lung transplant patients, whereas pneumonitis occurred in only 4 (4%), 0 had retinitis,[56] and only 1 patient had diarrhea and colonic involvement. Similarly, among 613 organ recipients, 93 patients (15%) developed tissue-invasive CMV infections, 17 of which (18%) involved the gastrointestinal tract.[75] Of the 14 patients with isolated gastrointestinal disease, most of whom had abdominal pain, 3 (21%) had colonic involvement, and only these 3 patients had diarrhea.

By contrast, in a placebo-controlled therapeutic trial of gastrointestinal CMV infection in bone marrow transplant patients in which less rigid entry criteria were used, the majority (30) of the 47 patients (64%) had diarrhea.[74] The CMV was cultured from the colon in only 2 patients (4%), however, and from the duodenum in 7 patients (15%). Moreover, despite inhibition of viral replication, endoscopic evaluation showed no significant improvement and symptoms were not significantly alleviated. Therefore, in contrast to the low rates of CMV-associated colitis and diarrhea in organ transplant patients, diarrheal symptoms in bone marrow transplant patients are common. These symptoms may not have been due, however, to CMV infection in many patients. Alternatively, the resolution of symptoms may require more than the suppression of the virus.

Overall, these results demonstrate that although reactivation of CMV may be very common in organ transplant patients, most infections are not severe.[49, 55, 58, 75, 76] Gastrointestinal involvement is usually not the principal manifestation. Colonic CMV disease is relatively uncommon but when present is often associated with diarrhea.[56, 75] Bone marrow transplant patients may have the added complication of GVHD, which may increase the risk of adenovirus and CMV disease and may also increase the frequency of nonviral intestinal symptoms.

HIV Disease

Enteric infections are among the most common manifestations of HIV infection, often representing the initial complaint leading to the diagnosis of HIV disease.[5, 33] Between 25 and 50% of patients with AIDS in developed countries and up to as many as 90% of those in developing nations such as Haiti and in some parts of Africa experience chronic diarrheal disease.[5, 33, 77–82] Patients at advanced stages of HIV infection are more likely to experience chronic diarrheal disease and weight loss and are more likely to have a pathogen identified, particularly a virus, than are those at earlier stages of infection (Table 4–4).[5, 26, 38, 83] Moreover, HIV-infected patients in developing countries[77, 82] and HIV-infected homosexual men may be more likely to have diarrheal disease than are intravenous drug users.[84]

In addition to these geographic and behavioral variables, a constellation of immune defects may contribute to the high rates of enteric infection in patients with HIV disease. Protection of mucosal tissues from infection requires the successful interaction of T lymphocytes, macrophages, and secretory immunoglobulin A (sIgA).[4] Nevertheless, the first line of immunologic defense, the mucosal barrier, may be compromised in patients with HIV infection. Chronic mucosal inflammation with partial villus atrophy is commonly present on histologic examination, independent of the presence or absence of symptoms or infection.[80, 85] The absorptive area is often decreased, as is villus height, and crypt depth is increased.[86] These functional abnormalities and the frequency of

TABLE 4–4. PREVALENCE OF ENTERIC VIRAL INFECTIONS IN HIV-INFECTED PATIENTS
WITH AND WITHOUT DIARRHEA

GROUP	REFERENCE	VIRUS	NO. INFECTED/NO. TESTED (%)	
			DIARRHEA	ASYMPTOMATIC
AIDS (Haiti)	Malebranche (1983)[77]	CMV	4/29 (14)	
		HSV	2/29 (7)	
AIDS (Australia)	Cunningham (1988)[26]	Coronavirus	1/69 (1)	1/55 (2)
		Rotavirus	21/116 (18)	
All HIV + (Australia)	Cunningham (1988)[26]	CMV†	3/68 (4)	0/55
		Adenoviruses	16/68 (24)	3/55 (5)
		Rotavirus	25/68 (37)	7/55 (13)
		Norwalk	1/68 (1)	1/55 (2)
AIDS (UK)	Dryden (1988)[230]	CMV	3/40 (8)	
		Rotavirus	0/100	
AIDS	Laughon (1988)[112]	CMV†	9/34 (26)	2/13 (15)
		HSV	8/20 (40)	7/38 (18)
		Adenovirus	0/29	0/20
		Rotavirus	1/29 (3)	1/20 (5)
		Coxsackieviruses	0/29	0/20
AIDS (Spain)	Miró (1988)[84]	CMV	6/30 (20)	
AIDS	Smith (1988)[38]	CMV	9/20 (45)	0/10
		HSV	1/20 (5)	0/10
		Rotavirus	0/20	0/10
All HIV +	Kaljot (1989)[83]	Norwalk virus	0/109	0/44
		Rotavirus	0/109	0/44
		Adenovirus*	5/109 (5)	2/44 (5)
AIDS	Rolston (1989)[231]	CMV	4/42 (10)	
AIDS (France)	Salmon (1990)[177]	Adenovirus	20/35 (57)	1/35 (3)
AIDS/ARC	Greenson (1991)[220]	CMV	1/22 (5)	0/13
AIDS	Janoff (1991)[175]	Adenovirus	5/67 (7)	0/10

NOTE: All studies performed in U.S. unless otherwise indicated.
*Only nonenteric adenoviruses (not types 40 or 41) detected.
†No biopsies performed, only culture of stool swabs or filtrates.
KEY: AIDS = acquired immunodeficiency syndrome, ARC = AIDS-related complex, CMV = cytomegalovirus, HIV = human immunodeficiency virus, HSV = herpes simplex virus.

oral and esophageal *Candida* infections suggest the presence of significant defects in the mucosal barrier.

The most striking immune defect in HIV-infected patients is dysregulation of cell-mediated immunity.[18, 31, 87, 88] The tropism of HIV for the pivotal regulatory cells of the immune system, CD4+ T lymphocytes, and the subsequent progressive dysfunction and destruction of these cells[87, 89] herald the onset of the profound immunosuppression that characterizes AIDS. The inability of CD4+ T cells to generate and focus a selective and effective immune response to these cell-associated pathogens allows viral infections, such as CMV and adenovirus, to reactivate and progress.

Control of CMV infections is dependent upon the activity of natural killer cells and cytotoxic T cells.[30, 90] Although these cells appear to be present in sufficient numbers in HIV-infected patients, their activity is impaired.[91-93] That the cytotoxic activity of these patients' cells can be enhanced by the addition of exogenous interleukin 2 (IL-2) or interferon-γ suggests that the defect resides in the capacity of cytokines to activate these cells, rather than in the cells themselves. In this regard, cytokine responses by mononuclear cells from HIV-infected patients may be impaired, including the production of interferon-γ[94] and, possibly, IL-2. These systemic defects of immune regulation and activation are probably reiterated in the intestinal mucosa, but these ideas await confirmation.

Immunologic evaluation of intestinal mucosal tissues from HIV-infected patients is based primarily on morphologic, rather than functional, studies. Comparable to findings with systemic lymphocytes, mucosal T cells from patients with HIV disease show a decreased ratio of CD4+ to CD8+ T lymphocytes among intestinal lamina propria lymphocytes.[95-100] These ratios derive from either a decreased or a normal number of CD4+ T cells in the presence of an increased proportion of CD8+ T cells. Mucosal T cells from HIV-infected patients also show decreased levels of expression of the activation marker IL-2 receptor (CD25),[100] compared with the high levels that characterize normal mucosal T cells.[101] The correlation between the functional activity of systemic and mucosal T cells in both

HIV-infected and control subjects is under investigation.

Both systemic and mucosal B cell defects are also present among patients with HIV disease[31, 102–106] but may play a less critical role than do T cells in the control of viral enteric infections. Therefore, patients with advanced HIV disease who develop serious enteric viral infections demonstrate multiple and severe defects in cell-mediated immunity and usually a compromise of barrier function. The persistence and progression of these defects over time place these patients at increasing risk of viral infection.

The majority of homosexual HIV-infected adults are at risk for CMV disease since most (>90%) show serologic evidence of prior CMV infection.[107] CMV is a principal pathogen, which remains latent for prolonged periods and can reactivate in the setting of impaired immune surveillance. In contrast, measles is not an important pathogen, since most patients also show serologic evidence of exposure to measles[108] but the virus does not reactivate. In addition, although HSV infections are common in these populations and their reactivation is common, they rarely cause significant pathologic change in the upper colon or small bowel, whereas CMV and adenoviruses may. In summary, as outlined in Table 4–2, the high rates of prior exposure to CMV, its ability to reactivate, and its tropism for multiple tissues, including all levels of the intestinal tract, account for the prominence of CMV as a cause of enteric viral infections in severely immunocompromised patients.

Table 4–2 also indicates that the identification of enteric pathogens in immunocompromised patients may be influenced by our ability to recognize them. Even with extensive, invasive, and expensive evaluations, no potential pathogens, whether viral or nonviral, are identified in 25 to 40% of HIV-infected patients with chronic diarrhea.[5, 33] Nevertheless, the proportion of cases of diarrhea in all settings that can now be associated with the presence of specific pathogens increased tremendously in the 1970s and 1980s. This improved diagnostic success has followed the introduction of improvements in staining methods and culture techniques and the introduction of enzyme immunoassays, fiberoptic endoscopes, molecular biologic techniques, and electron microscopy (EM). Data are accumulating on the epidemiology and biology of newer viruses (e.g., adenoviruses, coronaviruses, caliciviruses, astroviruses) in children and in both healthy and immunocompromised subjects.[2, 3, 71] Awareness of the presence of organisms such as Cryptosporidium, Microsporida,[109] and adenoviruses,[29, 103] through the use of the newer stains and EM has facilitated their recognition in tissue by routine light microscopy. The clinical correlate of these observations is that, despite the availability of these newer techniques, reports on the causes of diarrheal disease in HIV-infected patients in developing countries are conspicuously devoid of information on viral pathogens (see Table 4–4). The truly momentous advances in defining the range and pathogenesis of viral enteric infections will follow the development of diagnostic technology that is both sensitive and specific for the organisms sought as well as accessible to investigators and clinicians worldwide.

The factor listed in Table 4–2 that most dramatically affects the severity and sequelae of viral enteric infections in the immunosuppressed host is the availability of effective therapy. Among intestinal protozoal infections in patients with AIDS and diarrhea, G. lamblia is a relatively common cause but it is not a persistent problem, as the organism is easily eradicated with inexpensive and nontoxic therapy.[106] By contrast, Cryptosporidium is also common but may cause prolonged diarrhea, abdominal pain, and disability, owing to the unavailability of therapy. Some regimens, such as the use of hyperimmune bovine colostrum, show promise,[110] but a standardized product is not available. With viral infections, therapy with ganciclovir is often effective in limiting the symptoms and pathology of intestinal CMV infections in HIV-infected patients (Tables 4–5 and 4–6). Infections caused by ganciclovir-resistant CMV may now be treated effectively with foscarnet.[111] Both ganciclovir and foscarnet have, however, significant toxicity, are quite expensive, and often require continuous therapy. These factors may limit their use by immunosuppressed patients with HIV, particularly in developing countries. Nevertheless, the facts that effective antiviral agents have been developed and are available are very important and promising recent advances.

In summary, the increased risk for HIV-infected patients of viral enteric infections, particularly those caused by CMV, appears to be due to an accumulation of risk factors, summarized in Table 4–2. These risks include the presence of prolonged and severe dysfunction of cell-mediated immunity in the context of impaired barrier function and other immune defects. Moreover, patients with HIV disease have a high rate of prior exposure to CMV, a pathogenic virus that establishes an inducible latent infection with tropism for the intestinal tract. These infections can be identified by current diagnostic methods, and although the clinical syndrome produced by CMV in AIDS patients may be se-

TABLE 4–5. THERAPY OF ENTERIC VIRAL INFECTIONS IN THE IMMUNOCOMPROMISED HOST

AGENT	ROUTE	DOSE AND FREQUENCY	DURATION
CYTOMEGALOVIRUS			
Acute therapy			
Ganciclovir	IV	5 mg/kg q12h	14–21 d
Foscarnet	IV	60 mg/kg q8h	14–21 d
Chronic suppression*			
Ganciclovir	IV	5 mg/kg daily	Indefinitely
		6 mg/kg 5 d/wk	Indefinitely
Foscarnet	IV	90–120 mg/kg daily, over 2 h	Indefinitely
HERPES SIMPLEX PROCTITIS			
Acyclovir†	IV	5 mg/kg q8h	7–10 d
	PO	400 mg, 5 times per day (or 800 mg, as necessary)	7–10 d
Acyclovir-resistant HSV			
Foscarnet‡	IV	40 mg/kg q8h	10–42 d
Acyclovir‡	IV	1.5–2.0 mg/kg per hour	42 d
		Continuous infusion	

NOTE: *Adjustment for Renal Insufficiency.* Acyclovir dosage should be decreased for creatinine clearance (Cl$_{Cr}$) below 25 cc/min for oral and below 50 cc/min for IV doses. Ganciclovir dosage should be decreased for Cl$_{Cr}$ below 80 cc/min.

*Chronic suppression indicated for patients with AIDS due to high relapse rate. Chronic suppression with ganciclovir is supported by anecdotal data but not confirmed in controlled trials.

†Consider chronic suppression if necessary in AIDS patients with lowest dose that controls symptoms.

‡Not approved by the Federal Food and Drug Administration for this indication.

KEY: AIDS = acquired immunodeficiency syndrome, IV = intravenous, PO = per os (by mouth).

vere or even fatal, most cases are controllable with available therapy. These observations highlight the contributions of the host's immune status, the epidemiology and biology of the organism, and the role of technology in determining the clinical manifestations and outcome of viral enteric infections in immunocompromised patients.

The range of pathogens causing these intestinal symptoms is broad and includes bacterial, viral, and parasitic organisms. No specific cause is found in an appreciable proportion of these patients (15–50%).[33] A determined but sequential approach to identifying these pathogens is imperative, however, since the majority of pa-

tients initially have treatable infections.[33, 38, 84] Diagnosis of these infections may be challenging because polymicrobial enteric infections occur in nearly 10% of patients with HIV infection and diarrheal disease.[26, 112] In one study, multiple enteric viruses were identified in 11 of 37 HIV-infected patients with diarrhea (30%).[26] The frequency of enteric viral infections in HIV-infected patients is summarized in Table 4–4. The specific clinical syndromes associated with these infections are described later in this chapter.

Viral infections, such as those due to CMV, are likely to be chronic and unremitting in the absence of specific and prolonged therapy. The

TABLE 4–6. THERAPEUTIC TRIALS OF CMV COLITIS IN PATIENTS WITH HIV INFECTION

THERAPY	REFERENCE	NO. STUDIED	CLINICAL—NO. (%)			
			IMPROVED	STABLE	POOR RESPONSE*	RELAPSE
None	Collaborative group (1986)[163]	12	2 (17)			
Ganciclovir	Chachoua (1987)[165]	31	23 (74)			11/14‡ (79)
Ganciclovir	Laskin (1987)[164]	13	9 (69)			
Ganciclovir	Buhles (1988)[162]	31†	27 (87)			4/5 (80)
Ganciclovir	Dieterich (1988)[161]	46	35 (76)	7 (15)	4 (9)	13/24 (54)
Ganciclovir	Drew (1991)[166]	39†	33 (85)		6 (15)	
Ganciclovir	Dieterich (1993)[167]	32	20 (63)§		12 (38)	
Placebo		30	11 (37)		19 (63)	
Foscarnet	Nelson (1991)[111]	22	17 (77)		5 (23)‖	3/17 (18)

*Improvement primarily based on clinical response but also on colonoscopic and virologic results. Poor response includes progression of disease despite therapy, termination of therapy due to toxicity, and death.

†Includes patients with colitis or esophagitis[166] and gastritis or enteritis.[162]

‡Includes patients with retinitis, pneumonitis, or gastrointestinal disease.

§Compared with the placebo group, ganciclovir-treated patients showed significantly less fever, weight loss, and colonic inflammation after 14 days of therapy. No difference in diarrheal symptoms were noted between groups.

‖Four of 5 died within 10 days of beginning therapy.

intestinal manifestations of HIV infection include a complex array of symptoms, nutritional defects, morphologic and functional abnormalities, and infections in the gut during the course of HIV disease. The proposed mechanisms by which intestinal pathologic change evolves in HIV-infected patients are summarized in Table 4–7. These factors do not consistently show an independent or causal relationship with the clinical, structural, physiologic, and microbiologic intestinal findings, but each may contribute, alone or in combination, to intestinal symptoms. The high rates of intestinal symptoms and infections in patients with HIV disease reflect the struggle to maintain the integrity of our *milieu intérieur* in the face of microbial and immunologic challenges from without and within.

Primary Immunodeficiencies

Primary immunodeficiency syndromes result from intrinsic defects in production, maturation, or function of immune cells.[7, 113] They may be classified as affecting predominantly humoral responses, cell-mediated responses, or both, but the distinctions are not always clear in many patients and within clinically defined groups. The syndromes can be generally distinguished by the age at which symptoms most often begin, by the clinical manifestations and types of infections present, by the levels of immunoglobulins in serum, by the presence of immunoglobulin-bearing B cells in the circulation and lymphoid tissues, and by analysis of T-cell number and function, including delayed-type hypersensitivity (skin-test reactivity) and responses of T cells to stimulation in vitro. A history of infections in multiple sites on several occasions with common or atypical organisms beginning during infancy or in early adulthood suggests the presence of a primary immunodeficiency syndrome. Most common among the primary immunodeficiencies is impairment of antibody production without overt T-cell or cell-mediated immune defects. Clinically significant primary immunodeficiency syndromes are uncommon, occurring in approximately 1 in 10,000 live births.[114] Selective immunoglobulin A (IgA) deficiency is, however, much less unusual.

IgA Deficiency

Isolated deficiencies of IgA, characterized by serum levels below 5 mg per dl with normal levels of IgG and IgM and generally with normal cellular immunity and responses to antigens, are identified in 1 in 500 to 700 persons in the general population. IgA deficiency may result from chromosomal abnormalities or in association with congenital infections.[115] The number of circulating B cells, including those with membrane IgA, is normal, but B cells may be at an arrested stage of maturation.[116] Despite the frequency of IgA deficiency and the associated absence of mucosal IgA,[117] selective IgA deficiency is routinely associated neither with an increased risk of infection overall nor with viral enteric infections in particular.[118]

Several factors may contribute to the risk of infectious complications. Among IgA-deficient children, the frequency of pneumonia was higher in those with less than 5 mg of IgA per dl in serum compared with children with higher levels.[115] Moreover, symptomatic patients may have other immune defects, such as deficiencies in immunoglobulin G (IgG) subclasses, particularly IgG2.[119] The absence of symptoms in most IgA-deficient patients may be associated with the presence of corresponding increases in mucosal secretory immunoglobulin M (sIgM).[120] Although the complications of IgA deficiency may include both sinopulmonary bacterial infections[121] and noninfectious disorders (including the autoimmune gastrointestinal abnormalities pernicious anemia and gluten-sensitive enteropathy) in selected patients, serious and persistent viral enteric infections are unusual.

Common Variable Immunodeficiency

Common variable immunodeficiency (CVI) occurs in approximately 0.6 to 8.9 infants per 100,000 live births.[41, 122] In this heterogeneous group of patients of both sexes, the number and activity of B cells and T cells may be normal or

TABLE 4–7. PROPOSED PATHOGENIC MECHANISMS OF INTESTINAL DISEASE IN HIV-INFECTED PATIENTS

MECHANISM	REFERENCES
Overt enteric pathogens (bacterial, parasitic, fungal, viral, especially CMV)	5, 26, 33, 38, 112, 175, 218, 230, 231
Covert enteric pathogens (? adenovirus, Microsporida, other)	83, 109, 175, 220, 232, 233
Mucosal HIV infection	86, 211, 213, 234
Bacterial overgrowth in the small intestine	5, 38, 95, 235
Immune dysfunction (mucosal barrier; humoral, cellular)	5, 102, 106, 236
Combination of these mechanisms	

KEY: CMV = cytomegalovirus, HIV = human immunodeficiency virus.

decreased, but terminal B-cell differentiation is limited, resulting in depressed levels of IgG, immunoglobulin M (IgM), and IgA, and depressed humoral responses to antigenic challenge.[6, 41, 43] The production of IgM may be less severely affected. Cell-mediated immunity is grossly intact. The diagnosis of CVI is most often delayed until the second or third decade of life. Bacterial infections predominate at mucosal sites, particularly the lungs, sinuses, and intestinal tract.[43, 123]

Despite the high frequency of enteric symptoms, which occur in as many as 60% of patients, intestinal viral infections are not well described among adults with CVI.[43, 123] Diarrhea may be associated with infections with *G. lamblia*,[43, 45, 123, 124] pathogenic bacteria (including *C. jejuni*), or small bowel overgrowth.[28, 124] Autoimmune disease and intestinal nodular lymphoid hyperplasia are also common features.[28, 45, 125] Both children and adults with CVI experience severe and persistent systemic viral infections, such as enteroviruses, polio, and echoviruses, for which the intestinal tract is the portal of entry.[44, 126] Other than prolonged excretion of polio virus, however, these viruses are not associated with intestinal symptoms. Rotavirus infection has been reported in one child with CVI, and the acute infection resolved spontaneously within 10 days.[39]

X-Linked (Bruton's) Agammaglobulinemia

Boys with XLA come to medical attention with recurrent pyogenic bacterial infections after loss of maternal antibodies in infancy or early childhood. They show very low levels of all antibody classes and no antibody response to antigenic stimulation, and they are usually devoid of circulating B cells and of plasma cells in lymphoid tissue.[7, 113] T-cell number, subsets, and activity appear normal, although the frequency of primed T cells may be decreased.[127] Cell-mediated immunity and natural killer cell activity appear unimpaired.

Despite the absence of antibody production, gastrointestinal symptoms are relatively infrequent.[28] When present, symptoms may be associated with bacterial overgrowth in the small intestine, lactase deficiency, or *G. lamblia* infections.[45, 46] In a multicenter survey of XLA, 31 of 96 patients (32%) had experienced diarrhea, and 10 (10%) had chronic diarrhea.[40] Only 2 children (2%) had acute symptomatic rotavirus infections, which resolved with gammaglobulin therapy. Other investigators have suggested that enteric viral infections, although not frequently reported, may be both prolonged and more se-

vere among children with XLA than in those with other selective antibody deficiency syndromes.[39]

Transient Hypogammaglobulinemia of Infancy

Serum levels of IgG are lowest 3 to 6 months after birth, since maternal antibody is catabolized and the infant's immune system is developing in response to new antigenic stimuli. Transient hypogammaglobulinemia of infancy (THI) involves a relatively prolonged depression of serum IgG levels, but not of IgM or IgA, which reach normal by 2 years of age.[6, 113] The actual incidence of THI is unknown as is the rate of infectious complications. Chronic diarrheal symptoms among infants with THI may result from infections with *G. lamblia* or *C. difficile*.[47] One child with self-limited diarrhea due to rotavirus has been reported.[39]

Severe Combined Immunodeficiency

Infants with SCID show severe defects in both humoral and cellular immunity that result from abnormal development of T cells and, usually, of B cells. Levels of all antibody classes are low, as are the number of lymphocytes ($<1000/\mu l$), T cells, and, often, B cells. Infants who have SCID may show impaired growth and high mortality owing to recurrent bacterial, fungal, and viral infections that begin within the first few months of life. The syndrome typically manifests with oral thrush, recurrent pneumonia, and persistent diarrhea.[6, 113]

In contrast to patients with isolated antibody defects, these children experience high rates of enteric disease that is often of viral origin.[35, 39, 128-133] Among 12 patients with SCID, 9 children (75%) had 14 episodes of enteric viral infections.[35] Picornavirus-like or parvovirus-like viruses were identified in 5 children (56%), rotavirus in 4 (44%), "mini-reoviruses" in 3 (33%), and coxsackievirus A and adenoviruses each in 1 child (11%). Multiple pathogens were found in 3 of 11 episodes (27%). Similarly, 2 other boys with SCID and diarrhea are each reported to have excreted up to 5 viruses simultaneously.[128, 129] In both cases, these viruses were rotavirus, calicivirus, small round viruses, adenovirus, and astrovirus, which made the specific source of various symptoms difficult to discern.

Viral infections may be community-acquired or nosocomial.[35] Viral excretion in children with SCID is usually prolonged, continuing throughout hospitalization or until death.[35, 39, 130-133]

Symptoms and infection may last from 2 to more than 12 months, often despite the use of prophylactic or therapeutic systemic immunoglobulin[35] or breast milk containing pathogen-specific antibody.[39, 128] Viral excretion is usually associated with symptoms. That rotavirus has been identified in virtually all children with SCID and viral enteric pathogens may reflect the prevalence of rotavirus in the community and the availability of methods to detect it. Rotavirus induces relatively prolonged diarrheal symptoms, with higher rates of dehydration, hospitalization, and death in otherwise healthy children than those of other viral enteric pathogens.[134] These observations in healthy children highlight the potential impact of rotavirus as an important primary pathogen in these profoundly immunodeficient children.

Severe combined immunodeficiency is most often fatal within the first several years of life. Prolonged diarrhea, with malabsorption, other systemic infections, and growth impairment, contributes to the high mortality rate. Among 9 children with SCID who died, viral infections, particularly those of the herpesvirus group (herpes simplex, varicella-zoster virus, and cytomegalovirus), were the primary cause of death in 8 patients (89%) but often with concomitant viral enteritis. Enteric viral infections were the primary cause of death in 2 of these 8 children.[35] In the absence of effective antisecretory medications, antiviral therapy, or immune reconstitution, persistent viral infections and death ensue.[35, 39, 128, 129]

In summary, the rate of diarrhea among children with SCID is high and usually associated with viral pathogens. These infections may be due to multiple viruses, but rotaviruses appear to play a prominent role. Enteric viral infections are consistently symptomatic, and both symptoms and viral excretion are prolonged. Both morbidity and mortality are very high among these children.

SPECIFIC INFECTIONS

In the immunocompromised host, the intestinal tract may serve as a portal of entry for viral infections such as enteroviruses, including poliovirus, without being the primary focus of symptoms and pathologic change. Some intestinal viral infections, such as those due to CMV or adenoviruses, are more likely to be local manifestations of systemic infections, whereas others, such as rotavirus and herpes simplex virus, may be serious manifestations of localized infections. We will consider several enteric viral pathogens to compare their clinical syndromes in immunocompetent and immunocompromised patients.

Cytomegalovirus

Intestinal CMV disease is almost strictly an opportunistic infection in that virtually the only persons who manifest enteric symptoms are the immunocompromised. In the general population, exposure to CMV is common and increases with age. More than half of healthy adults have serologic evidence of prior CMV infection,[30, 135] but the majority of these primary infections were asymptomatic. Young adults may show a mononucleosis syndrome in association with primary CMV infection, with fever, nausea, abdominal pain, malaise, hepatitis, and mild diarrhea.[136, 137] These symptoms are self-limited and rarely associated with serious sequelae or organ damage. Recently, a small number of immunocompetent patients with CMV colitis was reported,[138] but the incidence is probably very low. Most primary infections with CMV evolve into a persistent latent phase during which the virus is not readily transmissible, although low levels of viral genome may be detected, and the host remains asymptomatic for life.[139] Therefore, among immunocompetent persons, primary CMV infection is most often asymptomatic or accompanied by transient symptoms, and clinically apparent reactivations are not well described. By contrast, among immunocompromised patients, CMV may cause severe and potentially fatal multiorgan disease after primary exposure or, more commonly, as a result of reactivation of latent infection.

Disseminated CMV infections have been reported in a variety of immunodeficient patient groups. Prominent among them are patients with HIV infection, as noted earlier, and recipients of organ transplants. Cytomegalovirus disease in patients with cancer occurs most often during chemotherapy, particularly if corticosteroids are included.[140, 141] Similarly, corticosteroids figure prominently in the presence of CMV disease in patients with rheumatologic and autoimmune disease.[72, 140, 142] Other uncommon and non–steroid-related conditions include trauma, burns, renal failure, and diabetes.[72] The clinical syndromes associated with CMV and the distribution of gastrointestinal lesions are comparable in each of these groups, including recipients of solid organ transplants (kidney, liver, heart, or heart and lung) and bone marrow transplants.

Among organ transplant patients, CMV infection is usually manifested within the first 4 months after operation.[30, 49, 63, 76] The reported rates of active CMV secondary infection were higher among 1328 transplant patients with prior exposure to the organism than the rates of primary infection among 1108 patients without prior exposure to CMV—73% compared with 44%, respectively.[30] Secondary infections may be reactivations or reinfections. The presence of CMV-specific antibody appeared to be a reliable marker of prior CMV in both the donor and the host. Despite high rates of productive infection,[30, 36, 52, 58, 76, 143–145] which include the development of viremia in as many as 50 to 70% of patients at some point after transplantation,[36] the majority of patients with active infection may be asymptomatic. Symptomatic infections are more common among renal transplant patients with primary, compared with reactivated, CMV infections (60–90% vs. 20–45%),[30, 36] but among other transplant patients, the clinical differences between primary and secondary infections are not so consistent.[146] Differences between studies and groups of transplant recipients may reflect the method and degree of immunosuppression, the underlying diseases of the patients, and the type of transplant.

The most common CMV-related symptoms in transplant patients are fever and hepatitis, often in association with neutropenia. Pneumonitis occurs in significantly less than 10% of kidney, liver, and heart transplant patients but in more than 30% of heart-lung transplant patients.[30] That bone marrow transplant patients also experience relatively high rates of CMV pneumonitis (17%) suggests that CMV is more likely to induce pathologic change in, or at least be isolated from, tissue that is already injured, as, for example, by GVHD, than in unaffected tissues. This hypothesis is supported by the observation that the presence of GVHD is a risk factor for CMV pneumonitis, but histopathologic confirmation is not available.

Among patients with invasive or serious CMV infections, involvement of the intestinal tract is relatively uncommon. Gastrointestinal CMV disease has been reported in 38 patients without either HIV infection or transplantation.[72] Many were receiving corticosteroids for cancer, collagen-vascular diseases, or chronic obstructive lung disease. The organism was identified in all areas of the intestinal tract, and CMV colitis appeared to be most severe and common in patients receiving immunosuppressive therapy for ulcerative colitis. Again, CMV infection and disease appeared to preferentially affect already inflamed tissues.[30, 147–151]

Among the transplant patients with visceral organs affected by CMV infection, gastrointestinal symptoms have been reported in 2.5 to 6.4% of patients with kidney transplants,[63, 75, 152] 2.8% of those with liver transplants,[75] and 2.7 to 16% in those with heart or heart and lung transplants.[56, 72, 75, 153] The entire length of the digestive tract may be involved, including the esophagus, stomach, small and large intestine, and less frequently, the anus. Among these sites, none predominates in all, nor in any specific, transplant groups. Although abdominal pain is commonly described with gastrointestinal CMV disease, diarrhea is not a prominent symptom because infection of the esophagus and stomach constitutes an appreciable proportion of cases; colonic involvement often presents with bleeding.[30, 56, 74]

Therapy is generally effective in organ transplant patients. Clinical response rates to ganciclovir therapy range from 60 to 100%,[56, 75, 152] death rates are low (0–7%), but relapse is common (20–40%) after discontinuation of therapy. Maintenance therapy is not routinely used in transplant patients, but higher relapse rates among HIV-infected patients with intestinal CMV do warrant chronic suppressive therapy. Diarrhea may be a more common symptom among bone marrow transplant patients with gastrointestinal CMV infection than among other transplant patients,[74] but the cause of the symptoms may be more difficult to discern. Perhaps as a result, positive response rates to ganciclovir in bone marrow transplant patients with intestinal CMV disease are less consistent than among patients with solid organ transplants.

Active CMV infection is also common among patients with HIV infection. Evidence of disseminated disease is identified in up to 90% of patients at autopsy.[154–156] At least 30% of patients experience severe disease during life, predominantly manifested as retinitis, gastrointestinal symptoms, and pneumonitis. Most symptomatic infections develop in patients with advanced HIV disease, with CD4+ T-cell counts below 100/μl. Unlike the case in transplant patients, CMV colitis is among the most common manifestations of invasive CMV disease in patients with HIV infection, occurring in 2 to 5% of all patients.[154, 156] CMV colitis may even be the presenting symptom that leads to the diagnosis of retroviral disease and AIDS in some patients.[157]

Symptoms and signs of serious intestinal CMV disease in HIV-infected patients most consistently include fever and weight loss, often with anorexia.[38, 156, 158, 159] Diarrhea may be intermittent or severe and watery or, less commonly, bloody. Abdominal pain and tenderness may be associated with rebound tenderness and abdominal distention. The combination of fever and bloody diarrhea in patients with AIDS is more suggestive of CMV colitis than of any of the multiple other causes of diarrhea.

Diagnosis of CMV colitis is based on endoscopic, histologic, and virologic examination of the involved tissue. Endoscopic evaluation of the colon usually shows erythema and inflammation (Fig. 4–1), often in association with erosions that may coalesce and evolve into frank ulcerations with hemorrhage.[38, 156, 160] Areas of mucosal damage may be separated by normal mucosa, although consistently normal-appearing mucosa is less suggestive of severe CMV disease. Deep ulcerations are most frequently identified in the upper gastrointestinal tract.[157, 159] The majority of diagnoses are made by evaluation of the left colon, but more than one third of cases are confined to the right colon. Small bowel infection may also induce enteritis and diarrheal symptoms.[38]

Microscopic examination shows chronic inflammatory cells in the small or large intestine associated with intranuclear inclusions (Fig. 4–2).[157] Mucosal ulceration may or may not be present. Intranuclear owl's-eye inclusions with a perinuclear halo, known as Cowdry's type A inclusions, are classic but not necessarily typical.[157] The presence of typical inclusions and the number of infected cells correlate with the severity of disease.[157, 159] Epithelial cells may be infected in conjunction with endothelial cells and lamina propria cells. Cells infected with CMV can be differentiated from those infected with adeno-

viruses by the presence of intracytoplasmic inclusions in the CMV-infected cells. Results of EM and immunocytochemical examination of paraffin sections help establish and confirm the diagnosis. Viral cultures of involved tissues are useful,[159] but isolation of CMV from the blood does not predict visceral disease. Owing to the high prevalence of CMV-specific IgG in the HIV-infected population and the infrequent rises of virus-specific IgM during reactivations, serologic diagnosis is not helpful. The diagnosis of invasive CMV disease, therefore, is predicated on the identification of infected cells from directly involved tissue by histologic examination in association with culture and immunocytochemical studies.

Therapeutic trials using ganciclovir in patients with AIDS and visceral CMV disease are summarized in Table 4–6. The majority of patients show a diminution of viral burden. Results of clinical and endoscopic evaluation generally show improvement,[161–167] although diarrheal symptoms do not invariably remit.[167] In some studies, it is difficult to distinguish the therapeutic effect of ganciclovir in patients with diarrhea and CMV colitis from its effect in those with CMV infection in other gastrointestinal sites.

Many difficulties emerge in maintaining a successful response to therapy. The cost of ganciclovir is high as are the support services necessary to continue its intravenous administration. Owing to the high rates of relapse after initial treatment, continuous maintenance therapy is most often required. Moreover, side effects of ganciclovir such as neutropenia are common, so therapy may be modified, discontinued, or augmented by granulocyte colony stimulating factor. Because of the emergence of ganciclovir-resistant strains of CMV,[168] therapy may become ineffective over time. Fortunately, foscarnet appears to be as effective as ganciclovir in the control of CMV colitis[111] and may have fewer side effects. Because invasive CMV disease occurs primarily in HIV-infected patients with advanced disease, control of HIV infection itself may help to limit the incidence and severity of CMV infections. The development of effective and lower priced drugs that can be taken orally will also be of appreciable benefit. Figures 4–1 through 4–5 illustrate the gross and histologic appearance of CMV and adenovirus infections.

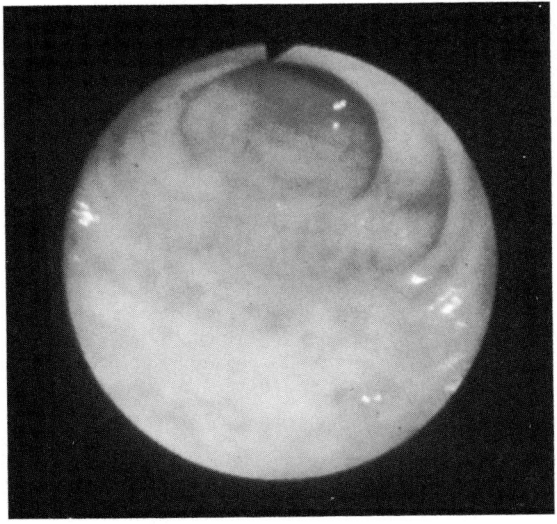

FIGURE 4–1.
Cytomegalovirus colitis with patches of erythema in a patient with AIDS. By colonoscopy. SOURCE: Courtesy of Dr Phillip D Smith.

Adenoviruses

As discussed in greater detail in Chapter 3, infections in otherwise healthy persons with adenoviruses, a large family of nonenveloped,

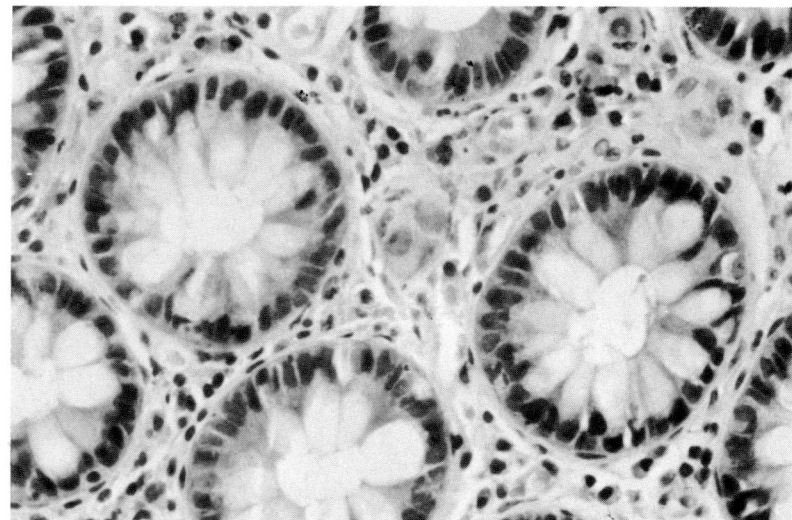

FIGURE 4–2.
Cytomegalovirus colitis with large intracellular inclusions. (Hematoxylin-eosin) SOURCE: Courtesy of Dr Steven Ewing.

double-stranded DNA viruses, are most often associated with acute respiratory symptoms, keratoconjunctivitis, and hemorrhagic cystitis.[169, 170] These infections of epithelial cells may occur as sporadic cases or in outbreaks, particularly among military recruits, suggesting that these viruses are highly infectious. Adenovirus infections associated with gastroenteritis, most often due to types 40 and 41, usually occur in young children in both temperate and tropical climates.[2, 169, 171]

In adults, enteric adenovirus infections have been described in the elderly[172] and in immunocompromised hosts. Among HIV-infected patients, adenoviruses have been cultured from multiple sources, including urine, lung, liver, stool, and intestinal tissues.[26, 29, 33, 83, 112, 171, 173–175] Unlike CMV, which is readily isolated from blood, adenoviruses are uncommonly recovered from blood.[176] Patients with advanced HIV disease are at the highest risk of disseminated and enteric adenovirus infections.[26] The controversy

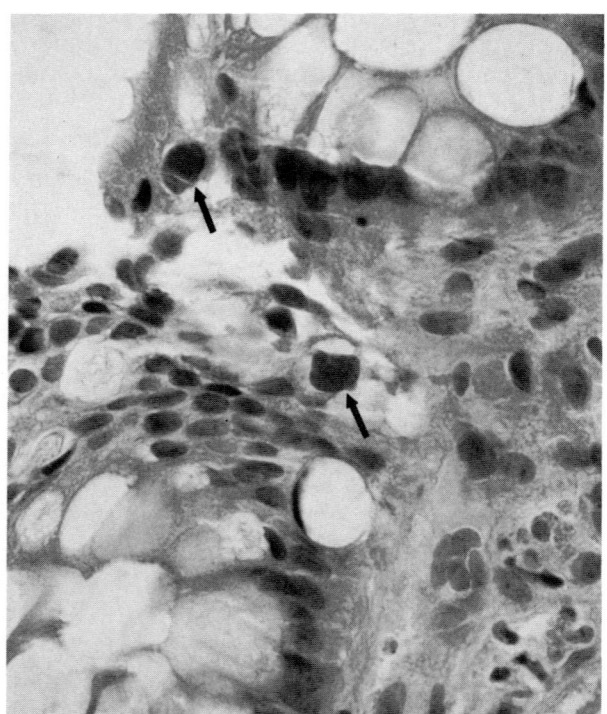

FIGURE 4–3.
A colonic biopsy from a patient with adenovirus colitis. Two epithelial cells contain large intranuclear inclusions *(arrows)* in an area of mucosal degeneration and necrosis. (Hematoxylin-eosin, ×600.) SOURCE: Courtesy of Dr. Jan Orenstein, Janoff EN, Orenstein JM, Manischewitz JF, Smith PD. Adenovirus colitis in the acquired immunodeficiency syndrome. Gastroenterology 1991;100:976–979.

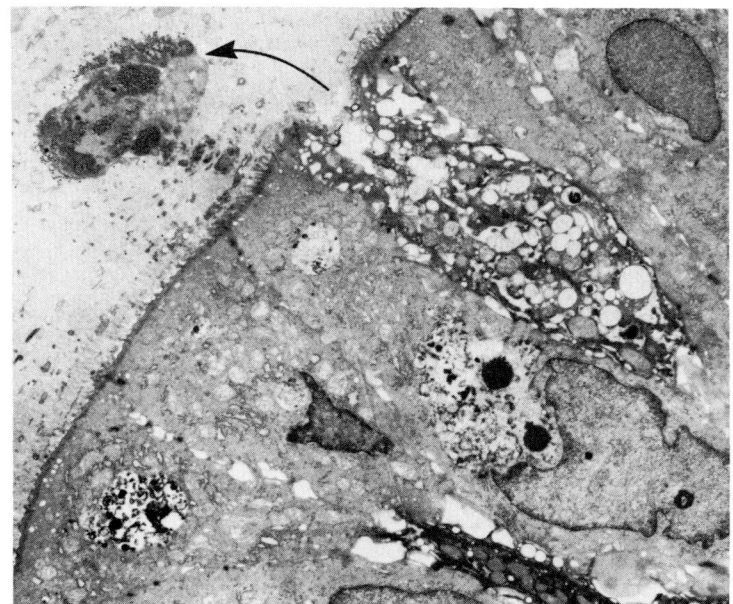

FIGURE 4–4.
Adenovirus colitis. Nucleus *(arrow)* filled with virions and extruded from infected cell into lumen. (×3400) SOURCE: Courtesy of Dr Jan Orenstein. Janoff EN, Orenstein JM, Manischewitz JF, Smith PD. Adenovirus colitis in the acquired immunodeficiency syndrome. Gastroenterology. 1991;100:976–979.

as to whether adenoviruses merely colonize intestinal tissues or actually cause enteric disease centers on the relative rates of identification of the viruses in patients with and without diarrhea. Three studies show higher rates in HIV-infected patients with diarrhea,[26, 175, 177] and three do not (see Table 4–4).[83, 112, 178] Similar to many other enteric pathogens (including rotaviruses, *G. lamblia,* and *Cryptosporidium*), adenoviruses may induce intestinal pathologic change in some patients but not in others.

Adenovirus infections have been shown to cause visceral disease, such as fulminant and fatal hepatic necrosis, in patients with AIDS or SCID and in transplant recipients.[29, 66, 179–182]

Nevertheless, despite reports of gastrointestinal hemorrhage with disseminated adenovirus infections, the colon is not a common site of adenovirus-associated symptoms and pathologic conditions.[29] Moreover, although adenoviruses can be isolated from at least 20% of AIDS patients, related signs may not be apparent. As recommended for CMV infections, the diagnosis of adenovirus colitis should be based on the identification of the virus by culture or EM examination of tissue and in the absence of copathogens. The presence of necrotic enterocytes and surrounding inflammation support the pathogenic role of the virus.

Only one study has relied solely on evaluation

FIGURE 4–5.
Adenovirus colitis. Classic crystalline array of hexagonal nucloids in the nucleus of a goblet cell. (×51,000) SOURCE: Courtesy of Dr Jan Orenstein. Janoff EN, Orenstein JM, Manischewitz JF, Smith PD. Adenovirus colitis in the acquired immunodeficiency syndrome. Gastroenterology. 1991;100:976–979.

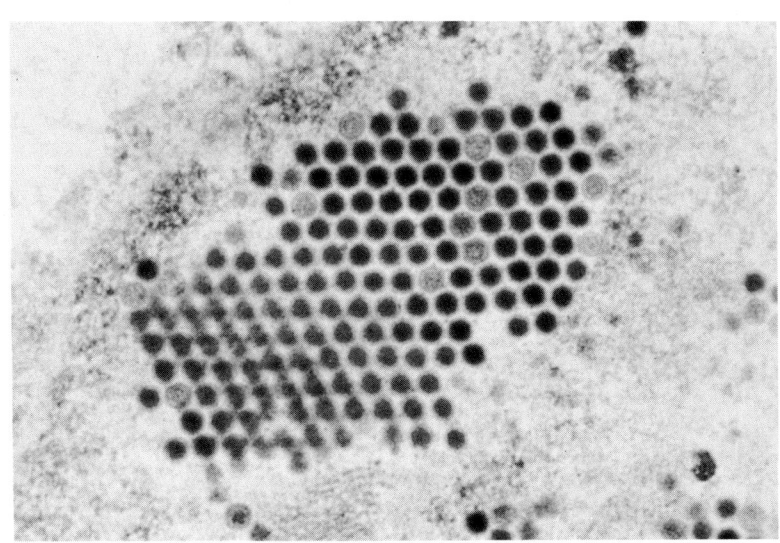

of tissue for the diagnosis of adenovirus colitis.[175] Adenovirus was identified in colonic tissue by transmission EM or culture in 5 of 67 HIV-infected homosexual men (7%) with chronic diarrhea (5 of 51 patients [10%] with AIDS), but in 0 of 10 asymptomatic control subjects. The infected mucosa, normal in 3 cases and mildly inflamed in 2, as shown by colonoscopic examination, showed foci of necrosis with chronic inflammatory cells and necrotic epithelial cells containing nuclear inclusions by light microscopy (see Fig. 4–3). These inclusions contained the crystalline array of typical hexagonal adenovirus particles by transmission electron microscopy (see Figs. 4–4 and 4–5). A second potential enteric pathogen, *Mycobacterium avium-intracellulare,* was identified concomitantly in only 1 patient. These data suggest that adenoviruses can cause intestinal pathologic conditions in some AIDS patients with diarrheal illness. More commonly, adenoviruses may also be excreted in many body fluids, including stools, from patients with advanced HIV infection, independent of the presence or absence of enteric symptoms. The diagnosis of adenovirus colitis, therefore, is predicated on the identification of the virus in inflamed tissue from symptomatic patients.

The presence of adenovirus in tissue may be missed or confused with the presence of CMV.[175, 183, 184] The viruses show similar tissue tropism, may be present simultaneously in severely immunocompromised patients,[29, 30, 185] and produce basophilic intranuclear inclusions in epithelial cells. The inclusions of adenoviruses may be amphophilic and fill the nucleus, whereas those of CMV often produce a characteristic owl's-eye appearance. Adenoviruses primarily infect epithelial cells, including goblet cells, whereas CMV is also commonly found in lamina propria endothelial cells and smooth muscle cells. The differences in cytopathic effects of adenoviruses and CMV in cell culture may not always be readily apparent, but the differentiation between the two viruses is readily made with species- and type-specific antisera. Electron microscopy is very useful in establishing the presence of adenovirus in tissue and in confirming other test results. Although serologic diagnosis using sera from immunocompromised patients is of limited value in adenovirus infections, these infections can be reliably identified using a combination of histologic studies for inclusions and inflammation with culture or EM examination of tissue.

The serotypes of adenoviruses identified in HIV-infected patients differ from those of otherwise healthy children with diarrhea. Of the six genera that comprise 47 serotypes and other new candidate types,[29, 176] those usually recovered from children, types 40 and 41,[171] are not found in stool from patients with AIDS. The AIDS patients excrete a wide range of serotypes, including those of subgenus D and new types.[29, 174, 176] Despite the primacy of subgenus D serotypes in stool isolates, no specific pathogenic role or epidemiologic significance for the serotype distribution has emerged.

Adenoviruses may produce disseminated infections in children with primary immunodeficiencies. Although hypogammaglobulinemia may be a risk factor,[186] most of these children have SCID.[29, 35, 128, 129, 187] The virus is typically isolated from multiple sites, and the serotypes are more diverse than are those from healthy children. Pneumonia and hepatitis are much more common syndromes than is diarrhea. Mortality with disseminated adenovirus infections in children with primary immunodeficiency is more than 50%.[29]

As in children with primary immunodeficiency, adenovirus-associated disease in recipients of organ and bone marrow transplants involves the lungs and liver more often than the intestinal tract.[29, 36, 66, 71] Adenoviruses are most often isolated within 4 months of transplantation.[68] Mortality appears to be a function, in part, of age. Disseminated disease is common with adenovirus infections in liver and bone marrow transplant patients (mean ages of 2 and 15 years, respectively), among whom the case fatality rates were 60% and 53%, respectively.[29] By contrast, renal transplant patients, who are older (mean age 35.6 years) and may require fewer immunosuppressive medications, are less likely to experience disseminated disease with adenovirus, resulting in a mortality of 18%.[29] The development of significant acute GVHD is related to the development of adenovirus infection and symptoms.[66, 71] Diarrheal disease attributable to adenovirus was not common in any study.

In summary, adenoviruses cause focal diarrheal disease primarily in healthy young children. The origin of defects of cell-mediated immunity that predispose patients to systemic adenovirus infections[29] include SCID,[29, 35, 128, 129, 187] malnutrition,[185] cancer, the use of corticosteroids, prematurity,[182] transplantation,[29, 36, 66, 71] and advanced HIV infection.[175, 176, 180, 181] These patients show a variety of clinical syndromes, often with disseminated infections and high mortality. Simultaneous infection with other opportunistic pathogens, particularly CMV, is common.[29, 66] Enteric symptoms are not a prominent feature in any group but are present in a limited subset. That children are exposed to adenoviruses early in life and that the viruses establish latency in lymphoid and renal cells suggests that most infections are reactivations.[66] Serotypes may be either those commonly found in the community or unusual serotypes, invoking the prospect that the viruses mutate in the immunocompromised host or that these patients may be more susceptible to atypical isolates. Prolonged excretion and identification of the virus from multiple sites are characteristics of adenovirus infections in immunodeficient patients. The presence of adenovirus in body fluids, however, is not consistently related to symptoms in the organ from which they are taken. Diagnosis of adenovirus-associated disease involves identification of the organism in tissue in the presence of local inflammation.

Rotavirus

Rotavirus is a leading cause of enteric infection in both immunocompetent[188] and immunocompromised young children,[35, 39, 133] producing substantial morbidity and mortality in both groups. Rotavirus is the leading cause of dehydration, hospitalization, and mortality among young children with diarrhea in the United States.[134, 189] The virus is identified in as many as half of otherwise healthy children younger than 3 years who have been hospitalized with acute gastroenteritis but is infrequently identified in stool samples from asymptomatic control children.[39] Similarly, among children with primary immunodeficiency, rotavirus is the organism most consistently associated with gastroenteritis but is infrequently found in asymptomatic immunodeficient children.[39] Although these infections resolve spontaneously within 1 to 2 weeks in immunocompetent children, they may induce prolonged symptomatic infections lasting longer than 6 weeks.[39]

Chronic diarrhea with rotavirus has been reported in children with SCID, THI, XLA, DiGeorge syndrome, and cartilage hair hypoplasia.[39, 128–133] These children may excrete typical or variant mutant strains of the virus. In the absence of immunoreconstitution of the host or passive antiviral immunotherapy, symptoms and excretion of the virus may last for many months and until the death of these children.

The youngest children with the most severe immunodeficiency (SCID or XLA) have prolonged infections, whereas children with THI or CVI have transient infections.[39] The severity of these rotavirus infections was suggested by the presence of viral antigen in sera from 3 of 4 immunodeficient children with diarrhea, but in 0 of 19 immunocompetent children with rotavirus-associated diarrhea. These observations suggest a defect in the barrier function of the intestinal mucosa of these children.[39] Neither children nor adults with CVI are predisposed to severe infections,[43, 123] whereas children with XLA may be.[39, 40] Children who have undergone bone marrow transplantation are not consistently at significant risk of rotavirus infection, perhaps because most are older than the children at highest risk, who are usually younger than 2 to 3 years.[66, 68] Nevertheless, gastroenteritis with rotavirus developed in 7 of 78 young adults (10%) with bone marrow transplantation, of whom 5 died.[71] Other than the two reports involving bone marrow transplant patients and AIDS patients in Australia,[26, 71] rotaviruses are not routinely identified in immunodeficient adults (see Table 4–1).[43, 123] These low rates may be due to lack of testing in adult populations, but the variation in rates between studies in immunodeficient adults is striking.

Immunotherapy is the primary approach for control of rotavirus infections in severely immunodeficient children (Table 4–8). Higher levels of preexisting neutralizing antibody rotavirus-specific IgA may correlate with resistance to infection,[190–192] and prior infection appears to confer at least partial immunity against reinfection or symptomatic infection. The role of antibody is highlighted by observations that, using preparations containing pathogen-specific antibody, these infections in immunodeficient children may be cured with human breast milk,[39] symptoms could be attenuated in low birth weight infants with oral administration of human gammaglobulin,[193] and nosocomial infections could be prevented with bovine colostrum.[194] Moreover, prevention of rotavirus infections in calves may be limited by suckling from immunized cows.[195] The cases summarized in Table 4–8 show that reconstituting the host's immune system actively by thymic reconstitution or passively with human immunoglobulin from serum or breast milk or hyperimmune bovine colostrum may provide control of these potentially serious infections in immunodeficient children. The challenge in passive immunotherapy is to provide sufficient quantities of standardized, reproducible lots of safe, tolerable (e.g., lactose-free), and effective therapy.

Herpes Simplex Virus

Herpes simplex virus causes blistering or ulceration of the lips, eyes, mouth, and skin, in-

TABLE 4–8. RESPONSE TO IMMUNOTHERAPY IN IMMUNOCOMPROMISED PATIENTS WITH DIARRHEA AND ROTAVIRUS INFECTION

UNDERLYING DISEASE	REFERENCE	NO. PATIENTS	AGE	DURATION OF SYMPTOMS	THERAPY	RESPONSE	COMMENTS
Cartilage hair hypoplasia	Wood (1988)[34]	1	18 mo	>7 mo	Human milk; IV/IM IgG	None	Astrovirus also detected
SCID	Saulsbury (1980)[39]	1	7 mo	Chronic	Human milk	Resolved	Relapsed, but then resolved on therapy
SCID	Booth (1982)[128]	1	7 mo	>3 mo	Human milk* (pooled, irradiated)	None	Died at 12 mo of disseminated adenovirus
SCID	Jarvis (1983)[35]	1	Child	months	Thymic reconstitution	Resolved	
XLA	Saulsbury (1980)[39]	1	19 mo	2 mo	Lactose-free human milk	Resolved	
XLA	Lederman (1985)[40]	2	Child	Acute	IV IgG	Resolved	

*Measurable antibody to rotavirus documented in human breast milk.

KEY: IV/IM IgG = intravenous/intramuscular pooled human IgG, SCID = severe combined immunodeficiency, XLA = X-linked agammaglobulinemia.

cluding the genital and perianal regions. Among otherwise healthy persons, HSV infections may be recurrent, but symptoms are relatively mild and transient. Among immunocompromised hosts undergoing chemotherapy for leukemia or receiving organ transplants, rates of reactivation are high (50% in both groups). These reactivated HSV infections are associated with buccal and oral lesions in most leukemic patients, but in only one third of renal transplant patients.[196] Among patients with HIV disease, however, HSV infections may be more invasive and severe and they may recur frequently, last longer, and heal more slowly. Other sites of infection include the pharynx, pancreas, and liver. Even among profoundly immunosuppressed patients, however, HSV is not a frequent cause of diarrhea or colitis,[5, 33, 38, 112] although ulcerative, necrotizing enteritis with perforation has been reported in a patient undergoing chronic steroid therapy.[197]

Among immunocompromised hosts, intestinal manifestations of HSV infection are most common in patients with HIV disease. Esophageal disease associated with HSV is discussed in Chapter 1. Chronic perianal HSV lesions and proctitis were among the first reported presentations of AIDS.[198] Symptoms include tenesmus, perianal pain, anal discharge, bleeding, and, less frequently, difficulties initiating urination. Examination reveals vesicles and progressive perianal ulcerations, often with rectal bleeding. Vesicles, ulcers, and bleeding may also be seen in the rectum and proximal sigmoid colon, and cultures show HSV type 2, at times with CMV.

Despite the invasive character of HSV infections in some immunocompromised patients and the inability to eradicate the infection, most symptoms and signs can be suppressed with antiviral therapy (see Table 4–5). Acyclovir (9-[(2-hydroxyethoxy)methyl]guanine), upon conversion from its mono- to its triphosphate derivative, inhibits replication of HSV types 1 and 2 and varicella-zoster virus by competitive inhibition of viral DNA polymerase.[199] Both intravenous and oral acyclovir shorten the time to resolution of mucocutaneous lesions compared with placebo,[200] and oral therapy is effective in preventing symptomatic lesions.[201]

Therapy may be complicated by the emergence of acyclovir-resistant organisms that show an absence of thymidine kinase or of its activity. Clinical isolates of acyclovir-resistant HSV are derived primarily from HIV-infected patients on prolonged courses of therapy for prophylaxis or chronic suppression.[202–206] Acute exacerbations of perirectal symptoms and signs that are no longer responsive to oral acyclovir owing to the development of resistance may respond to intravenous therapy with foscarnet[204–206] or to high dosages of acyclovir.[202] Relapses are typical after discontinuation of therapy.

Enterovirus

Prospective studies demonstrate that enteroviruses are not commonly the cause of acute enteric symptoms.[207] Immunodeficiency may predispose to infection, and to more severe infections, however, with systemic viruses that are acquired through an enteric route. Polioviruses, for example, are transmitted by intestinal routes and cause paralytic disease at a much higher rate among hypogammaglobulinemic patients than among immunocompetent subjects.[208, 209]

In the United States from 1980–1989, oral polio vaccine (OPV) was implicated as the source in 80 of 86 reported cases (93%) of paralytic polio; 5 were imported and none was endemic.[209] Of these vaccine-associated cases, 14 (18%) occurred in immunodeficient patients. The majority, 12 of 14 patients (86%), were hypogammaglobulinemic, 2 were being treated with steroids, and none was known to be infected with HIV. Only 9 patients had received OPV directly, and the subsequent diagnosis of hypogammaglobulinemia was previously unsuspected in all. Based on these data that an appreciable proportion of these cases occurred in immunodeficient patients, approximately half of whom were younger than 1 year, and that the incidence of primary immunodeficiency in children is approximately 1 case per 10,000 infants, the risk of vaccine-associated paralytic polio in immunodeficient infants (0.16%/yr) is estimated to be more than 2000 times higher than the risk in other infants receiving OPV.[209] These findings highlight the dramatic predisposition of immunodeficient patients to enteroviral infections, including those with attenuated vaccine strains. To date, HIV-infected patients do not appear to be at increased risk of enteroviral infections, particularly in association with enteric symptoms.[26]

Human Immunodeficiency Virus

The association between HIV infection and enteric disease is clear, but the pathogenesis of HIV-associated diarrhea is often obscure. Bacterial (*Salmonella* species, *C. jejuni*, *Shigella* species, and *M. avium* complex), viral (CMV and adenoviruses), fungal (such as *Histoplasma capsulatum*), and parasitic (especially *Cryptosporidium*, *Isospora belli*, *Enterocytozoon bieneusi* [Microsporida], and *G. lamblia*) enteric pathogens have been identified in the majority (50–85%) of HIV-infected patients with diarrhea.[5, 33, 38, 106, 112, 210] Nevertheless, no specific pathogen has been identified in an appreciable proportion of these patients (15–50%). In this setting, the role of HIV itself as an enteric pathogen is an intriguing and controversial concept.

Human immunodeficiency virus has been identified in intestinal tissues by direct culture, immunocytochemical study, and in situ hybridization in up to one third of patients tested.[86, 99, 211–213] Infected cells are found in the lamina propria of both colonic and duodenal specimens,[211, 212] and they may be found in the base of bowel crypts.[211] In the lamina propria, both macrophages and lymphocytes appeared to be infected. Nelson and colleagues and Levy and colleagues suggested that bowel neuroendocrine cells, such as enterochromaffin cells, were also infected,[211, 214] whereas Fox and colleagues found no evidence of HIV-infected cells outside of the lamina propria.[212] In vivo infection of columnar epithelial or goblet cells is not well documented, but in vitro, human colonic epithelial cell lines can be infected with several strains of HIV and can maintain productive infections.[215–217] Therefore, although the range of host cells infected is unclear, the presence of HIV in intestinal tissue and immune cells has been well documented. The clinical relevance of these findings is less well accepted.

Human immunodeficiency virus infection increases the susceptibility of infected patients to secondary enteric pathogens, but it may also have a direct role in inducing enteric symptoms. Diarrheal symptoms may occur during acute HIV infection.[218] These enteric symptoms may result directly from HIV infection of the bowel or may arise as an acute local response to systemic infection. Nevertheless, the virus has not been identified in intestinal tissues during acute infection. Attention has been directed to defining the effects of chronic HIV infection on intestinal function.

An early study suggested that HIV infection alone may be associated with enteric symptoms in patients in whom no traditional pathogen was identified, a condition referred to as AIDS enteropathy.[219] The impact of this study has been diminished by the identification of new potential pathogens, such as Microsporida, which may be responsible for the syndrome.[109] Nevertheless, independent of the presence or absence of other identifiable pathogens, patients with HIV infection demonstrate a range of morphometric and functional intestinal abnormalities. These abnormalities include lactase deficiency, malabsorption, small bowel atrophy, and defects in enterocyte maturation.[38, 85, 100, 220] That mucosal atrophy may be present without either diarrhea or identifiable pathogens suggests a role for HIV in its pathogenesis. However, these reports have shown no consistent correlation between the presence of HIV in tissue and enteric symptoms or between mucosal histologic change and symptoms in the presence or absence of other known pathogens.

The interaction between the intestinal tract and HIV is complex and multifactorial. The intestine may serve four important roles in the natural history and pathogenesis of HIV infection. First, it may be the site of entry of HIV into the body or the source of virus transmitted to others, since most HIV transmission occurs via mucosal routes among homosexual men and heterosexual men and women. In this capacity, HIV is not an opportunistic infection per se. Rather, HIV acts as a standard pathogen transmissible to normal tissues in immunocompetent hosts.[211, 221, 222] Second, in addition to its role in the transmission of HIV, the gastrointestinal tract probably serves as a reservoir of HIV infection. The intestinal tract is the largest immune organ, and lamina propria mononuclear cells are those most commonly detected with HIV.[212] Because lymphocytes routinely travel through the intestine en route to the lamina propria in distant mucosal immune tissues,[5, 28] HIV infection of the intestinal tract may augment infection in other sites. Third, HIV induces profound immune suppression both systemically and locally.[5, 93, 95, 97, 98, 102] As a result, HIV-infected patients are predisposed to a variety of routine and opportunistic pathogens that often produce severe, prolonged, and even fatal enteric infections. Fourth, HIV may play a direct role in inducing enteric symptoms after acute infection or later in the course of the disease. These concepts highlight the importance of defining the specific cells infected with HIV in the intestine and of determining the specific pathologic consequences of these infections in the gut. The intestine may serve as a major obstacle to controlling HIV infection, but it may also provide an avenue for preventing transmission of HIV.

APPROACH TO THERAPY OF ENTERIC DISEASE IN IMMUNOCOMPROMISED PATIENTS

Initial Management

Clinically, successful management of immunocompromised patients with enteric disease is dependent upon replenishing of fluids and nutrition, establishing a specific diagnosis, and attempting to reverse the degree of immunosuppression. As with any patient with diarrheal disease and independently of immune status, an appreciable proportion of the morbidity and mortality is a consequence of dehydration rather than of the primary pathology of the infection. In this regard, development and use of inexpensive but effective oral rehydration solutions for fluid and electrolytes have been of benefit to more children in developing countries than have many vaccines and antimicrobial agents.[223] If oral rehydration is not possible owing to nausea or vomiting, intravenous fluids are useful to reverse orthostatic changes and to restore fluid balance and urine output.

Once rehydration has been initiated, establishing the specific cause of the enteric symptoms is critical in the immunocompromised patient to avoid invasive and expensive diagnostic procedures and to prevent misdirected empirical therapy. In the clinical history, the duration and severity of symptoms are useful data for determining the need for more than supportive therapy. A history of recent travel may suggest more treatable pathogens (e.g., bacterial or parasitic) and a similar illness in the family may suggest a more transient and less ominous cause (e.g., Norwalk virus). Medications may induce malabsorption and steatorrhea (cholestyramine and clofibrate), intestinal hemorrhage or hematomas with pain and vomiting (anticoagulants), intestinal ischemia (oral contraceptives, nonsteroidal anti-inflammatory medications, digoxin), or transient ileus (cyclosporine).[224] The use of laxatives should be excluded. In association with the use of virtually any antibiotic and even after chemotherapy, *C. difficile* may induce mild diarrhea or severe colitis. Therefore, excluding reversible noninfectious and treatable nonviral causes of enteric symptoms provides a simple, cost-effective first step in the evaluation of the immunosuppressed patient with enteric symptoms (Table 4–9).

Another rationale for persevering in determining the specific cause for enteric symptoms in the immunodeficient patient is that the primary therapy for their underlying disease may also elicit serious enteric disease of noninfectious or nonviral origin. These complications may follow chemotherapy (e.g., ischemic colitis or necrotizing enterocolitis with granulocytopenia), radiation therapy, or bone-marrow transplantation GVHD[59] and include the occurrence of secondary bowel malignancies. Moreover, infectious and noninfectious syndromes may occur concurrently. *Clostridium difficile*–associated colitis, bacterial enteritis, or overgrowth of the small bowel may be associated with diarrhea in this setting. Similarly, enteric viral infections, particularly CMV, may accompany GVHD.[72] Given the complex co-incidence and interaction of noninfectious and infectious causes for intestinal symptoms in the immunocompromised host, identifying a specific cause is important for appropriate and effective management of these syndromes.

Initial management should not include empirical therapy of intestinal symptoms with antimicrobials. Because the range of enteric pathogens is extremely broad in immunocompromised patients, including bacterial, parasitic, fungal, and viral agents, empirical therapy is an unwarranted and unrewarding approach. Mis-

TABLE 4–9. DIAGNOSTIC EVALUATION OF IMMUNOCOMPROMISED PATIENTS WITH DIARRHEA

HISTORY

Underlying disease	Type of immunosuppression
Duration of symptoms	Travel history
Presence of fever, bloody stool	Medications

PHYSICAL EXAMINATION

Fever	Orthostatic signs (pulse, blood pressure)
Nutritional status (wasting)	Retinal examination (if suspecting CMV)

Abdominal pain (epigastric, lower abdominal, rebound, focal findings)

STOOL EXAMINATION

Culture for routine bacterial pathogens
  (e.g., *Campylobacter* spp, *Salmonella* spp, *Shigella* spp)
  (consider blood cultures in febrile HIV-infected patients)
Assay for *Clostridium difficile* cytotoxin
Culture for *C. difficile* organisms
Direct or concentrated specimen for ova and parasites or both (3 specimens)
Acid-fast stain of stool and parasitic examination
  (for *Cryptosporidium* spp, *Mycobacterium avium* complex [MAC], *Isospora belli*)
Modified trichrome stain for Microsporida[237]
Viral antigen detection (such as for rotavirus by enzyme-linked immunosorbent assay)
Viral detection by electron microscopy (for rotavirus, Norwalk, astrovirus)

ENDOSCOPIC EXAMINATION

Tissue inspection
  (e.g., for ulcers, nodules, pseudomembranes)
Biopsy culture
  Cytomegalovirus and MAC (duodenal and colonic tissue)
  Adenovirus and herpes simplex (colonic tissue)
  Bacterial cultures (duodenal tissue)
Biopsy histology
  Hematoxylin-eosin (cytomegalovirus, adenovirus, *Cryptosporidium*, *Isospora*)
  Giemsa *(Giardia)*
  Methenamine silver *(Histoplasma capsulatum)*
  Acid fast or Fite *(Cryptosporidium, Isospora*, MAC)
  Electron microscopy (Microsporida, adenovirus)
Duodenal fluid
  Culture for bacteria
  Examination for ova and parasites

SOURCE: Adapted from Janoff EN, Smith PD. Perspectives on gastrointestinal infections in AIDS. Gastroenterol Clin North Am. 1988; 17:451–463.

directed treatment may obscure the results of subsequent diagnostic techniques, may cause avoidable side effects, and may delay establishing the true cause and initiating proper therapy. Moreover, enteric pathogens in immunocompromised hosts are more often resistant to commonly used antimicrobial agents, including antiviral drugs, and viral pathogens may develop resistance during the course of therapy.[168, 203, 204] Therefore, a specific diagnosis should be made upon initial evaluation to initiate suitable treatment and to monitor appropriately the clinical and microbiologic response.

Defining the type of immunodeficiency present facilitates selecting the suitable tests for the most common organisms in specific patient groups (Tables 4–1 and 4–9). As described in Chapter 3 on enteric viral infections in the normal host and in Chapters 19 and 20 on diagnostic evaluations, newer methods have facilitated the detection of standard pathogens and the discovery of newer infectious agents.[1–3, 71] These assays include improved culture techniques, use of increasingly sensitive and specific enzyme-immunoassays, EM examination of stool, either direct EM or immune electron microscopy, in addition to light microscopy of intestinal biopsies. As a consequence of these advances, many enteric viral pathogens can be identified or excluded in patients at risk.

In addition to initiating fluid replenishment and establishing a specific diagnosis, the third priority in the initial approach to the immunocompromised patient with a documented serious viral infection is to attempt to limit the degree of immunosuppression. With HIV-infected patients, this may involve initiating or modifying antiretroviral therapy if possible. With the cancer patient, delaying or limiting the intensity of chemotherapy can be considered. With the transplant patient, administration of immunosuppressive therapy forces the physician perpetually to balance the risk of serious infection with the risk of organ or graft rejection. This quandary reinforces the value of establishing a specific diagnosis. For example, a serious infectious source of symptoms suggests a decrease in immunosuppressive therapy, often even at the risk, or even at the cost, of rejection (e.g., for renal transplants). By contrast, if GVHD is the source of symptoms, more aggressive immunosuppression may be indicated. These difficult clinical management problems are best decided with as complete a data base as possible and with an understanding of the pathogenesis and natural history of these enteric viral infections.

Long-Term Care

The development of specific antiviral agents has allowed prolonged survival in some immunocompromised patients with severe viral infections. Pharmacologic agents include acyclovir, ganciclovir, and foscarnet, and immune products include human serum IgG delivered orally or intravenously and immune human breast milk or colostrum as well as immune and hyperimmune bovine colostrum.[34, 35, 39, 40, 133, 194, 225, 226] The efficacy of selected agents is summarized in Tables 4–5, 4–6, and 4–8. Often, when no diagnosis is made or specific antiviral therapy is ineffective or unavailable, control of enteric symptoms becomes the goal. Antimotility agents (loperamide or opiate-based products) may be useful initially,[227, 228] but their efficacy may wane. Somatostatin analogs (octreotide) have been used in AIDS patients under these conditions with some limited success.[229] Bulk-forming agents may be administered to tolerance, although the actual volume loss may or may not be affected. Providing nutritional support, whether enteral or parenteral, may not enhance intestinal function. Therefore, the outcome for immunocompromised patients with viral enteric infections is dependent on the severity of the underlying disease and the susceptibility of the virus to spontaneous remission or available antiviral therapy.

ACKNOWLEDGMENTS

I thank Drs. Phillip D. Smith (University of Alabama School of Medicine, Birmingham AL) and Claire Pomeroy (Veterans Affairs Medical Center, University of Minnesota School of Medicine, Minneapolis MN) for thoughtful comments, Dr. Jan Orenstein for light and electron micrographs, and Ann Emery for excellent secretarial assistance. This work was supported in part by Veterans Affairs Research Service and National Institutes of Health grant AI31373.

REFERENCES

1. Greenberg HB, Matsui SM. Astroviruses and caliciviruses: Emerging enteric pathogens. Infect Agents Dis. 1992;1:71–91.
2. Christensen ML. Human viral gastroenteritis. Clin Microbiol Rev. 1989;2:51–89.
3. Blacklow NR, Greenberg HB. Viral gastroenteritis. N Engl J Med. 1991;325:252–264.
4. Elson CO, Kagnoff MF, Fiocchi C, et al. Intestinal immunity and inflammation: Recent progress. Gastroenterology. 1986;91:746–768.
5. Smith PD, Quinn TC, Strober W, et al. Gastrointestinal infections in AIDS. Ann Intern Med. 1992;116:63–77.
6. Rosen FS, Cooper MD, Wedgwood RJP. The primary immunodeficiencies. N Engl J Med. 1984;311:300–310.
7. Rosen FS, Cooper MD, Wedgwood RJP. The primary immunodeficiencies. N Engl J Med. 1984;311:235–242.
8. Keusch GT. Nutrition as a determinant of host response to infection and the metabolic sequelae of infectious diseases. In: Weinstein L, Fields BN, eds. Seminars in Infectious Disease, Vol 2. New York: Grune & Stratton; 1979:265–303.
9. Watson RR, McMurray DN. The effects of malnutrition on secretory and cellular immune processes. Crit Rev Food Sci Nutr. 1979;12:113–159.
10. Neumann CG, Lawlor GJ, Stiehm ER, et al. Immunologic response in malnourished children. Am J Clin Nutr. 1975;28:89.
11. Scrimshaw NS, Taylor CE, Gordon JE. Interactions of nutrition and infections. Am J Med Sci. 1959;237:367.
12. Sirisinha S, Suskind R, Edelman R, et al. Secretory and serum IgA in children with protein-calorie malnutrition. Pediatrics. 1975;55:166.
13. Casali P, Rice GPA, Oldstone MBA. Viruses disrupt functions of human lymphocytes: Effects of measles virus and influenza virus on lymphocyte-mediated killing and antibody production. J Exp Med. 1984; 159:1322–1327.
14. Hirsch RL, Griffin DE, et al. Cellular immune response during complicated and uncomplicated measles virus infections of man. Clin Immunol Immunopathol. 1984;31:1–12.
15. Joffee MI, Sukha RN, Rabson AR. Lymphocyte subsets in measles. J Clin Invest. 1982;72:77–80.
16. Monif GRG, Hood CI. Ileocolitis associated with measles (rubeola). Am J Dis Child. 1970;120:245–247.
17. Whittle HC, Dosseter J, et al. Cell-mediated immunity during natural measles infection. J Clin Invest. 1978;62:678–684.
18. Fauci AS. The human immunodeficiency virus: Infectivity and mechanisms of pathogenesis. Science. 1988;239:617–622.
19. Peterson PK. Host defense abnormalities predisposing the patient to infection. Am J Med. 1984;76:2–10.
20. Wilson CB. The cellular immune system and its role in host defense. In: Mandell GL, Douglas RGJ, Bennett JE. Principles and Practices of Infectious Diseases. 3rd ed. New York: Churchill Livingstone; 1990:101–128.
21. Ruskin J, McIntosh J, Remington JS. Studies on the mechanisms of resistance to phylogenetically diverse intracellular organisms. J Immunol. 1969;103:252–259.
22. Murray HW. Interferon-gamma, the activated macrophage, and the host defense against microbial challenge. Ann Intern Med. 1988;108:595–608.
23. Royer HD, Reinherz EL. T lymphocytes: Ontogeny, function, and relevance to clinical disorders. N Engl J Med. 1987;317:1136–1142.
24. Quinnan GV, Dirmani N, Rook AH, et al. Cytotoxic T cells in cytomegalovirus infection. N Engl J Med. 1982;307:7–12.
25. Murray HW, Scavuzzo D, Jacobs JL, et al. In vitro and in vivo activation of human mononuclear phagocytes by gamma interferon: Studies with normal and AIDS monocytes. J Immunol. 1987;138:2457–2462.
26. Cunningham AL, Grohman GS, Harkness J, et al. Gastrointestinal viral infections in homosexual men who were symptomatic and seropositive for human immunodeficiency virus. J Infect Dis. 1988;158:386–391.
27. Pomeroy C, Oken MM, Rydell RE, et al. Infection in the myelodysplastic syndromes. Am J Med. 1991; 90:338–344.
28. Brown WR, Strober W. Immunological diseases of the gastrointestinal tract. In: Samter M. Immunological Diseases. 4th ed. Boston: Little, Brown; 1988;1995–2033.
29. Hierholzer JC. Adenoviruses in the immunocompromised host. Clin Microbiol Rev. 1992;5:262–274.
30. Ho M. Cytomegalovirus: Biology and Infection. 2nd ed. New York: Plenum; 1991.
31. Lane HD, Masur H, Gelmann EP, et al. Correlation between immunologic function and clinical subpopulations of patients with the acquired immune deficiency syndrome. Am J Med. 1985;78:417–422.
32. Smith PD, Saini SS, Orenstein JM. Infections of the large intestine in the immunocompromised host. In: Phillips SF, Pemberton JH, Shorter RG. The Large Intestine: Physiology, Pathophysiology, and Disease. New York: Raven Press; 1991:437–444.
33. Janoff EN, Smith PD. Perspectives on gastrointestinal

infections in AIDS. Gastroenterol Clin North Am. 1988;17:451–463.

34. Wood DJ, David TJ, Chrystie IL, et al. Chronic enteric virus infection in two T-cell immunodeficient children. J Med Virol. 1988;24:435–444.

35. Jarvis WR, Middleton PJ, Gelfand EW. Significance of viral infection in severe combined immunodeficiency disease. Pediatr Infect Dis. 1983;2:187–192.

36. Zaia JA. Viral infections associated with bone marrow transplantation. Hematol Oncol Clin North Am. 1990;4:603–623.

37. Wingard JR, Chen DY, Burns WH, et al. Cytomegalovirus infection after autologous bone marrow transplantation with comparison to infection after allogeneic bone marrow transplantation. Blood. 1988;71:1432–1437.

38. Smith PD, Lane HC, Gill VJ, et al. Intestinal infections in patients with the acquired immunodeficiency syndrome (AIDS): Etiology and response to therapy. Ann Intern Med. 1988;108:328–333.

39. Saulsbury FT, Winkelstein JA, Yolken RH. Chronic rotavirus infection in immunodeficiency. J Pediatr. 1980;97:61–65.

40. Lederman HM, Winkelstein JA. X-linked agammaglobulinemia: An analysis of 96 patients. Medicine. 1985;64:145–156.

41. Yocum MW, Kelso JM. Common variable immunodeficiency: The disorder and treatment. Mayo Clin Proc. 1991;66:83–96.

42. MacCallum FO. The role of humoral antibodies in protection against and recovery from bacterial and virus infections in hypogammaglobulinaemia. Medical Research Council Special Report Series No. 310. London. Her Majesty's Stationery Office. 1971;310:72–85.

43. Cunningham-Rundles C. Clinical and immunologic analyses of 103 patients with common variable immunodeficiency. J Clin Immunol. 1989;9:22–33.

44. Misbah SA, Spickett GP, Ryba PCJ, et al. Chronic enteroviral meningoencephalitis in agammaglobulinemia: Case report and literature review. J Clin Immunol. 1992;12:266–270.

45. Ament ME, Ochs HD, Davis DD. Structure and function of the gastrointestinal tract in primary immunodeficiency syndromes: A study of 39 patients. Medicine. 1973;52:227–248.

46. LoGalbo PR, Sampson HA, Buckley RH. Symptomatic giardiasis in three patients with X-linked agammaglobulinemia. J Pediatr. 1982;101:78–80.

47. Perlmutter DH, Leichtner AM, Goldman H, et al. Chronic diarrhea associated with hypogammaglobulinemia and enteropathy in infants and children. Dig Dis Sci. 1985;30:1149–1155.

48. Melnick JL. Enteroviruses. In: Fields BN, Knipe DM, Chanock RM, et al. Virology. 2nd ed. New York: Raven Press; 1990:549–605.

49. Hofflin JM, Potasman I, Baldwin JC, et al. Infectious complications in heart transplant recipients receiving cyclosporine and corticosteroids. Ann Intern Med. 1987;106:209–216.

50. Dunn DL, Najarian JS. New approaches to the diagnosis, prevention, and treatment of cytomegalovirus infection after transplantation. Am J Surg. 1991;161:250–255.

51. Cates J, Chavez M, Laks H, et al. Gastrointestinal complications after cardiac transplantation: A spectrum of diseases. Am J Gastroenterol. 1991;86:412–416.

52. Dummer JS, Montero CG, Griffith BP, et al. Infections in heart-lung transplant recipients. Transplantation. 1986;41:725–729.

53. Gold JW, Yu B, Brigati D, et al. Disseminated adenovirus infection in marrow transplant unit patients. Clin Res. 1981;29:385A.

54. Gorensek MJ, Stewart RW, Key TF, et al. A multivariate analysis of the risk of cytomegalovirus infection in heart transplant recipients. J Infect Dis. 1988;157:515–522.

55. Gorensek MJ, Carey WD, Vogt D, et al. A multivariate analysis of risk factors for cytomegalovirus infection in liver-transplant recipients. Gastroenterology. 1990;98:1326–1332.

56. Kaplan CS, Petersen EA, Icenogle TB, et al. Gastrointestinal cytomegalovirus infection in heart and heart-lung transplant recipients. Arch Intern Med. 1989;149:2095–2100.

57. Keating MR, Wilhelm MP, Walker RC. Strategies for prevention of infection after cardiac transplantation. Mayo Clin Proc. 1992;67:676–684.

58. Kusne S, Dummer JS, Singh N, et al. Infections after liver transplantation: An analysis of 101 consecutive cases. Medicine. 1988;67:132–143.

59. McDonald GB, Shulman HM, Sullivan KM, et al. Intestinal and hepatic complications of human bone marrow transplantation. Gastroenterology. 1986;90:770–784.

60. Metselaar HJ, Weimar W. Cytomegalovirus infection and renal transplantation. J Antimicrob Chemother. 1989;23(suppl E):37–47.

61. Meyers WC, Harris N, Stein S, et al. Alimentary tract complications after renal transplantation. Ann Surg. 1979;190:535–542.

62. Meyers JD. Infection in bone marrow transplant recipients. Am J Med. 1986;81:27–38.

63. Peterson PK, Balfour HH Jr, Marker SC, et al. Cytomegalovirus disease in renal allograft recipients: A prospective study of the clinical features, risk factors and impact on renal transplantation. Medicine. 1980;59:283–300.

64. Peterson PK, Balfour HH Jr, Fryd DS, et al. Fever in renal transplant recipients: Causes, prognostic significance and changing patterns at the University of Minnesota Hospital. Am J Med. 1981;71:345–351.

65. Rubin RH. Impact of cytomegalovirus infection on organ transplant recipients. Rev Infect Dis. 1990;12(suppl 7):S754–S766.

66. Shields AF, Hackman RC, Fife KH, et al. Adenovirus infections in patients undergoing bone-marrow transplantation. N Engl J Med. 1985;312:529–533.

67. Townsend TR, Bolyard EA, Yolken RH, et al. Outbreak of coxsackie A1 gastroenteritis: A complication of bone-marrow transplantation. Lancet. 1982;1:820–823.

68. Wasserman R, August CS, Plotkin SA. Viral infections in pediatric bone marrow transplant patients. Pediatr Infect Dis J. 1988;7:109–115.

69. Willoughby RE, Wee S-B, Yolken RH. Non–group A rotavirus infection associated with severe gastroenteritis in a bone marrow transplant patient. Pediatr Infect Dis J. 1988;7:133–135.

70. Wreghitt T. Cytomegalovirus infections in heart and heart-lung transplant recipients. J Antimicrob Chemother. 1989;23(suppl E):49–60.

71. Yolken RH, Bishop CA, Townsend TR, et al. Infectious gastroenteritis in bone marrow transplant recipients. N Engl J Med. 1982;306:1010–1012.

72. Buckner FS, Pomeroy C. Cytomegalovirus disease of the gastrointestinal tract in patients without AIDS. Clin Infect Dis. 1993;17:644–656.

73. McDonald GB, Sale GE. The human gastrointestinal tract after allogeneic marrow transplantation. In: Sale GE, Shulman HM. The Pathology of Bone Marrow Transplantation. New York: Masson; 1984:77–103.

74. Reed EC, Wolford JL, Kopecky KJ, et al. Ganciclovir for the treatment of cytomegalovirus gastroenteritis in bone marrow transplant patients: A randomized pla-

cebo-controlled trial. Ann Intern Med. 1990;112:505–510.

75. Mayoral JL, Loeffler CM, Fasola CG, et al. Diagnosis and treatment of cytomegalovirus disease in transplant patients based on gastrointestinal tract manifestations. Arch Surg. 1991;126:202–206.

76. Paya CV, Hermans PE, Washington JA II, et al. Incidence, distribution, and outcome of episodes of infection in 100 orthotopic liver transplantations. Mayo Clin Proc. 1989;64:555–564.

77. Malebranche R, Arnoux E, Guerin JM, et al. Acquired immunodeficiency syndrome with severe gastrointestinal manifestations in Haiti. Lancet. 1983;2:873–878.

78. Colebunders R, Francis H, Mann JM, et al. Persistent diarrhea, strongly associated with HIV infection in Kinshasa, Zaire. Am J Gastroenterol. 1987;82:859–864.

79. DeHovitz JA, Pape JW, Boncy M, et al. Clinical manifestations and therapy of Isospora belli infection in patients with the acquired immunodeficiency syndrome. N Engl J Med. 1986;315:87–90.

80. Dworkin B, Wormser GP, Rosenthal WS, et al. Gastrointestinal manifestations of the acquired immunodeficiency syndrome: A review of 22 cases. Am J Gastroenterol. 1985;80:774–778.

81. Piot P, Quinn TC, Taelman H, et al. Acquired immunodeficiency syndrome in heterosexual population in Zaire. Lancet. 1984;1:65–69.

82. Serwadda D, Mugerwa RD, Sewankambo NK, et al. Slim disease: A new disease in Uganda and its association with HTLV-III infection. Lancet. 1985;1:849–852.

83. Kaljot KT, Ling JP, Gold JWM, et al. Prevalence of acute enteric viral pathogens in acquired immunodeficiency syndrome patients with diarrhea. Gastroenterology. 1989;97:1031–1032.

84. Miró JM, Mallolas J, Moreno A, et al. Infectious gastroenteritis with the acquired immunodeficiency syndrome (AIDS). Ann Intern Med. 1988;342, Letter.

85. Gillin JS, Shike M, Alcock N, et al. Malabsorption and mucosal abnormalities of the small intestine in the acquired immunodeficiency syndrome. Ann Intern Med. 1985;102:612–622.

86. Ullrich R, Zeitz M, Heise W, et al. Small intestinal structure and function in patients infected with human immunodeficiency virus (HIV): Evidence for HIV-induced enteropathy. Ann Intern Med. 1989;111:15–21.

87. Fauci AS, Schnittman SM, Poli G, et al. Immunopathogenic mechanisms in human immunodeficiency virus (HIV) infection. Ann Intern Med. 1991;114:678–693.

88. Spickett GP, Dalgleish AG. Cellular immunology of HIV-infection. Clin Exp Immunol. 1988;71:1–7.

89. Cohn ZA, Steinman RM. The immunological and infectious sequelae of the acquired immune deficiency syndrome. J Exp Med. 1988;168:2415–2423.

90. Rook AH. Interactions of cytomegalovirus with the human immune system. Rev Infect Dis. 1988;10(suppl 3):S460–S467.

91. Rook AH, Manischewitz JF, Frederick WR, et al. Deficient, HLA-restricted, cytomegalovirus-specific cytotoxic T cells and natural killer cells in patients with the acquired immunodeficiency syndrome. J Infect Dis. 1985;152:627–630.

92. Rook AH, Hooks JJ, Quinnan GV, et al. Interleukin-2 enhances the natural killer cell activity of acquired immunodeficiency syndrome patients through a γ-interferon–independent mechanism. J Immunol. 1985; 134:1503–1507.

93. Rook AH, Masur H, Lane HC, et al. Interleukin-2 enhances the depressed natural killer cell and cytomegalovirus specific cytotoxic activities of lymphocytes from patients with the acquired immunodeficiency syndrome. J Clin Invest. 1983;73:398–403.

94. Murray HW, Rubin BY, Masur H, et al. Impaired production of lymphokines and immune (gamma) interferon in the acquired immunodeficiency syndrome. N Engl J Med. 1984;310:883–889.

95. Budhraja M, Levendoglu H, Kocka F, et al. Duodenal mucosal T cell subpopulation and bacterial cultures in acquired immune deficiency syndrome. Am J Gastroenterol. 1987;82:427–431.

96. Dobbins WOI, Weinstein WM. Electron microscopy of the intestine and rectum in acquired immunodeficiency syndrome. Gastroenterology. 1985;88:738–749.

97. Rodgers VD, Fassett R, Kagnoff MF. Abnormalities in intestinal mucosal T cells in homosexual populations including those with the lymphadenopathy syndrome and acquired immunodeficiency syndrome. Gastroenterology. 1986;90:552–558.

98. Ellakany S, Whiteside TL, Schade RR, et al. Analysis of intestinal lymphocyte subpopulations in patients with acquired immunodeficiency syndrome (AIDS) and AIDS-related complex. J Clin Pathol. 1987;87:356–364.

99. Jarry A, Cortez A, René E, et al. Infected cells and immune cells in the gastrointestinal tract of AIDS patients: An immunohistochemical study of 127 cases. Histopathology. 1990;16:133–140.

100. Ullrich R, Zeitz M, Heise W, et al. Mucosal atrophy is associated with loss of activated T cells in the duodenal mucosa of human immunodeficiency virus (HIV)-infected patients. Digestion. 1990;46(suppl 2):302–307.

101. Zeitz M, Greene WC, Peffer NJ, et al. Lymphocytes isolated from the intestinal lamina propria of normal nonhuman primates have increased expression of genes associated with T-cell activation. Gastroenterology. 1988;94:647–655.

102. Kotler DP, Scholes JV, Tierney AR. Intestinal plasma cell alterations in acquired immunodeficiency syndrome. Dig Dis Sci. 1987;32:129–138.

103. Janoff EN, Wahl SM, Smith PD. Antibodies to human immunodeficiency virus-1 (HIV) in the small intestine are primarily IgG, not IgA. Gastroenterology. 1989;96:236A.

104. Jackson S. Secretory and serum IgA are inversely altered in AIDS patients. In: Macdonald TT, Challacombe SJ, Bland PW, et al. Advances in Mucosal Immunology. Lancaster: Kluwer Academic Publishers; 1990:665.

105. Janoff EN, Douglas JM, Gabriel M, et al. Class-specific antibody response to pneumococcal capsular polysaccharides in men infected with human immunodeficiency virus type 1. J Infect Dis. 1988;158:983–990.

106. Janoff EN, Smith PD, Blaser MJ. Acute antibody responses to Giardia lamblia are depressed in patients with the acquired immunodeficiency syndrome. J Infect Dis. 1988;157:798–804.

107. Quinnan GV Jr, Masur H, Rook AH, et al. Herpesvirus infections in the acquired immune deficiency syndrome. JAMA. 1984;252:72–77.

108. Janoff EN, Hardy WD, Smith PD, et al. Levels, specificity, and affinity of IgG specific for recall antigens in patients with HIV. J Immunol. 1991;147:2130–2135.

109. Orenstein JM, Chiang J, Steinberg W, et al. Intestinal microsporidiosis as a cause of diarrhea in human immunodeficiency virus–infected patients: A report of 20 cases. Hum Pathol. 1990;21:475–481.

110. Ungar BLP, Ward DJ, Fayer R, et al. Cessation of Cryptosporidium-associated diarrhea in an acquired immunodeficiency syndrome patient after treatment with hyperimmune bovine colostrum. Gastroenterology. 1990;98:486–489.

111. Nelson MR, Connolly GM, Hawkins DA, et al. Foscarnet in the treatment of cytomegalovirus infection of the esophagus and colon in patients with the acquired

immune deficiency syndrome. Am J Gastroenterol. 1991;86:876–881.

112. Laughon BE, Druckman DA, Vernon A, et al. Prevalence of enteric pathogens in homosexual men with and without acquired immunodeficiency syndrome. Gastroenterology. 1988;94:984–993.

113. Cooper MD, Butler JL. Primary immunodeficiency diseases. In: Paul WE. Fundamental Immunology. 2nd ed. New York: Raven Press; 1989:1033–1056.

114. Onorato IM, Markowitz LE, Oxtoby MJ. Childhood immunization, vaccine-preventable diseases and infection with human immunodeficiency virus. Pediatr Infect Dis J. 1988;6:588–595.

115. Plebani A, Ugazio AG, Monafo V, et al. Clinical heterogeneity and reversibility of selective immunoglobulin A deficiency in 80 children. Lancet. 1986;1:829–831.

116. Conley ME, Cooper MA. Immature IgA B cells in IgA-deficient patients. N Engl J Med. 1981;305:495–497.

117. McClelland DBL, Shearman DJC, Van Furth R. Synthesis of immunoglobulin and secretory component by gastrointestinal mucosa in patients with hypogammaglobulinemia or IgA deficiency. Clin Exp Immunol. 1976;25:103–111.

118. Doe WF. Immunodeficiency and the gastrointestinal tract. Clin Gastroenterol. 1983;12:839–853.

119. Oxelius VA, Laurell AB, Lindquist B, et al. IgG subclasses in selective IgA deficiency: Importance of IgG2-IgA deficiency. N Engl J Med. 1981;304:1476–1477.

120. Brandtzaeg P, Fjellander I, Geruldsen ST. Immunoglobulin M: Local synthesis and selective secretion in patients with immunoglobulin A deficiency. Science. 1968;160:789–791.

121. Ammann AJ, Hong R. Selective IgA deficiency: Presentation of 30 cases and a review of the literature. Medicine. 1971;50:223–236.

122. Ryser O, Morell A, Hitzig WH. Primary immunodeficiencies in Switzerland: First report of the national registry in adults and children. J Clin Immunol. 1988;8:479–485.

123. Hermans PE, Diaz-Buxo JC, Stobo JD. Idiopathic late-onset immunoglobulin deficiency. Am J Med. 1976;61:221–237.

124. Brown WR, Butterfield D, Savage D, et al. Clinical, microbiological, and immunological studies in patients with immunoglobulin deficiencies and gastrointestinal disorders. Gut. 1972;13:441–449.

125. Conley ME, Park CL, Douglas SD. Childhood common variable immunodeficiency with autoimmune disease. J Pediatr. 1986;108:915–922.

126. Wilfert CM, Buckley RH, Mohanakumar T, et al. Persistent and fatal central-nervous-system ECHO virus infections in patients with agammaglobulinemia. N Engl J Med. 1977;296:1485–1489.

127. Tedder TF, Crain MJ, Kubagawa H, et al. Evaluation of lymphocyte differentiation in primary and secondary immunodeficiency diseases. J Immunol. 1985;135:1786.

128. Booth IW, Chrystie IL, Levinsky RJ, et al. Protracted diarrhoea, immunodeficiency and viruses. Eur J Pediatr. 1982;138:271–272.

129. Chrystie IL, Booth IW, Kidd AH, et al. Multiple faecal virus excretion in immunodeficiency. Lancet. 1982;1:282.

130. Dolan KT, Twist EM, Horton-Slight P, et al. Epidemiology of rotavirus electrophorotypes determined by a simplified diagnostic technique with RNA analysis. J Clin Microbiol. 1985;21:753–758.

131. Pedley S, Hundley F, Chrystie I, et al. The genomes of rotavirus isolated from chronically infected immunodeficient children. J Gen Virol. 1984;65:1141–1150.

132. Eiden J, Losonsky GA, Johnson J, et al. Rotavirus RNA variation during chronic infection of immunocompromised children. Pediatr Infect Dis. 1985;4:632–637.

133. Losonsky GA, Johnson JP, Winkelstein JA, et al. Oral administration of human serum immunoglobulin in immunodeficient patients with viral gastroenteritis. J Clin Invest. 1985;76:2362–2367.

134. Ho M-S, Glass RI, Pinsky PF, et al. Diarrheal deaths in American children. JAMA. 1988;260:3281–3285.

135. Krech U. Complement-fixing antibodies against cytomegalovirus in different parts of the world. Bull World Health Organ. 1973;49:103–106.

136. Jordan MC, Roussear WE, Stewart JA, et al. Spontaneous cytomegalovirus mononucleosis. Ann Intern Med. 1973;79:153–160.

137. Klemola E. Cytomegalovirus infection in previously healthy adults. Ann Intern Med. 1973;79:267–268.

138. Surawicz CM, Myerson D. Self-limited cytomegalovirus colitis in immunocompetent individuals. Gastroenterology. 1988;94:194–199.

139. Ho M. Cytomegalovirus: Biology and Infection. 2nd ed. New York: Plenum Press; 1991.

140. Henson D. Cytomegalovirus inclusion bodies in the gastrointestinal tract. Arch Pathol. 1972;93:477–482.

141. Galloway P. Widespread cytomegalovirus infection involving the gastrointestinal tract, biliary tree, and gallbladder in an immunocompromised patient. Gastroenterology. 1984;87:1407.

142. Sackier JM, Kelly SB, Clarke D, et al. Small bowel haemorrhage due to cytomegalovirus vasculitis. Gut. 1991;32:1419–1420.

143. Singh N, Dummer JS, Kusne S, et al. Infections with cytomegalovirus and other herpesviruses in 121 liver transplant recipients: Transmission by donated organ and the effect of OKT3 antibodies. J Infect Dis. 1988;158:124–131.

144. Dummer JS, White LT, Ho M, et al. Morbidity of cytomegalovirus infection in recipients of heart or heart-lung transplants who receive cyclosporine. J Infect Dis. 1985;152:1182–1191.

145. Bombi JA, Cardesa A, Llebaria C, et al. Main autopsy findings in bone marrow transplant patients. Arch Pathol Med. 1987;111:125–129.

146. Meyers JD, Flournoy N, Thomas ED. Risk factors for cytomegalovirus infection after human marrow transplantation. J Infect Dis. 1986;153:478–488.

147. Powell RD, Warner NE, Levine RS, et al. Cytomegalic inclusion disease and ulcerative colitis. Am J Med. 1961;30:334–340.

148. Keren DF, Milligan FD, Strandberg JD, et al. Intercurrent cytomegalovirus colitis in a patient with ulcerative colitis. Johns Hopkins Med J. 1975;136:178–182.

149. Erye-Brook IA, Dundas S. Incidence and clinical significance of colonic cytomegalovirus infection in idiopathic inflammatory bowel disease requiring colectomy. Gut. 1986;27:1419–1425.

150. Swarbrick ET, Price HL, Kingham JGC, et al. *Chlamydia*, cytomegalovirus and *Yersinia* in inflammatory bowel disease. Lancet. 1979;2:11–12.

151. Sidi S, Graham JH, Razvi SA, et al. Cytomegalovirus infection of the colon associated with ulcerative colitis. Arch Surg. 1979;114:857–859.

152. Hrebinko R, Jordan ML, Dummer JS, et al. Ganciclovir for invasive cytomegalovirus infection in renal allograft recipients. Transpl Proc. 1991;23:1346–1347.

153. Merigan TC, Renlund DG, Keay S, et al. A controlled trial of ganciclovir to prevent cytomegalovirus disease after heart transplantation. N Engl J Med. 1992;326:1182–1186.

154. Drew WL. Diagnosis of cytomegalovirus infection. Rev Infect Dis. 1988;10(suppl 3):S468–S476.

155. Schooley RT. Cytomegalovirus in the setting of infec-

tion with human immunodeficiency virus. Rev Infect Dis. 1990;12(suppl 7):S811–S819.

156. Dieterich DT, Rahmin M. Cytomegalovirus colitis in AIDS: Presentation in 44 patients and a review of the literature. J Acquir Immune Defic Syndr. 1991;4(suppl 1):S29–S35.

157. Frances ND, Boylston AW, Roberts AH, et al. Cytomegalovirus infection in gastrointestinal tracts of patients infected with HIV-1 or AIDS. J Clin Pathol. 1989;42:1055–1064.

158. Kotler DP. Cytomegalovirus colitis and wasting. J AIDS. 1991;4(suppl 1):S36–S41.

159. Culpepper-Morgan JA, Kotler DP, Scholes JV, et al. Evolution of diagnostic criteria for mucosal cytomegalic inclusion disease in the acquired immune deficiency syndrome. Am J Gastroenterol. 1987;82:1264–1270.

160. Drew WL. Cytomegalovirus infection in patients with AIDS. Clin Infect Dis. 1992;14:608–615.

161. Dieterich DT, Chachoua A, Lafleur F, et al. Ganciclovir treatment of gastrointestinal infections caused by cytomegalovirus in patients with AIDS. Rev Infect Dis. 1988;10(suppl 3):S532–S537.

162. Buhles WC, Mastre BJ, Tinker AJ, et al. Ganciclovir treatment of life- or sight-threatening cytomegalovirus infection: Experience in 314 immunocompromised patients. Rev Infect Dis. 1988;10(suppl 3):S495–S506.

163. Collaborative DHPG Treatment Study Group. CDTS: Treatment of serious cytomegalovirus infections with 9-(1,3-dihydroxy-2-propoxymethyl) guanine in patients with AIDS and other immunodeficiencies. N Engl J Med. 1986;314:801–805.

164. Laskin OL, Cederberg DM, Mills J, et al. Ganciclovir for the treatment and suppression of serious infections caused by cytomegalovirus. Am J Med. 1987;83:201–207.

165. Chachoua A, Dieterich D, Krasinski K, et al. 9-(1,3-dihydroxy-2-propoxymethyl) guanine (ganciclovir) in the treatment of cytomegalovirus gastrointestinal disease with acquired immunodeficiency syndrome. Ann Intern Med. 1987;107:133–137.

166. Drew WL. Clinical use of ganciclovir for cytomegalovirus infection and the development of drug resistance. J AIDS. 1991;4(suppl 1):S42–S46.

167. Dieterich DT, Kotler DP, Busch DF, et al. Ganciclovir treatment of cytomegalovirus colitis in AIDS: A randomized, double-blind, placebo-controlled multicenter study. J Infect Dis. 1993;167:278–282.

168. Erice A, Chou S, Biron KK, et al. Progressive disease due to ganciclovir-resistant cytomegalovirus in immunocompromised patients. N Engl J Med. 1989;320:289–293.

169. Horwitz MS. Adenoviruses. In: Fields BN, Knipe DM, Chanock RM, et al. Virology. 2nd Ed. New York: Raven Press; 1990:1723–1740.

170. Edwards K, Thompson J, Paolini J, et al. Adenoviral infections in young children. Pediatrics. 1985;76:420–423.

171. Herrmann JE, Blacklow NR, Perron-Henry DM, et al. Incidence of enteric adenoviruses among children in Thailand and the significance of these viruses in gastroenteritis. J Clin Microbiol. 1988;26:1783–1786.

172. Hrdy DB. Epidemiology of rotavirus infection in adults. Rev Infect Dis. 1987;9:461–469.

173. deJong PJ, Valderrama G, Spigland I, et al. Adenovirus isolates from urine of patients with acquired immunodeficiency syndrome. Lancet. 1983;1:1293–1296.

174. Horwitz MS, Valderrama G, Hatcher V, et al. Characterization of adenovirus isolates from AIDS patients. Ann N Y Acad Sci. 1984;437:161–174.

175. Janoff EN, Orenstein JM, Manischewitz JF, et al. Ade-

novirus colitis in the acquired immunodeficiency syndrome. Gastroenterology. 1991;100:976–979.

176. Hierholzer JC, Wigand R, Anderson LJ, et al. Adenoviruses from patients with AIDS: A plethora of serotypes and a description of five new serotypes of subgenus D (types 43–47). J Infect Dis. 1988;158:804–813.

177. Salmon D, Garcia J, Leport C, et al. Isolation of adenovirus (ADV) from stools of AIDS patients with and without diarrhea. 6th International Conference of Immunocompromised Host Society; Peebles, Scotland, p 34, 1990. (Abstract 45.)

178. Somekh E, Berry CD, Ellison RT III, et al. Adenovirus isolation from the stool of HIV-infected patients. Chicago IL: 31st Interscience Conference on Antimicrobial Agents and Chemotherapy; 1991. Abstract.

179. Janner D, Petru AM, Belchis D, et al. Fatal adenovirus infection in a child with acquired immunodeficiency syndrome. Pediatr Infect Dis J. 1990;9:434–436.

180. Krilov LR, Kaplan MH, Frogel M, et al. Fatal adenovirus disease and human immunodeficiency virus infection. Pediatr Infect Dis J. 1990;9:753.

181. Krilov LR, Rubin LG, Frogel M, et al. Disseminated adenovirus infection with hepatic necrosis in patients with human immunodeficiency virus infection and other immunodeficiency states. Rev Infect Dis. 1990;12:303–307.

182. Zahradnik JM, Spencer MJ, Porter DD. Adenovirus infection in the immunocompromised patient. Am J Med. 1980;68:725–732.

183. Landry ML, Fong CK, Neddermann K, et al. Disseminated adenovirus infection in an immunocompromised host. Am J Med. 1987;83:555–559.

184. Parkin J, Tyms S, Roberts A, et al. "Cytomegalovirus" colitis: Can it be caused by adenovirus? Washington DC: III International Conference on AIDS; 1987. Abstract Th.8.3, p. 159.

185. Butler T, Dunn D, Colmer J. Concomitant intestinal adenovirus infection and pulmonary cytomegalovirus infection in children causing fatal enteritis and pneumonia. Trans R Soc Trop Med Hyg. 1992;86:298–300.

186. Siegal FP, Dikman SH, Arayata RB, et al. Fatal disseminated adenovirus 11 pneumonia in an agammaglobulinemic patient. Am J Med. 1981;71:1062–1067.

187. South MA, Dolen J, Beach DK, et al. Fatal adenovirus hepatic necrosis in severe combined immune deficiency. Pediatr Infect Dis. 1982;1:416–419.

188. Kapikian AZ, Flores J, Hoshino Y, et al. Rotavirus: The major etiologic agent of severe infantile diarrhea may be controllable by a "Jennerian" approach to vaccination. J Infect Dis. 1986;153:815–822.

189. Ho Mei-Shang, Glass RI, Pinsky PF, et al. Rotavirus as a cause of diarrheal morbidity and mortality in the United States. J Infect Dis. 1988;158:1112–1116.

190. Kapikian AZ, Wyatt RG, Levine MM, et al. Studies in volunteers with human rotaviruses. Dev Biol Stand. 1983;53:209–218.

191. Kapikian AZ, Wyatt RG, Levine MM, et al. Oral administration of human rotavirus to volunteers: Induction of illness and correlates of resistance. J Infect Dis. 1983;147:95–106.

192. Hjelt K, Grauballe PC, Paerregaard A, et al. Protective effect of preexisting rotavirus-specific immunoglobulin A against naturally acquired rotavirus infection in children. J Med Virol. 1987;21:39–47.

193. Barnes GL, Doyle LW, Hewson PH, et al. A randomized trial of oral gammaglobulin in low–birth-weight infants infected with rotavirus. Lancet. 1982;1:1371.

194. Davidson GP, Daniels E, Nunan H, et al. Passive immunisation of children with bovine colostrum containing antibodies to human rotavirus. Lancet. 1989;2:709–712.

195. Snodgrass DR, Fahey KJ, Wells PS, et al. Passive immunity in calf rotavirus infections: Maternal vaccination increases and prolongs immunoglobulin G' antibody secretion in milk. Infect Immun. 1980;28:344–349.
196. Greenberg MS, Friedman H, Cohen SG, et al. A comparative study of herpes simplex infections in renal transplant and leukemic patients. J Infect Dis. 1987;156:280–287.
197. Wasselle JA, Sedgwick JH, Dawson PJ, et al. Intestinal herpes simplex infection presenting with intestinal perforation. Am J Gastroenterol. 1992;87:1475–1477.
198. Siegal FP, Lopez C, Hammer GS, et al. Severe acquired immunodeficiency in male homosexuals, manifested by chronic perianal ulcerative herpes simplex lesions. N Engl J Med. 1981;305:1439–1444.
199. Derse D, Cheng Y-C, Furman PA, et al. Inhibition of purified human herpes simplex virus induced DNA polymerases by 9-(2-hydroxymethyl) guanine triphosphate. J Biol Chem. 1981;256:11447–11451.
200. Shepp DH, Newton BA, Dandliker PS, et al. Oral acyclovir therapy for mucocutaneous herpes simplex virus infections in immunocompromised marrow transplant recipients. Ann Intern Med. 1985;102:783–785.
201. Wade JC, Newton B, Flournoy N, et al. Oral acyclovir for prevention of herpes simplex virus reactivation after marrow transplantation. Ann Intern Med. 1984;100:823–828.
202. Engel JP, Englund JA, Fletcher CV, et al. Treatment of resistant herpes simplex virus with continuous-infusion acyclovir. JAMA. 1990;263:1662–1664.
203. Erlich KS, Mills J, Chatis P, et al. Acyclovir-resistant herpes simplex virus infections in patients with the acquired immunodeficiency syndrome. N Engl J Med. 1989;320:293–296.
204. Chatis PA, Miller CH, Schrager LE, et al. Successful treatment with foscarnet of an acyclovir-resistant mucocutaneous infection with herpes simplex in a patient with acquired immunodeficiency syndrome. N Engl J Med. 1989;320:297–300.
205. Erlich KS, Jacobson MA, Koehler JE, et al. Foscarnet therapy for severe acyclovir-resistant herpes simplex virus type-2 infections in patients with the acquired immunodeficiency syndrome (AIDS). Ann Intern Med. 1989;110:710–713.
206. Safrin S, Crumpacker C, Chatis P, et al. A controlled trial comparing foscarnet with vidarabine for acyclovir-resistant mucocutaneous herpes simplex in the acquired immunodeficiency syndrome. N Engl J Med. 1991;325:551–555.
207. Schreiber DS, Trier JS, Blacklow NR. Recent advances in viral gastroenteritis. Gastroenterology. 1977;73:174–183.
208. Wyatt HV. Poliomyelitis in hypogammaglobulinemics. J Infect Dis. 1973;128:802–806.
209. Strebel PM, Sutter RW, Cochi SL, et al. Epidemiology of poliomyelitis in the United States one decade after the last reported case of indigenous wild virus–associated disease. Clin Infect Dis. 1992;14:568–579.
210. Pape JW, Verdier R-I, Johnson WD Jr. Treatment and prophylaxis of Isospora belli infection in patients with the acquired immunodeficiency syndrome. N Engl J Med. 1989;320:1044–1047.
211. Nelson JA, Wiley CA, Reynolds-Kohler C, et al. Human immunodeficiency virus detected in bowel epithelium from patients with gastrointestinal symptoms. Lancet. 1988;1:259–262.
212. Fox CH, Kotler DP, Tierney AR, et al. Detection of HIV-1 RNA in the lamina propria of patients with AIDS and gastrointestinal disease. J Infect Dis. 1989;159:467–471.
213. Heise C, Dandekar S, Kumar P, et al. Human immunodeficiency virus infection of enterocytes and mononuclear cells in human jejunal mucosa. Gastroenterology. 1991;100:1521–1527.
214. Levy JA, Margaretten W, Nelson J. Detection of HIV in enterochromaffin cells in the rectal mucosa of an AIDS patient. Am J Gastroenterol. 1989;84:787–789.
215. Adachi A, Koenig S, Gendelman HE, et al. Productive, persistent infection of human colorectal cell lines with human immunodeficiency virus. J Virol. 1987;61:209–213.
216. Fantini J, Yahi N, Chermann J-C. Human immunodeficiency virus can infect the apical and basolateral surfaces of human colonic epithelial cells. Proc Natl Acad Sci U S A. 1991;88:9297–9301.
217. Fantini J, Yahi N, Baghdiguian S, et al. Human colon epithelial cells productively infected with human immunodeficiency virus (HIV) show an impaired differentiation and an altered secretion. J Virol. 1992;66:580–585.
218. Cooper DA, Gold J, Maclean P, et al. Acute AIDS retrovirus infection: Definition of a clinical illness associated with seroconversion. Lancet. 1985;1:537–540.
219. Kotler DP, Gaetz HP, Lange M, et al. Enteropathy associated with the acquired immunodeficiency syndrome. Ann Intern Med. 1984;101:421–428.
220. Greenson JK, Belitsos PC, Yardley JH, et al. AIDS enteropathy: Occult enteric infections and duodenal mucosal alterations in chronic diarrhea. Ann Intern Med. 1991;114:366–372.
221. Friedland GH, Klein RS. Transmission of the human immunodeficiency virus. N Engl J Med. 1987;317:1125–1135.
222. Vogt MW, Witt DJ, Craven DE, et al. Isolation patterns of the human immunodeficiency virus from cervical secretions during the menstrual cycle of women at risk for the acquired immunodeficiency syndrome. Ann Intern Med. 1987;106:380–382.
223. Avery ME, Snyder JD. Oral therapy for acute diarrhea. N Engl J Med. 1990;323:891–894.
224. Lewis JH. Gastrointestinal injury due to medicinal agents. Am J Gastroenterol. 1986;81:819–834.
225. Rump JA, Arndt R, Arnold A, et al. Treatment of diarrhoea in human immunodeficiency virus–infected patients with immunoglobulins from bovine colostrum. Clin Invest. 1992;70:588–594.
226. Matsumoto S, Watanabe T, Chiba S, et al. Oral administration of secretory immunoglobulin A and its clinical significance. Birth Defects: Original Article Series, March of Dimes Birth Defects Foundation 1983; 19:229–237.
227. Johanson JF, Sonnenberg A. Efficient management of diarrhea in the acquired immunodeficiency syndrome (AIDS): A medical decision analysis. Ann Intern Med. 1990;112:942–948.
228. Smith PD, Janoff EN. Infectious diarrhea in human immunodeficiency virus infection. Gastroenterol Clin North Am. 1988;17:587–598.
229. Cello JP, Grendell JH, Basuk P, et al. Effect of octreotide on refractory AIDS-associated diarrhea. Ann Intern Med. 1991;115:705–710.
230. Dryden MS, Shanson DC. The microbial causes of diarrhoea in patients infected with the human immunodeficiency virus. J Infect. 1988;17:107–114.
231. Rolston KV, Fainstein V, Bodey GP. Intestinal cryptosporidiosis treated with eflornithine: A prospective study among patients with AIDS. J Acquir Immune Defic Syndr. 1989;2:426–430.
232. Kotler DP, Francisco A, Clayton F, et al. Small intestinal injury and parasitic diseases in AIDS. Ann Intern Med. 1990;113:444–449.
233. Orenstein JM, Zierdt W, Zierdt C, et al. Identification

of spores of *Enterocytozoon bieneusi* in stool and duodenal fluid from AIDS patients. Lancet. 1990;336: 1127–1128.

234. Batman PA, Miller AR, Forster SM, et al. Jejunal enteropathy associated with human immunodeficiency virus infection: Quantitative histology. J Clin Pathol. 1989;42:275–281.

235. Belitsos PC, Greenson JK, Yardley JH, et al. Association of gastric hypoacidity with opportunistic enteric infec-

tions in patients with AIDS. J Infect Dis. 1992;166:277–284.

236. Ullrich R, Riecken E-O, Zeitz M. Human immunodeficiency virus–induced enteropathy. Immunol Res. 1991;10:456–464.

237. Weber R, Bryan RT, Owen RL, et al. Improved light-microscopical detection of microsporida spores in stool and duodenal aspirates. N Engl J Med. 1992;326:161–166.

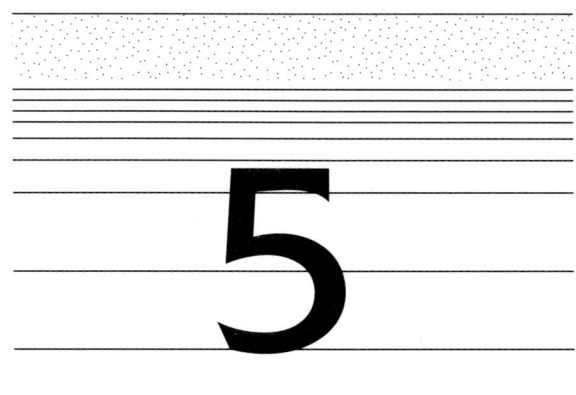

5

Approach to the Patient with Acute Bloody Diarrhea

PHILLIP I. TARR, M.D.

The patient presenting with acute bloody diarrhea frequently has a diagnosable enteric infection. Since the number of pathogens that cause these syndromes is limited they should be familiar to most gastroenterologists, but demographic factors may render some of these agents more common than others in clinical practice. This chapter reviews the mechanisms underlying the production of bloody diarrhea in otherwise normal hosts, the pathogens most frequently incriminated as causes of bloody diarrhea, the diagnostic and therapeutic approaches to these patients before and after the offending agent has been identified, and clinical and epidemiologic considerations pertaining to infectious bloody diarrhea. Each of the pathogens discussed in this chapter can cause both bloody and nonbloody diarrhea. Although many pathogens have on occasion been reported to cause bloody diarrhea, this chapter focuses only on those pathogens that commonly present with acute bloody diarrhea.

HISTORICAL ASPECTS

The clinical problem of bloody diarrhea has been noted since antiquity. In the Old Testa-

ment, the Philistine army was plagued by "emerods," or rectal outpouchings, from which the term hemorrhoids is derived. This plague caused considerable mortality among the Philistines, forcing them to relinquish the ark that they had stolen and taken to Ashdod.[1] While hemorrhoids are uncomfortable, embarrassing, and occasionally alarming, such retribution and restitution are unlikely to have been caused by hemorrhoids but rather by the rectal prolapse associated with shigellosis.

The early history of bloody diarrhea has been thoroughly reviewed by Davison.[2] Hippocrates first used the term dysentery, meaning trouble of the bowels, to describe the frequent passage of stools with blood and mucus. This definition helped to establish bloody diarrhea as a distinct medical problem but did not distinguish the many elements of its etiology.

In multiple post-Biblical military campaigns, dysentery rivaled ordinance as a cause of casualties. After the identification of *Shigella dysenteriae* in 1898, reviewed in Shiga,[3] bacteriologically confirmed shigellosis in troops in World War I, the Vietnam conflict, and the Persian Gulf War[4] has been indistinguishable from earlier descriptions of campaign dysentery and presumably has the same etiology.

The differentiation of amebic from bacillary dysentery was not easy. In 1860, Lambl reported fecal amebae in a child with fatal diarrhea, an observation confirmed by others during the late 1800s.[4] The presence of amebae in the stools of nondysenteric patients was at odds, however, with the observations of amebae in hepatic abscesses in patients dying of bloody diarrhea,[5] which corroborated the invasive and pathogenic potential of at least some strains of this protozoan.

Councilman and Lafleur settled the discrepancy between the observation of asymptomatic carriage of amebae or amebic dysentery and hepatic abscesses by proposing variable pathogenic potential of the amebae.[4] In 1898, Shiga identified the organism responsible for "diphtheritic dysentery."[3] This organism has subsequently been known as Shiga's bacillus, *Bacillus dysenteriae,* and *S. dysenteriae.* Shiga established the etiologic role of *S. dysenteriae* by demonstrating acquired agglutinins to this organism in patients recovering from dysentery, in whom the same organism was present in the stool during the acute illness. He also demonstrated the pathogenic role of this bacillus in a rabbit model. Soon afterward, Flexner discovered in the Philippines the second of four distinct *Shigella* species, now called *S. flexneri.*[6] It seems probable in retrospect that acute bloody diarrhea occurring in epidemics, without associated hepatic lesions, was probably bacillary in origin, but that endemic dysentery was probably caused by *Entamoeba histolytica.*

During the twentieth century, multiple additional pathogens have been established as causes of bloody diarrhea. These include bacteria (*Campylobacter, Yersinia, Salmonella,* enteroinvasive *Escherichia coli* [EIEC], enterohemorrhagic *E. coli* [EHEC], *Clostridium difficile, Clostridium perfringens,* and *Vibrio parahaemolyticus*) and parasites (*Balantidium coli* and *Schistosoma* species). Gastrointestinal bleeding without prominent diarrhea can be caused by viruses (herpes simplex virus, cytomegalovirus, adenovirus) and fungi (*Aspergillus* species), usually in the setting of severe immune impairment. Viral, fungal, and *C. difficile* gastrointestinal infections are covered in detail elsewhere in this book and are not addressed extensively in this chapter.

MECHANISMS OF BLOODY DIARRHEA

To produce grossly bloody diarrhea, a pathogen must traverse a mucosal epithelial membrane or produce a toxin that causes cell death, a cytotoxin. Colonic injury produces the red blood characteristic of dysentery, although pathogens that cause dysentery can also affect the small bowel and even the stomach. Vascular integrity is breached by microvascular hemorrhage secondary to inflammation, thrombosis, vascular invasion by the offending organism, or the cytocidal effects of its toxins. Noninvasive organisms elaborating secretory toxins, such as enterotoxigenic *E. coli* or *Vibrio cholerae,* do not cause bloody diarrhea.

Cellular Invasion

Invasion is more common in the pathogenesis of bloody diarrhea than is cytotoxin production. Before invasion, organisms must first contact the appropriate target cells. An example of a host structure that serves as a ligand for bacterial attachment and subsequent invasion is the β integrin family. These transmembrane glycoproteins are recognized by the invasin molecule of *Yersinia pseudotuberculosis* and *Yersinia enterocolitica.*[7] Invasin functions both as an adhesin to these integrins and as a molecule that allows an otherwise innocuous bacterium (*E. coli* HB101) to become invasive. After invasion of the mucosa, bloodstream penetration by the pathogen may or may not follow, despite the production of copious amounts of blood in the stool. For example, most cases of bacillary and amebic dysentery are limited to the colonic infection that is prominent clinically. *Shigella,* however, can cause bacteremia, and *E. histolytica* can be found in extraintestinal abscesses, but these complications are not related to the degree of dysentery. In fact, many patients with extraintestinal amebiasis have no recent history of dysentery.

Pathogenic events that follow invasion are poorly understood. Once some invasive pathogens breach the epithelium, replication and intracellular survival are necessary to cause disease. Alternatively, inflammatory reactions to nonreplicative stages (such as schistosomal egg granulomas) can also cause bloody diarrhea.

Cytotoxin Production

Noninvasive organisms can cause bloody diarrhea by the production of cytotoxins. Toxins of enteric pathogens can be grouped into two broad categories: secretory toxins, also called enterotoxins, of which cholera toxin is the best-studied example; and cytotoxins, of which Shiga toxin is the prototype. Secretory toxins produce no morphologic changes in their target cells but cause diarrhea by promoting electrolyte and water secretion and by inhibiting absorption of salt and water by the enterocyte. Cytotoxins cause cell death. It is not known for certain if cell death by itself is responsible for diarrhea in patients infected with cytotoxic bacteria, but the morphologic changes associated with cytotoxic noninvasive organisms (such as EHEC) are probably at least partially caused by the intraluminal effects of toxins on colonic mucosa.[8]

DIAGNOSIS AND THERAPY

General Considerations

The three most common diagnoses in patients with bloody diarrhea are infectious colitis, inflammatory bowel disease, and ischemic colitis. The history may provide some clues. Abrupt onset of illness, with nonbloody diarrhea followed by bloody diarrhea within 1 or 2 days, without prior constitutional symptoms such as weight loss or fever, suggests an infectious colitis of bacterial origin. Watery diarrhea for longer periods followed by bloody diarrhea suggests inflammatory bowel disease. Infectious proctitis is not usually confused with infectious colitis because proctitis is commonly accompanied by tenesmus, absence of diarrhea, and even constipation. Ischemic bowel disease typically presents as a left-sided colitis in an elderly patient.

Epidemiologic considerations in patients with acute bloody diarrhea include recent travel to areas where amebiasis or schistosomiasis, or both, are endemic, or where sanitary conditions are poor. These factors increase the risk of bacterial enteric infections. Apart from travel, it is futile to ask about epidemiologic risk factors such as food or water intake, because very few people consistently observe strictly hygienic diets. It is useful, however, to ask if any of the patient's contacts have experienced similar illnesses recently and to determine if the patient belongs to a group (daycare center, nursing home) in which this patient might be the sentinel case in an outbreak. Although a knowledge of the sexual practices of patients is not usually helpful in discerning the cause of bloody diarrhea, anal intercourse is a risk factor for enteric infection by a wide variety of pathogens that can cause bloody diarrhea.

When examining a patient with bloody diarrhea, the hydration status must be assessed, as with any fluid-losing gut infection. In children, postural hypotension is not a reliable finding because of the excellent sympathetic tone that

most children maintain, even when dehydrated. Tachycardia, postural tachycardia, and urine output are more reliable indicators, but even experienced observers frequently cannot assess accurately the extent of dehydration in infants and toddlers.[9]

Bloody diarrhea can be associated with disorders requiring surgical intervention. Intussusception can be confused with, or can accompany, infectious bloody diarrhea, especially in colitis caused by *Shigella* and EHEC. Perforations occur in salmonellosis, especially in typhoid fever, generally in the second or third week of infection. Toxic megacolon, indistinguishable from that seen in inflammatory bowel disease, can accompany shigellosis, amebiasis, and *C. difficile* infection. Bacteremia and extraintestinal seeding can occur in many cases of infectious colitis, sometimes with colonic organisms other than the offending enteric pathogen.

Laboratory Evaluation

If resources permit, that is, if the patient resides in a developed country, a bacterial stool culture should be obtained for all patients with acute bloody diarrhea. Bloody diarrhea increases the chance that bacterial culture will yield a pathogen.[10, 11] *Salmonella*, *Shigella*, *E. coli* O157, *Campylobacter*, *Yersinia*, and, if epidemiologically indicated, *V. parahaemolyticus*, should be sought in all patients. We also seek *C. difficile* toxin in such patients, whether or not antibiotics have recently been administered. To test for the presence of fecal leukocytes in patients with acute bloody diarrhea does little to assist in diagnosis because many patients infected with pathogens capable of causing bloody diarrhea do not have fecal leukocytes (Table 5–1).[12]

Some investigators have recommended the direct examination of stool using darkfield microscopy or the carbolfuchsin Gram stain to detect *Campylobacter*,[13] but these tests are not widely used.

Parasites should be sought if the physician is concerned that a patient's dysentery may be amebic or schistosomal in origin. *E. histolytica* is not confined to the tropics, but tropical travel is certainly a risk factor for amebiasis. Parasites rarely cause bloody diarrhea in North America.

Viral studies are rarely helpful in evaluating acute bloody diarrhea, unless the bloody diarrhea is part of a systemic hemorrhagic illness, such as Korean hemorrhagic fever, caused by *Hantavirus*. The isolation of a virus from a patient may not be relevant to the disorder being

TABLE 5–1. STOOL CULTURES CONTAINING FECAL LEUKOCYTES AMONG CULTURES POSITIVE
FOR SELECTED PATHOGENS

ORGANISM	PATIENTS WITH POSITIVE CULTURE	PATIENTS WITH FECAL LEUKOCYTES (%)
Campylobacter jejuni	114	56 (49.1)
Salmonella	95	40 (42.1)
Escherichia coli O157:H7	81	53 (65.4)
Shigella	36	26 (72.2)
Yersinia enterocolitica	27	13 (48.1)

NOTE: Pathogens isolated at Children's Hospital and Medical Center in Seattle, WA, 1985–1990.
SOURCE: Tarr PI, Clausen CR, Christie DL. Bacterial and protozoal gastroenteritis. Letter. Reprinted by permission of the New England Journal of Medicine (326:489, 1992).

evaluated, because many viruses are carried without symptoms, and prolonged fecal excretion can follow infection. Although herpes simplex virus can cause proctitis, and cytomegalovirus can occasionally cause a self-limited colitis, bloody diarrhea in immunocompetent hosts is not usually caused by viruses.

Serologic studies are of limited benefit in diagnosing and managing most cases of bloody diarrhea. By the time a patient's antibody level to a particular agent has risen, thereby suggesting a diagnosis, the illness has usually been diagnosed by stool studies, or it has resolved. An exception is the use of serology in patients with suspected amebic or schistosomal colitis, both of which may be difficult to diagnose by fecal examination.

Fecal antigen studies are limited to detecting *C. difficile* toxin, especially in smaller laboratories without access to tissue culture facilities.[14] Toxin phenotype analysis on fresh stool samples or on culture supernatants is a research tool for the detection of EHEC.

Bacteremia due to bloody diarrhea occurs most frequently in salmonellosis and less frequently in campylobacteriosis, shigellosis, and yersiniosis. Blood cultures should be obtained on all febrile, immunocompromised, or very young (less than 6 months of age) patients with bloody diarrhea. A complete blood count and differential white cell count sometimes reveal a relative "bandemia," or increase in neutrophils, especially in band forms, associated with shigellosis, or they can serve as a baseline in patients with infection caused by *S. dysenteriae* or *E. coli* O157. Electrolyte studies, renal function tests, and urinalysis can guide therapy in cases of severe dehydration or oliguria.

gery. We recommend a plain film of the abdomen if patients have severe abdominal pain, are less than 2 months of age, or appear toxic. For example, bloody diarrhea might be the manifestation of necrotizing enterocolitis in an infant or intussusception in an older child, both of which might be suggested by radiographs. Thumbprinting, suggestive of bowel wall edema, is seen in hemorrhagic colitis caused by *E. coli* O157 as well as in other conditions such as inflammatory bowel disease and ischemia. Toxic megacolon can occur in shigellosis, amebiasis, pseudomembranous colitis, and fulminant ulcerative colitis. Surgery is usually warranted, whatever the cause. Perforations can occur in typhoid fever, but this occurs later in the illness.

Patients with bloody diarrhea and findings on physical examination suggesting acute appendicitis should be evaluated by diagnostic ultrasound. Bloody diarrhea rarely implies a surgical emergency if abdominal films do not suggest toxic megacolon, perforation, or intussusception. However, if reproducible tenderness in the right lower quadrant suggests a focal process, the physician must exclude appendicitis. Diagnostic ultrasound is helpful in establishing bacterial ileocecitis, a disorder that resembles acute appendicitis but can be caused by many organisms that can also cause bloody diarrhea.[15, 16]

Barium enema should be performed only if reason exists to believe that a treatable disorder (in particular, an intussusception) will be found on this examination. Our hesitancy to perform this study is due to our concern about increasing toxemia in *E. coli* O157 or *Shigella* infections, precipitating perforations in amebiasis, or obscuring parasites in microscopic examinations of the stool.

Radiologic Investigations

Radiologic studies can be useful in detecting complications of bloody diarrhea requiring sur-

Sigmoidoscopy and Colonoscopy

Colonoscopic examination of the colon in acute bloody diarrhea is safe and can be useful, but this procedure is rarely necessary before the results of the microbiologic studies are known. Most laboratories can examine stool daily for parasites, and culture results for bacterial enteric pathogens and detection of *C. difficile* toxin should be known within 2 working days. If a cause is not then apparent, sigmoidoscopy and mucosal biopsy can frequently identify ischemic changes (minimal inflammatory changes, superficial mucosa that is disproportionately necrotic compared with deeper portions), pseudomembranes, and acute self-limited colitis.[17]

The setting in which bloody diarrhea occurs can influence the diagnostic approach. For example, an otherwise healthy child or young adult with the abrupt onset of painful bloody diarrhea should be evaluated first by stool culture. More invasive workup should be deferred until the results of microbiologic studies are known. Sigmoidoscopy would be used earlier in an elderly patient who develops bloody diarrhea after several days of hospitalization, especially if antibiotics have been administered. The yield of bacterial stool cultures for standard enteric pathogens in patients who develop diarrhea in hospitals is exceedingly low,[18] whereas the frequency of *C. difficile* infection in this setting is much higher. Sigmoidoscopy can be useful in differentiating these entities. If we suspect that bloody diarrhea is caused by a fastidious pathogen in spite of negative findings of stool cultures, we obtain mucosal biopsies at various points along the colon and, if entered, the terminal ileum, for bacterial culture.[19]

Differential Diagnosis

The differential diagnosis of acute bloody diarrhea consists of acute surgical abdominal problems, especially intussusception, which may be related to infection; sigmoid or cecal volvulus; toxic megacolon, caused by infectious and inflammatory colitis; and perforation. Abdominal radiographs can help detect these disorders. If any doubt exists as to their presence, surgical consultation should be obtained. Occasionally, bleeding from an anal fissure due to straining at stool during diarrhea caused by noninvasive and nontoxic pathogens, confuses the picture. Acute infectious colitis and inflammatory bowel disease can be present simultaneously.[20] Inflammatory bowel disease can be exacerbated by a superimposed enteric infection. Hence, we recommend stool cultures for enteric pathogens including *C. difficile* in patients experiencing flares of inflammatory bowel disease.

Empirical Therapy

Patients with acute bloody diarrhea are often in pain, appear toxic, and present a compelling case for immediate therapy. The appeal of this approach is undeniable because physicians wish to treat an infection as rapidly as possible to hasten clearance of the pathogen and prevent complications. It is difficult to determine when bacteremia begins, which would mandate antibiotic therapy for some enteric pathogens. Significant reasons for caution exist, however, in administering antibiotics empirically. First, it is impossible in most cases to distinguish enteric infection caused by *Campylobacter, Salmonella, Shigella,* or *E. coli* O157, each of which might mandate a different therapy. Second, antibiotics may be contraindicated, as in the case of diarrhea caused by *E. coli* O157 (in the author's opinion); may prolong the carrier state, as in nontyphoidal salmonellosis[21]; or may be ineffective entirely, as in yersiniosis.[22] Third, oral antibiotics might not reach the colon or might not be absorbed because of the vomiting that frequently accompanies these infections. Finally, enteric pathogens have a remarkable ability to develop resistance to a wide variety of antimicrobial agents, and the promiscuous dispensing of antibiotics increases this problem. In sum, we do not recommend empirical therapy for bloody diarrhea, unless the patient has been in recent contact with another patient with diarrhea caused by a culture-proven pathogen for which antibiotics are indicated.

Antimotility agents should not be given to patients with bloody diarrhea that is possibly infectious in origin.

Specific Therapy

After a bacterial or protozoal infection is diagnosed in a patient with acute bloody diarrhea but before sensitivities are known, the physician must consider antibiotic resistance patterns of the pathogen on a probability basis. Because resistance patterns change rapidly, especially for *Salmonella* and *Shigella,* the most recent antibiotic recommendations should be sought. Travel history is important in this regard, because imported enteric pathogens are more likely to be resistant than are domestic strains. Before starting to administer antibiotics, blood cultures should be drawn. A spinal tap should be considered if the host is an infant or an immunocompromised patient or if the organism is *Salmonella,* in which metastatic infection is possible.

Antibiotic sensitivities are usually reported 24 hours after a bacterial pathogen is identified and are not obtained for parasites. The ideal antibiotic is safe, efficacious, and inexpensive, and has a narrow spectrum. Safety is a function of the host's age and associated medical history. For example, quinolones are active against most bacterial enteric pathogens and are tolerated well but are not considered safe for children less than 18 years because of theoretical osteotoxicity. Efficacy is not ensured by merely matching the sensitivity of the organism to the antibiotic chosen. One must also consider the route of administration and penetration into various body compartments. For example, a neonate with salmonellosis should be treated with a parenteral antibiotic capable of penetrating the central nervous system because of the potential for meningitis in this age group. Oral amoxicillin, although better absorbed than ampicillin, is less desirable in uncomplicated shigellosis because its intracolonic concentration is lower than that of ampicillin. Cost considerations extend beyond medication charges. Administration expenses, side effects, patient compliance, reduction of days of incapacitation, and elimination of excretion must all be taken into account. Cost-benefit analyses of various therapies have not been performed for bloody diarrhea as they have been for traveler's diarrhea.[23]

EPIDEMIOLOGY AND INFECTION CONTROL

Important infection control matters should be considered in patients with bloody diarrhea. The physician must be concerned with the source of the infection and other persons who might have been infected with the offending agent prior to the consultation and must take steps to reduce the risk of transmission.

It is often difficult to determine the source of infection, which is usually foodborne. Many enteric pathogens are so ubiquitous that any attempt to detect a source is futile. For example, most retail poultry is colonized with *Campylobacter*.[24] Considering the high rate of colonization, it is surprising that more enteric infection does not occur. Also, recall bias is common in dramatic illnesses such as bloody diarrhea, with patients recalling events and oral intake very well for the day of the first symptom but overlooking exposures occurring several days earlier, when it is more likely that the vehicle containing the pathogen was actually ingested. In addition, the

recovery of pathogens from food is difficult, even in many epidemiologically verified point-source outbreaks.[25] Therefore, we generally do not recommend microbiologic studies on leftover food, unless the food was clearly incriminated in an outbreak. Person-to-person transmission of each of the bacterial enteric pathogens occurs, and "rounding up the usual (food) suspects" in sporadic cases allows a real culprit, such as a human carrier, to be overlooked.

Identifying the vehicle of transmission of enteric pathogens is easier in outbreaks than in sporadic cases. Such outbreaks, if discerned early, provide extensive data for epidemiologic investigations conducted by the proper authorities. The most important question for the physician to ask is whether the patient has recently been around others with similar symptoms. If the answer is no, the patient or family should be advised that if any similar cases do become known, the physician who treats these additional cases should contact the physician treating the index case. Continuing point-source outbreaks can be investigated early, and further transmission halted, by early notification of public health authorities. Many bacterial enteric pathogens are reportable to these authorities, and microbiology laboratories usually assume this function, but the reporting may occur well after an outbreak is over.

Patients with bloody diarrhea are infectious to others, and they may have in their vicinity an asymptomatic carrier who could spread the offending pathogen to additional susceptible hosts. Because of the considerable morbidity and potential mortality caused by the pathogens that precipitate bloody diarrhea, we stress the importance of observing hygienic practices until the organism has been cleared. Such practices include thorough hand washing by patients and caregivers, use of separate eating utensils, temporary removal from group settings such as daycare centers, and avoidance of contact with immunocompromised patients. Because prolonged fecal excretion can follow infection, we continue these precautions until stool cultures indicate clearance of the pathogen.

Of the bacterial enteric pathogens discussed later in this chapter, we recommend carrier screening only for households and institutional contacts of patients with *Salmonella* because of the high rate of asymptomatic carriage of this organism and because of the adverse consequences of infection in a variety of hosts, including pregnant women, immunocompromised individuals, and infants.

CAMPYLOBACTER

History and Microbiology

Campylobacter is a genus of nonmotile, gram-negative curved rods. A member of this genus was first isolated from the blood of sheep abortuses in 1909[26] and was designated *Vibrio fetus* because of its microscopic resemblance to *V. cholerae*. In 1947, the first human isolates of *V. fetus* were obtained from blood cultures of women in the middle trimester of pregnancy. The species was subsequently designated *Campylobacter* (campylo = curved, and bacter = rod) because of biochemical characteristics different from those of vibrios.

It was not until 1957 that *Campylobacter* organisms were first suspected of causing enteric disease, when King isolated "related vibrios" (actually *C. fetus*) from the blood of infants with bloody diarrhea.[26] The first isolation of organisms of this genus from human stool was accomplished by Dekeyser and coworkers in 1972,[27] and confirmed by Skirrow[28] and Blaser and coworkers.[29]

Over a dozen *Campylobacter* species exist, but the most common human pathogens are *C. jejuni* and *C. fetus. C. fetus*, which has four subspecies (*C. fetus*, subspp. *fetus, intestinalis, veneralis,* and *jejuni*), rarely causes gastrointestinal illness. *C. jejuni,* however, frequently causes bloody diarrhea and is rarely isolated from extraintestinal sites. This organism is difficult to grow because of its prolonged generation time, preference for growth at 42°C with low oxygen (5%) and carbon dioxide (10%) tension, and selective growth disadvantage against other enteric bacteria. Despite these difficulties, however, *C. jejuni* is among the most frequently isolated bacterial enteric pathogens.

Epidemiology

C. jejuni infection occurs worldwide. Asymptomatic carriage occurs more frequently in developing countries than in industrialized nations.[30, 31] Most bacterial enteric infections have a peak incidence in preschool children, but *C. jejuni* infection is unique in having a second peak in young adults.[32]

C. jejuni is ubiquitous, and it is difficult to determine the vehicle of infection.[33] Many wild and domesticated animals excrete *C. jejuni* organisms during and after symptomatic and asymptomatic infection. Food of animal origin, including unpasteurized milk and cheese, is contaminated with *C. jejuni* bacteria at very high rates.[24] Animal excreta may also contaminate soil and water with *C. jejuni*. These multiple sources make it difficult to identify the origin of *Campylobacter* in most human infections and should compel us to reinforce good hygiene in handling potentially contaminated foods. *C. jejuni* infection occurs most frequently in the summer.[32] Person-to-person transmission occurs and usually affects children who are not yet toilet trained. Infection from food handlers appears to be uncommon.[33]

Mechanisms of Pathogenesis

Campylobacter jejuni is susceptible to gastric acid.[34] After traversing the stomach, *C. jejuni* organisms multiply in the neutral proximal small bowel. Tissue damage, secondary to invasion of epithelial cells, is first apparent in the jejunum, ileum, and colon. The colonoscopist can see edema, erythema, small ulcerations, friability, and granularity. Biopsies of the colon demonstrate acute colitis, with prominent neutrophilic infiltration of the epithelium and superficial ulcerations. The mucin is depleted, and crypt abscesses are present. The lamina propria is edematous. Granulomas are not seen. Resolution occurs over the course of several weeks.[35–37] Of course, these findings are not specific to colitis caused by *C. jejuni*.

Virulence mechanisms of *C. jejuni* have eluded molecular cloning. Animal and tissue culture experiments have, however, demonstrated cytotoxic,[38, 39] enterotoxigenic,[40] and invasive[41] activity in *C. jejuni*. Considerable variability exists in pathogenic potential of different strains and host susceptibility to infection.[42]

Clinical Presentation

C. jejuni can be carried asymptomatically, but infections caused by this organism usually present as severe diarrhea that is frequently bloody. The incubation period is usually from 2 to 4 days. Headache, myalgia, and fever frequently precede the diarrhea. Fever may be as high as 40°C (104°F) or may be absent. The colitis may be severe. Toxic megacolon may develop in rare cases.

C. jejuni colitis is usually self-limited and lasts a week. Up to 20% of patients have illnesses lasting longer than 1 week, and between 5 and 10% of patients have apparent relapses.[43]

Campylobacteriosis may present with the pseudoappendicular syndrome, similar to that found with *Y. enterocolitica*. This complication occurs less frequently in campylobacteriosis than in yersiniosis. If appendicitis is suspected, an exploratory laparotomy should not be delayed pending cultures because of the several days necessary to establish a definite microbiologic diagnosis of *Campylobacter* infection. Most infants and children aged more than 1 year who are infected with *C. jejuni* have bloody diarrhea and fever.[44, 45]

Diagnosis

No clues distinguish *Campylobacter* colitis from other colon infections, making stool cultures necessary to establish the diagnosis. Because other bacterial enteric pathogens can produce symptoms that mimic *C. jejuni* infection, we do not recommend restricting bacterial enteric cultures to *Campylobacter*. In most centers, *C. jejuni* is the most common bacterial enteric pathogen. Because the ability to recover *C. jejuni* might vary among laboratories and from day to day in the course of an illness, cultures should be repeated if the suspicion of campylobacteriosis persists despite a negative stool culture.

Although rarely used, microscopy (darkfield examination, carbolfuchsin Gram stain) is useful in predicting the patients who are likely to demonstrate *Campylobacter* on stool culture when vibrio-like organisms are detected.[13] Microscopy is most useful when employed early in illness, when fecal excretion of *C. jejuni* is maximal, and it should be performed on specimens less than 2 hours old.

We recommend that blood cultures be performed if patients with enterocolitis are at risk for complicated bacteremia with *Campylobacter* or are still febrile or toxic when the stool cultures are reported positive for *C. jejuni*.

Therapy

Antibiotic treatment of *C. jejuni* infection is usually not necessary because the patient is often improved by the time the results of the stool culture are known. Patients at risk of dissemination have traditionally been treated with erythromycin, which will probably hasten clearance of the organism from the feces.[46, 47] However, no evidence suggests hat erythromycin therapy, if initiated after the *C. jejuni* infection is diagnosed, improves the clinical course.[47] If erythromycin is administered at the time a patient presents for medical attention, the course of *C. jejuni* infection may be favorably affected.[48] We do not recommend this approach, however, because of our concern that the symptoms may be caused by some other organism that is indistinguishable clinically from *C. jejuni*, in which case antibiotic use is either inefficacious or contraindicated, and the symptoms would be inappropriately treated.

Erythromycin resistance to *C. jejuni* has been reported,[49] and the quinolones have emerged as the drug class of choice for *Campylobacter* infections, at least in adults. Resistance to quinolones by *Campylobacter* has, however, been reported after short-course therapy for diarrhea.[50]

Septicemic patients should be treated with at least two parenteral antibiotics until susceptibility results are known. Gentamicin, chloramphenicol, or a third-generation cephalosporin is a reasonable adjunct to erythromycin.

Extraintestinal Complications

Metastatic infections with *C. jejuni* are rare. Bacteremia is probably underdiagnosed, because blood cultures are infrequently drawn from patients evaluated for diarrhea and because *C. jejuni* bacteremia usually clears spontaneously. Patients with bacteremia and a sustained clinical course should be investigated for a focus of deep infection. Immunocompromised patients may have bacteremia without prominent enterocolitis. Pregnant women usually handle *C. jejuni* infection well, with minimal risk to the fetus. Bacteremia does not have to be treated if the patient is improving by the time the positive blood culture is reported, but a second blood culture should be obtained.

Most patients recover completely from *C. jejuni* infections, but a small minority with the HLA-B27 haplotype develop a reactive arthritis, and an even smaller number develop Guillain-Barré syndrome. Death is rare and usually occurs in debilitated or compromised hosts.

Infection Control Measures

We recommend confirmation that the *C. jejuni* is cleared from the stools before patients return to group settings, especially daycare. Erythromycin, which hastens clearance, might be useful in rendering patients less infectious, but as noted earlier, its ability to improve the clinical course is questionable. Secondary cases from person-to-person spread are apparently rare.[33]

ENTEROHEMORRHAGIC *ESCHERICHIA COLI*

History and Microbiology

In 1977, Konawalchuk and coworkers[51] described *E. coli* with the ability to produce a toxin, verotoxin (VT), lethal for Vero (African green monkey kidney) cells. These strains were designated verotoxigenic *E. coli* (VTEC). In 1983, Riley and coworkers[52] reported the isolation of *E. coli* O157:H7 from the stools of patients in two clusters of cases of painful bloody diarrhea that was usually unaccompanied by fever. This disorder was termed hemorrhagic colitis. *Escherichia coli* O157:H7 was shown to produce a toxin to cultured eukaryotic cells that was neutralized by antibody to Shiga toxin.[53]

Also in 1983, Karmali reported that children with hemolytic-uremic syndrome (HUS) had detectable verotoxic activity in their stools and developed antibodies that neutralized this toxicity as they recovered. *Escherichia coli* elaborating verotoxin was also recovered from many of these children.[54] These three observations formed the basis for an expanding body of knowledge of this newly discovered class of diarrheagenic *E. coli*.

Cytotoxic *E. coli* organisms capable of causing hemorrhagic colitis in humans have been described as enterohemorrhagic *E. coli* (EHEC). However, the designation of a particular serotype as an EHEC is difficult. First, multiple serotypes of *E. coli* are capable of producing cytotoxins, but a substantially smaller number have been implicated in disease.[55, 56] Second, *E. coli* with toxin genes are ubiquitous in food products[57–60] but are not usually *E. coli* O157. Third, in HUS, the disease most easily recognized as being caused by an EHEC, *E. coli* O157 is implicated in a large majority of cases if stool is cultured early in illness[61] or if serologic studies are performed.[62, 63] The frequency with which *E. coli* O157 is recovered from the stool of patients is at least partially related to its unusual sorbitol-negative phenotype,[64] which distinguishes this organism from other coliforms on appropriate indicator media (sorbitol-MacConkey agar). A 1992 report from Germany describing sorbitol-fermenting *E. coli* O157 may augur difficulty in detecting this serotype, however, if such strains are found elsewhere.[65] To identify other potential EHEC organisms, colonies must be probed with cytotoxin genes or tested for cytotoxin production. Some cytotoxic *E. coli* other than *E. coli* O157 are likely to be capable of causing bloody diarrhea in humans and therefore deserve the designation EHEC.[66]

In addition to its inability to ferment sorbitol, *E. coli* O157 has several other unusual phenotypes. These include its inability to produce β-glucuronidase and to ferment rhamnose.[67] These phenotypes are not so frequently exploited in clinical laboratories, however, as is sorbitol negativity. Most cytotoxic *E. coli* O157 possess the H7 flagellar antigen, but some strains are nonmotile or possess flagellar antigens that cannot be typed.

Epidemiology

Microbiologically diagnosed enteric infection with *E. coli* O157 most frequently occurs in children less than 5 years of age and in the elderly, according to the only two population-based studies reported by the early 1990s.[68, 69] The source in most clusters of cases has been of bovine food origin.[52, 70–72] Cattle are a reservoir for this pathogen,[73–79] but a wide variety of retail foods are contaminated with *E. coli* O157, including beef products, pork, and poultry.[80]

Despite the association between beef consumption and *E. coli* O157 in point-source outbreaks, this pathogen can be transmitted from person to person[81] and acquired from drinking water.[82] Most cases of *E. coli* O157 infection occur sporadically, and attempts to identify a source would be futile in almost all of these cases.

Mechanisms of Pathogenesis

Escherichia coli O157 is the most readily diagnosed and best-studied EHEC. Hence, all subsequent discussion in this chapter concerns this serotype.

Escherichia coli O157 possesses one or two cytotoxin genes, which encode VT I and VT II. Verotoxin I is nearly identical with Shiga toxin, the principal extracellular cytotoxin of *S. dysenteriae*.[83] Verotoxin II is approximately 58% homologous to VT I at both the amino acid and the nucleotide level.[84] Verotoxins I and II are also called Shiga-like toxins (SLTs) I and II, respectively, because of their similarity to Shiga toxin. The confusing nomenclature used to describe *E. coli* O157 and other *E. coli* organisms capable of producing cytotoxins includes EHEC, VTEC, SLT-producing *E. coli* (SLTEC), and cytotoxin-producing *E. coli*. The author prefers the use of the term cytotoxin-producing *E. coli* if an organism produces a cytotoxin for eukaryotic cells, SLTEC if that isolate has genes homologous to SLT I or II, and EHEC if a cytotoxin-producing isolate has a firm link to human disease.

The cytotoxins produced by *E. coli* O157 bind to globotriosyl ceramide on eukaryotic cell surfaces through their B subunits.[85, 86] After internalization, these toxins inhibit target cell protein synthesis by the *N*-glycosidation function of the A subunit of the toxin acting at A4324 in the 23S ribosomal subunit.[87] Shiga toxin is toxic to cultured colonic epithelial cells,[8] and SLT I and II presumably have the same activity. Shiga-like toxins I and II are toxic to cultured human umbilical vein endothelial cells. Shiga-like toxin II is apparently the more pathogenic toxin, as measured by risk for development of renal lesions in mice[88, 89] or HUS in children[91–93] Almost all *E. coli* O157 produce SLT II, and approximately two thirds of these produce SLT I. Very few strains produce only SLT I.[91, 92] The evidence that SLT I can precipitate HUS is derived from the occurrence of HUS after *S. dysenteriae* infection in Bangladesh.[94]

E. coli O157 organisms adhere to epithelial cells in a localized pattern similar to the pattern displayed by enteropathogenic *E. coli* (EPEC),[95] but the molecular mechanisms through which this adherence is mediated are unknown.

E. coli O157 strains induce actin aggregation in epithelial cells to which they adhere, another phenotypic similarity to EPEC. *E. coli* O157 possesses the *eae* gene that encodes a transmembrane protein responsible for this phenomenon.[96, 97] This gene product probably plays a role in the attaching and effacing lesions seen in animals infected with EPEC and *E. coli* O157. Whether the presence or absence of this gene accounts for the variable pathogenicity among cytotoxin-producing *E. coli* is not known.

Because of the severe disease caused by *E. coli* O157, it is not possible to conduct human volunteer studies to learn more about its pathogenesis. Colonoscopic examination and biopsies have demonstrated prominent right- and left-sided colonic pathology (edema, friability, microulceration of the mucosa, superficial inflammation with variable abnormalities of the lamina propria and crypts, and occasional pseudomembranes),[98] and ultrasound has detected small bowel abnormalities consistent with bacterial ileocecitis.[16]

Clinical Presentations

The two most comprehensive studies of diseases caused by *E. coli* O157 have been performed by MacDonald and coworkers[68] and Ostroff and coworkers,[69] who gleaned clinical data from large population bases—one, a health maintenance organization, and the other, a statewide disease reporting system, both in Washington State. A summary of the combined symptoms reported in these two studies demonstrates that diarrhea is always present and is bloody in 96% of the patients. Associated symptoms include cramping abdominal pain (93%), nausea (58%), and vomiting (39%). On the basis of restaurant-associated outbreaks, the interval between ingestion and the first symptoms is 3 to 4 days, on average.[99]

Generally, bloody diarrhea is preceded by nonbloody diarrhea by 1 day, and fever, when present, is either low grade or short-lived.[68, 69] Nonbloody diarrhea can occur,[68, 69, 99] as can asymptomatic and postsymptomatic carriage of *E. coli* O157.[100, 101]

Diarrhea caused by *E. coli* O157 organisms lasts approximately 1 week. As the diarrhea abates, microangiopathic hemolytic anemia can become manifest in an undetermined proportion of patients. In children, the postdiarrheal vascular and renal derangements have been termed HUS. In patients in whom cerebral manifestations are prominent, this disorder closely resembles thrombotic thrombocytopenic purpura (TTP).

Diagnosis

Identification of *E. coli* O157 in stool is facilitated by its unusual sorbitol-negative phenotype. All stools from patients with acute bloody diarrhea should, therefore, be cultured on sorbitol-MacConkey agar. Non–sorbitol-fermenting colonies are tested for the *E. coli* O157 antigen using the rapid latex particle agglutination test.[102] Serologic tests for the H7 antigen are not usually employed in clinical laboratories. The detection of other cytotoxic *E. coli* organisms is not possible in most clinical laboratories.

E. coli O157 can also be preliminarily identified by an immunofluorescence test on sorbitol-negative colonies,[103] and infection can be suggested by seroconversion.[62, 63] Serology is not available, however, in clinical laboratories.

Therapy

Most *E. coli* O157 organisms are sensitive to a wide range of antibiotics, but, for several reasons, we do not recommend therapy.[104] First, the organism is rapidly cleared from the stool of patients. Even patients with HUS do not usually have positive findings for this pathogen by the time of presentation with microangiopathic hemolytic anemia. Second, most of the cytotoxin is associated with the bacterial cell, and lysis or damage of the *E. coli* O157 in the gastrointestinal tract might make more toxin available for systemic absorption. Third, many patients with *E. coli* O157 infection have vomiting and intestinal edema. Orally administered agents might not reach therapeutic levels in the colon, which is probably the site of the heaviest burden of *E. coli* O157 organisms. Analysis of drug use in several outbreaks suggested that administration of antibiotics might risk progression of hemorrhagic colitis to HUS.[72, 105] In these studies, however, antibiotics were administered at the discretion of physicians, and a bias was likely in prescribing therapy to the sicker patients, who might have been more likely to develop HUS in any case. Cimolai and coworkers reported that antimotility agents, but not antibiotics, posed a risk for progression of occasional cases of hemorrhagic colitis to HUS.[106]

Extraintestinal Complications

Hemolytic-uremic syndrome is the major extraintestinal complication of enteric infection with *E. coli* O157. On average, this disorder is manifested 1 week after the onset of diarrhea and consists of nonimmune hemolytic anemia, thrombocytopenia, and renal failure and occurs in approximately 10% of children infected with *E. coli* O157. Subclinical HUS no doubt goes undetected in a larger number of patients.

We recommend a complete blood count and urinalysis on the fourth or fifth day of illness caused by *E. coli* O157, especially if the patient is in an age group with a high risk of developing HUS or TTP (less than 10 or more than 60 years of age). Severe hematologic or urinary abnormalities require immediate hospitalization, assiduous fluid management, and blood product support.

Bacteremia[107] and hemorrhagic cystitis and balanitis[108] with *E. coli* O157 have each been reported once. Bacteriuria can also occur, but rarely.[108, 109]

Infection Control Measures

Escherichia coli O157 infection should be considered highly communicable, even though the exact secondary case rate and infectious dose are unknown. Careful hand washing after contact with infected patients is warranted. All food of animal origin should be assumed to be infectious. Patients should not return to daycare or other group settings where transmission to others can occur if they are unable to control their defecation, nor should they return until a stool culture is negative for *E. coli* O157. We recommend that a follow-up stool culture be performed 1 week after the first positive culture to assess clearance if hygiene is likely to be a problem.

ENTEROINVASIVE *ESCHERICHIA COLI*

History and Microbiology

Enteroinvasive *E. coli* (EIEC) causes dysentery by invading colonic epithelial cells. The association between *E. coli* and bloody diarrhea was first recognized in American soldiers and British children in the 1940s.[110, 111] *E. coli* serotype O124 was eventually implicated as the cause of the illness, which was initially thought to be caused by *Shigella*.

In addition to producing a syndrome indistinguishable from dysentery caused by *Shigella*, EIEC organisms have many other similarities to this genus. Shigella bacteria are closely related phylogenetically to all *E. coli* bacteria, and EIEC organisms display several phenotypes that are even more similar to those of *Shigella* than to those of other *E. coli*. For example, EIEC organisms, unlike most *E. coli* organisms, are lysine decarboxylase–negative, are usually nonmotile, frequently do not ferment lactose,[112] are positive in the Sereny test, and show antigenic identity with multiple *Shigella* serovars.[113] The organisms of EIEC belong to a limited number of serotypes (O28ac, O29, O112ac, O124, O136, O143, O144, O152, and O164, O167).[113, 114]

Epidemiology

EIEC organisms are difficult to identify using standard microbiologic techniques, and most microbiologists overlook lactose-nonfermenting organisms if they are not of the *Salmonella, Shigella,* or *Yersinia* genus. Hence, the epidemiology of EIEC in general populations is poorly understood. At least one epidemic, however, was foodborne.[115] In etiologic studies of diarrhea in defined populations in developing countries, EIEC organisms are found to be present when sought with DNA diagnostic techniques.[116]

Mechanism of Pathogenicity

The central pathogenetic mechanism of EIEC is apparently its ability to invade epithelial cells. Toxins have not been consistently identified. The ability to invade epithelial cells is highly correlated with the presence of a 140 MDa plasmid, which is also found in *Shigella* species.[117] Considerable homology exists between the 140 MDa plasmids of EIEC and the large plasmid found in shigellae.[117, 118]

Clinical Presentation

The most striking manifestations of EIEC infections are related to colonic epithelial cell invasion. Patients have fever, low-volume bloody diarrhea, and, frequently, inflammatory cells in their feces. Patients infected with EIEC most closely resemble patients infected with *Shigella,* and it is this presentation that causes EIEC to be sought in patients with dysentery from whom shigellae are not isolated. Because of the difficulty in identifying EIEC, these pathogens are not routinely sought except in epidemiologic studies or suggestive clinical settings. Therefore, the full spectrum of disease due to EIEC is not known and may be broader than initially suspected. For example, when sought using DNA probes, EIEC organisms were determined to cause some cases of traveler's diarrhea.[119] Most patients with outbreak-associated EIEC infection do not have bloody diarrhea.[111, 115]

Diagnosis

The possibility of infection with EIEC should be considered in patients with febrile dysenteric syndromes if standard enteric pathogens are not found in stool culture. Copious lactose-nonfermenting *E. coli* organisms would be one clue to diagnosis, but some EIEC do ferment lactose and would be missed by screening on Mac-Conkey plates.[112] Tissue culture or the Sereny test[120] to identify EIEC is definitive, but these tests are hardly practical in diagnostic laboratories. Diagnosis is often academic, because antibiotics may be administered empirically after nonproductive stool microbiologic studies are performed.

Therapy

Controlled trials for treatment of EIEC infection have not been performed. The current sensitivities of EIEC to antibiotics are unknown. If infection with EIEC is confirmed or strongly suspected after the results of microbiologic investigations are known, the treatment used for *Shigella* is recommended for EIEC.

Extraintestinal Complications

The extent to which extraintestinal complication and postinfectious sequelae occur with EIEC is unknown. More extensive data on these complications will be available after better techniques of diagnosis have become available.

Infection Control Measures

It is not known how often EIEC organisms are spread from person to person or by contaminated food. Clusters of cases of bloody diarrhea, with or without an identifiable agent, should be reported to appropriate public health authorities. The duration of carriage after infection and the frequency of asymptomatic carriage are unknown.

SALMONELLA

History and Microbiology

Salmonella is a non-lactose-fermenting genus of the family Enterobacteriaceae, as is *Shigella.* Unlike shigellae, however, salmonellae produce hydrogen sulfide and are almost always motile. They have various somatic (O) and flagellar (H) antigens, as do *E. coli* bacteria. More than 2000 O-H combinations of *Salmonella* have been identified. Instead of the numerical designation of serotypes assigned to *E. coli,* unique *Salmonella* O-H serotypes are given names (e.g., *S. heidelberg, S. typhimurium*) that have historical but not clinical significance. This taxonomy is misleading, because these 2000 serotypes belong to one of only several species. The use of names instead of numbers suggests a speciation that has no basis in phylogenetic fact.

Of all the schemes proposed for *Salmonella* nomenclature, we prefer to divide the genus into three species: *S. typhi, S. choleraesuis,* and *S. enteritidis. S. typhi* infects only humans, causes typhoid fever, and has no additional serotypes. *S. choleraesuis* can infect humans but is much better adapted to swine, and it too consists of only one serotype. *S. enteritidis* is a species that is composed of multiple serotypes, each named rather than numbered, and it can infect both humans and animals. Unless a *Salmonella* is designated *S. typhi* or *S. choleraesuis*, it should be assumed that it is a serotype of *S. enteritidis*.

The genus *Salmonella* was first discovered by Theobald Smith, working under Daniel Salmon in the Federal Bureau of Animal Industry in 1885.[121] Soon after their description, it became apparent that salmonellae were responsible for a wide range of human enteric and systemic illnesses, including diarrhea, enterocolitis, abscesses, septicemia, meningitis, and typhoid fever. Salmonellae are an increasingly common cause of human disease in developed countries. Their persistence in animals poses challenges for veterinary microbiologists.

Epidemiology

Unlike *S. typhi*, which is adapted only to humans and is rarely recovered in developed countries, the organisms of all other *Salmonella* species colonize a wide range of animals. Contaminated poultry and eggs are the most frequent sources of human infection, but beef, pork, dairy products, and pet reptiles are also vehicles of transmission. Food handlers carrying salmonellae are apparently rare sources of infection,[122] the notoriety of Typhoid Mary notwithstanding.

Salmonellae are recovered most frequently from children less than 5 years of age, and in the summer and autumn. The number of cases of salmonellosis has been increasing steadily during the past several decades.[123] In the United States, *Salmonella* has been estimated to be responsible for 18,000 annual hospitalizations, 500 deaths, and 50 million dollars in medical costs.[124]

Infections spread in institutions when an asymptomatic carrier or patient with enterocolitis is introduced, with caretakers transmitting the organism from resident to resident. Food, instruments,[125] and fomites cause institutional outbreaks.[126] Hospital-acquired salmonellosis has a particularly high mortality rate because of the compromised immune systems or the young or old age of many of the patients or both these factors.

Mechanisms of Pathogenesis

Salmonella produces disease by one definitely known mechanism (cellular invasion) and one postulated mechanism (enterotoxin production). *S. typhi* is the prototype of the invasive strain. This species causes typhoid fever (enteric fever) and only rarely causes enterocolitis. Dissemination by multiple *Salmonella* strains is possible and can occur with strains that cause bloody diarrhea.

Colonization of the gastrointestinal tract occurs only after ingestion of relatively large numbers of organisms, because salmonellae are sensitive to gastric acid.[127–129] Conditions in which gastric acidity is reduced or gastric emptying time is delayed predispose to salmonellosis. Once *Salmonella* leaves the stomach, it must compete with the normal flora. In animals, prior antibiotic administration increases susceptibility to *Salmonella*.[130, 131]

In the small bowel, investigators have postulated that salmonellae preferentially invade M cells in the ileum and then invade the underlying Peyer's patch. After breaching the mucosa, salmonellae are phagocytosed by monocytes within Peyer's patches, and, depending on the strain and the host, disseminate within monocytes to various sites. Most strains of *Salmonella* probably remain confined to Peyer's patches or local lymph nodes, but for some strains, classically *S. typhi*, dissemination is the rule rather than the exception. Dissemination with a wide variety of serotypes is common in infants less than 3 months old.[132] In most cases, dissemination is asymptomatic, although suppurative infection of any organ can occur. Frequent sites of seeding include the liver, biliary tree, spleen, meninges, bone, and bone marrow. *Salmonella* persists in the biliary tree, and stool cultures that can become negative for *Salmonella* within a few days of illness can become positive again when organisms are reintroduced to the small bowel from the bile.

Infections with *S. typhi*, and to a lesser extent *S. paratyphi*, *S. schottmuelleri*, and *S. hirschfeldii*, follow an enteric fever pattern. Dissemination is common, and ileal lymphoid proliferation at the site of the original invasion is prominent during the first 7 to 14 days of infection. During this time, perforation can occur secondary to pressure effects of the hypertrophied lymphoid tissue, and intestinal and systemic symptoms are prominent and occur simultaneously (fever, malaise, constipation, diarrhea, headache, abdominal pain, chills, emesis, and cough).

Most strains do not cause enteric fever, and some strains cause few or no gastrointestinal symptoms. For example, *S. choleraesuis* invades the intestinal epithelial cell without causing diarrhea, but causes metastatic infection. Most *Salmonella* strains, however, cause diarrhea, which may or may not be bloody, with potential clinical or subclinical dissemination and clearance of infection.

The mechanisms of diarrhea and colonic hemorrhage in salmonellosis, beyond the physical consequences of invasion, are unknown. Enterotoxigenic activity[133] has been postulated for *Salmonella*, but the gene or genes responsible for this phenotype have eluded cloning.

Clinical Presentations

Salmonellosis has an incubation period between 6 hours and 2 days. Self-limited symptoms of the upper gastrointestinal tract and systemic symptoms predominate at first and include nausea, vomiting, myalgia, and headache. The initial diarrheal stools are nonbloody and remain so in most cases. Fluid loss may be voluminous. Accompanying abdominal pain is usually periumbilical or infraumbilical.[121]

A variable proportion of patients with salmonellosis have frankly bloody diarrhea. The blood may merely tinge watery stools or may cause them to resemble dysenteric stools. In the latter case, tenesmus and small volume stools may occur. Fever is usually mild (38–39°C, 100.4–102.2°F) and is lower than the fever in shigellosis. Rarely, toxic megacolon occurs.[134] Bacteremia occurs in an unknown number of cases. Because it is usually self-limited and without extraintestinal seeding, bacteremia is probably underdiagnosed.

Untreated nontyphoidal salmonellosis usually lasts approximately 1 week. The duration of the carrier state depends on the age of the infected patient. Children less than 5 years of age carry nontyphoidal *Salmonella* strains approximately 12 weeks on average, whereas adults clear the organism after a shorter period, approximately 4 weeks.[135]

Diagnosis

Salmonellosis is diagnosed by culturing the appropriate body substance. Stool cultures are the logical first diagnostic approach, but physicians should be aware that an interval between enterocolitis and establishment of the carrier state may exist when stool cultures are negative for *Salmonella*. Before starting antibiotics, blood cultures should be obtained for all patients with suspected or proven salmonellosis if they are immunosuppressed or less than 6 months of age. In children less than 6 months of age, spinal taps and cerebrospinal fluid cultures should be performed. Cultures of suppurative extraintestinal sites (abscesses, mesenteric lymph nodes, bone marrow, cerebrospinal fluid) should be performed as indicated on clinical grounds.

Once *Salmonella* is identified, it is important to determine whether the isolate is *S. typhi*, because antibiotics are efficacious in typhoid fever. As noted earlier, however, *S. typhi* is rare in the United States, and bloody diarrhea during typhoid fever is even more rare. Sensitivity studies should be performed on all isolates so that appropriate empirical therapy can be started if metastatic complications ensue. We do not recommend routine blood cultures in hosts who are at low or negligible risk of developing metastatic infection with nontyphoidal strains of *Salmonella*.

Therapy

Antimicrobial use in salmonellosis is controversial; the vast majority of cases in normal hosts are self-limited, antibiotics have not been conclusively shown to be efficacious in mitigating the symptoms caused by *Salmonella*, and some,[21] but not all,[136] authorities believe that antibiotics prolong the carrier state. Because *Salmonella* excretion is common after *Salmonella* enterocolitis, especially in children, prolongation of excretion increases the prevalence of carriers, which is estimated at 200,000 at any given time in the United States alone.[135] Reducing this reservoir of *Salmonella* excretors should be an important public health priority, and interventions that increase this pool should be avoided.

In those circumstances in which the risk of prolonging *Salmonella* carriage is exceeded by the risk of extraintestinal metastatic infection, we do recommend treatment. Such patients include infants less than 6 months old, in whom most cases of *Salmonella* meningitis occur, and patients with hemoglobinopathies, cancer, or acquired immunodeficiency syndrome (AIDS).

As mentioned earlier, *S. typhi* should always be treated, and this recommendation extends to *S. choleraesuis*, which frequently causes metastatic infection. *S. typhi* and *S. choleraesuis* rarely cause bloody diarrhea. Serotypes of *S. enteritidis* that cause enterocolitis have a variable tendency to colonize sites other than blood, and the decision to treat should be based on the risk factors presented by the host. Empirically administered antibiotics often need to be chosen prior to the availability of results of antibiotic sensitivity tests. If the patient has been in contact with someone else who is known to be excreting *Salmonella* organisms, the sensitivities of the organism from the probable index case may be usefully reviewed, and the antibiogram used to guide initial therapy. If metastatic infection is a possibility, we recommend either intravenous ampicillin and chloramphenicol or a third-generation cephalosporin. In infants, a drug that can penetrate the central nervous system must be chosen, at least until the results of the cerebrospinal fluid culture are known. Sensitivity testing is crucial because of the frequent resistance of this organism to antibiotics.

The optimal duration of therapy for systemic salmonellosis is unknown. Intravenous antibiotics should be continued for at least a week if uncomplicated bacteremia is established in a host at risk for metastatic infection. Suppurative collections should be drained, if possible.

Treatment of severe typhoid fever with high-dose dexamethasone is efficacious in reducing the mortality of this disease,[137] although it presents some risk of increasing the relapse rate.[138] Intestinal perforations during typhoid fever should be treated by surgery.[139] Gastrointestinal hemorrhage in typhoid fever, which is not to be confused with the bloody diarrhea of enterocolitis, should be treated conservatively unless there is intestinal perforation.

Considerable interest has arisen in the use of the quinolones for the treatment of *Salmonella* infections in patients old enough to take them safely.[140] These drugs are tolerated well, and most *Salmonella* species are sensitive to their antibacterial effect. High intraintestinal concentrations of drugs are achieved after oral administration. Furthermore, the quinolones also achieve high levels in monocytes and bile, two reservoirs for *Salmonella* during dissemination and chronic carriage. However, resistance of *Salmonella* to quinolones has emerged.[141] Moreover, Neill[142] and Wiström[142a] and their colleagues have demonstrated that *Salmonella* carriage was not eliminated by quinolones. Hence, it is our belief that the quinolones offer no advantage over older less expensive agents and should not be used in the absence of risk for metastatic infection.

In children less than 6 months of age, the risk of meningitis persists if the organism is carried, even if the acute episode of enterocolitis resolves without metastatic infection. Therefore, we recommend the administration of an oral antibiotic, usually amoxicillin, on a daily basis until the child is 6 months old, providing the isolate is sensitive to the drug chosen. Few data exist to support this practice, but we believe that the minimal risk and cost of daily antibiotic therapy to maintain some circulating microbicidal activity are small compared with the serious consequences of *Salmonella* meningitis.

Extraintestinal Complications

As described earlier, the most important extraintestinal complication of *Salmonella* enterocolitis is metastatic infection. Meningitis is the most dreaded of these complications and tends to occur most frequently in children less than 6 months of age. Once established, *Salmonella* meningitis can be difficult to eradicate.

Suppurative complications with *Salmonella* infection can occur anywhere in the body. The most frequent extraintestinal infections include osteomyelitis and osteoarthritis, especially in patients who have hemoglobinopathies or are immunosuppressed; arteritis, especially with underlying atherosclerotic disease; urinary tract infections; hepatic and splenic abscesses other than biliary colonization, which is very common; abdominal abscesses; and endocarditis and pericarditis.

Several nonsuppurative extraintestinal complications may accompany salmonellosis. These include reactive arthritis and a migratory polyarthritis that occurs approximately 10 days after the onset of diarrhea and is usually found in HLA-B27–positive patients. The arthritis can persist for months. In addition, a subset of these patients will also have urethritis or conjunctivitis or both. Reactive arthritis is much more common than pyogenic arthritis in salmonellosis. Cases of HUS after *S. typhi* infection have also been reported.[143]

Infection Control Measures

The most important infection control measures for salmonellosis are an awareness that this organism is ubiquitous in our food and the prevention and recognition of the postsymptomatic and asymptomatic carrier states. Physicians should caution patients at particular risk of developing complicated salmonellosis that no food of animal origin is free of *Salmonella,* even apparently uncracked eggs. Food should be cooked well to kill organisms, and hands and utensils should be washed thoroughly after coming in contact with these uncooked foods.

Vaccination[144] should be offered to people who are in contact with a human carrier of *S. typhi* or who are anticipating travel to an area where typhoid fever is endemic. Another efficacious vaccine consisting of the *S. typhi* Vi polysaccharide antigen[145] is not yet approved for human use in the United States.

As discussed earlier, treatment of uncomplicated nontyphoidal salmonellosis usually does not warrant the use of antibiotics, because the carrier state might be prolonged. *S. typhi* is the species most frequently associated with chronic carriage, but the temporary carrier state should be assumed in all patients infected with salmonella, and hygienic infection control measures should be emphasized. Unless the infected patient has an occupation in which passage to susceptible hosts is possible, follow-up cultures are not recommended. Follow-up cultures may be affected by the fact that fecal excretion can be intermittent and antimicrobial therapy can delay the appearance of *Salmonella* organisms in the stool. Hence, 2 or 3 negative coprocultures a week apart and at least 3 weeks after antibiotics have been stopped are necessary to certify that a patient is no longer carrying *Salmonella*. We recommend screening for carriers in contacts of a documented case of salmonellosis if they might be in a position to pass the organism to a host whose disease has a high likelihood of progressing to systemic complications.

Attempts to eradicate the carrier state have been variably successful. Although quinolones might be disappointing in preventing or treating temporary carriage of nontyphoidal *Salmonella*, some successful cures, perhaps coincidental, have been reported.[140] Amoxicillin or ampicillin for prolonged periods (6 weeks) is efficacious in patients without cholelithiasis.[146] A regimen of rifampin and trimethoprim-sulfamethoxazole (TMPSMX) has also been used successfully with typhoidal and nontyphoidal strains of *Salmonella*.[147] Follow-up cultures are mandatory to confirm clearance, and cholecystectomy is sometimes required to end the carrier state.

SHIGELLA

History and Microbiology

Shigella species have probably caused human disease since ancient times and continue to do so.[148] Early in this century, it became apparent that the genus *Shigella*, named after Kiyoshi Shiga, who first isolated *S. dysenteriae*, is composed of four species: *S. dysenteriae*, *S. flexneri*, *S. boydii*, and *S. sonnei* (also called *Shigella* groups A, B, C, and D, respectively). Each species has several serotypes. Prior to World War I, *S. dysenteriae* was the predominant isolate worldwide. Subsequently, *S. flexneri* (named after Simon Flexner, who discovered this species in the Philippines before 1900)[6] was isolated more frequently than any of the other *Shigella* species. In mid-century, the epidemiology again shifted, with *S. sonnei* becoming the most frequently isolated species in industrialized countries.

Shigella genus is a member of the Enterobacteriaceae family and is closely related to the *Escherichia* genus. Phenotypically, *Shigella bacteria* differ from most *E. coli* in their slow fermentation of lactose and their nonmotility.

Epidemiology

Shigella infections occur worldwide. Their frequency in developed parts of the world has declined dramatically during this century, but since the mid-1980's the number of cases of shigellosis reported to the Centers for Disease Control in Atlanta has increased, and outbreaks of shigellosis occur fairly frequently.[148] It is estimated that shigellosis in the United States is severely underreported.

The ability of *Shigella* to survive the acidic conditions of the stomach no doubt contributes to the low dose necessary to cause infection that is characteristic of this genus. For example, DuPont and coworkers were able to cause shigellosis in human volunteers challenged with as few as 10 organisms.[149] The epidemiologic implications of this small inoculum include high attack rates of shigellosis in institutionalized or military settings, ease of person-to-person spread, and high secondary attack rates when an index case is present in a family or group.

Worldwide, *S. dysenteriae* infection has a tendency to occur in pandemics. Peaks and troughs of the incidence of dysentery have been noted for several centuries in England,[2] probably because of waxing and waning of population immunity.

Person-to-person spread is probably the most important mode of transmission of *Shigella*, but foodborne outbreaks and contaminated water sources have been identified.

Mechanisms of Pathogenesis

Members of the *Shigella* genus display two phenotypic traits (invasion and toxin production) that are believed to be significant in their virulence. *Shigella* organisms invade epithelial cells, producing superficial epithelial cell death. Invasion of epithelial cells is probably responsible for the intense colonic inflammatory reaction and the high fevers seen in patients who have shigellosis. Invasion and virulence for *Shigella* species are associated with proteins encoded by a large plasmid, as is the case with EIEC.[117] Interestingly, however, invasion of guinea pig keratoconjunctiva[120] has been the traditional measure of virulence, but this phenotype depends on a chromosomal rather than a plasmid locus.

Shiga toxin elaborated by *S. dysenteriae* is an additional virulence factor produced by strains of serotype 1 of this species. Shiga toxin has several effects on cells that could potentiate the symptoms caused by epithelial cell invasion. Shiga toxin is an *N*-glycosidase, inhibiting protein synthesis in eukaryotic cells by cleavage of the 60S ribosomal subunit at the A 4324 nucleotide.[87] Purified toxin causes net secretion in rabbit ileal loops.[150, 151] The toxin also kills colonic epithelial cells[8] and cultured human umbilical vein endothelial cells, suggesting that HUS might result from absorbed toxin produced by *S. dysenteriae*[94] and by *E. coli* organisms that elaborate similar toxins.

Escherichia coli that produce toxins similar to Shiga toxin[83, 84] provide indirect evidence of the role of Shiga toxin in human disease. These *E. coli* organisms do not invade epithelial cells[152] but are capable of causing enteric illness with bloody diarrhea and HUS, as is *S. dysenteriae*. Infections with these noninvasive toxigenic *E. coli* bacteria are generally associated with little or no fever.[68, 69]

Even though Shiga toxin almost certainly plays some pathogenetic role in *S. dysenteriae* type 1 infections and might be responsible for the virulence of this strain compared with that of other shigellae, additional virulence mechanisms independent of the toxin remain. For example, Shiga toxin deletion mutants of *S. dysenteriae* retain some cytotoxicity.[153]

Toxins have been described in species of *Shigella* other than *S. dysenteriae* serotype 1,[154–156] and investigators have proposed that toxin production is related to the clinical manifestations of infection by these various strains. These toxins have yet to be isolated chemically or cloned, however, and until they are characterized at a molecular level, their role in disease remains a matter for speculation.

Clinical Presentations

The manifestations of enteric infection with *Shigella* are somewhat species-dependent. *S. dysenteriae* and *S. flexneri* usually cause dysenteric illness, and *S. sonnei* frequently causes non-bloody, self-limited diarrhea. Typically, patients with shigellosis are febrile and have malaise and watery diarrhea for 1 or 2 days before bloody diarrhea ensues. This progression is postulated to derive from the sequential effects of infection as the organism descends the gastrointestinal tract. In some patients, especially children, the neurologic manifestations of shigellosis are striking and can consist of obtundation, delirium, or seizures. Because these signs present before dysentery but are concomitant with fever, a spinal tap may be necessary to exclude meningitis.

As the bloody diarrhea evolves, colonic manifestations of shigellosis become pronounced. The distal colon is most severely affected.[157] Microscopic findings include edema, capillary congestion, neutrophilic infiltration, goblet cell depletion, epithelial and erythrocyte shedding, and crypt abscesses. Capillary thromboses and superficial necrosis of the epithelium are also occasionally seen. The histopathologic findings correlate well with the colonoscopic observations.[157]

After 1 or 2 days, the stool volume decreases, but the urgency increases, and tenesmus can be painful. The abdomen is frequently tender and distended, and patients are listless. Rectal prolapse may occur, especially in children.

In severe cases of shigellosis, toxic megacolon and perforation can occur. Obstruction is an ominous complication of shigellosis.[158] Shigellaemia is documented in approximately 4–7% of patients,[159, 160] but its frequency is probably higher than appreciated. The fatality rate of reported cases of *Shigella* bacteremia has been high.[161, 162] Interestingly, gram-negative bacteremia in shigellosis is likely to be caused by non-*Shigella* enteric flora.[160, 163] If left untreated, *Shigella* infections cause persistent intestinal symptoms for approximately 1 week, although the duration of illness ranges from 1 day to 1 month.[164] The duration of enteric illness with *S. sonnei* is shorter (2–3 days).[165]

Diagnosis

Shigella organisms are usually sought by microbiology laboratories when a stool culture is requested. The most common screening techniques involve placement of a small aliquot of stool on MacConkey agar as well as the more selective *Salmonella-Shigella* (SS) agar. Lactose-nonfermenting colonies isolated from these plates are subsequently tested for other biochemical characteristics of *Shigella* and serogrouped with *Shigella* antisera.

Fecal leukocytes are usually, but not always, present in shigellosis, and absence of this finding should not eliminate *Shigella* from consideration as a cause of a patient's bloody diarrhea.[12]

In contrast to their viability in the human host, *Shigella* organisms are difficult to isolate if stool is left unplated for too long. If a long interval between specimen collection and plating is unavoidable, an appropriate transport medium (Cary-Blair medium) is useful. Cup specimens plated directly are preferable to specimens submitted on swabs. If swabs are used to obtain fecal specimens, however, we suggest that they be inserted well proximal to the anal verge, to the extent that the cotton tip disappears.

Therapy

Shigellosis is one of the few bacterial diarrheas in which antibiotic therapy is of unequivocal benefit when administered at the time the positive culture results are reported to the physician. Even if patients are improving by the time a positive result is known, we recommend therapy to reduce fecal excretion in convalescence.

Ampicillin and TMP/SMX have been the preferred drugs to treat shigellosis because of their efficacy, safety, and low cost. Oral ampicillin is preferred over oral amoxicillin because of the higher intracolonic levels of the less well-absorbed ampicillin. Unfortunately, resistance to ampicillin and TMP/SMX is increasing, and therapy must be guided by patterns of current resistance reported for the strain identified, taking into account the probable locale of acquisition, because strains from developing countries tend to be more resistant to antibiotics.

Alternative regimens include nalidixic acid (to which resistance has also been reported), the quinolones, third-generation cephalosporins, tetracyclines, nonabsorbable aminoglycosides, and furazolidone. Tetracycline or quinolones should not be given to children less than 9 or 18, respectively, or to pregnant women, because of potential tooth discoloration with tetracycline and osteotoxicity with quinolones. A single dose of 2.5 g of tetracycline may be as efficacious as a longer course,[166] even for strains resistant to the antibiotic.

Extraintestinal Complications

Shigella can cause bacteremia and, in very rare cases, seed distant sites. Generally, however, bacteremia during shigellosis results in either spontaneous clearance or a septic syndrome with a high mortality, rather than metastatic infection, as with *Salmonella*. In fact, most deaths during acute shigellosis are caused by septicemia.[167]

Systemic toxemia during shigellosis is manifested by alterations in CNS function. Children are more likely to develop the neurologic abnormalities of lethargy, delirium, and seizures. It is not certain if seizures in children with shigellosis are independent of the nearly universal fever that accompanies this disorder. Nonetheless, the combination of seizures and high fever in the setting of bloody diarrhea strongly suggests a diagnosis of shigellosis.

Shigellosis is associated with hematologic complications and sequelae. The leukemoid reaction is the most common hematologic abnormality in shigellosis and was detected in approximately 4% of hospitalized patients in Bangladesh,[168] where this finding predicted a poor outcome. Neutropenia can also occur, as well as a "relative bandemia." Usually the blood loss in the stool is not severe enough to cause anemia.

Hemolytic-uremic syndrome is the most dramatic hematologic disturbance after *Shigella* infection. This abnormality is usually associated only with *S. dysenteriae* infection,[94] but a few cases have followed *S. flexneri* infections.[165] The onset of diarrhea is followed by HUS in approximately 1 week. Postshigellosis HUS carries a higher mortality than does HUS after enteric infection with cytotoxic *E. coli*, probably because *S. dysenteriae* infection occurs in areas of the world where the transfusions and dialysis needed to treat HUS are prohibitively expensive.

Massive vascular collapse (Ekiri syndrome) with cerebral manifestations and death after a brief course of shigellosis occurs in children but is fortunately very rare.[169]

Shigellosis complications that are immunologically mediated include keratoconjunctivitis, sterile arthritis, and an HLA-B27–associated Reiter's syndrome.

Infection Control Measures

Patients should not return to groups in which person-to-person spread might lead to secondary cases until it is confirmed that they have cleared their infecting strain. In persistent carriers, we have used ampicillin, TMP/SMX, and oral gentamicin (2.5 mg/kg/dose, given 3 times a day for a week) in sequential attempts to eradicate this organism.

YERSINIA ENTEROCOLITICA

History and Microbiology

Yersiniae are motile (at 25°C), lactose-nonfermenting coccobacilli, and *Yersinia* belongs to the Enterobacteriaceae family. Of the three *Yersinia* species, *Y. enterocolitica* and *Y. pseudotuberculosis* produce prominent enteric infection, and *Y. pestis* causes the plague. This genus was overlooked as an enteric pathogen for the first half of this century. Gradually, however, pseudotuberculosis in animals and mesenteric adenitis and pseudoappendicitis in humans were attributed to *Y. pseudotuberculosis,* and *Y. enterocolitica* was detected in diarrheal stools that did not yield *Salmonella* or *Shigella*.[170] Although still relatively uncommon in North America, *Y. enterocolitica* is recovered commonly from patients in Northern Europe and is the only *Yersinia* species to cause bloody diarrhea, although it does so in only a minority of cases.[171-173]

Y. enterocolitica can be characterized by biochemical phenotypes, phage typing, plasmid analysis, and O (somatic) and H (flagellar) antigen serotyping. The most commonly used epidemiologic tool is O serotyping, and the 0:3, 0:8, and 0:9 serotypes predominate in human disease.

Epidemiology

Y. enterocolitica occurs worldwide but is reported more frequently in cold climates. The northern Europe incidence exceeds the North American incidence. European cases occur most often in the fall and winter[170] and are sporadic. In nature, pathogenic serotypes are most often found in swine, raw milk, and water, and these vehicles are the probable sources for most sporadic and outbreak-associated cases of yersiniosis.[170]

Mechanisms of Pathogenesis

The ability of *Y. enterocolitica* to invade epithelial cells is relevant to its pathogenicity. Invasion is chromosomally mediated.[174] *Yersinia* organisms do not multiply in epithelial cells,[175] but do replicate in Peyer's patches in animals.[176-179] *Y. enterocolitica* grows best at neutral pH,[179] suggesting that reduced gastric acidity and gastrectomy are risk factors for yersiniosis.

Regional lymphatic spread occurs after *Y. enterocolitica* multiplies in Peyer's patches, and it is at this point that a picture of pseudoappendicitis and mesenteric adenitis can occur. In some hosts, systemic dissemination can occur, with resultant bacteremia and metastatic infection.

Y. enterocolitica possesses several interesting virulence mechanisms. In *Y. enterocolitica*, outer membranes confer resistance to phagocytosis[180, 181]

and lysis mediated by complement.[182-184] *Y. enterocolitica* utilizes siderophores produced by other bacteria to incorporate iron, which is important for its virulence.[185, 186] Its chromosomally encoded enterotoxin, which resembles *E. coli* heat-labile toxin, probably does not play a role in pathogenesis.[170]

Clinical Presentation

Y. enterocolitica most often causes enterocolitis, with diarrhea (32–86% of cases), abdominal pain (61–100% of cases), and fever (53–100% of cases).[170] Bloody diarrhea is present in up to one quarter of the patients.[170] Additional symptoms include nausea, vomiting, pharyngitis, arthralgia, and erythema nodosum. Nonsuppurative peritoneal inflammation in yersiniosis has resulted in laparotomies for suspected acute abdomen. Pharyngitis commonly accompanies *Y. enterocolitica* infection. *Y. enterocolitica* infection has an incubation period of between 1 and 11 days, and symptoms last between 1 and 2 weeks. Organisms are excreted for an average of 6 weeks after an infection in childhood.[171]

Symptomatic bacteremia usually occurs in patients with iron overload, chronic liver disease, diabetes mellitus, alcoholism, and malnutrition and is associated with a high mortality rate.[187, 188] The actual incidence of bacteremia in yersiniosis is unknown, but no doubt it occurs more frequently than it is detected. This conclusion is supported by detection of asymptomatic bacteremia in apparently healthy blood donors.[189] The pseudoappendicular syndrome (pseudoappendicitis) occurs most frequently among teenagers and young adults, and enterocolitis tends to occur in younger children.

Diagnosis

If *Y. enterocolitica* is suspected, the microbiology laboratory should be so advised, especially if it does not routinely attempt to detect this pathogen, so that appropriate selective media or cold enrichment techniques can be used on the specimen. Suppurative mesenteric nodes discovered at laparotomy should be cultured for *Y. enterocolitica* as well as for *E. coli* and *Streptococcus*. Blood cultures should be obtained from febrile patients, especially if they are at high risk of bacteremia or if signs or symptoms suggest metastatic infection. Serologic diagnosis is possible at reference centers, but its use is limited. Antibodies to *Yersinia* antigens occur in the absence of a history of *Yersinia* infection, and cross-reactions may occur between this organism and other bacteria. Also, *Yersinia* organisms that are detected in stool cultures after long incubation times may not be relevant to the disease being evaluated. These are probably commensal organisms, with little, if any, virulence.[190]

Treatment

Yersinia organisms are susceptible to a wide variety of antibiotics, including TMP/SMX, aminoglycosides, tetracyclines, chloramphenicol, quinolones, and third-generation cephalosporins, but they are resistant to penicillin, ampicillin, and first-generation cephalosporins. Their sensitivity has not, however, been translated into efficacious treatment. For example, children with *Y. enterocolitica* enterocolitis receiving TMP/SMX responded at the same rate as those receiving placebo in a double-blind control study. Therapy was administered late in the course, however, on average 12 days after the onset of symptoms.[22] Despite the lack of demonstrated efficacy, most clinicians do prescribe TMP/SMX or a quinolone to patients with diagnosed *Y. enterocolitica* infection. Metastatic infections are also treated with antimicrobial therapy. Because of its high mortality rate, *Yersinia* septicemia is usually treated with two antibiotics pending sensitivity testing. Cephalosporins are usually avoided, and parenteral aminoglycosides, tetracycline, chloramphenicol, or TMP/SMX are recommended.

The pseudoappendicular syndrome does not require a laparotomy, but if doubt remains as to the presence of appendicitis, surgery should not be deferred until the results of cultures are reported.

Extraintestinal Complications

At the time of the acute enterocolitis, local spread to mesenteric lymph nodes and distal abscess formation can occur. Few *Y. enterocolitica* infections, however, spread beyond the gastrointestinal tract to other areas, including the tonsils.

Postinfectious complications have been documented best in Scandinavia and consist of reactive arthropathy and erythema nodosum. Sterile polyarticular arthritis occurs 1 or 2 weeks after the onset of diarrhea. *Yersinia* antigens have been detected in these joints.[191] Patients with HLA-B27 haplotype seem to be at particular risk of developing this reactive arthropathy.

Other autoimmune disorders attributed to *Y. enterocolitica* include Reiter's syndrome, myocarditis, glomerulonephritis, and thyroid dysfunction.[170]

Infection Control Measures

Public health authorities should be notified if patients with documented *Y. enterocolitica* infection report similar illnesses among contacts. Follow-up stool cultures should be obtained before patients, especially children, return to settings where additional people may become infected.

ENTAMOEBA HISTOLYTICA

History and Microbiology

E. histolytica causes amebic dysentery. This protozoan was first proved to be pathogenic in 1875 by Loesch,[2] who induced bloody diarrhea in dogs fed stools from patients with dysentery. As described in the introduction to this chapter, the differentiation between bacillary and amebic dysentery was a major microbiologic advance.

E. histolytica is in the pseudopod-forming subphylum of Protozoa. There are multiple additional nonpathogenic *Entamoeba* species, including *E. hartmanni*, *E. polecki*, *E. coli*, and *E. gingivalis*. Multiple zymodemes, or distinct isoenzyme patterns, with variable pathogenic potential exist within *E. histolytica*. Cysts of *E. histolytica* average 12 μ in diameter and contain one to four nuclei. Excystation occurs in the small bowel, and the resulting trophozoite, which averages 25 μ in diameter, contains only one nucleus. Both forms may be excreted, but trophozoites degenerate rapidly, whereas cysts may remain viable for months. Cysts are resistant to gastric acidity and digestive enzymes, but trophozoites are not. Cysts, therefore, are the infective form of this parasite.

Epidemiology

E. histolytica is found worldwide, but clinical amebiasis is manifest chiefly in tropical countries and regions where sanitation is inadequate. Humans are the main reservoir. Asymptomatic cyst passers, especially food handlers, are significant sources of infection. Fecal-oral transmission occurs by sexual contact or by inadequate disposal of fecal waste. The 40,000 deaths attributable to amebiasis each year make this the third leading parasitic cause of death, behind malaria and schistosomiasis.

Mechanisms of Pathogenesis

E. histolytica is a lytic pathogen. In the colon, which is the principal site of gastrointestinal pathology, direct contact of the parasite with tissue causes mucosal destruction. The mechanism of cytotoxicity is uncertain. Trophozoites can destroy leukocytes, resulting in release of proteolytic enzymes by neutrophils, with secondary tissue destruction.[192, 193] In axenic cultures, *E. histolytica* has not been documented to produce a cytotoxin.[194, 195] Direct contact with target cells by the parasite is crucial, however, for cytopathic effect. The Gal/Gal Nac lectin through which *E. histolytica* adheres to target cells is required for toxicity, and, in fact, this lectin, when purified, is itself a cytotoxin.[196]

Death of target cells after adherence of *E. histolytica* or addition of the purified lectin appears to be associated with sustained elevation of intracellular calcium. Phorbol esters and protein kinase C activators augment parasite cytotoxicity. *E. histolytica* produces a pore-forming protein that might contribute to the rise in intracellular calcium.[197, 198] The parasite also produces numerous proteolytic enzymes, including an acid[199] and a neutral proteinase,[200] cathepsin B,[201] collagenase,[202] β-glucosaminidase,[203] and neuraminidase,[204] which might contribute to the destruction of connective tissue and mucus, allowing amebic ulcers to become established and permitting the parasites to enter the circulation. Sonicates of *E. histolytica* and whole trophozoites cause intestinal secretion.[205–207]

The pathogenicity of *E. histolytica* also seems to be affected by the colonic milieu. Bacteria phagocytosed by trophozoites and anaerobic conditions increase virulence.[208] None of these potential virulence mechanisms, however appealing its role might seem in pathogenesis, is useful in separating pathogenic from nonpathogenic zymodemes.

Clinical Presentation

Experimental amebiasis can be induced with 2000–4000 cysts. The incubation period has been estimated to be between 1 and 3 weeks.[209, 210] Most often, amebic infection of the gastrointestinal tract is asymptomatic, especially in temperate parts of the world, and seems to

be correlated with the isoenzyme pattern (zymodeme) of the strain.[211] In fact, it has been estimated that approximately 10% of the world's population is infected with *E. histolytica*,[212] but only 10% of these patients are symptomatic in the course of a year.

The most common manifestation of amebiasis is bloody diarrhea. Onset is usually gradual during a period of several weeks. Diarrhea without blood can occur but is rare, and occult blood in the stool is usually present even when the diarrhea is not bloody. In fact, rectal bleeding can occur without prominent diarrhea, especially in children. Abdominal pain is common. Weight loss occurs in approximately half of the patients with amebic dysentery, but fever is reported in only one third.

Amebic dysentery rarely presents as fulminant colitis, but when it does, it can be rapidly fatal. The most common setting of fulminant colitis is in severely malnourished immunosuppressed patients, such as patients taking corticosteroids, pregnant women, or infants.[213] Colonic perforation, which may be multiple, occurs in most of these cases. Toxic megacolon can also occur secondary to amebic colitis and may be precipitated by steroids.

Amebic infection of the colon can also cause a chronic nonbloody diarrheal syndrome, lasting several years, with symptoms suggesting either inflammatory bowel disease or giardiasis.[214] A self-limited syndrome resembling irritable bowel syndrome can follow amebic dysentery. Ulcerative postdysenteric colitis, which consists of persistent bloody diarrhea with mucous discharge, does not respond to amebicidal therapy. This disorder, which can also present as a granulomatous colitis with fistula formation, is rare and very difficult to treat.

Diagnosis

The observation of either *E. histolytica* trophozoites or cysts in freshly passed stool establishes a diagnosis of intestinal amebiasis. The efficiency of detection of *E. histolytica* varies considerably from laboratory to laboratory.[215] Therefore, physicians should continue to suspect amebiasis if the patient is epidemiologically at risk and the symptoms are appropriate, because a misdiagnosis of inflammatory bowel disease could be disastrous if steroids were given to a patient with amebic dysentery.

Factors that decrease the yield of stool examination for *E. histolytica* include the administration of barium, bismuth, tetracycline, erythromycin, antacids, laxatives, or soap or hypertonic enemas, and delay in mounting or fixing the specimen. Examination of multiple specimens increases the yield of positive findings in stool studies, because only about one third of infected patients are identified by examination of a single specimen. Axenic culture for *E. histolytica* has not yet found its way into clinical practice, even though it has a theoretically higher yield of positive findings than does direct examination of the stool.

Instrumentation can help diagnose amebic dysentery and differentiate it from other infectious colitides and ulcerative colitis. Punctate hemorrhages and variably sized ulcers, ranging from several millimeters to 1 to 2 cm in diameter, can be seen in the rectosigmoid. In fulminant colitis, larger and confluent ulcerations are seen. Amebic ulcers are covered with a yellow exudate at their centers and are usually surrounded by hyperemic borders. Results of sigmoidoscopic examination can be normal early in the illness. Occasionally, the only ulcerations are in the cecum and ascending colon.[213]

Microscopic examination of samples obtained during sigmoidoscopy augments the gross observation of the colonic mucosa because classic ulcerations may not be seen. If *E. histolytica* infection is considered possible, the colonoscopist should aspirate exudate, preferably by a plastic tube, and the aspirated material should be examined as soon as possible for trophozoites. Biopsies of inflamed areas may show the characteristic flasklike ulcer on histologic examination, with ragged edges hanging over an area of cytolysis. Additional histologic findings include capillary thromboses, hemorrhages, and necrosis. Parasites, if present, are located at the base of the ulcer. Inflammatory changes are usually not present, probably because of the leukocytolytic effect of *E. histolytica*. Secondary bacterial infection can occur and may obscure the pathologic findings.

Serology can be quite helpful in excluding *E. histolytica* as the cause of the bloody diarrhea. Antibodies directed against *E. histolytica* appear approximately 1 week after infection is manifest, and, given the gradual onset of invasive amebiasis, are usually detectable at the time medical attention is sought. Generally, the more invasive the amebiasis, the higher the likelihood that antibodies are present.[216] Samples from patients without symptoms or with minimally invasive amebiasis are usually nonreactive in standard serologic studies. Antibodies detected in the indirect hemagglutination assay may remain positive for many years after invasive amebiasis, so a positive result from serologic studies should be interpreted cautiously if a patient has ever been at risk for amebiasis. We recommend serologic studies to rule out amebiasis before performing a colectomy on patients with presumed ulcerative colitis and before starting steroids if a patient could plausibly be suffering from amebic dysentery, even if the results of stool tests for ova and parasites are negative.

Perforation of the colon is not rare in acute amebiasis and may occur at multiple sites. The colonic tissue may be fragile. Therefore, barium studies, which are not generally helpful, should be undertaken only after consideration of amebiasis as a possible cause for enteric symptoms, and sigmoidoscopy or colonoscopy should be performed carefully to reduce the risk of perforation.

Therapy

Multiple approaches exist to treat amebiasis, and therapy consists of agents active against *E. histolytica* in its three venues: the intestinal lumen (diloxanide furoate, paromomycin, diiodohydroxyquin), the bowel wall (tetracycline, erythromycin), and the liver (chloroquine). Metronidazole, tinidazole (not available in the United States), emetine, and 2-dehydroemetine are active against *E. histolytica* at all sites. The location of the infection, that is, which, if any, extraintestinal sites are involved, and the side effects of the drugs must both be considered. The efficacies of most regimens are between 80 and 95%. Ravdin's proposed regimens for treating amebiasis are given in Table 5–2.[213] These recommendations differ slightly from another widely used protocol published in the *Medical Letter*.[217]

Debate surrounds the concept of treatment for asymptomatic cyst passers. Most of the strains involved have nonpathogenic zymodemes, which are of little threat to the carrier or contacts, and many patients, such as male homosexuals or patients residing in an area in which *E. histolytica* is endemic, are likely to become reinfected. Although the stability of zymodeme expression raises concern,[218] it is a controversial topic.[219] Also, many patients with apparently asymptomatic infection have antibodies to *E. histolytica*, suggesting that some degree of invasion has occurred to stimulate the development of an immune response.[220] Furthermore, colitis and hepatic abscess can present after many years of asymptomatic carriage.[220] Therefore, we concur with Ravdin and coworkers,[213] Krogstad,[221] and Martinez-Palomo[209] that asymptomatic *E. histolytica* infection should be treated.

Several principles of therapy warrant elabora-

TABLE 5–2. THERAPEUTIC REGIMENS FOR THE TREATMENT OF *ENTAMOEBA HISTOLYTICA* AMEBIASIS

TYPE	EFFICACY (%)
Cyst Passers	
Diloxanide furoate, 500 mg tid for 10 d	87–96
Paromomycin, 30 mg/kg/d in 3 divided doses for 5–10 d	85–90
Tetracycline, 250 mg qid for 10 d, then diiodohydroxyquin, 650 mg tid for 20 d	95
Metronidazole, 750 mg tid for 10 d	90
Invasive Rectocolitis	
Metronidazole, 750 mg tid for 5–10 d	>90
Or 2.4 g qd for 2–3 d	>90
Or 50 mg/kg × 1 dose	86
Plus diloxanide furoate or paromomycin	
Tetracycline, 250 mg qid for 15 d, plus chloroquine (base), 600 mg, 300 mg, then 150 mg tid for 14 d	94
Dehydroemetine, 1–1.5 mg/kg/d for 5 d plus diloxanide furoate or paromomycin	90
Liver Abscess	
Metronidazole, 750 mg tid for 5–10 d or 2.4 mg qd for 1–2 d plus diloxanide furoate or paromomycin	95
Dehydroemetine, 1–1.5 mg/kg/d for 5 d plus diloxanide furoate or paromomycin	90
Chloroquine (base), 600 mg qd for 2 d, 300 mg base qd for 2–3 wk (can be added to other regimens)	60

NOTE: All dosages are for oral administration except that for dehydroemetine, which is administered intramuscularly; metronidazole can be used intravenously.

SOURCE: Ravdin JI, Petri WA. Entamoeba histolytica (amebiasis). In: Mandell GL, Douglas RG, Bennett JE, eds. Principles and Practice of Infectious Diseases. New York: Churchill-Livingstone; 1990:2036–2049.

tion. First, encysted forms of the parasite are eradicated by luminal agents such as diloxanide furoate, paromomycin, and diiodohydroxyquin. Metronidazole should be followed or accompanied by one of these three drugs. The recommended dose of metronidazole (750 mg po 3 times a day for 10 days) frequently causes gastrointestinal symptoms that may limit patient compliance. Abbreviated therapy with metronidazole[222] and with tinidazole[223] is reportedly effective. Metronidazole can be administered intravenously, if necessary. Diloxanide furoate is available only through the Centers for Disease Control. Tinidazole is not available and diiodohydroxyquin is difficult to obtain in the United States. Chloroquine is added to the antiamebic regimen in severely ill patients, but no evidence of synergy exists with this agent. It does, however, provide some extra coverage in rare situations of metronidazole failure. Cure should be ascertained by follow-up stool examination for parasites, because no regimen is 100% effective.

Surgery in acute intestinal amebiasis has a small diagnostic role, and attempts to resect perforated or severely inflamed bowel often fail, because the fragile infected colon is not amenable to suturing. Toxic megacolon, however, is not treatable pharmacologically, and colectomy must be performed.

Extraintestinal Complications

The most common extraintestinal complications of amebiasis are liver abscess, which may be complicated by rupture into the peritoneum, and intrathoracic extension with empyema, hepatobronchial fistula, or pericarditis. Lung and brain abscesses can occur but are much less common than are hepatic abscesses. Although amebic abscesses can present concomitantly with diarrhea, they are more commonly manifest without a history of bloody diarrhea. Metastatic amebic infection should be considered in the context of bloody diarrhea only if pressure effects caused by a potential abscess exist. Chemotherapy for amebic dysentery, which would include an agent active against parasites in the bowel wall, is usually adequate for extraintestinal infection. Hence, we do not recommend imaging of the liver or other organs in patients with intestinal amebiasis to detect extraintestinal abscesses without symptoms.

The rare complication of genitourinary amebiasis results from spread of infection from fecal sources. It is manifested as rectovaginal fistulae, granulomatous fissures, or ulcers.[213] Biopsy is diagnostic, and excision is not necessary because pharmacologic therapy is efficacious.

Infection Control Measures

Amebiasis can be prevented by avoiding food and water sources that are potentially contaminated with fecal matter. If this is not possible, boiling water is recommended, because halogenation is not completely amebicidal. Fresh vegetables are best disinfected with soap and by soaking in acetic acid or vinegar. This is often not practical for the traveler.

Anal-oral sexual practices should be discouraged to decrease transmission in susceptible populations. Hygienic practices in institutionalized populations should be encouraged. Eradication of the carrier state, both asymptomatic and postsymptomatic, is important.

MISCELLANEOUS AND RARE CAUSES OF BLOODY DIARRHEA (*BALANTIDIUM COLI*, *SCHISTOSOMA* SPECIES, *CLOSTRIDIUM PERFRINGENS* TYPE C, *AEROMONAS* SPECIES, *VIBRIO PARAHAEMOLYTICUS*)

Several unusual causes of bloody diarrhea should be kept in mind if classic diagnostic bacteriology and parasitology fail to identify a causative agent in specific cases or if peculiar epidemiologic or clinical risk factors are present. Usually, special investigations must be requested or performed by the physician to detect these pathogens in regions where there is a low frequency of these infections.

Balantidium coli

Balantidium coli, a parasitic protozoan, causes balantidiasis, which resembles amebiasis. Patients may be asymptomatic or have the same spectrum of illness as in *E. histolytica* infection, ranging from mild diarrhea to frank dysentery. Swine are the natural reservoir for *B. coli*, but the source of human infection is unknown. Foodborne and person-to-person transmission can occur.[224]

Diagnosis of *B. coli* infection is usually made by examination of formed stools for cysts or diarrheal stools for trophozoites. On biopsy, the parasite is observed in the mucosa and submucosa of the colon. Groups of parasites form "nests," with progression to abscess and ulcer formation. Metastatic infection in the liver occurs but is extremely rare.[224]

B. coli infection must be considered in patients with symptoms resembling dysentery caused by *E. histolytica*, because treatment of the two infections is somewhat different. Ten days of tetracycline in patients 9 years of age or older is the drug course of choice. A 20-day course of iodoquinol or a 5-day course of metronidazole is an alternative therapy.[217]

Schistosomiasis

Schistosomes are trematodes that belong to three medically significant species: *Schistosoma haematobium*, which infects the veins of the urinary bladder, and *S. mansoni* and *S. japonicum*, which infect the intestinal veins. Eggs produced by copulating worms invade locally, working their way through the intestinal wall, and are expelled in the feces. Embolic eggs lodge in distal organs, especially the liver in the case of *S. mansoni* and *S. japonicum*. The host's reaction to these eggs produces the pathologic conditions characteristic of schistosomiasis, including cirrhosis and portal hypertension.

Intestinal inflammatory reaction to transmurally migrating eggs can produce a colitis, with occasional frank dysentery. Diagnosis of *S. japonicum* or *S. mansoni* infection is usually by identification of schistosomal eggs in the stool or by rectal biopsy. *S. japonicum* is more likely to produce symptomatic intestinal disease than is *S. mansoni*, because it produces 10 times as many eggs as does the former species. Usually, dysenteric symptoms are manifested in the first 2 months of infection, the acute stage. Chronic inflammation of the colon, however, can result in polyps, papillomas, and fibrosis. Blood and pus secondary to this inflammation or sloughing of a polypoid mass can occasionally mimic dysentery in the chronic stage of schistosomiasis.[225]

Schistosomiasis is contracted by transdermal penetration by cercariae, the free-living form of *Schistosoma* species excreted by snails in fresh water in affected parts of the world (Asia for *S. japonicum;* Africa, South America, and certain regions of the Caribbean and the Middle East for *S. mansoni;* and Africa for *S. haematobium*). Patients who have resided in these regions should be considered at risk for schistosomiasis, if less exotic causes of bloody diarrhea are excluded. Empirical treatment should be considered prior to diagnosis if a patient might have acute schistosomiasis, because the risk of developing granulomas and inflammatory reaction to embolic eggs in the central nervous system[226] is severe compared with the low risk of therapy. Praziquantel is the drug of choice for schistosomiasis. It is safe, inexpensive, and efficacious.

Aeromonas Species

Aeromonas species are of controversial pathogenicity.[227] The organisms of this genus are aquatic gram-negative bacilli and belong to one of three species (*A. hydrophila*, *A. caviae*, and *A.*

sobria). They are most frequently associated with watery diarrhea[227, 228] but have been found in the stools of patients with colitis from whom other enteric pathogens were not isolated.[229] No correlation exists between the virulence of *A. hydrophila* and the clinical syndromes in humans infected with this species.[230] The antibiotic most frequently used to treat infections with aeromonads, if no other pathogens can be found to explain the enteric illness, is TMP/SMX.

Clostridium perfringens Type C

Clostridium perfringens type C causes a severe gastrointestinal infection characterized by obstructive intestinal symptoms and bloody diarrhea.[231] Infections caused by this agent have been given various names, including pigbel in children in Papua New Guinea,[232] darmbrand in post–World War II Germany,[233] and enteritis necroticans.[234] This disorder usually follows a meal containing an excess of protein in chronically undernourished children, and *C. perfringens* type C is frequently isolated from affected loops of small bowel. This organism produces clostridial β toxin, and survivors have antibodies to this toxin.

Most symptoms begin between several hours and several days after ingestion of the precipitating food.[232] In Papua New Guinea, pigbel is frequently manifested as abdominal distention and diarrhea, which progresses to signs and symptoms of abdominal sepsis and bowel necrosis. In a recent series from a refugee camp in Thailand, bloody diarrhea was prominent.[231] Antibiotics and small bowel resection are the only therapy in established cases,[235] but mortality remains high.[231] Immunoprophylaxis in endemic areas is achieved with intramuscular vaccination with *Clostridium* β toxoid.[236]

Diagnosis on clinical grounds in endemic areas is not difficult, given a fairly typical presentation in most cases and familiarity with this entity by health care workers. Enteritis necroticans can occur sporadically, however, in industrialized countries,[237] where this infection is unusual. Patients with enteritis necroticans in this setting have usually had chronic illnesses or alcoholism. Diagnosis is usually made at laparotomy by pathologic examination of the resected specimen. *C. perfringens* type C is difficult to detect in feces, because it is phenotypically identical to ambient nonpathogenic *C. perfringens*, and detection of β toxin requires mouse lethality tests and specific protection with antisera to β toxin.

Vibrio parahaemolyticus

Vibrio parahaemolyticus, a noncholera *Vibrio*, is acquired from eating insufficiently cooked fish or seafood. It may cause a choleralike illness, with profuse watery diarrhea, as well as a dysenteric illness, with pus and blood in the diarrhea. Ulcerations may be seen on proctosigmoidoscopy, and patients may be febrile and in a toxic condition. If suspected, *V. parahaemolyticus* as well as other *Vibrio* species can be detected by inoculation of the stool on thiosulfate citrate bile salts sucrose (TCBS) agar, but this medium is not used routinely in most microbiology laboratories unless the physician requests that *Vibrio* be sought.[238, 239]

REFERENCES

1. I Samuel 5.
2. Davison WC. A bacteriological and clinical consideration of bacillary dysentery in adults and children. Medicine. 1992;1:389–510.
3. Shiga K. The trend of prevention, therapy and epidemiology of dysentery since the discovery of its causative organism. N Engl J Med. 1936;215:1205–1211.
4. Hyams KC, Bourgeois AL, Merrell BR, et al. Diarrheal disease during Operation Desert Shield. N Engl J Med. 1991;325:1423–1428.
5. Osler W. On the amoeba coli in dysentery and in dysenteric liver abscess. Johns Hopkins Hosp Bull. 1890;1:53–55.
6. Flexner S. On the etiology of tropical dysentery. Phila Med J. 1900;vi:414–424.
7. Isberg RR, Leong JM. Multiple β₁ chain integrins are receptors for invasin, a protein that promotes bacterial penetration into mammalian cells. Cell. 1990;60:861–871.
8. Moyer MP, Dixon PS, Rothman SW, Brown JE. Cytotoxicity of Shiga toxin for primary cultures of human colonic and ileal epithelial cells. Infect Immun. 1987;55:1533–1535.
9. Mackenzie A, Barnes G, Shann F. Clinical signs of dehydration in children. Lancet. 1989;2:605–607.
10. Guerrant RL, Sheilds DS, Thorson SM, et al. Evaluation and diagnosis of acute infectious diarrhea. Am J Med. 1985;78(suppl 6B):91–98.
11. DeWitt TG, Humphrey KF, McCarthy P. Clinical predictors of acute bacterial diarrhea in young children. Pediatrics. 1985;76:551–556.
12. Tarr PI, Clausen CR, Christie DL. Bacterial and protozoal gastroenteritis. N Engl J Med. 1992;326:489. Letter.
13. Thorson SM, Lohr JA, Dudley S, Guerrant RL. Value of methylene blue examination, dark-field microscopy, and carbol-fuchsin Gram stain in the detection of *Campylobacter enteritis*. J Pediatr. 1985;106:941–943.
14. Peterson LR, Holter JJ, Shanholtzer CJ, et al. Detection of *Clostridium difficile* toxins A (enterotoxin) and B (cytotoxin) in clinical specimens. Am J Clin Pathol. 1986;86:208–211.
15. Puylaert JBCM, Vermeijden RJ, van der Werf SDJ, et al. Incidence and sonographic diagnosis of bacterial ileocaecitis masquerading as appendicitis. Lancet. 1989; 2:84–86.

16. Tarr PI, Weinberger E, Hatch EI Jr, Christie DL. Bacterial ileocecitis caused by *Escherichia coli* 0157:H7. J Pediatr Gastroenterol Nutr. 1992;14:261–263.

17. Surawicz CM, Belic L. Rectal biopsy helps to distinguish acute self-limited colitis from idiopathic inflammatory bowel disease. Gastroenterology. 1984;86:104–113.

18. Siegel DL, Edelstein PH, Nachamkin I. Inappropriate testing for diarrheal diseases in the hospital. JAMA. 1990;263:979–982.

19. Rich EJ, McDonald RA, Christie DL. *Yersinia pseudotuberculosis:* Report of a case with endoscopic findings. J Pediatr Gastroenterol Nutr. 1990;10:413–415.

20. Rubin RH, Weinstein L. Clinical features of Salmonellosis. In: Salmonellosis: Microbiologic, Pathologic, and Clinical Features. New York: Stratton Intercontinental Medical Book Corporation; 1977:43–94.

21. Aserkoff B, Bennett JV. Effect of antibiotic therapy in acute salmonellosis on the fecal excretion of salmonellae. N Engl J Med. 1969;281:636–640.

22. Pai CH, Gillis F, Tuomanen E, Marks MI. Placebo-controlled double-blind evaluation of trimethoprim-sulfamethoxazole treatment of *Yersinia enterocolitica* gastroenteritis. J Pediatr. 1984;104:308–311.

23. Reves RR, Johnson PC, Ericsson CD, DuPont HL. A cost-effectiveness comparison of the use of antimicrobial agents for treatment or prophylaxis of traveler's diarrhea. Arch Intern Med. 1988;148:2421–2427.

24. Blaser MJ. *Campylobacter*. In: Farthing MJG, Keusch GT, eds. Enteric Infection: Mechanisms, Manifestations, and Management. New York: Raven Press; 1989:299–316.

25. Bean NH, Griffin PM, Goulding JS, Ivey CB. Foodborne disease outbreaks: 5-year summary, 1983–1987. MMWR CDC Surveill Summ. 1991;39:ss-1:15–23.

26. King EO. Human infections with *Vibrio fetus* and a closely related *Vibrio.* J Infect Dis. 1957;101:119–136.

27. Dekeyser P, Gossuin-Detrain M, Butzler JP, Sternon J. Acute enteritis due to related *Vibrio:* First positive stool cultures. J Infect Dis. 1972;125:390–392.

28. Skirrow MB. *Campylobacter* enteritis: A "new" disease. Br Med J. 1977;2:9–11.

29. Blaser MJ, Berkowitz ID, LaForce FM, et al. *Campylobacter* enteritis: Clinical and epidemiologic features. Ann Intern Med. 1979;91:179–185.

30. Rajan DP, Mathan VI. Prevalence of *Campylobacter fetus* subsp. *jejuni* in healthy populations in southern India. J Clin Microbiol. 1982;15:749–751.

31. Glass RI, Stoll BJ, Huq MI, et al. Epidemiologic and clinical features of endemic *Campylobacter jejuni* infection in Bangladesh. J Infect Dis. 1983;148:292–296.

32. Riley LW, Finch MJ. Results of the first year of national surveillance of *Campylobacter* infections in the United States. J Infect Dis. 1985;151:956–959.

33. Cowden J. *Campylobacter:* Epidemiological paradoxes. Br Med J. 1992;305:132–133.

34. Blaser MJ, Hardesty HL, Powers B, Wang WLL. Survival of *Campylobacter fetus* subsp. *jejuni* in biological milieus. J Clin Microbiol. 1980;11:309–313.

35. Lambert ME, Schofield PF, Ironside AG, Mandal BK. *Campylobacter* colitis. Br Med J. 1979;1:857–859.

36. Guandalini S, Cucchiara S, de Ritis G, et al. *Campylobacter* colitis in infants. J Pediatr 1983;102:72–74.

37. Van Spreeuwel JP, Duursma GC, Meijer CJLM, et al. *Campylobacter* colitis: Histological immunohistochemical and ultrastructural findings. Gut. 1985;26:945–951.

38. Yeen WP, Puthucheary SD, Pang T. Demonstration of a cytotoxin from *Campylobacter jejuni.* J Clin Pathol. 1983;36:1237–1240.

39. Johnson WM, Lior H. Cytotoxic and cytotonic factors produced by *Campylobacter jejuni, Campylobacter coli,* and *Campylobacter laridis.* J Clin Microbiol. 1986;24:275–281.

40. Klipstein FA, Engert RF. Properties of crude *Campylobacter jejuni* heat-labile enterotoxin. Infect Immun. 1984;45:314–319.

41. Duffy MC, Benson JB, Rubin SJ. Mucosal invasion in *Campylobacter* enteritis. Am J Clin Pathol. 1980;73:706–708.

42. Black RE, Levine MM, Clements ML, et al. Experimental *Campylobacter jejuni* infection in humans. J Infect Dis. 1988;157:472–479.

43. Blaser MJ. *Campylobacter* species. In: Mandell GL, Douglas RG, Bennett JE, eds. Principles and Practice of Infectious Diseases. New York: Churchill Livingstone; 1990:1649–1658.

44. Karmali MA, Fleming PC. *Campylobacter* enteritis in children. J Pediatr. 1979;94:527–533.

45. Anders BJ, Lauer BA, Paisley JW. *Campylobacter* gastroenteritis in neonates. Am J Dis Child. 1981;135:900–902.

46. Pitkänen T, Pettersson T, Pönkä A. Effect of erythromycin on the fecal excretion of *Campylobacter fetus* subspecies *jejuni.* J Infect Dis. 1982;145:128.

47. Anders BJ, Lauer BA, Paisley JW, Reller LB. Double-blind placebo controlled trial of erythromycin for treatment of *Campylobacter* enteritis. Lancet. 1982;1:131–132.

48. Salazar-Lindo E, Sack RB, Chea-Woo E. Early treatment with erythromycin of *Campylobacter jejuni*–associated dysentery in children. J Pediatr. 1986;109:355–360.

49. Ryan CA, Blaser MJ, Taylor DN, Echeverria P. Characterization of erythromycin resistance in isolates of *Campylobacter jejuni* and *Campylobacter coli* from domestic- and foreign-acquired human infections, AIDS patients, and poultry. Antimicrob Agents Chemother. In press.

50. Goodman LJ, Trenholme GM, Kaplan RL, et al. Empiric antimicrobial therapy of domestically acquired acute diarrhea in urban adults. Arch Intern Med. 1990;150:541–546.

51. Konowalchuk J, Speirs JI, Stavric S. Vero response to a cytotoxin of *Escherichia coli.* Infect Immun. 1977;18:775–779.

52. Riley LW, Remis RS, Helgerson SD, et al. Hemorrhagic colitis associated with a rare *Escherichia coli* serotype. N Engl J Med. 1983;308:681–685.

53. O'Brien AD, Lively TA, Chen ME, et al. *Escherichia coli* O157:H7 strains associated with haemorrhagic colitis in the United States produce a *Shigella dysenteriae* 1 (Shiga) like cytotoxin. Lancet. 1983;1:702. Letter.

54. Karmali MA, Steele BT, Petric M, Lim C. Sporadic cases of haemolytic-uraemic syndrome associated with fecal cytotoxin and cytotoxin-producing *Escherichia coli* in stools. Lancet. 1983;1:619–620.

55. Karmali MA. Infection by verocytotoxin-producing *Escherichia coli.* Clin Microbiol Rev. 1989;2:15–38.

56. Griffin PM, Tauxe RV. The epidemiology of infections caused by *Escherichia coli* O157:H7, other enterohemorrhagic *E. coli,* and the associated hemolytic uremic syndrome. Epidemiol Rev. 1991;13:60–98.

57. Samadpour M, Liston J, Ongerth JE, Tarr PI. Evaluation of DNA probes for detection of Shiga-like-toxin-producing *Escherichia coli* in food and calf fecal samples. Appl Environ Microbiol. 1990;56:1212–1215.

58. Suthienkul O, Brown JE, Seriwatana J, et al. Shiga-like-toxin-producing *Escherichia coli* in retail meats and cattle in Thailand. Appl Environ Microbiol. 1990;56:1135–1139.

59. Read SC, Gyles CL, Clarke RC, et al. Prevalence of verocytotoxigenic *Escherichia coli* in ground beef, pork, and chicken in southwestern Ontario. Epidemiol Infect. 1990;105:11–20.

60. Sekla L. Verotoxin-producing *Escherichia coli* in ground beef in Manitoba. Can Med Assoc J. 1990;143:519–521.

61. Tarr PI, Neill MA, Clausen CR, et al. *Escherichia coli* O157:H7 and the hemolytic uremic syndrome: Importance of early cultures in establishing the etiology. J Infect Dis. 1990;162:553–556.

62. Chart H, Smith HR, Scotland SM, et al. Serological identification of *Escherichia coli* O157:H7 infection in haemolytic uraemic syndrome. Lancet. 1991;337:138–140.

63. Bitzan M, Moebius E, Ludwig K. High incidence of serum antibodies to *Escherichia coli* O157 lipopolysaccharide in children with hemolytic-uremic syndrome. J Pediatr. 1991;119:380–385.

64. Wells JG, Davis BR, Wachsmuth IK, et al. Laboratory investigation of hemorrhagic colitis outbreaks associated with a rare *Escherichia coli* serotype. J Clin Microbiol. 1983;18:512–520.

65. Gunzer F, Bohm H, Russmann H, et al. Molecular detection of sorbitol-fermenting *Escherichia coli* O157 in patients with hemolytic uremic syndrome. J Clin Microbiol. 1992;30:1807–1810.

66. Lopez EL, Diaz M, Grinstein S, Devoto S. Hemolytic uremic syndrome and diarrhea in Argentine children: The role of shiga-like toxins. J Infect Dis. 1989;160:469–475.

67. Chapman PA, Siddons CA, Zadik PM, Jewes L. An improved selective medium for the isolation of *Escherichia coli* O157. J Med Microbiol. 1991;35:107–110.

68. MacDonald KL, O'Leary MJ, Chen ML, et al. *Escherichia coli* O157:H7, an emerging gastrointestinal pathogen: Results of a one-year, prospective, population-based study. JAMA. 1988;259:3567–3570.

69. Ostroff SM, Kobayashi JM, Lewis JH. Infections with *Escherichia coli* O157:H7 in Washington state: The first year of statewide disease surveillance. JAMA. 1989;262:355–359.

70. Belongia E, MacDonald KL, Parham GL, White KE. An outbreak of *Escherichia coli* O157:H7 colitis associated with consumption of precooked meat patties. J Infect Dis. 1991;164:338–343.

71. Ryan CA, Tauxe RV, Hosek GW, et al. *Escherichia coli* O157:H7 diarrhea in a nursing home: Clinical, epidemiological, and pathological findings. J Infect Dis. 1986;154:631–638.

72. Carter AO, Borczyk AA, Carlson JAK, et al. A severe outbreak of *Escherichia coli* O157:H7–associated hemorrhagic colitis in a nursing home. N Engl J Med. 1987;317:1496–1500.

73. Duncan L, Mai V, Carter A, et al. Outbreak of gastrointestinal disease: Ontario. Can Dis Wkly Rep. 1987;13:5–8.

74. Martin ML, Shipman LD, Wells JG, et al. Isolation of *Escherichia coli* O157:H7 from dairy cattle associated with two cases of haemolytic uraemic syndrome. Lancet. 1986;2:1043. Letter.

75. Wells JG, Shipman LD, Greene KD, et al. Isolation of *Escherichia coli* serotype O157:H7 and other Shiga-like toxin-producing *E. coli* O157:H7 from dairy cattle. J Clin Microbiol. 1990;29:985–989.

76. Borczyk AA, Karmali MA, Lior H, et al. Bovine reservoir for verotoxin-producing *Escherichia coli* O157:H7. Lancet. 1987;1:98. Letter.

77. Chapman PA, Wright DJ, Norman P. Verotoxin-producing *Escherichia coli* infections in Sheffield: Cattle as a possible source. Epidemiol Infect. 1989;102:439–445.

78. Montenegro MA, Bulte M, Trumpt T, et al. Detection and characterization of fecal verotoxin-producing *Escherichia coli* from healthy cattle. J Clin Microbiol. 1990;28:1417–1421.

79. Orskov F, Orskov I, Villar JA. Cattle as reservoir of verotoxin-producing *Escherichia coli* O157:H7. Lancet. 1987;2:276. Letter.

80. Doyle MP, Schoeni JL. Isolation of *Escherichia coli* O157:H7 from retail fresh meats and poultry. Appl Environ Microbiol. 1987;53:2394–2396.

81. Karmali MA, Arbus GS, Petric M, et al. Hospital-acquired *Escherichia coli* O157:H7 associated haemolytic uraemic syndrome in a nurse. Lancet. 1988;1:526. Letter.

82. Herwaldt BL, Craun GF, Stokes SL, Juranek DD. Waterborne-disease outbreaks, 1989–1990: MMWR CDC Surveill Summ. 1991;40:ss–3:1–13.

83. Calderwood SB, Auclair F, Donohue-Rolfe A, et al. Nucleotide sequence of the Shiga-like toxin genes of *Escherichia coli*. Proc Natl Acad Sci U S A. 1987;84:4364–4368.

84. Jackson MP, Neill RJ, O'Brien AD, et al. Nucleotide sequence analysis and comparison of the structural genes for Shiga-like toxin I and Shiga-like toxin II encoded by bacteriophages from *Escherichia coli* 933. FEMS Microbiol Lett. 1987;44:109–114.

85. Lingwood CA, Law H, Richardson S, et al. Glycolipid binding of purified and recombinant *Escherichia coli* produced verotoxin in vitro. J Biol Chem. 1987;262:8834–8839.

86. Waddell T, Head S, Petric M, et al. Globotriosyl ceramide is specifically recognized by the *Escherichia coli* verocytotoxin 2. Biochem Biophys Res Commun. 1988;152:674–679.

87. Endo Y, Tsurugi K, Yutsudo T, et al. Site of action of a vero toxin (VT2) from *Escherichia coli* O157:H7 and of Shiga toxin on eucaryotic ribosomes. Eur J Biochem 1988;171:45–50.

88. Tesh VL, Samuel JE, Perera LP, et al. Evaluation of the role of Shiga and Shiga-like toxins in mediating direct damage to human vascular endothelial cells. J Infect Dis. 1991;164:344–352.

89. Louise CB, Obrig TG. Shiga toxin-associated hemolytic uremic syndrome: Combined cytotoxic effects of Shiga-toxins and lipopolysaccharide (endotoxin) on human vascular endothelial cells in vitro. Infect Immun. 1992;60:1536–1543.

90. Wadolkowski EA, Sung LM, Burris JA, et al. Acute renal tubular necrosis and death of mice orally infected with *Escherichia coli* strains that produce Shiga-like toxin type II. Infect Immun. 1990;58:3959–3965.

91. Scotland SM, Willshaw GA, Smith HR, et al. Properties of strains of *Escherichia coli* belonging to serogroup 0157 with special reference to production of vero cytotoxins VT1 and VT2. Epidemiol Infect. 1987;99:613–624.

92. Tarr PI, Neill MA, Clausen CR, Newland JW. Genotypic variation in pathogenic *Escherichia coli* O157:H7 isolated from patients in Washington, 1984–1987. J Infect Dis. 1989;159:344–347.

93. Ostroff SM, Neill MA, Lewis JH, et al. Toxin genotypes and plasmid profiles as determinants of systemic sequelae in *Escherichia coli* O157:H7 infections. J Infect Dis. 1989;160:994–998.

94. Koster F, Levin J, Walker L, et al. Hemolytic-uremic syndrome after shigellosis. N Engl J Med. 1978;298:927–933.

95. Knutton S, Baldwin T, Williams PH, et al. Actin accumulation at sites of bacterial adhesion to tissue culture cells: Basis of a new diagnostic test for enteropathogenic and enterohemorrhagic *Escherichia coli*. Infect Immun. 1989;57:1290–1298.

96. Yu J, Kaper JB. Cloning and characterization of the *eae* gene of enterohaemorrhagic *Escherichia coli* O157:H7. Mol Microbiol. 1992;6:411–417.

97. Beebakhee G, Louie M, De Azavedo J, Brunton J. Cloning and nucleotide sequence of the *eae* gene homologue from enterohemorrhagic *Escherichia coli* O157:H7. FEMS Microbiol Lett. 1992;91:63–68.

98. Griffin PM, Olmstead LC, Petras RE. *Escherichia coli* O157:H7–associated colitis. A clinical and histological study of 11 cases. Gastroenterology. 1990;99:142–149.

99. Griffin PM, Ostroff SM, Tauxe RV, et al. Illnesses associated with *Escherichia coli* O157:H7 infections: A broad clinical spectrum. Ann Intern Med. 1988;109:705–712.

100. Ratnam S, March SB, Sprague WD. Are humans a source of *Escherichia coli* O157:H7, the agent of hemorrhagic colitis? N Engl J Med 1986;315:1612–1613.

101. Pai CH, Ahmed N, Lior H, et al. Epidemiology of sporadic diarrhea due to verocytotoxin-producing *Escherichia coli:* A two-year prospective study. J Infect Dis. 1988;157:1054–1057.

102. Chapman PA. Evaluation of commercial latex slide test for identifying *Escherichia coli* O157:H7 associated with hemorrhagic colitis. J Clin Pathol. 1988;42:1109–1110.

103. Tison DL. Culture confirmation of *Escherichia coli* serotype O157:H7 by direct immunofluorescence. J Clin Microbiol. 1990;28:612–613.

104. Tarr PI, Neill MA, Christie DL, Anderson DE. *Escherichia coli* O157:H7 hemorrhagic colitis. N Engl J Med. 1988;318:1697.

105. Pavia AT, Nichols CR, Green DP, et al. Hemolytic-uremic syndrome during an outbreak of *Escherichia coli* O157:H7 infection in institutions for mentally retarded persons: Clinical and epidemiologic observations. J Pediatr. 1990;116:544–551.

106. Cimolai N, Carter JE, Morrison BJ, et al. Risk factors for the progression of *Escherichia coli* O157:H7 enteritis to hemolytic-uremic syndrome. J Pediatr. 1990;116:589–592.

107. Krishnan C, Fitzgerald VA, Dakin SJ, et al. Laboratory investigation of outbreak of hemorrhagic colitis caused by *Escherichia coli* O157:H7. J Clin Microbiol. 1987;25:1043–1047.

108. Gransden WR, Damm MAS, Anderson JD, et al. Haemorrhagic cystitis and balanitis associated with verotoxin-producing *Escherichia coli* O157:H7. Lancet. 1985;2:150. Letter.

109. Harris AA, Kaplan RL, Goodman LJ, et al. Results of a screening method used in a 12-month stool survey for *Escherichia coli* O157:H7. J Infect Dis. 1985;152:775–777.

110. Ewing WH, Gravatti JL. *Shigella* types encountered in the Mediterranean area. J Bacteriol. 1947;53:191–195.

111. Hobbs BC, Thomas MEM, Taylor J. School outbreak of gastro-enteritis associated with a pathogenic paracolon bacillus. Lancet. 1949;2:530–532.

112. Toledo MRF, Trabulsi LR. Correlation between biochemical and serological characteristic of *Escherichia coli* and results of the Sereny test. J Clin Microbiol. 1983;17:419–421.

113. Cheasty T, Rowe B. Antigenic relationships between the enteroinvasive *Escherichia coli* O antigens O28ac, O112ac, O124, O136, O143, O152, and O164, and *Shigella* antigens. J Clin Microbiol. 1983;17:681–684.

114. Gross RJ, Thomas LV, Cheasty T, et al. Enterotoxigenic and enteroinvasive *Escherichia coli* strains belonging to a new O group, 0167. J Clin Microbiol. 1983;17:521–523.

115. Marier R, Wells JG, Swanson RC, et al. An outbreak of enteropathogenic *Escherichia coli* foodborne disease traced to imported French cheese. Lancet. 1973;2:1376–1378.

116. Echeverria P, Sethabutr O, Serichantalergs O, et al. *Shigella* and enteroinvasive *Escherichia coli* in households of children with dysentery in Thailand. J Infect Dis. 1992;165:144–147.

117. Hale TL, Sansonetti PJ, Schad PA, et al. Characterization of virulence plasmids and plasmid-associated outer membrane proteins in *Shigella flexneri, Shigella sonnei,* and *Escherichia coli.* Infect Immun. 1983;40:340–350.

118. Sansonetti PJ, d'Hauteville H, Formal SB, Toucas M. Plasmid-mediated invasiveness of "Shigella-like" *Escherichia coli.* Ann Microbiol (Paris). 1982;133:351–355.

119. Wanger AR, Murray BE, Echeverria P, et al. Enteroinvasive *Escherichia coli* in travelers with diarrhea. J Infect Dis. 1988;158:640–642.

120. Sereny B. Experimental keratoconjunctivitis shigellosa. Acta Microbiol Hung. 1957;4:367–376.

121. Hook EW. Salmonella species (including typhoid fever). In: Mandell GL, Douglas RG, Bennett JE, eds. Principles and Practice of Infectious Diseases. New York: Churchill Livingstone; 1990:1700–1716.

122. Cruickshank JG, Humphrey TJ. The carrier food handler and nontyphoidal salmonellosis. Epidemiol Infect. 1987;98:223–230.

123. CDC, Outbreak of *Salmonella enteritidis* infection associated with consumption of raw shell eggs, 1991. MMWR. 1992;41:369–372.

124. Cohen ML, Tauxe RV. Drug-resistant *Salmonella* in the United States: An epidemiologic perspective. Science. 1986;234:964–969.

125. O'Connor BH, Bennett JR, Alexander JG, et al. Salmonellosis infection transmitted by fibreoptic endoscopes. Lancet. 1982;2:864–866.

126. Baine WB, Gangarosa EJ, Bennett JV, Barker WH Jr. Institutional salmonellosis. CDC News. 1973;128:357–360.

127. Hook EW. Salmonellosis: Certain factors influencing the interaction of *Salmonella* and the human host. Bull N Y Acad Med. 1961;37:499–512.

128. Hornick RB, Greisman SE, Woodward TE, et al. Typhoid fever: Pathogenesis and immunologic control, Part I. N Engl J Med. 1970;283:686–691.

129. Hornick RB, Greisman SE, Woodward TE, et al. Typhoid fever: Pathogenesis and immunologic control, Part II. N Engl J Med. 1970;283:739–746.

130. Miller CP, Bohnhoff M. Changes in the mouse's enteric microflora associated with enhanced susceptibility to *Salmonella* infection following streptomycin treatment. J Infect Dis. 1963;113:59–66.

131. Bohnhoff M, Miller CP, Martin WR. Resistance of the mouse's intestinal tract to experimental *Salmonella* infection. J Exp Med. 1964;120:817–828.

132. Hyams JS, Durbin WA, Grand RJ, Goldmann DA. *Salmonella* bacteremia in the first year of life. J Pediatr. 1980;96:57–59.

133. Candy DCA, Stephen J. Salmonella. In: Farthing MJG, Keusch GT, eds. Enteric Infection: Mechanisms, Manifestations, and Management. New York: Raven Press; 1989:289–298.

134. Mandal BK, Mani V. Colonic involvement in salmonellosis. Lancet. 1976;1:887–888.

135. Buchwald DS, Blaser MJ. A Review of human salmonellosis, Part II: Duration of excretion following infection with nontyphi *Salmonella.* Rev Infect Dis. 1984;6:345–356.

136. Nye FJ. Do antibiotics really prolong *Salmonella* excretion? J Antimicrob Chemother. 1981;7:215–216.

137. Hoffman SL, Punjabi NH, Kumala S, et al. Reduction of mortality in chloramphenicol-treated severe typhoid fever by high-dose dexamethasone. N Engl J Med. 1984;310:82–88.

138. Cooles P. Adjuvant steroids and relapse of typhoid fever. J Trop Med Hyg. 1986;89:229–231.

139. Archampong EQ. Operative treatment of typhoid perforation of the bowel. Br Med J. 1969;3:273–276.

140. Asperilla MO, Smego RA Jr, Scott LK. Quinolone antibiotics in the treatment of *Salmonella* infections. Rev Infect Dis. 1990;12:873–889.

141. Cherubin CE, Eng RHK. Quinolones for the treatment of infections due to *Salmonella.* Rev Infect Dis. 1991;13:343–344.

142. Neill MA, Opal SM, Heelan J, et al. Failure of ciprofloxacin to eradicate convalescent fecal excretion after acute salmonellosis: Experience during an outbreak in health care workers. Ann Intern Med. 1991;114:195–199.

142a. Wiström J, Jertborn M, Ekwall E, et al. Empiric treatment of acute diarrheal disease with norfloxacin. Ann Intern Med. 1992;117:202–208.

143. Baker NM, Mills AE, Rachman I, Thomas JEP. Haemolytic uremic syndrome in typhoid fever. Br Med J. 1974;2:84–87.

144. Keitel WA, Robbins JA. Prevention and treatment of typhoid fever. Semin Pediatr Infect Dis. 1992;3:49–53.

145. Acharya IL, Lowe CU, Thapa R, et al. Prevention of typhoid fever in Nepal with the Vi capsular polysaccharide of Salmonella typhi. N Engl J Med. 1987;317:1101–1104.

146. Nolan CM, White PC Jr. Treatment of typhoid carriers with amoxicillin. JAMA. 1978;239:2352–2354.

147. Freerksen E, Rosenfeld M, Freerksen R, Krüger-Thiemer M. Treatment of chronic salmonella carriers. Chemotherapy. 1977;23:192–210.

148. Lee LA, Shapiro CN, Hargrett-Bean N, Tauxe RV. Hyperendemic shigellosis in the United States: A review of surveillance data for 1967–1988. J Infect Dis. 1991;164:894–900.

149. DuPont HL, Levine MM, Hornick RB, Formal SB. Inoculum size in shigellosis and implications for expected mode of transmission. J Infect Dis. 1989;159:1126–1128.

150. Keusch GT, Grady GF, Mata LJ, McIver J. The pathogenesis of Shigella diarrhea. J Clin Invest. 1972;51:1212–1218.

151. Fuchs G, Mobassaleh M, Donohue-Rolfe A, et al. Pathogenesis of Shigella diarrhea: Rabbit intestinal cell microvillus membrane binding site for shigella toxin. Infect Immun. 1986;53:372–377.

152. Cantey JR, Moseley SL. HeLa cell adherence, actin aggregation, and invasion by nonenteropathogenic Escherichia coli possessing the eae gene. Infect Immun. 1991;59:3924–3929.

153. Neill RJ, Gemski P, Formal SB, Newland JW. Deletion of the Shiga toxin gene in a chlorate-resistant derivative of Shigella dysenteriae type 1 that retains virulence. J Infect Dis. 1988;158:737–741.

154. Keusch GT, Jacewicz M. The pathogenesis of shigella diarrhea: Part VI, Toxin and antitoxin in Shigella flexneri and Shigella sonnei infections in humans. J Infect Dis. 1977;135:552–556.

155. Prado D, Cleary TG, Pickering LK, et al. The relation between production of cytotoxin and clinical features in shigellosis. J Infect Dis. 1986;154:149–155.

156. Bartlett AV III, Prado D, Cleary TG, Pickering LK. Production of Shiga toxin and other cytotoxins by serogroups of Shigella. J Infect Dis. 1986;154:996–1002.

157. Speelman P, Kabir I, Islam M. Distribution and spread of colonic lesions in shigellosis: A colonoscopic study. J Infect Dis. 1984;150:899–903.

158. Bennish ML, Azad AK, Yousefzadeh D. Intestinal obstruction during shigellosis: Incidence, clinical features, risk factors, and outcome. Gastroenterology. 1991;101:626–634.

159. Duncan B, Fulginiti VA, Sieber OF, Ryan KJ. Shigella sepsis. Am J Dis Child. 1981;135:151–154.

160. Struelens MJ, Patte D, Kabir I, et al. Shigella septicemia: Prevalence, presentation, risk factors, and outcome. J Infect Dis. 1985;152:784–790.

161. Martin T, Habbick BF, Nyssen J. Shigellosis with bacteremia: A report of two cases and a review of the literature, Pediatr Infect Dis. 1983;2:21–26.

162. Morduchowicz G, Huminer D, Siegman-Igra Y, et al. Shigella bacteremia in adults. Arch Intern Med. 1987;147:2034–2037.

163. Haltalin KC, Nelson JD. Coliform septicemia complicating shigellosis in children. JAMA. 1965;192:441–443.

164. DuPont HL. Shigella species (bacillary dysentery). In: Mandell GL, Douglas RG, Bennett JE, eds. Principles and Practice of Infectious Diseases. New York: Churchill Livingstone; 1990:1716–1722.

165. Keusch GT, Bennish M. Shigella. In: Farthing MJG, Keusch GT, eds. Enteric Infection: Mechanisms, Manifestations, and Management. New York: Raven Press; 1989:265–282.

166. Pickering LK, DuPont HL, Olarte J. Single-dose tetracycline therapy for shigellosis in adults. JAMA. 1978;239:853–854.

167. Bennish ML, Wojtyniak BJ. Mortality due to shigellosis: Community and hospital data. Rev Infect Dis. 1991;13 (suppl 4):S245–S251.

168. Butler T, Islam MR, Bardhan PK. The leukemoid reaction in shigellosis. Am J Dis Child. 1984;138:162–165.

169. Sakamoto A, Kamo S. Clinical, statistical observations on Ekiri and bacillary dysentery: A study of 785 cases. Ann Paediat. 1956;186:1–18.

170. Cover TL, Aber RC. Yersinia enterocolitica. N Engl J Med. 1989;321:16–24.

171. Marks MI, Pai CH, Lafleur L, et al. Yersinia enterocolitica gastroenteritis: A prospective study of clinical, bacteriologic, and epidemiologic features. J Pediatr. 1980;96:26–31.

172. Tacket CO, Ballard J, Harris N, et al. An outbreak of Yersinia enterocolitica infections caused by contaminated tofu (soybean curd). Am J Epidemiol. 1985;121:705–711.

173. Snyder JD, Christenson E, Feldman RA. Human Yersinia enterocolitica infections in Wisconsin. Am J Med. 1982;72:768–774.

174. Portnoy DA, Moseley SL, Falkow S. Characterization of plasmids and plasmid-associated determinants of Yersinia enterocolitica pathogenesis. Infect Immun. 1981;31:775–782.

175. Devenish JA, Schiemann DA. HeLa cell infection by Yersinia enterocolitica: Evidence for lack of intracellular multiplication and development of a new procedure for quantitative expression of infectivity. Infect Immun. 1981;32:48–55.

176. Carter PB. Pathogenicity of Yersinia enterocolitica for mice. Infect Immun. 1975;11:164–170.

177. Pai CH, Mors V, Seemayer TA. Experimental Yersinia enterocolitica enteritis in rabbits. Infect Immun. 1980;28:238–244.

178. Skurnik M, Poikonen K. Experimental intestinal infection of rats by Yersinia enterocolitica 0:3. Scand J Infect Dis. 1986;18:355–364.

179. Aulisio CCG, Hill WE, Stanfield JT, Sellers RL Jr. Evaluation of virulence factor testing and characteristics of pathogenicity in Yersinia enterocolitica. Infect Immun. 1983;40:330–335.

180. Lian CJ, Pai CH. Inhibition of human neutrophil chemiluminescence by plasmid-mediated outer membrane proteins of Yersinia enterocolitica. Infect Immun. 1985;49:145–151.

181. Tertti R, Eerola E, Lehtonen OP, et al. Virulence-plasmid is associated with the inhibition of opsonization in Yersinia enterocolitica and Yersinia pseudotuberculosis. Clin Exp Immunol. 1987;68:266–274.

182. Pai CH, DeStephano L. Serum resistance associated with virulence in Yersinia enterocolitica. Infect Immun. 1982;35:605–611.

183. Perry RD, Brubaker RR. Vwa+ phenotype of Yersinia enterocolitica. Infect Immun. 1983;40:166–171.

184. Balligand G, Laroche Y, Cornelis G. Genetic analysis of

virulence plasmid from a serogroup 9 *Yersinia enterocolitica* strain: Role of outer membrane protein P1 in resistance to human serum and autoagglutination. Infect Immun. 1985;48:782–786.
185. Perry RD, Brubaker RR. Accumulation of iron by yersiniae. J Bacteriol. 1979;137:1290–1298.
186. Robins-Browne RM, Prpic JK. Effects of iron and desferrioxamine on infections with *Yersinia enterocolitica*. Infect Immun. 1985;47:774–779.
187. Bouza E, Dominguez A, Meseguer M, et al. *Yersinia enterocolitica* septicemia. Am J Clin Pathol. 1980;74:404–409.
188. Rabson AR, Hallett AF, Koornhof HJ. Generalized *Yersinia enterocolitica* infection. J Infect Dis. 1975;131:447–451.
189. Update: *Yersinia enterocolitica* bacteremia and endotoxin shock associated with red blood cell transfusions—United States, 1991. MMWR. 1991;40:176–178.
190. Van Noyen R, Vandepitte J, Wauters G, Selderslaghs R. *Yersinia enterocolitica:* Its isolation by cold enrichment from patients and healthy subjects. J Clin Pathol. 1981;34:1052–1056.
191. Granfors K, Jalkanen S, Von Essen R, et al. Yersinia antigens in synovial-fluid cells from patients with reactive arthritis. N Engl J Med. 1989;320:216–221.
192. Tsutsumi V, Mena-Lopez R, Anaya-Velazquez F, Martinez-Palomo A. Cellular bases of experimental amebic liver abscess formation. Am J Pathol. 1984;117:81–91.
193. Salata RA, Ravdin JI. The interaction of human neutrophils and *Entamoeba histolytica* increases cytopathogenicity of liver cell monolayers. J Infect Dis. 1986;154:19–26.
194. Ravdin JI, Croft BY, Guerrant RL. Cytopathogenic mechanisms of *Entamoeba histolytica*. J Exp Med. 1980;152:377–390.
195. Ravdin JI, Guerrant RL. Role of adherence in cytopathogenic mechanisms of *Entamoeba histolytica*. J Clin Invest. 1981;68:1305–1313.
196. Ravdin JI, Moreau F, Sullivan JA, et al. Relationship of free intracellular calcium to the cytolytic activity of *Entamoeba histolytica*. Infect Immun. 1988;56:1505–1512.
197. Young JDE, Young TM, Lu LP, et al. Characterization of a membrane pore-forming protein from *Entamoeba histolytica*. J Exp Med. 1982;156:1677–1690.
198. Lynch EC, Rosenberg IM, Gitler C. An ion-channel forming protein produced by *Entamoeba histolytica*. EMBO J. 1982;1:801–804.
199. Scholze H, Werries E. A weakly acidic protease has a powerful proteolytic activity in *Entamoeba histolytica*. Mol Biochem Parasitol. 1984;11:293–300.
200. Keene WE, Petitt MG, Allen S, McKerrow JH. The major neutral proteinase of *Entamoeba histolytica*. J Exp Med. 1986;163:536–549.
201. Lushbaugh WB, Hofbauer AF, Pittman FE. *Entamoeba histolytica:* Purification of cathepsin B. Exp Parasitol. 1985;59:328–336.
202. Muñoz MDL, Calderón J, Rojkind M. The collagenase of *Entamoeba histolytica*. J Exp Med. 1982;155:42–51.
203. Werries E, Nebinger P, Franz A. Degradation of biogene oligosaccharides by β-N-acetylglucosaminidase secreted by *Entamoeba histolytica*. Mol Biochem Parasitol. 1983;7:127–140.
204. Udezulu IA, Leitch GJ. A membrane-associated neuraminidase in *Entamoeba histolytica* trophozoites. Infect Immun. 1987;55:181–186.
205. Udezulu IA, Leitch GJ, Bailey GB. Use of indomethacin to demonstrate enterotoxic activity in extracts of *Entamoeba histolytic* trophozoites. Infect Immun. 1982;36:795–801.
206. McGowan K, Kane A, Asarkoff N, et al. *Entamoeba histolytica* causes intestinal secretion: Role of serotonin. Science. 1983;221:762–764.

207. Feingold C, Bracha R, Wexler A, Mirelman D. Isolation, purification, and partial characterization of an enterotoxin from extracts of *Entamoeba histolytica* trophozoites. Infect Immun. 1985;48:211–218.
208. Bracha R, Mirelman D. Virulence of *Entamoeba histolytica* trophozoites. J Exp Med. 1984;160:353–368.
209. Martinez-Palomo A. *Entamoeba histolytica*. In: Farthing MJG, Keusch GT, eds. Enteric Infection: Mechanisms, Manifestations, and Management. New York: Raven Press; 1989:318–396.
210. Beaver PC, Jung RC, Sherman HJ, et al. Experimental *Entamoeba histolytica* infections in man. Am J Trop Med Hyg. 1956;5:1000–1009.
211. Sargeaunt PG, Williams JE, Grene JD. The differentiation of invasive and non-invasive *Entamoeba histolytica* by isoenzyme electrophoresis. Trans R Soc Trop Med Hyg. 1978;72:519–521.
212. Walsh JA. Problems in recognition and diagnosis of amebiasis: Estimation of the global magnitude of morbidity and mortality. Rev Infect Dis. 1986;8:228–238.
213. Ravdin JI, Petri WA. *Entamoeba histolytica* (amebiasis). In: Mandell GL, Douglas RG, Bennett JE, eds. Principles and Practice of Infectious Diseases. New York: Churchill Livingstone; 1990:2036–2049.
214. Haider Z, Rasul A. Chronic non-dysenteric intestinal amoebiasis: A review of 159 cases. J Pakistan Med Assoc. 1975;25:75–78.
215. Krogstad DJ, Spencer HC Jr, Healy GR, et al. Amebiasis: Epidemiologic studies in the United States, 1971–1974. Ann Intern Med. 1978;88:89–97.
216. Patterson M, Healy GR, Shabot JM. Serologic testing for amoebiasis. Gastroenterology. 1980;78:136–141.
217. Drugs for parasitic infections. Med Lett Drugs Ther. 1992;34:17–26.
218. Mirelman D, Bracha R, Wexler A, Chayen A. Changes in isoenzyme patterns of a cloned culture of nonpathogenic *Entamoeba histolytica* during axenization. Infect Immun. 1986;54:827–832.
219. Clark CG, Cunnick CC, Diamond LS. *Entamoeba histolytica:* Is conversion of "nonpathogenic" amebae to the "pathogenic" form a real phenomenon? Exp Parasitol. 1992;74:307–314.
220. Banerjee RN, Sahani AL, Nag AK, et al. A longitudinal study of intestinal amoebiasis. J Assoc Phys Ind. 1976;24:83–88.
221. Krogstad DJ. Isoenzyme patterns and pathogenicity in amebic infection. N Engl J Med. 1986;315:390–391. Editorial.
222. Powell SJ, Wilmot AJ, Elsdon-Dew R. Single and low dosage regimens of metronidazole in amoebic dysentery and amoebic liver abscess. Ann Trop Med Parasitol. 1969;63:139–142.
223. Lasserre R, Jaroonvesama N, Kurathong S, Soh CT. Single-day drug treatment of amebic liver abscess. Am J Trop Med Hyg. 1983;32:723–726.
224. Brown HW, Neva FA. Intestinal and luminal protozoa. In: Brown HW, Neva FA, eds. Basic Clinical Parasitology. 5th ed. Norwalk, CT: Appleton-Century-Crofts; 1983:23–44.
225. Brown HW, Neva FA. Trematoda. In: Brown HW, Neva FA. Basic Clinical Parasitology. 5th ed. Norwalk, CT: Appleton-Century-Crofts; 1983:205–212.
226. Scully RE, Mark EJ, McNeely BU. Case 21-1985. N Engl J Med. 1985;312:1376–1383.
227. Namdari H, Bottone EJ: *Aeromonas* species: Pathogens of aquatic inhabitants with a human host range. Clin Microbiol Newslett. 1991;13:113–120.
228. Deodhar LP, Saraswathi K, Varudkar A. *Aeromonas* spp and their association with human diarrheal disease. J Clin Microbiol. 1991;29:853–856.
229. Gracey M, Burke V, Robinson J. *Aeromonas*-associated gastroenteritis. Lancet. 1982;2:1304–1306.

230. Morgan DR, Johnson PC, DuPont HL, et al. Lack of correlation between known virulence properties of *Aeromonas hydrophila* and enteropathogenicity for humans. Infect Immun. 1985;50:62–65.

231. Johnson S, Echeverria P, Taylor DN, et al. Enteritis necroticans among Khmer children at an evacuation site in Thailand. Lancet. 1987;2:496–500.

232. Murrell TGC, Walker PD. The pigbel story of Papua New Guinea. Trans R Soc Trop Med Hyg. 1991;85:119–122.

233. Jeckeln E. Uber Darmbrand. Dtsch Med Wochenschr. 1947;72:105–108.

234. Zeissler J, Rassfeld-Sternberg L. Enteritis necroticans due to *Clostridium welchii* type F. Br Med J. 1949;1:266–269.

235. Shann F, Lawrence G. The medical management of enteritis necroticans (pigbel). Papua New Guinea Med J. 1979;22:18–23.

236. Lawrence GW, Lehmann D, Anian G, et al. Impact of active immunisation against enteritis necroticans in Papua New Guinea. Lancet. 1990;336:1165–1167.

237. Severin WP, de la Fuente AA, Stringer MF. *Clostridium perfringens* type C causing necrotizing enteritis. J Clin Pathol. 1984;37:942–944.

238. Guerrant RL. Principles and syndromes of enteric infection. In: Mandell GL, Douglas RG, Bennett JE, eds. Principles and Practice of Infectious Diseases. New York: Churchill Livingstone; 1990:837–851.

239. Carpenter CCJ. Other pathogenic vibrios. In: Mandell GL, Douglas RG, Bennett JE, eds. Principles and Practice of Infectious Diseases. New York: Churchill Livingstone; 1990:1646–1649.

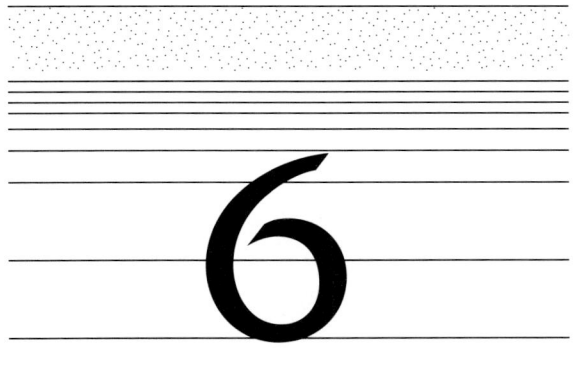

6

Clostridium difficile–Associated Disease

LYNNE McFARLAND, M.S., Ph.D.

The gastrointestinal tract contains a complex milieu of interacting organisms whose populations may shift dramatically in response to antibiotics, other medications, or the introduction of new organisms. The most common result of the disruption of colonic equilibrium is diarrhea. Depending on the specific inciting agent, diarrhea can be observed in 1 to 25% of patients. Approximately one third of cases of antibiotic-associated diarrhea (AAD) and nearly all cases of pseudomembranous colitis (PMC) are due to a spore-forming anaerobe, *Clostridium difficile.*[2]

Clostridium difficile is an opportunistic organism that may result in a variety of clinical manifestations. Most commonly, the target organ is the gastrointestinal tract, and the outcome of infection may range from asymptomatic carriage to diarrhea that may progress to colitis, toxic megacolon, or death. Extra-intestinal *C. difficile* infections have been reported infrequently. *Clostridium difficile* is the most frequent cause of hospital-acquired diarrhea reported for inpatients and a common cause of chronic recurrent diarrhea-causing colitis found in outpatients.

HISTORICAL PERSPECTIVE

The elucidation of *C. difficile* as an etiologic agent required the synthesis of research from three separate fields: clinical medicine, microbiology, and animal pathology. Discoveries in these fields were made at different periods. After decades of work, researchers finally fit all the pieces of the puzzle together (Table 6–1).

On the clinical side, the earliest report of *C. difficile* was in 1893, when Finney described a 22-year-old woman who had a resection of a tumor in the gastric pylorus. She died on her 15th postoperative day and was found to have pseudomembranes in her colon upon autopsy.[3] Subsequently, the finding of pseudomembranes was sporadically associated with cases of ischemic cardiovascular insufficiency, colonic obstruction, heavy metal intoxication, sepsis, shock, spinal fracture, and uremia, although it was not a common infection.[4]

In the 1950s, after the introduction of the broad-spectrum antibiotics chloramphenicol and tetracycline, the incidence of AAD began to rise. When the increase of AAD was noted,

TABLE 6–1. MAJOR HISTORICAL LANDMARKS IN *Clostridium difficile* RESEARCH

TIME	CLINICAL MEDICINE	ETIOLOGIC AGENT	ANIMAL MODELS
1893	Finney describes first case of pseudomembranous colitis (PMC) (postsurgical)	Unknown	No work
1935	Sporadic cases of PMC	Hall & O'Toole report *Bacillis difficilis* causes death in lab animals Found in healthy neonates	
1940–1950	Antibiotics introduced; antibiotic-associated PMC sporadic cases	*Staphylococcus aureus* suspected *B. difficilis* remains laboratory curiosity	1943 Hambre reports penicillin lethal for guinea pigs; cause unknown
1960s	Lincomycin & clindamycin introduced; antibiotic-associated diarrhea (AAD) increases	1962 Smith & King rename *B. difficilis* to *Clostridium difficilis*	1969 Small uses hamster as model for lincomycin-based colitis
1974	Tedesco reports outbreak of clindamycin-associated PMC (10%) and AAD (21%)	Hafiz's thesis on *C. difficile* Widespread in nature Produces a lethal toxin for animals Not associated with human disease	Green proposes latent viral infection as cause for animal lethality due to CPE associated with animal organ samples
1977	Price & Davis describe different types of PMC lesions	Search for virus uncovers the toxin: Larson finds heat labile toxin (from patients with PMC) capable of causing CPE on tissue culture; no viral particles or bacteria found; toxin mediated?	Bartlett shows similar histology in hamsters as in Price's descriptions; links Larson's CPE and transfers disease hamster to hamster in cell-free preparations; shows vancomycin protective in hamsters
1978		CPE neutralized by gas gangrene antiserum (5 clostridial species) by Bartlett, George, Fekety Responsible clostridium was *C. sordellii* (but not found in PMC patients)	
1979		Bartlett finds *C. sordellii* cross-reacts with *C. difficile* George develops selective media (CCFA), which grows *C. difficile* Chang describes classic cytotoxin assay Taylor & Bartlett partially purify cytotoxin	Allo, Silva & Fekety prevent clindamycin colitis in hamsters by *C. sordellii* antitoxin
1980	Burton first reports hospital outbreak	Taylor & Bartlett report two toxins exist	
1981	Kim reports environmental detection of *C. difficile* in ICU	Taylor & Banno purify enterotoxin (toxin A), distinct from cytotoxin	Wilson finds normal hamster cecal flora prevents antibiotic associated cecitis
1982	George describes prevalence of *C. difficile* in various populations	Sullivan, Pellett, & Wilkins characterize toxins A & B Justus describes a motility-altering virulence factor	Sullivan & Libby find the 2 toxins cause fetal cecitis in hamsters
1984			Arnon observes IV or intraperitoneal injection of toxins A & B in monkeys caused lethargy, then death
1985		Wilkins describes pathophysiology of the 2 toxins	
1986	Bender reports first nursing home outbreak Heard finds outbreak in hospital due to distinct strain type X		
1988		Rothman describes immunologic & structural properties of toxins A & B	Corthier reports nontoxigenic clones may arise from toxigenic clones
1989	McFarland describes nosocomial transmission by hospital personnel & roommates & via environmental sites of identical *C. difficile* strains	New commercial kits for identification available	

Staphylococcus aureus was believed to be the cause because of its frequent isolation in the stools of these patients and the prompt response of these patients to therapy with vancomycin. The role of *S. aureus* may have been spuriously assigned; although it was the most common nosocomial pathogen at the time, it is now considered to be normal in the intestinal flora in 15 to 30% of healthy persons.[5]

Clindamycin was introduced in the 1960s to treat anaerobic infections. Its increased use refocused attention on the etiology of PMC, because the disease was beginning to be reported more frequently, and *Staphylococcus* was not isolated in these cases.

Interest waned until 1974, when Tedesco and colleagues reported an unacceptably high rate of adverse reaction to the most commonly prescribed antibiotic for the treatment of anaerobic infections. In 200 patients receiving clindamycin, an unexpected finding was the development of serious diarrhea in 21% of the patients; most startlingly, 10% of these patients developed pseudomembranous colitis.[6] Studies of the stools from these patients revealed the presence of a cytotoxic factor on tissue culture monolayers that was believed to be due to a virus or a toxin from an unknown source. If clindamycin was to continue to be useful as an antibiotic, this finding had to be explained.

The second track of research was in the field of microbiology. In 1935, an organism identified as *Bacillus difficilis* (so named because it was difficult to cultivate) was reported initially by Hall and O'Toole as a component organism in the normal flora of newborn infants.[7] These investigators noted that this bacterium caused neurologic symptoms and frequently mortality in guinea pigs or rabbits. Since it was found in healthy neonates, it was erroneously thought not to be pathogenic in humans. *Bacillus difficilis* remained a laboratory curiosity, and its role in AAD was not determined until later. In 1974, a review by Hafiz described *C. difficile* as a bacterium widely found in nature, with most strains producing a toxin lethal to animals.[8] It was not, however, associated with the clinical disease reported by Tedesco.

The third track of research centered on the investigation into the unexplained death of some animals after exposure to penicillins and lincomycin. Between 1940 and 1960, investigators proposed a variety of causes but could not determine the reason for this mortality in animals. In 1974 Green showed cytotoxic changes in tissue culture monolayers inoculated with specimens from dead animals exposed to penicillins. Green hypothesized that a latent viral infection was being reactivated by the antibiotics.[9]

It was not until 1977 that Bartlett and others linked the research found in these three vital areas of research. Bartlett showed that the clindamycin-induced colitis in hamsters could be serially transferred using cecal contents. Only one strain of *Clostridium* that was isolated from these hamsters could induce the identical illness in other hamsters. The ability of the cell-free supernatant to produce the same illness suggested that a toxin was also present. This strain was identified as *C. difficile*.[10] The final link was forged in 1977, when Larson and colleagues described a cytotoxic factor present in the stools of patients with PMC.[11]

Fekety found that stool filtrates from 2 patients with antibiotic-associated colitis (AAC) caused a cytopathic effect (CPE) on human fibroblast cell culture. Hamsters injected with fecal filtrates from the patients developed a toxic syndrome and died within 48 hours. The CPEs were neutralized with gas gangrene antitoxin composed of antitoxin from five clostridial species.[12]

Most of the causal pathway for *C. difficile* was known, but parts of it were located in diverse areas of research. The synthesis of this information was not achieved until work with the hamster model integrated the observations that the lesions in patients with PMC described by Tedesco were caused by the cytopathic toxin (and not a virus) reported by Green and produced by the organism described by Hafiz. Once these observations were synthesized, the pattern was evident.

Since that time, the characterization of the epidemiology, transmission, diagnosis, and treatment of *C. difficile* infection has been of great importance. *Clostridium difficile* has been found to be highly associated with factors that perturb the normal intestinal flora, and it is now the leading cause of nosocomial outbreaks of diarrhea and colitis.

DISEASE SPECTRUM

Prevalence

Clostridium difficile organisms are present in the normal colonic flora in 2 to 5% of the general adult population, but the prevalence increases when a person is hospitalized or exposed to antibiotics (Table 6–2). *Clostridium difficile* is usually associated with a variety of gastrointestinal infections, ranging from simple diarrhea to PMC. In adults, *C. difficile* has been

TABLE 6–2. FREQUENCY OF *Clostridium difficile* DISEASE IN VARIOUS PATIENT POPULATIONS

	PREVALENCE (%)	INCIDENCE
Pseudomembranous colitis in adults	1–8	0
Colitis in adults	0.7	1–3/100,000
Diarrhea in adults	3–22	8–80/1000
Adult carrier	11–18	13/100
Adult inpatient (mixed clinical status)	21–26	10–30/100
Adult outpatients, healthy	1–3	ND
Healthy neonates	15–100	ND
Healthy infants	9–14	
Cancer chemotherapy	18	ND
Cystic fibrosis patients	22–50	

KEY: ND = not determined.
SOURCE: Compiled from references 2, 19, 53, 60, 64, 65, 144, 145, 166–176.

found to account for 15 to 20% of all cases of AAD, 50 to 70% of AAC, and 90 to 100% of PMC.[1] In neonates *C. difficile* is found fairly frequently, but symptomatic disease itself is rare.

Carriage

A recent finding is the high rate of asymptomatic colonization of *C. difficile* in patients who fail to develop any symptomatic disease. *Clostridium difficile* can be isolated in patients without apparent effect in 1 to 5% of normal healthy adults, 30 to 75% of neonates, 9 to 14% of healthy infants less than 1 year old, and 10 to 36% of adult inpatients experiencing no diarrheal symptoms.[1, 4, 13–15] In the majority of colonized hosts, asymptomatic carriage does not progress to symptomatic disease, but carriers have been shown to transmit their strain to other hospitalized patients who may develop disease.[2]

Clostridium difficile Diarrhea

Diarrhea is the most common symptom observed in patients with *C. difficile*. Diarrhea may be generally defined as a change from the patient's normal bowel habit with three or more loose stools a day for at least 2 consecutive days. The three principal *C. difficile* diseases in which this may be the presenting symptom are, as has already been noted, AAD, AAC, and PMC, often referred to simply as diarrhea, colitis, and PMC, respectively.

Antibiotic-Associated Diarrhea

Antibiotic-associated diarrhea can be defined as diarrhea associated with recent antibiotic use with no evidence of colitis. The range of incidence of AAD is broad and dependent on numerous factors. Generally, the incidence of AAD varies from 3 to 30 in 100 admissions among hospitalized patients.[2, 16, 17] This rate varies by the type of antibiotic given, for example, antibiotics that inhibit normal intestinal anaerobic flora have higher rates; the dose of antibiotic given, and perhaps the duration; and host factors such as age, and concurrent illnesses and surgeries. In the earliest report of a hospital outbreak, 21% of 200 consecutive patients receiving clindamycin developed diarrhea.[6] Antibiotic-associated diarrhea was observed in 10 to 25% of patients receiving clindamycin and 5 to 10% receiving ampicillin.[18] In a study of 399 hospitalized patients, 103 patients developed

AAD, for an overall incidence of AAD of 26 in 100, and *C. difficile* was attributed to approximately 25% of all reported cases of AAD.[2] Route of antibiotic may also be significant, but all routes of administration (oral, intravenous [IV], intramuscular [IM], and topical) have been implicated at various times. The lowest prevalence (0.01%) of AAD associated with *C. difficile* was reported by Ramirez-Ronda in 1974, before selective, enhanced media were used for *C. difficile* isolation.[16] More commonly, rates range from 5 to 26% in general medicine patients, depending on the risk factors present in the population studied; including types of prescribed antibiotics, endemic rate of *C. difficile* infection at admitting hospital or nursing home, occurrence of an outbreak, type of *C. difficile* assay used, and degree of expertise of microbiology laboratory.[18] McFarland and colleagues reported an incidence of AAD associated with *C. difficile* of 7.1 in 100 per year in patients receiving antibiotics.[2] Riley and colleagues reported an incidence of *C. difficile* AAD of 15 in 100 per 6 months.[19] *Clostridium difficile* was isolated from diarrheal stools of 873 of 4793 patients (18%) receiving antibiotics in Sweden. The majority of these patients were more than 70 years of age, and the higher rates were associated with cephalosporins and lincosamides.[20]

The severity of the condition may range from a nuisance diarrhea, which resolves as soon as the inciting antibiotic is stopped, to a distressful diarrhea, which may occur 20 to 30 times a day and last as long as 2 to 3 months, without therapy.[6] In patients with AAD, the clinical symptoms are mild, and the average duration of diarrhea is 8 to 10 days.[21] The incubation period may be 1 to 10 days after the inciting antibiotic is started (early onset) or, more frequently (66% of cases), symptoms may be delayed until 2 to 6 weeks after the antibiotic is discontinued (late onset). Even though AAD is thought of as a benign diarrhea, symptoms may persist for 4 weeks or longer, if untreated. When the stool of AAD patients is cultured, only 11 to 33% have positive findings for *C. difficile*. The majority of AAD is due to other causes that remain undiscovered to date.[1, 2] Patients with AAD rarely complain of fever or abdominal distress and do not commonly have leukocytosis.

Antibiotic-Associated Colitis

Antibiotic-associated colitis is a diagnosis that includes patients with a recent antibiotic exposure of 6 weeks or less who are experiencing diarrhea with evidence of a nonspecific inflammatory reaction seen with colonic biopsy but with no apparent pseudomembranes. Endoscopic examination may reveal erythema, friability, hyperemia, or frank hemorrhage.[4] The incidence of AAC ranges from 1–3/100,000 in outpatients to 1/100 to 1/1000 in inpatient populations.[22] In patients with AAC, severe symptoms are more commonly reported. Patients with AAC often have a rapid onset of watery or mucus-containing diarrhea, a frequency of up to 10 to 20 times a day, and a duration of diarrhea longer than 4 weeks, if untreated. Abdominal pain and tenderness, low-grade fever ranging from 100 to 102°F (37.7–38.8°C), and leukocytosis are also more frequent in AAC than in AAD.[1] Infrequently, peripheral leukocyte counts may exceed 50,000 per mm^3 or fevers higher than 106°F (41.1°C) may occur. In 45 to 50% of patients, leukocytosis or fecal white blood cells also may be found. In 20% of patients with AAC, occasional blood is found in the stool.[1]

When the stool of AAC patients is cultured, 60 to 75% have positive findings for *C. difficile* or for cytotoxin. Diagnosis of *C. difficile* is complicated by its similarity to bacterial dysentery, ulcerative colitis, and intra-abdominal sepsis.[18] Occasionally, a right-sided AAC has been reported, which is associated with ampicillin use.

Pseudomembranous Colitis

At the extreme end of the disease spectrum is PMC. Diagnosis can be definitively determined only when pseudomembranes are observed with a sigmoidoscopic or colonoscopic examination.

The prevalence of PMC ranges from 0.1 to 10.1% of inpatients receiving high-risk antibiotics (cephalosporins or penicillins). Interestingly, no factor consistently predicts which patients develop PMC rather than AAD or AAC. Many cases of PMC occur sporadically among outpatients, but PMC may also become evident in hospitalized patients and nursing home residents.[1]

The symptoms are remarkably similar to those of AAC cases. The majority of PMC patients have watery diarrhea (90–95%), and the remainder report bloody diarrhea, which develops 1 to 4 weeks after antibiotic therapy. Abdominal cramps, leukocytosis, anorexia, and fever ranging from 102 to 104°F (38.8–40.0°C) are reported in approximately 80% of cases of PMC, and hypoalbuminemia is seen in as many as 25% of the cases.[1] Physical examination reveals mild abdominal distention and tenderness, except in the rare cases of toxic megacolon and perforation. Fecal leukocytes are observed in 30 to 66% of patients with PMC.[23] The incubation period may be rapid, occurring 1 to 5 days after antibiotics begin, or delayed, occurring 1 to 5 weeks after antibiotic cessation. Duration of the initial episode of PMC may be from 1 to 3 weeks, if untreated.

In untreated cases of PMC, recovery has been reported within 7 days, if the initiating antibiotic was stopped. If the diagnosis is delayed and antibiotics are continued, the disease is more severe and may last as long as 3 weeks. Delayed diagnosis has been associated with fulminant colitis or perforation.[6] Mortality from PMC ranges from 0 to 75% in the absence of treatment.[6, 24, 25]

Complications of PMC are due to protein-losing enteropathy, colonic perforations, toxic megacolon, severe fluid loss, and electrolyte imbalances.[18]

Recurrent Disease

Recurrent episodes of *C. difficile* disease are observed in 20 to 66% of patients with diarrhea, colitis, or PMC.[26] Patients who suffer one recurrence often continue to have further episodes that fail standard therapies.[27–30]

The factors that may predict patients with higher risk for developing recurrent episodes are largely unknown. The ability of *C. difficile* to sporulate and recolonize the intestine after antibiotic cessation may rest on the ability of the spores to survive in pouches and diverticula in the intestine of some patients. Other patients may become reinfected with *C. difficile* from exogenous sources after antimicrobials have been stopped and before normal flora of the bowel becomes reestablished. One study showed that the second episode was caused by a strain different from the original *C. difficile* infecting strain.[31] In some cases, the recurrence may have been stimulated by initiation of systemic chemotherapy.[32]

Other Gastrointestinal Conditions

Although the principal clinical symptoms associated with *C. difficile* infection are abdominal pain and diarrhea, several other effects on the intestinal processes have been reported.

Protein-Losing Enteropathy

Malnutrition has been noted in patients with chronic recurrent *C. difficile* disease. Protein-losing enteropathy has been associated with 12 of 12 patients with PMC, 6 of 14 patients (43%)

with *C. difficile* diarrhea, and 50% of nursing home patients.[33, 34] The diagnosis of protein-losing enteropathy should be considered in all *C. difficile*–infected patients and its course followed closely, especially in nursing home patients, in whom malnutrition can have devastating results.

Inflammatory Bowel Disease

Several early studies attempted to link *C. difficile* with the etiology of inflammatory bowel disease (IBD) owing to the isolation of *C. difficile* in a few patients with chronic IBD.[35–37] The relationship between *C. difficile* and IBD has been obscured by the high use of antibiotics in these patients. When IBD patients who were not receiving antibiotics were studied, no significant association with *C. difficile* was found.[38] *Clostridium difficile* has been found frequently in patients with IBD, but the *C. difficile* organisms may be carried without a causative role or they may have a role in provoking exacerbations of IBD. Treatment with vancomycin generally alleviates the acute diarrhea and eliminates *C. difficile*, but the underlying chronic bowel disease persists.[4]

Toxic Megacolon

Toxic megacolon is characterized by massive dilatation of the entire colon, fever, and abdominal distress, necessitating surgical intervention in 65 to 71% of cases, but still resulting in a high mortality rate (35%).[39] Toxic megacolon may occur, if infrequently, as a complication of *C. difficile*–associated PMC, and diarrhea may or may not be present. The existence of PMC is often unsuspected and may be detected only at surgery.[40]

Acute Abdomen

Occasionally, *C. difficile*–positive patients may present with symptoms of an acute abdomen (distention, pain, fever, leukocytosis) with little or no diarrhea as the first symptoms of PMC. In a series of 6 patients with this presentation, all were shown to have pseudomembranes and were treated with IV metronidazole with a good response.[41]

Extracolonic Infection

On very rare occasions, *C. difficile* infections have been reported in body sites other than the gastrointestinal tract.

Reactive Arthritis

Sterile arthritis is a documented sequela of infection with *Shigella*, *Salmonella*, *Yersinia*, and *Campylobacter*, occurring 2 to 3 weeks after the onset of diarrhea. There are 11 cases of reactive oligoarthritis in the literature that have developed after a *C. difficile* infection.[42] When patients were treated with vancomycin for the *C. difficile* infection, the arthritis resolved. Interestingly, most patients (73%) possessed the HLA-B27 allele that has been associated with other causes of reactive arthritis.[42]

Chronic Osteomyelitis

On rare occasions, osteomyelitis has been associated with *C. difficile* cultured from pus, bone, and aspirated material. Patients respond well to vancomycin.[43, 44]

Neurologic Effects

Clostridium difficile is known to be lethal to experimental animals that develop hindlimb paralysis or seizure activity when moribund, and changes in electrocardiogram (ECG) show arrhythmias on intravenous infusion of *C. difficile* toxin in rabbits.[45] The pathologic consequences of the fatal injection of *C. difficile* toxin (lethargy, hypotonia, hypothermia, and, after 3 to 8 hours, cessation of breathing, leading to death) were similar to those of infants dying of sudden infant death syndrome (SIDS). Although initially suggestive of an intriguing hypothesis, no further data on this correlation have been reported.

Septicemia

Fewer than 10 patients have been reported to have *C. difficile* septicemia with and without intestinal symptoms. High mortality (83%) occurs when *C. difficile* organisms are found in the blood.[46]

Abscesses

Pancreatic and splenic abscesses have been reported sporadically in the absence of gastrointestinal disease.[47, 48] One case of primary infection of ascitic fluid with a toxigenic strain of *C. difficile* was reported by De Leeuw and colleagues. The patient had no diarrhea or any evidence of colitis, and the only *C. difficile* grown from her stool was nontoxigenic. She was successfully treated with two courses of metronidazole.[49]

Hemolytic-Uremic Syndrome

The hemolytic-uremic syndrome (HUS) is a distinct clinical entity described by renal failure, microangiopathic hemolytic anemia, and thrombocytopenia. Patients with HUS usually present with bloody diarrhea but, rarely, with pseudomembranes. A reported complication of typhoid, shigellosis, infection with verotoxin-producing *Escherichia coli*, HUS has infrequently been associated with toxin-producing *C. difficile*.[50] Because the majority of patients with *C. difficile*–associated HUS are children, a causal role is suspect. *Clostridium difficile*–associated PMC may possibly activate or exacerbate hemolytic-uremic syndromes, but further data are needed for confirmation.

PATHOPHYSIOLOGY

The production of *C. difficile* disease is a multifactorial process that involves four main factors. First, "colonization resistance" is disrupted by antibiotics, other medications, or medical procedures. Second, once loss of the protective barrier of normal flora occurs, exposure to *C. difficile* from a variety of sources leads to colonization of the colon. Third, the presence of *C. difficile* exposes the colonic lumen to virulence factors (enterotoxin or cytotoxin) that produce the symptoms of diarrhea and colitis. The fourth factor, rather than a stage in the disease process, is a combination of risk factors that determines the likelihood and severity of the disease, including the host's age and underlying disease and immunologic status.[15, 51]

Disruption of Colonization Resistance

One of the roles of normal intestinal flora is to inhibit colonization of other species of organisms, a phenomenon termed colonization resistance. This beneficial role was not fully appreciated until research into AAD showed distinct shifts of normal flora in these patients.[52, 53] The mechanism of colonization resistance may be through the production of inhibitory fatty acids, toxin-degrading proteases, nutrient competition, the competition for attachment sites, or a combination of these factors.[54] The influence of antibiotics and other medications on *C. difficile* disease may be to kill or suppress normal flora to such an extent that the colonization resistance is neutralized and *C. difficile* is free to reproduce and cause toxigenic diarrhea. The specific organisms that are responsible for colonization resistance have not been determined, although anaerobic bacteria seem to play a major role. *Lactobacillus* and group D enterococci were specifically shown to be highly inhibitory toward *C. difficile* in vitro.[55] Antibiotics that result in *C. difficile* disease frequently have been shown to be the antibiotics that have a profound effect on the normal colonic flora.[56]

Colonization by Various Sources of *Clostridium difficile*

C. difficile infection may arise from one endogenous source or a multitude of exogenous sources, ranging from other patients to contaminated environmental sites. The majority of infections are acquired within the hospital environment, when the patient, ill with a disease requiring antibiotics, is exposed to spores or vegetative *C. difficile* organisms dormant in the hospital environment and becomes colonized.

Nosocomial Transmission

HOSPITALS

Sporadic outbreaks of *C. difficile* disease in hospital patients were first reported in 1978 and have increased in frequency since that time (Table 6–3). These outbreaks have provided valuable clues in discovering the mode of transmission, routes of infection, and risk factors for *C. difficile* disease. In nosocomial clusters, the sources of *C. difficile* infection often are not found, but in a few cases the source has been determined. Savage and Alford reported transmission between 2 patients due to a shared contaminated commode chair.[57] Mogg and colleagues traced transmission in an outbreak of PMC to a contaminated sigmoidoscope.[24]

Clostridium difficile may be an endogenous infection, since 2 to 5% of newly admitted patients with no recent prior hospitalization carry *C. difficile* as normal flora. Exposure to risk factors or medications that disrupt colonization resistance allows the disease to become symptomatic. Far more frequently, the *C. difficile* infection is acquired from an exogenous source (Table 6–4). The routes of infection may include person-to-person transmission or indirect transmission via contaminated fomites, such as commode chairs, bathroom or sink surfaces, floors, bedrailings, call buttons, or any shared environmental surface.[2]

Hospital personnel may transmit *C. difficile* to susceptible patients by transient hand carriage. Kim and Fekety and their coworkers found that

TABLE 6–3. NOSOCOMIAL OUTBREAKS OF *Clostridium difficile* DISEASE

YEAR	DISEASE	POPULATION	NO. INFECTED	TRANSMITTED	REFERENCE
1974	Pseudomembranous colitis (PMC), colitis	Hospital inpatients	10	Unknown	Tedesco[6]
1979	PMC	Inpatients	66	Sigmoidoscope	Mogg[24]
1979	PMC	Hospital inpatients	Unkn	Unknown	Price[148]
1981	PMC, diarrhea	Hospital inpatients	8	Unknown	Greenfield[177]
1982	Diarrhea	Neonates	Unkn	Person-to-person	Larson[69]
1982	PMC	ICU	2	Environment	Walters[62]
1982	Diarrhea	Surgical wards	62	Person-to-person	Burdon[70]
1983	Colitis	Hospital	2	Commode chair	Savage[57]
1986	Diarrhea	Nursing home	54	Unknown	Bender[74]
1986	Diarrhea	Oncology ward	35	Epidemic strain X, Environment	Heard[169]
1987	PMC	Hospital	23	Person-to-person	Nolan[178]
1988	Diarrhea	Hospital ward	10	Environment, Sluice room	Testore[179]
1989	Diarrhea	Orthopedic ward	6	Environment?	McKay[180]
1989	Diarrhea	ICU	8	Environment?	Foulke[181]
1989	PMC, diarrhea, and carriers	Orthopedic ward	5	Unknown	Degl'Innocenti[182]

between 13 and 15% of hospital personnel had positive findings on cultures for *C. difficile* in the stool yet remained without symptoms, and 2% of these personnel had a small number of *C. difficile* organisms on their hands.[58, 59] Other studies of hospital personnel have found low rates of colonization (1.5–2.8%), but the rate escalates dramatically (59%) after caring for an infected *C. difficile* patient.[2, 60] Roommates of colonized patients may also be a target of infection. In one study, 25% of patients who had previously had negative findings acquired *C. difficile* after 48 hours of sharing a room with an infected roommate, and 87% of the roommates were shown to have acquired the identical strain.[2] Outbreaks in daycare settings have also been reported, in which the same strain of *C.*

difficile was isolated from the hands of the children and the teachers.[61] Transient hand carriage is one common mode of nosocomial transmission of *C. difficile* infection.

Clostridium difficile is an efficient nosocomial pathogen owing to the ease of its transmission and its persistence in the hospital environment in conjunction with the exposure to a susceptible population, that is, patients receiving antibiotics. Several studies have shown the wide variety of environmental sites that become contaminated with *C. difficile* spores once a colonized patient is admitted into the room.[2, 58, 59] In addition, the isolation rates of *C. difficile* organisms from environmental sites increase dramatically once infected patients are located in a room or an outbreak occurs in a hospital (see

TABLE 6–4. TRANSMISSION OF NOSOCOMIAL *Clostridium difficile*

SOURCE	FREQUENCY POSITIVE *C. difficile* (%)	ASSOCIATED WITH	INVESTIGATOR
ENDOGENOUS	2.0–5.0	Healthy adults	McFarland, 1989
EXOGENOUS			
Hospital personnel	1.5	Endemic stool carriage	Gerding, 1986
	2.8	Pre–*C. difficile* patient contact	McFarland, 1989
	59.0	Post–*C. difficile* patient contact	McFarland, 1989
Patient roommate	25.0	Infected roommate	McFarland, 1989
Environmental sites	2.8	No *C. difficile* patients in ICU	Kim, 1981
	11.0	*C. difficile* patient in ICU	
	6.8	No symptomatic patients	Fekety, 1981
	19.0	Symptomatic *C. difficile* patients	
	4.9	*C. difficile* carrier	Malamou-Ladas, 1983
	14.0	*C. difficile* symptomatic	Heard, 1986
	31.4	*C. difficile* colitis outbreak	Kaatz, 1988
	8.0	No *C. difficile* patients	McFarland, 1989
	29.0	*C. difficile* carriers only	
	49.0	*C. difficile* symptomatic	

Table 6–3). In survival experiments, the number of *C. difficile* organisms that had been inoculated into a vacant hospital room decreased by 90% in 24 hours, but spores were detectable for as long as 5 months afterward.[58, 59] Other investigations have shown that environmental cultures continue to produce positive findings for 7 to 10 weeks after an outbreak.[62, 63]

Although *C. difficile* is found in the soil, raising concern that fresh vegetables may transmit spores to susceptible patients, investigators have failed to isolate *C. difficile* organisms from food or food preparation areas in the hospital.[2, 58, 59]

Neonates frequently acquire *C. difficile* in the hospital within the first weeks of life.[64–66] *Clostridium difficile* may be passed from the mother to the infant at birth, but evidence for vertical transmission has been contradictory. Hafiz and colleagues found that 71% of women in a clinic for sexually transmitted diseases carried *C. difficile* organisms in the vagina, but only 18% of women from a family planning clinic had positive findings on vaginal cultures.[67] Al-jumaili and colleagues took vaginal swabs from women in labor just before delivery and failed to isolate *C. difficile* from any of the 35 women, yet 7% of the neonates born to these women had positive cultures on the first day of life.[68] Larson and colleagues also failed to find any positive vaginal isolates in 16 mothers whose babies produced positive results on culture. Of 17 stool specimens taken from mothers of babies with positive findings, only one specimen also had positive findings.[69] A major source for neonatal *C. difficile* may be in the environment of the nursery.

The differentiation of strains of *C. difficile* is valuable as a tool to document the transmission and spread of this organism within the hospital. Several methods have been used, including immunoblot profiles, antibiotic sensitivity patterns, plasmid profiles, and immunologic fingerprinting by means of counterimmunoelectrophoresis (CIE).[62, 70–73] These methods have demonstrated that outbreaks in the hospital were generally of one strain.

EXTENDED CARE FACILITIES

Clostridium difficile outbreaks have been reported in nursing homes, and controlling their transmission may prove to be a problem. In 1986, Bender and colleagues reported an outbreak in which one third of patients acquired *C. difficile*, 34% of the patients with toxin-positive cultures developed diarrhea, and 38% died.[74] Since then, more outbreaks have been reported, with high mortality observed in those patients who develop *C. difficile* disease.[75]

Virulence Factors

Once a host is colonized with *C. difficile*, production of toxins and other virulence factors causes the cellular disruption and diarrhea characteristic of the disease.

Enterotoxin

In 1981, Taylor and colleagues reported the separation of a distinct toxin (called toxin A) from the cytotoxin (toxin B).[76] The next year, Sullivan and colleagues separated cytotoxin from enterotoxin using ion-exchange chromatography and began to characterize the differences between the two *C. difficile* toxins.[77] Toxin A is not a classic enterotoxin in that it produces a hemorrhagic exudate containing inflammatory debris and serum, rather than a clear liquid.[78] Toxin A was found to be an extremely large toxin molecule (MW 308,000), heat and acid labile, and weakly cytopathic on most cell lines (3–200 ng/ml minimum dose). Several cell lines (F9, PTF9-63, P19) are more susceptible to enterotoxin and show cytotoxic effects with as little as 2 μg of enterotoxin.[78] The enterotoxin induces intestinal fluid accumulation in rabbit ligated ileal loops, an acute inflammatory response, and hemorrhagic edema, and it is weakly cytotoxic.[79]

The structure of toxin A is thought to be an aggregate of smaller components that share a common subunit with toxin B.[80, 81] A binding site for toxin A was located on hamster and rabbit brush borders and discovered to be a trisaccharide with a Gal (α) 1-3Gal β 1-4GlcNAc terminal end.[82] This trisaccharide is not present on the human brush border cells, but the human receptor site appears to contain a similar oligosaccharide. No similar receptor for cytotoxin was found on brush borders.[82] Enterotoxin also was found to hemagglutinate rabbit erythrocytes and bovine thyroglobulin at 4°C, but not at 37°C.[82] The hemagglutination is due to the enterotoxin binding on the sugar sequence (described earlier) located on the surface of the rabbit erythrocytes.

MECHANISM

The mechanism of injury produced by the enterotoxin involves direct epithelial cell damage as well as recruitment of inflammatory cells (Table 6–5). Enterotoxin binds to a glycoprotein receptor on brush border membranes, causes direct epithelial cell damage, and attracts inflammatory cells. Once toxin A is bound to the cell, the toxin is internalized and changes in the actin-myosin cytoskeleton lead to cell re-

TABLE 6–5. CHARACTERISTICS OF THE TOXINS OF *Clostridium difficile*

CHARACTERISTIC	ENTEROTOXIN (TOXIN A)	CYTOTOXIN (TOXIN B)
Primary action	Enterotoxic	Cytotoxic
Molecular weight range	308,000 (440,000–600,000)	270,000 (107,000–550,000)
Stability	Heat & acid labile	Heat & acid labile
	Inactivated by proteases	Inactivated by proteases
	Inactivated by pH = 2	Inactivated by pH = 2
Pathology	Lethal for mice (LD_{50} = 26 ng)	Less lethal for mice (LD_{50} = 1.5 μg)
	Intestinal fluid secretion	No increase in fluid secretion
	Vascular permeability increased	Vascular permeability increased
	Hemorrhagic enteritis	Hemorrhagic enteritis only at high concentrations
	Causes rounding of cells	Rounding of cells (1000× more than toxin A)
Binding site	Trisaccharide on outer brush border membranes	Binds to lower layers of mucosa
	Penetrates undamaged intestinal mucosa	No effect on undamaged intestinal mucosa
Mechanism	Binds to brush border membranes	Binds to lower layers in mucosa
	Stimulates endocytosis	
	Does not activate adenylate cyclase	Activates guanylate cyclase
	Disorganization of cell structure; nucleus shifted its polar location	Actin microfilament disruption Cell structure disorganized
	Opening of tight junction between rounded cells	Opening of tight junction between rounded cells
	Serum, proteins, & fluids leak into lumen	Serum, proteins, fluid leak into lumen
	Diarrhea results	Penetration of toxins into lower layers of mucosa
	Attracts PMC by releasing leukotriene β4 from epithelial cells or resident macrophages	
	Intracellular calcium increase	
	Attracts circulating neutrophils	
	Inflammatory mediators released	

SOURCE: Compiled from references 78, 80, 81, 83, 183, 184.

traction and rounding, accompanied by marginalization of the nucleus at a polar location.[83] Enterotoxin stimulates intracellular calcium release, which alters epithelial cell permeability without initially causing cell death.[84] The rounding of the cells, especially at the perijunctional ring, enhances tight junction permeability between the cells, allowing for the leakage of fluids and soluble components into the colonic lumen. In addition, deeper cell layers are exposed to the toxins from the lumen.[85] The pseudomembranes indicative of PMC are composed of neutrophils, coagulated serum proteins, mucus, and cellular debris. Once enterotoxin binds to the brush borders of epithelial cells, the inflammatory cells are attracted by the release of inflammatory mediators (leukotrienes, cytokines, and histamines). The intensity of the inflammatory response results in additional cellular damage and increased permeability observed in the toxin-damaged lamina propria.

Cytotoxin

By contrast, toxin B was found to be a potent cytotoxin, causing cytopathic effects at pico-

gram levels (1.5–5.0 pg/ml) but not inducing intestinal fluid accumulation, and it is much less lethal than toxin A (see Table 6–5).[77, 78] Cytotoxin appears to act in a manner similar to that of enterotoxin in that cytotoxin modifies the cells by disaggregating actin filaments and modifying actin-binding proteins.[83] The disruption of the cellular structure causes the cells to become rounded (Fig. 6–1).

Observations of the effects of these two toxins in animal models (hamsters, mice, and rats) showed that the toxins act synergistically.[86] When either purified enterotoxin or purified cytotoxin was given alone, no biologic effects were noted. Intragastric injection of toxin B caused fluid accumulation and hemorrhage only when small amounts of toxin A were coadministered or the cecum was bruised beforehand. Lyerly and colleagues hypothesized that toxin A must cause initial tissue damage and that toxin B acted upon deeper intestinal layers.[86]

Nontoxigenic strains of *C. difficile* have been infrequently isolated in diseased patients and asymptomatic carriers.[51, 87] Fluit and colleagues tested 39 toxigenic strains and 20 nontoxigenic

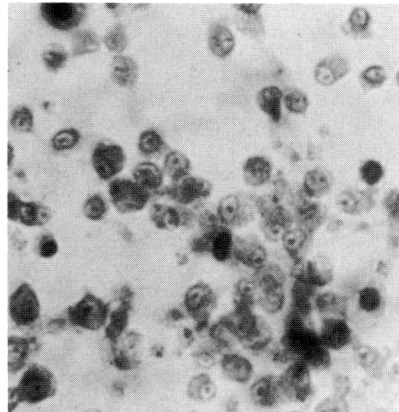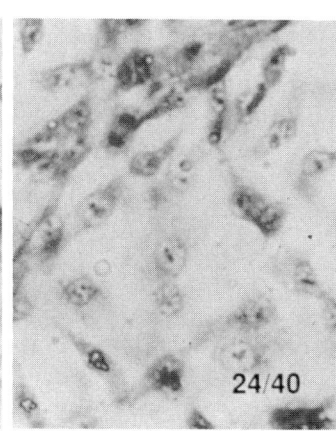

FIGURE 6–1.
Cytopathic effect of cytotoxin from *Clostridium difficile* on tissue culture monolayers. *A*, A monolayer with *C. difficile* cytotoxin and rounded fibroblastic cells; *B*, monolayer with no cytotoxin. (Courtesy of Dr Robert Fekety. Dept Infectious Diseases, University of Michigan, Ann Arbor.) [See also Color Plate 1]

strains, but only the toxigenic strains showed positive toxin A or B polymerase chain reactions.[88] No strains were found to produce only one of the toxins; either toxins A and B were coproduced or no toxins were found of either type. Nontoxigenic strains may perhaps lack the genes for toxin A and B, or a regulatory gene sequence or promoter may be lacking or inhibited. Interestingly, these nontoxigenic strains may be useful in reseeding the colon, since nontoxigenic strains are protective in mouse models of overgrowth by toxigenic strains of *C. difficile*.[89]

Risk Factors

A variety of factors increase the risk of infection and disease in hosts colonized with *C. difficile*.

Antibiotics

Specific antibiotics may predispose patients to acquire *C. difficile*, and yet, for reasons unknown, the asymptomatic carriage does not progress to clinical disease. A study of single intravenous prophylactic antibiotics given before surgery showed variation in carriage rates depending on whether the antibiotic was a cephalosporin (23.0%) or mezlocillin (3.3%) or whether the patient received no presurgical antibiotic (0%), but other studies failed to show an association with antibiotics and asymptomatic carriage.[15, 90]

Although virtually every type of antibiotic has been implicated in cases of *C. difficile* disease, antibiotics frequently associated with *C. difficile* diarrhea are clindamycin, ampicillin, and cephalosporins.[4, 18, 91] Both oral and parenteral routes of administration give rise to AAD, and no dose-response relationship is apparent in *C. difficile*

infections.[4] Diarrhea has been associated with other agents less frequently, for example, other penicillins, erythromycin, sulfamethoxazole-trimethoprim, and tetracycline.[92, 93] Broad-spectrum antibiotics such as clindamycin result in a longer duration of increased susceptibility to *C. difficile* colonization than do other antibiotics (cefuroxime and ampicillin), but almost every oral antibiotic has been associated with *C. difficile* disease.[94] *C. difficile* disease occasionally occurs in the absence of antibiotics and is presumably associated with factors described in the preantibiotic era, such as insulin-dependent diabetes mellitus, hepatic or renal failure, cystic fibrosis, cancer chemotherapy, and the recovery period after gastrointestinal tract surgery.[1, 22, 95]

Gastrointestinal Manipulations

A variety of procedures that affect the intestinal microbial flora predispose patients to infections with *C. difficile*. These procedures include repeated enemas, insertion of a nasogastric tube for longer than 2 days, and gastrointestinal tract surgery.[51, 96]

Similarly, medications given to decrease intestinal motility may produce an increase in the severity of symptoms. In a study by Trnka and LaMont, patients given atropine sulfate with diphenoxylate hydrochloride (Lomotil) or codeine for AAD had more pronounced diarrhea than did patients who did not receive these medications.[4] In addition, cathartics such as castor oil and vegetable oil given to hamsters increased intestinal motility and were protective against *C. difficile* enterocolitis.[5]

Age

Although the prevalence of positive cultures for *C. difficile* is highest in children younger than 2 years old, disease itself develops infrequently in this age group.[68, 97] Cases of pediatric PMC (age range 5 d to 17 yr) have been reported with a high case mortality rate (20%) owing to a delay in specific therapy because *C. difficile* was not a suspected pathogen in children.[98] The incidence of *C. difficile*–associated disease increases with age. Nash and colleagues found that 62% of patients with symptoms were older than 60 years of age.[99] In a survey made in Sweden from 1980 to 1982, 63% of patients were older than 60 years of age, but all age groups were represented.[20] In addition to increased antibiotic use in older patients, the presence of intestinal neoplasms, intestinal surgery, or other factors that influence the ability of the immune system to mount an effective response increases the susceptibility of older patients to this disease.[95, 96, 100]

Gender

A higher frequency of *C. difficile* disease has been reported to exist in women. A study by Pierce and colleagues showed that 60% of patients with AAC were female,[96] and Aronsson and colleagues reported that females had positive assays for cytotoxin 1.8 times as often as males.[20] These gender differences may reflect the differences in the use of broad-spectrum antibiotics to treat urogenital infections in women. Another study failed to find a significant difference in the gender distribution of patients with *C. difficile* disease.[51]

Cancer Chemotherapy

Patients who are undergoing chemotherapy for cancer and who have had no antibiotic exposure may be at increased risk of *C. difficile* disease.[101] Morris and colleagues surveyed 22 inpatients with malignant hematologic disorders who reported diarrhea; 36% were found to be harboring *C. difficile*.[100] Diarrhea resolved with vancomycin therapy, strengthening the association between *C. difficile* infections and AAD in patients with leukemia. Milligan and Kelly reported 5 fatal cases of PMC associated with *C. difficile* in patients with leukemia.[102] An increased incidence of *C. difficile*–associated disease in patients with leukemia may be caused by associated neutropenia. Neutrophils have been shown to inactivate toxin B in vitro; hence, patients with neutropenia may be more susceptible to *C. difficile* infections.[4] Neutropenic patients differ in their clinical presentation of AAC in that diarrhea and pseudomembranes are often absent, but ascites, jaundice, and severe necrotizing colitis are found.[103]

Renal Disorders

A variety of renal disorders have been associated with *C. difficile* infections.[104] Peiken and colleagues reported a case of PMC in a patient with membranoproliferative glomerulonephritis who had no antibiotic exposure.[105] Renal disorders may be associated with *C. difficile* infections as a result of changes in bowel flora that have been seen in patients with uremia when the serum creatinine concentration was greater than 6 mg/dl.[106]

DIAGNOSIS OF *Clostridium difficile* DISEASE

Unfortunately, the signs and symptoms of *C. difficile* disease are not sufficiently distinctive to allow a diagnosis based solely on clinical presentation. An accurate diagnosis must be based on four factors: microbiologic laboratory assays indicating the presence of *C. difficile* or its toxins; clinical symptoms with confirmation of colitis by sigmoidoscopy when appropriate; exclusion of other causes of diarrhea; and presence of risk factors, such as antibiotic use, advanced age, or procedures that disrupt normal bowel flora. If a patient has been hospitalized for more than 2 days, has been exposed to antibiotics, and develops diarrhea, the first diagnostic test should be for *C. difficile*. Normal stool pathogens (parasites, *Shigella*, *Salmonella*) are not found to be the most frequent causes of nosocomial diarrhea in the absence of specific outbreaks of infection due to those organisms.[107] *Clostridium difficile* is the prevalent agent of nosocomial diarrhea, especially in patients who have had antibiotic therapy.[2, 108, 109]

Microbiologic Cultures

Clostridium difficile is a fastidious anaerobic bacterium that must be cultured into anaerobic conditions quickly. Failure to culture *C. difficile* organisms from patients who are actually infected may be due to delays in transport or processing of the specimens. Fresh stool or rectal swabs held in an anaerobic transport medium should be cultured and incubated anaerobically within 1 to 3 hours or refrigerated if processing will be delayed.[110] Studies have shown that cytotoxin titers decrease over several days when held at 22 to 27°C and that freezing stools decreases the viability counts of *C. difficile*.[111, 112]

The search for an assay for *C. difficile* that is

both highly accurate and rapid has not been an easy task. The most sensitive procedures require either 2 to 3 days' processing time or specialized laboratory equipment not available at all hospitals. The most rapid assays suffer from a lack of specificity and may lead to erroneous diagnosis if not confirmed by other assays. The most sensitive and specific tests for the isolation of *C. difficile* organisms include selective plate or enrichment broth cultures followed by a confirmatory identification test.

Cultures for *Clostridium difficile*

Selective and Differential Media. The lack of selective and differential media hindered the association of *C. difficile* infection with clinically apparent disease for many years. In 1979 George and colleagues developed a cefoxitin-cycloserine-fructose agar (CCFA) that selectively inhibited the growth of other enteric anaerobes and allowed *C. difficile* to be differentiated from other clostridia.[113] After 24 to 48 hours' incubation in anaerobic conditions on the CCFA medium, *C. difficile* colonies appear yellowish white, emit golden yellow fluorescence under ultraviolet light, have a distinctive "elephant house" odor, and have a ground-glass appearance under magnification.[114] Unfortunately, these characteristics are not unique to *C. difficile*.

Efforts to improve the selectivity of the medium have included lowering the level of cycloserine, adding sheep erythrocytes, and adding 0.1% sodium taurocholate.[115–117] *Clostridium difficile* colonies impart a greenish hue to the blood agar, and taurocholate increases the isolation rate by stimulating spore germination. The limits of detection of solid plate medium (<1000 *C. difficile* organisms per ml or g of stool) renders it insensitive in detecting low concentrations of *C. difficile* organisms typically found in carriers or environmental samples.[114] In laboratories that do not have access to selective media, methods such as heat- or alcohol-shocked broths have been used to select for spores, but they are not differential for *C. difficile*.[118, 119]

Broth Cultures. To increase the detection rate of *C. difficile*, some clinical laboratories also inoculate stool into a selective enrichment broth containing sodium taurocholate and particular antibiotics with an incubation of 72 hours at 35°C. The broth culture allows lower levels of *C. difficile* colonization to be detected and additional spores to germinate.[117] Studies using broth cultures have been reported to have an increased recovery rate, ranging from 18 to 24%, over plate cultures alone.[111, 120] The advantages of using a broth culture are its increased

ability to detect lower levels of *C. difficile* organisms and its use as a confirmatory identification method using gas liquid chromatography (GLC) methods. Production of isocaproic acid and other fatty acids has been used to identify *C. difficile*, resulting in high rates of sensitivity (61–99.6%) and specificity (95–99%).[111, 120–122]

Biochemical Panels. Another highly sensitive way to identify *C. difficile* is the use of biochemical panels that use purified cultures and fermentation patterns to determine species identification. Head and Ratnam compared 4 biochemical panels and found different sensitivities depending on the kit used: 77.9% for AN-Ident (Analytab Products, Plainview NY), 88.6% for RapID-ANA (Innovative Diagnostic Systems, Decatur GA), 90.9% for Minitek Anaerobe II (BBL Microbiology Systems, Cockeysville MD), 95.5% for API 20A (Analytab Products, Plainview NY).[123]

Gas-Liquid Chromatography. Studies of other methods to detect *C. difficile* have also included use of species-specific oligonucleotide probes for ribosomal ribonucleic acid (rRNA) of *C. difficile*, a dot immunobinding assay, and other improved GLC techniques.[124–126] Microbiologic culture is still the most accurate assay for the detection of *C. difficile*, but the disadvantages are its 24- to 48-hour processing time and the requirement for anaerobic microbiologic techniques.

Latex Agglutination Assay. In hospitals and clinics with limited laboratory facilities, the rapid latex agglutination assay (LAT) has been used. The LAT was initially marketed to detect the enterotoxin, but Lyerly and Wilkins and their colleagues, who were working on purifying the enterotoxin, reported that it did not detect purified enterotoxin but rather another *C. difficile* protein.[79, 127, 128] This protein was later found to be a glutamate dehydrogenase that is also found in other bacterial species.[129] Although the LAT maintains its role as an initial, rapid screening test for *C. difficile*, caution must be exercised because the LAT is falsely positive for other bacteria (*Clostridium sporogenes*, *Peptostreptococcus anaerobius*, *Bacteroides asaccharolyticus*, *Salmonella enteritidis*, *Shigella boydii*), and parasites (*Blastocystis hominis* and *Giardia lamblia*).[130, 131] False-positive findings reportedly range from 1 to 32%, and the sensitivity of the latex assay ranges from 68 to 90%.[109, 125, 131]

The frequency of positive findings for *C. difficile* cultures is dependent upon the severity of the disease (Table 6–6). Most patients (86–100%) with PMC have positive *C. difficile* cultures, and the majority of AAC patients are found to carry *C. difficile* (60–85%). In patients

TABLE 6–6. FREQUENCY OF POSITIVE DIAGNOSTIC TESTS FOR *Clostridium difficile*

Clostridium difficile POSITIVE	CULTURE	CYTOTOXIN	ENTEROTOXIN
Carriers	10–46%	2–25%	ND
Diarrhea	11–33%	2–25%	62%
	92%	88%	
	75%	66%	
		15–25%	
Colitis	60–75%	32–44%	ND
	85%	90%	
		50–75%	
Pseudo- membranous colitis	86–100%	83–100% 57%	
Healthy neonates	29–62%	40–100% 27%	ND

KEY: ND = not determined, PMC = pseudomembranous colitis.
SOURCE: Compiled from references 1, 114, 144, 185.

with simple colonization or benign diarrhea, approximately one half have positive findings for *C. difficile.*

Toxin Assays

Cytotoxin. The cytotoxin assay detects toxins capable of causing a cytopathic effect (CPE) in tissue culture cell lines after 24 to 48 hours' incubation. The choice of cell lines is wide because the CPE of *C. difficile* cytotoxin is evident in many cell lines.[112, 132] For the cytotoxin assay to be specific, neutralization tests using *Clostridium sordellii* antitoxin, which cross-reacts with the *C. difficile* cytotoxin, must be used as a negative control, and diluted stool (1:10–1:100) should be used because undiluted stool is cytopathic on most cell lines. Cytotoxin is readily detected in diluted stool because the limit of detection has been found to be 3–5 ng/ml, but it has been discovered that as little as 1 to 2 pg (10^{-12} g) can result in cell rounding in some cell lines.[1, 4, 51] A sample of the stool is homogenized, centrifuged, and filtered, and then the cell-free supernatant is added to the cell monolayer and incubated for 24 to 48 hours. Positive cytotoxin samples show a rounding of the cells and a thinning of the cytoplasmic projections used for adherence to the plastic plate (see Fig. 6–1). Negative cytotoxin samples and the control with *C. sordellii* antitoxin show the normal rounded cells. The disadvantages of the cytotoxin assays are that they are not standardized, since different procedures and cell lines and varying fecal concentrations are used; not all laboratories test for specificity using *C. sordellii* antitoxin neutralization; and the choice of

added antibiotics and growth media may affect the production of cytotoxin.[133] Although the cytotoxin assay is portrayed as the "gold standard" for the diagnosis of *C. difficile* disease, the limitations of this assay arise from the significant number of cytotoxin-positive cultures in patients who carry *C. difficile* but who are asymptomatic, and conversely, the significant number of patients who have *C. difficile* disease but produce cytotoxin-negative findings.[51, 87] The disadvantages of tissue culture assays are that they require specialized facilities, the assay cost of $30 to $40 is high, and results have a 24- to 48-hour turnaround time.

Other methods for cytotoxin detection include counterimmunoelectrophoresis (CIE), latex particle agglutination (LPA), and enzyme-linked immunosorbent assay (ELISA), but all these developing assays either lack high sensitivities or are highly technical procedures. The CIE method has been found to have a high rate of false-positive (24–33%) and false-negative (15–75%) findings by several researchers and thus has not been pursued as an accurate method.[134, 135] The LPA test had a positive predictive value of only 68% compared with cytotoxin tissue culture assays.[136] The ELISA assays for cytotoxin are sensitive to 0.1 ng of toxin, but sensitivity may range from 80 to 85%.[137]

The cytotoxin assay becomes more closely correlated with disease as the severity of symptoms increases (see Table 6–6). Interestingly, the titer of stool cytotoxin is not predictive of the severity of disease and is not a useful diagnostic tool for physicians.[51, 138, 139] In patients with PMC, 57 to 100% have positive cytotoxin assays; in patients with AAC, 32 to 90% have positive cytotoxin assays; in patients with AAD, 2 to 88% have positive results; and asymptomatic carriers can have 2 to 25% positive findings.[140] Negative cytotoxin assays may be true negatives or they may be the result of poor specimen processing, for example, a delayed transport time or titers below detection levels.

Enterotoxin. Lack of a useful assay for enterotoxin has hindered examination of this toxin in the pathogenesis and prevalence of *C. difficile* disease. Early assays for enterotoxin were entirely for research laboratories and used the ELISA method, with sensitivity ranging from 80 to 98.6% and specificity of 96 to 100%.[137, 141, 142] The limits of ELISA tests are approximately 0.2 mg/ml.[51] Other research tools for detecting the presence of *C. difficile* include the use of a rapid and inexpensive dot immunobinding assay (C. diff-CUBE (Difco Laboratories, Ann Arbor MI) and toxin probes for the detection of enterotoxin. In one study, the dot immunobinding assay agreed with 92% of the positive cytotoxin assay results and 88% of the LAT assays.[125] Gene-specific probes for toxin A have been used that detect only toxin A–producing *C. difficile* strains and have limited value if the patient is infected with an enterotoxin-negative strain of *C. difficile*.[143] The main disadvantages of ELISA and probes are the expense, the high degree of technical expertise required, and the 48-hour delay until results are obtained. Several commercial kits for enterotoxin that have been tested are rapid (<3 h) in processing time and easy to use, but their accuracy varies with their ability to correlate well with standard cytotoxin assays. Holter and colleagues tested 179 samples using the VIDAS CDA (Vitek Systems, Hazelwood MO) test and found a 70% correlation with positive cytotoxin assays, a sensitivity of 62%, and a specificity of 75%, but a positive predictive value of only 44%.[144] Doern and others tested another rapid (2.5 h) enzyme immunoassay kit (Premier *C. difficile*–Toxin A, Meridian Diagnostics, Cincinnati OH) and compared the results to cytotoxin assays. Sensitivity ranged from 61 to 68%, and specificity ranged from 99.5 to 100%.[145]

Until an accurate and sensitive enterotoxin assay is available commercially and tested widely in large populations, the predictive value and prevalence of enterotoxin relative to *C. difficile* remain undetermined.

Colonoscopic Examination

Antibiotic-associated diarrhea is defined as diarrhea with no histologic abnormalities seen by microscopy. Examination by colonoscopy of patients with AAC may reveal areas of edema, hyperemia, friability, or frank hemorrhage. Areas of inflammation may be observed in all or part of the colon with rectal sparing reported in only 10 to 20% of the patients.[146]

The site of infection in the colon may be proximal, distal, or universal. Earlier studies in which AAC was diagnosed with a sigmoidoscope may have missed lesions beyond the range of the scope. For this reason, the use of a flexible sigmoidoscope or colonoscope is recommended for diagnosis.[146] The symptoms and histologic changes are common to *C. difficile* infections and IBD such as Crohn's disease and ulcerative colitis. Unlike ulcerative colitis, which usually extends proximally from the rectum, distribution of inflammatory sites in AAC is patchy, and the rectum may be spared.[147] Discriminating criteria of *C. difficile* infections include the association with antibiotics, the resolution of diarrhea

in response to vancomycin, and the lack of response to corticosteroids.[5, 91]

The principal criterion that differentiates AAC from antibiotic-associated PMC is the presence of pseudomembranes in the colon in PMC. Diagnosis is made by sigmoidoscopic or colonoscopic examination. Raised white-yellow-green adherent plaques 2 to 8 mm in diameter up to as large as 20 mm are observed. Coalescence of several plaques may produce the classic pseudomembrane. The plaques are made of fibrin, mucin, polymorphonuclear neutrophil leukocytes (PMN), and epithelial debris. The mucosa between plaques may appear normal, slightly hyperemic, or edematous. Histologic examination reveals that the lamina propria of the mucosal layer is infiltrated with inflammatory cells.

The spectrum of pathologic changes has been divided into three categories.[148] The mildest form of PMC disease (type I) shows focal necrosis with PMN infiltrates and eosinophilic exudate restricted to the interglandular surface epithelium and the lamina propria. Summitlike "volcano" lesions are observed that result from the eruption of PMN and fibrin from the necrotic focus. The summitlike lesions occur immediately beneath the surface epithelium between glandular openings. The lamina propria may contain eosinophilic material and debris. The summitlike lesions of PMC occur adjacent to normal mucosa with a minimum of inflammatory changes (Fig. 6–2). Crohn's disease and ulcerative colitis rarely exhibit these summitlike lesions, but the mucosa is more inflamed and damaged than in PMC disease.

In the second category of PMC disease (type II), well-defined groups of disrupted glands have been distended by mucin and PMN cell infiltrate. As much as half the superficial epithelial lining may be gone. The damaged glands are surrounded by epithelial debris, fibrin, mucus, and PMNs, and a convergent pseudomembrane begins to appear. The inflammatory changes are limited to the superficial layers of the lamina propria. The areas between focal eruptions and plaque formation still appear normal.

In the most severe stage of PMC disease (type III), the inflammatory changes have progressed deeper into the lamina propria, and complete structural mucosal necrosis is seen (Fig. 6–3). Plaques merge to become a confluent layer of pseudomembrane (Fig. 6–4). When a confluent pseudomembrane is present, distinguishing it from other necrotic forms of colitis may be difficult. The yellow appearance of the necrotic

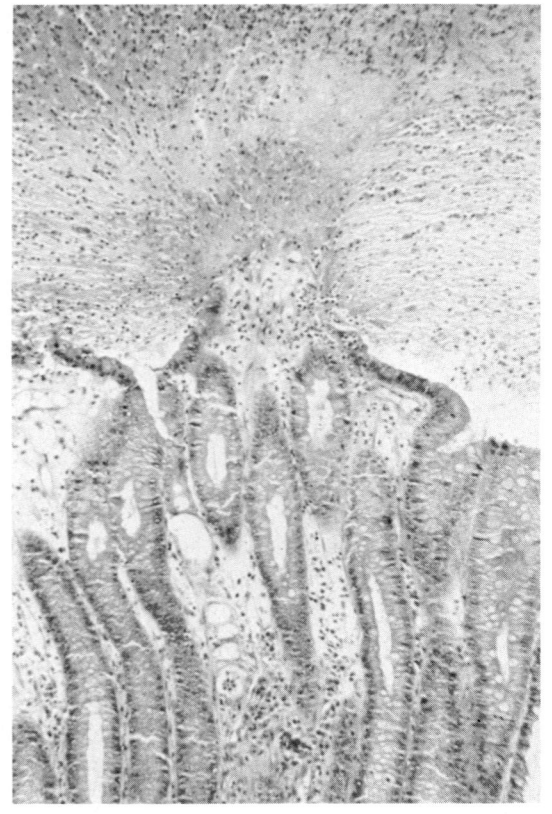

FIGURE 6–2.
Summitlike lesion noted in a rectal biopsy from a patient with
C. difficile colitis. (Courtesy of Dr Christina Surawicz. Dept of
Medicine, University of Washington, Seattle.) [See also Color
Plate 1]

mucosa can mimic other forms of ischemic colitis and is not by itself diagnostic of PMC.

The proper diagnosis is contingent upon the
use of a flexible sigmoidoscope or colonoscope

due to the presence of rectal sparing.[149] In addition, the small local plaques of type I PMC
can easily be missed by sigmoidoscopic examination. Seppala and colleagues found characteristic plaques in 31% of patients with suspected
PMC using a sigmoidoscope, but 85% were diagnosed if a colonoscopic examination was performed.[146] In a study of 96 patients with suspected PMC, pseudomembranes were found in
32 of 66 patients (48%) examined by a rigid
sigmoidoscope, 2 of 5 patients (40%) by colonoscopic examination, and only 5 of 25 patients
(20%) examined by a rigid proctoscope.[60]

Plain abdominal films are not valuable in the
diagnosis of *C. difficile* disease. Positive findings
are observed only in cases of severe PMC associated with toxic megacolon. Typical features
are mucosal thickening and ''thumbprinting,''
but these features are also seen with ischemia or
IBD. Computed tomographic (CT) scans of the
abdomen or radionuclide tests, such as indium-
labeled leukocyte or gallium citrate scans, can
be helpful in some patients.[22] Barium enemas
are not a useful diagnostic tool for PMC, since
the mucosal changes are too superficial to be
detected, and this procedure is liable to have a
detrimental effect in patients with toxic megacolon.

Exclusion of Other Causes

Other known causes of diarrhea and colitis
must be excluded without fail when diagnosing
C. difficile disease. These other causes may be
other infectious agents or an acute episode of a
chronic condition, or they may be drug-induced
or procedure-related. Infectious agents that pro-

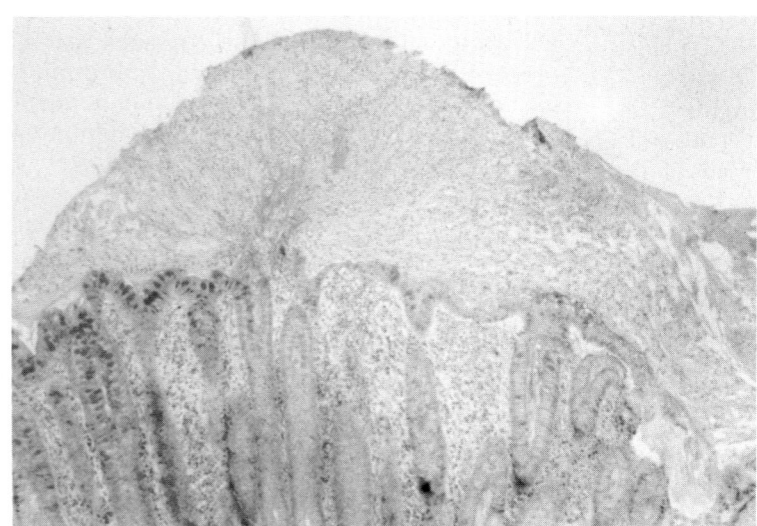

FIGURE 6–3.
Histologic appearance of pseudomembrane. (Courtesy of Dr Christina Surawicz.
Dept of Medicine, University of Washington, Seattle.) [See also Color Plate 1]

duce clinically similar colitis profiles include *Shigella, Salmonella, Campylobacter, Candida* and *Escherichia coli* (O157:H7) and other amebic, fungal, or viral agents.[150–152]

Colitis or diarrhea may also be induced by a wide variety of medications, including alcohol, gold, vasopressin, salicylates, cyclosporine, and methotrexate, or by disinfectant solutions used for cleaning endoscopes.[150, 153] As many as 10% of colitis cases have been associated with nonsteroidal anti-inflammatory drugs and not with *C. difficile*.[150, 153] Patients who chronically use enemas (soap, phosphate, or sorbitol) have developed colitis.[150] Chronic conditions may also cause acute episodes of diarrhea that are clinically similar to *C. difficile* disease, such as Crohn's disease, collagenous colitis, diverticulitis, and ischemic colitis.[150]

If *C. difficile* is found to be associated with these causes, determining the real inciting agent responsible for the colitis or diarrhea may be difficult, since *C. difficile* may be causing the disease or may simply be present without causing symptoms.

TREATMENT

Six strategies of treatment of *C. difficile*–associated disease have been used: discontinuation

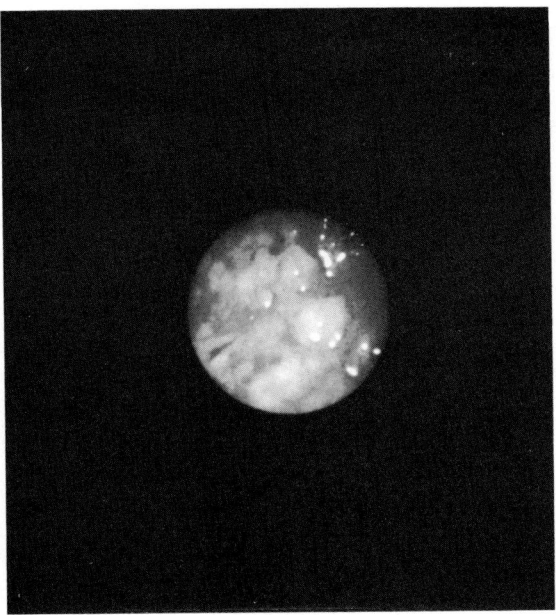

FIGURE 6–4.
Gross appearance of pseudomembrane in a patient with *C. difficile*–associated pseudomembranous colitis. (Courtesy of Dr Christina Surawicz. Dept of Medicine, University of Washington, Seattle.) [See also Color Plate 1]

of the inducing agent, use of antibiotic therapy directed against *C. difficile*, use of resin binders, replacement of the normal colonic flora, use of biotherapeutic agents, and antitoxin therapy.

The aggressiveness of treatment for *C. difficile* disease is dependent upon the severity of symptoms. Asymptomatic carriers are not generally treated, because most patients do not progress to symptomatic disease.[2] The major threat posed by carriers is as a source of nosocomial transmission to other, susceptible patients.

For uncomplicated diarrhea, a conservative approach is recommended, consisting of cessation of the inciting antibiotic and oral rehydration to compensate for fluid loss. In approximately one third of untreated cases of AAD, the diarrhea resolves in 7 to 28 days.[154] Mild diarrhea may be controlled with bismuth subsalicylate.[155]

In patients with moderate diarrhea (1–2 L/d) and low-grade fever of 100 to 101°F (37.8–38.3°C), either metronidazole or vancomycin can be given to eradicate *C. difficile* organisms. Metronidazole was given by Cherry and colleagues to patients in a dosage of 2 g a day by mouth for 10 days. They found that symptoms resolved in 1 to 5 days with a relapse rate of only 15%.[156] Metronidazole has the advantage of being less expensive than vancomycin. A typical course of treatment (1.5–2.0 g/d for 10 d) ranges in price from $5 to $90, compared with a 10-day course of 125 mg qid of vancomycin, which costs approximately $115 to $150.[22] In contrast to vancomycin, metronidazole is absorbed well after oral administration, and the obtainable fecal concentration is much lower than that of vancomycin. The clinical relevance of this observation is uncertain, inasmuch as comparative trials have shown vancomycin and metronidazole to be equally effective. A randomized clinical trial by Teasley and colleagues found that 2 of 42 patients (5%) given metronidazole and none of the 52 patients given vancomycin failed to respond to therapy, but that the relapse rate was higher for vancomycin (11% vs 4%) than with metronidazole.[28] Disadvantages of metronidazole therapy are the adverse reactions associated with its use. Nausea, vomiting, and an unpleasant metallic taste are common, and peripheral neuropathy has reportedly been associated with prolonged use of metronidazole.

Vancomycin, which has been extensively studied, is absorbed poorly when given orally, and high fecal concentrations (2000–5000 µg/ml) are found in patients given 2 g a day.[157] All strains of *C. difficile* are sensitive to vancomycin in vitro at concentrations of 16 µg/ml or less.

The symptoms of diarrhea and abdominal pain and the patient's fever usually decline within 48 hours of institution of vancomycin therapy, and most diarrheal symptoms completely resolve in 2 to 15 days.[158] Bartlett's treatment of 189 patients with 2 g a day of vancomycin showed an initial effectiveness of 97%.[18] Initial response rates have ranged from 95 to 100% in most studies.[4] Recurrences of disease (in 2–21 days, with a median of 6 days) after discontinuation of vancomycin are found in 12 to 24% of patients who have received treatment, and multiple relapses were reported in 11% of patients.[4, 158]

The recommended initial dose for vancomycin is 125 mg qid for 10 days given orally. Higher doses (500 mg qid) were not shown to be more effective and are significantly more expensive.[158] When oral antibiotics cannot be given, intravenous metronidazole or vancomycin may be given, but the effectiveness is uncertain.[159] Owing to the comparable effectiveness of metronidazole and vancomycin, vancomycin is generally reserved for patients with colitis, PMC, or recurrent disease.

Bacitracin has been used to treat these infections, but little experience with this drug has been published. Although limited studies have shown it to be as effective as vancomycin or metronidazole, the disadvantages of its unpleasant taste and production of nausea have argued against its use.[27]

Teicoplanin (200 mg, tid for 1 d, bid for 8 d) was compared with vancomycin (500 mg qid for 10 d) in 47 patients with *C. difficile* disease. All patients initially responded, but 3 of the 23 vancomycin patients (13%) suffered recurrences, and none of the patients in the teicoplanin group had a recurrence.[160] Further clinical trials using teicoplanin may determine whether this glycopeptide antibiotic could be a useful alternative treatment to vancomycin or metronidazole.

Anion-exchange resins (colestipol and cholestyramine) have been shown to bind both toxin A and toxin B of *C. difficile*, but conflicting estimates of the effectiveness are reported in the literature.[161] Anion-exchange resins (4 g tid po) probably should be used only in patients with mild diarrhea until more convincing evidence of efficacy in severe cases is obtained.

Since *C. difficile* disease is a result of the disruption of normal colonic bowel flora, an early attempt at treatment was the use of fecal enemas.[162] The marginal effectiveness combined with the low patient acceptance has limited this form of treatment. In addition, the risk of transferring unapparent pathogens from donor to recipient is not a trivial issue.

Another potential mode of therapy involves reseeding the susceptible colon with protective bacterial flora after antibiotic therapy has been stopped. Certain species of bacteria are reportedly inhibitory to *C. difficile* and have been used to reseed the colon.[163] One commercial preparation (Lactinex; Hynson, Westcott & Dunning, Baltimore MD) containing lactobacilli was not found to be effective in preventing amoxicillin-induced diarrhea.[164] *Lactobacillus* GG containing yoghurt was found to reduce erythromycin-associated diarrhea in a small study.[165] *Saccharomyces boulardii* has been shown to be effective in preventing antibiotic-associated diarrhea when taken in conjunction with the antibiotics that may predispose a patient to the development of diarrhea. In one study of 180 patients, 22% of the placebo-treated group developed diarrhea, while only 9.5% of the *S. boulardii*–treated group developed AAD.[56] *Saccharomyces boulardii* was also used as an adjunct treatment with vancomycin in patients with relapsing PMC and successfully prevented further recurrences in 85% of those patients in an open study.[30]

The use of antitoxin for the treatment of PMC has been studied only in animal models. In studies using hamsters, *Clostridium sordellii* antitoxin (which cross-reacts with toxins A and B) was not effective in treating enterocolitis.[18] The development of a toxoid to toxins A and B may be of value, but to date no such toxoid is available.

Optimal treatment of *C. difficile* disease must be tailored to the severity of the clinical illness. If the patient is only mildly ill, the inciting antibiotic can be discontinued and replaced with an antibiotic not often associated with *C. difficile* diseases. In the milder cases of diarrhea or colitis, the offending agent should be stopped and therapy with metronidazole or vancomycin started. If the patient has symptomatic PMC, vancomycin should be given. Careful attention to fluid and electrolyte replacement is needed. For patients experiencing recurrent episodes of *C. difficile* diarrhea due to PMC, the range of treatment is wide. A second course of either vancomycin or metronidazole is usually successful. Tapering or pulsed doses of either antibiotic have been used when *C. difficile* eradication has proved recalcitrant. The addition of biotherapeutic agents to help stabilize normal bowel flora and reestablish colonization resistance may prove to be an exciting adjunct to antibiotic treatments.

PREVENTION

The key to preventing *C. difficile* disease is to disrupt the epidemiologic transmission and promptly treat symptomatic patients to limit dissemination of *C. difficile* into the environment. Person-to-person transmission may be diminished by decreasing the number of infected sources and instituting proper infection control practices. Interventions involving the establishment of universal body substance procedures have resulted in the control of outbreaks in hospitals. Patients who have poor hygiene or are incapacitated should receive special attention by the hospital staff to prevent cross-infection of adjacent patients. Proper and thorough hand-washing techniques by hospital personnel are critical, because studies indicate that hand carriage of *C. difficile* may be a means of transmission of infection to susceptible patients. Alternatively, interventions using vinyl gloves in one study showed a decrease of *C. difficile* diarrhea from 7.7 of 1000 discharged patients to 1.5 of 1000, indicating the effectiveness of breaking the chain of transmission as a control mechanism for *C. difficile* in the hospital.[13]

Indirect transmission through contaminated environmental sites must be controlled by proper decontamination methods that destroy the vegetative cells and, more importantly, the spores of *C. difficile*. Once an outbreak occurs in a hospital, the wide environmental contamination by *C. difficile* spores through its many routes of transmission allows this pathogen to become entrenched as an endemic nosocomial organism that may result in recurring outbreaks. At the end of an outbreak, it is necessary to decontaminate the environment thoroughly. The spores generally are resistant to the quaternary ammoniacal or phenolic agents used as routine disinfectants. A 2% solution of alkaline glutaraldehyde or phosphate-buffered alkaline hypochlorite solution (1600 ppm) has been found to be effective in killing *C. difficile* spores. Caution must be exercised with both these compounds, since glutaraldehyde has been found to be carcinogenic, and hypochlorite solutions may be corrosive to some surfaces. Potential environmental sources of *C. difficile*, such as shared bathrooms, commode chairs, nasogastric suction devices, and sigmoidoscopic equipment, should be cleaned and disinfected between uses.[59] Any piece of equipment that has been exposed to the colonic flora must be sterilized between uses.

Finally, more judicious use of broad-spectrum antibiotics may prevent cases of *C. difficile* disease. In institutions where these infections are highly prevalent, an antibiotic audit leading to measures to control antibiotic use more carefully may be of value.

REFERENCES

1. Bartlett JG. *Clostridium difficile*: Clinical considerations. Rev Infect Dis. 1990;12:S243–S251.
2. McFarland LV, Mulligan ME, Kwok RY, Stamm WE. Nosocomial acquisition of *Clostridium difficile* infection. N Engl J Med. 1989;320:204–210.
3. Finney JMT. Gastro-enterostomy for cicatrizing ulcer of the pylorus. Johns Hopkins Med J. 1893;4:53–55.
4. Trnka YM, LaMont JT. *Clostridium difficile* colitis. Adv Intern Med. 1984;29:85–107.
5. Terplan K, Paine JR, Sheffer J, et al. Fulminating gastroenterocolitis caused by staphylococci. Gastroenterology. 1953;24:476–509.
6. Tedesco FJ, Barton RW, Alpers DH. Clindamycin-associated colitis. Ann Intern Med. 1974;81:429–433.
7. Hall IC, O'Toole E. Intestinal flora in new-born infants, with a description of a new pathogenic anaerobe: *Bacillus difficilis*. Am J Dis Child. 1935;49:390–402.
8. Hafiz S. *Clostridium difficile* and its toxins. Leeds, UK: University of Leeds; 1974, PhD dissertation.
9. Green RH. The association of viral activation with penicillin toxicity in guinea pigs and hamsters. Yale J Biol Med. 1974;47:166–181.
10. Bartlett JG, Chang TW, Gurwith M, et al. Antibiotic-associated pseudomembranous colitis due to toxin-producing clostridia. N Engl J Med. 1978;298:531–534.
11. Larson HE, Parry JV, Price AB, et al. Undescribed toxin in pseudomembranous colitis. Br Med J. 1977;1:1246–1248.
12. Fekety R. Blazevic DJ, McCarty LR, and Morello JA, eds. Antibiotic-Associated Colitis: Clinical Microbiology Newsletter. Boston: GK Hall; 1978.
13. Johnson S, Gerding DN, Olson MM, et al. Prospective, controlled study of vinyl glove use to interrupt *Clostridium difficile* nosocomial transmission. Am J Med. 1990;88:137–140.
14. George RH. The carrier state: *Clostridium difficile*. J Antimicrob Chemother. 1986;18:47–58.
15. McFarland LV, Surawicz CM, Stamm WE. Risk factors for *Clostridium difficile* carriage and *C. difficile*–associated diarrhea in a cohort of hospitalized patients. J Infect Dis. 1990;162:678–684.
16. Ramirez-Ronda CH. Incidence of clindamycin-associated colitis: Comments and corrections. Ann Intern Med. 1974;81:860.
17. Brause BD, Romankiewicz JA, Gotz V, et al. Comparative study of diarrhea associated with clindamycin and ampicillin therapy. Am J Gastroenterol. 1980;73:244–248.
18. Bartlett JG. Antibiotic-associated colitis: Dis Mon. 1984;30:1–54.
19. Riley TV, Bowman RA, Carroll SM. Diarrhoea associated with *Clostridium difficile* in a hospital population. Med J Aust. 1983;1:166–169.
20. Aronsson B, Mollby R, Nord CE. Antimicrobial agents and *Clostridium difficile* in acute enteric disease: Epidemiological data from Sweden, 1980–82. J Infect Dis. 1985;151:476–481.
21. Bartlett JG. AAPMC. Hosp Pract (Off Ed). 1981;16:85–95.
22. Silva J. Update of pseudomembranous colitis. West J Med. 1989;151:644–648.

23. Suppaiah L. Pseudomembranous colitis induced by *Clostridium difficile.* Crit Care Nurse. 1988;8:65–72.

24. Mogg GAG, Keighley MRB, Burdon DW, et al. Antibiotic-associated colitis: A review of 66 cases. Br J Surg. 1979;66:738–742.

25. Parasakthi N, Puthucheary SD, Goh KL, et al. *Clostridium difficile* associated diarrhoea: A report of seven cases. Singapore Med J. 1988;29:504–507.

26. McKay I, Coia JE, Poxton IR. Typing of *Clostridium difficile* causing diarrhoea in an orthopaedic ward. J Clin Pathol. 1989;42:511–515.

27. Young GP, Ward PB, Bayley N, et al. Antibiotic-associated colitis due to *Clostridium difficile:* Double blind comparison of vancomycin with bacitracin. Gastroenterology. 1985;89:1038–1045.

28. Teasley DG, Gerding DN, Olson MM, et al. Prospective randomized trial of metronidazole versus vancomycin for *Clostridium difficile* diarrhea and colitis. Lancet. 1983;1:1843–1846.

29. Kimmey MB, Elmer GW, Surawicz CM, et al. Prevention of further recurrences of *Clostridium difficile* colitis with *Saccharomyces boulardii.* Dig Dis Sci. 1990;35:897–901.

30. Surawicz CM, McFarland LV, Elmer G, et al. Treatment of recurrent *Clostridium difficile* colitis with vancomycin and *Saccharomyces boulardii.* Am J Gastroenterol. 1989;84:1285–1287.

31. Johnson S, Adelmann A, Clabots CR, et al. Recurrences of *Clostridium difficile* diarrhea not caused by the original infecting organism. J Infect Dis. 1989;159:340–343.

32. Satin AJ, Harrison CR, Hancock KC, et al. Relapsing *Clostridium difficile* toxin-associated colitis in ovarian cancer patients treated with chemotherapy. Obstet Gynecol. 1989;74:487–489.

33. Bennett RG, Greenough WB III: *Clostridium difficile* diarrhea: A common—and overlooked—nursing home infection. Geriatrics. 1990;45:77–87.

34. Rybolt AH, Bennett RG, Laughon BE, et al. Protein-losing enteropathy associated with *Clostridium difficile* infection. Lancet. 1989;1:1353–1355.

35. Bartlett JG. *Clostridium difficile* and IBD. Gastroenterology. 1981;80:863–865.

36. LaMont JT, Trnka YM. Therapeutic implications of *Clostridium difficile* toxin during relapse of chronic inflammatory bowel disease. Lancet. 1980;1:381.

37. Bolton RP, Sherriff RJ, Read AE. *Clostridium difficile* associated diarrhea: A role in IBD? Lancet. 1980;1:383.

38. Meyers S, Mayer L, Bottone E, et al. Occurrence of *Clostridium difficile* toxin during the course of inflammatory bowel disease. Gastroenterology. 1981;80:697–700.

39. Morris JB, Zollinger RM, Stellato TA. Role of surgery in antibiotic-induced pseudomembranous enterocolitis. Am J Surg. 1990;160:535–539.

40. Burke GW, Wilson ME, Mehrez IO. Absence of diarrhea in toxic megacolon complicating *Clostridium difficile* pseudomembranous colitis. Am J Gastroenterol. 1988;83:304–307.

41. Triadafilopoulos G, Hallstone AE. Acute abdomen as the first presentation of pseudomembranous colitis. Gastroenterology. 1991;101:685–691.

42. Hannonen P, Hakola M, Mottonen T, et al. Reactive oligoarthritis associated with *Clostridium difficile* colitis. Scand J Rheumatol. 1989;18:57–60.

43. Riley TV, Karthigasu KT. Chronic osteomyelitis due to *Clostridium difficile.* Br Med J. 1982;284:1217–1218.

44. Incavo SJ, Muller DL, Krag MH, et al. Vertebral osteomyelitis caused by *Clostridium difficile:* A case report and review of the literature. Spine. 1988;13:111–113.

45. Arnon SS, Mills DC, Day PA, et al. Rapid death of infant rhesus monkeys injected with *Clostridium difficile* toxins A and B: Physiologic and pathologic basis. J Pediatr. 1984;104:34–40.

46. Gerard M, Defresne N, Van der Auwera P, et al. Polymicrobial septicemia with *Clostridium difficile* in acute diverticulitis. Eur J Clin Microbiol Infect Dis. 1989;8:300–302.

47. Saginur R, Fogel R, Begin L, et al. Splenic abscess due to *Clostridium difficile.* J Infect Dis. 1983;147:1105.

48. Sofianou DC. Pancreatic abscess caused by *Clostridium difficile.* Eur J Clin Microbiol Infect Dis. 1988;7:528–529.

49. De Leeuw P, de Mot H, Dugernier T, et al. Primary infection of ascitic fluid with *Clostridium difficile.* J Infect. 1990;21:77–80.

50. Rooney N, Variend S, Taitz LS. Haemolytic uraemic syndrome and pseudomembranous colitis. Pediatr Nephrol. 1988;2:415–418.

51. McFarland LV, Elmer GW, Stamm WE, et al. Correlation of immunoblot type, enterotoxin production, and cytotoxin production with clinical manifestations of *Clostridium difficile* infection in a cohort of hospitalized patients. Infect Immun. 1991;59:2456–2462.

52. Marr JJ, Sans MD, Tedesco FJ. Bacterial studies of clindamycin-associated colitis. Gastroenterology. 1975;69:352–358.

53. Van der Waaij D. The ecology of the human intestine and its consequences for overgrowth by pathogens such as *Clostridium difficile.* Annu Rev Microbiol. 1989;43:69–87.

54. Wilson KH, Perini F. Role of competition for nutrients in suppression of *Clostridium difficile* by the colonic microflora. Infect Immun. 1988;56:2610–2614.

55. Rolfe RD, Helebian S, Finegold SM. Bacterial interference between *Clostridium difficile* and normal fecal flora. J Infect Dis. 1981;143:470–475.

56. Surawicz CM, Elmer GW, Speelman P, et al. Prevention of antibiotic-associated diarrhea by *Saccharomyces boulardii:* A prospective study. Gastroenterology. 1989;96:981–988.

57. Savage AM, Alford RH. Nosocomial spread of *C. difficile.* Infect Control. 1983;4:31–33.

58. Kim KH, Fekety R, Batts DH, et al. Isolation of *C. difficile* from the environment and contacts of patients with AAC. J Infect Dis. 1981;143:42–44.

59. Fekety R, Kim KH, Brown D, et al. Epidemiology of AAC: Isolation of *C. difficile* from the hospital environment. Am J Med. 1981;70:906–908.

60. Gerding DN, Olson MM, Peterson LR, et al. *C. difficile*-associated diarrhea and colitis in adults. Arch Intern Med. 1986;146:95–100.

61. Kim K, Dupont HL, Pichering LK. Outbreaks of diarrhea associated with *C. difficile* and its toxin in daycare centers: Evidence of person-to-person spread. J Pediatr. 1983;102:376–382.

62. Walters BAJ, Stafford R, Roberts RK, et al. Contamination and crossinfection with *C. difficile* in intensive care unit. Aust N Z J Med. 1982;12:255–258.

63. Mulligan ME, Rolfe RD, Finegold SM, et al. Contamination of a hospital environment by *Clostridium difficile.* Curr Microbiol. 1979;3:173–175.

64. Viscidi R, Willey S, Bartlett JG. Isolation rates and toxigenic potential of *C. difficile* isolates from various patient populations. Gastroenterology. 1981;81:5–9.

65. Malamou-Ladas H, O'Farrell S, Nash JQ, et al. Isolation of *C. difficile* from patients and the environment of hospital wards. J Clin Pathol. 1983;36:88–92.

66. Cooperstock M. *Clostridium difficile* in infants and children. In: Rolfe R, Finegold S, eds. *Clostridium difficile:* Its Role in Intestinal Disease. San Diego: Academic Press; 1988:45–64.

67. Hafiz S, Morton RS, McEntergart MG, et al. *C. difficile*

in the urogenital tract of men and women. Lancet. 1975;1:420–421.

68. Al-jumaili IJ, Shibley M, Listman AH, et al. Incidence and origin of *C. difficile* in neonates. J Clin Microbiol. 1984;19:77–78.

69. Larson HE, Barclay FE, Honour P, et al. Epidemiology of *C. difficile* in infants. J Infect Dis. 1982;146:727–733.

70. Burdon DW. *C. difficile*: The epidemiology and prevention of hospital-acquired infection. Infection. 1982;10:203–204.

71. Wust J, Sullivan NM, Hardegger U, et al. Investigation of an outbreak of AAC by various typing methods. J Clin Microbiol. 1982;16:1096–1101.

72. Poxton IR, Aronsson B, Mollby R, et al. Immunochemical fingerprinting of *Clostridium difficile* strains isolated from an outbreak of antibiotic-associated colitis and diarrhea. J Med Microbiol. 1984;17:317–324.

73. Mulligan ME, Peterson LR, Kwok RYY, et al. Immunoblots and plasmid fingerprints compared with serotyping and polyacrylamide gel electrophoresis for typing *Clostridium difficile*. J Clin Microbiol. 1988;26:41–46.

74. Bender BS, Laughon BE, Gaydos C, et al. Is *Clostridium difficile* endemic in chronic-care facilities? Lancet. 1986;2:11–13.

75. Thomas DR, Bennett RG, Laughon BE, et al. Postantibiotic colonization with *Clostridium difficile* in nursing home patients. J Am Geriatr Soc. 1990;38:415–420.

76. Taylor NS, Thorne GM, Bartlett JG. Comparison of two toxins produced by *Clostridium difficile*. Infect Immun. 1981;34:1036–1043.

77. Sullivan NM, Pellett S, Wilkins TD. Purification and characterization of toxins A and B of *Clostridium difficile*. Infect Immun. 1982;34:1032–1040.

78. Tucker KD, Carrig PE, Wilkins TD. Toxin A of *Clostridium difficile* is a potent cytotoxin. J Clin Microbiol. 1990;28:869–871.

79. Banno Y, Kobayashi T, Kono H, et al. Biochemical characterization and biologic actions of two toxins (D-1 and D-2) from *Clostridium difficile*. Rev Infect Dis. 1984;6:S11–S21.

80. Lyerly DM, Phelps CJ, Toth J, et al. Characterization of toxins A and B of *Clostridium difficile* with monoclonal antibodies. Infect Immun. 1986;54:70–76.

81. Kamiya S, Yamakawa K, Ogura H, et al. Recovery of spores of *Clostridium difficile* altered by heat or alkali. J Med Microbiol. 1989;28:217–221.

82. Krivan HC, Clark GF, Smith DF, Wilkins TD. Cell surface binding site for *Clostridium difficile* enterotoxin: Evidence for a glycoconjugate containing the sequence Gal alpha 1-3Gal beta 1-4GlcNAc. Infect Immun. 1986;53:573–581.

83. Fiorentini C, Malorni W, Paradisi S, et al. Interaction of *Clostridium difficile* toxin A with cultured cells: Cytoskeletal changes and nuclear polarization. Infect Immun. 1990;58:2329–2336.

84. Pothoulakis C, Sullivan R, Melnick DA, et al. *Clostridium difficile* toxin A stimulates intracellular calcium release and chemotactic response in human granulocytes. J Clin Invest. 1988;81:1741–1745.

85. Hecht G, Pothoulakis C, LaMont JT, Madava JL. *Clostridium difficile* toxin A perturbs cytoskeletal structure and tight junction permeability of cultured human intestinal epithelial monolayers. J Clin Invest. 1988;82:1516–1524.

86. Lyerly DM, Saum KE, MacDonald DK, et al. Effects of *Clostridium difficile* toxins given intragastrically to animals. Infect Immun. 1985;47:349–352.

87. Lashner BA, Todorczuk J, Sahm DF, et al. *Clostridium difficile* culture-positive toxin-negative diarrhea. Am J Gastroenterol. 1986;81:940–943.

88. Fluit AC, Wolfhagen MJHM, Verdonk GPHT, et al. Nontoxigenic strains of *Clostridium difficile* lack the genes for both toxin A and toxin B. J Clin Microbiol. 1991;29:2666–2667.

89. Wilson KH, Sheagren JN. Antagonism of toxigenic *Clostridium difficile* by nontoxigenic *Clostridium difficile*. J Infect Dis. 1983;147:733–736.

90. Privitera G, Scarpellini P, Ortisi G, et al. Prospective study of *Clostridium difficile* intestinal colonization and disease following single-dose antibiotic prophylaxis in surgery. Antimicrob Agents Chemother. 1991;35:208–210.

91. George WL, Rolfe RD, Finegold SM. *Clostridium difficile* and its cytotoxin in feces of patients with antimicrobial agent-associated diarrhea and miscellaneous conditions. J Clin Microbiol. 1982;15:1049–1053.

92. Gantz NM, Zawacki JK, Dickerson WJ, et al. PMC associated with erythromycin. Ann Intern Med. 1979;91:866–867.

93. McKinley MD, Troncale F, Sangree MH, et al. AAC: Clinical and epidemiological features. Am J Gastroenterol. 1982;77:77–81.

94. Larson HE, Borriello SP. Quantitative study of antibiotic-induced susceptibility to *Clostridium difficile* enterocecitis in hamsters. Antimicrob Agents Chemother. 1990;34:1348–1353.

95. Cudmore MA, Silva J, Fekety R, et al. *C. difficile* colitis associated with cancer chemotherapy. Arch Intern Med. 1982;142:333–335.

96. Pierce PF, Wilson R, Silva J, et al. AAPMC: An epidemiologic investigation of a cluster of cases. J Infect Dis. 1982;145:269–274.

97. Vesikari R, Isolauri E, Maki M, et al. *C. difficile* in young children. Acta Paediatr Scand. 1984;73:86–91.

98. Zweiner RJ, Belknap WM, Quan R. Severe pseudomembranous enterocolitis in a child: Case report and literature review. Pediatr Infect Dis J. 1989;8:876–882.

99. Nash JQ, Chattopadhyay B, Honeycombe J, et al. *C. difficile* and cytotoxin in routine faecal specimens. J Clin Pathol. 1982;35:561–565.

100. Morris G, Jarvis WR, Nuñez-Montiel OL, et al. *C. difficile* colonization and toxin production in a cohort of patients with malignant hematologic disorders. Arch Intern Med. 1984;144:967–969.

101. Fainstein V, Bodey GP, Fekety R. Relapsing PMC associated with cancer chemotherapy. J Infect Dis. 1981;143:865.

102. Milligan DW, Kelly JK. PMC in a leukaemia unit: A report of five fatal cases. J Clin Pathol. 1979;32:1237–1243.

103. Rampling A, Warren RE, Berry PJ, et al. Atypical *Clostridium difficile* colitis in neutropenic patients. Lancet. 1982;1:162. Letter.

104. Bruce D, Ritchie C, Jennings LC, et al. *C. difficile* associated colitis: Cross infection in predisposed patients with renal failure. Johns Hopkins J Med. 1982;151:1–9.

105. Peiken SR, Galdibini J, Bartlett JG. Role of *C. difficile* in a case of nonantibiotic associated PMC. Gastroenterology. 1980;79:948–951.

106. Rifkin GD, Fekety FR, Solva J. Antibiotic-induced colitis implication of a toxin neutralised by *Clostridium sordellii* antitoxin. Lancet. 1977;2:1103–1106.

107. Siegel DL, Edelstein PH, Nachamkin I. Inappropriate testing for diarrheal diseases in the hospital. JAMA. 1990;263:979–982.

108. Walker RC, Ruane PJ, Rosenblatt JE, et al. Comparison of culture, cytotoxicity assays and enzyme-linked immunosorbent assay for toxin A and toxin B in the diagnosis of *Clostridium difficile*–related enteric disease. Diagn Microbiol Infect Dis. 1986;5:61–69.

109. Peterson LR, Olson MM, Shanholtzer CJ, Gerding DN. Results of a prospective, 18-month clinical evaluation

of culture, cytotoxin testing, and culturette brand (CDT) latex testing in the diagnosis of *Clostridium difficile*–associated diarrhea. Diagn Microbiol Infect Dis. 1988;10:85–91.

110. McFarland LV, Coyle MB, Kremer WH, Stamm WE. Rectal swab cultures for *Clostridium difficile* surveillance studies. J Clin Microbiol. 1987;25:2241–2242.

111. Bowman RA, Riley TV. Laboratory diagnosis of *Clostridium difficile*–associated diarrhoea. Eur J Clin Microbiol Infect Dis. 1988;7:476–484.

112. Chang T-W, Lavermann M, Bartlett JG. Cytotoxicity assay in antibiotic-associated colitis. J Infect Dis. 1979;140:765.

113. George WL, Sutter VL, Citron D, et al. Selective and differential medium for isolation of *Clostridium difficile*. J Clin Microbiol. 1979;9:217–219.

114. McFarland LV, Stamm WE. Review of *Clostridium difficile*–associated diseases. Am J Infect Control. 1986;14:99–109.

115. Willey SH, Bartlett JG. Cultures for *Clostridium difficile* in stools containing a cytotoxin neutralized by *C. sordellii* antitoxin. J Clin Microbiol. 1979;10:880–884.

116. Wilson KH, Kennedy MI, Fekety FR. Use of sodium taurocholate to enhance spore recovery on a medium selective for *Clostridium difficile*. J Clin Microbiol. 1982;15:443–445.

117. O'Farrell S, Wilks M, Nash JQ, et al. A selective enrichment broth for the isolation of *Clostridium difficile*. J Clin Pathol. 1984;37:98–99.

118. Borriello SP, Honour P. Simplified procedure for the routine isolation of *Clostridium difficile* from faeces. J Clin Pathol. 1981;34:1124–1127.

119. Clabots CR, Gerding SJ, Olson MM, et al. Detection of asymptomatic *Clostridium difficile* carriage by an alcohol shock procedure. J Clin Microbiol. 1989;27:2386–2387.

120. Johnson LL, McFarland LV, Dearing P, et al. Identification of *Clostridium difficile* in stool specimens by culture-enhanced gas-liquid chromatography. J Clin Microbiol. 1989;27:2218–2221.

121. Potvliege D, Labbe M, Yourassowsky E. GLC as screening test for *Clostridium difficile*. Lancet. 1981;2:1105.

122. Borriello SP. GLC and *Clostridium difficile*. Lancet. 1981;2:1283.

123. Head CB, Ratnam S. Comparison of API ZYM system with API AN-Ident, API 20A, Minitek Anaerobe II, and RapID-ANA systems for identification of *Clostridium difficile*. J Clin Microbiol. 1988;26:144–146.

124. Wilson KH, Blitchington R, Hindenach B, et al. Species-specific oligonucleotide probes for rRNA of *Clostridium difficile* and related species. J Clin Microbiol. 1988;26:2484–2488.

125. Woods GL, Iwen PC. Comparison of a dot immunobinding assay, latex agglutination, and cytotoxin assay for laboratory diagnosis of *Clostridium difficile*–associated diarrhea. J Clin Microbiol. 1990;28:855–857.

126. Cundy KV, Willard KE, Valeri LJ, et al. Comparison of traditional gas chromatography (GC), headspace GC, and the microbial identification library GC system for the identification of *Clostridium difficile*. J Clin Microbiol. 1991;29:260–263.

127. Kamiya S, Nakamura S, Yamakawa K, et al. Evaluation of a commercially available latex immunoagglutination test kit for detection of *Clostridium difficile* D-1 toxin. Microbiol Immunol. 1986;30:177–181.

128. Lyerly DM, Wilkins TD. Commercial latex test for *Clostridium difficile* toxin A does not detect toxin A. J Clin Microbiol. 1986;23:622–623.

129. Lyerly DM, Barroso LA, Wilkins T. Identification of the latex test–reactive protein of *Clostridium difficile* as glutamate dehydrogenase. J Clin Microbiol. 1991;29:2639–2642.

130. Lyerly DM, Ball DW, Toth J, Wilkins TD. Characterization of cross-reactive proteins detected by Culturette Brand Rapid Latex Test for *Clostridium difficile*. J Clin Microbiol. 1988;26:397–400.

131. Qadri SM, Akhter J, Ostrawski S, et al. High incidence of false positives by a latex agglutination test for the diagnosis of *Clostridium difficile* associated colitis in compromised patients. Diagn Microbiol Infect Dis. 1989;12:291–294.

132. Bowman RA, Riley TV. Isolation of *Clostridium difficile* from stored specimens and comparative susceptibility of various tissue cell lines to cytotoxin. FEMS Microbiol Lett. 1986;34:31–35.

133. Haslam SC, Ketley JM, Mitchell TJ, et al. Growth of *Clostridium difficile* and production of toxins A and B in complex and defined media. J Med Microbiol. 1986;21:293–297.

134. Levine HG, Kennedy M, LaMont JT. Counterimmunoelectrophoresis vs. cytotoxicity assay for the detection of *Clostridium difficile* toxin. J Infect Dis. 1982;145:398.

135. Jarvis W, Nunez-Montiel O, Thompson F, et al. Comparison of bacterial isolation, cytotoxin assay and counter immunoelectrophoresis for the detection of *Clostridium difficile* and its toxin. J Infect Dis. 1983;147:778.

136. Shahrabadi MS, Bryan LE, Gaffney D, et al. Latex agglutination test for detection of *Clostridium difficile* toxin in stool samples. J Clin Microbiol. 1984;20:339–342.

137. Laughon BE, Viscidi RP, Godvin SL, et al. Enzyme immunoassays for detection of *Clostridium difficile* toxins A and B in faecal specimens. J Infect Dis. 1984;149:781–788.

138. Church J, Fazio VW. The significance of quantitative results of *Clostridium difficile* cultures and toxin assays in patients with diarrhea. Dis Colon Rectum. 1985;28:765–769.

139. Vernet A, Corthier G, Dubos-Rarmare F, et al. Relationship between levels of *C. difficile* toxin A and toxin B and cecal lesions in gnotobiotic mice. Infect Immun. 1989;57:2123–2127.

140. McFarland LV. The epidemiology of *Clostridium difficile* infections. View Dig Dis. 1990;22:19–24.

141. Lyerly DM, Sullivan NM, Wilkins TD. Enzyme-linked immunosorbent assay for the *Clostridium difficile* toxin A. J Clin Microbiol. 1983;17:72–78.

142. Aronsson B, Granstrom M, Mollby R, et al. Enzyme immunoassay for detection of *Clostridium difficile* toxins A and B in patients with antibiotic-associated diarrhoea and colitis. Eur J Clin Microbiol. 1985;4:102–107.

143. Wren BW, Clayton CL, Castledine NB, et al. Identification of toxigenic *Clostridium difficile* strains by using a toxin A gene-specific probe. J Clin Microbiol. 1990;28:1808–1812.

144. Holter JJ, Shanholtzer CJ, Willard KE, et al. Comparisons of VIDAS CDA assay with *C. difficile* culture, cytotoxin and latex test in patients who had and who did not have *C. difficile*–associated disease. Chicago IL: ICAAC; Abstract #725, 1991.

145. Doern GV, Coughlin RT, Pickett M, et al. Clinical laboratory comparison of four *C. difficile* toxin assays. Chicago IL: Interscience Conference on Antimicrobial Agents and Chemotherapy; Abstract #722, 1991.

146. Seppala K, Hjelt L, Sipponen P. Colonoscopy in the diagnosis of AAC: A prospective study. Scand J Gastroenterol. 1981;16:465–468.

147. Miller PD, LaMont JT. Antibiotic-induced diarrhea. Pract Gastroenterol. 1989;13:45–51.

148. Price AB, Davies DR. PMC. J Clin Pathol. 1977;30:1–12.

149. Rubesin SE, Levine MS, Glick SN, et al. Pseudomembranous colitis with rectosigmoid sparing on barium studies. Radiology. 1989;170:811–813.

150. Whitehead R. Colitis: Problems in definition and diagnosis. Virchows Arch A Pathol Anat Histopathol. 1990;417:187–190.

151. Griffin PM, Olmstead LC, Petras RE. *Escherichia coli* 0157:H7–associated colitis: A clinical and histological study of 11 cases. Gastroenterology. 1990;99:142–149.

152. Danna PL, Urban C, Bellin E, et al. Role of candida in pathogenesis of antibiotic-associated diarrhoea in elderly inpatients. Lancet. 1991;377:511–513.

153. Fortson WC, Tedesco FJ. Drug-induced colitis: A review. Am J Gastroenterol. 1984;79:878–883.

154. Bartlett JG. Treatment of antibiotic-associated colitis. Rev Infect Dis. 1984;6:S235–S241.

155. Chang T-W, Dong M-Y, Gorbach SL. Effect of bismuth subsalicylate on *Clostridium difficile* colitis in hamsters. Rev Infect Dis. 1990;12:S57–S58.

156. Cherry RD, Portnoy D, Jabbari M, et al. Metronidazole: An alternate therapy for antibiotic-associated colitis. Gastroenterology. 1982;82:849–851.

157. Silva J, Batts DH, Fekety R, et al. Treatment of *C. difficile* colitis and diarrhea with vancomycin. Am J Med. 1981;71:815–821.

158. Fekety R, Silva J, Kauffman C, et al. Treatment of antibiotic-associated *Clostridium difficile*-colitis with oral vancomycin: Comparison of two dosage regimens. Am J Med. 1989;86:15–19.

159. Oliva SL, Guglielmo BJ, Jacobs R, et al. Failure of intravenous vancomycin and intravenous metronidazole to prevent or treat antibiotic-associated pseudomembranous colitis. J Infect Dis. 1989;159:1154–1155.

160. De Lalla F, Privitera G, Rinaldi E, et al. Treatment of *Clostridium difficile*-associated disease with teicoplanin. Antimicrob Agents Chemother. 1989;33:1125–1127.

161. Ariano RE, Zhanel GG, Harding GKM. The role of anion-exchange resins in the treatment of antibiotic-associated pseudomembranous colitis. Can Med Assoc J. 1990;142:1049–1051.

162. Bowden TA, Mansberger AR, Lykins LE. Pseudomembranous enterocolitis: Mechanism for restoring flora homeostasis. Am Surg. 1981;47:178–183.

163. Tvede M, Rask-Madsen J. Bacteriotherapy for chronic relapsing *Clostridium difficile* diarrhoea in six patients. Lancet. 1989;1:1156–1160.

164. Tankanow RM, Ross MB, Ertel IJ, et al. A double-blind, placebo-controlled study of the efficacy of Lactinex in the prophylaxis of amoxicillin-induced diarrhea. DICP Ann Pharmacother. 1990;24:382–384.

165. Siitonen S, Vapaatalo H, Salminen S, et al. Effect of *Lactobacillus* GG yoghurt in prevention of antibiotic associated diarrhoea. Ann Med. 1990;22:57–59.

166. Munro R, Foldes M, Morris G. An evaluation of a rapid latex test for the diagnosis of *Clostridium difficile*-associated diarrhea. Pathology. 1988;20:349–352.

167. DiPersio JR, Varga FJ, Conwell DL, et al. Development of a rapid enzyme immunoassay for *Clostridium difficile* toxin A and its use in the diagnosis of *C. difficile*-associated disease. J Clin Microbiol. 1991;29:2724–2730.

168. Varki NM, Aquino TI. Isolation of *Clostridium difficile* from hospitalized patients without antibiotic-associated diarrhea or colitis. J Clin Microbiol. 1982;16:659–662.

169. Heard SR, O'Farrell S, Holland D, et al. The epidemiology of *Clostridium difficile* with use of a typing scheme: Nosocomial acquisition and cross-infection among immuno-compromised patients. J Infect Dis. 1986;153:159–162.

170. Gerard M, Defresne N, Daneau D, et al. Incidence and significance of *Clostridium difficile* in hospitalized cancer patients. Eur J Clin Microbiol Infect Dis. 1988;7:274–278.

171. Foulke GE, Silva J Jr. *Clostridium difficile* in the intensive care unit: Management problems and prevention issues. Crit Care Med. 1989;17:822–826.

172. Johnson S, Clabots CR, Linn FV, et al. Nosocomial *Clostridium difficile* colonisation and disease. Lancet. 1990;336:97–100.

173. Johnson S, Gerding DN, Olson MM, et al. Prospective, controlled study of vinyl glove use to interrupt *Clostridium difficile* nosocomial transmission. Am J Med. 1990;88:137–140.

174. Delmee M, Verellen G, Avesani V, et al. *Clostridium difficile* in neonates: Serogrouping and epidemiology. Eur J Pediatr. 1988;147:36–40.

175. Wu TC, McCarthy VP, Gill VJ. Isolation rate and toxigenic potential of *Clostridium difficile* isolates from patients with cystic fibrosis. J Infect Dis. 1983;148:176.

176. Welkon CJ, Long SS, Thompson CM Jr, et al. *Clostridium difficile* in patients with cystic fibrosis. Am J Dis Child. 1985;139:805–808.

177. Greenfield C, Burroughs A, Szawathowski M, et al. Is pseudomembranous colitis infectious? Lancet 1981;i:371–372.

178. Nolan NPM, Kelly CP, Humphreys JFH, et al. An epidemic of pseudomembranous colitis: Importance of person to person spread. Gut 1987;28:1467–1473.

179. Testore GP, Pantosti A, Cerquetti M, et al. Evidence for cross-infection in an outbreak of *Clostridium difficile*-associated diarrhoea in a surgical unit. J Med Microbiol 1988;26:125–128.

180. McKay I, Coia JE, Poxton IR. Typing of *Clostridium difficile* causing diarrhoea in an orthopaedic ward. J Clin Pathol 1989;42:511–515.

181. Foulke GE, Silva J Jr. *Clostridium difficile* in the intensive care unit: Management problems and prevention issues. Crit Care Med 1989;8:822–826.

182. Degl'Innocenti R, De Santis M, Berdondini I, Dei R. Outbreak of *Clostridium difficile* diarrhoea in an orthopaedic unit: Evidence of phage-typing for cross-infection. J Hosp Infect 1989;13:309–314.

183. Heyman M, Corthier G, Lucas F, et al. Evolution of the caecal epithelial barrier during *Clostridium difficile* infection in the mouse. Gut. 1989;30:1087–1093.

184. Triadafilopoulos G, Pothoulakis C, Weiss R, et al. Comparative study of *Clostridium difficile* toxin A and cholera toxin in rabbit ileum. Gastroenterology. 1989;97:1186–1192.

185. Church J, Fazio VW. The significance of quantitative results of *Clostridium difficile* cultures and toxin assays in patients with diarrhea. Dis Colon Rectum. 1985; 28:765–769.

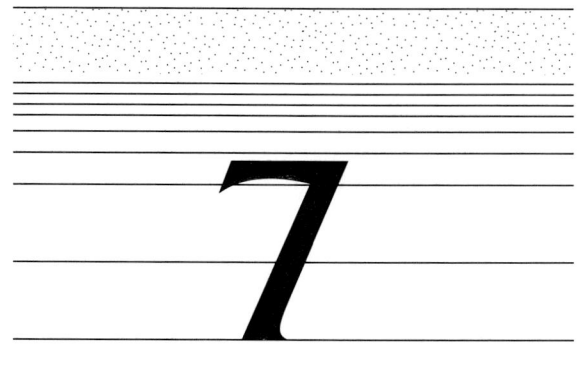

7

Parasites of the Small Intestine

JOHN H. CROSS, Ph.D.

The small intestine is a repository for more than 20 different species of animal parasites, consisting of nematodes, cestodes, trematodes, and protozoa. The small intestine in adult humans may vary from 12 to 20 feet in length, and certain parasites have an affinity for a particular location or for the entire small intestine. The parasites in the small bowel usually feed on chyme, or intestinal debris, essentially competing with the host for food. Others may feed on tissue or tissue juices and blood and are considered more pathogenic. Most parasites cause little or no disease, but some may provoke severe illness and death. All small intestinal parasites should be considered potentially pathogenic, however, and should be eliminated. This chapter considers some of the more common worms and protozoa, with brief presentations on those of lesser significance.

ASCARIASIS

Parasite

Ascaris lumbricoides is the largest of the intestinal nematodes and also has the distinction of

being the most common parasite of humans. The worm is elongated, cylindrical, and tapered at both ends; females measure 20 to 35 cm in length and 3 to 6 mm in diameter, males are 15 to 30 cm by 2 to 4 mm in diameter. The male posterior end is curved and houses the copulatory spicule. The cuticle or outer skin is striated with two lateral lines. The color of the parasite varies from yellow to white with a pinkish hue. As adults, most *A. lumbricoides* parasites reside in the lumen of the jejunum.

After mating, female worms deposit eggs, which pass in the fecal stream. When female worms predominate and only one or two males are present, many of the eggs found in feces are unfertilized. When the sex ratio is balanced, most eggs are fertilized. One female worm may produce as many as 240,000 eggs per day. Under optimal conditions of warm (28–30°C) moist shady soil, the fertilized eggs embryonate in 10 to 14 days. The larva that develops within the egg is able to withstand many chemicals and adverse climatic conditions. Embryonation is able to continue even in eggs stored in 10% formalin, and motile larvae within eggs have been observed in fecal specimens stored for several years. The eggs are ingested by humans and hatch within a few hours in the jejunum by the action of enzymes from the larvae with assistance from gastric and duodenal digestion. The larva penetrates the jejunal mucosa, and passes

The opinions or assertions contained herein are the author's own and are not to be construed as official or reflecting the views of the United States Department of Defense or the Uniformed Services University of the Health Sciences.

to the liver by the portal vessels and then to the lungs. Migration to the lung takes 3 to 4 days, and after 2 to 3 weeks the parasite penetrates the alveolar air sacs, migrates up the tracheo-bronchial tree, and is coughed up and swallowed. The fourth-stage larva reaches the small intestine and develops into an adult, copulates, and reproduces. The prepatent period is 60 to 75 days. Adult worms may live for 12 to 18 months, with females producing as many as 87 million eggs in a lifetime.

Source of Infection

Ascariasis occurs in areas with a warm climate and poor sanitation. In most endemic areas children acquire infection by ingesting soil (pica) that is fecally contaminated, and adults acquire infections by eating contaminated vegetables. Eggs may be carried into the home on feet after walking through contaminated areas. Water is another source of infection. In some areas, eating vegetables or ground-fruit from land irrigated with untreated sewage water leads to infection. Promiscuous defecation by children and adults is a main source of infection as well as the use of night soil to fertilize vegetables. There are also reports of neonatal transmission.[1]

Clinical Manifestation

The disease associated with *A. lumbricoides* infection is considered in two distinct stages: that attributed to larval migration and that associated with adult worm infection. Little reaction to the migrating larval stages occurs during a first-time infection, but in subsequent exposures, serious reactions may occur in hypersensitized individuals. Generalized symptoms may be present, with urticaria, angioneurotic edema, and bronchospasms as well as elevated immunoglobulin E serum (IgE) levels. Infection with large numbers of larvae may cause liver problems, hepatitis, hepatomegaly, jaundice, and biochemical changes. Blood and serous exudate may fill alveoli on larval penetration, and coughing may result. Löffler's syndrome may develop in such cases. On occasion, larvae are known to migrate to other locations, such as the nasolacrimal duct.[2]

Most infections with adult worms are asymptomatic, but on occasion a single worm may migrate into extra-intestinal locations and cause symptoms. Worms may erratically enter small orifices, leading to obstruction. Erratic ascariasis is not uncommon, with worms migrating from the anus, nose, and mouth. Internally, the parasite is known to migrate into vital organs, such as the liver, pancreas, and lungs. Surgical complications have been reported in which abdominal complications included intestinal obstruction, perforation of the appendix, and migration into the biliary tree or into the peritoneal cavity.[3] Hepatic abscesses have also been reported. Erratic ascariasis may be provoked by illness, fever, general anesthesia, and certain medications. Male worms respond to stimuli more often than do female worms. A bolus of worms may cause blockage of the intestine at the ileocecal valve, especially in children. Untreated obstructions lead to gangrene of the bowel, perforation, and peritonitis. Volvulus and intussusception can result from infections. Large numbers of worms may lead to nutritional problems and malabsorption of protein, fats, and carbohydrates owing to decreased transit time resulting from increased peristalsis caused by the worms. Poor nutrition affects acquired immunity, and consequently infected persons are more susceptible to infection.

Although most infections are asymptomatic, vague abdominal discomfort and acute cramping in the midabdomen with anorexia and insomnia are reported in children. Diarrhea and weight loss may also occur. Morbidity is usually associated with intensity of infection, and since intensity decreases with age, children suffer from this disease more often than do adults.

Pathology

At first, few pathologic changes occur with migrating larvae, but in sensitized individuals larvae migrating through the liver may cause inflammatory lesions with subsequent infection. Intense tissue reactions may occur, including inflammation and granulomatous lesions in the lungs as a result of infections with large numbers of worms. Infiltration of eosinophils, epithelioid cells, and macrophages is possible. Charcot-Leyden crystals are formed along with increased mucus production and bronchial spasms. This combination of conditions has been called *Ascaris* pneumonitis, and at times larvae are found in sputum.

Adult worms do not usually cause much pathologic disturbance unless they become erratic and migrate out of the orifices or into vital organs or they block the bile ducts. Various nutritional problems are suspected when the worms are present, but direct evidence to suggest that the parasite is responsible is slight.

Diagnosis

Making a clinical diagnosis of ascariasis is difficult, since the symptoms are similar to those caused by other parasitic infections. Larval and adult worms passed from the nose, mouth, or anus as well as in sputum and feces are easily recognized. The parasitologic diagnosis, however, is usually made by detecting eggs in the feces. Three types of eggs may be found: the typical fertilized egg, the unfertilized egg, and the decorticated fertilized egg. Regular fertilized eggs are 55 to 75 by 35 to 50 μm and have thick shells with a bile-stained prominent outer albuminoid mamillated coat (Fig. 7–1). Decorticated fertilized eggs are 30 to 40 μm in diameter and lack mamillation (Fig. 7–2). Unfertilized eggs are 85 by 45 μm, contain an unorganized mass, and are of irregular shape with a bumpy outer coat (Fig. 7–3). The eggs are usually abundant, and a direct microscopic examination of a fecal smear is all that is necessary for their visualization. Concentration techniques, such as flotation, sedimentation, and formalin–ethyl acetate centrifugation, or the Kato-Katz technique, are useful in light infections. (Diagnostic techniques are described elsewhere.[4]) Radiographic examination of the intestinal tract may reveal parallel cylindrical filling defects that may show a stringlike shadow of barium in the worm's intestine. In obstructions, abdominal films may show the outline of interlocking worms. Serologic tests are available but are not considered reliable.

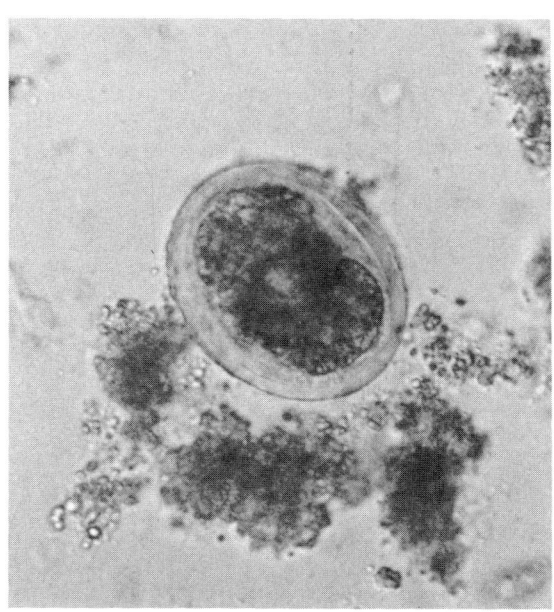

FIGURE 7–2.
Decorticated egg of *Ascaris lumbricoides* (30–40 μm). [See also Color Plate 2]

Treatment

A number of anthelminthics are available for the treatment of intestinal ascariasis. Since some anthelminthics may cause the parasite to migrate, a patient with a history of erratic ascariasis should probably be treated initially with pyrantel pamoate, given orally in a single dose of 11

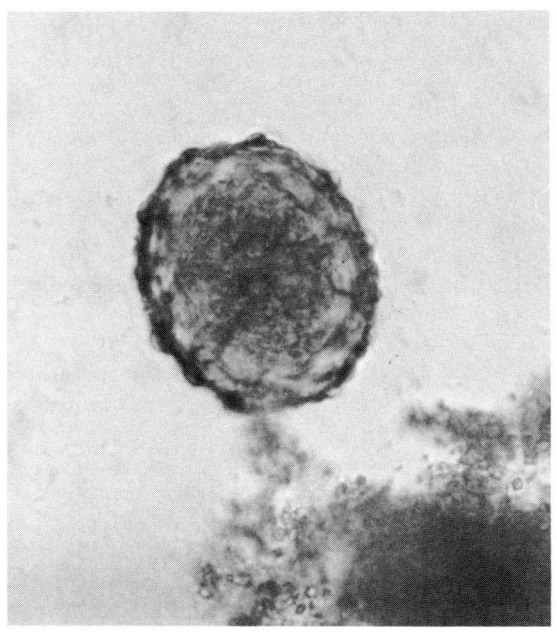

FIGURE 7–1.
Regular fertilized egg of *Ascaris lumbricoides* (55–75 × 35–50 μm). [See also Color Plate 2]

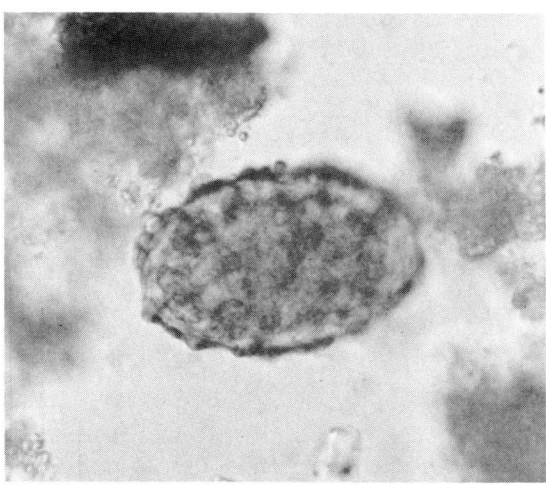

FIGURE 7–3.
Unfertilized egg of *Ascaris lumbricoides* (85 × 45 μm). [See also Color Plate 2]

mg/kg or a maximum of 1 g, or levamisole, given in a single oral dose of 150 mg for adults or 3 mg/kg for children. In most endemic areas, where multiple helminthic infections are common, the initial treatment can be followed by 100 mg of mebendazole taken orally twice daily for 3 days. Mebendazole is effective in the treatment of trichuriasis, hookworm, and enterobiasis. Albendazole and ivermectin are also effective anthelminthics but are not available in the United States. Retreatment is often necessary, especially in endemic areas. Most anthelminthics are not effective in cases of extra-intestinal ascariasis, but mebendazole, albendazole, and ivermectin may have some value since they are known to affect helminths in tissue. The drugs may have to be given in higher dosages for longer periods to be effective against larvae in the liver, lungs, and intestinal mucosa.

Piperazine salts in a dose of 150 mg/kg may be given by a nasogastric tube in cases of incomplete intestinal obstruction. Smaller doses of 65 mg/kg can be given every 12 hours for 6 doses. Cases of complete obstruction with signs of acute abdomen require surgery. Biliary ascariasis can be treated conservatively with intravenous fluids, antispasmodics, and anthelminthics or by removal of the worm by endoscopic retrograde cholangiopancreatography (ERCP)[5] or by surgery.

Epidemiology

Ascariasis occurs in one fifth of the world's population. Children are most often infected, with infections decreasing with age. Males and females are equally infected, but in surveys among 7000 inhabitants of 23 villages in Northern Luzon in the Philippines, 59% of the males and 63% of the females were infected.[6] In some villages of Indonesia, infection rates were nearly 90%.[7] The highest prevalence rates are in tropical countries with warm moist climates year-around; 40% of the world's infections are estimated to be in Asia.[8] Most infections in children are acquired by eating dirt, and adults acquire infections from vegetables or water. In Jamaica children are estimated to ingest 6 to 20 *A. lumbricoides* eggs per year.[9] The intensity of infection, however, has been estimated to be six adult worms per person.[10] With over 1 billion people infected worldwide, this suggests a world population of *A. lumbricoides* eggs of more than 6 billion. If half these worms are female, each producing 240,000 eggs per day, 720 trillion eggs could be deposited in the environment daily. Fortunately, not all the eggs complete development; many are destroyed in the soil because of environmental factors, including temperature, moisture, oxygen, pH, and the presence of organic matter and antagonistic organisms such as fungi that attack *A. lumbricoides* eggs.

Human behavior influences prevalence and intensity of infection, as does population density, occupation, and ethnic factors. The prevalence of ascariasis is higher in low socioeconomic classes. Generally, children from poor families are more often infected with more worms than are children from higher income families. Improvement in the standard of living and sanitation reduces infections. Predisposition of persons to either heavy or light *A. lumbricoides* infections is also recognized. Persons heavily infected with parasites have been demonstrated to become heavily reinfected after treatment, both individuals and families. Factors responsible for this may be genetic, environmental, behavioral, nutritional, or combinations of these factors.[11, 12]

Seasonal variation occurs in some countries, causing fluctuations in prevalence ratios that are higher in warm moist months and lower when temperatures decrease or when the weather is drier. Eggs may survive for years in countries like India but would be unable to survive in the soil in the colder months in European countries.

Prevention and Control

Ascariasis is classified as a "dooryard infection." Infected children playing in areas around their homes indiscriminately defecate and constantly seed the soil with *A. lumbricoides* eggs. In rural areas this may occur in the schoolyard. If this practice could be eliminated, parasite prevalence rates would decrease dramatically. Although outhouses and water-seal toilet facilities are available in some rural areas, people do not like to use them because of the bad odors that eventually develop. In such areas, even adults defecate in the fields. When sanitary conditions improve, parasitic diseases decrease.

Night soil continues to be used to fertilize vegetables and other crops in China, parts of Europe, and other places. Human feces and night soil are not usually composted long enough to destroy the rugged *A. lumbricoides* eggs. Changing these cultural habits is difficult but necessary in any successful eradication program.

In countries such as Japan and Korea, control programs were successful by eliminating the use of night soil, improving sanitation, educating the population, and instituting mass-treatment campaigns, especially among schoolchildren. Many anthelminthics have been used, with mebendazole being the most effective since it is active against hookworm and whipworm as well as *A. lumbricoides*. In a pilot study conducted in a Philippine village in an attempt to eradicate soil-transmitted helminths by periodic mass treatment with mebendazole, the prevalence of ascariasis was reduced from 78% to less than 1% in 3 years (JHC and V Basaca-Sevilla, M.D., unpublished data, 1977). Community-based programs are the best approach for prevention and control of ascariasis and other soil-transmitted parasitoses.

HOOKWORM INFECTION AND DISEASE

No other helminthic infection is of greater significance to the health and welfare of the human race than hookworm. The parasite has been a scourge to humankind in the warmer parts of the world at least since diseases were first documented. Hippocrates in the 5th century BC noticed that people with intestinal disturbances ate stones and earth, a practice known as pica. Historically, the pallor of miners has been noted, and gold was once thought to give miners the same color as the metal they sought. No one suspected anemia caused by hookworm until centuries later, when anemia was recognized in men working on tunnels in Europe. Hookworm anemia has subsequently been called miner's disease. In the early part of the twentieth century, the Rockefeller Sanitary Commission began hookworm eradication programs. In rural southern United States, more than 2 million people were infected. The parasitosis is still present but is considered a rarity, except in some remote rural areas. No other parasite, essentially insidious, year after year for generations saps the vitality and undermines the health and efficiency of whole communities, especially in the developing world. Hookworm is the second most common parasitosis worldwide, with over 1 billion infections estimated.

Parasite

Two major hookworm species infect humans, and a number of related species that infect animals may occasionally invade humans. *Necator americanus* and *Ancylostoma duodenale* are endemic to most warm moist areas of the world;

N. americanus is more common in Asia, the Americas, Africa, Australia, and the Pacific islands; *A. duodenale* is found in Africa, India, China, Japan, and parts of Australia and South America. Both species are found together in several parts of the world. These two species are discussed fully in this chapter, but mention is made of others that occasionally infect humans.

Females of both species measure 10 to 13 mm in length, but *N. americanus* is more slender, being 0.2 to 0.5 mm compared with *A. duodenale*, which is 0.6 to 0.7 mm in width. Males of *N. americanus* measure 6 to 8 by 0.2 to 0.3 mm, and those of *A. duodenale* are 8 to 11 by 0.4 to 0.5 mm. The mouth or buccal capsule of *N. americanus* worms has two pairs of cutting plates, and that of *A. duodenale* has two pairs of teeth. The males of both species have a bell-shaped bursa, with that of *N. americanus* being longer than it is wide and that of *A. duodenale* wider than it is long. The bursa is used to attach to females during copulation. It has fingerlike rays that are characteristic for each species. The females of both species are slender, with the vulva midventrally located. In copulation the male wraps the bursa around the area of the female vulva and inserts a pair of copulatory spicules. A cement substance is secreted as a holdfast, to ensure deposition of spermatozoa. Eggs pass from the female worm into the intestinal stream and out with the feces. The eggs are in early cleavage when passed, and they embryonate in 2 to 3 days. Under the right environmental conditions, a first-stage or rhabditiform larva emerges from the egg and feeds on bacteria. The larva has a long narrow buccal cavity, a flask-shaped muscular esophagus, and a small inconspicuous genital primordium. Within a few days, the larva sheds the cuticle and develops into a second stage. Within a week, the larva molts again and develops into a slender nonfeeding third stage, or filariform larva. This is the infective stage at which the larva migrates to the top of the soil and waits for a human host.

After penetrating through breaks in the skin or under scales, fissures, or hair follicles, larvae enter venules, are carried to the heart and lungs, and break out into the alveoli. The third-stage larva of *A. duodenale* remains unchanged as it passes from the lung up the pulmonary tree and is swallowed. The third-stage larva of *N. americanus*, however, requires development in the lung before completing migration. The worms reach sexual maturity in the small intestine, attach to the mucosa, suck blood, and reproduce. The prepatent period is about 5 weeks. Females of *N. americanus* produce 5000 to 10,000 eggs per day, and *A. duodenale* 10,000 to 25,000. Infections persist for 2 to 6 years and as long as 13 years.[12b]

Source of Infection

Most hookworm infections occur in people who walk barefooted over infected areas. The larvae cluster in groups on the soil surface, are thigmotropic, and often enter the skin between the toes. The parasites can enter any skin surface that they contact. *Necator americanus* can enter humans only by the percutaneous route, but *A. duodenale* may also enter by the oral route. Water and vegetables contaminated with *A. duodenale* infective-stage larvae are also sources of infection. Evidence also suggests transmammary transmission with *A. duodenale*.[13]

Clinical Manifestation

Skin penetration by larvae may cause a dermatitis, or ground itch, at the site of entrance. Intense itching is accompanied by edema, erythema, and infiltration of neutrophils and eosinophils. A papulovesicular eruption develops later and lasts for 1 to 2 weeks. This reaction occurs in young children born of mothers from endemic areas and expatriates exposed to infections for the first time. The reaction becomes more severe with heavy infections.

Filariform larvae reach the lung in 24 hours, and their migration from the pulmonary capillaries into the alveoli may result in minute hemorrhages and eosinophilic and leukocytic infiltration. In heavy infections, pneumonitis may develop, but the symptoms are mild compared with those of *A. lumbricoides* infections. In Japan, a syndrome called Wakana disease is described in which *A. duodenale* infection is acquired by ingestion of contaminated vegetables. The larvae go directly to the lung and cause nausea and vomiting as well as pulmonary symptoms of dyspnea, cough, and hypereosinophilia. Chest radiographs show a patchy infiltration.

Adult worms attach to the duodenum or upper jejunum by the mouth and, with the cutting plates or teeth, lacerate the tissue and suck blood. Old established infections with a stable population of worms may be asymptomatic, but a recent infection in a person for the first time may produce abdominal pain, nausea, vomiting, diarrhea with bloody mucus, Charot-Leyden crystals, and a peripheral eosinophilia. Continuous blood loss occurs at sites of attachment, which is probably due to anticoagulants secreted by the worms. Symptoms are said to appear with the presence of 30 *A. duodenale* or 100 *N. americanus* worms. Blood losses are estimated to be an average of 0.15 ml and 0.03 ml per day per worm for *A. duodenale* and *N. americanus*, respectively. Daily blood loss can reach 13 ml for the former and 8 ml for the latter in heavy infections.

Continuous blood loss over a period of time results in iron and protein depletion and in hookworm disease, anemia, and hypoalbuminemia. The severity depends on the number of worms and on the host's nutritional and immune status. A plethora of symptoms are associated with hookworm diseases, the most common being lassitude, shortness of breath, palpitations, syncope, peripheral or generalized edema, impotence, pale mucosa and conjunctiva, facial puffiness, low-grade fever, pica, tachycardia, cardiac murmur, and other signs of high-output cardiac state. Congestive heart failure and ascites may also occur. Patients often appear well, even with hemoglobin levels as low as 2 g/dl. Although many have hookworm infection, disease only occurs in relatively few. Most disease occurs in children and in adult farmers with exceptionally heavy worm burdens.

Pathology

Penetration of larvae into the skin causes ground itch, but secondary bacterial infection introduced by the larvae or continuous scratching is responsible for the tissue reaction.

Pulmonary reactions are rare, with coughing, dyspnea, and wheezing usually occurring in those who live in nontropical areas. Larvae produce minute focal hemorrhages. Chest radiographs reveal patchy fluffy opacities in areas of pneumonitis. Sputum may contain Charcot-Leyden crystals and eosinophils. The most serious lung manifestations are associated with ingested larvae, causing Wakana disease in Japan. Onset is acute with pharyngeal itching, coughing, dyspnea, wheezing, urticaria, nausea, and vomiting. The pulmonary reactions may be caused by active movement of the larvae through the arterioles.

Intestinal symptoms often resemble those associated with gastric ulcer and are caused by the attachment of the adult worms to the intestinal mucosa. Small erosive lesions, hemorrhages, tissue cytolysis, and neutrophilic responses result. The worms suck blood and plasma vigorously and often abandon one site and move to another, leaving the old site oozing blood and plasma. Long-term infections with many worms lead to iron deficiency anemia, and blood loss correlates with degree of anemia. Nutritional and immune factors are also associated with protein loss. Pathologic changes may occur in the bone marrow as a result of blood loss. Liver function may change as a result of anemia along with a reduced capacity for albumin synthesis. Fatty deteriorations of heart, liver, and kidney may also develop.

Diagnosis

Hookworm disease in tropical endemic areas is usually suspected in persons with a microcytic hypochromic anemia and eosinophilia. A stool examination usually reveals the presence of hookworm eggs (Fig. 7–4). The eggs are ovoid, 65 by 40 μm, and thin-shelled, and freshly passed feces contain 4 to 8 cells. Direct fecal smears examined microscopically usually reveal eggs, but in light infections, one of the concentration methods can be used, such as Kato thick smear, formalin–ethyl acetate concentration, or flotation with ZnSO$_4$. Intensities of infection can be measured by use of the Stoll or Kato-Katz methods. Stools may also be cultured by the Harada-Mori test-tube and charcoal Petri dish methods, and microscopic examination of larvae can aid in speciation of the hookworm. (Laboratory techniques are described elsewhere.[4])

Rhabditiform larvae are 0.3 by 17 μm and may be found in feces if the stool specimen is permitted to remain in the laboratory for some hours prior to examination. The larvae can be differentiated from those of *Strongyloides stercoralis* rhabditiform larvae by the presence of a long buccal capsule and an indistinct genital primordium. *Strongyloides stercoralis* larvae have a short buccal cavity and large genital primordium.

Treatment

Hookworm disease should be treated with 50 to 100 mg of ferrous sulfate daily along with a high protein diet and vitamins. This regimen should be continued until 3 months after hemoglobin levels reach 10 to 12 g/dl. In patients with severe anemia, blood transfusions and intravenous iron supplements may be required.

One of many anthelminthics can be given: mebendazole, in 100 mg doses given orally bid for 3 days; pyrantel pamoate, given in a single 11 mg/kg oral dose; albendazole, at 200 mg a day for 3 days; levamisole, in a single 150 mg dose for adults, and for children, 3 mg/kg. Both 5g of bephenium hydroxynaphtholate, in 1 day for *A. duodenale* or 5 g for 3 days for *N. americanus* and 0.1 mg/kg of tetrachloroethylene for a maximum dosage of 5 ml are alternative drugs, but they cause more side effects. Stools should be examined after 2 weeks to determine if retreatment is necessary.

Epidemiology

Hookworm disease occurs in nearly all tropical and subtropical countries. Transmission is particularly successful in areas with warm moist climates and in places where the soil is loose and sandy. Infections are more common in rural farming areas, where sanitation is poor and defecation indiscriminate and the population does not wear shoes. Prevalence rates may be as high as 90% in some regions, and in Sichuan Province in China, 50% of the 100 million inhabitants are infected with *A. duodenale* or *N. americanus* or both. Night soil is used to fertilize vegetables, tea plants, and even mulberry trees, and many of the farmers tend the crops barefooted. In some parts of China, infant deaths have been reported because of the use of diapers that are packed with sand or dirt so as to require changing only every few days. The soil often contains hookworm larvae that invade the skin of the infants. In most countries, however, infants and children are less often infected with hookworm than adults, but infection rates increase with age. In the Philippines, infection rates average 35%, with *N. americanus* the more

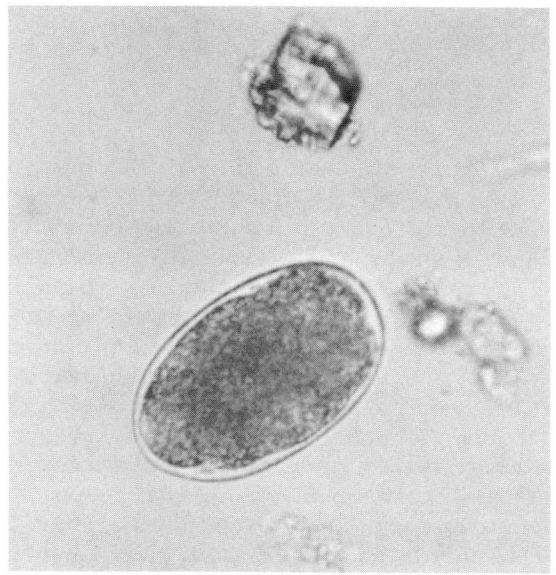

FIGURE 7–4.
Hookworm egg (65 × 40 μm). [See also Color Plate 2]

prevalent of the two species.[6] In Indonesia, the prevalence of hookworm averages 59%.

Rainfall is an important determinant of the locales in which hookworm is endemic. The larvae require a water film to migrate vertically to the soil surface. Dryness kills the larvae. Temperatures of 26–32°C (79–90°F) are best for development of the larvae; they perish in cold soil.

Arrested development of the larvae occurs with *A. duodenale* infection. In this state, termed hypobiosis, larvae remain someplace in the body in a dormant state for an extended time before completing development. The phenomenon may be triggered by seasonal and climatic factors.[14]

Data on morbidity and mortality are not available. Most persons do not have symptoms from hookworm infection, but death can result from severe hookworm disease.

Prevention and Control

The prevention and control of hookworm infection and disease is essentially the same as that for ascariasis. In addition to improvement in sanitation and education, the wearing of shoes has been shown to lower infection rates. Habits, customs, and beliefs must change, such as the cessation of the use of night soil and sand diapers in China. Mines and plantations develop high infection rates because of the practice of using one area for defecation. The use of latrines would benefit these places.

Predisposition for hookworm infection has also been demonstrated. Those with heavy hookworm infections easily become heavily reinfected after treatment.[15]

Mass-treatment campaigns are being carried out worldwide to reduce and eliminate hookworm infections. In one effort in the Philippines, after 3 years of periodic treatment with mebendazole, hookworm was nearly eradicated. The prevalence rate was reduced from 33.0% to 0.3% and remained at about 1.0% for the following 5 years. The continuous use of mebendazole dramatically suppressed the development of the parasite in this village (JHC and V Basaca-Sevilla, M.D. unpublished data, 1977).

Prevention and control of hookworms as well as other parasites will not be achieved until populations in endemic areas change their habits.

Zoonotic Hookworms. Two species of hookworm that are considered natural parasites of dogs and cats occasionally infect humans. *Ancylostoma ceylonicum* occurs in cats and other felines in Southeast and South Asia and has been reported in humans in the Philippines, Taiwan,

and India. It must be distinguished from *A. duodenale* and *N. americanus* in humans in the Far East.

Ancylostoma caninum is a common parasite of dogs worldwide and has been reported on rare occasions in humans. Recently, however, *A. caninum* has been incriminated in an epidemic of eosinophilic enteritis in Queensland, Australia.[16]

STRONGYLOIDIASIS

Although more than 50 species of *Strongyloides* have been reported to infect humans, only two are considered significant in human health, *S. stercoralis* and *S. fuelleborni*. *Strongyloides stercoralis* is the more common nematode, since it has a widespread distribution in tropical and subtropical areas. *Strongyloides fuelleborni*, by contrast, has been reported in Africa and Papua New Guinea. Some doubt exists, however, as to whether the parasite in Papua New Guinea is the same as that found in Africa.

Strongyloides stercoralis was first reported in French troops returning from Vietnam, the former French Indochina. The troops were suffering from Cochin China diarrhea, and tiny worms were recovered from the feces and from the intestines at autopsy. The parasite was first called *Anguillula stercoralis* (little eel) and later renamed *S. stercoralis*. In French-speaking countries the disease is now called anguillulosis.

The parasite is unusual in that it has both parasitic and free-living life cycles. It may internally autoinfect its host, become disseminated throughout the body, and cause death. Its ability to autoinfect the host makes it a very dangerous parasite.[17]

Parasite

The geographic distribution of *S. stercoralis* is similar to that of hookworm, and it too is found in areas with a warm moist climate year-round. The parasite is known in free-living and parasitic stages that are morphologically quite distinct. Only parasitic females are known; no males exist in the parasitic life cycle. The female reproduces parthenogenetically. Parasitic females are rarely recovered from antemortem specimens and live in tunnels in the mucosa of the duodenum and jejunum. The females measure 1.5 to 2.5 mm by 30 to 50 μm. The body is attenuated anteriorly, very slender, and transparent. The anterior portion contains a long cylindrical esophagus and a long straight intestine. The vulva is in the posterior third of the body, and the paired uteri contain embryonated thin-shelled eggs. The eggs are deposited in the intestinal epithelium, where they hatch. The eggs are not usually seen, since they hatch soon after release from the female. The first-stage larvae are passed in the feces and develop into second-stage, then into infective third-stage filariform larvae, which penetrate the skin of the next host. During passage down the intestine, some larvae molt into filariform larvae, penetrate the intestinal epithelium, migrate, and develop into adult females in the intestine; this process is known as internal autoinfection. Some first-stage larvae, after passing out of the host with the feces, develop into rhabditoid free-living adult males and females that mate, and the female produces eggs that hatch, releasing rhab-ditiform larvae in the soil. These larvae develop into the infective stage or into new free-living adult worms.

The rhabditiform larva is approximately 250 by 15 μm, has a small buccal cavity, a bulbous esophagus, and a large genital primordium (Fig. 7–5). The filariform larva is 500 by 15 μm and has a nonbulbous esophagus that extends about one third of the length of the worm. The tail is notched (Fig. 7–6). Free-living adults have a rhabditiform appearance; the females are 1 mm in length by 60 μm in diameter and the males are 750 by 45 μm.

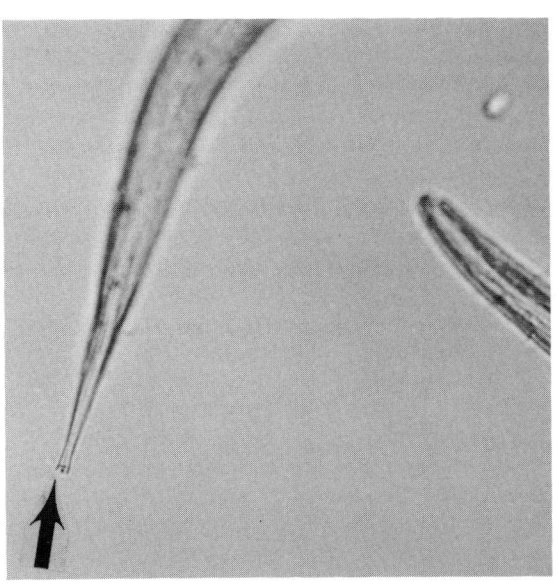

FIGURE 7–6.
Filariform larva of *Strongyloides stercoralis*, showing posterior end with notch in the tail *(arrow)*. The larvae may measure 500 × 15 μm.

Source of Infection

The source of infection is similar to that of hookworm: contact of the host with fecally contaminated soil and penetration of filariform larvae into the skin. In most endemic areas defecation is indiscriminate and personal hygiene poor. Person-to-person transmission of infections occur in institutions, especially in those housing the mentally handicapped. A few cases of transmission among homosexual men have been reported. Transmission was high among Allied prisoners of war in Southeast Asia during World War II, where prison camps were located in warm, wet, tropical and subtropical regions, conditions that foster perpetuation of the organism's life cycle. Evidence also exists of trans-mammary transmission from infected mothers to nursing infants. Since transplant recipients are immunosuppressed, transmission may occur by donor organs that carry *S. stercoralis* larvae.[18]

Clinical Manifestation

Strongyloidiasis is an unusual disease with a wide range of manifestations. Most infections are asymptomatic, but in some patients the disease may produce acute symptoms, develop into a chronic state, or lead to disseminated strongyloidiasis and death. The prepatent period is approximately 3 weeks, but cutaneous lesions,

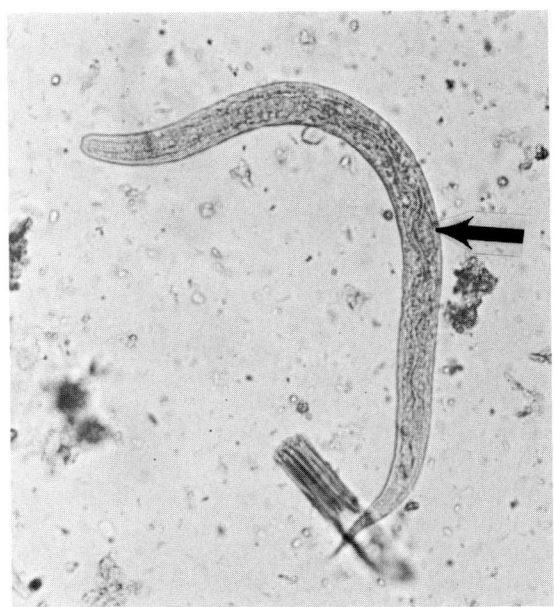

FIGURE 7–5.
Rhabditiform larvae of *Strongyloides stercoralis* (250 × 15 μm); note small buccal capsule and large genital primordium *(arrow)*. [See also Color Plate 2]

such as edema, erythema, urticaria, and petechiae, may develop soon after larval penetration of the skin. The presence of worms in the lungs may cause cough, shortness of breath, wheezing, fever, and pulmonary infiltration with eosinophilia. Pulmonary opacities may be seen on chest radiographs, and peripheral eosinophilia develops. Adult worms entering the intestinal mucosa cause diarrhea, and epigastric and abdominal pain. Heavy infections may produce vomiting, malabsorption, steatorrhea, weight loss, and edema. Obstruction may be due to paralytic ileus with edema of the small bowel.

Chronic strongyloidiasis may continue for 35 to 40 years, giving rise to periodic episodes of cutaneous and gastrointestinal symptoms; some individuals, however, remain asymptomatic. Dermal lesions occur at irregular intervals and appear as urticarial eruptions or wheals on the buttocks and around the waist. An urticarial serpiginous lesion may extend from the perianal region to the gluteal and abdominal skin in some individuals. This sign is pathognomonic for strongyloidiasis, is due to autoinfection by filariform larvae, and is called larva currens or racing larva, since the larva and lesion move at a rate of several centimeters per hour. This is unlike cutaneous lesions caused by *Ancylostoma braziliense,* dog hookworm, larvae, which move slowly. Larva currens may last for 1 to 2 days or reappear at a later time. The cutaneous lesions may occur periodically for years[19] and are usually associated with infections with Southeast Asian strains of the parasite.[20] A variety of gastrointestinal symptoms may develop and periodically consist of cramping lower abdominal pain, intermittent diarrhea, nausea, vomiting, anorexia, weight loss, and pruritus ani. The disease may be associated with gastric bleeding[21] and jejunal perforation.[22] Arthritis and uveitis are also reported in patients with long-term infections with *S. stercoralis.* These symptoms may also be associated with human T-cell leukemia virus type 1 (HTLV-1) infection.[23] In an earlier publication, however, a correlation between an *S. stercoralis* carrier state with antibodies to HTLV-1 was observed in Japan.[24] A later report suggested that, owing to the immunomodulating effects of the retroviral infection and the parasite, patients with both infections are at risk for overwhelming strongyloidiasis as well as T-lymphocyte hemopathy. *Strongyloides stercoralis* is thought to be a cofactor for retroviral replication and leukemogenic power.[25] Other clinical manifestations associated with chronic strongyloidiasis are rheumatic, psychiatric, neurologic, respiratory, urinary, and septicemic.[26]

Some people may have asymptomatic strongyloidiasis for many years without being aware of the disease. Such is the case of the Allied military in prison camps in Southeast Asia in World War II. In later life, many of these veterans became immunocompromised because of malignancies or the use of corticosteroid therapy for various illnesses. Under these conditions rhabditiform larvae in the patients transform into filariform larvae, enter the tissue, and become disseminated throughout the body. The worm population increases rapidly, and through autoinfection the patient develops hyperinfection.

Organ transplant recipients are also at risk for disseminated strongyloidiasis since they must be immunosuppressed to receive the organ. The infection can be transmitted from the donor organ, or the recipient may have had a subclinical infection. The filariform larvae are carried by the bloodstream to every organ, especially the lungs. Patients present with severe enteritis resulting in malabsorption or a protein-losing enteropathy, pulmonary changes, bronchitis, pneumonia, and pleural effusion, cough, wheezing, or dyspnea. A mucopurulent sputum or blood-tinged sputum often contains rhabditiform larvae. Their presence indicates that larvae had been retained in the lung, where they matured and completed the life cycle. A high fever, pneumonia, or meningitis and death may result from a gram-negative septicemia. Disseminated strongyloidiasis is a result of a depressed cellular immunity, but few persons with acquired immunodeficiency syndrome (AIDS) have been reported with strongyloidiasis. In Africa, where both conditions exist, few reports document both diseases in the same patient.

Pathology

The pathogenesis of strongyloidiasis is apparently related to the host-parasite relationship. Cellular immunity plays an important role in keeping the parasite under control. When cellular immunity is affected by disease or immunosuppressive therapy, the parasite is able to multiply internally and become disseminated. When filariform larvae enter the skin, an inflammatory reaction develops, with lymphocytic and eosinophilic infiltration. In larva currens, biopsies have not revealed the presence of larvae, but perivascular infiltrates of mononuclear cells and scanty eosinophils have been seen.

Larvae migrating through the lungs may cause eosinophilic infiltration related to immediate hypersensitivity reactions. With massive infections resulting from autoinfection, however, pneumonia or hemorrhage may occur. Migrating larvae may carry bacteria from the intestines to the lungs, setting up secondary bacterial infections, which appear as patchy pulmonary infiltrates. Pulmonary abscesses may also develop on rare occasions.

The pathologic condition in chronic uncomplicated strongyloidiasis is usually confined to the duodenum and jejunum. The mucosa may be edematous and covered with mucus. The adult female worms, larvae, and, at times, eggs may be found in the crypts. Histologic changes may include a cellular infiltration consisting of eosinophils and mononuclear cells. Reactions around worms may be seen in the lamina propria. In more severe cases, mucosal atrophy, flattening of the villi, and, in long-standing infections, fibrotic changes with ulcerative enteritis may result.

In disseminated strongyloidiasis, larvae can be found in tissue of any organ, causing similar changes and secondary bacterial infections. No reaction is also a possibility, depending on the degree of immunosuppression. In many cases of hyperinfection, the eosinophil and IgE levels, which are usually elevated with *S. stercoralis* infections, are normal.

Diagnosis

The parasitologic diagnosis of strongyloidiasis requires detecting the presence of *S. stercoralis* larvae or adults in feces, sputum, or duodenal aspirates. On rare occasions, larvae may be found in the blood.[27] A clinical diagnosis is difficult to make, but the presence of elevated IgE and eosinophilia and a history of travel to an endemic area are suggestive. Direct microscopic examination of the stools may reveal rhabditiform larvae or, in the case of constipated stool, filariform larvae. Fecal concentration methods also recover larvae. Stool cultures are useful, either the Harada-Mori filter paper test-tube technique or charcoal cultures followed by baermannization of the culture. If strongyloidiasis is suspected and larvae cannot be found by routine methods, several cultures should be carried out for a week to rule out infection. Charcoal culture and baermannization is considered the most sensitive technique, but a 1991 publication promotes the use of an agar method for the detection of *S. stercoralis*.[28] (Specific diagnostic techniques are described elsewhere.[4])

If stools are consistently negative, duodenal fluid may be examined by obtaining material by intubation and aspiration or by duodenal string capsule.[29] Small intestine tissue biopsy is not very reliable. Sputum is usually examined directly for the parasite by smearing the material on a glass slide and examining it microscopically. Radiologic methods usually show duodenal and jejunal dilations, rigidity, and mucosal edema. In severe disease, strictures may be found, and in advanced stages, fibrosis, narrowing, and diminished peristalsis.

Serologic methods have been found to be of value in the diagnosis. An enzyme-linked immunosorbent assay (ELISA), an immunofluorescent antibody, and an IgE-mediated skin test have all been found reliable in most patients,[17] and in a report of testing former Far East prisoners of war, the ELISA was found sensitive and specific.[30] Antigen for the serologic tests was prepared from cultured filariform larvae.

The rhabditiform larvae of *S. stercoralis* must be differentiated from those of hookworm and other nematodes. They can be distinguished by noting either the short buccal cavity and large genital primordium of the rhabditiform larvae of *S. stercoralis* (see Fig. 7–5) or the long buccal cavity of hookworm larvae. The filariform larvae of *S. stercoralis* have a notch in the tail that differentiates them from hookworm and other larvae (see Fig. 7–6).

Treatment

All cases of strongyloidiasis should be treated, and the drug of choice is thiabendazole, given in 25 mg/kg doses twice daily for 2–3 days. The patient should be followed, and routine examinations made in 6 to 12 months to ensure elimination of the parasite. Retreatment is often necessary. The side effects of thiabendazole include nausea, vomiting, malaise, dizziness, and headache. Albendazole and ivermectin are also reported to have an effect on *S. stercoralis* but are not available in the United States for human use.

In severe complicated strongyloidiasis, patients may need intravenous fluids as well as thiabendazole given in 25 mg/kg doses for 7 days. In immunosuppressed patients, when the parasite is difficult to eliminate, anthelminthic treatment may have to be repeated at monthly intervals. The dosage of the immunosuppressant should be reduced if possible. Specific antibiotics are given in cases of septicemia.

Epidemiology

Strongyloidiasis is endemic in regions with a warm moist climate and substandard sanitary conditions. The most highly endemic areas are in Asia, Africa, and Latin America, with endemic foci in the southern parts of Europe and the United States. Data on prevalence rates and age and gender distribution throughout the world are not satisfactory because routine stool examinations do not always reveal the presence of the parasite. In studies in Asia using the Harada-Mori filter paper test-tube technique, less than 1% of the stools examined in surveys in Indonesia and the Philippines were positive for larvae.[7] In other regions of the world, however, infection rates are reported to be as high as 25%.[31] Estimates range from 50 to 100 million infections worldwide. Evidence of strain variations in the parasite is suggested by the development of the free-living cycle and strain involvement in disseminated strongyloidiasis. In particular, variations in strains may exist in Southeast Asia.

Humans are the primary reservoirs for *S. stercoralis* organisms. Although infections can develop in dogs, cats, and monkeys, the role of these animals in the spread of the parasitosis is not clear. Animal handlers working with infected animals run the risk of infection.

Endemic areas have a warm climate with adequate light and moisture year-round. Where the soil remains moist, the larvae do not dry out. Direct sunlight dries out the larvae. Certain amounts of oxygen and an acid pH are also required for larval development. In sandy or relatively loose soil the larvae are able to crawl easily.

Certain population groups are more prone to infection than others. Miners and plantation workers often become infected because of indiscriminate defecation in the working environment. Military personnel and missionaries may become infected when assigned to endemic areas and, because of the nature of the assignment, come into contact with contaminated soil. Mental hospital patients are exposed to a variety of parasitic infections because of careless deposition of feces in the hospital environment. People who do not wear shoes are easily infected in endemic areas. Transmammary transmissions are reported, but the frequency of this and of waterborne transmission of larvae require further study.

Prevention and Control

Strongyloidiasis can be controlled by improving sanitary conditions and disposing of feces properly. The construction of latrines and dissemination of education on the importance of their use aid in the control of all parasitoses. The wearing of shoes prevents infections of farmers and others working in endemic areas. Individuals who travel into endemic regions should be examined for infection after returning home. Persons with high eosinophilia should be examined parasitologically and serologically for the parasite, particularly if they are to receive immunosuppressive therapy. Similarly, organ donors and recipients should be tested for possible infections. Animals found infected should be treated. All infected persons should be treated and followed for several months to ensure elimination of the parasite.

Strongyloides fuelleborni. *Strongyloides fuelleborni* is a zoonotic parasite endemic in equatorial Africa and Papua New Guinea. Monkeys are reservoir hosts in Africa, but apparently in Papua New Guinea only humans are reservoirs and transmission is human-to-human. The parasite is similar to that of *S. stercoralis*, but the life cycle gives no evidence of autoinfection. Eggs are similar to hookworm eggs but rounder and smaller, are passed in the feces, develop in the soil, and release the rhabditiform larvae. The parasite has a free-living cycle, and filariform larvae penetrate the skin and migrate through the body to the intestine. Transmammary transmission from mother to child occurs; larvae have been found in mothers' milk. Infections are more common in children than in adults. Rash develops on second infections. Cough, anorexia, malaise, abdominal pain, and diarrhea occur 3 weeks after exposure to infection. In Papua New Guinea, the infections occur in younger children more often than in older children and adults. This parasite may cause a fatal illness, with the development of abdominal distention, respiratory distress, and generalized edema. It has been called swollen belly disease in Papua New Guinea. Infections can be treated with thiabendazole. Transplantation centers drawing patients from endemic areas must examine donors and recipients carefully for occult strongyloidiasis prior to initiating immunosuppressants and transplantations.[32]

INTESTINAL CAPILLARIASIS

Capillaria philippinensis is the latest intestinal nematode parasite to be found to cause disease and death in humans. The parasite was described as a species in 1968 after being found to be a cause of an epidemic of gastroenteritis in the Philippines. Nearly 100 people died by the time the epidemic subsided in the early 1970s. By the early 1990s, nearly 1900 cases of intestinal capillariasis were confirmed, and the disease remains endemic in certain areas of the Philippines as well as Thailand. There have been reports of only 1 to 3 cases each from Japan, Korea, Taiwan, Iran, and Egypt.

Parasite

Capillaria philippinensis is a small nematode related to *Trichuris trichiura* and *Trichinella spiralis.* Characteristic of the group, *C. philippinensis* has a long stichosome that consists of stichocytes that surround the esophageal tube at the thin anterior end. The posterior half of the worm is the wider half and contains the intestines and reproductive organs. The male ranges in length from 1.3 to 3.9 mm and has a long copulatory spicule of 230 to 300 μm at the posterior end. Females range in length from 2.5 to 5.3 mm. The vulva is at the end of the stichosome, and the uterus may contain thick-shelled bi-operculated eggs with mucoid coat, thin-shelled eggs with a mucoid coat, or embryos.

The life cycle of the parasite has been determined experimentally in animals[33] and is assumed to be similar in humans. Eggs passed in feces reach water by indiscriminate defecation in or near the water or in fields from which the feces are washed into water bodies by torrential tropical rains. Eggs embryonate in water in 5 to 10 days, and, after ingestion by small freshwater fish, they hatch, and the emerged larvae grow into infective stages in 3 weeks. When the fish is eaten raw, *C. philippinensis* larvae mature into adult males and females in 12 to 14 days in the small intestine. After mating, the females produce larvae, and they, in turn, mature, and the second generation of females produce eggs that pass in the feces. The prepatent period is 25 to 26 days. Autoinfection continues by means of a few larviparous female worms that are always present, resulting in hyperinfection. In experimental infections in Mongolian gerbils, 2000 to 5000 worms were recovered after infections with two larvae from fish.[33]

Source of Infection

As far as is known, infections are acquired by eating small freshwater fish. A variety of fish have been experimentally infected in the Philippines and Thailand, and larvae from the fish infected monkeys and Mongolian gerbils.[34]

Clinical Manifestation

The presence of large numbers of parasites in the intestine (200,000 in 1 L of bowel fluid in 1

patient at autopsy) initially causes abdominal pain, diarrhea, and borborygmi. The disease progresses, with voluminous watery stools passed, 5 to 10 times a day and malaise, anorexia, vomiting, and weight loss. The disease progresses over months, and the patients exhibit muscle wasting and weakness, hypotension, distant heart sounds, gallop-rhythm and pulsus alternans, abdominal distention and tenderness, edema, and anasarca, or hyporeflexia. Excretion of xylose is decreased, and the patient exhibits hypokalemia, hypocalcemia, hypoproteinemia, and a protein-losing enteropathy. Fats and sugars are malabsorbed. Serum immunoglobulin levels are altered with increases in IgE and decreases in IgG, IgM, and IgA.[35, 36]

Pathology

The parasite is located primarily in the jejunum but may be found elsewhere in the small intestine. The worms enter the crypts, which become atrophic. The villi are flattened and denuded. The mucosal glands are denuded, and the lamina propria is infiltrated with plasma cells, lymphocytes, macrophages, and a few neutrophils and eosinophils. Other organs are also affected by malnutrition and hypokalemia.[37] Electron microscopic examination of jejunal biopsies and gerbil intestines showed complete loss of adhesion specialization and widespread separation of the epithelial cells. Gerbil epithelium showed microulceration, compressive degeneration of cells, mechanical compression, and the presence of a thick layer of electron-dense homogeneous material at the tip of the larva in the tissue. The separation of cells and ulcerations caused by parasite secretions are considered responsible for the fluid, electrolyte, and protein loss.[38]

Diagnosis

A clinical diagnosis based on symptoms can be made in known endemic areas, but a definitive diagnosis is made by identification of *C. philippinensis* eggs, larvae, or adults in feces. The parasite may also be found in duodenal or jejunal aspirates or biopsied material. Repeated stool examinations may be required in some cases. The eggs are 36 to 45 by 21 μm, are characteristic in shape, bipolar plugs and mucoid coat but not size (Fig. 7–7) and must be differentiated from eggs of *T. trichiura.*

Treatment

In severe cases, treatment consists of electrolyte replacement, an antidiarrheal, and an

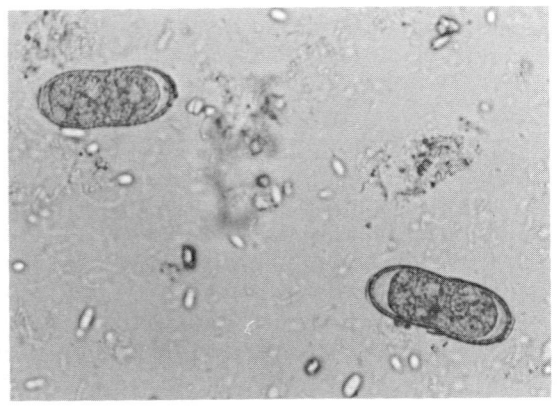

FIGURE 7–7.
Egg of *Capillaria philippinensis* (36–45 × 21 μm); note flattened bipolar plugs. [See also Color Plate 2]

anthelminthic. Thiabendazole is effective but causes side effects. Mebendazole at dosages of 400 mg per day in 2 divided doses for 20 days is recommended. Albendazole, if available, requires 10 days of treatment at 400 mg per day in 2 divided doses. Parasites disappear from the stools in 3 to 4 days, and most patients are asymptomatic after a week. Long-term treatment with an effective anthelminthic is required because of the worm's ability to multiply in the host. Relapses often result from incomplete treatment.

Epidemiology

Small freshwater or brackish water fish are intermediate hosts. These fish are usually eaten by birds, and birds have been experimentally infected with the parasite. Migratory fish-eating birds are considered natural hosts, and they disseminate the parasite along their migratory pathway to cause sporadic widespread dissemination of the parasite. Most human infections have occurred in the Philippines and Thailand, where people routinely eat freshwater fish raw. In most other areas, patients have also eaten raw fish. Many species of fish and birds may be involved in the natural life cycle of the parasite. In the Philippines, infections have occurred among the Ilocano populations of Northern Luzon, particularly middle-aged men who are fishermen or farmers. Twice as many males as females have had the disease. Males more often than females eat raw fish.[34]

Prevention and Control

Infections could be prevented by educating indigenous populations concerning the hazards of eating raw fish. The treatment of all infected persons is advised in areas where sanitation is poor and defecation indiscriminate.

TRICHINOSIS

Trichinosis, caused by nematodes of the genus *Trichinella*, is usually not considered a disease of the small intestine. People suffering from the disease consult their doctors only after experiencing muscle soreness and edema of the upper eyelid, symptoms that usually appear after the worms leave the intestine. Gastrointestinal symptoms occur early in the infection with adult *T. spiralis* parasites or, possibly, with those of one of the more recently recognized species of *Trichinella*, *T. pseudospiralis*, *T. nelsoni*, *T. nativa*, and *T. britovi*.[38b] Trichinosis is widely distributed and considered to be primarily a disease of temperate regions, with a few cases reported in some tropical areas, such as northern Thailand and parts of Africa.

Parasite

The worms have features characteristic of the trichurids: slender anterior and wider posterior portions, stichocytes, and stichosome. The females are 2 to 4 mm by 60 to 100 μm, and the males are 1.0 to 1.5 mm.

Humans acquire infections by eating uncooked muscle from animals, most commonly wild or domestic pigs. *Trichinella* larvae are encysted in the meat, and upon ingestion the larvae are digested from the cyst and pass to the small intestine, where they burrow beneath the epithelium and lie above the lamina propria. After 2 to 3 days, the larvae molt four times and develop into adults. The males die a week after copulation occurs and the viviparous females discharge larvae, which enter the circulation and are carried throughout the body. The larvae may enter any tissue but survive only in striated muscle. The adult females remain in the mucosa for several weeks and finally die.

Source of Infection

Trichinella species are found in a wide variety of carnivorous animals, with rats considered a primary reservoir for *T. spiralis* and pigs the main source of human infection. Wild animal meat, however, is of increasing importance, especially bears and wolverines. Horse meat was the source of an outbreak in France.[39] In most cases, the meat is eaten raw or only partially cooked.

Clinical Manifestation

Most infections in humans are asymptomatic, with the severity depending on the number of larvae in the ingested meat. The earliest symptoms are associated with the development of adult worms in the small intestine and usually occur within 1 week of eating infected meat. The symptoms include fever, anorexia, abdominal pain, nausea, weight loss, and diarrhea. The symptoms are easily confused with those of other gastrointestinal infections, especially in light infections. In heavy infections, the symptoms may be severe and persist for weeks. Once the larvae begin migration, other symptoms develop, such as muscle and joint pain, anorexia, emaciation, fever, dyspnea, periorbital edema, and eosinophilia. Neurologic and myocardial complications may also develop with heavy infections.

Pathology

The immune status of the host, previous exposure, and allergic responses all play a role in the pathogenesis of trichina infections. During the intestinal phase of the life cycle, the adult worms in the mucosa induce edema, hyperemia, increased mucus secretions, and eosinophilic infiltration. The adult worms are gradually expelled as the inflammatory reaction develops. Toxins elaborated by the migrating larvae may contribute to the pathophysiologic process, but evidence for this effect is not conclusive.

The primary pathologic condition associated with trichinosis results from penetration of the migratory larvae into the striated muscles and other tissues.

Diagnosis

Arriving at a definitive diagnosis of the gastroenteritis associated with trichina infection is difficult. Biopsy of the small intestine or intubation rarely reveals infections. Larvae and adult worms may pass in the feces, but recovery of these worms is extremely unlikely. A recent history of eating raw or partially cooked infected meat is helpful in making a presumptive diagnosis. Differentiation based on clinical manifestations is not reliable. Serologic tests are available, but antibodies to the parasite are usually not detectable until 3 to 4 weeks after exposure to infection. Antigen detection techniques may be available in the future.

Treatment

Since trichinosis is not usually diagnosed during the intestinal phase, treatment is rarely given. If it is diagnosed, 25 mg per day of thiabendazole twice a day for 7 days is the recommended anthelminthic to eliminate adult worms from the intestines. Mebendazole, in doses of 200 mg twice a day for 4 days and 10 mg/kg of pyrantel pamoate for 4 days are also reported effective. Early treatment during the intestinal phase affects production of larvae and prevents muscle invasion. Steroids may be given to alleviate symptoms.

Epidemiology

In past years, when people fed garbage that contained meat scraps to domestic pigs, pork and pork products were the main source of human trichinosis. The practice has nearly stopped in North America, and, although pork remains a source of infection, wild animal meat is increasing in importance. In the late 1940s, on average 400 cases of trichinosis and 10 to 15 deaths in the United States were reported for each year, but between 1982 and 1986, the average had declined to 57 infections per year with 3 deaths. The highest incidence of trichinosis was in Alaska, with the highest number of cases being in the northeast of that state. Domestic swine remain the most common source of infection, but cases associated with wild swine, bear meat, and walrus have increased. Many of the cases of trichinosis have been among recent emigrants from Southeast Asia, who have the habit of eating raw pork. Ground beef adulterated with pork is also a source of infection.[40] In Europe, horse meat imported from the United States has been incriminated in one epidemic.[39] Rats are a source of infection for pigs in some pig-farming areas. Other species of *Trichinella* are found in wild animal populations. *Trichinella nelsoni* is maintained in equatorial Africa in the bush pig, warthog, jackal, hyena, leopard, and lion. *Trichinella nativa* is found in northern temperate regions, infecting especially Arctic polar bears and walruses, since this species of *Trichinella* is resistant to freezing. Neither *T. nelsoni* nor *T. nativa* is highly infective to rats and pigs. *Trichinella pseudospiralis* has not been reported in humans and appears to be a parasite only of birds and not of humans. This species is characterized by the absence of a cyst around muscle larvae.

Prevention and Control

Infections can be controlled by eating only cooked meat, especially pork and wild animal meat. Freezing meat at $-15°C$ (5°F) for 20 days, or $-23°C$ ($-9.4°F$) for 10 days renders it safe. Freezing of meat from Arctic animals may, however, be ineffective. Garbage fed to pigs should be boiled for 30 minutes. Control of rodent populations around pig farms contributes to the control of trichinosis. Farmers and hunters should be educated about the dangers of feeding wild game to pigs. Beef should not be ground in a meat grinder after pork has been processed, except after a thorough cleaning. Automated ELISA testing of swine sera could be carried out at the time of slaughter and all seropositive swine examined parasitologically for infection. If trichinosis were found, the carcass would have to be condemned. Gamma irradiation at 30 krad has been found to be an effective way to sterilize trichina larvae in pork and could be used to control infections in highly endemic areas.

ANISAKIASIS

Anisakiasis is a relatively newly recognized disease that was first reported from the Netherlands in the early 1960s and later from other parts of the world. The disease is caused by the larval stage of a marine ascarid of the family Anisakidae. The adult worms are found in whales, seals, porpoises, and other marine mammals. The larval stages are found in the flesh of marine fish, and humans acquire the infection by eating an intermediate host raw.

Parasite

Third-stage larvae of *Anisakis simplex* and *Pseudoterranova decipiens* are the usual anisakids found in humans. *Anisakis simplex* larvae are 20 to 35 mm in length and 0.3 to 0.6 mm in width and white or milky in color. The larvae of *P. decipiens* measure 25 to 50 mm in length and 0.3 to 1.2 mm in width and are yellowish brown.

Adult worms are found in the stomachs of marine mammals, and the eggs produced pass in the feces into the ocean. First-stage then second-stage larvae develop in the egg, and after hatching from the egg, the larvae are eaten by small marine crustaceans. After they have developed into the third stage, the larvae are infective to squid and a variety of marine fish. The larvae may pass from squid to fish or fish to fish along the predatory chain. When an infected fish or squid is eaten by a marine mammal, the parasite develops into an adult in the stomach.

Source of Infection

Humans acquire *A. simplex* infection by eating raw herring, salmon, mackerel, cod, or squid. Infection from *P. decipiens* is acquired from cod, halibut, flatfish, and red snapper. Traditional raw fish dishes, such as green herring, ceviche, salmon prepared as lomilomi, sushi and sashimi, and uncooked, poorly pickled, or smoked fish are also able to transmit the infection. The larvae are in the fish muscle, and if the muscle is not cooked or pickled sufficiently, the parasite can emerge from the muscle and penetrate the gastrointestinal mucosa.

Clinical Manifestation

The parasite most often enters the stomach and, at times, the small intestine but rarely the large intestine. The parasites of *A. simplex*, more often than those of *P. decipiens*, invade the intestinal mucosa, usually the distal ileum. One to 5 days after an infecting meal, abdominal pain, nausea, vomiting, and possibly diarrhea are experienced. Slight fever and leukocytosis with eosinophilia may occur. Occult blood may be present in the stool.

Pathology

The entrance of the larva into the intestinal mucosa elicits a foreign-body reaction around the worm, with cellular infiltration and proliferation of neutrophils with a few eosinophils and giant cells. In a few days, the submucosa becomes edematous with a massive infiltration of eosinophils, lymphocytes, monocytes, neutrophils, and plasma cells. An abscess develops that is characterized by necrosis and hemorrhagic and eosinophilic infiltration. Worms can be found in early lesions but are eventually destroyed by the inflammatory reaction. Tunnels and burrows have been found in stomach mucosa and submucosa, and some observers have hypothesized that secreted protease from the parasite may be involved in the degradation of host tissue macromolecules to allow tunnel formation.[41]

Diagnosis

The diagnosis of anisakiasis is difficult to make, except in countries where the disease is well recognized, as it is in Japan and the Netherlands. In acute infections, the worms can be seen by endoscopic examination, but the diagnosis is made after a histologic examination of surgically removed tissue. Worms seen histologically reveal cross-sections of worms and typical Y-shaped lateral cords. Serologic tests may be useful in the presumptive diagnosis; ELISA, immunofluorescence, and radioallergosorbent test (RAST) methods have been found of value. The disease must be differentiated from other causes of acute abdomen, such as stomach ulcer, neoplasms or cholelithiasis, appendicitis, ileus, and regional enteritis.

Treatment

Endoscopic removal of the worm is the recommended treatment. In many cases, however, surgery is required. In Japan, endoscopy is widely used, especially for gastric infections. Anthelminthics have not been evaluated, but mebendazole and albendazole are promising possibilities worth testing. The vomiting of worms has been reported, and patients who do so require no treatment.

Epidemiology

Most cases of anisakiasis have been reported from Europe, especially the Netherlands, and are associated with pickled herring. Japan, however, has documented the most infections. The Japanese enjoy raw marine fish prepared as sushi and sashimi. The larvae are found in the fish viscera and musculature. Some investigators believe that after the fish is caught, larvae from the viscera migrate to the muscles. The disease was not recognized prior to World War II, and some believe that the introduction of large refrigerated fishing boats may be responsible for the development of the parasitosis. Fish are caught in large numbers and refrigerated until reaching port. During this time, the larvae migrate from the viscera to the muscles. The worms are hardy and can withstand cold conditions for extended periods of time.

The parasites of *A. simplex* are usually responsible primarily for gastrointestinal Anisakidae infections, but *P. decipiens* is noninvasive and gives rise to "tingling throat," and the worms are often coughed up. The worm is known as the cod worm. Reports of anisakiasis are increasing in the United States with the increase in eating fish raw, Japanese style.

Prevention and Control

Anisakiasis can be prevented by eating only cooked marine fish and squid. Larvae are killed at temperatures above 60°C (140°F) or by freezing at −20°C (−4°F) for 24 hours. Smoking temperatures are not high enough to kill the larvae in tissue, and neither salt-curing nor microwave cooking is reliable. In the Netherlands, the incidence of disease has been reduced by freezing herring. The increase in the seal population along the Pacific Coast of the United States presents an increased threat of anisakiasis.

TAENIASIS

Adult cestodes, or tapeworms, are parasites of the intestinal tract of vertebrates. They are flat, segmented, hermaphroditic worms that lack a digestive tract and absorb their food through the integument. The worm's body is divided into three regions, scolex or head, neck, and strobila, which consists of immature, mature, and gravid proglottids, or segments. Except for one species, *Hymenolepis nana*, all tapeworms infecting humans require either one intermediate host or two. The most important of the human intestinal cestodiases are the cyclophyllidean species of *Taenia*, *T saginata*, the beef tapeworm, and *T. solium*, the pork tapeworm. They are endemic throughout most of the world wherever people eat raw beef and pork and where sanitation is poor.

Parasite

Adult *T. saginata* and *T. solium* worms reside in the jejunum, and both are very long, those of *T. saginata* being 1 to 4 m and those of *T. solium* 2 to 4 m. The worms of *T. saginata* may have 1000 to 2000 proglottids, but *T. solium* has 1000 or fewer. The number of uterine branches in the gravid proglottids differs in the two worms; those of *T. saginata* being 12 or more and those of *T. solium* fewer than 12. The scolex of a *T. solium* worm has a rostellum, which is armed with rows of hooklets. The rostellum is lacking in *T. saginata*, but the scolex of both has 4 suckers.

These two species of *Taenia* produce eggs that are indistinguishable from one another. The eggs are round, 30 to 40 μm in diameter, and have a thick radially striated shell containing an embryo with 6 hooklets (Fig. 7–8). The eggs are passed individually in feces or in gravid proglottids that detach from the strobilae and pass from the host. When ingested by the intermediate host, the eggs hatch, and the hexacanth embryos, or oncospheres, migrate to the muscles of the animal. These larvae subsequently develop into fluid-filled translucent cysts with an invaginated scolex and are called cysticerci. When humans eat the infected beef or pork raw or undercooked, the cysticercus ruptures in the small intestine, and the scolex everts and attaches to the mucosa. The parasites reach sexual maturity, and egg production begins in 10 to 12 weeks. The parasite may live in the intestines for as long as 20 years.

On some occasions, humans become infected with eggs of *T. solium* either by ingestion of food or water that contains eggs or gravid proglottids or by reverse peristalsis. Reverse peristalsis has not been confirmed as a means of transmission in humans but is suspected. Infection with the larval stage of *T. solium* is called cysticercosis and may be a life-threatening disease when the larvae encyst in the central nervous system (CNS) or other vital organs.

Source of Infection

Taeniasis saginata is acquired by humans by eating raw beef or beef that is not completely cooked. Similarly, taeniasis solium is acquired by eating raw or inadequately cooked pork or pork products. These parasites are host specific, with adult worms developing only in humans. The cysticercus larva of *T. saginata* develops in bovids, but *T. solium* cysticerci can develop in a variety of animals, including humans.

Clinical Manifestation

Usually only one tapeworm is present in the intestine, but occasionally two or more *T. saginata* worms are found, and possibly both species are present at one time. Most infected persons are asymptomatic and are unaware of the infection until spontaneous passage of proglottids through the anus or in the feces. The most common symptom is the movement of segments through the rectum and out the anus, causing intense itching in the perianal area. Abdominal pain, nausea, anorexia or increased appetite, weight loss, headache, and constipation or diarrhea may be present. Allergic manifestations are also reported, including urticaria, pruritus or other skin condition, eosinophilia, and elevated IgE levels. The worms may also cause intestinal, appendiceal, biliary, or pancreatic obstructions, resulting in an acute abdomen requiring surgery. Abdominal pain and nausea are more common in the morning and are relieved by eating breakfast.

Symptoms associated with cysticercosis vary with the degree of infection and location of the cyst. Parasites in the sucutaneous tissue or muscle are asymptomatic, but those in the CNS can cause a plethora of symptoms.

Pathology

One tapeworm in the small intestines usually causes little pathology and the infection is asymptomatic. Attachment of the scolex, especially that of *T. solium*, may cause local irritation. Infection with two or more worms increases the possibility of intestinal and appendiceal obstruction and invasion of the parasite or its proglottids into pancreatic and bile ducts. The absorption of toxic substances produced by the worms may be responsible for systemic manifestations. The worms may induce a moderate eosinophilia.

Diagnosis

Eggs of various *Taenia* species are indistinguishable and may or may not be found in feces

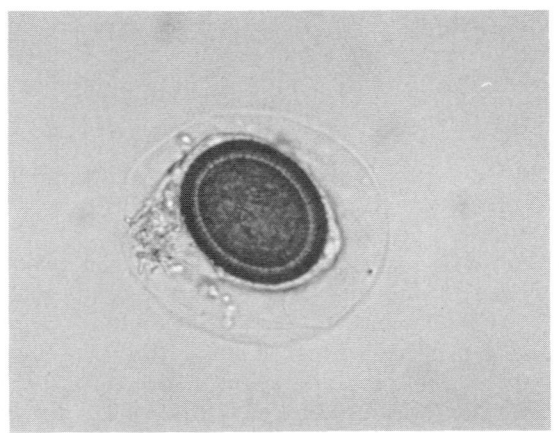

FIGURE 7–8.
Taenia sp egg (30–40 μm) with striated shell; note retention of large embryonic membrane.

of infected persons. The eggs, when found, are characteristic of the genus (see Fig. 7–8) and may be present in stools on the perianal skin. Cellophane tape swabs or paddle-shaped swubes may be used to recover eggs from the perianal area. The finding of white, often motile, 1 to 2 cm proglottids passing out of the anus confirms the diagnosis. These proglottids are more commonly found for *T. saginata* than for *T. solium*. The proglottids can be differentiated by injecting India ink into the uterus and counting the branches thus revealed. If the uterus is heavily laden with eggs, the ink is not necessary and the branches can be visualized by viewing the proglottid between two glass slides held up to a light.

Serologic tests for intestinal taeniasis are not reliable. A 1990 report, however, describes an ELISA that captures antigens, which has been developed to detect coproantigens.[42]

Treatment

The drug of choice is praziquantel given in a single dose of 10 to 20 mg/kg after a light meal. A purge 1 to 2 hours after treatment is recommended for taeniasis solium. Side effects are not common with praziquantel. Niclosamide, an alternative drug, may be given in a single dose of 2 g in chewable tablets. Children are given reduced dosages of 0.5 to 1.0 g once. Mebendazole or albendazole, given in doses of 300 to 400 mg a day for 3 to 4 days, is also reported effective.

The stools should be examined for the scolex. If the scolex is not removed, the strobila can regenerate and the parasite become reestablished. Patients should be followed and reexamined after 6 weeks and retreated if necessary. In some endemic areas, the patients may be reinfected after treatment.

Cysticercosis can be treated with 50 mg/kg of praziquantel given in 3 divided doses for 14 days. Albendazole is an alternative and may be given at a dosage of 15 mg/kg in 3 doses for 30 days. Corticosteroids may be used to suppress inflammatory responses induced by destruction of the cyst.

Epidemiology

Both *T. saginata* and *T. solium* parasites are found in all parts of the world. Prevalence rates are not known, but approximately 3 million *T. solium* and 45 million *T. saginata* infections are estimated. Beef tapeworm is highly prevalent in parts of Europe, Africa, and Asia, and it is occasionally reported in the United States. Infections of *T. solium* and cysticercosis are problems in Mexico and other Latin American countries, parts of Europe, China, India, and Africa. They are rare in the United States.

Infections are associated with the eating of raw pork and beef. Steak tartare, raw ground beef, is a favored dish in Europe and America, as is raw pork in Southeast Asia. On Taiwan, *T. saginata* infection is acquired by eating wild boar and some strains of domestic pig. Studies are under way to determine whether this Taiwanese infection actually is due to a strain of *T. saginata* or to a new species.

Animals acquire the infection by eating human feces containing eggs or proglottids. This occurs in areas of poor sanitation and also in areas where pastureland may be contaminated by sewage effluents used for irrigation and fertilization.[43] In Asia and Latin America, pigs are permitted to roam freely, and, when available, they eat human feces.

Prevention and Control

Improved sanitation, protection of bovids and porcines from exposure to human excrement, and thorough cooking of beef and pork prevent human infections, as will freezing their meat at −20°C (−4°F) for 12 hours. Smoking or pickling in brine is not adequate to kill cysticerci in meat. The use of sewage on pastures should be discouraged, since even treated sewage may contain viable eggs. Treatment of all infected persons is required in all control programs. Once developed, automated serologic tests could be used at packing houses to detect infected animals. Irradiation techniques to sterilize beef and pork may be available in the future.

HYMENOLEPIASIS

Hymenolepids are the smallest cestodes that infect humans. *Hymenolepis nana*, the dwarf tapeworm, and *H. diminuta*, the rat tapeworm, are parasites of rodents as well as of humans, and insects serve as their intermediate hosts. The infections are more common in children than in adults worldwide.

Parasites

Hymenolepis nana is unique in that infection with this parasite can be transmitted directly by the egg or by ingestion of fleas or beetles infected with the larval cysticercoids. The *H. nana* parasite when passing through an intermediate host may belong to a subspecies, *H. nana fraterna*, a rodent parasite that infects humans. A parasite of the species *H. nana*, however, is transmitted person-to-person. *Hymenolepis diminuta* parasites require a grain beetle intermediate host to complete the life cycle.

A tapeworm of *H. nana* is 15 to 40 mm by 0.5 to 1.0 mm. The scolex has four suckers and four rows of hooklets on the rostellum. The neck is long and slender, and the proglottids wider than they are long. Gravid proglottids disintegrate in the intestine and release eggs containing a hexacanth embryo; the eggs measure 35 to 52 μm (Fig. 7–9). The embryo is enclosed in a membrane that possesses two polar thickenings with 4 to 8 polar filaments. The eggs are infectious to humans when passed in the feces. Therefore, unlike the situation with other tapeworms, an intermediate host is not necessary for transmission of the parasites. Once the egg is in the intestine, the oncosphere enters the lymph channels of the villi, and after 5 to 6 days, a cysticercoid larva emerges into the lumen of the small intestine. The worm matures and releases eggs in 20 to 30 days. Eggs ingested by insects release oncospheres, which develop into cysticercoid larvae when the insect is eaten by humans, and the larvae develop directly in the intestines without entering the villi. Rodent strains of the parasite do not easily develop in humans.

Hymenolepis diminuta is the larger worm of the two, being 10 to 60 by 3 to 5 mm. The scolex lacks hooklets on the rostellum, and the proglottids are also wider than they are long. Eggs are passed and eaten by insects. Insect intermediate hosts are necessary for the development of

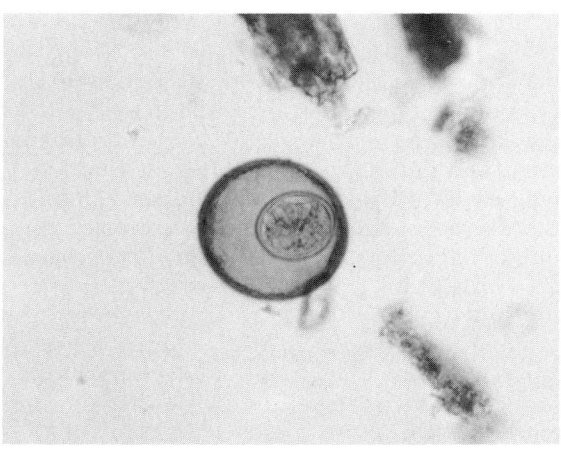

FIGURE 7–10.
Hymenolepis diminuta egg (60–86 μm).

the cysticercoid larvae. When the insect, usually a rat flea or grain beetle, is eaten, the larva is released and develops into an adult in 3 weeks. The eggs are yellowish brown, spherical, and 60 to 86 μm in diameter (Fig. 7–10). The oncosphere in the egg is surrounded by a large clear area, and the embryonic membrane has no polar filaments. Infections are short-lived in humans, but reinfection is common.

Source of Infection

Person-to-person infection occurs with the human strain of *H. nana* by the fecal-oral route. Rodent strains are transmitted by the accidental ingestion of insects in uncooked cereal or flour. The transmission of the *H. diminuta* parasite is only by the accidental ingestion of an infected insect in dried grain, fruit, or other food.

Clinical Manifestation

Similar to other parasitoses, light hymenolepid infections are usually asymptomatic. Heavy infections, however, may cause nonspecific symptoms of diarrhea, loss of appetite, abdominal pain, headache, generalized weakness, and, at times, epileptoid convulsions, instability, eosinophilia, and keratoconjunctivitis. Infection by 3000 or more *H. nana* worms causes symptoms, but infections of fewer than 1000 may simply cause diarrhea. The *H. diminuta* worm causes little disease, except possibly diarrhea.

Pathology

Developing *H. nana* cysticercoids damage villi, and large numbers invading the tissue are

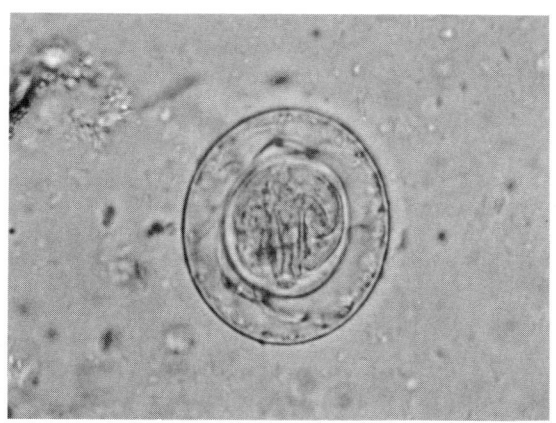

FIGURE 7–9.
Hymenolepis nana egg (35–52 μm).

responsible for the enteritis. Host reactions to worm secretions and excretions contribute to the clinical manifestations. Once absorbed, the products are able to reach the brain and eyes. The worm products provoke necrotic ulceration of the conjunctiva and cornea. Host immunity and nutrition may regulate worm numbers.

Diagnosis

Eggs are present in the feces and can be detected microscopically either directly or after concentration of fecal samples. Perianal specimens on cellophane tape swabs or paddle-shaped swubes may also reveal *H. nana* eggs. Multiple stools should be examined on alternate days, since eggs are not consistently passed but dependent on the periodic rupture and release of eggs by gravid proglottids.

Treatment

Praziquantel given in a single dose of 25 mg/kg or a single dose of 2 g of niclosamide followed by 1 g daily for 6 days is recommended. The pediatric dose is the same for praziquantel, but for niclosamide, ½ the adult dose. Heavy infections may require retreatment after 10 days. Patients should be reexamined several times during a period of 3 months. The entire family of the patient may also have to be treated.

Epidemiology

The *H. nana* cestode is the most common tapeworm in North America, especially in children in areas with poor sanitation. Epidemics are reported among populations inhabiting institutions such as orphanages, mental hospitals for the retarded, or refugee camps, where fecal contamination is common. The parasite is transmitted to humans by the fecal-oral route and on rare occasion by accidental ingestion of insects. In surveys carried out in Indonesia and the Philippines, *H. nana* and *H. diminuta* were rarely found,[7] but in 158 children from a Taiwan offshore island, 19% were found to be infected with *H. nana* tapeworms.[44] In a report on Ethiopian refugees in Israel in the mid-1980s, 21% of more than 5000 stools contained *H. nana* eggs.[45] Some murine strains of *H. nana* can develop in humans, and pet mice, rats, hamsters, and gerbils could be the source of human infection.

The tapeworms of *H. diminuta* are only occa-sionally found in humans, except in China, where it is not uncommon. The definitive hosts are rats, mice, and other murine species, and transmission is by the ingestion of beetles or fleas infected with the parasite in the cysticercoid stage. The larvae of beetles are also infected with the cysticercoids and are accidentally ingested by humans in dry cereal, grains, flour, and dried fruit.

Prevention and Control

Infections can be prevented by the improvement of environmental and personal hygiene. Mass chemotherapy is necessary in institutions with many infected children. Pet rodents should also be treated, and household rodents should be eliminated, since their feces and fleas can serve as sources of infection.

DIPHYLLOBOTHRIASIS

A number of pseudophyllidean tapeworms of the genus *Diphyllobothrium* parasitize the small intestines of humans. Most are reported only rarely from various parts of the world except *D. latum*, the fish tapeworm or broad tapeworm, which is widespread in the temperate and subarctic areas of the Northern Hemisphere. Two less commonly reported species are *D. pacificum* from Peru and Chile and *D. nikonkaiense* in Japan. Some closely related parasites are the cause of sparganosis in humans.

Parasite

The cestode of *D. latum* is one of the largest to infect humans, being 2 to 15 m in length and a maximum of 20 mm in width. The scolex, or bothrium, is 2 by 1 mm and has dorsal and ventral sucking grooves. The strobila has 3000 to 4000 proglottids, with each gravid proglottid having male and female sex organs and uteri filled with eggs. The uterine pore is midventral and discharges eggs continuously.

Eggs passed in the feces reach cool fresh water and mature in 10 to 14 days into a ciliated hexacanth larva called a coracidium. The coracidium leaves the egg through the opened operculum and swims freely in the water until ingested by the first intermediate host, a crustacean species of copepod. It develops into a procercoid larva in the body cavity, and the infected copepod is eaten by the second intermediate host, a fish. The procercoid migrates from the fish intestines to the muscles and develops into a plerocercoid larva or sparganum. When the fish is eaten raw by the final host, the plerocercoid larva develops into an adult in the intestines in 3 to 5 weeks and produces large numbers of eggs. Worms are known to live in humans for 10 years or more.

Source of Infection

A *D. latum* infection is acquired by the ingestion of freshwater fish or fish products such as roe or liver. Dietary habits differ worldwide, and sources of infection vary with the habits. Some people enjoy pickled fish, others salted or smoked fish. Salted burbot is a delicacy in Finland. Liver of burbot is a Russian favorite. Gefilte fish is an important source of transmission of this parasite among Jewish populations in Europe and the United States. Jewish housewives often become infected by tasting the fish before or during cooking. In Minnesota and Michigan, people of Scandinavian origin eat raw or pickled fish.

Some broad tapeworms are also acquired by eating marine fish. *Diphyllobothrium cordatum* infection occurs in Greenland, and *D. pacificum* in Peru is acquired by eating marine fish prepared as ceviche. The Japanese dish of raw fish prepared as sushi causes diphyllobothriasis in California. Fresh salmon, walleyed pike, sand pike, yellow perch, rainbow trout, and ruff are known second intermediate hosts. Frozen fish shipped to nonendemic areas is known to transmit infections.

Clinical Manifestation

Most cases of diphyllobothriasis are asymptomatic. The patient is usually unaware of the infection until passage of a series of spent proglottids in the stool or vomitus. In a study in Finland of nearly 300 nonanemic patients, the reported symptoms were fatigue and weakness, desire for salt, dizziness, numbness of extremities, and diarrhea, with some patients reporting epigastric pain and fever.

About 2% of the people infected with *D. latum* tapeworm develop anemia, and about 40% have low serum vitamin B_{12} levels. The anemia results from the competition between the parasite and host for vitamin B_{12}. Most patients are elderly and have reduced intrinsic factor, and the worms are usually located in the jejunum. More than one worm can be involved. The vitamin B_{12} concentration in expelled worms has been found to be high.

Symptoms of CNS involvement may occur, causing weakness, numbness, and dizziness along with paresthesia and disturbances of mobility and coordination. Central scotomata secondary to optic atrophy occur occasionally. The anemia may also be accompanied by fever and glossitis, by edema due to hypoalbuminemia, and by hemolytic jaundice.

Pathology

Although the presence of such a large worm in the intestine would be expected to cause serious disease, disease is rare. More than one worm may cause intestinal obstruction. The presence of the parasite in the upper jejunum is responsible for decreased absorption of vitamin B_{12}. Folate absorption may be diminished, and levels of ascorbic acid, thiamine, and riboflavin decreased. Anemia develops after 3 to 4 years of infection. The parasites may excrete toxic materials, which, when absorbed, are responsible for the neurologic manifestations.

The hematologic profile is characterized by macrocytes and megaloblastic anemia with leukopenia, thrombocytopenia, and increased hemolysis.

Diagnosis

Large numbers of eggs are produced by the worms and can easily be found upon direct microscopic examination of feces. The eggs are large, being 60 by 40 μm, yellowish brown, and thin-shelled, with an operculum and knob at the aoperculated end (Fig. 7–11). Concentration of specimens may be necessary for diagnosis in

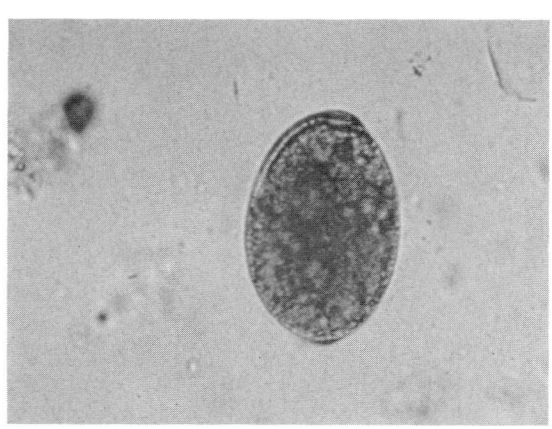

FIGURE 7–11.
Egg of *Diphyllobothrium latum* (60 × 40 μm).

early infections, when fewer eggs are produced. Proglottids may occasionally be found in feces or in vomit. If the proglottids are intact, they can easily be identified, being broader than they are long and having a large rosette uterus.

Treatment

Praziquantel, given in one dose of 10 to 20 mg/kg, or niclosamide, in a single dose of 2 g, is an effective treatment. The dosages are reduced one half for children. Side effects, if any, are minimal and transient. Vitamin B_{12} and folic acid may also be given after expulsion of the worm.

The patient should be examined weekly for a month to ensure expulsion of the worm. If the scolex remains in the intestine, the parasite will regenerate.

Epidemiology

Diphyllobothrium latum is usually found in the cool climates of Asia, Europe, and North America. Humans and a variety of other carnivores are reservoirs for infection: dogs, cats, pigs, bears, seals, sea lions, and foxes. The total number of human cases of infection was estimated to be over 9 million in 1973, with 5 million in Europe, 4 million in Asia, and 100,000 in North America. Important endemic zones include countries bordering the Baltic Sea (Scandinavia, Finland, areas of Russia, and Siberia) and Alaska. Scattered cases are reported elsewhere in the world, but many of them may have been based on misidentification of eggs. The parasitosis was once highly endemic in the Great Lakes region of North America, but reports indicate that it is no longer a problem. *Diphyllobothrium pacificum* is reported from Chile and Peru.

Many copepod species of *Cyclops* and *Diaptomus* are first intermediate hosts and are indigenous to most natural bodies of fresh water. These small crustaceans are eaten by fish, which serve as second intermediate hosts. The most common host for plerocercoids are pike *(Esox)*, perch *(Perca)*, burbot *(Lota)*, salmon *(Salmo* and *Oncorhynchus)*, and trout *(Salmo* and *Salvelinus)*.

Infected animal feces contaminate lakes and other fresh water, and in many endemic areas, humans defecate directly into freshwater bodies, thereby seeding the waters with eggs. Dietary habits are responsible for human infections. The preference for eating raw or undercooked, smoked, or pickled fish is respon-

sible for transmission to humans. The popularity of raw fish prepared as sashimi, sushi, or ceviche is increasing in the United States, exposing those who eat it to risk. Slightly frozen fish can also be a source of infection.

Prevention and Control

Human infection can be prevented by changing dietary habits and by eating only thoroughly cooked fish. Preventing fish infections would be difficult, since infected wildlife populations could not be prevented from contaminating the waters that harbor the fish. Raw sewage should not be permitted to be pumped into water where susceptible fish may be present. Ships traversing water bodies should treat sewage before permitting it to leave the ship.

Freezing fish at $-18°C$ (0°F) for 24 hours or $-10°C$ (14°F) for 72 hours prevents infection. Education regarding the tasting of fish during preparation as well as detection and treatment of all infected persons would control infections.

INTESTINAL TREMATODIASES

More than 50 species of trematodes, or flukes, are parasites of the intestines. Nearly all are associated with water, and all use a molluscan intermediate host in their life cycles. Although foci of trematode infections occur worldwide, the most highly endemic areas are in the Far East. The intestinal trematodiases are associated with dietary habits, and although infections can cause severe illness in some people, most trematodes are not considered serious pathogens. A few of the more important intestinal trematodes are considered here in generalities; all of these trematodes are diecious, the worm having both male and female sex organs.

Fasciolopsiasis. *Fasciolopsis buski* is indigenous to China, Taiwan, Thailand, Laos, Bangladesh, India, and, more recently, Indonesia. Reports of infection are usually from endemic areas.

Fasciolopsis buski is the largest intestinal fluke of humans. It is thick and fleshy, measuring 20 to 75 mm by 8 to 20 mm. It has an oral and a ventral sucker. It has two intestinal ceca, two branched testes that occupy most of the body, a central ovary, and a coiled uterus.

Eggs are passed in the feces and must reach water; a ciliated larva, a miracidium, develops in 3 to 7 weeks. The larva emerges and swims in the water in search of a specific planorbid snail. A sporocyst develops in the snail that releases rediae, which produce daughter rediae. Cercariae are formed in the latter, escape, and leave the snail. The cercariae encyst on aquatic plants or any other hard surface and become metacercaria. When aquatic plants are eaten uncooked, the metacercariae excyst in the small intestine, attach to the mucosa, and develop into adults in 3 months. The worms may live for 6 months or more.

The presence of a large number of worms causes morbidity. Bleeding, inflammation, ulceration, and excess mucus secretions may occur as well as obstruction or abdominal distention, hunger pains, increased appetite, and diarrhea. Absorption of parasite secretions or excretions may be toxic, causing generalized edema, ascites, nausea, vomiting, and possibly cachexia and leukocytosis with eosinophilia. Death can occur in massive infections owing to toxemia.

Characteristic symptoms in patients in endemic areas may suggest fasciolopsiasis, but the diagnosis is confirmed by finding eggs in the feces. The eggs are large, being 130 to 140 by 80 to 85 μm, thin-shelled, and operculated (Fig. 7–12). The eggs must be differentiated from other trematode eggs, such as *Fasciola hepatica* and *Echinostoma* species.

The drug of choice for treatment is praziquantel, 75 mg/kg divided into 3 doses in 1 day. Niclosamide may also be used, in a single dose of 2 g for adults and 1 to 1.5 g for children.

Humans and pigs are the most common reservoir hosts for fasciolopsiasis. Feces from these hosts reach water bodies containing planorbid snails and freshwater plants. Common among these aquatic plants are water caltrop, water chestnut, water bamboo, water lily, water hyacinth, and watercress. Any aquatic plant in endemic areas can be a source of infection if eaten uncooked. Many infections are acquired while peeling plant nuts with the teeth, thus releasing metacercariae encysted in the husk. Children are more often infected than are adults because they eat freshwater caltrop on their way to and from school.

Infections can be prevented by controlling fecal contamination of water used to raise food plants and by treating all infected persons and pigs. In some endemic areas, the prevalence of infection was altered by changing pig-raising practices. Instead of water plants, pigs were fed commercial food preparations. Urbanization and industrialization have eradicated fasciolopsiasis from some areas of Taiwan.

Heterophyiasis. A number of tiny trematodes of the genus *Heterophyes* infect humans, but the most common is *Heterophyes heterophyes*. Another equally important heterophyid is *Metagonimus yokogawai*. Most heterophyid infections are reported from the Far East except *H. heterophyes*, which is also reported from the Middle East, Mediterranean countries, and parts of Africa. *Metagonimus yokogawai* is reported only in Asian populations.

The heterophyids are tiny worms 1 to 2 mm long. Seen microscopically, they have oral and ventral suckers with tegumentary spines around the oral sucker. The eggs are small, being 27 to 30 by 15 to 17 μm, operculated, ovoid, and yellowish to brown (Fig. 7–13). Eggs of heterophyids are difficult to differentiate by species. The eggs contain a miracidium when laid and

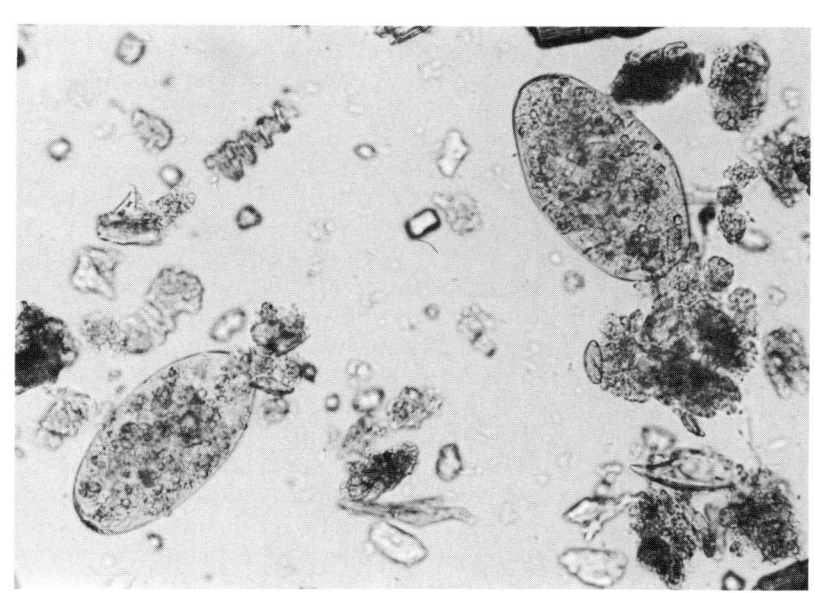

FIGURE 7–12.
Egg of *Fasciolopsis buski* (130–140 × 80–85 μm).

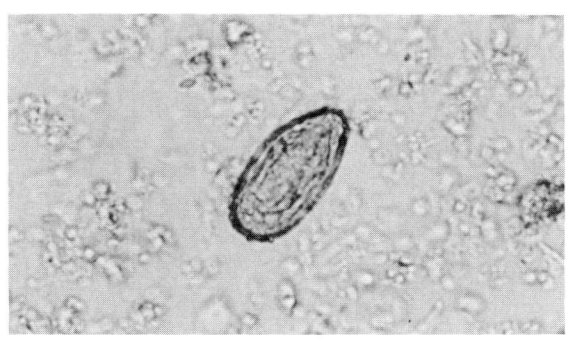

FIGURE 7–13.
Heterophyid egg (27–30 × 15–17 μm).

hatch after being eaten by the snail intermediate host. Development in the snail is similar to that of other trematodes, and the resulting cercariae encyst in freshwater fish. When the fish is eaten raw or undercooked, the metacercariae are digested from the fish tissue and then excyst, and the tiny parasites develop into adults in the small intestine in 1 to 2 weeks.

Worms in the jejunum and upper ileum may cause mild inflammation and necrosis. With heavy infections, chronic diarrhea, upper abdominal pain, anorexia, nausea, vomiting, abdominal tenderness, and peptic ulcer–like symptoms may be present. The tiny eggs may filter through the intestinal wall and be carried by the lymphatics or venules to ectopic locations, such as the heart and CNS. Deaths have been known to occur when eggs are lodged in the myocardium.

Infections can be diagnosed by finding eggs in feces, but species identification of the parasite can be made only from worms recovered from feces after treatment. In endemic areas, such as Thailand, a number of species of heterophyids may be found after treatment.[46] Praziquantel, 75 mg/kg given in 3 divided doses in 1 day, is the recommended treatment.

Many species of snails serve as first intermediate hosts. Mullet species of fish are second intermediate hosts for *H. heterophyes* in Egypt, and in Japan minnows serve as hosts. Trout and salmon are frequent sources for *M. yokogawai* infections in Japan and Korea. In some areas, heterophyid metacercariae are also found in frogs. Dogs, cats, and other fish-eating vertebrates also serve as definitive hosts.

A change of eating habits would prevent infections. Health education on the dangers of eating raw and undercooked or improperly salted or pickled fish would control infections.

Echinostomiasis. Echinostomes are small intestinal parasites of birds and some mammals primarily in Asia. A few species are reported in humans in the Philippines, Indonesia, Malaysia, Thailand, China, Japan, Korea, India, Egypt, Romania, and Russia, but infection rates are usually low. *Echinostoma ilocanum* is reported from the Ilocano areas of northern Luzon in the Philippines, where as much as 40% of the population is infected. In surveys conducted throughout the Philippines, 3% of more than 30,000 stools examined were positive for echinostome eggs.[6]

The flukes are elongated, 5 to 15 by 1 to 2 mm, with tapering rounded ends. The worms have a collar of spines in two rows around the oral sucker, a characteristic of the group. Eggs pass from the worms with feces, and in water a miracidium develops within the egg in 2 weeks. Larvae enter specific snails, develop, and release cercariae, which search out second intermediate hosts to penetrate and form metacercariae. Many aquatic animals serve as second intermediate hosts: snails, clams, fish, crustaceans, frogs, and tadpoles. When these animals are eaten uncooked, the metacercariae excyst and develop into adults in the jejunum. Reservoir hosts include humans, birds, rats, dogs, cats, and pigs.

The flukes attach to the intestinal mucosa and may cause shallow ulcers and a mild inflammatory response. Most infections are asymptomatic, but heavy infections may be accompanied by diarrhea and abdominal pain. Most infections are brief, and reinfection is common, especially in *E. ilocanum* areas of the Philippines.

The diagnosis is made by finding eggs in the feces. These are operculated, thin-shelled, and of variable size from 59 to 137 μm by 53 to 82 μm (Fig. 7–14). The eggs are similar to those of *F. buski*. Praziquantel is used for treatment, given in doses similar to those given for other intestinal trematodiases.

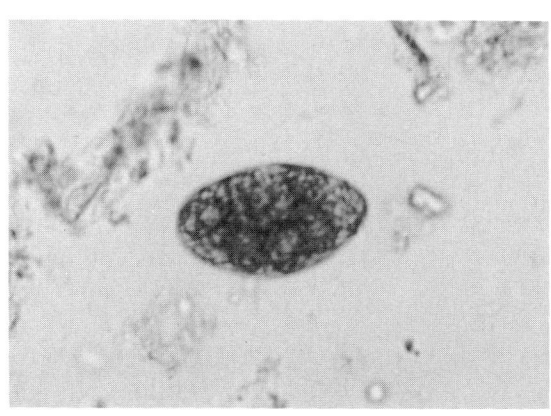

FIGURE 7–14.
Echinostomal egg (59–137 × 53–82 μm).

Infections can be prevented by changing eating habits and by cooking all aquatic animal life before it is eaten. In the Philippines, infections are acquired by eating *Pila* species of snails, which are found in rice fields during the rainy season. In the Lindu Lake region of Sulawesi, Indonesia, *Echinostoma lindoensis* was once endemic and acquired by eating clams. The parasite has now vanished because *Talapia* species of fish was introduced into the lake, and the fish ate the larval stages of the clam.

Other Trematodiases. A number of other flukes are reported in humans, but they usually cause little disease. Some of these are *Fabricola seoulensis* in Korea, *Phaneropsolus bonnei* and *Prosthodendrium molenkampi* in Thailand and Indonesia, and *Plagiorchis* species throughout the same region. Praziquantel is used for treatment.

GIARDIASIS

Giardia lamblia was probably the first parasite to be visualized. Antony van Leeuwenhoek described motile animalcules in his own diarrheic stool in 1681 using his primitive microscope. Lambl in 1859 found the parasite in the stool of children and the genus *Lamblia* was given to the organisms by Blanchard in 1888. The parasite is also known as *Lamblia intestinalis* or *Giardia duodenalis*, and it was not considered a serious pathogen until recent years. Giardiasis is now the most common waterborne pathogenic intestinal protozoan disease in the United States. During 1989 and 1990, *G. lamblia* was implicated as the cause of 7 of 12 waterborne disease outbreaks for which an agent was identified.[47] The parasite has a worldwide distribution with highest prevalence in areas with poor sanitation. In developed countries, infections lead to what has been called beaver fever or backpacker's diarrhea.

Parasite

The trophozoite of the protozoan *G. lamblia* inhabits the duodenum and upper jejunum and attaches itself to the mucosal surface by an adhesive disk. The organism is pear-shaped and measures 12 to 15 μm in length and 5 to 9 μm at the widest portion. A pair of nuclei is present in the anterior half, and basal bodies lie between the anterior poles of the nuclei. Four pairs of flagellae originate from the basal bodies, one pair on the ventral surface and three pairs along the periphery (Fig. 7–15). The flagellae provide motility, producing a tumbling

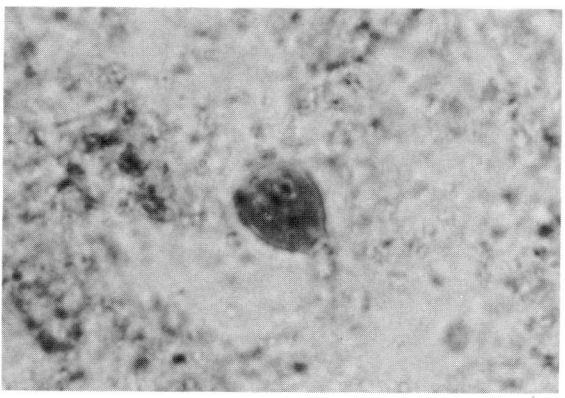

FIGURE 7–15.
Trophozoite of *Giardia lamblia* (12–15 × 5–9 μm).

motion or a descending wave motion like that of a falling leaf. In stained preparations, the organism gives the appearance of a face with two large eyes and a median body resembling a nose. The cyst is elliptical and 6 to 12 by 6 to 10 μm (Fig. 7–16). It may contain 2 or 4 nuclei, and the flagellae are retracted into axonemes. A median body and curved fibrils may also be present. The cell cytoplasm often shrinks away from the cyst wall. Little of the structure can be seen in unstained preparations under high-power microscopy. Scanning and transmission electron microscopy present greater details.

When ingested with food or water, the cyst is first acted upon by stomach acid but then passes to the duodenum, where the trophozoite emerges in an alkaline environment. The tetranucleated organism immediately divides into two daughter trophozoites by binary fission.

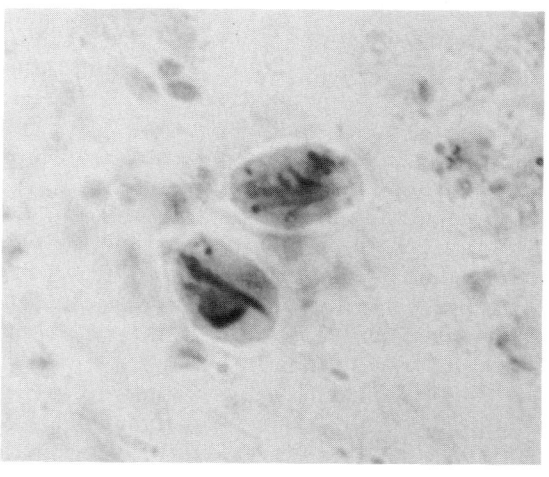

FIGURE 7–16.
Cyst of *Giardia lamblia* (6–12 × 6–10 μm).

Bile and biliary lipids stimulate the growth and multiplication of the organism. The organisms continue to multiply and colonize in the upper small intestine. The trophozoites eventually undergo encystation in the proximal small intestine and colon, and the cyst is excreted with the feces. In cases of diarrhea, trophozoites are passed in the feces, but they do not survive outside of the bowel.

Source of Infection

Transmission is only by cysts, since trophozoites are destroyed in the environment and, if ingested, would be killed by gastric acid. The organism may be transmitted directly by person-to-person contact or indirectly by the ingestion of fecally contaminated food or water. Giardiasis may be spread by infected feces from animal reservoirs when feces have contaminated natural untreated water sources. Because of sexual practices, transmission also occurs between male homosexuals. Institutionalized persons are also at risk and poor sanitation perpetuates infection.

Clinical Manifestation

The majority of persons infected with G. lamblia protozoa are asymptomatic. Those infected with pathogenic strains experience an explosive diarrhea 1 to 2 weeks after exposure. The stool is foul-smelling, has a greasy appearance at times, and floats. Diarrhea may be accompanied by nausea, weight loss, foul-smelling sulfuric belching, anorexia, flatulence, and abdominal cramping in the epigastric region. The acute symptoms may persist for weeks or months, causing a weight loss, with mucosal dysfunction leading to steatorrhea and malabsorption.

Pathology

The factors associated with clinical giardiasis are not completely understood. The strain of the parasite and the patient's age, previous exposure, and immune status are probably involved. Mechanical injury to the microvilli of the mucosal cells caused by the adhesive disk of giardia, may also occur. Studies have shown mucosal changes from normality through partial and nearly total villus atrophy. The villi may appear normal by light microscopy, but damage can be seen by transmission electron microscopy.[48] The parasite was once thought to physi-

cally occlude the surface of the intestinal mucosa, preventing absorption of nutrients. Later investigators demonstrated, however, that the trophozoites attach at the bases of the intestinal villi and occasionally at the distal villi, where absorption of nutrients occurs. Thus mechanical occlusion of the mucosal surface is an unlikely explanation for either the diarrhea or the malabsorption associated with giardiasis.[49] Steatorrhea was also thought to be caused by the ability of G. lamblia to deconjugate bile salts, but later studies have shown that the parasite does not deconjugate bile salts. Bacterial overgrowth, enterotoxin secretions, and pancreatic and biliary dysfunction have also been implicated but not proved as causes of steatorrhea.

Children are infected more often than adults, which suggests that immunity may be acquired with age or that better hygiene practices may protect adults. Secretory IgA, however, may play a role in protection against infections. The parasite has been reported to invade the intestinal mucosa, and in some patients invasion is correlated with symptoms. This correlation has been documented infrequently. The parasite has been reported in the bile ducts, gallbladder, and pancreas. Symptomatic patients usually display villus atrophy, crypt hypertrophy, epithelial cell damage, increased epithelial mitoses, and cellular infiltrations. Giardia antigens may be responsible for local mucosal inflammatory reactions that result in epithelial damage.

Diagnosis

A clinical diagnosis of giardiasis is difficult to make, since other diseases often manifest similar symptoms. Although abdominal tympany, hyperactive bowel sounds, and diffuse mild tenderness are suggestive of giardiasis, the definitive diagnosis is demonstration of G. lamblia cysts or trophozoites in feces. Cysts are found in formed stools, and trophozoites in soft or watery stools. Direct and concentration methods and microscopic examination usually reveal the parasite. From 3 to 5 stool specimens collected during 6 to 10 days may be required to find the organism. Stool specimens can also be preserved in polyvinyl alcohol (PVA), and smears stained with trichrome stain or hematoxylin. (Diagnostic techniques are described elsewhere.[4])

Material from the duodenum may be examined when the parasitosis is suspected and the stools are negative. Fluid from the bowel can be aspirated by a duodenal tube or by the string capsule, or Entero-test. The collected specimen can be placed on a microscope slide with a coverglass on top and viewed through a microscope. Actively moving trophozoites are usually found in the duodenal fluid. Tissue collected by duodenal biopsy may also be examined for the parasite. If the parasite cannot be demonstrated, but giardiasis is still suspected, empirical treatment may be given. A number of *G. lamblia* antigen detection techniques have been developed and are now available commercially for the examination of parasite antigens in the feces.[50] A variety of serologic tests are also available but do not contribute much to the diagnosis.

Treatment

Quinacrine, given in 100 mg doses for adults and 2 mg/kg tid for children tid for 7 days, is effective in the treatment of giardiasis. The possible side effects of this drug are intestinal upset, headache, and yellow urine. Unfortunately, quinacrine is unavailable at present in many areas. Alternatives are metronidazole, given in 250 mg doses tid for 5 days, or furazolidone, in 100 mg doses qid for 7 days for adults, less for children. Side effects may also be experienced with these drugs. Tinidazole and ornidazole are also effective and their treatment periods are shorter, but these drugs are not available in the United States. The nitroimidazole drugs metronidazole, tinidazole, and ornidazole are not considered safe for use during pregnancy. Treatment with these compounds should be given only when the symptoms are severe and treatment would benefit the patient. Quinacrine has a lower potential risk to the fetus and is suggested for use in pregnancy if treatment is required. Since treatment failures occur, patients should have follow-up stool examinations after 4 to 6 weeks, and 3 separate stool specimens taken every other day should be examined.

Epidemiology

Giardiasis is a major waterborne disease in the United States. Between 1989 and 1990, waterborne giardiasis was reported in 697 persons from four states. Four outbreaks were associated with community water systems and three with noncommunity systems. In six of the seven outbreaks, surface water supplies were implicated, and in the seventh, water was from a spring. Six of the outbreaks were associated with water treatment deficiencies. Breakdowns in water purification systems have been associated with outbreaks of infection in communities. Inadequate chlorination and technical failure in filtered water systems are usually responsible.[47]

Wild animals are often infected with various *Giardia* species. Beavers are infected with a species that is indistinguishable from human *G. lamblia*, and feces from this animal contaminate surface waters and have been incriminated as a source of infection for campers and hikers, especially in the Rocky Mountains. Dogs and cats are also suspected sources of infection in homes. Travelers to St. Petersburg, Russia, often return home with *G. lamblia* infections, and outbreaks of giardiasis have been reported from India and the United Kingdom. The fecal-oral route of transmission is known to occur in children and infants in nurseries, in institutions, and within families. Oral-anal sexual practices are responsible for transmission among male homosexuals. Foodborne outbreaks are rare.

Prevention and Control

All persons known to be infected with *G. lamblia* should be treated. Community water suppliers should maintain water treatment facilities to ensure reliable filtration and disinfection, by chlorination, of the water supply. Water from surface sources should be boiled or chlorinated before drinking. Commercially available purification tablets are available and effective when adequate dosages are used and sufficient time is allowed for the chemicals to work. Higher dosages should be used for cold water. Sanitary standards should be imposed in nurseries and institutions where the disease is known to occur. Tests for the parasite in water supplies are available but unreliable. A DNA probe for the detection of the organism in water systems has been described and may be available in the future.[51]

ISOSPORIASIS

Isosporiasis is caused by a coccidian protozoan, *Isospora belli*. In the past the disease was reported only sporadically, but with the occurrence of AIDS, reports of the parasitosis are increasing. Two closely related species of coccidia are *Sarcocystis hominis* and *Sarcocystis suihominis*, but reports of infections are rare. *Cryptosporidium* species are also coccidia, but they are parasites of both the small and large intestines (see Chapter 10). The parasites are found worldwide, with the highest prevalence of *I. belli* reported from South America, Haiti, Africa, and

Southeast Asia. *Isospora belli* is considered to be an opportunistic parasite in the immunocompromised. (See also Chapter 25.)

Cyclospora species is a newly described coccidian-like parasite reported to cause diarrhea in travelers (Peru and Nepal), immunocompromised patients, and immunocompetent individuals exposed to contaminated water supplies.[52, 53]

Parasite

Isosporiasis is acquired by ingestion of an oocyst of *I. belli* in food or water contaminated with human feces. The oocyst is elliptical, 20 to 33 by 10 to 15 μm, and has a thin translucent cyst wall. A mature oocyst contains two sporocysts, each with two sporozoites. After being ingested, the sporozoites are released, enter epithelial cells, and undergo schizogony. Resulting merozoites enter new epithelial cells to continue schizogony, and others become sexual gametocytes. Microgametocytes produce male microgametes, which fertilize female macrogametocytes, which, in turn, form unsporulated oocysts. These oocysts sporulate in the feces and become infective.

Sarcocystis hominis and *S. suihominis* infections are acquired by humans by eating raw or undercooked beef or pork containing muscle cysts with bradyzoites. The bradyzoites invade intestinal cells and develop into gametocytes. Oocysts are produced by gametogony and are passed in the feces. The oocysts initially produce two sporocysts with four sporozoites each, but the two sporocysts rupture from the oocyst in the feces. The sporozoites are ingested by cows or pigs, the sporozoites are released, enter the intestinal wall, and find their way to the vascular epithelium, where they undergo schizogony in the endothelial cells. Merozoites from the schizont enter striated muscle cells of the animal, initiate cell formation, and produce bradyzoites by endodyogony. A mature muscular cyst is formed after several months. Sarcocysts can also develop in human muscles following ingestion of sporocysts.

Source of Infection

Humans acquire isosporiasis or sarcocystosis by ingestion of sporocysts or oocysts in fecally contaminated water or food.

Clinical Manifestation

Most infections are asymptomatic, and infections generally remain unknown unless sporocysts are found in the feces. Symptomatic isosporiasis is accompanied by diarrhea, abdominal pain, flatulence, malaise, anorexia, weight loss, fever, headache, and in most patients eosinophilia with the stool containing Charcot-Leyden crystals, mucus, and undigested food. Symptoms may continue as long as the intestinal asexual cycle continues. Most of the symptoms subside after a few weeks, except in AIDS patients, in whom infection becomes chronic. Malabsorption, steatorrhea, weight loss, and electrolyte imbalance in chronic infections can lead to death. Intestinal *S. hominis* and *S. suihominis* infections usually lead to a self-limiting gastroenteritis. When humans acquire sarcocystosis, myositis may result, accompanied by local swelling, fever, and eosinophilia.

Pathology

Isospora belli–infected intestinal cells are usually destroyed, and an atrophic mucosa, shortened villi, hypertrophic crypts, and cellular infiltration into the lamina propria occur. Extraintestinal isosporiasis has been reported involving the lymph nodes in an AIDS patient.[54] Sarcocystosis in humans causes little tissue damage, but inflammation follows disintegration of the cyst. Muscle necrosis with cellular infiltration may occur.

Diagnosis

Since sporocysts are usually scanty, numerous stool specimens may have to be examined microscopically or after concentration by zinc sulfate or sugar flotation or by formalin–ethyl acetate concentration. Fecal smears can also be examined, and the parasites visualized with Kinyoun's acid-fast staining. Intestinal mucosal biopsies and examination of duodenal aspirates may also reveal infection. *Sarcocystis hominis* and *S. suihominis* sporocysts are rarely found in feces, but muscle biopsy can reveal sarcocysts.

Treatment

Isosporiasis can be treated with trimethoprim-sulfamethoxazole (TMP-SMX), in doses of 160 mg of TMP and 800 mg of SMX qid for 10 days then bid for 3 weeks. AIDS patients are treated indefinitely with TMP-SMX at lower dosages or weekly with pyrimethamine-sulfadoxine. Nitrofurantoin or furazolidone may also be used. Sarcocystosis treatment is unsatisfactory, but corticosteroids may be useful in treating the muscular inflammation. Treatment for enteric infection is not satisfactory, but TMP-SMX may be helpful if the diagnosis is made.

Epidemiology

Isosporiasis is most common in children, especially those in tropical areas living under poor sanitary conditions. Male homosexuals are often infected with *I. belli.* High prevalence rates are also reported from Haiti. The parasite is opportunistic, often causing disease in immunosuppressed patients and persons with AIDS. The parasite also has been known to cause epidemics among institutionalized persons.

Sarcocystis infections are acquired by humans from eating raw beef or pork containing muscle sarcocysts. Humans may acquire muscle forms of the parasite after ingestion of sporocysts in animal or human feces, usually in food or water.

Prevention and Control

Isosporiasis can be prevented by improvement of sanitation, eating only washed and thoroughly cooked food, and drinking safe water. *Sarcocystis* infections can be prevented by eating only thoroughly cooked meat or meat that has been frozen at $-20°C$ ($-4°F$) for at least 24 hours.

REFERENCES

1. Chu W-G, Chen P-M, Huang C-C, et al. Neonatal ascariasis. J Pediatr. 1972;81:783–785.
2. Cunhua MC, Veloudios A, Dantas PEC, et al. Obstruction of the nasolacrimal duct by *Ascaris lumbricoides.* Ophthal Plast Reconstruct Surg. 1989;5:141–143.
3. Ochoa B. Surgical complications of ascariasis. World J Surg. 1991;15:222–227.
4. Ash LR, Orihel TC. Parasites: A Guide to Laboratory Procedures and Identification. Chicago: American Society of Clinical Pathologists; 1987.
5. Tabbaa MI, Marshall JB. Endoscopic balloon catheter extraction of *Ascaris lumbricoides* from the biliary tree. Gastrointest Endosc. 1988;34:272–274.
6. Cross JH, Basaca-Sevilla V. Biomedical Surveys in the Philippines. U.S. Naval Medical Research Unit No. 2 SP-47, 1984:1–117.
7. Cross JH, Basaca-Sevilla V. Intestinal parasitic infection in Southeast Asia. Southeast Asian J Trop Med Public Health. 1981;12:262–274.
8. Crompton DWT. The prevalence of ascariasis. Parasitol Today. 1988;4:162–169.
9. Wong MS, Bundy DAP, Golden MHN. The rate of ingestion of *Ascaris lumbricoides* and *Trichuris trichiura* eggs in soil and its relationship to infection in two children's homes in Jamaica. Trans R Soc Trop Med Hyg. 1991;85:89–91.
10. World Health Organization: Prevention and control of intestinal parasitic infections. Geneva: WHO; Tech Rep Ser No. 749: 1987.
11. Anderson RM. The population dynamics and epidemiology of intestinal nematode infections. Trans R Soc Trop Med Hyg. 1986;80:686–696.
12. Forrester JE, Scott ME, Bundy DAP, et al. Predisposition of individuals and families in Mexico to heavy infection with *Ascaris lumbricoides* and *Trichuris trichiura.* Trans R Soc Trop Med Hyg. 1990;84:272–276.
12b. Intestinal protozoan and helminthic infections. Report of a WHO Scientific Group. WHO Tech Rep Ser 666. Geneva: World Health Organization: 1981.
13. Yu SH, Shen WX. Hookworm infection and disease in China. In: Schad GA, Warren KA. Hookworm Disease: Current Status and New Directions. New York: Taylor and Frances; 1990:44–54.
14. Schad GA, Chowdhury AB, Dean CG, et al. Arrested development in hookworm infection: An adaptation to a seasonal unfavorable external environment. Science. 1973;180:502–504.
15. Schad GA, Anderson EM. Predisposition of hookworm infection in humans. Science. 1985;228:1537–1540.
16. Prociv P, Croese J. Human eosinophilic enteritis caused by dog hookworm *Ancylostoma caninum.* Lancet. 1990;335:1299–1302.
17. Neva FA. Biology and immunology of human strongyloidiasis. J Infect Dis. 1986;153:397–406.
18. Stone WJ, Schaffner W. *Strongyloides* infections in transplant recipients. Semin Respir Infect. 1990;5:58–64.
19. Leighton PM, MacSween HM. *Strongyloides stercoralis*: The cause of an urticarial-like eruption of 65 years' duration. Arch Intern Med. 1990;150:1747–1748.
20. Genta RM, Gomes MC. Pathology. In: Grove DI. Strongyloidiasis: A Major Roundworm Infection of Man. New York: Taylor and Francis; 1989:105–132.
21. Dees A, Batenburg PL, Umar HM, et al. *Strongyloides stercoralis* associated with a bleeding gastric ulcer. Gut. 1990;31:1414–1415.
22. Kennedy S, Campbell RM, Lawrence JE, et al. A case of severe *Strongyloides stercoralis* infection with jejunal perforation in an Australian ex-prisoner-of-war. Med J Aust. 1989;150:92–93.
23. Patey O, Bouhali R, Breuil J, et al. Case report: Arthritis associated with *Strongyloides stercoralis.* Scand J Infect Dis. 1990;22:233–236.
24. Nakada K, Kohakura M, Komoda H. High incidence of HTLV antibody in carriers of *Strongyloides stercoralis.* Lancet. 1984;17:633.
25. Neisson-Vernant C, Edouard A. Malignant strongyloidiasis and the HTLV-1 virus. Revue du Praticien 1990;40:2127–2128.
26. Grove DI. Clinical Manifestations. In: Grove DI. Strongyloidiasis: A Major Roundworm Infection of Man. New York: Taylor and Francis; 1989:155–173.
27. Onuigbo MAC, Ibeachum GI. *Strongyloides stercoralis* larvae in peripheral blood. Trans R Soc Trop Med Hyg. 1991;85:97.
28. Koga K, Kasuya S, Khamboonruang D, et al. A modified agar plate method for detection of *Strongyloides stercoralis.* Am J Trop Med Hyg. 1991;45:518–521.
29. Vighi G, Schroeder J, Gallo C, et al. 'Enterotest' and *Strongyloides stercoralis.* Lancet. 1989;15:156–157.
30. Bailey JW. A serological test for the diagnosis of *Strongyloides* antibodies in ex Far East prisoners of war. Ann Trop Med Parasitol. 1989;83:241–247.
31. Pawlowski ZS. Epidemiology, prevention and control. In: Grove DI. Strongyloidiasis: A Major Roundworm Infection of Man. New York: Taylor and Francis; 1989:233–250.
32. DeVault GA Jr, King JW, Rohr MS, et al. Opportunistic

infections with *Strongyloides stercoralis* in renal transplantation. Rev Infect Dis. 1990;12:653–671.

33. Cross JH, Banzon T, Singson C. Further studies on *Capillaria philippinensis*: Development of the parasite in the Mongolian gerbil. J Parasitol. 1978;64:208–213.

34. Cross JH, Bhaibulaya M. Intestinal capillariasis in the Philippines and Thailand. In: Croll N, Cross JH. Human Ecology and Infectious Diseases. New York: Academic Press; 1983:103–136.

35. Whalen GE, Strickland GT, Cross JH, et al. Intestinal capillariasis—a new disease in man. Lancet. 1969;1:13–16.

36. Rosenberg EB, Whalen GE, Bennich H, et al. Increased circulating IgE in a new parasitic disease—human intestinal capillariasis. N Engl J Med. 1970;283:1148–1149.

37. Fresh JW, Cross JH, Reyes V, et al. Necropsy findings in intestinal capillariasis. Am J Trop Med Hyg. 1972;21:169–173.

38. Sun SC, Cross JH, Berg HS, et al. Ultrastructural studies of intestinal capillariasis *Capillaria philippinensis* in human and gerbil hosts. Southeast Asian J Trop Med Public Health. 1974;5:524–533.

38b. Pozio E, La Rosa G, Murrell KD, Lichtenfels JR. Taxonomic revision of the genus *Trichinella*. J Parasitol. 1992;78:654–659.

39. Dupouy-Camet J, Bougnoux ME, Ancelle T, et al. Antigenic characteristics of two strains of *Trichinella spiralis* isolated during the horsemeat-related outbreaks in 1985 in France. Parasitol Res. 1988;75:79–80.

40. Bailey TM, Schantz PM. Trends in the incidence and transmission patterns of trichinosis in humans in the United States: Comparisons of the periods 1975–1981 and 1982–1986. Rev Infect Dis. 1990;12:5–11.

41. Sakanari JA, McKerrow JH. Identification of the secreted neutral proteases from *Anisakis simplex*. J Parasitol. 1990;76:625–630.

42. Allen JC, Avila G, Garcia Noval J, et al. Immunodiagnosis of taeniasis by coproantigen detection. Parasitology. 1990;101:473–477.

43. Ayres RM, Stott R, Mara DD, et al. Wastewater reuse in agriculture and the risk of intestinal nematode infection. Parasitol Today. 1992;8:32–35.

44. Chung PR, Cross JH. Prevalence of intestinal parasites in children on a Taiwan offshore island determined by the use of several diagnostic methods. J Formos Med Assoc. 1975;74:411–418.

45. Nahmias J, Greenberg Z, Djerrasi L, et al. Mass treatment of intestinal parasites among Ethiopian immigrants. Isr J Med Sci. 1991;27:278–283.

46. Radomyos P, Bunnag D, Harinasuta T. Worms recovered in stools following praziquantel treatment. Arzneimittelforschung/Drug Res. 1984;34:1215–1217.

47. Herwaldt BL, Craun GF, Stokes SL, Juranek DD. Waterborne-disease outbreaks, 1989–1990. MMWR CDC Surveillance Summaries. 1991;40:1–21.

48. Farthing MJG. *Giardia lamblia*. In: Farthing MJG, Keusch GT. Enteric Infection: Mechanism, Manifestations and Management. London: Chapman and Hall Medical; 1989:397–413.

49. Smith PD: *Giardia lamblia*. In: Walzer PD, Genta RM. Parasitic Infections in the Compromised Host. New York: Marcel Dekker; 1989:343–384.

50. Addiss DG, Mathews HM, Stewart JM, et al. Evaluation of a commercially available enzyme-linked immunosorbent assay for *Giardia lamblia* antigen in stool. J Clin Microbiol. 1991;29:1137–1142.

51. Abbaszadegan M, Gerba CP, Rose JB. Detection of *Giardia* cysts with a cDNA probe and applications to water samples. Appl Environ Microbiol. 1991;57:927–931.

52. Ortega YR, Sterling CR, Gilman RH, et al. *Cyclospora* species—a new protozoan pathogen of humans. N Engl J Med. 1993;328:1308–1312.

53. Hoge CW, Shlim DR, Rajah R, et al. Epidemiology of diarrhoeal illness associated with coccidian-like organism among travellers and foreign residents in Nepal. Lancet. 1993;341:1175–1179.

54. Restrepo C, Macher AM, Radany EH. Disseminated extraintestinal isosporiasis in a patient with acquired immune deficiency syndrome. Am J Clin Pathol. 1987;87:536–542.

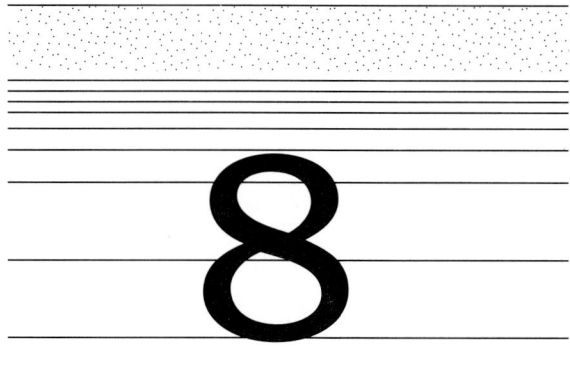

Gastrointestinal Mycobacterial Disease

LOWELL S. YOUNG, M.D.

The mycobacteria include some of humanity's oldest and most feared microbial pathogens. Peritonitis and enteritis were common entitities in hospital wards before the advent of effective tuberculosis chemotherapy prior to World War II.[1] Indeed, tuberculous involvement of the gut or the peritoneum often entered into the clinician's differential diagnosis of fever and abdominal pain. Disseminated tuberculosis involving the peritoneum or solid organs like the liver or spleen still poses an important clinical problem in third world countries.[2] This recent experience from medical centers in third world countries has contributed to our understanding of tuberculous peritonitis and enteritis.[3]

Tuberculosis is resurgent throughout the world; this phenomenon is related, in part, to the uncontrolled spread of human immunodeficiency virus 1 (HIV-1) infection in much of Asia, South America, and Africa.[4] Thus, tuberculous involvement of the gut and of the peritoneum is likely to stage a clinical resurgence not only in these geographic areas, but also in North America and Europe.

In modern medical centers providing care for acquired immunodeficiency syndrome (AIDS) patients in North America and western Europe, the atypical mycobacteria, and *Mycobacterium avium* complex organisms in particular, are important causes of symptoms and decreased survival.[4, 5] Previously considered a rare cause of disseminated disease, *M. avium* complex organisms are now the most common bacterial pathogens in patients with AIDS[6] and have a special predilection for the gastrointestinal tract. Indeed, it is believed that these organisms, widely distributed throughout nature, are acquired primarily via the gastrointestinal route.[5] Involvement of the gut seems to be a prelude to disseminated disease.

The inflammatory bowel diseases remain major diagnostic and therapeutic enigmas in gastroenterology. Whipple's disease, a relatively uncommon disorder, had previously been attributed either to fastidious organisms or to atypical mycobacteria.[7] That controversy has finally been resolved with modern molecular microbiologic techniques, and a newly characterized organism has been identified as the cause of Whipple's disease.[8] However, a role for atypical mycobacteria in inflammatory bowel disease has long been postulated by some experts, based on the similarities between human inflammatory bowel disease (specifically, Crohn's disease) and Johne's disease in cattle, which is caused by *Mycobacterium paratuberculosis*.

With renewed interest in the treatment of tuberculosis as well as the challenge posed by *M. avium* organisms complicating AIDS, new forms of chemotherapy have been developed in an attempt to treat a wide variety of mycobacterial disease processes.

GASTROINTESTINAL TUBERCULOSIS

Tuberculosis can involve any portion of the gastrointestinal tract from the tongue to the anus[2] (Table 8–1 provides a summary of sites reported in one review). Tuberculous enteropathy is presumably secondary to infection that follows the swallowing of infectious secretions. Swallowed infectious secretions are probably the major causal mechanism leading to gastrointestinal disease, but fewer than 50% of modern cases are associated with an active pulmonary focus. The other probable pathogenic mechanism involves rupture of, or disease extension from, a tuberculous lymph node. Because lymphadenopathy can represent reactivation of infection, the primary infection may have occurred many years earlier. Tuberculous ulcerations of the tongue or the oropharynx that heal very poorly were noted in the older literature. Infection of the esophagus may be acquired by swallowing infected secretions, but it can be associated with adjacent caseating lymphadenitis and development of a tracheoesophageal fistula. Chronic ulcerations of the stomach have been reported in tuberculosis; in such instances, the radiologic appearance has mimicked that of neoplastic infiltration. Pyloric ulcers or tuberculomas may actually result in obstruction in a manner not dissimilar to that caused by a malignant or benign ulcer of the duodenum. Inflammation of the small intestine can lead to perforation, obstruction, fistula formation, and massive hemorrhage. The severe cachexia of disseminated tuberculous disease may be a manifestation of malabsorption.

Involvement of the cecum is perhaps the most common or typical gastrointestinal manifestation of tuberculous enteropathy. Symptoms can include abdominal pain, diarrhea, intermittent obstruction, hemorrhage, and severe wasting. Because of the inflammatory granulomatous response, radiologic imaging studies may suggest a hyperplastic or neoplastic process. Involvement of the colon can also result in multiple ulcerations. Anal tuberculosis with development of abscesses, fistulas, and fistulas between abscesses was known earlier to clinicians and can still occur today. Involvement of the pancreas, biliary tree, and liver is common, with granulomatous hepatitis being one of the more important syndromes. Elevation of the serum alkaline phosphatase is a typical finding in tuberculosis of the gastrointestinal tract. As a result of intestinal involvement, mesenteric nodes may become infected and hypertrophic. Lymphadenitis may cause abdominal pain, fever, and even palpable masses, with subsequent gastrointestinal obstruction.

Tuberculous Peritonitis

Tuberculous involvement of the peritoneum is a chronic form of peritonitis. It is usually thought to be secondary to dissemination or miliary disease, but the primary focus, such as the lungs or the intestines, is not always evident. Some cases are probably due to reactivation of latent peritoneal tuberculosis in foci that originated from dissemination of acute disease. The pathogenesis of tuberculous peritonitis is thought to involve rupture of caseous abdominal lymph nodes.[9] Direct spread may also occur from an initial focus in the intestine or fallopian tube or from an abscess that abuts the peritoneal cavity. Bacteremic seeding of the peritoneum is also a possible pathogenetic mechanism. The association with active pulmonary disease may be as high as 50%,[10] but in other series, the prevalence of coexisting pulmonary infection is lower. In some regions, such as the Middle East or Africa, 2 to 2.5% of all hospital admissions are related to tuberculosis of the gastrointestinal tract.[11]

Histopathologically, granulomatous inflammation involves both the visceral and parietal peritoneum. Normally smooth visceral and peritoneal surfaces become studded with miliary tu-

TABLE 8–1. SITES OF INVOLVEMENT WITH GASTROINTESTINAL TUBERCULOSIS IN 46 PATIENTS

SITE	PATIENTS (%)
Esophagus	2
Stomach	7
Duodenum	2
Small intestine	28
Ileocecal region	24
Colon	28
Anorectal	9*

*Includes 1 patient with involvement of both the rectum and ileum.

SOURCE: Gilinsky NH, Marks IN, Kottler RE, Price SK. Abdominal tuberculosis: A ten-year review. S Afr Med J. 1983;64:849–857.

bercles. Additionally, ascites is often present, with an increase in peritoneal fluid protein concentration, a lymphocyte predominance in the differential leukocyte count, and a glucose concentration of less than 30 mg/dl. Diagnosis is made by culturing the ascitic fluid in large volumes (eg, 1 L), and this is preferably done by concentrating the fluid with a membrane filter (see Chapter 19) or by centrifugation to obtain a bacterial cell pellet. More rapid diagnostic approaches include biopsy of the peritoneum with a hook-type of biopsy needle. Laproscopic approaches, which are being used increasingly, will detect peritoneal studding and fibrin adhesions, which are thought to be characteristic of this complication.

Although ascites usually accompanies tuberculous peritonitis, resolution of the process following treatment results in a decrease in the ascites and the development of fibrous adhesions, producing firm matting together of the small intestines and omentum.

Symptoms include chronic abdominal pain, fever, generalized malaise, and ascites. The clinical onset of disease can be very insidious, with anorexia, weakness, and weight loss. Some observers have described the distended abdomen as characteristically doughy in consistency, but this has not been mentioned frequently in recent reports. Tuberculous peritonitis can be totally asymptomatic, presumably on the basis of miliary dissemination with incidental peritoneal loci.

Chest radiographs have been normal in approximately one third to three quarters of patients with tuberculous peritonitis. If there is an associated finding outside of the abdomen, it is usually a pleural effusion. The spectrum of the disease ranges from totally asymptomatic involvement of the abdomen with studding on the peritoneum discovered accidentally, such as during elective surgery, to an abrupt clinical syndrome that mimics acute bacterial peritonitis, characterized by chills, fever, and rebound abdominal tenderness. There may be problems in differential diagnosis if patients have coexisting Laennec's cirrhosis.

Tables 8–2 and 8–3 summarize an abundance of information from Gilinsky and associates[2] on clinical aspects and laboratory findings in abdominal tuberculosis. Weight loss, abdominal pain, and distention are nonspecific and could easily be due to tumor. Only half of the patients in this series were febrile, and a minority had diarrhea or rectal bleeding. Anemia and hypoalbuminemia were the most common laboratory findings—emphasizing the nonspecificity of common tests that physicians may order.

In diagnosis, the tuberculin test has not been helpful, with a reported range in positivity in patients with abdominal tuberculosis of between 30% and 100%, but often less (see Table 8–3). The peritoneal fluid is exudative, with a lymphocyte predominance in a peritoneal leukocyte count ranging from between 500 to 2000 cells/mm[3.] Early in the clinical course, however, there may be a neutrophil predominance in peritoneal fluid. Acid-fast staining of peritoneal fluid is only occasionally positive (see Table 8–3). With respect to other diagnostic approaches, Table 8–4, adapted from al-Quorain and colleagues,[3] indicates that the most common abdominal abnormality in patients with abdominal tuberculosis is hepatomegaly detected by computed tomographic (CT) scanning or ultrasonography. However, these imaging abnormalities were no more common than hepatomegaly detected by physical examination.

TABLE 8–2. PHYSICAL SIGNS AND SYMPTOMS IN 125 PATIENTS WITH ABDOMINAL TUBERCULOSIS

	INTESTINAL (46 PS) %	NODAL (8 PS) %	PERITONEAL (71 PS) %	TOTAL (125 PS) %
Weight loss	83	100	76	76
Abdominal pain	80	56	61	68
Abdominal distension	33	25	89	64
Fever (>37.2°C)	50	63	63	58
Ascites	15	13	85	54
Vomiting	50	25	28	36
Diarrhea	48	38	14	28
Intraabdominal mass present	35	88	17	28
Peripheral lymphadenopathy	20	13	18	18
Constipation	20	13	15	17
Rectal bleeding/melena	15	0	0	6

KEY: PS = patients.
SOURCE: Gilinsky NH, Marks IN, Kottler RE, Price SK. Abdominal tuberculosis: A ten-year review. S Afr Med J. 1983;64:849–857.

TABLE 8–3. INVESTIGATIVE FINDINGS IN 125 PATIENTS WITH ABDOMINAL TUBERCULOSIS

	PERCENT OF 46 PATIENTS WITH INTESTINAL TB	PERCENT OF 8 PATIENTS WITH NODAL TB	PERCENT OF 71 PATIENTS WITH PERITONEAL TB	PERCENT OF 125 PATIENTS TOTAL
Anemia*	67	75	75	72
RBC sedimentation rate				
15–40 mm/hr	15	13	20	18
>40 mm/hr	57	75	68	64
Albumin level <30 g/L	52	38	56	54
Chest radiograph†				
Active tuberculous disease	50	38	41	44
Inactive or normal	33	50	46	42
Abnormal barium study	74	38	7	34
AFB in sputum/pleural fluid	24	—	20	20
Tuberculin skin test				
Positive	13	—	18	15
Negative	13	25	10	12
Fistulas	15	—	1	6

*Hemoglobin concentration less than 13.5 g/dl in males and less than 12.5 g/dl in females.
†Performed in 107 patients.
KEY: AFB = acid-fast bacilli, RBC = red blood cell, TB = tuberculosis.
SOURCE: Gilinsky NH, Marks IN, Kottler RE, Price SK. Abdominal tuberculosis: A ten-year review. S Afr Med J. 1983;64:849–857.

INFLAMMATORY BOWEL DISEASE—WHIPPLE'S DISEASE

Almost a hundred years ago, a single report by Dr. George Whipple described a syndrome of migratory polyarthritis, malabsorption, weight loss, diarrhea, and mesenteric lymphadenopathy.[7] Subsequently called Whipple's disease, this systemic syndrome has been associated with periodic acid–Schiff (PAS)–positive inclusions in macrophages that infiltrated the lamina propria of the intestinal wall. Rod-shaped microorganisms, visualized by light and subsequently by electron microscopy, corresponded to the PAS-positive materials seen in stained tissue sections. Despite many attempts to grow an organism reproducibly, a variety of culture techniques have been unsuccessful. Whipple's original concept was that there was a similarity between this disorder and gastrointestinal mycobacterial infection. *Nocardia*-like organisms, *M. avium* complex, *M. paratuberculosis,* and *Rhodococcus equi* have been associated with illnesses resembling Whipple's disease in animals or in patients infected with HIV. Using molecular biologic techniques, the bacillus of Whipple's disease has been identified by sequencing its 16-S ribosomal RNA.[8] The polymerase chain reaction was used to identify an organism which, by phylogenetic analysis, is a gram-positive actinomycete that is not closely related to any known genus. This organism has subsequently been named *Tropheryma whippelii* gen. nov. sp. nov. The actinomycetes, as a group, are variably acid-fast in their staining characteristics.

Attempts to treat Whipple's disease and other inflammatory bowel disorders with antibiotics have led to variable success, but some patients have experienced notable improvement. Controlled studies, particularly of broad-spectrum antibiotics versus "specific" antimycobacterial agents, are lacking.

MYCOBACTERIUM AVIUM COMPLEX—A GASTROINTESTINAL AND SYSTEMIC PATHOGEN COMPLICATING THE ACQUIRED IMMUNODEFICIENCY SYNDROME

The term *Mycobacterium avium* complex refers to a relatively diverse group of slow-growing bacilli, largely of environmental origin, that stain positively with the Ziehl-Neelsen acid-fast stain.[5] Prior to the AIDS pandemic, these organisms were considered to be primarily veterinary pathogens. Besides infecting birds, they were known to cause important and economically serious diseases in domesticated livestock and in a wide variety of nondomesticated animals as well. Following World War II, some patients in tuberculosis sanitariums were found to have pulmonary disease caused by these nontuberculous mycobacteria.[5] These organisms, like many mycobacteria, reside within phagocytic cells, and hence the designation *M. intracellulare.* The organism is also known as the Battey bacillus, for the institution where this syndrome of nontuberculous mycobacterial pulmonary disease was initially described. *M. intracellulare,* as well as

TABLE 8–4. ULTRASONIC FINDINGS COMPARED WITH CT SCAN FINDINGS IN PATIENTS WITH ABDOMINAL TUBERCULOSIS

FINDING	ULTRASOUND 44 PATIENTS (%)	CT SCAN 29 PATIENTS (%)
Normal	11	24
Hepatomegaly	43	31
Ascites	16	21
Splenomegaly	30	17
Mass in right iliac fossa	9	14
Mass in pancreas	11	10
Para-aortic lymphadenopathy	9	14

SOURCE: al-Quorain AA, Facharzt SMB, Satti MB, et al. Abdominal tuberculosis in Saudi Arabia: A clinicopathological study of 65 cases. Am J Gastroenterol. 1993;88:75–79.

organisms previously classified as *M. avium,* have been found to be sufficiently similar to be grouped microbiologically within the *M. avium–M. intracellulare* complex, often referred to as the MAC.

Organisms of the MAC are found widely throughout nature. Besides their isolation from mammalian sources, these organisms, which resist standard water-purification procedures and chlorination, can be readily cultured from natural and treated urban water supplies. In addition, they have been found to be laboratory contaminants, even in microbiologic diagnostic reagents, hence giving false-positive results.

The association between the MAC and AIDS was recognized shortly after the initial description of AIDS.[12] MAC infection was recognized to be systemic. Indeed, at autopsy, organ involvement was diffuse and, with the advent of appropriate microbiologic techniques, most patients with systemic involvement were found to be bacteremic.

The source and pathogenetic events leading to the dissemination of MAC in AIDS patients remains in question. Prior to the AIDS epidemic, most of the MAC cases were of a pulmonary nature, but the respiratory route for infection with MAC is probably not as likely as the gastrointestinal route (ie, ingestion). The recovery of *M. avium* from respiratory secretions of AIDS patients has been related to subsequent dissemination, but usually those pulmonary secretions were obtained during the evaluation of lung infiltrates in patients who were bronchoscoped in order to diagnose pneumocystis pneumonia.[13] The aerosolization of water that contains the organism remains a theoretical mode of spreading MAC, but clinically, primary *M. avium* pneumonia in AIDS patients is quite rare. In contrast, the symptoms of diarrhea and abdominal pain are very common in patients with AIDS. Some of our earlier observations and those of Damsker and Bottone[14] established a positive predictive relationship between the recovery of MAC from gastrointestinal secretions (duodenal aspirates, stool cultures) and the subsequent development of systemic disease by organisms of the same serotype. This sequence suggests that MAC organisms are ingested from abundant environmental sources and swallowed, then colonize the gut, where they cause localized infection or enteropathy at an early stage, prior to bloodborne dissemination. This postulated pathogenetic mechanism correlates with studies in immunosuppressed animals, in which feeding of organisms to rodents has led to disseminated disease.[15]

Clinical Syndrome of MAC Disease in AIDS Patients

With MAC infection, gastroenteropathy or the more serious systemic disease is usually a late complication of AIDS. By 'late,' we refer to an opportunistic infection that characteristically develops at low CD4 helper T lymphocyte counts (fewer than 50 cells/mm^3). Patients with levels of 50 CD4$^+$ lymphocytes per cubic millimeter^3 of blood have a 20 to 30% chance of developing disseminated MAC disease in each succeeding year, and the likelihood of this complication increases as the lymphocyte count declines.[16]

Patients with AIDS are often symptomatic from concurrent infectious processes. Because the signs and symptoms of MAC infection are nonspecific, this complication should be anticipated by performing chest radiographs, assessing the CD4$^+$ lymphocyte count, and obtaining conventional cultures of body fluids. The signs and symptoms of MAC disease are summarized in Table 8–5. When HIV-infected patients with fever, weight loss, diarrhea, and wasting have relatively low CD4 lymphocyte counts and no other identifiable opportunistic infection source, the odds of culturing *M. avium* from stool or from blood exceed 80%. However, stool culture is not recommended because of the large burden of other organisms that must be suppressed in such samples prior to the isolation of MAC on selective media. In addition to fever and abdominal pain, many patients with MAC disease have nausea, vomiting, and intractable cramping abdominal pain. Ileal volvulus and intestinal obstruction have been described in this infection.[17] Hepatosplenomegaly is common, as is

TABLE 8–5. *MYCOBACTERIUM AVIUM* CLINICAL SYNDROME IN AIDS PATIENTS

Early symptoms
  Fever
  Lymphadenopathy
  Lung infiltrates
Late symptoms
  Fever
  Severe fatigue, malaise
  High fever, chills, drenching night sweats
  Weight loss
  Diarrhea
  Organomegaly
  Abdominal pain (intestinal intussusception)
  Anorexia
Laboratory findings in the late syndrome
  Anemia
  Liver function abnormalities, especially elevated
    alkaline phosphatase
  Neutropenia
  Granulomas in bone marrow, liver

retroperitoneal lymphadenopathy. The laboratory abnormalities that accompany MAC involvement of the viscera include an elevated plasma alkaline phosphatase, but this may not necessarily be accompanied by parallel increases in hepatic aminotransferases.

In one endoscopic study, of patients in whom fine white mucosal nodules were visualized, 88% had biopsy-proven gastrointestinal involvement by MAC.[18] Malabsorption was also documented in a majority of patients with MAC and diarrhea by a D-xylose absorption test.[18] Involvement of the colon, appendix, and perirectal areas is also common. In these areas, as well as in the esophagus, erosions associated with MAC infiltration are common. Gastrointestinal radiographs can reveal dilation and thickening of mucosal folds of the intestine, which is accompanied by mesenteric lymph node hypertrophy.

Small intestinal biopsies reveal histiocytic and mycobacterial infiltration that resembles bovine paratuberculosis (Johne's disease) or Whipple's disease[19] (Figs. 8–1 through 8–3).

The diagnosis of gastrointestinal MAC disease is most convincingly made by endoscopy and biopsy. However, from a clinical viewpoint, bacteremia in association with abdominal and gastrointestinal symptoms is almost certain to reflect initial gastrointestinal involvement. Although organisms may be found in stool by selective culture techniques, such tests are time consuming and expensive. Simple acid-fast staining of stool or diarrheal secretions in AIDS patients may reveal mycobacteria, but species determination will be needed to confirm the

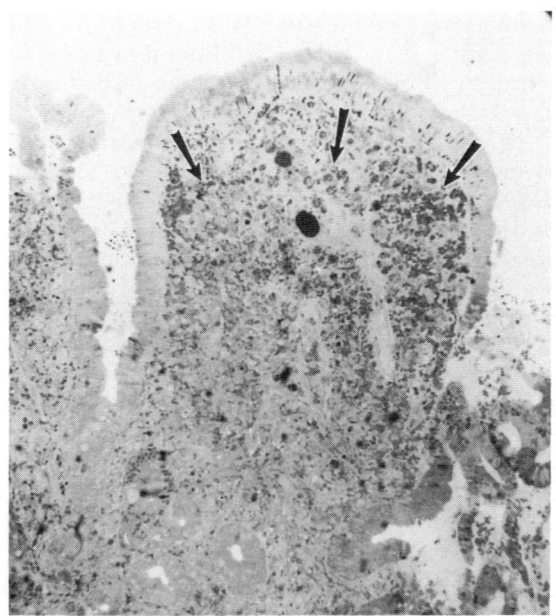

FIGURE 8–1.
Endoscopic duodenal biopsy from an AIDS patient with intestinal *Mycobacterium avium-intracellulare* infection. This villus is broadened and its lamina propria is filled with engorged macrophages *(arrows)*. (Plastic-embedded section, toluidine blue stain, × 120). SOURCE: Courtesy of Dr. Robert L. Owen.

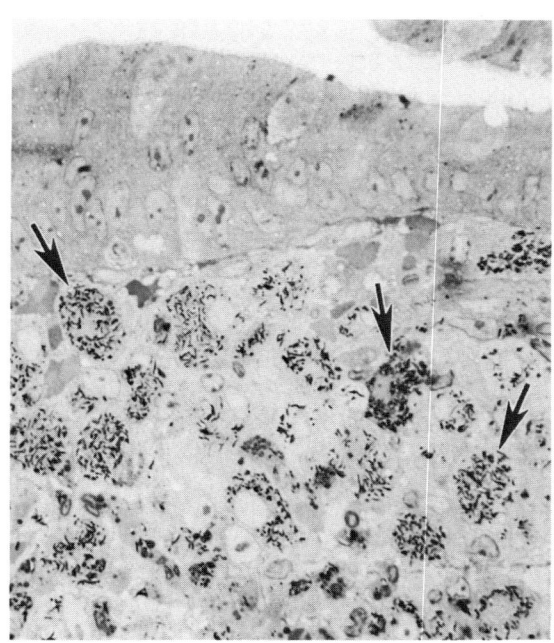

FIGURE 8–2.
Mycobacteria fill the cytoplasm of macrophages *(arrows)* in the lamina propria of a duodenal villus in an AIDS patient with diarrhea and wasting. (Plastic-embedded section, toluidine blue stain, × 880). SOURCE: Roth RI, Owen RL, Keren DF, Volberding PA. Intestinal infection with *Mycobacterium avium* in acquired immune deficiency syndrome (AIDS): Histological and clinical comparison with Whipple's disease. Dig Dis Sci. 1985;30:497–504.

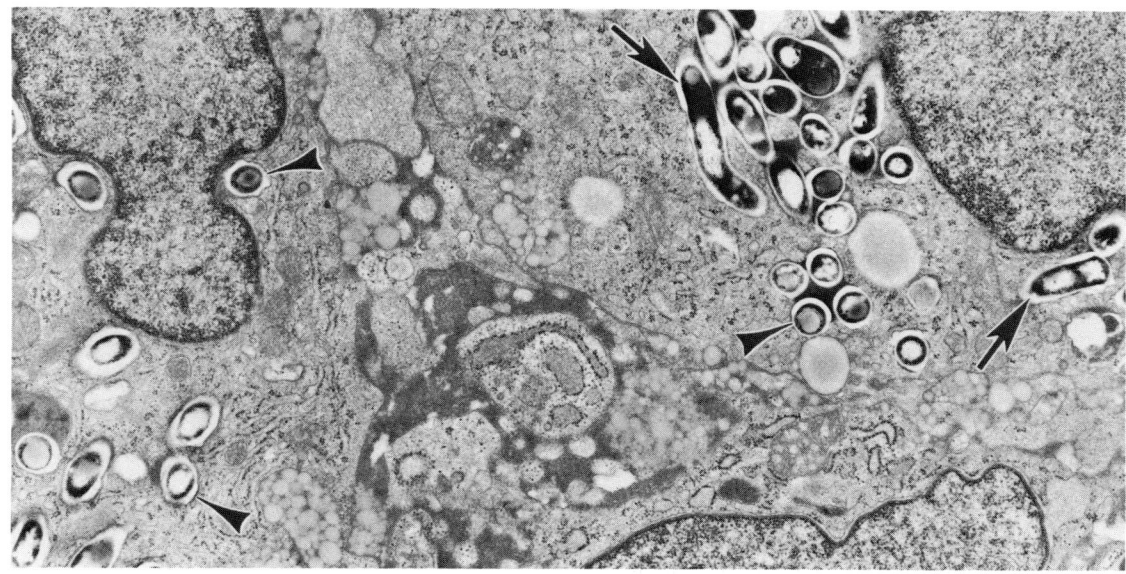

FIGURE 8–3.
Electron micrograph showing mycobacteria with rod-like, longitudinal profiles *(arrows)* and round, cross-sectional profiles *(arrowheads)* within the cytoplasm of duodenal villus macrophages. (Lead citrate and uranyl acetate stains, × 13,600). SOURCE: Roth RI, Owen RL, Keren DF, Volberding PA. Intestinal infection with *Mycobacterium avium* in acquired immune deficiency syndrome (AIDS): Histological and clinical comparison with Whipple's disease. Dig Dis Sci. 1985;30:497–504.

presence of MAC (Table 8–6). From a clinical viewpoint, however, most of the organisms thus identified by stool smears will be organisms of the MAC. For blood cultures, the most sensitive and rapid techniques involve systems that concentrate and lyse macrophages and their leukocytes, thus releasing viable intracellular organisms so that their growth may be detected by radiorespirometric methods (BACTEC Johnston Laboratories, Cockeysville, MD).

TREATMENT OF MYCOBACTERIAL DISEASE

The mainstays of treatment of *M. tuberculosis* are the drugs isoniazid (INH) and rifampin. To-

TABLE 8–6. MYCOBACTERIAL SPECIES KNOWN TO CAUSE DISSEMINATED NONTUBERCULOUS MYCOBACTERIAL INFECTION IN AIDS PATIENTS

SPECIES	NUMBER	(%)
M. avium complex	1906	(96.1)
M. kansasii	57	(2.9)
M. gordonae	11	(0.6)
M. fortuitum	5	(0.3)
M. chelonae	5	(0.3)
Total	1984*	(100.0)

*An additional 285 isolates were reported without speciation.
SOURCE: Horsburgh CR Jr, Selik RM. The epidemiology of disseminated mycobacterial infection in the acquired immunodeficiency syndrome. Am Rev Respir Dis. 1989;139:4–7.

gether with aminoglycosides (streptomycin, kanamycin, and amikacin), these are among the most potent antimycobacterial drugs. The advantages of INH and rifampin are that they may be taken orally for long periods of time without the nephrotoxicity and ototoxicity of the aminoglycosides. Until the advent of the AIDS pandemic, recommendations for the treatment of pulmonary tuberculosis also included a third drug, pyrazinamide, added to INH and rifampin. The rationale for the use of pyrazinamide was that during the early course of antituberculous treatment (eg, within the first 2 months), there was a rapid sterilizing effect of pyrazinamide; this drug appeared to work even in the low pH environment of tuberculous cavities. Much of the emphasis in the treatment of pulmonary tuberculosis has been on the development of short-course regimens that facilitate oral outpatient therapy and bring about rapid clinical improvement in a nonhospital setting. Some authorities have also substituted ethambutol for pyrazinamide at the end of the initial 2 months of treatment, reasoning that ethambutol, although perhaps not as active as pyrazinamide initially, can potentiate the effects of other antimycobacterial agents.

The above recommendations were fairly standard until the advent of the AIDS pandemic. Patients are now appearing who have multiple drug-resistant (MDR) organisms. By MDR, we refer to strains of *M. tuberculosis* that can grow

TABLE 8–7. DRUG SUSCEPTIBILITIES OF PATHOGENIC NONTUBERCULOUS MYCOBACTERIA

SPECIES	SUSCEPTIBLE	RESISTANT	INTERMEDIATE
M. kansasii	RMP, EMB	PZA	INH, SM
M. marinum	RMP, EMB	INH, PZA	SM
M. avium complex	None	INH, RMP, SM, PZA	Cycloserine, EMB
M. fortuitum	None	INH, RMP, EMB	Capreomycin
M. chelonae		SM, PZA	

KEY: RMP = rifampin, EMB = ethambutol, SM = streptomycin, PZA = pyrazinamide, INH = isoniazid.
SOURCE: Wallace JM, Hannah JB. *Mycobacterium avium* complex infection in patients with the acquired immunodeficiency syndrome: A clinicopathologic study. Chest. 1988;93:926–932.

in the presence of both INH and rifampin. Where suspicion of MDR tuberculosis exists, at least two more antimycobacterial agents are advocated in addition to INH, rifampin, and pyrazinamide.[20] Extensive clinical trials have not yet been carried out to identify the most appropriate additional drugs. However, drugs such as ofloxacin or ciprofloxacin and ethionamide have commonly been added in the clinical setting when there was concern about the development of MDR.

With respect to the MAC, it has long been appreciated that these organisms are more resistant to conventional antimycobacterial agents than is *M. tuberculosis*. Indeed, at drug concentrations achieved clinically, MAC is resistant to most of the commonly used agents (Table 8–7).[21] As a direct consequence of the AIDS pandemic, efforts have been under way to develop newer agents that would be more more active against *M. avium*. Table 8–8 lists some of these drugs and the doses that have been used. Clinical trials summarizing drug efficacy and the treatment of *M. avium* disease have been pub-

lished with increasing frequency.[4, 5] Most of these trials include multiple-drug regimens, from which it has been difficult to draw any firm conclusions about individual drug activity.

It may be convenient to consider patients in two groups: those who have serious systemic disease and severe clinical symptoms, where intravenous therapy may be necessary; and a second and larger group of patients, who have clinical symptoms such as fever, weight loss, and diarrhea, but who can still tolerate oral medications. For those individuals who are more ill, drugs such as amikacin and rifampin should be given intravenously. However, the mainstay of both oral and parenteral regimens should probably be one of the newer macrolides, in view of the convincing clinical evidence of their efficacy.[22] Both azithromycin and clarithromycin given in doses of 500 mg to 2 g per day have been shown to decrease the bacteremia of MAC disease while also ameliorating symptoms. However, resistance to these agents develops in a matter of months, so the clinical question is what additional agent or agents should be added to the

TABLE 8–8. ANTIMICROBIAL AGENTS USEFUL FOR TREATING *MYCOBACTERIUM AVIUM* COMPLEX INFECTION

DRUG	RECOMMENDED ADULT DOSE*	NOTABLE ADVERSE REACTIONS
Aminoglycosides		Otoxicity, nephrotoxicity
Amikacin	10–15 mg/kg qd†	
Streptomycin	15–20 mg/kg qd†	
Macrolides		Nausea, abdominal pain, diarrhea, hepatoxicity
Clarithromycin	500–1000 mg bid	
Azithromycin	500 mg qd†	
Quinolones		Nausea, abdominal pain, diarrhea
Ciprofloxacin	500–750 mg bid	Light-sensitive rash
Ofloxacin	500 mg bid	Anxiety, insomnia
Rifamycins		Rash, hepatoxicity
Rifampin	600 mg qd†	Neutropenia, orange urine
Rifabutin	450–600 mg qd	Neutropenia, orange urine, uveitis
Other compounds		
Ethambutol	15–25 mg/kg qd	Nausea, abdominal pain, changes in visual acuity
Clofazimine	50–100 mg qd	Skin hyperpigmentation, nausea, abdominal pain

*All drugs are administered by mouth, with the exception of the aminoglycosides (intravenous or intramuscular).
†May administer twice daily, depending on patient convenience and side effects.

TABLE 8–9. RECOMMENDATIONS FOR
TREATING *MYCOBACTERIUM AVIUM* BACTEREMIA
IN AIDS PATIENTS

Severe symptomatic disease and poor oral intake
Intravenous: amikacin + rifampin
Oral: ethambutol + macrolide (either
azithromycin or clarithromycin)
Symptomatic disease, adequate oral intake
Essential: macrolide + ethambutol
Probably beneficial: clofazimine, rifabutin
If diarrhea present: ciprofloxacin or ofloxacin

macrolide in order to enhance the mycobacterial activity without fostering the development of resistance? Ethambutol appears to potentiate the effect of other antimycobacterial agents and is probably an important companion to macrolide treatment. Another agent (clofazimine) is slower in onset and has some unpleasant side effects, but may add to long-term suppression of mycobacterial growth.

The agents listed in Table 8–8 are those that have been subjected either to previous or ongoing clinical trials. The use of antibiotics in patients who already have diarrhea poses an important clinical challenge, because patients who have AIDS may have multiple concurrent processes. Diarrhea could be a result of mycobacteria infecting the gut wall, or infection with *Cryptosporidium parvum,* cytomegalovirus, or *Clostridium difficile* (see Chapter 25). Of the agents listed in Table 8–8, almost all that are administered via the oral route achieve much higher concentrations in the gastrointestinal tract than in the blood. Thus, their effect in diarrheal syndromes might be greater than their effect on bacteremic MAC infection. In particular, we recommend the use of a quinolone such as ciprofloxacin or ofloxacin in situations where diarrhea has been linked to acid-fast organisms in the stool. Although these fluoroquinolones have borderline activity against *M. avium* bacteremia, the high intestinal concentrations that they achieve may be sufficient to inhibit MAC organisms in the gastrointestinal tract. The larger, currently unanswered question is how to achieve effective antibiotic levels inside macrophages, where the mycobacteria replicate and persist.

Table 8–9 summarizes recommendations for treatment of *M. avium* bacteremia in AIDS patients.

REFERENCES

1. Gonnella JS, Hudson EK. Clinical patterns of tuberculous peritonitis. Arch Intern Med. 1966;117:164–169.
2. Gilinsky NH, Marks IN, Kottler RE, Price SK. Abdominal tuberculosis: A ten-year review. S Afr Med J. 1983;64:849–857.
3. al-Quorain AA, Facharzt SMB, Satti MB, et al. Abdominal tuberculosis in Saudi Arabia: A clinicopathological study of 65 cases. Am J Gastroenterol. 1993;88:75–79.
4. Young LS. The Garrod Lecture: Mycobacterial diseases in the 1990s. J Antimicrob Chemother. 1993;32:179–194.
5. Bermudez LE, Inderlied CB, Young LS. *Mycobacterium avium* complex in AIDS. Curr Clin Top Infect Dis. 1992;12:257–281.
6. Horsburgh CR Jr, Selik RM. The epidemiology of disseminated nontuberculous mycobacterial infection in the acquired immunodeficiency syndrome (AIDS). Am Rev Respir Dis. 1989;139:4–7.
7. Graham DY, Markesich DC, Yoshimura HH. Mycobacteria and inflammatory bowel disease. Gastroenterology. 1987;92:436–442.
8. Relman DA, Schmidt TM, MacDermott RP, Falkow S. Identification of the uncultured bacillus of Whipple's disease. N Engl J Med. 1992;327:293–301.
9. Fitzgerald JM, Menzies RI, Elwood RK. Abdominal tuberculosis: A critical review. Dig Dis. 1991;9:269–281.
10. Pettengell KE, Larsen C, Garb M, et al. Gastrointestinal tuberculosis in patients with pulmonary tuberculosis. Q J Med. 1990;74:303–308.
11. Nafeh MA, Medhat A, Abdul-Hameed AG, et al. Tuberculous peritonitis in Egypt: The value of laparoscopy in diagnosis. Am J Trop Med Hyg. 1992;47:470–477.
12. Zakowski P, Fligiel S, Berlin GW, Johnson L Jr. Disseminated *Mycobacterium avium-intracellulare* infection in homosexual men dying of acquired immunodeficiency. JAMA. 1982;248:2980–2982.
13. Jacobson MA, Hopewell PC, Yajko DM, et al. Natural history of disseminated *Mycobacterium avium* complex infection in AIDS. J Infect Dis. 1991;164:994–998.
14. Damsker B, Bottone EJ. *Mycobacterium avium–Mycobacterium intracellulare* from the intestinal tracts of patients with the acquired immunodeficiency syndrome: Concepts regarding acquisition and pathogenesis. J Infect Dis. 1985;151:179–180.
15. Bermudez LE, Petrofsky M, Kolonoski P, Young LS. An animal model of *Mycobacterium avium* complex disseminated infection after colonization of the intestinal tract. J Infect Dis. 1992;165:75–79.
16. Nightingale SD, Byrd LT, Southern PM, et al. Incidence of *Mycobacterium avium-intracellulare* complex bacteremia in human immunodeficiency virus-positive patients. J Infect Dis. 1992;165:1082–1085.
17. Cappell MS, Hassan T, Rosenthal S, Mascarenhas M. Gastrointestinal obstruction due to *Mycobacterium avium-intracellulare* associated with the acquired immunodeficiency syndrome. Am J Gastroenterol. 1992;87:1823–1827.
18. Gray JR, Rabeneck L. Atypical mycobacterial infection of the gastrointestinal tract in AIDS patients. Am J Gastroenterol 1989; 84:1521–1524.
19. Roth RI, Owen RL, Keren DF, Volberding PA. Intestinal infection with *Mycobacterium avium* in acquired immune deficiency syndrome (AIDS). Histological and clinical comparison with Whipple's disease. Dig Dis Sci. 1985;30:497–504.
20. Wolinsky E. Statement of the tuberculosis committee of the Infectious Diseases Society of America. Clin Infect Dis. 1993;16:627–628.
21. Wallace JM, Hannah JB. *Mycobacterium avium* complex infection in patients with the acquired immunodeficiency syndrome: A clinicopathologic study. Chest. 1988;93:926–932.
22. Young LS, Inderlied CB, Bermudez LE. Antimycobacterial activity. In: Neu H, Young LS, Zinner SH, eds. The New Macrolides, Azalides, and Streptogramins: Pharmacology and Clinical Applications. New York: Marcel Dekker; 1993:183–186.

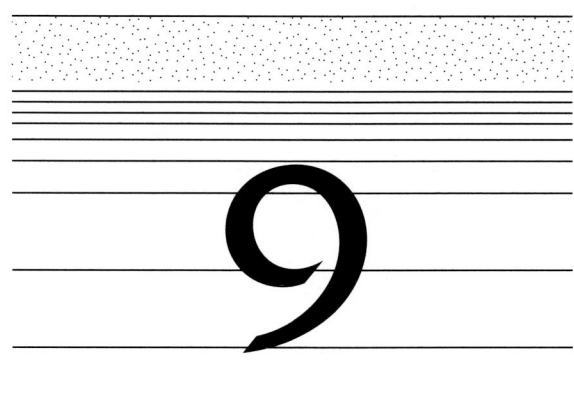

Fungal Infections of the Gastrointestinal Tract

JACK D. SOBEL, M.D.

JOSÉ A. VAZQUEZ, M.D.

Fungi are ubiquitous in nature, in association with plants, mammals, and insects. Accordingly, humans are continually exposed to multiple genera of fungi by various routes but particularly by the ingestion of food, allowing colonization of the gastrointestinal (GI) tract. Depending on the interaction between host mucosal defense mechanisms and fungal virulence factors, colonization may be transient or persistent or local disease may ensue.

Of the various pathogenic fungi, yeasts of the *Candida* species constitute the dominant fungal genus responsible for human GI tract diseases, and hence the major focus of this chapter is candidiasis, although brief discussions of GI tract diseases caused by other genera of fungi are also included (Table 9–1).

GASTROINTESTINAL CANDIDIASIS

Hippocrates is credited with first describing oral thrush in debilitated individuals,[1] and nineteenth-century authorities such as Trousseau[2] and Parrot[3] recognized that thrush invariably arose as a consequence of preexisting illness. The ini-

tial discovery of the organism that causes thrush was not made until 1839, when Langenbeck[4] described a fungus in buccal aphthae in a case of typhus. It was left to Berg in 1846[5] to establish a cause-and-effect relationship between the fungus and oral lesions. In 1875, Haussmann demonstrated that the causal agents of oral and vaginal thrush were the same.[6] Zenker, in 1862, provided the first report of systemic candidiasis, ascribing the etiology to the same fungus thought to be responsible for thrush. The taxonomic confusion accompanying the above observations continued until 1923, when Berkhout[7] proposed the genus name *Candida,* separating the genus from the universal *Monilia* genus of molds that affect fruit and vegetables.

Ecology and Epidemiology of Gastrointestinal Candidiasis

The digestive tract, especially the esophagus and the crop, is the most frequent source of yeast isolation in the majority of animals.[8] Although most species of *Candida* have been isolated from the GI tract of almost all animals, *Candida albicans* organisms have been recovered

TABLE 9–1. FACTORS PREDISPOSING TO FUNGAL INFECTION OF GASTROINTESTINAL TRACT

DISEASE	PREDISPOSING FACTOR
Candidiasis	Age, hospitalization, debility,
Diarrhea (?)	antibiotic therapy
Noninvasive	
Invasive	Granulocytopenia, hematologic malignancy, AIDS, chronic mucocutaneous candidiasis, corticosteroid or immunosuppressive therapy
Zygomycosis	Diabetes mellitus, hematologic malignancy, granulocytopenia, corticosteroid therapy
Aspergillosis	Hematologic malignancy, neutropenia
Histoplasmosis	Residence in endemic area
Paracoccidiodomycosis	Residence in endemic area Occupation involving contact with endemic area

SOURCE: Chretien JH, Garagusi VF. Current management of fungal enteritis. Med Clin North Am. 1982;66:675–687.

from a far wider range of animal hosts than those of any other *Candida* species. *C. albicans* is also the species with the highest prevalence among human yeast isolates and is the principal opportunistic yeast pathogen in most warm-blooded animals. Do-Carmo-Sousa concluded that *C. albicans* and *Candida glabrata* (*Torulopsis*) are obligatory animal saprophytes, whereas other non-*albicans Candida* species function as facultative saprophytes being recovered from sources other than animal.[9] *Candida* species are frequently found in the hospital environment in food and air and on floors and other surfaces. Moreover, *Candida* can be found on the hands of hospital personnel, and nosocomial spread among patients has been traced to personnel carriage.[10] Patients colonized with *Candida* species act as carriers and may contaminate their immediate environment with yeasts, but the contamination does not usually spread far. Because *C. albicans* organisms survive poorly on dry surfaces, transmission of *C. albicans* from one individual to another via dry fomites is a route of only limited consequence. Wade and Schimpff have reported yeasts, particularly *Candida* species, in hospital foods, especially juices and soups.[11]

Symptomatic GI candidiasis arises in subjects who are colonized with *Candida* and predisposed by illness, debility, or local reduction in host resistance to an overgrowth of their own indigenous yeast flora. Carriage rates vary according to anatomic site, a variety of local human host factors, and sampling methods used to measure *Candida* colonization. The overall prevalence of *Candida* GI tract colonization is significantly lower in normal individuals than in patients with a variety of disorders. *Candida* species are most frequently isolated from the oral cavity and are detected in approximately 31 to 55% of healthy individuals.[8] A peak frequency of oral yeast colonization is found in infants up to 18 months of age, with a lower frequency in older children and adults, increasing once more in healthy middle-aged and elderly subjects, among whom incidence may be related to the wearing of dentures.[12, 13] Colonization occurs more frequently in sick persons and especially among those requiring hospitalization than in healthy ones. Colonization rates vary with severity of illness and duration of hospitalization.

Estimates of yeast concentrations indicate that healthy colonized subjects have on average 300 to 500 CFU/ml of saliva, with a diurnal as well as day-to-day variation. Imprint culture techniques in dental subjects show that the tongue is the oral site most densely populated with yeasts, followed by the palate and buccal mucosa. Enhanced yeast carriage is associated with poor oral hygiene.[14]

Yeast isolation from feces is slightly lower than from oral culture, with a median of 23% in healthy individuals and 38% in hospitalized patients.[8] Some studies reveal a prevalence as high as 65%,[15] and 60 to 80% of isolated yeasts are *C. albicans*. Estimates of yeast concentrations in feces indicate a range of 10^1 to 10^3 CFU/g in normal subjects,[15] which is sufficiently low to make isolation difficult. Higher concentrations of 10^4 CFU/g have been reported, with even higher concentrations when the patient is treated with antibiotics.[16] Data on yeast carriage in less accessible regions of the GI tract are scanty. Most studies do, however, indicate a high carriage rate in the stomach and small intestine, with point-prevalence rates similar to those observed in the oropharynx.[8]

Candida albicans organisms usually account for 70 to 80% of oral isolates. *Torulopsis glabrata* and *Candida tropicalis* each account for approximately 5 to 8%, and other species occur only rarely.[17, 18] The lower GI tract, particularly the anorectal region, usually has a lower percentage of *C. albicans* isolates.

Occasionally, more than one species from a single specimen and more than one *C. albicans* strain are also reported.[8] The prevalence of multiple species is usually less than 10%, and combinations of *C. albicans* with *T. glabrata, Candida krusei* or *C. tropicalis* are those most commonly described. In the past, epidemiologic studies were hampered by the lack of a reliable typing system to distinguish among different strains of

C. albicans. Serotyping lacks sensitivity, and biotyping lacks reproducibility. In spite of these limitations, biotyping has shown that most individuals who carry *C. albicans* as a commensal organism or as a pathogen tend to carry the identical biotype simultaneously in different anatomic sites,[8] and most patients carry their own unique strains. Occasionally, however, two or more different biotypes or strains are found at different sites in the same person.[19] No difference in the distribution frequency of biotypes is found when colonizing organisms are compared with pathogenic isolates. Although most patients do not acquire the organism from the hospital environment, nosocomial acquisition does occur.[20]

Factors Predisposing to Gastrointestinal Candidiasis

A variety of host and exogenous factors, both localized and systemic, increase the prevalence of the carriage and population levels of *Candida* organisms in the GI tract and are conducive to the transformation from the colonizing and carrier blastoconidial phase to the more virulent hyphal phase of the organism (Table 9–2). Antifungal agents, although suppressing most commonly found GI tract yeasts, are eventually associated with yeast superinfection in the form of colonization by relatively more resistant strains of *C. albicans* and especially by more resistant, non-*albicans Candida* species. The severity and extent of *Candida* infections are likely to increase with the number and severity of predisposing factors.

AGE

The association of thrush with neonates dates back to the time of Galen.[21] Studies by Taschdjian and Kozinn showed that most cases of oral infection within the first few days of life arise primarily because of maternal contamination of the neonates with yeast from the birth canal.[22, 23] Other routes of transmission exist, however, including cross infection in neonatal intensive care units. The vulnerability of neonates to *Candida* infection stems from the immaturity of their anti-*Candida* defense mechanisms, including a lack of secretory immunoglobulin A (sIgA), deficient colonization resistance due to lack of protective bacterial flora, depressed cell-mediated immunity, and, possibly, the influence of maternal reproductive hormones.

Although the elderly are more likely to develop oral candidiasis, whether this is the direct effect of age is unclear, since multiple other factors simultaneously interact or contribute to oral candidiasis, including the increased frequency of underlying diseases and their treatments and the loss of dentition and use of dentures.

INNATE IMMUNITY

Chronic mucocutaneous candidiasis (CMC) is an uncommon syndrome that includes a variety of defects in the afferent and efferent arms of the cell-mediated immunity (CMI) response to *Candida* antigen.[24, 26] Most often this syndrome is associated with defects in either T-helper or T-suppressor cell function. The syndrome may be recessively inherited, idiopathic, associated with multiple endocrinopathies, or the result of a thymoma. Patients present with chronic, often intractable, mucosal candidiasis characterized by severe oral thrush and other cutaneous manifestations as a result of loss of normal T-cell response to *Candida* antigens. The role of T cells in the normal GI mucosal defense mechanism against *Candida* infection is highlighted by the frequent occurrence of oral[26, 27] and esophageal[28–30] candidiasis in patients with acquired immunodeficiency syndrome (AIDS). After human immunodeficiency virus (HIV) infection, oral carriage of yeasts and risk of mucosal invasion increase in frequency in patients with progressive reduction in cluster designation 4 (CD4) cells.[31, 32] The anti-*Candida* protective mechanism of T cells at a mucosal level is in-

TABLE 9–2. FACTORS PREDISPOSING TO GASTROINTESTINAL CANDIDIASIS

HOST FACTORS
AGE
Infants, the elderly
DEBILITY
IMMUNITY
Mucocutaneous candidiasis
Acquired immunodeficiency syndrome
DIABETES MELLITUS
OTHER ENDOCRINOPATHIES
DISRUPTION OF MUCOSAL INTEGRITY
Mucositis or ulceration due to chemotherapy
Radiation
Denture wearing
Trauma or surgery
Ischemia
Neoplasms
EXOGENOUS FACTORS
DIETARY
High intake of refined sugar, avitaminosis
ANTIMICROBIAL THERAPY
IMMUNOSUPPRESSIVE THERAPY
Corticosteroids, immunosuppressives
MICROBIAL SYNERGY
DURATION OF HOSPITALIZATION

completely understood, but investigations have shown that cytokines, especially gamma-interferon, inhibit transformation of *Candida* blastoconidia to the more invasive hyphal phase.[33]

Candida infections associated with other immune defects have been described in patients with primary and secondary hypogammaglobulinemia,[34] including a case of putative *Candida* gastroenteritis in a patient with sIgA deficiency.[35]

The role of phagocytic cells in GI tract mucosal defense against *Candida* is emphasized by the high prevalence of *Candida* mucositis in patients with granulocytopenia.[36, 37] Absence of neutrophils and monocytes not only predisposes patients to mucosal candidiasis but also is associated with *Candida* invasion of the gut wall and subsequent candidiasis. Similarly, qualitative neutrophil dysfunction is associated with superficial and deep candidiasis, as, for example, in patients with chronic granulomatous disease[38] or myeloperoxidase deficiency.[39]

DIABETES MELLITUS

Higher than normal frequencies of yeast carriage in the oral cavity[40] and feces[41] have been reported in diabetics. In addition, elevated concentrations of yeast are found in oral samples. Poorly controlled diabetics often present with thrush, perianal rash, and pruritus. The mechanism by which diabetes increases host susceptibility to candidiasis is incompletely understood. Segal and colleagues demonstrated increased in vitro adherence of *Candida* to exfoliated buccal and vaginal epithelial cells, facilitating colonization[42]; moreover, high tissue glucose levels favor growth of *Candida* in diabetics. Insulin-deficient diabetics, especially when acidotic, show impaired polymorphonuclear neutrophil leukocyte (PMN) phagocytic and fungicidal activity.[43]

OTHER ENDOCRINOPATHIES

Oral candidiasis is associated with endocrine disorders other than diabetes, including hypothyroidism, hypoparathyroidism,[44, 45] hypoadrenocorticism,[46] and paradoxically, Cushing's syndrome.[47] The association between candidiasis with multiple endocrinopathies and defective CMI as part of the chronic mucocutaneous syndrome is particularly common. The convergence of such a diverse group of endocrine deficiencies in a common manifestation such as oral candidiasis is not likely to reflect a direct hormone-receptor interaction but, rather, is more likely to reflect a common unrecognized immunodeficiency.

DIETARY FACTORS

Several investigators have suggested that a high carbohydrate diet, especially of refined sugar, favors multiplication of yeast in the gut resulting in higher carriage rates,[48] particularly in the oral cavity.[49] Direct evidence for the effects of high carbohydrate on *Candida* overgrowth and symptomatic infection in vivo is minimal. Gorbach and colleagues, in fact, reported a lower concentration of yeast in the stools of healthy volunteers fed a high carbohydrate diet.[50] Malnutrition augments *Candida* carriage and infection, but multiple factors operate to result in this susceptibility. Hypovitaminosis A has been postulated as predisposing to chronic mucocutaneous candidiasis,[49] as have a variety of other nutritional deficiencies, including vitamins C and B complex and folic acid and selenium.[49] The role of iron deficiency in predisposing patients to mucocutaneous candidiasis is highly controversial, although Jenkins and colleagues found no evidence for iron deficiency associated with oral thrush.[51]

LOCAL TRAUMA

Oral thrush is common after irradiation of head and neck cancer and is a frequent complication of chemotherapy-induced mucositis. In denture stomatitis, palatal inflammation appears to develop as a result of *Candida* overgrowth in the occluded space between denture and palate. Numerous authors have reported a higher oral yeast carriage among denture wearers[19] and those who use orthodontic appliances.

ANTIMICROBIAL AGENTS

The most commonly reported cause of higher than normal GI yeast carriage rate, population levels, and symptomatic oral candidiasis is the use of antibiotics. No antimicrobial agent is free from this common side effect. Certain broad-spectrum agents, notably tetracyclines and β-lactam agents, are considered more likely to encourage yeast overgrowth.[52, 53] Drugs active against gram-negative anaerobic bacteria are particularly prone to promote *Candida* overgrowth in the intestine, since these population-dominant bacteria are mainly responsible for the colonization resistance of the bowel. The prevalence of symptomatic GI tract superinfection with *Candida* is, however, generally low (<2%) after antibiotic use, even in hospitalized patients, in whom distinguishing among several contributory factors is often difficult.[54] Several studies of the mid-1970s indicate that tetracyclines are no more likely to enhance *Candida* overgrowth than are other antibiotics.[54]

Elimination of bacterial competition is almost certainly the mechanism by which antibiotics affect *Candida* numbers in vivo. No reliable studies exist demonstrating that antibiotics directly stimulate growth of *C. albicans* organisms,[55] although antibiotics may enhance growth in natural fluids such as saliva.

CORTICOSTEROID THERAPY

Several surveys have shown a high oral yeast prevalence in patients receiving corticosteroids,[56] and many animal experimental studies have found that corticosteroids increase susceptibility to local, superficial, invasive, and disseminated *Candida* infections. Corticosteroids exert both dose-dependent anti-inflammatory and immunosuppressive effects, increasing the risk of symptomatic mucosal infections and facilitating gut invasion. *C. albicans* possesses an intracellular steroid-binding protein receptor, with high specificity for corticosterone and progesterone.[57] This finding suggests that steroids may directly affect *C. albicans* infection, although this has been difficult to prove in the laboratory.

Steroids used in aerosol inhalers for therapy of bronchial asthma have been associated with oropharyngeal candidiasis.[58] Several studies found an incidence of 1 to 17% of oral thrush in steroid-aerosol users, but others found no increase in this complication.[59] Most studies have described increased oral yeast carriage, but many of the patients had previously received systemic corticosteroids. Vogt, in a 1979 review of the literature, determined that the long-term risk of developing oropharyngeal candidiasis was 4 to 13%, but that the benefits of the aerosol therapy far outweighed the risks.[59]

HISTAMINE BLOCKERS

An association between histamine (H_2) blockers, yeast, and gastric ulcers has been described.[60, 61] These H_2 blockers have been thought to aggravate *Candida* invasion of gastric ulcers and to cause gastric candidiasis at a distance from the ulcer site. Histamine blockers are thought to encourage yeasts to perforate ulcers, inducing peritonitis. (See section on gastric candidiasis.) In spite of numerous anecdotal observations, case-control studies have not been carried out. Moreover, the hypothesis that H_2 blockers, by raising pH, facilitate growth of *Candida* organisms has not been proved, since *Candida* thrives in vitro over a pH range of 3 to 8, and most species, especially *C. albicans*, grow at a pH of 2 or below.[62] Hence, pH per se is unlikely to affect carriage rate, growth, or survival of *C. albicans* organisms over the range of acidity naturally found in the human stomach, bowel, and oral cavity.

MALIGNANCY

Gastrointestinal tract colonization has been studied most extensively in patients with acute leukemia and in bone marrow transplant recipients. In a study of 91 patients with acute leukemia, cultures taken upon admission revealed that 47% of patients were colonized by *C. albicans*, 14% by *T. glabrata*, and 18% by other species.[63] In a later study of 89 patients, *C. albicans* organisms were recovered from the stools of 54% and *C. tropicalis* organisms from 17%.[64] An autopsy study of patients with hematologic malignancy and disseminated candidiasis revealed that the stomach and intestines were more frequently colonized by *C. tropicalis* than by *C. albicans* and that *C. tropicalis* was more likely to involve the entire GI tract. *Candida tropicalis* was also more likely to penetrate into the submucosa and cause vascular invasion.[64] An animal model has suggested that *C. tropicalis* organisms are more capable of invading through damaged GI mucosa than are those of *C. albicans*.[65] Eras and colleagues, in reviewing GI candidiasis in 2517 autopsy examinations of cancer patients,[66] identified GI infection in 4%. Although the esophagus was the organ most often involved, the stomach was infected in 23%, the bowel in 7%, and multiple sites in 28%. The overall frequency of infection of the lower GI tract was 0.6% in solid tumor patients but reached 30.0% in patients with leukemia and lymphoma. Several additional studies in cancer patients revealed GI candidiasis in excess of 50%.[67]

Pathogenesis of Candidiasis in the Gastrointestinal Tract

Epidemiologic studies suggest that humans are exposed repeatedly to *Candida* organisms in food and other sources. Point-prevalence studies reveal that at any given time, in 30 to 55% of subjects *Candida* organisms can be identified in the GI tract. The natural history of this commensal normal colonization over weeks, months, and years is poorly understood, primarily because previous longitudinal studies were severely handicapped by the absence of a reliable typing system to differentiate among various strains of *C. albicans*. Nevertheless, one may reasonably conclude that *Candida* colonization is almost universal. Among colonized individuals, the most frequently found species is *C. albicans,* and no unique strains of *C. albicans* with specific GI tract tropism have been identified. Moreover, commensal yeasts in the GI tract appear to exist, at least on a short-term basis, in some symbiotic relationship with the natural bacterial flora of the gut. Under these circumstances, the most notable characteristic of commensal yeast in asymptomatic individuals is its small size in comparison with the enormous indigenous bacterial flora.

Commensal yeasts are also characteristically found in vivo in the blastospore phase and tend to be associated with the lumen rather than the mucosa. The normal outcome of the introduction of *Candida* organisms into the GI tract depends on the interplay of yeast virulence factors. These factors establish the presence of yeasts in the GI tract by colonization, and allow their persistence and possible expansion in the gut despite defense mechanisms aimed at preventing colonization or maintaining low numbers of yeast commensals. These naturally occurring anti-*Candida* defense mechanisms are highly complex and efficient and have been the subject of many in vitro and experimental animal studies.[68–72] Factors operating to maintain low numbers of *Candida* organisms are shown in Table 9–3. Natural defense mechanisms include the normal protective function of the GI tract bacterial flora and intact CMI. Cell-mediated immunity has been recognized only since the appearance of AIDS, but the mechanism of normal CD4 cell function in preventing oropharyngeal and esophageal candidiasis is not known. Most of the attention of investigators has been focused on the normal bacterial flora's offering effective colonization resistance and maintaining low numbers of ungerminated yeast. As shown in Table 9–2, the normal GI flora profoundly antagonize and suppress *Candida* growth by anaerobiosis, prolongation of lag phase and doubling time, competition for growth-limiting nutrients, production of inhibitors that limit substrate availability, and elaboration of inhibitor substances,[71, 72] including short-chain fatty acids and deconjugated bile acids. Apart from its growth inhibition role, the normal flora acts to prevent the adherence of *Candida* organisms to mucosal receptor sites, thus preventing mucosal association and colonization. An association with mucosa would allow *Candida* organisms to persist in the gut despite severely depressed growth. Animal studies indicate that the mainstay of anti-yeast resistance is not *Escherichia coli* but the dominant anaerobic bacterial flora.

In spite of the efficiency of the natural anti-*Candida* defense mechanisms, any of the factors described in Table 9–2 can induce clinical infection by facilitating the growth of colonizing strains of *Candida* as well as by enhancing transformation of the relatively virulent yeast phase to the more invasive hyphal form (Fig. 9–1). This transformation results in an expanded population of germinated, more virulent, opportunistic pathogens capable of inducing mucosal disease, primarily by causing superficial invasion of epithelial cells. The symptoms caused by *Candida* infection in the GI tract are related primarily to tissue invasion, although hypersensitivity mechanisms and possibly by-products of *Candida* growth may induce functional abnormalities. In the presence of mucositis, GI tract ulceration, or other forms of loss of integrity of the mucosa, a portal of entry is available for pathogens to invade deeply, with the potential to translocate to the bloodstream, causing candidemia and disseminated candidiasis. The process by which yeasts transmigrate the wall of the digestive tract and gain access to the circulation is known as persorption and has been demonstrated in animals and humans.[73, 74] Yeasts have been recovered within 30 minutes from the livers of dogs orally challenged with *C. albicans* and within hours from the blood of an adult human subject who ingested 10^{12} *C. albicans* cells.[75] It appears that persorption occurs primarily in the small bowel. In rhesus monkeys, *Candida* species selectively transmigrates the jejunum but not the stomach or the colon.[74] Persorption is facilitated by mucosal damage, and

TABLE 9–3. REGULATION OF *Candida albicans* POPULATION IN NORMAL GASTROINTESTINAL TRACT

Natural intestinal and bowel motility (adherence)
Mucus production and flow (adherence)
Suppression of *Candida* growth by endogenous microflora by
  Anaerobiosis
  Prolongation of lag phase and doubling time
  Competition for growth-limiting nutrients
  Production of inhibitors that limit substrate availability
  Elaboration of inhibitor substance
Inhibition of mucosal association (adherence) by endogenous microflora
  Competition for adhesin receptor sites
  Blocking mucosal access
  Production of substances that modify *Candida* adhesins on host receptors
Inhibition of transformation in hyphal phase
  Cell-mediated immunity and lymphocyte function
Adherence inhibited by secretory sIgA
Natural mucosal anti-*Candida* histidine-containing peptides

SOURCE: Kennedy MJ. Regulation of *Candida albicans* populations in the gastrointestinal tract: Mechanisms and significance in GI and systemic candidiasis. Curr Top Med Mycol. 1989;3:315–402.

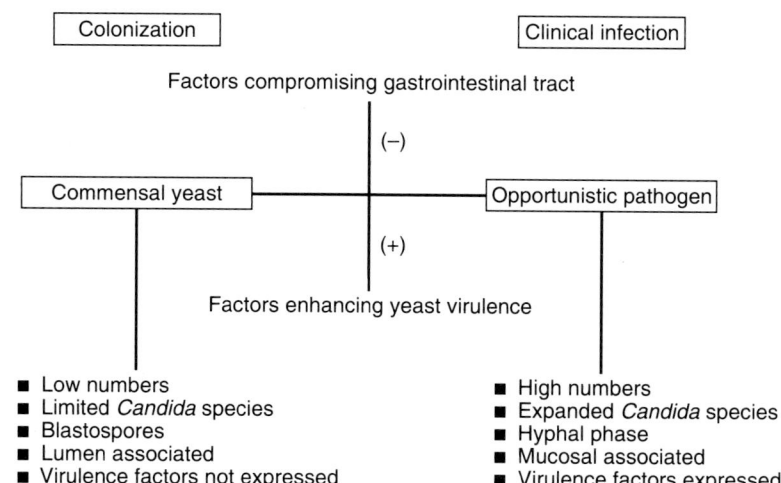

FIGURE 9–1.
Pathogenesis of gastrointestinal candidiasis.

ulceration facilitates tissue invasion and infection.[71, 72]

Oropharyngeal Candidiasis

Oral thrush has been known since the time of Hippocrates,[1] who referred to it as aphtha. Von Rosenstein in 1771 described thrush lesions as resembling "a membrane of lard."[76] Several clinical forms of oral candidiasis exist (Table 9–4); the most common and widely recognized is thrush, also called acute pseudomembranous candidiasis.

Oral Thrush

Thrush is most common among infants, the elderly, and the terminally ill.[77, 78] It occurs in association with serious underlying conditions, including diabetes, leukemia, neoplasia, and AIDS. A comprehensive list of predisposing factors can be found in Table 10–2. Persistent oral thrush in infants may be the first manifestation of childhood AIDS or CMC. Thrush may be a complication of steroid aerosol inhalers and possibly psychotropic drugs and is also common in patients receiving irradiation for head and neck cancer.[79]

Oral thrush is a particular problem in cancer patients receiving chemotherapy. Samonis et al. reported that 28% of patients who were not receiving antifungal prophylaxis developed oropharyngeal candidiasis.[80] In a similar immunocompromised hospitalized population, Yeo observed thrush in 57% of patients.[81] Patients at greatest risk of developing oral candidiasis included those who were being treated with adrenal corticosteroids, those with prolonged granulocytopenia, and those colonized with *Candida* species.[81] Approximately 80 to 90% of patients with AIDS develop oral candidiasis at some stage. The presence of oral candidiasis in persons at risk for AIDS should alert the physician to possible HIV infection. Sixty percent of HIV-positive patients develop an AIDS-related infection or Kaposi's sarcoma within 2 years of the appearance of oral candidiasis.

PATHOGENESIS

C. albicans is the species responsible for the overwhelming majority of cases of oral thrush.[19] The ability of *C. albicans* to adhere to buccal epithelial cells is critical in establishing oral colonization. *Candida albicans* adheres better in vitro to epithelial cells than do non-*albicans Candida* species. Adherence is enhanced by germ tube formation. After colonization of the oral cavity, *Candida* organisms may persist for months or years in low numbers with no mani-

TABLE 9–4. CLINICAL FORMS OF OROPHARYNGEAL CANDIDIASIS

Thrush
Chronic atrophic stomatitis—Denture stomatitis
Angular cheilitis
Chronic hyperplastic candidiasis (*Candida* leukoplakia)
Midline glossitis—Median rhomboid glossitis
Acute atrophic candidiasis
Chronic mucocutaneous candidiasis (CMC)

festation of inflammation. The low number of colonizing organisms is the result of effective antifungal host defense mechanisms in the oral cavity. Resistance is provided by an intact epithelial surface, a normal indigenous background flora, anti-*Candida* IgA in salivary secretions,[82] and natural anti-*Candida* histidine-containing peptides in saliva.[83] Low salivary flow rates correlate with higher prevalence rates of yeasts. Genetic typing of *Candida* strains obtained from AIDS patients with oral and esophageal candidiasis produces the same distribution-frequency curve in the AIDS patients as in healthy subjects, suggesting that AIDS-associated candidiasis is not caused by unique or particularly virulent strains but probably results from defects in host defense mechanisms.

Symptoms of thrush are extremely variable, ranging from nil to complaints of a sore, painful mouth, burning tongue, and dysphagia with involvement of the hypopharynx. Frequently, however, severe objective changes are unaccompanied by symptoms. Clinical signs include diffuse erythema and white patches that appear as discrete lesions on the surfaces of the buccal mucosa, throat, tongue, and gums. With some difficulty, the plaques can be wiped off, revealing a raw, erythematous, and sometimes bleeding base. Constitutional signs of infection are absent, as are signs of regional lymphadenopathy.

Oral thrush impairs the quality of life and may result in a reduction in fluid or food intake. The most serious complication of untreated oropharyngeal candidiasis is extension to the esophagus, fungemia, and disseminated candidiasis.

DIAGNOSIS

In spite of the characteristic clinical picture, physical signs are insufficient to allow a reliable diagnosis. Oral lesions that resemble candidiasis occur with severe mucositis accompanying chemotherapy, reflecting tissue necrosis and mixed bacterial infection.[84] Oropharyngeal *Candida* infections can complicate herpes simplex infection or leukoplakia. Diagnosis requires mycologic confirmation, which can be rapidly achieved by 10% potassium hydroxide microscopic examination. Cultures are not essential for diagnostic purposes and, even when found to be positive, do not distinguish between colonization and true infection.

PATHOLOGY

The plaques in oral thrush comprise necrotic material and desquamated epithelial cells, penetrated by *C. albicans* hyphae and yeast cells, which continue their invasion into the stratum corneum but rarely penetrate beyond the stratum spinosum.[85] Depending on the presence or absence of neutropenia, the accompanying inflammatory response ranges from minimal to heavy infiltration with PMNs.

TREATMENT

Gentian violet, introduced as a thrush treatment in 1925, is generally less successful than modern antifungals.[86] Therapy with a topical agent such as nystatin or amphotericin B is effective, but tolerance and compliance are usually a problem. Furthermore, many of the effective topical antimycotics such as nystatin have been replaced by more active and rapidly acting drugs such as azoles; clotrimazole and miconazole have shown results superior to those of nystatin.[86] Nystatin has been the time-honored treatment for oral thrush in otherwise healthy adults and infants. Its limitations include its bitter taste and, more important, its lack of efficacy in severely immunocompromised patients. Azole antifungals have replaced nystatin for treatment of oral candidiasis in AIDS. Clotrimazole in 10 mg troches administered 5 times a day has been highly successful in treating mild to moderate oropharyngeal candidiasis,[87, 88] and patient compliance has been reported as excellent. Ketoconazole 200 mg daily was the first oral systemic imidazole antifungal agent used and is highly effective even in debilitated patients, including those with malignancy or AIDS.[89] Ketoconazole has also been highly effective in the mucocutaneous candidiasis syndrome.[90] Clinical cure rates in excess of 80% have been achieved with daily ketoconazole administered for 10 to 14 days.[89, 90] Ketoconazole therapy has, however, been limited by fears of hepatotoxicity and concerns about the reliability of gastric absorption, especially in patients receiving H_2-blockers. Accordingly, the newer triazoles, itraconazole and fluconazole, with markedly improved safety profiles have become extremely popular, especially for patients with severe oropharyngeal candidiasis. Fluconazole given in dosages of 50 to 100 mg daily has been compared with clotrimazole or ketoconazole in several open, placebo-controlled, double-blind studies.[91–94] In the studies reported, most of the patients had underlying hematologic and solid tumor malignancy or HIV infection. Although most studies of fluconazole efficacy used an initial loading dose of 200 mg followed by 100 mg daily, success has been achieved with 50 mg daily.[91] Studies indicate that clinical recovery is achieved in 80% of those treated, in spite of severe underlying disease, but complete mycologic cure is more difficult to attain.

In a study of 71 patients, 61 of whom had antibody to HIV, a regimen of 50 mg daily of fluconazole was used.[96] In 42 symptomatic patients, including a few patients with proven esophagitis, clinical recovery was achieved in 7 days (range: 5–20 d). Yeast colonization was monitored by quantitative buccal cultures. On completion of therapy, 79% of those treated had less than 15 CFU per swab. Only 48% had completely negative cultures at the end of therapy. All patients with HIV infection experienced a relapse of oropharyngeal candidiasis within 30 days. No adverse reactions were reported other than mild diarrhea or nausea in a few patients. A striking feature of fluconazole therapy is the rapidity of response, usually within 10 days with 50 mg of fluconazole daily and within 5 days with the higher dose of 200 mg daily even in the most intractable forms of thrush associated with AIDS and CMC.[91] Similar but slower cure rates have been described with both ketoconazole[96] and clotrimazole troches[87] in patients with solid tumors. All published studies revealed that fluconazole was at least equal in efficacy and in some studies superior to clotrimazole or ketoconazole.[94, 95] Overall, clinical response rates indicate that clinical failure is rare. Eighty percent or more of the patients are clinically cured, with an additional 10 to 15% experiencing considerable improvement. It is important to recognize that the endpoint or goal of antimycotic therapy in oral thrush is rapid relief of symptoms and the prevention of complications and early relapse immediately following cessation of therapy. The goal is not to achieve sterilization of the oral cavity. Mycologic eradication is rarely achieved, although routing cultures may become negative for *Candida* toward the end of a standard course of therapy. Even in patients with negative findings on culture, low numbers of yeast persist below the threshold of detection of swab cultures. This is, in part, the consequence of the use of fungistatic azole agents.

The newer triazoles, itraconazole and fluconazole, have demonstrated an improved safety profile, but they have to be used cautiously because, as with ketoconazole, pharmacologic interactions occur with azoles, as with several other agents administered concomitantly in immunocompromised patients, including phenytoin and cyclosporine.[97]

Several concerns have been raised about the widespread use of the more potent oral triazoles, which in the average case of oral candidiasis offer only minor advantages. These concerns include drug interactions, side effects, increased expense, and risk of development of resistance. Several studies have documented the selection of *T. glabrata,* a pathogenic, less susceptible species of yeast in patients treated with ketoconazole for prolonged periods. *C. albicans* resistance to ketoconazole is rare,[90] but both clinical failure and in vitro resistance of *C. albicans* has been observed increasingly with the widespread and often indiscriminate use of fluconazole (P. Dupont, M.D., Pasteur Institute, personal communication, 1991). Although the recommended dosage for fluconazole is 100 mg daily, many clinicians have observed a therapeutic efficacy with 50 mg daily, and although this regimen is less expensive, the potential for low-dosage regimens to contribute to resistance selection is of concern.

Clinical relapse is not uncommon, particularly in patients with persistent underlying immunodeficiency, as in AIDS or CMC. Relapse appears to be dependent on duration of therapy and may occur earlier after ketoconazole than after fluconazole therapy.[96] After several recurrences of symptomatic thrush in AIDS, many clinicians prescribe maintenance chemosuppressive prophylaxis. Stevens and colleagues documented the protective effect of 100 mg of fluconazole daily in preventing thrush in AIDS patients.[98] The most appropriate long-term strategy in the management of such patients has not been investigated thoroughly. The use of intermittent versus continuous long-term therapy needs to be compared, as does the need to establish the minimum effective dose that will not select for resistant strains of *C. albicans.* Although intermittent fluconazole prophylaxis, given in dosages of 150 mg or 200 mg weekly, reduces the frequency of thrush in AIDS patients,[99] it does not provide complete protection, and recurrent oral thrush can be anticipated in 10 to 20% of patients.[99, 100] Apart from the use of azole prophylaxis in AIDS and CMC, azole drugs have been shown to prevent oral thrush in neutropenic patients with cancer.[80] Prospective randomized studies indicate that *Candida* oropharyngitis is less common in neutropenic patients receiving clotrimazole prophylaxis.[101] Ketoconazole, itraconazole, and fluconazole all reduce the attack rate of symptomatic oral thrush in neutropenic leukemia patients.[80] Ketoconazole, however, is not effective in preventing candidemia. Two studies utilizing fluconazole 400 mg daily in profoundly neutropenic bone marrow transplant and leukemia patients demonstrated exceptional protective efficacy in these high-risk patients.[102, 103] Fluconazole also reduced the frequency of systemic candidiasis. Although fluconazole given in 50 to 100 mg dosages daily may be effective in preventing oral thrush in this high-risk population, this dosage cannot be relied on to prevent candidemia.[80, 98]

Chronic Atrophic Stomatitis—Denture Stomatitis

This form of oral candidiasis is thought to be the most common form of *Candida*-associated disease. Although often asymptomatic, some patients may complain of soreness and burning of the mouth. The characteristic presenting signs are chronic erythema and edema of the portion of the palate that comes into contact with dentures. Lower dentures are rarely involved. Associated angular cheilosis is commonly present.

Denture stomatitis was recorded in 24 to 60% of denture wearers[104] and is several-fold more frequent in females than in males. The association between *Candida* and denture stomatitis is now well documented,[106] with the detection of *Candida* by culture or microscopy in over 90% of subjects. Even in the absence of signs or symptoms, the prevalence of oral yeast is invariably higher than normal in denture wearers. Maximum concentrations of yeast are found on the denture-fitting surface. Yeast readily adheres to plastic objects, including orthodontic appliances.

Histologically, denture stomatitis lesions reveal parakeratosis and vacuolation, with neutrophilic infiltration in the upper spinous layer and lymphocyte infiltration of deep spinous layers. Notably, no evidence of fungal penetration is present.[106] Given the lack of fungal invasion and the lack of exudative features characteristic of oral thrush, the pathogenesis remains unclear. Although the wearing of dentures leads to an increased carriage rate and high concentrations of yeast in the enclosed space between prosthesis and palate, the frank exudative lesions of thrush do not usually develop. Instead, diffuse erythema appears and suggests that *Candida* is capable of inducing pathology by more than one route. Elaboration of proteases and phospholipases may possibly induce inflammation. No changes or aberrations in salivary or serum anti-*Candida* immunoglobulins or CMI have been documented.[8] Similarly, no unique virulence characteristic has been identified in the yeast. Notably, *T. glabrata* yeast has been found in 15 to 30% of all species isolated, a much higher prevalence than normally found in the mouth.[8] Successful management of denture stomatitis is easily achieved by the use of oral nonabsorbable antimycotics such as nystatin or clo-

trimazole, denture disinfection, and patient education, emphasizing the importance of not wearing dentures continuously. The dentures can be brushed in tap water and removed before retiring.

Angular Cheilitis—Perlèche

The conditions of angular cheilitis and cheilosis are characterized by soreness, erythema, and fissuring at the corners of the mouth. Cheilitis may accompany oral thrush or denture stomatitis[107] or may appear in the absence of oral disease. Vitamin deficiency and iron-deficiency anemia are also associated with cheilitis. Angular cheilitis frequently responds to topical antifungals,[108] but this response alone does not demonstrate a direct cause-and-effect relationship, and many consider *Candida* yeasts to be primarily secondary colonizers.

Chronic Hyperplastic Candidiasis (*Candida* Leukoplakia)

Oral white patches, or leukoplakia, are discrete transparent to whitish raised lesions of variable size found on the inner surface of the cheeks and, less frequently, the tongue. These lesions are found predominantly in males and are highly associated with smoking. Although most examples of leukoplakia are not related to *Candida* infection, *Candida* invasion of the lesions has been observed in biopsies from 6 to 90% of cases,[108, 109] often in association with neutrophilic infiltration. Although leukoplakia lesions are thought to be premalignant, no association between *Candida* and dysplasia or malignancy is known. Biopsy of *Candida*-related leukoplakia lesions reveals parakeratosis and epithelial hyperplasia, with *Candida* invasion restricted to the upper layers of epithelium. Pathologic changes analogous to those seen in human leukoplakia have been produced on the rat tongue and hamster cheek by *Candida* infections. Although some leukoplakias respond to prolonged topical therapy with antimycotics, most do not and require diagnostic biopsies and surgical resection.[106]

Midline Glossitis—Median Rhomboid Glossitis, Acute Atrophic Stomatitis

Median rhomboid glossitis refers to symmetric lesions of the center dorsum of the tongue characterized by loss of papillae and erythema. Owing to the isolation of *Candida* from these lesions, *Candida* yeast has been suspected of being responsible for the syndrome[110] rather than merely functioning as an innocent by-stander. The pathologic role of *Candida* yeast in this syndrome remains unresolved in spite of occasional histologic smears showing *Candida* hyphae invading tissues, a finding that most likely represents secondary infection only. Nevertheless, repeated oral dosing of tetracycline-treated rats with *C. albicans* may lead to chronic oral colonization and development of chronic midline atrophic tongue lesions.[111] Similar findings have been produced in diabetic rats.[8]

Candida has been incriminated in a variety of acute atrophic oral syndromes that are characterized by a raw or sore tongue, especially after antibiotic administration.[112] This self-limiting entity, although common, has not been shown to be due to primary or secondary *Candida* infection in spite of positive smears or cultures. Similarly, the role of *Candida* in causing the burning mouth syndrome remains unsettled, since *Candida* can be expected to be cultured in 20 to 50% of patients, and this syndrome is of multifactorial etiology.[113] Anecdotal reporting suggests that patients do occasionally improve after nystatin therapy.[19]

Candida Esophagitis

In contrast to the skin and the oral and enteric mucosa, where infection is common and caused by a wide variety of pathogens, including some that are site-specific, the esophagus is not usually a site of infection. Virtually all infections of the esophagus are caused by a small group of opportunistic pathogens that frequently coinfect the epithelial surface in compromised hosts. Thus, esophagitis invariably occurs in predisposed individuals.

Candida species are by far the most common cause of esophagitis and, after the oropharynx, the esophagus is the most common site of GI candidiasis. Autopsy studies of patients with systemic candidiasis detected esophageal involvement in 28 to 56% of cases and gastric involvement in 23 to 35%.[66, 114, 115] The prevalence of *Candida* esophagitis has increased mainly because of the frequency of this entity in AIDS as well as the increased number of organ transplant, cancer, and severely immunocompromised patients.

Pathogenesis

Candida microorganisms are seldom cultured from the esophageal surface and reach the esophagus contained in oral secretions. *Candida albicans* is the species implicated in the majority of patients with esophagitis, although Walsh and Merz found a high prevalence of *C. tropicalis* organisms in patients with malignancy and disseminated candidiasis.[64] In contrast to oral candidiasis, little is known about host and yeast factors operative in the pathogenesis of esophageal candidiasis, and experimental models have not been established. It is likely, however, that the usual yeast virulence factors and defects in host defense mechanism operate. Esophageal candidiasis in an HIV-positive patient may be the first manifestation of AIDS. In cancer patients, factors predisposing to esophagitis include previous exposure to radiation, recent cytotoxic chemotherapy, recent antibiotic therapy, corticosteroid therapy, and neutropenia.[116] The high prevalence of esophagitis in AIDS patients indicates the critical role of CMI in normally protecting the esophagus from *Candida* invasion. *Candida* esophagitis occurs later in the natural history of AIDS and almost invariably at a lower CD4 count.[117] Histologic sections of esophagitis lesions reveal yeast hyphae forms in the mucosal epithelium accompanied mainly by a PMN response similar to that seen in oral thrush.

Clinical Features

Candida esophagitis presents most commonly with dysphagia, odynophagia, and retrosternal pain. Constitutional findings, including fever, occasionally occur; vomiting and hematemesis are rare. Occasionally, epigastric pain is the dominant symptom. Even before AIDS, a male to female predominance was noted.[118–120] Most patients have underlying hematologic malignancies or AIDS or have recently undergone transplantation. Although esophagitis may arise as an extension of oropharyngeal candidiasis, in more than two thirds of published reports, the esophagus was the only site involved and was more often encountered in the distal two thirds than in the proximal third of the esophagus. An occasional feature of *Candida* esophagitis in AIDS patients is the complete lack of symptoms in spite of extensive objectively noted esophageal involvement.[121] Physical findings vary in distribution, character, and severity. Kodsi and colleagues classified *Candida* esophagitis on the basis of endoscopic appearance.[119] They characterized type I cases as having a few white or beige plaques, up to 2 mm in diameter. In type II, plaques are more numerous and larger than 2 mm in diameter. In these milder grades, plaques may be hyperemic or edematous, but no ulceration is present. Type III esophagitis involves confluent linear and nodular elevated plaques with hyperemia and frank ulceration,

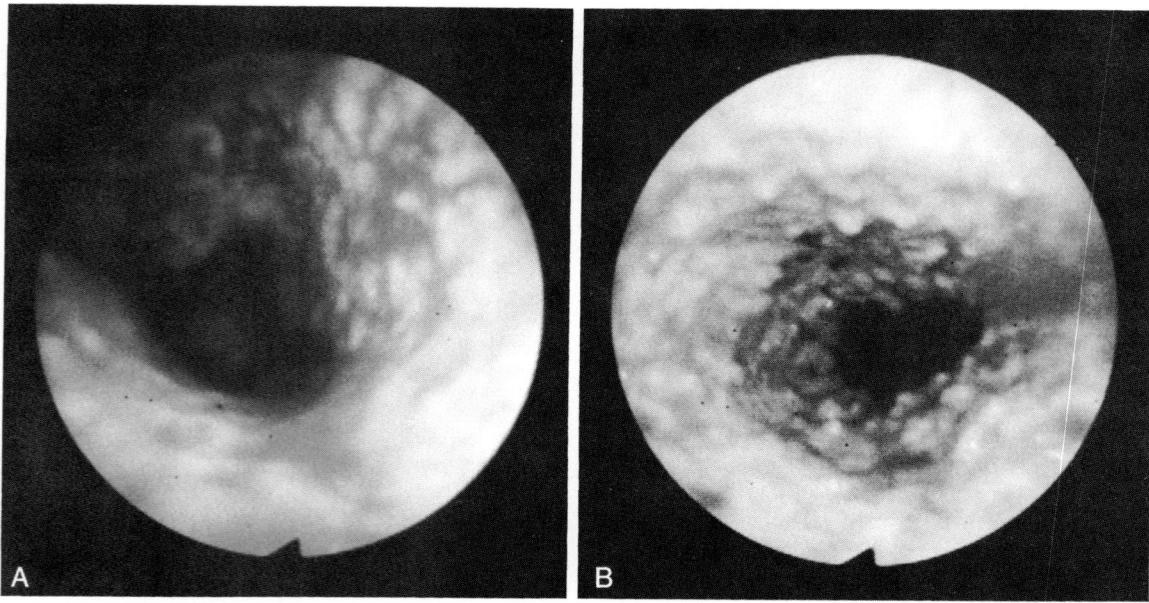

FIGURE 9–2.
A, intense congestion, erythema, and white exudative plaques, which have become confluent in B. [See also Color Plate 3]

and Type IV has, in addition, increased friability of the mucosa and occasional narrowing of the lumen.

Rare complications of esophagitis include fungal bezoar formation, perforation,[122] aortic-esophageal fistula formation,[123] and, rarely, extensive necrosis destroying the entire esophageal mucosa. In neutropenic patients, *Candida* esophagitis may lead to candidemia, and, when extensive ulceration is present, it also provides a portal of entry for bacteria, resulting in bacteremia.

Diagnosis

Reliable diagnosis can be made only by histologic evidence of tissue invasion in biopsy material. Nevertheless, less conclusive evidence than that provided by histologic examination is accepted as a basis for initiating anti-*Candida* therapy. Although useful for demonstrating the presence of *Candida* within an esophageal lesion, smear or culture techniques do not provide sufficient evidence to distinguish *Candida* the commensal from *Candida* the invasive pathogen. Although esophageal brushings are highly sensitive in diagnosing esophagitis, specificity is not high with this procedure nor is the positive predictive value, since the presence of *Candida* hyphae together with squamous cells in esophageal brushings is just as compatible with commensal colonization as with invasive infec-

tion. In the absence of biopsy material, radiologic features previously formed the basis for diagnosis. A barium contrast radiograph of the upper GI tract in *Candida* esophagitis frequently reveals shaggy mucosal irregularities and nodular filling defects.[124, 125] With increase in severity, the nodular pattern becomes extensive, giving a cobblestone appearance. Peristaltic abnormalities are common.[126] Infrequently, discrete ulceration and stenosis are seen. Unfortunately, the sensitivity of barium swallow is relatively low, and radiologic abnormalities are often absent in mild-to-moderate esophagitis,[124] especially in patients with AIDS.[126] Accordingly, radiology has been displaced by endoscopy,[116] which not only provides rapid and high-sensitivity diagnosis but also is the only reliable method of differentiating the various causes of esophagitis. The characteristic endoscopic appearance is of yellow-white plaques on erythematous background, with varying degrees of ulceration (Fig. 9–2). White plaques and pseudomembranes are not exclusive in *Candida* infection, and frequently erythema in the absence of plaques may be due to candidiasis.

Radionuclide tests are of little value in the diagnosis of *Candida* esophagitis, and no serologic tests diagnose invasive esophageal candidiasis reliably. Differential diagnosis includes radiation sickness, reflux esophagitis or cytomegalovirus and herpes simplex virus infection, often in combination.

Treatment

Oral nystatin and clotrimazole are of value only in very mild forms of esophageal candidiasis.[127] Intravenous (IV) miconazole,[128] although effective, has unacceptable toxicity and, given the alternatives available, should no longer be used. Ketoconazole, given in 200 mg doses twice daily, was the first oral systemic imidazole agent shown to be effective in *Candida* esophagitis,[129] providing superior results in comparison with those of oral clotrimazole. The limitations of ketoconazole include side effects such as hepatotoxicity, problems with gastric absorption, and the lack of a parenteral form for patients unable to swallow. Accordingly, in spite of the advances provided by ketoconazole, the more severe forms of esophagitis require therapy with IV amphotericin B. Low-dosage IV amphotericin B, from 0.15 to 0.3 mg/kg or 10 to 20 mg per day for 10 days, is often sufficient for moderate disease.[130, 131] For severe esophagitis, however, conventional dosages of 0.3 to 0.6 mg/kg for 10 to 14 days is necessary. Oral and IV fluconazole have now become an integral part of the management of *Candida* esophagitis. Oral fluconazole enjoys a superior safety profile compared with ketoconazole, has superior gastric absorption, and when necessary can be given IV. Studies of fluconazole compared with clotrimazole and ketoconazole reveal high cure rates that are superior to those encountered with imidazoles, together with more rapid action.[132, 133] Given the high success rate achieved with fluconazole, IV amphotericin B is usually reserved for endoscopically proven cases that have failed fluconazole therapy. Oral flucytosine, given in divided doses of 100 to 150 mg/kg per day, although effective, is rarely prescribed because of the tendency for resistance to develop.

In spite of rapid response to antimycotic therapy, AIDS patients are at high risk of developing symptomatic recurrences of either oropharyngeal or esophageal candidiasis.[134–136] Accordingly, most clinicians, after a single episode of *Candida* esophagitis, begin secondary prophylaxis with oral maintenance suppressive therapy, using either ketoconazole or fluconazole. Several studies are currently in progress to determine the optimal effective dosage and frequency of administration of these agents.

Gastric Candidiasis

Since the normal gastric microbial flora is derived from oropharyngeal secretions, saliva, and food, *Candida* organisms are, not surprisingly, a normal component of gastric flora, albeit in lower numbers. Factors previously mentioned that enhance the oral carriage rate of *Candida* organisms can be expected to similarly increase gastroduodenal colonization with *Candida* species. The role of acid in influencing gastric carriage rates of *Candida* remains controversial since yeast thrive at a wide range of pH and have been found to proliferate and germinate in vitro at a pH of less than 2.0. Histamine blockers have not been shown unequivocally to increase *Candida* virulence. *Candida* infections of the stomach, both superficial and deep, have been documented far less often than those in the esophagus, implying relatively greater gastric mucosal resistance to *Candida* infection. For the most part, *C. albicans* usually invades preexisting gastric lesions, particularly gastric ulcers, both benign and malignant, as well as sites of gastric resection. Other mucosal lesions, such as those caused by chemical injury, acute leukemia, and cancer chemotherapy, have also been associated with infection.[137] *Candida* organisms were found at histologic examination in 24 of 72 consecutive patients (33%) who had undergone surgical resection for gastric ulcers.[138]

Thrushlike lesions of the stomach are rarely seen on endoscopic examination,[139–143] but, when found, they are most frequently superimposed directly on preexisting gastric ulcers or gastritis, irrespective of the cause of the primary gastric pathology. In patients with AIDS and *Candida* esophagitis, gastric thrush is rare. When symptoms such as epigastric pain, nausea, and vomiting are present, establishing the role attributable to candidiasis, if any, is extremely difficult. Most patients are asymptomatic, but if they do experience symptoms, they are those of the associated abnormality, not of the *Candida* esophagitis.

Accordingly, a spectrum exists that ranges from *Candida* colonization only, in which *Candida* is found on routine culture; to more extensive superficial overgrowth of *Candida,* recognized by histologic examination of the surface of the ulcer; to histologically confirmed mucosal invasion. Most frequently, yeasts are seen mainly in the superficial exudate. When peptic ulcers perforate, not surprisingly *Candida* is occasionally cultured from the peritoneal fluid. Holmström and colleagues in 1978 found yeast in 22 of 30 patients (73%) when the peptic ulcer was cultured directly, indicating a strong natural tendency for yeasts to colonize and occasionally invade peptic ulcers, a tendency that is not likely to be altered by H_2 blockers.[144] Most authors believe that yeast colonization or invasion is not responsible for impaired healing of gastric ulcers when the latter are appropriately treated.[145, 146] Nevertheless, Neeman and colleagues reported that in 5 of 7 elderly patients (71%) who had *Candida* infection of benign gastric ulcers, therapy with antacids and cimetidine failed to produce improvement. Replacing cimetidine with nystatin resulted in healing after 4 weeks.[147] The addition of amphotericin B to an antiulcer regimen was effective in a similar group of patients.[148] Clear-cut evidence indicates that yeast invasion contributes to perforation, although histologic study not infrequently demonstrates transmural extension of hyphal elements in excised gastric surgical specimens. Information about the need for, or efficacy of, antifungal therapy for gastric candidiasis is scanty. After perforation of an ulcer or in the presence of histologic evidence of *Candida* tissue invasion, systemic antifungal therapy is indicated. Colonization of ulcers or gastritis mucosa requires no therapy.

Candida Enterocolitis and Diarrhea Syndromes

Autopsy surveys of adults with hematologic malignancy and other debilitating diseases including AIDS show that enteric and colonic mucosal invasion by *Candida* yeast does occur.[113–115] Rarely, *Candida* species and *T. glabrata* have been associated with invasive necrotizing enterocolitis in neonates,[149] causing sepsis. Infection of the small bowel was found at autopsy in 22 of the 109 patients (20%) with GI candidiasis reported by Eras and colleagues, but the infection was limited to the small bowel in only 4 patients.[66] The most common abnormality was ulceration of the mucosa, which led to penetration into the submucosa in some patients. *Candida* ulceration is frequently associated with tumor masses. Another rare manifestation includes small white mucosal patches that can be recognized under endoscopic examination.[150] The most common symptoms attributed to invasive intestinal candidiasis are nausea, abdominal pain, and diarrhea. Nevertheless, a substantial proportion of neutropenic patients who are discovered to have extensive *Candida* ulcerations of the stomach or intestine at autopsy examination manifest no symptoms of this infection antemortem.

Although *Candida* is clearly not a specific cause of sprue, its association with other forms of diarrhea remains highly controversial. Kozinn and Taschdjian reported that *C. albicans* mycelial forms were common in watery or mucoid feces from neonates and concluded that the presence of hyphal forms in feces was pathognomonic for *Candida*-induced diarrhea in infants.[151] Although numerous investigators have shown a high prevalence of *Candida* in feces in children with diarrhea,[152, 153] these observations alone are insufficient to establish a causal role for fungi, since this may merely reflect increased yeast proliferation in pathologically altered intestinal contents.[154a] In an experimental rabbit model, intestinal infection with *Candida* was associated with depressed disaccharidase (lactase) activity.[154b] Stained sections of duodenal mucosa did not show candidal invasion. Other investigators have postulated that *Candida* may not be a primary cause of diarrhea, but that its subsequent proliferation in abnormal bowel contents allows the yeast to perpetuate the diarrheal process as a secondary mechanism[152, 154] in patients with immunodeficiency[144] and preexisting inflammatory bowel disease. *Candida albicans* has been shown to inhibit GI tract absorption of sugar in rats in vivo, and Burke and Gracey in an experimental rat model described a net increase in secretion of water into the gut of protein-deficient animals.[155]

Gupta and Ehrinpreis reported in 1990 what they considered to be *Candida*-associated or -induced diarrhea developing during hospitalization.[156] Diarrhea developed in 10 elderly, malnourished, critically or chronically ill patients. The diarrhea was secretory in nature, characterized by frequent watery stools, usually without blood, mucus, tenesmus, or abdominal pain. All the patients had received therapy with multiple antibiotics or chemotherapeutic agents. Diarrhea was often severe, leading to dehydration, prerenal azotemia, hyperchloremic metabolic acidosis, and electrolyte imbalance. Colonoscopic examination failed to reveal evidence of colitis. Diagnosis of *Candida*-associated diarrhea was made by excluding other infectious inflammatory conditions and other causes of secretory diarrhea, negative results on colonoscopic examination, culture of *Candida* species, and dramatic response to a short course of oral nystatin. Yeast forms were visualized in 8 of 10 patients on Gram stain of stool. Gupta and Ehrinpreis's study is, however, limited by the absence of a placebo-treated control group and by the lack of quantitative fungal cultures and information on the accompanying bacterial flora. Nevertheless, the possibility of intestinal overgrowth of yeast as a cause of diarrhea in the hospitalized elderly requires further attention and clarification of the causal mechanism. A recent study of yeast in antibiotic-associated diarrhea similarly found *Candida* overgrowth as a treatable cause in approximately 30% of elderly subjects.[157] No evidence has been found that *Candida* species contribute to diarrheal disease in patients with AIDS.

Allergic reactions to *Candida* fungus have also been suggested as being responsible for *Candida*-associated diarrhea.[158] Alexander considered that, in patients who had positive stool cultures for *C. albicans* and who had suffered from diarrhea for more than 1 month after antibiotic therapy, the diarrhea was caused by gut hypersensitivity to the fungus[158] Holti reported on 56 patients who had cutaneous hypersensitivity to yeast antigens and from whose stools *C. albicans* and *C. tropicalis* had been isolated. In 2 of these patients, the symptoms were reproduced by ingestion of *C. albicans* antigens. Nystatin treatment and yeast-free diets resulted in some clinical improvement of their mucous colitis.[159]

The significance of *Candida* as a noninvasive cause of GI symptoms remains controversial. In spite of the aforementioned evidence suggesting that *Candida* species can cause diarrhea, the evidence is marginal at best. Numerous patients with *Candida* overgrowth and diarrhea have been treated with antifungal therapy, resulting in suppression of the fungal overgrowth but no improvement in the diarrhea.[160]

Candida Cholecystitis

Candida species are occasionally cultured from bile or gallbladder tissue taken at the time of biliary surgery, both elective and emergent.[161] Yeasts have been found as clinical isolates in 0 to 2% of cholecystectomies.[162] In most instances, the positive cultures for *Candida* are similar to those of bactobilia in which bile is no longer sterile, complicating bile duct obstruction, cholelithiasis, obstructive jaundice, and biliary strictures in the elderly and especially in diabetic subjects. In these instances, *Candida* organisms may be isolated in pure culture or as part of polymicrobial cultures. The role of *Candida* species in contributing to acute or chronic cholecystitis, if any, is unknown. Occasionally *Candida* is isolated in pure culture from purulent material aspirated from a distended inflamed gallbladder, suggesting a pathogenic role, especially when histologic examination reveals hyphal invasion of gallbladder mucosa and wall. Usually, the presence of *Candida* in bile or gallbladder tissue is discovered only after cholecystectomy. In asymptomatic, non-neutropenic patients who have undergone uncomplicated cholecystectomy, the addition of antifungal therapy is not recommended, since the cholecystectomy and removal of obstruction constitute the definitive curative procedures for a process confined to the gallbladder. By contrast, postcholecystectomy patients with associated extrabiliary candidiasis or candidemia, especially in the presence of neutropenia, should be treated with systemic antifungal agents. Complicated *Candida* biliary tract infections requiring specific therapy and surgery include hepatic or common duct obstruction, fungus ball formation, gangrenous cholecystitis, *Candida* cholangitis, and subhepatic biliary abscess formation. Systemic amphotericin B has been used, achieving therapeutic concentrations of 2.5 μg/ml in bile. No reports of azole use in this rare entity are available.[163]

More common, and controversial, is the isolation of *Candida* from bile that drains through postoperative T tubes and other drains, and from diverting bile stents placed to facilitate internal and external bile drainage following obstructive neoplastic involvement of the biliary system. Frequently, positive cultures for *Candida* reflect colonization of the drainage systems only and require no therapy. In the febrile patient with candidemia, therapy is not controversial and merits immediate administration of amphotericin B. The difficult patient is the noncandidemic individual with antibiotic-resistant fever in whom antifungal therapy is contemplated. A trial of therapy may be reasonable after every effort has been made to exclude other causes, including peribiliary infected collections. Another limiting factor is the inability of antifungal therapy to sterilize bile in the presence of obstruction and a foreign body such as a catheter or stent. Antifungal therapy may control sepsis and achieve temporary sterilization of bile, but inevitably relapse, with accompanying positive *Candida* cultures, occurs.

Acalculous cholecystitis is a rarely recognized secondary complication of disseminated candidiasis, although gallbladder involvement has been reported in 10 to 20% of cases. In a report of 109 fatal cases of disseminated candidiasis in children, Hughes found that gallbladder involvement occurred in 10%.[114]

Chronic Mucocutaneous Candidiasis

Chronic mucocutaneous candidiasis is a syndrome in which multiple superficial sites, particularly mouth, facial skin, and fingernails, are infected with *Candida* simultaneously over a period of months or years. This syndrome is not a single disease entity, but it is the consequence of multiple possible defects in anti-*Candida* host defenses. The final outcome is chronic superficial *Candida* infection at anatomic sites where *Candida* normally resides as a commensal.

Because of the confusion arising from disparate clinical, genetic, and immunologic features seen in patients with CMC, attempts have been made to classify CMC, recognizing that some forms develop in infancy and childhood and other forms begin only in adult life. Initial clinical classifications[112, 164, 165] have given way to a newer classification on the basis of hereditary factors as well as clinical factors.[164] Group 1 comprises cases of familial CMC with autosomal recessive inheritance. Group 2 generally contains the most severely affected cases, in which familial factors are unknown or obscure. Group 3 comprises cases of CMC associated with endocrinopathy in which autosomal recessive inheritance is a question; Group 3 has also been called *Candida* endocrinopathy syndrome or autoimmune polyendocrinopathy candidiasis syndrome. Group 4 contains the adult-onset CMC cases. This classification fails to include the occasional cases demonstrating autosomal dominant transmission. Other authors have classified patients on the basis of T-cell function.[8]

CLINICAL FEATURES

In most cases, regardless of age or type, the earliest *Candida* lesion to appear is oral thrush or chronic pseudomembranous oral candidiasis only.[166] In addition to thrush and angular cheilitis, lip fissures may develop and infection may spread to involve the esophagus and larynx. In postmenarchal females, *Candida* vaginitis may supervene, but it is not a common feature.

Persistent onychia and paronychia are nearly as common as oral lesions. The fingernail lesions vary from discoloration and dystrophy of the nails to crusting and hyperkeratotic hornification. Skin lesions, when present, are found mainly on the face, neck, ears, and shoulders, but occasionally involve the scalp and groin. Milder forms consist of mild erythema as background to brown dry areas of desquamation. In severe forms, there are hyperkeratotic crusts or *Candida* granulomas producing severe disfigurement. These findings invariably occur in the idiopathic infant- or juvenile-onset cases and, rarely, in association with endocrinopathies or mature-onset cases.

Onset of CMC is within the first year of life in nonendocrinopathic cases, and between the first and ninth year when associated with endocrinopathies. Approximately 90% of all cases of CMC have their onset before the age of 20 years, approximately one third are associated with endocrinopathies. Hypoparathyroidism is the most common endocrine dysfunction associated with CMC, followed by Addison's disease and hypothyroidism. Diabetes mellitus is rare in CMC. A striking feature of CMC is the lack of candidemia and disseminated candidiasis; CMC can persist for many years.

Chronic mucocutaneous candidiasis is most often associated with defects in CMI. A variety of *Candida* antigen-specific defects have been described. The most common abnormality, a negative cutaneous hyposensitive delayed reaction to *Candida* antigen, is evident in more than 80% of patients tested (controls: 16 to 37%) regardless of clinical type of CMC. About 70% of patients tested showed defective in vitro lymphocyte blastogenesis in response to *Candida* antigen.[167] The nature of the T-cell defect has not been clarified. Fischer and Durandy and colleagues identified a subpopulation of T-suppressor cells that inhibit T-helper cell function in response to *Candida* mannoproteins.[168, 169] These same authors reported a serum inhibitory factor in CMC that suppressed T-cell function. The majority of patients with CMC have normal or high serum levels of antibodies to *Candida*, and no consistent or common B-cell dysfunction has been reported.

Frequently CMC is associated with autoantibodies and manifestations of autoimmune disease in patients with endocrinopathy. Antiparathyroid, antiadrenal, and antithyroid antibodies are common. It is apparent that, given the diversity of clinical findings and immunologic abnormalities that are present, no unifying theory exists that encompasses all aspects of CMC. Nevertheless, it would appear that the unique susceptibility to superficial candidiasis is the common endpoint and that defective T-cell function leading to candidiasis can arise by a variety of defects, including those of serum inhibitors and suppressor T cells. Impaired T-cell function may, by deregulation, facilitate the formation of autoantibodies that lead to the endocrinopathies. Furthermore, a component of T-cell dysfunction in CMC is often reversible, with improvement in immunological parameters following clinical remission achieved by antimycotic therapy.

The availability of oral azoles, specifically ketoconazole, has revolutionized the treatment of patients with CMC. Parenteral miconazole and amphotericin B, although effective, cannot be given long-term. Ketoconazole induces long treatment-free remissions of CMC and can be used continuously or intermittently in cases requiring long-term therapy.[170] During the 1980s, although a variety of therapeutic immunological approaches aimed at improving CMI were attempted, they produced inconsistent results and only moderate success in comparison with those of oral azole therapy.

GASTROINTESTINAL DISEASE FROM FUNGI OF OTHER GENERA

Zygomycosis

Zygomycosis is an infection caused by the fungi of the orders Mucorales and Entomophthorales. These organisms are ubiquitous and generally saprophytic, rarely causing disease in the immunocompetent host.[171] Zygomycosis is the third most common cause of invasive fungal infection in cancer patients.[172] The most common agent of zygomycosis is *Rhizopus arrhizus (R. oryzae),* which tends to produce an acute and rapidly fatal infection, mucormycosis, despite early diagnosis and treatment. These organisms have a predilection for invading major blood vessels, with ensuing ischemia, infarction, and necrosis of the adjacent tissues and with the production of black pus. The Zygomycetes species have a propensity to infect the acidotic, usually diabetic, patient but may infect patients with acidosis secondary to uremia, diarrhea, and aspirin abuse. At additional risk are patients receiving glucocorticoids or deferoxamine therapy and those who have granulocytopenia or have undergone splenectomy.[173, 174] Mucormycosis has five major clinical forms: rhinocerebral, pulmonary, abdominopelvic and gastric (GI), primary cutaneous, and disseminated. Each is associated with various abnormalities in host defense mechanisms.[175]

Gastrointestinal zygomycosis is uncommon and usually results from the ingestion of the organism by malnourished individuals or patients with chronic renal failure or underlying GI tract disease. The most common underlying conditions include kwashiorkor, amebiasis, uremia, typhoid fever, and gastric neoplasms. The major defect leading to GI tract zygomycosis is the disruption in mucosal integrity, as, for example, peptic ulcer, which subsequently leads to deeper invasion of the GI tract by the fungi.[176] Infection most commonly affects the stomach and colon, producing necrotic ulcerations with ischemia and gangrene.[177] Occasionally, zygomycosis is responsible for benign colonization of gastric ulcer without causing invasion.[178] More frequently, however, these pathogens cause mucosal infiltration and vascular invasion but invariably in the presence of preexisting mucosal disease. The presentation of mucosal infiltrations and tissue invasion closely mimics malignancy, with symptoms persisting after appropriate therapy. Accordingly, the diagnosis is usually made only after surgical resection.[178]

Infections of the ileum have also been described.[179, 180] One patient who had no underlying illness developed multiple ulcerations in the ileum after treatment of bacterial peritonitis with antimicrobials and steroids.[179] Kahn described a patient who developed gastric mucormycosis associated with a nasogastric tube.[180] In the majority of cases, dyspepsia, abdominal pain, and diarrhea are present. Occasionally, vomiting and frank GI tract bleeding ensue. Perforation of the GI tract may occur, resulting in peritonitis. The fungal pathogens may extend from the gut lumen to the gallbladder, liver, pancreas, and spleen. As with other types of mucormycosis, GI involvement is usually rapidly progressive, resulting in death within a few days. Systemic mucormycosis usually begins in the lungs but may also originate from the GI tract[181] and may spread to the CNS, producing infarction with abscess formation. The disseminated form of infection is seen primarily in patients with hematologic malignancy and, in addition to involving lungs and the CNS, frequently spreads hematogenously to the liver, spleen, kidney, heart, and skin.[181] Disseminated mucormycosis from a GI source is not uncommon.[182]

In most cases the diagnosis is made at surgery or postmortem. Several authors have suggested that the presence of these fungi in gastric aspirates or stool may be a useful diagnostic tool. Diagnostic confirmation, however, depends on biopsy demonstration of fungi invading tissue structures.

Successful treatment of zygomycosis requires a high index of clinical suspicion for rapid diagnosis. Mortality rates as high as 85% have been documented. Treatment requires reversal of underlying condition when possible; surgical removal of the affected tissue, which frequently includes multiple operations; and intravenous amphotericin B. Since the fungus is relatively resistant, high dosages are needed, usually in the range of 1.0 to 1.5 mg/kg per day. The optimal duration of therapy is unknown, but in most studies, a total dose of 2 to 4 g has been used. Using this aggressive therapeutic approach, several authors have demonstrated slightly improved outcome in their patients with rhinocerebral zygomycosis, the fulminant form of the disease,[183, 184] but the prognosis with GI tract zygomycosis remains poor. When invasive zygomycosis complicates peptic ulcer disease, in the absence of severe immunosuppression, surgical resection is frequently curative.

Hyalohyphomycosis

Hyalohyphomycosis is an important and increasingly prevalent array of fungal infections. These saprophytic fungi are normally found in the soil. They are nondematiaceous molds with colorless hyaline walls that have emerged as a cause of opportunistic fungal infection in the immunocompromised host. The most common causal agents in this group include *Fusarium moniliforme, Fusarium solani, Fusarium oxysporum, Chrysosporium* species, *Geotrichum candidum, Monosporium inflatum, Monosporium apiospermum, Scopulariopsis acremonium, Scopulariopsis brevicaulis, Scopulariopsis candida, Paecilomyces* species, and *Pseudallescheria boydii.*[185]

Fusarium species, the most common of this group, are important plant pathogens and common soil fungi.[186] Systemic disease following the ingestion of cereals contaminated with *Fusarium* species was initially associated with aplastic anemia and death after exposure to contaminated grain.[187] During World War II, up to 1 million people were poisoned by contaminated grain. Today, the most common form of disease is due to bloodstream dissemination. In most instances, the disseminated disease caused by these normally innocuous organisms occurs in severely immunocompromised patients. These patients often have an underlying hematologic malignancy and receive intensive chemotherapy accompanied by profound and prolonged neutropenia. Similarities to aspergillosis in presenting manifestations and tissue histology frequently confound diagnosis.[187]

The GI tract is usually involved as a result of disseminated disease during fungemia. Manifestations include oral ulcerative lesions on the hard palate as well as necrotic ulcerations extending from the esophagus to the large bowel. These fungi have the propensity for vascular invasion, as do *Aspergillus* and Zygomycetes species; accordingly, necrotic ulcers are usually accompanied by underlying thrombosis of adjacent blood vessels. On occasion, the necrotic bowel ulcerations perforate, producing fungal peritonitis with associated systemic infection. Fungal cultures are required for final identification of the organism because of the many clinical and histologic similarities with *Aspergillus.* Unlike those of *Aspergillus, Fusarium* species are cultured from the blood in approximately 70% of cases of disseminated disease, and the appearance of new skin lesions that evolve from erythema to necrosis is an important diagnostic clue to disseminated fusariosis. The mortality rate associated with fusariosis is still greater than 95%, despite intensive antifungal therapy and surgical resection of the infected tissue. The status of the host's defense mechanisms, underlying disease, and severity of dissemination are all important factors in the final prognosis.[187]

An important factor affecting survival is the susceptibility of these molds to antifungal agents. *Fusarium* isolates are frequently resistant to flucytosine (5-fluorocytosine), to many of the azoles, and occasionally to amphotericin B.[185, 187] Preliminary studies with liposomal amphotericin B, which may be given in higher doses and reduced toxicity, have shown promise.[188] One report, describing the successful treatment of a *Fusarium* infection in a severely immunocompromised child, documented evidence of synergy between amphotericin B and rifampin together with granulocyte transfusions.[188a]

Aspergillosis

Aspergillus species are found worldwide and are ubiquitous in the environment. Approximately 600 species are recognized, of which *A. fumigatus* is the most frequent cause of disease in humans, followed by *A. flavus, A niger,* and occasionally *A. terreus.* Aspergilli are molds that reproduce by means of spores termed conidia. Invasive infection is rare unless a marked immunodeficiency is present. *Aspergillus* species are frequently isolated from hospital ventilation systems and areas near hospital construction or renovation.[172] *Aspergillus* is the second most common cause of fungal disease in cancer patients.[189] In general, infection occurs in severely immunocompromised hosts, particularly in patients with prolonged and profound neutropenia secondary to chemotherapy or in patients with neutrophil dysfunction due to corticosteroid therapy.[190] Similarly, patients with chronic granulomatous disease may present with invasive aspergillosis because of the inability of their phagocytes to generate microbicidal substrates.[191] Less frequently, patients with alcoholic cirrhosis, collagen vascular diseases, and postinfluenza infection are also at risk of developing invasive aspergillosis,[192, 193] and even nonimmunocompromised hosts may develop disseminated aspergillosis.[194]

Inhalation of the spores from the environment is believed to be the most frequent route of infection. Accordingly, upper respiratory tract infection of the sinuses and pulmonary diseases are the major sequelae of *Aspergillus* infection. Invasion from a cutaneous source, such as central venous catheters, may also occur. As with other molds, *Aspergillus* organisms also have a tendency toward vascular invasion, producing thrombosis, ischemia, infarction, and tissue necrosis. The clinical manifestations are varied and depend on the route of infection and the underlying disease. Most infections are initiated in the lungs, then subsequently disseminate via the bloodstream to other tissues including the CNS, kidneys, eyes, skin, liver, and spleen.

Gastrointestinal involvement is common. In an autopsy series of 98 patients with invasive aspergillosis, 21 patients had GI tract infection.[195] The stomach, esophagus, small intestine, and colon were all sites of invasion. The lesions extended from the mucosa into the muscularis.[195] Vascular invasion with resultant thrombosis and infarction may lead to GI tract hemorrhage and, in some cases, perforation with secondary polymicrobial peritonitis. Fever is universally present and unresponsive to broad-spectrum antimicrobials. The definitive diagnosis of aspergillosis is difficult. No reliable serologic tests are available. Several authors have suggested a correlation between the presence of an *Aspergillus* antigen in the serum, urine, or bronchoalveolar lavage fluid and invasive pulmonary aspergillosis.[196] Unfortunately *Aspergillus* species are rarely cultured from blood.

Therapy for invasive disease is still inadequate. Mortality rates range from 50 to 100%, depending primarily on the underlying disease.[197] According to Denning and Stevens in their extensive review of invasive aspergillosis, the mortality rate in bone marrow transplant patients with pulmonary or cerebral aspergillosis or both was 95%, regardless of therapy.[197] The administration of flucytosine appears to lower the mortality in neutropenic patients who have not undergone a transplant.[197] The mainstay of therapy for invasive aspergillosis is still IV amphotericin B, with dosages ranging from 0.6 to 1.5 mg/kg per day for the duration of neutropenia for a total dose of 1.5 to 4.0 g. *Aspergillus* species are relatively insensitive to amphotericin B; thus results are poor. Lipid complex amphotericin B, which facilitates the administration of much higher dosages of amphotericin with fewer side effects, has shown highly encouraging results in preliminary studies of refractory aspergillosis.[198] Itraconazole, an experimental triazole, has demonstrated efficacy in patients with pulmonary aspergilloma, chronic necrotizing pulmonary aspergillosis, and invasive aspergillosis.[199] Surgical therapy, either alone or in combination with antifungal chemotherapy, may be useful in selected patients with localized disease. A crucial factor in optimizing therapy is the removal of the immunosuppression whenever possible.[200] If patients are diagnosed and treated early, the response rates may reach 50%. The response rate in invasive aspergillosis in neutropenic patients depends on the return to normal of the neutrophil number.[201]

Cryptococcosis

Cryptococcus neoformans, a species of encapsulated yeast, is an important opportunistic fungal pathogen in humans. It is the second most common fungal infection in AIDS patients and the most frequent cause of disseminated fungal infection. Infection is acquired through inhalation of the yeast, producing an initial asymptomatic pulmonary infection in the normal host. The most common clinical form of the disease is a subacute progressive meningitis, followed by pulmonary infection.

Although cryptococcal organisms have been isolated from stool specimens, the GI tract is rarely affected. Several reports exist of oral and esophageal ulcerations due to cryptococci seen primarily in HIV-positive patients.[202] The diagnosis of GI tract disease is made by tissue biopsy and visualization of yeast cells in affected tissues. Fungal cultures should also be carried out to exclude other fungal pathogens. The standard therapeutic regimen for acute cryptococcal infection in HIV-negative individuals is still the combination of amphotericin B in a dosage of 0.3 mg/kg per day plus flucytosine in the dosage of 37.5 mg/kg every 6 hours for 6 weeks. This regimen was found to be effective in 85% of cryptococcal meningitis cases and produced more rapid sterilization of the cerebrospinal fluid than did monotherapy.[203] Because of severe and persistent immunosuppression and high relapse rates in HIV-positive patients, maintenance therapy with 200 mg of fluconazole a day has been very effective in preventing recurrent cryptococcal infection.[204] Studies are currently under way that use a shorter, 2-week, initial course of amphotericin B, both with and without flucytosine in acute cryptococcal infection, followed by maintenance therapy with either fluconazole or itraconazole. Optimal therapy for localized GI tract infection has not been established.

Histoplasmosis

Histoplasma capsulatum is a dimorphic fungus with worldwide distribution. It is the source of the most common systemic endemic mycosis in the United States and is found primarily in the central regions of the country from the Gulf Coast to the Great Lakes. The fungus grows readily in soil containing a high nitrogen content, particularly in soil enriched by bird and bat guano. Because of their moderate temperatures and shady areas, the fertile river valleys of Ohio and Mississippi harbor the fungus.[205] In-

238   Fungal Infections of the Gastrointestinal Tract

habitants of these endemic regions are probably repeatedly infected and are generally asymptomatic. Areas most frequently associated with *H. capsulatum* include caves, chicken coops, bird roosts, decayed wood piles, dead trees, chimneys, and old buildings. Spores are inhaled, reach the bronchioles or alveoli, and germinate after 48 to 72 hours, producing the yeast form of the fungus. After inhalation of few to a moderate number of spores, the pulmonary event is asymptomatic. Heavy inhalation of spores results in symptomatic illness, even in the immunocompetent or immune individual. In a small percentage of individuals, a more severe form of progressive pulmonary infection or disseminated disease may occur. These patients are often infants with immature immunity, individuals immunosuppressed secondary to chemotherapy or steroids, or patients with HIV infection.[206, 207]

The clinical syndromes associated with *H. capsulatum* include acute self-limited syndrome, disseminated histoplasmosis, chronic pulmonary histoplasmosis, mediastinal granulomata, and fibrosing mediastinitis. The acute syndrome in the normal host is generally mild and is manifested by fever, headaches, chills, cough, and chest pain in at least two thirds of patients.[208] The results of chest radiographs are normal in most cases. Because the disease is usually self-limited, treatment is unnecessary. Gastrointestinal histoplasmosis usually appears as part of disseminated disease and is acquired by the hematogenous route.

The disseminated form is uncommon and may be fatal, with greater risk among blacks, males, and individuals less than 1 year and more than 54 years of age.[209] The severity of the disease depends on the degree of involvement of the reticuloendothelial system (RES), and it may be subdivided into five classes. The acute, or infant, type of disseminated disease has a high degree of RES involvement and is found predominantly in infants and but rarely in adults. GI tract symptoms including nausea, vomiting, and diarrhea are common. Fever is uniformly present, as is severe hepatosplenomegaly. Frequently, superficial ulcerations of the oral mucosa are present. In the second form of disease, subacute disseminated histoplasmosis, RES is only moderately involved. This subtype is seen primarily in adults. Manifestations are usually due to the development of focal lesions in various organ systems accompanied by fever. Gastrointestinal tract involvement is very common. Deep oropharyngeal ulcerations with rolled edges are present in more than 25% of cases.[209] Intestinal ulceration is common, occa-

sionally leading to perforation and peritonitis.[210] Autopsy studies reveal GI tract involvement in 70% of cases and oropharyngeal involvement in 67% of cases. Hepatosplenomegaly is almost always present. The third form of disseminated disease occurs in adults, is more chronic, and has the mildest degree of RES involvement. Manifestations are generally mild, chronic, and occasionally intermittent. In this form, oropharyngeal ulcerations are the predominant findings and are due to focal granulomatous lesions. Gradual weight loss, fatigue, and weakness are the most common complaints. Hepatosplenomegaly, intestinal ulceration, and interstitial pneumonitis are rare.[211]

In AIDS patients with disseminated histoplasmosis, the syndrome is often acute and severe, with associated shock, respiratory failure, and disseminated intravascular coagulation present in 33% of cases.[212] The oropharyngeal mucosa is rarely involved; few cases of GI tract involvement exist and those are primarily of the colon.[213] An extensive 1988 review by Johnson and colleagues reported that only 4% of AIDS patients had GI tract involvement.[214] By contrast, in a more recent series of disseminated histoplasmosis in AIDS patients, Driks and colleagues detected GI involvement, especially colonic, by biopsy in 70% of patients, although GI symptoms were present in approximately 10% of patients.[215]

When GI involvement occurs in histoplasmosis, pulmonary symptoms are uncommon and GI symptoms predominate.[216] Fever is less common than it is in other forms of dissemination. The most common lesions are a mass or ulcers, which often mimic inflammatory bowel disease or carcinoma. Terminal ileal involvement predominates in one third of cases. Accordingly, in the immunosuppressed patient, GI histoplasmosis must be considered, even in a patient from a nonendemic region who presents with lesions resembling carcinoma or inflammatory bowel disease. Nevertheless, GI tract involvement in AIDS patients is invariably part of disseminated disease and may present at any GI site, including esophagus, stomach, and small and large bowel.

Diagnosis of disseminated disease depends on the demonstration of the fungus in cultured material from blood, urine, bone marrow, liver, or other affected tissue. Frequently, organisms are found within well-formed granulomata. The histologic examination of Giemsa-stained sections reveals small intracellular yeastlike *H. capsulatum* organisms within lamina propria macrophages. Scrapings of oropharyngeal ulcerations are frequently positive on stains and always positive on biopsy. Skin testing is not diagnostically useful. Serologic study is useful, using complement fixation tests for the yeast-phase antigens. A titer of 1:32 or greater or a 4-fold increase is evidence of active or recent infection. In GI histoplasmosis, the complement fixation test is positive in approximately 75% of cases. Therapy for disseminated disease is required since the mortality of untreated infection ranges from 83 to 93%, whereas the mortality with therapy is between 7 and 23%.[217] Amphotericin B is the drug of choice for fulminant disease, and patients should receive at least 35 mg/kg total dosage. In AIDS patients, because relapse is predictable and occurs in more than 90% of cases, maintenance therapy with amphotericin B, oral ketoconazole, or oral itraconazole is recommended for use indefinitely. In non–life-threatening disease, amphotericin B has been replaced by the oral azoles ketoconazole and itraconazole. Both of these agents are highly effective against GI tract histoplasmosis.[209]

Histoplasmosis can also produce a mediastinal granuloma syndrome. In this syndrome associated with *H. capsulatum*, enlarged lymph nodes obstruct and encroach upon important mediastinal structures, usually in patients with active disease, even years after primary infection. The esophagus is frequently affected, producing symptoms of esophageal motility dysfunction, obstruction, or perforation. Treatment with amphotericin B is often useful, but surgical resection of the fibrotic mass may be required. Fibrosing mediastinitis, a rare complication of mediastinal histoplasmosis, is a late inflammatory reaction. The most common manifestations are superior vena cava syndrome and tracheobronchial obstruction.[218] Esophageal obstruction is seen in 2 to 5% of cases. No form of therapy is effective, and surgery is hazardous.

Blastomycosis

Blastomyces dermatitidis is a species of dimorphic round budding yeast with daughter cells that form a bud with a broad base. *Blastomyces* is known to cause epidemics of infection but is also endemic to certain geographic regions. The yeast is found worldwide, but the majority of cases within the US are found along the Mississippi and Ohio river valleys.[171] The precise ecology and epidemiology of this organism have been perplexing because of the difficulty in isolating the organism from the environment. Infection begins with the inhalation of spores into the lung, followed by control of the infectious process by the lung phagocytes.[219] Blastomycosis usually produces pulmonary, cu-

taneous, and osseous disease. Involvement of the GI tract, although rare, is usually manifested as lesions in the mouth and oropharyngeal area.[219] Gastrointestinal disease distal to the oropharynx is very rare and is usually due to disseminated infection.[219]

Diagnosis of GI tract blastomycosis necessitates the isolation of the organism by culture and histopathologic examination of the suspected lesion. Amphotericin B has been considered the primary mode of therapy for all types of blastomycosis. The newer therapeutic regimens that use ketoconazole have been shown to be effective in mild to moderate infection.[220] Amphotericin B is used for severe infection and CNS infection or to treat those patients who have an intolerance for ketoconazole. Most authors currently recommend 1.5 to 2.5 g of amphotericin B given IV. The relapse rate of patients treated with amphotericin B is less than 10%. Studies indicate superior therapeutic results with itraconazole with an improved safety profile compared with ketoconazole.

Paracoccidioidomycoses

Paracoccidioides brasiliensis is a species of dimorphic fungus that grows as mycelium in nature and as yeastlike form in tissue. It is found only in certain areas of Central and South America, with Brazil at the center of the endemic region. The organism grows readily in areas with moderate temperatures, high humidity, and rich vegetation.[221] Unique among systemic mycoses, the disease is more common in men than in women (15:1) and has long periods of latency, in some cases up to 30 years.[222]

As with other endemic mycoses, infection is acquired when conidia are inhaled into the lungs. Infection results in a chronic granulomatous process that begins with an asymptomatic pulmonary infection. The fungus can also disseminate outside the lungs to form ulcerative granulomata in other organs. Predominant sites of extrapulmonary dissemination include skin, mucous membranes, lymph nodes, adrenal glands, intestines, spleen, and liver. The oropharyngeal lesions begin as vesicles or papules that then ulcerate; this condition is termed moriform stomatitis. The ulcerative lesions have a characteristic rolled border with a white exudative base and small hemorrhagic dots. The lesions initially are painless and spread gradually, forming large vegetations. In severe cases, the lesions may advance and extend into deeper tissues, causing destruction of the uvula and hard palate. The tongue frequently thickens and develops granulomatous nodules. Involvement of the lymph nodes draining the affected area is common, with frequent suppuration, drainage, and sinus tract formation. Diagnosis is suspected clinically in endemic areas and confirmed by the isolation of the yeast form from affected tissues. Serologic examination using gel immunodiffusion has produced positive results in 95% of patients.[223] Ketoconazole at a dosage of 200 to 400 mg per day for a prolonged period, usually 12 to 18 months, is the treatment of choice.[224] Triazoles such as itraconazole and fluconazole have been extremely successful in producing remission of disease with even less toxicity.[225] Sulfadiazine or a long-acting sulfonamide may also be used as therapy, but the length of treatment should be at least 5 to 6 years to prevent relapses. Amphotericin B may also be used for the severe cases but is not curative by itself.

Coccidioidomycosis

Coccidioides immitis is a dimorphic fungus found predominantly in the southwestern United States and northern Mexico. Infection is usually acquired by inhalation of arthroconidia, which are readily aerosolized. In the host, the arthroconidia enlarge and form spherules, which are large septate structures containing endospores. The endospores are then released and form new spherules.[171]

Predisposing factors that may lead to dissemination of infection include pregnancy; age less than 5 years and greater than 50 years; and Philippine, Asian, or African descent.[226] Primary pulmonary infection is asymptomatic in approximately 60% of cases. In the symptomatic cases, evidence of pulmonary infection is frequent, with associated cutaneous lesions. Most acute infections resolve without therapy over a period of several weeks. In 10% of symptomatic patients, chronic pulmonary lesions persist. Gastrointestinal coccidioidomycosis is rare. Weisman and colleagues reported a case of GI infection in the setting of massive chylous ascites and extensive abdominal lymphatic involvement.[227] Coccidioidal peritonitis has also been reported on several occasions, but most of these infections were incidental findings at surgery and did not require antifungal therapy.[228]

REFERENCES

1. Hippocrates' Epidemics. Book 13. Adams F, trans. Baltimore: Williams & Wilkins; 1939.
2. Cormack Jr trans. and ed., Trousseau Lectures on Clinical Medicine: Delivered at Hôtel-Dieu, Paris. London: New Sydenham Society; 1869;2.
3. Parrot J. Cliniques des noruveaux-nés l'athrepsie: Leçons recuelliés par Dr. Troisier. Paris: G Masson; 1877.
4. Langenbeck B. Auffingung von Pilzer aus der Schleimhaut der Speiseröhre einer Typhus-Leiche. Neue Not Geb Natur-u-Heilk (Froorief). 1939;12:145–147.
5. Berg FT. GM Torsk hos Barn. Stockholm: LJ Hjerta; 1846.
6. Haussmann D. Parasites de organes sexuels femeil-les de l'homme et de quelques animaux avec une notice sur développement de l'*Oidium albicans* Robin. Paris: JB Baillière; 1875.
7. Berkhout CM: De Schimmelgeschlachter Monilia, Oidium, Vospora, en Torula. Utrecht, Netherlands: University of Utrecht; 1923. Dissertation.
8. Odds FC. *Candida* and Candidosis: A Review and Bibliography. 2nd ed. London: Baillière Tindall; 1988:67.
9. Do-Carmo-Sousa L. Distribution of yeasts in nature. In: Rose AH, Harrison JS. The Yeasts. London: Academic Press; 1969;1:79–105.
10. Vazquez JA, Beckley A, Sobel JD, et al. Comparison of restriction enzyme analysis versus pulsed-field gradient gel electrophoresis as a typing system for *Candida albicans*. J Clin Microbiol. 1991;29:962–967.
11. Wade JC, Schimpff SC. Epidemiology and prevention of *Candida* infections. In: Bodey GP, Fainstain V. Candidiasis. New York: Raven Press; 1985:111–133.
12. Marples MJ. Microbiological studies in Western Samoa: Part II, The isolation of yeast-like organisms from the mouth. Trans R Soc Trop Med Hyg. 1960;54:166–170.
13. Smith BJ, Pman AP, Arblasto PG. Incidence of *Candida* in hospital in-patients and the effects of antibiotic therapy. Br Med J. 1966;1:208–210.
14. Cambon M, Pétavy AF, Guillot J, et al. Etude de la fréquence des protozoaires et des levuires isolés du parodonte chez 509 sujets. Pathol Biol (Paris). 1979;27:603–606.
15. Cohen R, Roth FJ, Delgado F, et al. Fungal flora of the normal human small and large intestine. N Engl J Med. 1969;280:638–641.
16. Sakata H, Fujita K, Yahioka H. The effects of antimicrobial agents on the fecal flora of children. Antimicrob Agents Chemother. 1986;29:225–229.
17. Mackenzie DWR. Yeast from human sources. Sabouraudia. 1962;1:8–15.
18. Stenderup A, Pedusen GT. Yeasts of human origin. Acta Pathol Microbiol Scand. 1962;54:462–472.
19. Odds FC. Ecology and epidemiology of candidiasis. In: Odds FC. Candida and Candidosis: A Review and Bibliography. 2nd ed. London: Baillière Tindall; 1985:89.
20. Fox BC, Mobley HL, Wade JC. The use of a DNA probe for epidemiological studies of candidiasis in immunocompromised hosts. J Infect Dis. 1989;159:488–493.
21. Galen. Des remedius parabilibus I–III. In: Kuhn CG. Opera Omnia. Hildersheim: George Olms; 1965.
22. Kozinn PJ, Taschdjian CL, Weiner HM. Incidence and pathogenesis of neonatal candidiasis. Pediatrics. 1958;21:421–429.
23. Taschdjian CL, Kozinn PJ. Laboratory and clinical studies on candidiasis in the newborn infant. J Pediatr. 1957;50:426–433.
24. Rothschild H, Wilson M, Lopez M, et al. An immunological investigation of a family with chronic mucocutaneous candidiasis. Int Arch Allergy Appl Immunol. 1976;52:291–296.
25. Sams WM Jr, Tomzzo JL, Snyderman R, et al. Chronic mucocutaneous candidiasis. Am J Med. 1979;67:948–959.
26. Beta PG. Pathology of some of the opportunistic infections in acquired immune deficiency syndrome (AIDS). Pathologica. 1985;77:67–75.
27. Chandler FW. Pathology of the mycoses in patients

with the acquired immune deficiency syndrome (AIDS). Curr Top Med Mycol. 1986;1:1–23.

28. Fauci AS, Macher AM, Long DL, et al. Acquired immunodeficiency syndrome: Epidemiologic, clinical, immunological and therapeutic considerations. Ann Intern Med. 1984;100:96–106.

29. Jaffe HW, Bergman DJ, Selik RM. Acquired immune deficiency syndrome in the United States: The first 1000 cases. J Infect Dis. 1983;148:339–345.

30. Stenderup A, Schonheyder H. Mycoses complicating AIDS. Microbiol Sci. 1984;1:219–223.

31. Melbye M, Schonheyder H, Kesters L, et al. Carriage of oral C. albicans associated with a high number of circulating suppressor T Lymphocytes. J Infect Dis. 1985;52:1356–1357.

32. Schonheyder H, Melbye M, Biggar RJ, et al. Oral yeast flora and antibodies to Candida albicans in homosexual men. Mykosen suppl. 1984;27:539–544.

33. Kalo-Klein A, Witkin SS. Prostaglandin E_2 enhances and gamma interferon inhibits germ tube formation in Candida albicans. Infect Immun. 1990;58:260–262.

34. Claman HN, Hartley TF, Merrill D. Hypogammaglobulinemia, primary and secondary: Immunoglobulin levels in 125 patients. J Allergy. 1966;38:215–225.

35. Strober W, Krakauer R, Kaeveman HL, et al. Secretory component deficiency. N Engl J Med. 1976;294:351–356.

36. Bodey GP. Candidiasis in cancer patients. Am J Med. 1984;77:13–19.

37. Walsh TJ, Gray WC. Candida epiglottitis in immunocompromised patients. Chest. 1987;91:482–485.

38. Kim MH, Rodey GE, Good RA. Defective candidacidal capacity of polymorphonuclear leukocytes in chronic granulomatous disease of childhood. J Pediatr. 1969;75:300–303.

39. Lehrer RI. Antifungal effects of peroxidase systems. J Bacteriol. 1969;99:361–365.

40. Topper-James L, Aldred MJ, Walker DM. Candidal infections and populations of Candida albicans in mouths of diabetics. J Clin Pathol. 1981;34:706–711.

41. Barlow AJE, Chattaway FW. Observations on the carriage of Candida albicans in man. Br J Dermatol. 1969;81:103–106.

42. Segal E, Sotoka A, Schechter A. Correlative relationship between adherence of Candida albicans to human vaginal epithelial cells in vitro and candidal vaginitis. J Med Vet Mycol. 1984;22:191–200.

43. Wilson RM, Reeves WG. Neutrophil phagocytosis and killing in insulin-dependent diabetes. Clin Exp Immunol. 1986;63:478–484.

44. Sutptin A, Albright F, McCure DJ. Five cases of idiopathic hypoparathyroidism associated with moniliasis. J Clin Endocrinol. 1943;3:625–630.

45. Spinner MW, Blizzard RM, Childs B. Clinical and genetic heterogeneity in idiopathic Addison's disease and hypoparathyroidism. J Clin Endocrinol. 1968;28:795–804.

46. Podolsky S, Ferguson BD. Fatal systemic candidiasis following treatment of Addisonian crisis in a juvenile diabetic. Diabetes. 1970;19:438–444.

47. Giombetti R, Hagstrom JWC, Landey S, et al. Cushing's syndrome in infancy: A case complicated by monilial endocarditis. Am J Dis Child. 1971;122:264–266.

48. Cormane RH, Goolings WRO. Factors influencing the growth of Candida albicans. Sabouraudia. 1963;3:52–63.

49. Samaranayake LP. Nutritional factors and oral candidosis. J Oral Pathol. 1986;15:61–65.

50. Gorbach SL, Nahas L, Lerner PJ. Studies of intestinal microflora: Effects of diet, age, and periodic sampling on numbers of fecal microorganisms in man. Gastroenterology. 1967;53:845–855.

51. Jenkins WM, MacFarlane TW, Ferguson NM. Nutritional deficiency in oral candidiasis. Int J Oral Surg. 1977;6:204–210.

52. Seelig MS. The role of antibiotics in the pathogenesis of Candida infections. Am J Med. 1966;40:887–917.

53. Fitzpatrick JJ, Topley HE. Ampicillin therapy and Candida overgrowth. Am J Med Sci. 1966;252:310–313.

54. Caldwell JR, Cluff LE. Adverse reactions to antimicrobial agents. JAMA. 1974;230:77–80.

55. Winner HI, Hurley R. Candida albicans. London: Churchill; 1964.

56. Johnson RD, Chick EW, Johnston NS. Asymptomatic quantitative increase of Candida albicans in the oral cavity: Predisposing factors. South Med J. 1967;60:1244–1247.

57. Loose DS, Feldman D. Characterization of a unique corticosterone-binding protein in Candida albicans. J Biol Chem. 1982;257:4925–4930.

58. Clayton RM, Soutal CA, Stanford CF, et al. Double-blind trial comparing two dosage schedules of beclomethasone aerosol in bronchial asthma. Lancet. 1974;2:303–307.

59. Vogt FC. The incidence of oral candidiasis with use of inhaled conticosteroids. Ann Allergy. 1979;43:205–210.

60. Boero M, Pera A, Andruilli A, et al. Candida overgrowth in gastric juice of peptic ulcer subjects and short- and long-term treatment with H_2-receptor antagonists. Digestion. 1983;28:158–163.

61. Neeman A, Kadish U. Candidal infection of benign gastric ulcer. Gastroenterology. 1984;87:1406–1407.

62. Johnson SAM, Guzman MG, Aguilera CT. Candida albicans: Effects of amino-acids, glucose, pH, chlortetracycline dibasic sodium, calcium phosphates, and anaerobic and aerobic conditions on its growth. Arch Dermatol. 1954;70:49–60.

63. Sanford GR, Metz WG, Wingard JR, et al. The value of fungal surveillance cultures as predictors of systemic fungal infections. J Infect Dis. 1980;142:503–509.

64. Walsh TJ, Merz WG. Pathologic features in the human alimentary tract associated with invasiveness of Candida tropicalis. Am J Clin Pathol. 1986;85:498–502.

65. Wingard JR, Dick JD, Metz WG, et al. Pathogenicity of Candida tropicalis and Candida albicans gastrointestinal inoculation in mice. Infect Immun. 1980;29:808–813.

66. Eras P, Goldskin MJ, Sherlock P. Candida infections of the gastrointestinal tract. Medicine. 1972;51:367–379.

67. Maksymiuk AW, Thongprosert S, Hopfer R, et al. Systemic candidiasis in cancer patients. Am J Med. 1984;77:20–27.

68. Liljemark WF, Gibbons RJ. Suppression of Candida albicans by human oral streptococci in gnotobiotic mice. Infect Immun. 1973;8:846–849.

69. Pope LM, Cole GT. SEM studies of adherence of Candida albicans to the gastrointestinal tract of infant mice. Scanning Electron Microsc. 1981;3:73–80.

70. Savage DC. Microbial ecology of the gastrointestinal tract. Annu Rev Microbiol. 1977;31:107–133.

71. Kennedy MJ. Candida albicans adhesions. In: Curr Top Med Mycol. 1988;2:73–169.

72. Kennedy MJ. Regulation of Candida albicans populations in the gastrointestinal tract: Mechanisms and significance in GI and systemic candidiasis. Curr Top Med Mycol. 1989;3:315–402.

73. Fisher V. Intestinal absorption of viable yeast. Proc Soc Exp Biol Med. 1980;28:948.

74. Stone HH. Studies in the pathogenesis, diagnosis and treatment of Candida sepsis in children. J Pediatr Surg. 1974;9:127–134.

75. Krause W, Matheis H, Wulf K. Fungemia and funguria after oral administration of Candida albicans. Lancet. 1969;1:598–599.

76. Rosen Von Rosenstein N. Underãtrelse on Barns Sjukdomar och Deras Botemedal. Stockholm: Wenneberg and Nordstrom; 1771.

77. Boggs DR, Williams AF, Howell A. Thrush in malignant neoplastic disease. Arch Intern Med. 1961;107:354–360.

78. Finlay IG. Oral symptoms and *Candida* in the terminally ill. Br Med J. 1986;292:592–593.

79. Silverman S Jr, Luangjarmekorn L, Greenspan D. Occurrence of oral *Candida* in irradiated head and neck cancer patients. J Oral Med. 1984;39:194–196.

80. Samonis G, Rolston K, Karl C, et al. Prophylaxis of oropharyngeal candidiasis with fluconazole. Rev Infect Dis. 1990;12(suppl 3):369–373.

81. Yeo E, Alvarado T, Fainstein V. Prophylaxis of oropharyngeal candidiasis with clotrimazole. J Clin Oncol. 1985;3:1668–1671.

82. Epstein JB, Kimura LH, Menard TW, et al. Effects of specific antibodies on the interaction between the fungus *Candida albicans* and human oral mucosa. Arch Oral Biol. 1982;27:469–474.

83. Pollock JJ, Denepitiya L, Mackay BJ, et al. Fungistatic and fungicidal activity of human parotid salivary histidine-rich polypeptides on *Candida albicans*. Infect Immun. 1984;44:702–707.

84. Smith JMB, Meech RJ. The polymicrobial nature of oropharyngeal thrush. N Z Med J. 1984;97:335–336.

85. Letiner T. Oral thrush or acute pseudomembranous candidiasis: A clinical-pathologic study of 44 cases. Oral Surg. 1964;18:27–37.

86. Kozinn PJ, Taschdjian CL, Dragutsky D, et al. Therapy of oral thrush: A comparative evaluation of gentian violet, mycostatin and amphotericin B. Monogr Ther. 1957;2:16–24.

87. Yap BS, Bodey GP. Oropharyngeal candidiasis treated with a troche form of clotrimazole. Arch Intern Med. 1979;139:656–657.

88. Schectiman LB, Funaro L, Robin T, et al. Clotrimazole treatment of oral candidiasis in patients with neoplastic disease. Am J Med. 1984;76:91–94.

89. Hughes WT, Bartley DL, Patterson GG. Ketoconazole and candidiasis: A controlled study. J Infect Dis. 1983;147:1060–1063.

90. Horsburgh CR Jr, Kirkpatrick CH. Long-term therapy of chronic mucocutaneous candidiasis with ketoconazole: Experience with 21 patients. Am J Med. 1983;74(suppl 1B):23–29.

91. Hay RJ. Overview of studies of fluconazole in oropharyngeal candidiasis. Rev Infect Dis. 1990;12(suppl 3):334–337.

92. Meunier F, Aoun M, Gerard M. Therapy of oropharyngeal candidiasis in the immunocompromised host: A randomized double-blind study of fluconazole vs ketoconazole. Rev Infect Dis. 1990;12(suppl 3):364–368.

93. DeWit S, Weerts D, Gooscens H. Comparison of fluconazole and ketoconazole for oropharyngeal candidiasis in AIDS. Lancet. 1989;1:746–748.

94. Laine L, Detler RH, Conteas CN, Tirazon C, et al. Fluconazole compared with ketoconazole for the treatment of Candida esophagitis in AIDS. Ann Int Med. 1992; 117:655–660.

95. Dupont B, Drouhet C. Fluconazole in the management of oropharyngeal candidiasis in a predominantly HIV antibody-positive group of patients. J Med Vet Mycol. 1988;26:67–71.

96. Meunier-Carpentier F, Cruciani M, Klastersky J. Oral prophylaxis with miconazole or ketoconazole of invasive fungal disease in neutropenic cancer patients. Eur J Cancer Clin Oncol. 1983;19:43–48.

97. Baciewicz AM, Self TH, Bekemer WB. Update on rifampin drug interactions. Arch Intern Med. 1987;147:565–568.

98. Stevens DA, Greene I, Lang OS. Thrush can be prevented in patients with AIDS and the acquired immunodeficiency syndrome–related complex. Arch Intern Med. 1991;151:2458–2464.

99. Leen CLS, Dunbar EM, Ellis ME, et al. Once weekly fluconazole to prevent recurrence of oropharyngeal candidiasis in patients with AIDS and AIDS-related complex: A double-blind placebo-controlled study. J Infect. 1990;21:55–60.

100. Lavilla Paz GA, Valencia ME, Pintado V, et al. Fluconazole preventative therapy for *Candida* esophagitis in AIDS. Florence, Italy: Sixth International Conference on AIDS. Abstract. 1990▼B 466.

101. Owens NJ, Nightingale CH, Schweizen RT, et al. Prophylaxis of oral candidiasis with clotrimazole troches. Arch Intern Med. 1984;144:290–296.

102. Goodman JL, Winston DJ, Greenfield RA, et al. Does fluconazole prevent fungal infections in patients undergoing bone marrow transplantation? Results of a randomized controlled trial. N Eng J Med. 1992; 326:845–851.

103. Winston DJ, Islam Z, Buell D, et al. Fluconazole prophylaxis of fungal infections in acute leukemia patients: Results of a placebo-controlled, double-blind multi-center trial. Chicago: 31st Interscience Conference on Antimicrobial Agents and Chemotherapy. 1991;6:99. Abstract.

104. Budtz-Jorgensen E, Stenderup A, Grabowski M. An epidemiological study of yeasts in elderly denture wearers. Community Dent Oral Epidemiol. 1975;3:115–119.

105. Cawson RA, Lehner T. Chronic hyperplastic candidiasis—candidal leukoplakia. Br J Dermatol. 1968;80:9–16.

106. Ritchie GM, Fletcher AM, Main DMG, et al. The etiology, exfoliative cytology and treatment of denture stomatitis. J Prosthet Dent. 1969;22:185–200.

107. Cawson RA. Denture sore-mouth: Part II, The role of *Candida*. Dent Pract Dent Rec. 1965;16:138–142.

108. Russotto SB. The role of *Candida albicans* in the pathogenesis of angular cheilosis. J Prosthet Dent. 1980; 44:243–246.

109. Daftary DK, Mehta FS, Gupta PC. The presence of *Candida* in 723 oral leukoplakias among Indian villagers. Scand J Dent Res. 1972;80:75–79.

110. Cernéa P, Crépy C, Kuffer R, et al. Aspects peu connus des candidoses buccales. Rev Stomat Chir Maxillofac. 1965;66:103–138.

111. Russel C, Jones JH, Gibbs AAC. The carriage of *Candida albicans* in the mouth of rats treated with tetracycline briefly or for a prolonged period. Mycopathologica. 1976;58:125–129.

112. Lehner T. Classification and clinico-pathological features of *Candida* infections in the mouth. In: Winner H, Hurley R. Symposium on *Candida* Infections. Edinburgh: Livingstone; 1966:119–137.

113. Lamey PJ, Lamb AB. Prospective study of etiological factors in burning mouth syndrome. Br Med J. 1988;296:1243–1246.

114. Hughes WT. Systemic candidiasis: A study of 109 fatal cases. Pediatr Infect Dis. 1982;1:11–18.

115. Grutin JG, Sanson J. Mycotic infections in leukemic patients at autopsy. Cancer. 1963;6:61–73.

116. Wheeler RR, Peacock JE Jr, Cruz JM. Esophagitis in the immunocompromised host: Role of esophagoscopy in diagnosis. Rev Infect Dis. 1987;9:88–96.

117. Stevens DA. Fungal infections in AIDS patients. Br J Clin Pract. 1990;44(suppl. 71):11–22.

118. Jensen KB, Stenderup A, Thomsen JB. Esophageal moniliasis in malignant neoplastic disease. Acta Med Scand. 1964;175:455–459.

119. Kodsi BE, Wickiemisinghe PC, Kozinn PJ. *Candida*

esophagitis: A prospective study of 27 cases. Gastroenterology. 1976;71:715–719.

120. Scott BB, Jenkins D. Gastro-oesophageal candidiasis. Gut. 1982;23:137–139.

121. Clotet B, Grijol M, Parro B, et al. Asymptomatic esophageal candidiasis in AIDS-related complex. Ann Intern Med. 1986;105:145.

122. Sehhat S, Hazeghi K, Bajoghli M. Oesophageal moniliasis causing fistula formation and lung abscess. Thorax. 1976;31:361–364.

123. Lefkowitz M, Elsas LJ, Levine RJ. *Candida* infection complicating peptic esophageal ulcer: Infection in an aortic-esophageal fistula. Arch Intern Med. 1964;113: 672–675.

124. Athey PA, Goldstein HM, Dodd GD. Radiologic spectrum of opportunistic infections of the upper gastrointestinal tract. Am J Roentgenol. 1977;129:419–424.

125. Pagani JJ, Libshitz HI. Radiology of *Candida* infections. In: Bodey GP, Fainstain V. *Candidiasis.* New York: Raven Press; 1981:71–84.

126. Bier SJ, Keller RJ, Kmvisky BA, et al. Esophageal moniliasis: A new radiographic presentation. Am J Gastroenterol. 1985;80:734–737.

127. Ginsburg CH, Braden GL, Tauber AL. Oral clotrimazole in the treatment of esophageal candidiasis. Am J Med. 1981;71:891–894.

128. Rutgeerts L, Verhaegen H. Intravenous miconazole in the treatment of chronic esophageal candidiasis. Gastroenterology. 1977;72:316–318.

129. Fazio RA, Wickiemesinghe PC, Arsura EL. Ketoconazole treatment of *Candida* esophagitis: A prospective study of 12 cases. Am J Gastroesterol. 1983;78:261–264.

130. Medoff G, Dismukes WE, Meade RH III, et al. A new therapeutic approach to *Candida* infections: A preliminary report. Arch Intern Med. 1972;130:241–245.

131. Bennet JE. Diagnosis and management of candidiasis in the immunosuppressed host. Scand J Infect Dis. 1978;16(suppl):83–86.

132. Dewit S, Urbain D, Rahir F, et al. Efficacy of oral fluconazole in the treatment of AIDS-associated esophageal candidiasis. Eur J Clin Microbiol Infect Dis. 1991;10:503–505.

133. Gil A, Lavilla P, Valencia ME, et al. Fluconazole treatment of esophageal candidiasis in AIDS patients. Medicina Clinica 1992; 918:612–617.

134. Tavitian A, Raufman JP, Rosenthal LE, et al. Ketoconazole-resistant *Candida* esophagitis in patients with AIDS. Gastroenterology. 1986;90:443–445.

135. Glatt AE, Chirgwin K, Landesman SH. Treatment of infections associated with human immunodeficiency virus. N Engl J Med. 1986;18:1439–1448.

136. Selik RM, Starcher ET, Curran JW. Opportunistic diseases reported in AIDS patients: Frequencies, associations, trends. AIDS. 1988;1:175–182.

137. Khuroo MS, Naik SR, Sehgal SC, et al. *Candida* infection of the upper gastrointestinal tract super-added upon chemical injury with acids. Am J Gastroenterol. 1979;72:276–281.

138. Katzenslerin AL, Maksem J. Clinical infections of gastric ulcers: Histology, incidence and clinical significance. Am J Clin Pathol. 1979;71:137–141.

139. Gaylorf SF. Gastric Candidiasis. JAMA. 1979;241:791.

140. Gillespie PE, Green PHR, Barrett PJ, et al. Gastric candidiasis. Med J Austr. 1978;1:228–229.

141. Minoli G, Terruzzi V, Rossini A. Gastroduodenal candidiasis occurring without underlying disease: Report on 2 cases. Endoscopy. 1979;11:18–22.

142. Nelson RS, Bruni HC, Goldstein HM. Primary gastric candidiasis in uncompromised subjects. Gastrointest Endosc. 1975;22:92–94.

143. Piken E, Dwyer R. Gastric Candidiasis. JAMA. 1978; 240:2181–2182.

144. Holmström B, Wallensten S, Frisk A. Presence of fungi in gastric and duodenal ulcers. Acta Clin Scand. 1978; 117:215–220.

145. DiFebo G, Miglioli M, Calo G, et al. *Candida albicans* infections of gastric ulcer—frequency and correlation with medical treatment: Results of multicenter study. Dig Dis Sci. 1985;30:178–181.

146. Minoli G, Temuzzi V, Butti GC, et al. Invasive candidiasis does not complicate short-term cimetidine treatment of duodenal ulcer. Gastrointest Endosc. 1987;33: 227–228.

147. Neeman A, Avidoe I, Kadis U. Candidal infection of benign gastric ulcers in aged patients. Am J Gastroenterol. 1984;75:211–213.

148. Vilotte J, Toutoungi M, Loquillard A. Ulcers gastriques colonisés par *Candida.* Nouv Presse Med. 1981;10: 1471–1474.

149. Bailey JE, Kliegman RM, Annable WL, et al. *T. glabrata* sepsis appearing as necrotizing enterocolitis and endophthalmitis. Am J Dis Child. 1984;183:965–966.

150. Joshi SN, Garvin PJ, Sunwoo YC. Candidiasis of the duodenum and jejunum. Gastroenterology. 1981;80: 829–833.

151. Kozinn PJ, Taschdjian CL. Enteric candidiasis: Diagnosis and clinical considerations. Pediatrics. 1962;30:71–85.

152. Alam SA, Tahir M, De MN. *Candida* as a cause of diarrhoea in children. Bangladesh Med Res Counc Bull. 1977;3:32–36.

153. Sunato, Suharyono, Gracey M. Gastrointestinal candidiasis in malnourished children with diarrhea. Pediatr Indonesiano 1980;20:117–129.

154a. Garagusi VF, Chretien JH. Diarrhea caused by *Candida.* Lancet. 1976;1:697–698.

154b. Bishop RF, Barnes GL. Depression of lactase activity in the small intestine of infant rabbits by *Candida albicans.* J Med Microbiol. 1974;7:259–261.

155. Burke V, Gracey M. An experimental model of gastrointestinal candidiasis. J Med Microbiol. 1980;13: 103–110.

156. Gupta TP, Ehrinpreis MN. *Candida* associated diarrhea in hospitalized patients. Gastroenterology. 1990;98: 780–785.

157. Danna PL, Urban C, Bellin E, et al. Role of *Candida* in pathogenesis of antibiotic-associated diarrhea in elderly inpatients. Lancet. 1991;337:511–514.

158. Alexander JG. Allergy in the gastrointestinal tract. Lancet. 1975;2:1264.

159. Holti G. Candida allergy. In: Winner HI, Hurley R, eds. Proceedings of Symposium on *Candida* Infections. London: Livingstone Press; 1966;78–81.

160. Cooper TW. Secretory diarrhea and candidal overgrowth: Cause and effect? J Infect Dis. 1991;164:823.

161. Morris AB, Sands ML, Shiraki M, et al. Gallbladder and biliary tract candidiasis: Nine cases and review. Rev Infect Dis. 1990;12:483–488.

162. Gupta NM, Chaudhary A, Telwas P. Candidal obstruction of the common bile duct. Br J Surg. 1985;72:13.

163. Adamson PC, Rinaldi MG, Pizzo PA, et al. Amphotericin B in the treatment of *Candida* cholecystitis. Pediatr Infect Dis. 1989;8:408–411.

164. Wells RS. Chronic mucocutaneous candidiasis: A clinical classification. Proc R Soc Med. 1973;66:801–802.

165. Hermans PE, Ritts RE. Chronic mucocutaneous candidiasis. Its association with immunologic and endocrine abnormalities. Minn Med. 1970;53:75–80.

166. Shama SK, Kirkpatrick CH. Dermatophytosis in patients with chronic mucocutaneous candidiasis. J Am Acad Dermatol. 1980;2:285–294.

167. Holt PJ, Higgs JM, Munro J, et al. Chronic mucocutaneous candidiasis: A model for the investigation of cell mediated immunity. Br J Clin Pract. 1972;26:331–336.

168. Fischer A, Ballett JJ, Griscelli C. Specific inhibition of in vitro *Candida* induced lymphocyte proliferation by polysaccharide antigens present in the serum of patients with chronic mucocutaneous candidiasis. J Clin Invest. 1978;62:1005–1013.

169. Durandy A, Fischer A, LeDeist F, et al. Mannan-specific and Mannan-induced T-cell suppressive activity in patients with chronic mucocutaneous candidiasis. J Clin Immunol. 1988;7:400–410.

170. Hay RJ, Clayton YM. The treatment of patients with chronic mucocutaneous candidiasis and *Candida* onychomycosis with ketoconazole. Clin Exp Dermatol. 1982;7:155–162.

171. Rippon JW. Medical Mycology: The Pathogenic Fungi and the Pathogenic Actinomycetes. 3rd ed. Philadelphia: WB Saunders 1988:681–713.

172. Devita VT, Hellman S, Rosenberg, SA. Cancer: Principles and Practice of Oncology. 2nd ed. Philadelphia: JB Lippincott; 1985:1963–1998.

173. Ingram CW, Sennesh J, Cooper JN, et al. Disseminated Zygomycosis. Report of 4 cases and review. Rev Infect Dis. 1989;5:741–754.

174. Windus DW, Stokes TJ, Julian BA, et al. Fatal *Rhizopus* infections in hemodialysis patients receiving deferoxamine. Ann Intern Med. 1987;107:678–680.

175. Rinaldi MG. Zygomycosis—systemic fungal infections: Diagnosis and treatment II. Infect Dis Clin North Am. 1989;3:19–41.

176. Parfrey NA. Improved diagnosis and prognosis of mucormycosis. A clinico-pathologic study of 33 cases. Medicine. 1986;65:113–123.

177. Neame P, Rayner D. Mucormycosis: A report on 22 cases. Medicine. 1986;65:113–123.

178. Thomson SR, Bado PG, Taams M, et al. Gastrointestinal mucormycosis. Br J Surg. 1991;78:952–954.

179. Calle S, Klatsky S. Intestinal phycomycosis (mucormycosis). Am J Clin Pathol. 1966;45:264–277.

180. Kahn LB. Gastric mucormycosis: Report of case with review of the literature. S Afr Med J. 1963;39:1265–1269.

181. Satire AA, Sila MD, Mahgoub S, et al. Systemic phycomycosis. Br Med J. 1971; 1:440.

182. Meyer RD, Rosen P, Armstrong D. Phycomycosis complicating leukemia and lymphoma. Ann Intern Med. 1972;77:871–879.

183. Hamill R, Oney LA, Crane LR. Successful therapy for rhinocerebral mucormycosis with associated bilateral brain abscesses. Ann Intern Med. 1983;143:581–583.

184. Woods KF, Hanna BJ. Brainstem mucormycosis in a narcotic addict with eventual recovery. Am J Med. 1986;80:126–128.

185. Rinaldi MG. Emerging opportunist—Systemic fungal infections: Diagnosis and treatment II. Infect Dis Clin North Am. 1989;3:65–76.

186. Booth C. The Genus *Fusarium*. Kew, Surrey, England. Mycological Institute; 1971:1–69.

187. Anaisse E, Kantarjian H, Ro J, et al. The emerging role of *Fusarium* infections in patients with cancer. Medicine. 1988;67:77–83.

188. Lopez-Berestein G, Fainstein V, Hopfer R, et al. Liposome amphotericin B for the treatment of fungal infections in patients with cancer: A preliminary report. J Infect Dis. 1985;151:704–710.

188a. Barrios NS, Kirkpatrick DV, Murciano A, et al. Successful treatment of disseminated Fusarium infection in an immunocompromised child. Am J Ped Hem Oncol. 1990;12(3):319–324.

189. Gold JWM. Opportunistic fungal infections in patients with neoplastic disease. In: Brown AE, Armstrong D. Infectious Complications of Neoplastic Disease. New York: York Medical Books; 1985:111–121.

190. Rinaldi MG. Invasive aspergillosis. Rev Infect Dis. 1983;5:1061–1077.

191. Levitz SM. Aspergillosis—Systemic fungal infections: Diagnosis and treatment II. Infect Dis Clin North Am 1989;3:1–18.

192. Hovender JL, Nicklason F, Barnes RA. Invasive pulmonary aspergillosis in non-immunocompromised patients. Br Med J. 1991;302:583–584.

193. Horn CR, Wood NC, Hughes JA. Invasive aspergillosis following post-influenzal pneumonia. B J Dis Chest. 1983;77:407–410.

194. Cook DJ, Achong MR, King DEL. Disseminated aspergillosis in an apparently healthy patient. Am J Med. 1970;88:74–76.

195. Young RC, Bennett JE, Vogel CL, et al. Aspergillosis: The spectrum of the disease in 98 patients. Medicine. 1970;49:147–173.

196. Rogers TR, Haynes KH, Barnes RD. Value of antigen detection in predicting invasive pulmonary aspergillosis. Lancet. 1990;336:210–213.

197. Denning DW, Stevens DA. Antifungal and surgical treatment of invasive aspergillosis: Review of 2,121 published cases. Rev Infect Dis. 1990;12:1147–1201.

198. Lopez-Berestein G, Feinstein V, Hopfer R, et al. Liposomal amphotericin B for treatment of systemic fungal infections in patients with cancer: A preliminary study. J Infect Dis. 1985;151:704–710.

199. Dupont B. Itraconazole therapy in aspergillosis: Study in 49 patients. J Am Acad Dermatol. 1990;23:607–614.

200. Kinder RB, Jourdan MH. Disseminated aspergillosis and bleeding colonic ulcers in a renal transplant patient. J R Soc Med. 1985;78:338–339.

201. Armstrong D. Problems in management of opportunistic fungal diseases. Rev Infect Dis. 1989;11(suppl 7):1591–1599.

202. Vandepitte J. Clinical aspects of cryptococcoses in patients with AIDS. In: Vanden-Bossche H. Mycoses in AIDS Patients. New York: Plenum Press; 1989:115–122.

203. Bennett JE, Dismukes WE, Duma RJ, et al. A comparison of amphotericin B alone and combined with flucytosine in the treatment of cryptococcal meningitis. N Engl J Med. 1979;301:612–131.

204. Bozzette S, Larson R, Chiu J. A placebo controlled trial of maintenance therapy with fluconazole after treatment of cryptococcal meningitis in the acquired immunodeficiency syndrome. N Engl J Med. 1991;324:580–584.

205. Furcolow ML. Environmental aspects of histoplasmosis. Arch Environ Health 1965;10:4–10.

206. Mandell W, Goldberg DM, Neu HC. Histoplasmosis in patients with the acquired immunodeficiency syndrome. Am J Med. 1986;81:974–978.

207. Davies SF, Khan M, Sarosi G. Disseminated histoplasmosis in immunologically suppressed patients. Am J Med. 1978;64:94–100.

208. Goodwin RA, Loyd JE, Des Prez RM. Histoplasmosis in the normal host. Medicine. 1981;60:1–33.

209. Slama TG. Histoplasmosis: Changing concepts in diagnosis and therapy. Infect Med. 1991;1:5–6, 47–51.

210. Brett MT, Kwan JTC, Bending MR. Cecal perforation in a renal transplant patient with disseminated histoplasmosis. J Clin Pathol. 1988;41:992–995.

211. Goodwin RA, Shapiro JL, Thurman GH, et al. Disseminated histoplasmosis. Medicine. 1981;59:1–33.

212. Wheat LJ, Slama TG, Zeckel ML. Histoplasmosis in the acquired immunodeficiency syndrome. Am J Med. 1985;78:203–210.

213. Graybill JD. Histoplasmosis and AIDS. J Infect Dis. 1988;158:623–626.

214. Johnson PC, Kardori N, Najjer AF, et al. Progressive disseminated histoplasmosis in patients with acquired

immunodeficiency syndrome. Am J Med. 1988;85:152–158.

215. Driks MR, Gupta MR, McKinsey DS, et al. Gastrointestinal histoplasmosis in patients with AIDS: Atlanta: Proceedings of the 30th Interscience Conference on Antimicrobial Agents and Chemotherapy. A1272;1990. Abstract.

216. Cappell MS, Mandell W, Grimes MM, et al. Gastrointestinal histoplasmosis. Dig Dis Sci 1988;33:353–360.

217. Sarosi GA, Voth DW, Dahl BH, et al. Disseminated histoplasmosis: Results of long-term follow-up. Ann Intern Med. 1971;75:511–516.

218. Wheat LJ. Histoplasmosis—Systemic fungal infections: Diagnosis and Treatment I. Infect Dis Clin North Am. 1988;2:841–859.

219. Bradsher RW. Blastomycosis—Systemic fungal infections: Diagnosis and Treatment I. Infect Dis Clin North Am. 1988;2:877–898.

220. Saag MS, Dismukes WE. Treatment of histoplasmosis and blastomycosis. Chest. 1988;98:848–851.

221. Restrepo A. The ecology of *Paracoccidioides brasiliensis*:

A puzzle still unsolved. J Med Vet Mycol. 1985;23:323–334.

222. Restrepo A, Robledo M, Giraldo R, et al. The gamut of paracoccidioidomycosis. Am J Med. 1976;61:33–42.

223. Restrepo A. Immune response to *P. brasiliensis* in human and animal hosts. In: McGinnis MR. Current Topics in Medical Mycology. New York: Springer-Verlag; 1987;2:239–277.

224. Restrepo A, Gomez I, Cano LE, et al. Treatment of paracoccidioidomycosis. Am J Med. 1983;74(suppl. B):48–52.

225. Restrepo A, Gomez I, Robledo J, et al. Itraconazole in the treatment of paracoccidioidomycosis: A preliminary report. Rev Infect Dis. 1987;9(suppl 1):51–56.

226. Ampel NM, Wieden MA, Galgiani, JN. Coccidioidomycosis: Clinical update. Rev Infect Dis. 1989;6:897–910.

227. Weisman IM, Moreno AJ, Parker AL. Gastrointestinal dissemination of coccidiodomycosis. Am J Gastro. 1986;81:589–593.

228. Cuen KTK. Coccidioidal peritonitis. Am J Clin Pathol. 1983;80:514–516.

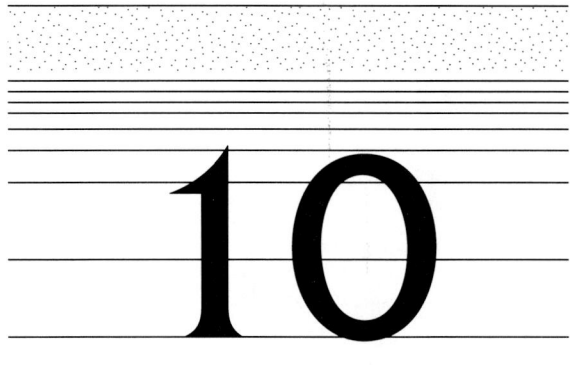

Colonic Parasitic Diseases

J. GORDON FRIERSON, M.D.

One of the most fascinating aspects of parasitology, and indeed of all infectious disease, is the tropism of parasites. Some parasites invade the colon, some prefer the small bowel, some the liver, and so forth. Immediately, a fundamental question is raised: Why is the colon singled out by some parasites? Unfortunately, the molecular mechanisms that control this tropism are not fully understood. Our account of what transpires must therefore be descriptive in nature: in due time further research will illuminate the fundamental biologic questions.

We focus here on aspects of parasitic infections only as they pertain to the colon, with the understanding that some infections, such as schistosomiasis, involve other parts of the body as well.

PROTOZOAL INFECTIONS

Amebiasis

Organism and Epidemiology

The term amebiasis refers to infection with *Entamoeba histolytica*, a protozoan found in both a cyst and a trophozoite form. The infection is acquired through ingestion of the cyst form, which occurs via fecally contaminated food or water, by contaminated fingers, or by oral-anal sexual contact. The cyst resists gastric digestion and passes to the lower small bowel, where excystation occurs. Then, through division, each cyst gives rise to eight trophozoite forms, which inhabit the colon. The trophozoites measure from 10 to 60 μm in diameter, are uninucleate, have pseudopodia, and are further identified by four characteristics: their unidirectional motility; the presence of a clear zone between the granular cytoplasm and the pseudopodial membrane; their ability to ingest erythrocytes; and their nuclear structure (Fig. 10–1). Some trophozoites, through as yet undetermined stimuli, transform to cysts. Cysts range in size from 10 to 20 μm. Immature cysts have one nucleus, a mass of glycogen, and dark-staining chromatoid bodies. Mature cysts have four nuclei, and the glycogen and chromatoid bodies have disappeared (Fig. 10–2). Both trophozoites and cysts may be passed with stool, but the trophozoites are fragile and do not contribute to transmission. Ingestion of these cysts by another host completes the cycle.

Although the organism may be found anywhere in the world, the first case of infection was reported from northern Russia. The prevalence of infection increases as the degree of sanitation decreases, and it is thus most prevalent in countries where sanitary conditions are poor. Practices such as using human excreta for fertilizer and lack of hand washing contribute

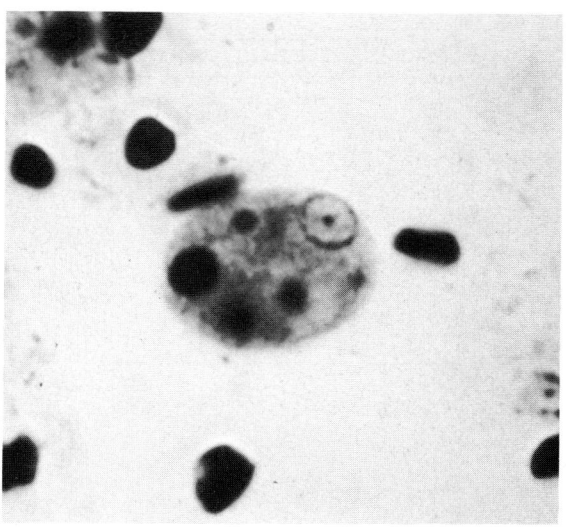

FIGURE 10–1.
Trophozoite of *E. histolytica* stained with iron hematoxylin. Note the ingested erythrocyte and nucleus with central karyosome.

to its spread. Spread within households is common. Waterborne outbreaks have occurred but seem not to be common. Amebiasis has also been a problem in the gay community because of oral-anal sexual practices. Outbreaks have occurred in certain institutional settings such as mental hospitals, where fecal contamination occurs. Flies and roaches are presumed to contribute to transmission, though direct evidence is scanty.

Amebic cysts are quite sensitive to drying but can survive for as long as a month in moist environments at cool temperatures. They are killed quickly at temperatures above 50°C (122°F) and below −5°C (23°F), and are killed immediately by boiling water. They have been recovered from the feces and vomitus of flies and roaches. One study found cysts to remain viable under fingernails for up to 45 minutes.

Pathogenesis and Pathology

The mere presence of *E. histolytica* organisms in the colon does not necessarily signify active disease or even any detectable pathologic condition. Whether the trophozoite invades the colonic mucosa depends on a number of factors. Host-related factors are still under study but are thought to include the number and type of colonic bacterial flora, the composition of the mucous barrier, the nutritional status of the host, the status of cellular immune defenses, and other physiologic factors, such as pregnancy.[1] Clinical observations that support these theories

are the improvement in symptoms seen with nonamebicidal antibiotics, the exacerbation of disease with steroids,[2] and the severity of disease during pregnancy[3] and in the newborn.[4] Anecdotal evidence indicates that recovery from amebic hepatic abscess provides resistance to future invasive disease.[3] Both circulating antibodies and cellular immune responses are generated during infection, though the exact role they play in protective immunity is still under investigation.

Parasite-related factors have received much attention, but a complete composite picture of a pathogenic strain of ameba has not yet been worked out. By studying mobility bands of isoenzymes on thin layer starch-gel electrophoresis, Sargeaunt was able to list different zymodemes (*zymo* = enzyme, *deme* = population), or patterns, that characterized populations of *E. histolytica*. Certain zymodemes were seen in amebae isolated from diseased patients, and other zymodemes from asymptomatic carriers, the correlation being remarkably constant.[5] Whether these zymodemes are genetically determined, and therefore true markers of pathogenicity, or phenotypic representations subject to change under certain conditions is controversial.[6] Conversion from nonpathogenic to pathogenic zymodemes has been accomplished in the laboratory under specified conditions. In addition, amebae with pathogenic zymodemes have been found in asymptomatic patients. This group, however, tends to have positive serologic tests, suggesting that invasion has occurred and has healed or is subclinical. Evidence for a genetic difference between pathogenic and nonpathogenic strains is the finding that each has a distinctly different gene coding for cysteine pro-

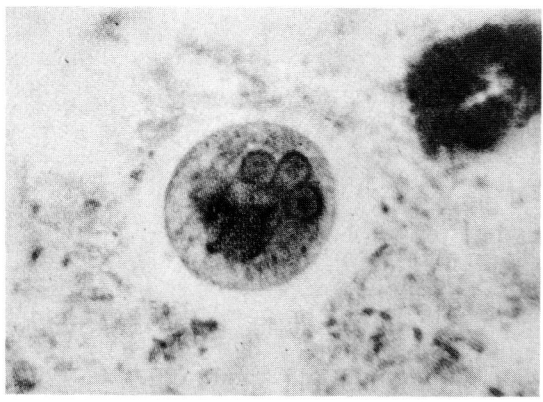

FIGURE 10–2.
Early mature cyst of *E. histolytica*. Three of the four nuclei are visible. Residua of the glycogen and chromatoid bodies are present.

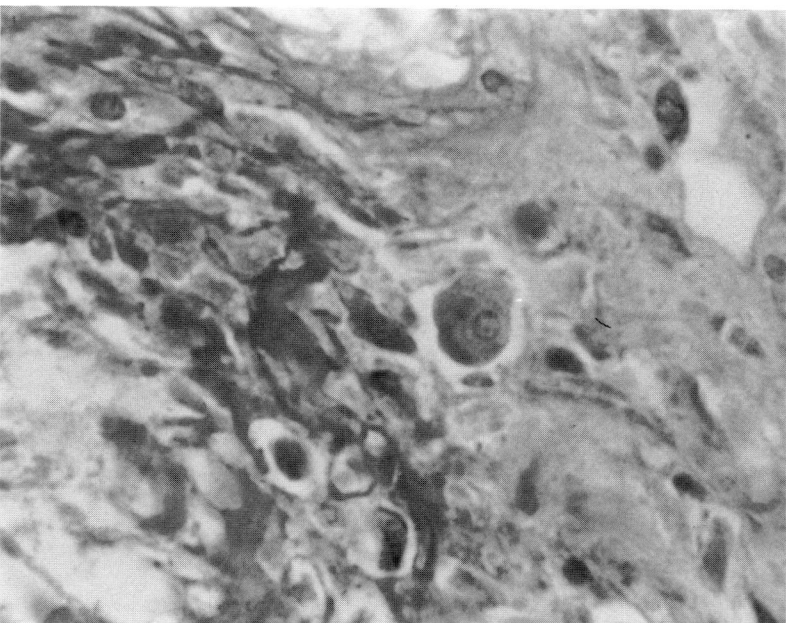

FIGURE 10–3.
Detail of base of amebic ulcer in the colon. On the left is the ulcer crater, with a trophozoite of *E. histolytica* advancing into the deeper tissues. Note absence of inflammatory cells around it. SOURCE: Original slide by William C. Schraft, New Rochelle, NY from A Pictorial Presentation of Parasites, edited by Herman Zaiman. Valley City, ND.

tease, a virulence factor.[7] In addition, correlation between strains identified as pathogenic by DNA probes and by zymodeme analysis has been good, though published numbers are still small.[8] Whether zymodeme analysis is reliable enough to allow a decision regarding treatment is not yet clear, and the technique remains a research tool.[9]

Certain strains that are morphologically distinct from invasive *E. histolytica* have been isolated from asymptomatic patients. They are able to grow in lower temperatures and are tolerant of hypotonic conditions, suggesting that they belong to another species. These strains are referred to collectively as Laredo strains, because the first was isolated from a patient in Laredo TX.

Pathogenic *E. histolytica* organisms employ a variety of mechanisms to enhance tissue invasion. These include secretion of proteolytic enzymes, phagocytosis, cytotoxicity and cytolysis.[10] Amebae also contain adhesins that enable them to adhere to the colonic epithelial cells, a process that is apparently a prerequisite to destructive enzymatic activity.

Amebic colitis is an ulcerative disease. The ulcers, beginning as small areas of necrosis in the colonic mucosa, are presumably caused by enzymatic activity of the trophozoites. In their earliest stage they appear only as tiny areas of mucosa denuded of mucus, with local necrosis of epithelial cells, a few amebae in the lamina propria, and a mild inflammatory response.[11] The ulcers gradually enlarge and tend to be undermined at the edges, producing the char-

acteristic flask or bottleneck ulcer, which extends to the submucosa. The base of the ulcer is covered with necrotic cellular debris and fibrin. The ulcers are round and have smooth edges that may be slightly elevated or undermined. The mucosa between ulcers is relatively spared, producing the smooth, round, punched-out appearance seen through the sigmoidoscope.[12] They vary in size from a couple of millimeters to several centimeters and may be few in number or so numerous as to be almost confluent. One often sees trophozoites infiltrating the tissues surrounding the ulcerated area, but they are not usually accompanied by inflammatory cells (Fig. 10–3). Ulcers may be found anywhere in the colon but are most common in the cecum, followed by the sigmoid, descending colon, and rectum. The transverse colon, being relatively spared, accounts for only approximately 10% of cases. Involvement of the appendix has been described with varying frequency. The terminal ileum is only rarely involved. In severe cases, ulcers become confluent, and the smaller areas of spared mucosa, because of hyperemia and edema, may assume a polypoid appearance. In the most severe instances, the ulcers may cover the entire colonic wall and extend through the muscle layers to the serosa.[13, 14]

A lesion of a different type is the ameboma (Fig. 10–4). This is a proliferative response of the host to the organism and tends to be associated with disease of relatively long duration. The ameboma appears as a mass, usually in conjunction with an ulcer, and is composed histo-

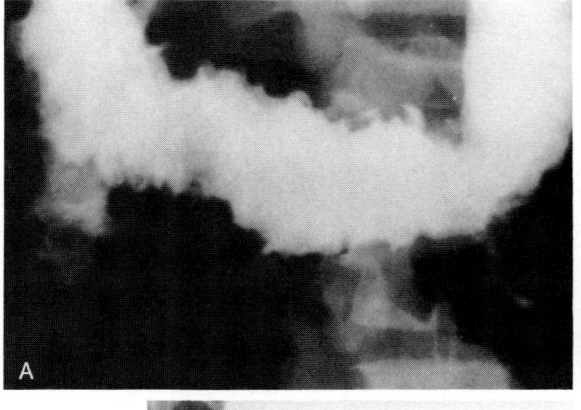
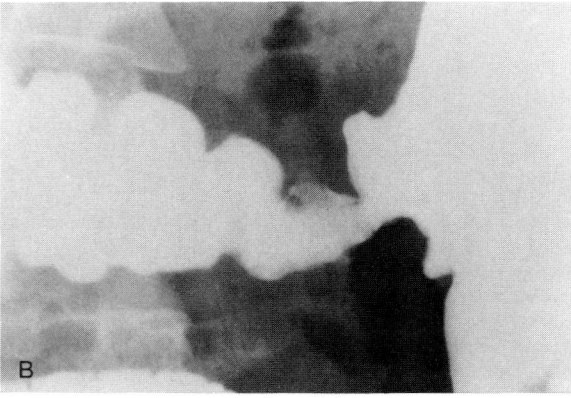
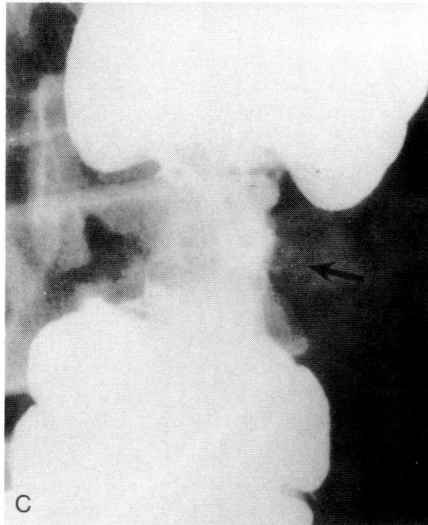

FIGURE 10–4.
Varieties of amebic disease seen on radiographs. *A*, Severe amebic colitis, showing extensive ulcerations, thumbprinting, and spasm. *B*, Ameboma of the distal transverse colon, partly treated. Note tapering edges, especially proximally. *C*, The arrow indicates an apple core–like lesion of transverse colon in a 25-year-old returnee from Vietnam. Indistinguishable from carcinoma by radiograph. SOURCE: *A*, Courtesy of Dr Philip E. Palmer, University of California, Davis. *B,C*, Reeder MM, Palmer PE. The Radiology of Tropical Diseases with Epidemiological, Pathological and Clinical Correlation. Baltimore: Williams & Wilkins, 1981 B, p 22, C, p 29.

logically of granulation tissue with round cell infiltration and giant cells. Fibrous tissue is absent or uncommon. The cause of this proliferative response is not known. Amebomas are seen most commonly in the cecum and rectum, and they occur in approximately 1% of cases.

Complications. The most frequent complication of amebic colitis is perforation, which occurs most often in the cecum, followed by the rectosigmoid. It often occurs as a slow leak, producing a localized peritonitis or abscess or both. If associated with diffuse colitis and multiple areas of deep ulceration, however, the picture is catastrophic and associated with generalized peritonitis. Paracolic abscess may occur. Less commonly, perforation into another organ may occur. Hemorrhage is possible but rare and usually associated with erosion of a blood vessel. Strictures are also uncommon, but when found, are usually, like the ameboma, due to proliferative granulation tissue rather than to fibrosis.

Toxic megacolon, a rare but serious complication, is associated with extensive confluent ulcerations and is usually of full-thickness involvement. The colon becomes dilated, atonic, friable, and shaggy, and perforation may occur.

Extraintestinal Disease. The most common extraintestinal target is the liver. (Disease of the liver and the pleuropericardial spaces is discussed in Chapter 17.) Cutaneous amebiasis is usually seen in the perianal or genital area or at the site of a draining hepatic abscess. Pathologic conditions that one sees include ulceration of the superficial skin, with varying degrees of necrosis and debris in the base and the presence of trophozoites in the leading edges of the ulcer. Amebic involvement may extend to the genitourinary tract. Amebic abscesses are rarely found in the brain and even more rarely in the spleen.

Clinical Findings

The clinical presentation of amebic colitis runs a gamut from absence of symptoms to fulminant disease. The picture is clouded by the fact that identification of strains as pathogenic or nonpathogenic has not generally been possible. Thus, a patient with amebae and mild symptoms may in fact be passing a nonpathogenic *E. histolytica* strain, with symptoms generated from another source.

When true disease can be identified, the incubation period varies from as little as 4 days to as much as 1 year. Not uncommonly amebae may be found in the stool sometime before the onset of clinical disease. Mild cases are characterized by mild diarrhea, cramps or abdominal discomfort, and often some mucus and perhaps some blood in the stool. Malaise and anorexia may be present. Low-grade fever is possible but not common in mild cases. More severe cases show an intensification of these symptoms, with greater degrees of diarrhea, usually of the dysenteric variety, having blood and mucus rather than being watery; more cramps; low-grade to moderate fever; weight loss; and anorexia. Presentations of even greater severity include dehydration, severe abdominal pain, and hypotension. Extensive blood loss is unusual. Amebic colitis tends to run a subacute or chronic course, whereas bacterial diarrheas are more likely to have an abrupt onset and acute course. Other clinical presentations include the complications of localized or generalized peritonitis and appendicitis. Abdominal distention due to toxic megacolon is a rare but ominous sign.

The results of physical examination in asymptomatic carriers and mildly ill people are usually normal. With more severe illness, one sees varying degrees of abdominal tenderness, especially in the lower quadrants, and a mass may be palpable if an ameboma is present. Peritoneal signs suggest impending perforation. Chronic cases may show varying degrees of pallor and wasting. In amebic dysentery, a tender liver is a possibility, which in former times gave rise to the term amebic hepatitis. This tenderness appears related to nonspecific toxic factors and poor nutrition, as a general infiltration of the liver with amebae has never been found. A liver abscess, may, of course, be present to account for this tenderness (see Chapter 17).

Laboratory findings are relatively nonspecific. In mild cases, the leukocyte count and hemoglobin levels are generally normal, with some elevation in leukocytes being common in more severe disease. Eosinophilia is not seen. The white blood cell count is raised and shifted to the left in liver abscess, making it hard to distinguish amebic abscess from bacterial abscess.

Diagnosis

STOOL EXAMINATION

Stool examination is the most common way of demonstrating *E. histolytica*. Identification of

E. histolytica is difficult, the organism often being mistaken for white blood cells or for other amebae, and vice versa.[15] Therefore, the clinician must be assured of a competent laboratory for proper identification. It is customary to collect 3 stools during a period of several days since amebic cysts may be shed intermittently. In a nondysenteric patient, a light saline purge such as phosphosoda administered before collecting the third stool sample is recommended. In more severe cases, the organisms are easier to find. Since trophozoites survive only a short time outside the intestine, a specimen should be examined within 30 minutes of passage, or a preservative should be used. A favored preservative has been polyvinyl alcohol (PVA), although it is now falling into disuse because of its mercury content. A suitable substitute is a sodium acetate-formalin-acetic acid mixture. Both these methods, using trichrome or iron hematoxylin stains, allow proper identification of trophozoites to be made. Concentration techniques to detect scanty organisms are possible with these preservatives. Other methods for concentration utilize formalin-ether or formalin–ethyl acetate. A zinc flotation method can be used, but the concentration method is favored because helminth eggs can be detected with the latter.[16] The merthiolate-iodine-formalin concentration method is favored by some investigators for field work.[17] Ideally, a smear of fresh or preserved stool and a concentrated specimen should both be examined.

Many agents, including barium contrast agents, antibiotics, antiparasitic drugs, antacids, nonsaline laxatives such as castor oil or mineral oil, bismuth, kaolin, and enema products can inhibit the growth of amebae or interfere with their laboratory identification. Thus, if amebiasis is suspected, stools should be collected before these agents are employed, or else the patient should wait until at least 2 weeks after the use of antibiotics, antiparasitic agents, or barium radiographs, and perhaps 1 week after the use of other products before collecting stools. The exact sensitivity of microscopic stool examination has not been studied in recent years, so exact figures cannot be given. Old data and current experience suggest however, that 85 to 90% of cases can be diagnosed when 3 properly collected stools are examined by an experienced technician. Examination of 3 additional stool samples raises the identification rate by a few more percentage points. Stool examinations are positive in less than 50% of cases of amebic liver abscess.

Other stool findings are suggestive but nonspecific. Uncomplicated amebic colitis demonstrates a relative paucity of stool leukocytes in contrast to the number found in bacterial dysentery. Charcot-Leyden crystals may be seen but are not diagnostic. If flecks of mucus are seen, they should be examined in the fresh state for trophozoites. Erythrocytes are common. *Entamoeba histolytica* can be cultured, but many laboratories are not equipped to do so and the diagnostic yield is not demonstrably better.[18]

Enzyme-linked immunosorbent assay (ELISA) methods have been developed to detect amebic antigen in the stool, thus obviating the tedious microscopic techniques.[19] Results have been satisfactory, but the techniques are not yet in wide use. More recently, a deoxyribonucleic acid, (DNA) hybridization probe has been used,[20] but it is still in the investigational stage.

ENDOSCOPY

Endoscopic examination may be helpful in diagnosis. The availability of the flexible sigmoidoscope and colonoscope has added a new dimension to the diagnosis of bowel disease. The entire colon is now accessible for biopsy, making the diagnosis of amebiasis of the right colon and of amebomas easier. The ability to examine scrapings of surface mucus is lost with these instruments, however, and the use of the rigid sigmoidoscope should be considered when amebiasis is suspected. Asymptomatic and mildly symptomatic patients seldom present findings on endoscopic examination. In moderately to severely affected patients, however, sigmoidoscopy may allow visualization of one or more ulcers, though their absence does not exclude amebiasis since only the proximal colon may be involved. The finding of discrete, smooth, round ulcers with only slight elevation of the borders and relatively normal mucosa between them is suggestive and typical of amebiasis but not diagnostic. In some cases, larger ulcers with shaggy edges may be seen. Severe cases may demonstrate a confluence of ulcers or shagginess of the mucosa or both. In diagnosing amebiasis with the sigmoidoscope, the physician should have a microscope or laboratory readily available. Scraping the surface of ulcers with a firm instrument, not a cotton swab, through the rigid sigmoidoscope followed by microscopic examination often yields the organism. The mucus should be examined directly in a drop of saline. *Entamoeba histolytica* organisms are easily identified by their unidirectional motility, the presence of ingested erythrocytes, and the clear space between granular cytoplasm and cell membrane. Biopsy of the edges of an ulcer may also show the parasite, but organisms have also been absent from biopsy specimens in documented cases. Ethanol fixation and staining with either periodic acid–Schiff (PAS) or fluorescent antibody enhances the sensitivity of biopsies.[21]

RADIOLOGY

Radiologic examination may be helpful, but the findings are frequently nondiagnostic. Furthermore, since barium may interfere with proper stool examination, its use should be deferred until stool collections are completed. Flat plate radiologic examination is generally nonspecific, though toxic megacolon, (a rare condition) is easily seen. Barium enema is likely to produce normal findings in mild cases and in more severe cases shows evidence of ulceration in the form of multiple spicules or outright ulceration, spasm, diminished distensibility, loss of haustral markings, and perhaps areas of narrowing (see Fig. 10–4A). Severe edema may produce "thumbprinting." The cecum is involved in a high percentage of cases, and early in the disease it loses its clear silhouette, becoming hazy and indistinct. The transverse colon tends to be spared. In more advanced cases, the bowel wall becomes less distensible, may develop deeper ulcers, and appears more tubular, and the cecum takes on a V- or cone-shaped deformity.[22–24] Amebomas may be detected as a mass by barium enema but cannot reliably be differentiated from carcinoma (Fig. 10–4B, C). Helpful differential signs, however, are the presence of tapered rather than shelflike edges of the lesion, the presence of multiple lesions, the maintenance of an intact mucosa over the mass, the lack of actual bowel obstruction, less rigidity of the bowel, and obvious improvement after antiamebic therapy.[22, 25] Double-contrast barium enema has been reported to give better definition to mucosal ulcerations, enhancing diagnostic sensitivity.[26] (For imaging of the liver, see Chapter 17.)

SEROLOGY

A variety of serologic tests are available. They are of limited value in the evaluation of amebic colitis since their sensitivity decreases with decreasing severity of disease and the parasite is usually not hard to find in more severe cases. Serologic tests are essential, however, in differentiating amebic from bacterial liver abscesses, being positive in about 95% of the former and rarely positive in the latter. The most sensitive test is the indirect hemagglutination (IHA) assay, which may be considered a reference standard. Unfortunately, it is technically difficult to perform and available mainly through the federal Centers for Disease Control in Atlanta and some other reference laboratories. It is highly sensitive, but titers may remain elevated for years, making it hard in some instances to distinguish between past and present disease. It is positive in about 85 to 90% of cases of amebic dysentery, dropping to somewhere between 5 and 25% in mild cases. Other, more widely available tests are the counterimmunoelectrophoresis and gel-immunodiffusion tests. These tests also produce positive results in more than 90% of amebic liver abscess cases and generally suffice in the evaluation of such cases. They are also likely to produce positive findings in cases of amebic dysentery but lose reliability in milder disease. In addition, they appear to measure different antibodies than does the IHA assay since they become negative within a few months after cure of amebiasis, whereas the IHA results may remain positive for up to 20 years. Although ELISA tests have also been developed,[27, 28] they are less widely available.

Serologic tests are more helpful clinically in the evaluation of liver disease. In cases of bowel disease, they are most helpful in evaluating masses that could be amebomas, for which serologic tests are positive in at least 90% of cases, and in evaluating inflammatory bowel disease in which stool examinations have produced negative findings or are of doubtful accuracy owing to poor collection, inexperienced laboratory, or other such factors.[29] Proper stool examinations supplemented by endoscopic evaluation and scrapings or biopsy or both are still the mainstay of diagnosis. Serologic testing is occasionally helpful, however, if such examinations produce negative results or if the use of corticosteroids is contemplated.

Treatment

A number of drugs are available for the treatment of amebiasis, and the exact regimen used depends on the clinical state of the patient, the availability of certain drugs, and the experience of the physician. Broadly speaking, the drugs can be divided into those that act only within the lumen of the bowel, that is, the intraluminal amebicides, and those that act systemically. (The discussion presented here is augmented in Chapter 17.)

INTRALUMINAL AMEBICIDES

Iodoquinol. A halogenated oxyquinoline, iodoquinol (diiodohydroxyquinoline) is available generically or as Yodoxin. It acts only within the lumen since only 1% is absorbed. It has few side effects, and these are limited to mild gastrointestinal complaints. Patients sensitive to iodine should avoid it, and its safety in pregnancy is not established. Rare cases of optic atrophy have been reported after excessive dosages but not with conventional dosages.

Paromomycin. A poorly absorbed aminoglycoside paromomycin is available as Humatin. Although generally tolerated well, it may cause diarrhea and occasionally anorexia and nausea. Extensive ulcerative disease may lead to greater absorption, and it probably should be avoided in these cases. It is considered safe in pregnancy when treating mild to moderate disease.

Diloxanide furoate. An esterified agent, diloxanide furoate is hydrolyzed to the active form diloxanide in the intestine. Diloxanide is absorbed, but the delayed esterification allows enough diloxanide to reach the large intestine to make it useful as an intraluminal agent.[30] It is an effective agent for asymptomatic and mildly symptomatic disease. Its principal side effect is flatulence, other gastrointestinal side effects being less common. It is not recommended in pregnancy because of lack of knowledge concerning teratogenicity. In the United States it is available as Furamide but only from the Parasitic Disease Drug Service of the Centers for Disease Control.

TISSUE AMEBICIDES

Metronidazole. This drug is absorbed well and eliminated primarily through hepatic metabolism. It is rapidly amebicidal and is the drug of choice for most cases in which tissue levels of a drug are needed. Because of its efficient absorption, it is less effective within the bowel lumen and should be supplemented with an intraluminal amebicide in treating bowel disease. Common side effects at dosages used are nausea, headache, dizziness, paresthesias, and a metallic taste in the mouth, with gastrointestinal complaints being less frequent. Patients should be cautioned against alcohol since the drug has an effect similar to that of disulfiram (Antabuse), and it may potentiate the action of Coumadin. It has been found to be carcinogenic in rodents and mutagenic in bacteria, but extensive clinical use of the drug has failed to reveal any obvious carcinogenic properties in humans.[31] Nevertheless, caution should be exercised in its use during pregnancy.

Tinidazole. This is another nitroimidazole related to metronidazole but available only outside the United States. Its pharmacology and side effects are similar to those of metronidazole, but it seems to work a little more effectively, and treatment times are about half those of metronidazole.

Emetine. This salt of an ipecac alkaloid is rapidly amebicidal and was once the tissue amebicide of choice. It must be given intramuscularly and can cause local inflammation. The drug is excreted by the kidney, but a portion is excreted during several weeks, and prolonged administration results in accumulation and toxicity. Its most important side effect is cardiac toxicity, with cardiac arrhythmias, tachycardia, precordial pain, and hypotension being possible manifestations. Other side effects include muscular weakness, myalgias, nausea, vomiting, and diarrhea.[32] Because of its toxicity, it is now generally reserved for severe cases, in which it may be used in conjunction with metronidazole. If used, the patient should be hospitalized and receive daily electrocardiograms or cardiac monitoring. One mg/kg up to a maximum of 65 mg can be given daily in 1 or 2 divided doses for no more than 10 days. Although rarely needed, at least 6 weeks should pass before more is given. It has poor activity within the bowel lumen, is less effective against cysts than against trophozoites, and where bowel disease exists needs to be supplemented with an intraluminal agent.

Dehydroemetine. This drug is similar to emetine but has somewhat less cardiac toxicity. The same precautions need to be observed. It is available only through the Centers for Disease Control (404) 639–3670.

Chloroquine. This agent is weakly amebicidal but is absorbed well and concentrated in the liver. It has therefore been used to some extent against hepatic amebiasis but is not helpful against amebic colitis.

Tetracycline and Erythromycin. These antibiotics are only weakly amebicidal, but their use often results in alleviation of colitis. Tetracycline, when used in conjunction with an intraluminal amebicide, is relatively effective in mild disease. Erythromycin also has a mitigating effect and has been recommended as a temporizing measure for use in pregnancy.

Treatment Regimen by Type of Amebiasis

Dysenteric Amebiasis. The dysenteric form of amebiasis should be considered an invasive disease and treated with an agent acting systemically and an intraluminal agent to eliminate any organisms remaining in the bowel lumen. A common choice is metronidazole, in a dosage of 750 mg given 3 times daily for 5 to 10 days, followed by iodoquinol, given in a dosage of 650 mg 3 times daily for 20 days.[33–35] A full 10 days of metronidazole tends to produce the disagreeable side effects listed above, and use for a period closer to 5 days usually suffices for bowel disease. Outside the United States, tinidazole is a good alternative and perhaps even a little more effective.[36, 37] Emetine and dehydroemetine are also very effective but seldom used owing to their toxicity. The response to these agents is dramatic, and a lack of improvement after 24 hours should raise the question of an incorrect diagnosis or the presence of a concomitant disease.

Mildly Symptomatic Disease. Cases in which blood in the stool, fever, leukocytosis and significant abdominal pain or tenderness are absent may be treated as above but will also respond to other approaches. Good success has been achieved with diloxanide furoate alone, given in a dosage of 500 mg 3 times daily for 10 days.[38, 39] The drug is tolerated well, with the major side effect being flatulence. In the United States the major drawback is the necessity of obtaining the drug from the Centers for Disease Control. Another approach is to use paromomycin alone in a dosage of 25 to 30 mg/kg in 3 divided doses for 10 days.[40, 41] The main side effect is diarrhea, which is seldom severe enough to force the discontinuation of this therapy. Yet another approach is to use tetracycline, in a dosage of 250 mg given 4 times daily for 2 weeks and followed by iodoquinol, given in 650-mg doses 3 times daily for 20 days.[35, 42] Although data on this regimen are scantier, it is considered acceptable.

Asymptomatic Amebiasis. The asymptomatic patient with *E. histolytica* organisms in the stool presents a controversial problem. Limited clinical studies, including one using colonoscopy, suggest that asymptomatic patients are not experiencing invasive disease and do not have more symptoms than do controls.[43, 44] More extensive data are available for the homosexual community, showing the apparent benignity of amebae in this group.[45] Epidemiologic studies using zymodeme analysis have shown a consistent relationship between certain zymodemes and the presence or absence of disease, as described earlier, and homosexuals and asymptomatic individuals almost always have nonpathogenic zymodemes.[5] Another group of patients has been reported, however, who have pathogenic zymodemes, are asymptomatic, and are distinguished from those with nonpathogenic zymodemes only by elevated serologic titers. These titers suggest that invasive disease is indeed present but at a subclinical level, or that invasive disease at some time in the past has resolved spontaneously.[46] These observations, along with the finding that zymodemes are subject to change under certain laboratory conditions,[47] thereby suggesting that under proper conditions they might change in the patient, have led to the recommendation that all patients with amebic infestation, even if asymptomatic, be treated.[6, 48] Other clinicians believe that asymptomatic patients, especially if homosexual (a group of patients among whom zymodeme analysis has shown a consistent nonpathogenic pattern), need not be treated.[45] This author believes that, considering the safety of drugs for this stage of disease, all cases should be treated with a luminal agent, iodoquinol, paromomycin, or diloxanide furoate, as noted above.

For the most reliable results, one should wait 4 weeks after treatment to obtain follow-up stool examinations.

Amebomas. The presence of amebomas should be treated as invasive disease, as discussed earlier, with metronidazole and iodoquinol being the preferred regimen.

Perforation. Especially with peritonitis, perforation should be treated also with intravenous metronidazole or intramuscular emetine or even both along with appropriate surgical measures and antibiotics. Adams and MacLeod[33] classify perforations into two types. The first type is a sudden perforation in a patient not already severely ill. This type may be treated by surgery, since the bowel is not severely diseased and can be handled. The second type progresses slowly in a patient with severe colitis and presents a difficult surgical problem since the bowel is often very fragile, and gross spillage may result from surgical manipulation.

Amebic Appendicitis. A rare condition, amebic appendicitis is almost never recognized before surgery and often not detected in routine pathologic examination.[49] Appendectomy together with treatment for invasive disease is recommended for this entity.

Prevention

Since amebiasis is acquired through practices allowing fecal-oral transmission, prevention is aimed at eliminating these activities. Proper disposal of excrement, proper sewage treatment or disposal, adequate water purification, identification and treatment of infected food handlers, and appropriate hand washing are all important measures. In areas of high transmission, vegetables should be cooked at least to boiling, and

all fruits should be peeled by the consumer before eating. Flies can probably transmit the infection and should be eliminated by the use of proper screening and insecticides.

Boiling water kills amebic cysts immediately. Water can also be safely treated with tetraglycine hydroperiodide tablets, such as Potable-Aqua, though this leaves a significant aftertaste. Other methods of water purification include addition of 5 drops of tincture of iodine to each quart of water and letting it stand 30 minutes, addition of a saturated iodine solution, and filtration through an iodine-resin filter. Cysts are relatively resistant to chlorine but can be destroyed by hyperchlorination.

Individuals engaged in oral-anal sexual activities should receive appropriate counseling and education. In high-risk populations such as male homosexuals, identification and treatment of carriers are sensible measures. Control of amebiasis in an institution such as a home for mentally retarded is difficult and may require varying combinations of treatment and casefinding.[50]

The use of medications for prophylaxis of amebic infection is not recommended. The risk of amebiasis in a reasonably prudent American traveler is low, being on the order of 1%, and the effectiveness of such an approach has not been established by proper trial.

Entamoeba polecki

Entamoeba polecki is an ameba found in the intestine of monkeys and pigs. It is seen infrequently in humans, though in Papua New Guinea it is reported to be common. The trophozoites resemble those of *E. histolytica* but are differentiated from them by having poor directional motility, a nuclear structure intermediate between that of *E. histolytica* and *E. coli,* and uninucleate cysts. Transmission is effected through the cyst stage. Most cases of *E. polecki* infection are asymptomatic, but diarrhea has been attributed to the parasite. Most drugs are ineffective, but diloxanide furoate (Furamide, available only from the Centers for Disease Control) in combination with metronidazole has proved effective.[51]

Dientamoeba fragilis

Organism and Epidemiology

Although *Dientamoeba fragilis* resembles an ameba, it contains flagellum-like structures and is classified with the trichomonads. Its complete life cycle and mode of transmission are unknown. In the human, it is found only as an ameboid organism, usually in a binucleate form considered to be an arrested telophase. Attempts to infect humans and monkeys with cultured organisms have failed. No cyst form has been identified. A related organism, *Histomonas meleagridis*, is transmitted to turkeys inside a nematode egg, raising the possibility that transmission to humans occurs in some similar way. *Dientamoeba fragilis* has been found to be more frequent than expected in populations with pinworm, and structures resembling dientamoebae have been seen in pinworm eggs, but direct transmission by this route has yet to be proved.[62]

Pathogenesis and Clinical Findings

The organisms of *D. fragilis* are found in the crypts and lumen of the colon. No invasive pathologic condition has been described. Many cases are asymptomatic, but many patients have diarrhea. In an individual case, it is hard to know whether symptoms relate to the parasite, though relief of symptoms with treatment is presumptive supporting evidence. Symptoms described include nonbloody diarrhea, abdominal cramps, bloating, flatulence, fatigue, nausea, and weight loss. In a few cases, small ulcerations have been seen on sigmoidoscopic examination, but usually no pathologic condition is visible.[53, 54]

Diagnosis and Treatment

The diagnosis of *D. fragilis* infection is made by finding the organism on stool examination. Stools preserved in PVA and stained with trichrome or iron hematoxylin give the best results. Routine blood count and laboratory findings are usually normal. Radiography is not helpful, and no serologic test exists. For treatment 650 mg of iodoquinol, given 3 times daily for 20 days, is usually successful. Other regimens include 500 mg of paromomycin, given 3 times daily for 5 to 7 days, and 250 mg of tetracycline given 4 times daily for 7 days.

Balantidium coli

Organism and Epidemiology

Balantidium coli is the only ciliated protozoan to parsitize humans. The organism is large and is seen in two size ranges: from 42 to 60 μm and from 90 to 120 μm in length. Conjugation always occurs between the small and large individuals. They are ciliated and have a funnel-shaped cytostome at one end and two nuclei. A cyst form exists that has a thick refractile wall.

The infection has been reported worldwide but is uncommon. It may occur in outbreaks and is seen most often where pigs and humans are in close contact. It has been found in a large variety of mammals. Transmission from pigs is presumed when there is appropriate contact and from other animals, especially rats, if no human-pig contact is present. Human-to-human transmission seems to be rare. The cyst is the infective form and is ingested through contaminated food or water. The cysts can live for weeks in moist stool. After excystation, the trophozoites invade the colonic wall or live in the lumen. Cyst formation occurs as the organisms are passed out.

Pathology and Clinical Findings

Invasion of the colon by *B. coli* organisms produces ulcerations of the mucosa, and one finds numerous trophozoites and much inflammatory response in the submucosa. The overall appearance of *B. coli* infection resembles that of amebic dysentery, though hourglass ulcerations are less common in balantidiasis (Fig. 10–5) than in amebic dysentery. Areas of intervening normal or only mildly inflamed mucosa may be seen. The cecum and sigmoid are the areas most common affected. The appendix may be affected.

The clinical picture may range from the asymptomatic state to fulminant dysentery, with varying stages in between. The majority of patients are asymptomatic or mildly symptomatic. The milder end of the spectrum may include chronic mild diarrhea with alternating constipation, cramps, mucus in the stool, and perhaps weight loss. More severe symptoms include blood or pus in the stool, nausea, weakness, and greater abdominal pain. Perforation and hemorrhage are rare complications. Symptoms may persist for years.[55, 56]

Diagnosis and Treatment

The diagnosis is made by finding the parasite in the stool. It is almost always present in the trophozoite form. Sigmoidoscopic examination may show ulcers as previously described. Treatment consists of 500 mg of tetracycline, given 4 times daily for 10 days,[56] or 650 mg of iodoquinol, given 3 times daily for 20 days. Metronidazole has been reported as effective[57] and only partly effective.[56]

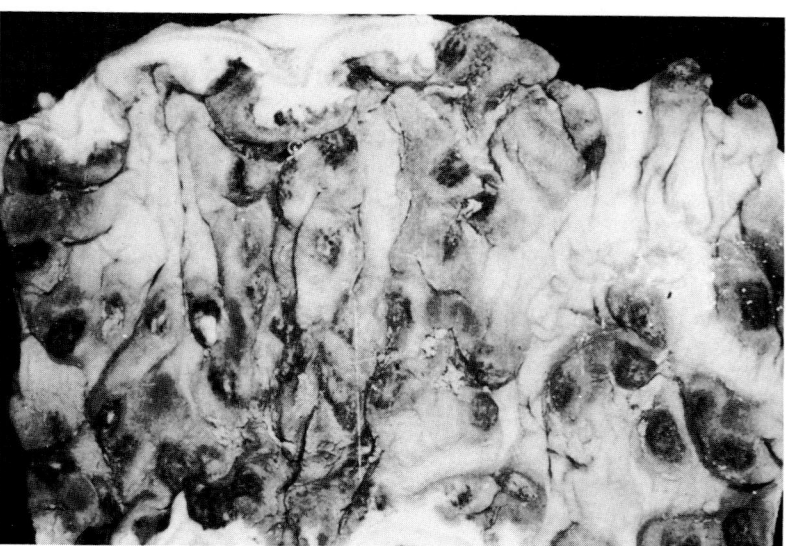

FIGURE 10–5.
Colon specimen showing ulcerations of *Balantidium coli*. SOURCE: Original slide by R. E. Kuntz, Laboratory of Parasitic Diseases, NIH, Bethesda, MD from A Pictorial Presentation of Parasites, edited by Herman Zaiman, Valley City, ND.

Miscellaneous Protozoa Found in Stool

Blastocystis hominis

The parasite *Blastocystis hominis*, formerly considered a harmless yeast, has more recently been said to be a protozoan. Its final classification is not yet settled. It is found fairly frequently in stool examinations, both in symptomatic and asymptomatic patients. Because of its detection in cases of diarrhea, it has been implicated by some as a causal agent. Patients with the parasite may also complain of flatulence, nausea, and bloating. No invasive disease has been described.

A 1991 review argues for considering *B. hominis* a pathogen.[58] Another review found no convincing evidence implicating *B. hominis* as a disease agent.[59] An investigation of asymptomatic cases with this parasite indicated that, when thoroughly investigated, almost all cases had another demonstrable cause for symptoms.[60] These data suggest that when faced with this parasite in a symptomatic patient, the clinician should look further for an etiology. If none can be found on repeated stool examination and other pertinent investigations, then treatment can be considered.

Metronidazole and iodoquinol have both been used against *B. hominis* infestation, but in this author's experience they are not always effective. No treatment trials have been published, and whether to treat this infection remains a controversial issue.

Other Intraluminal Protozoa

The following protozoa are frequently found on stool examination. They are considered nonpathogens and do not require treatment. If found in a symptomatic patient, another cause for the symptoms should be sought.

AMEBAE

Entamoeba hartmanni. This ameba is distinguished from *E. histolytica* only by its smaller size. Proper identification therefore requires examination by an experienced technician. The trophozoites are less than 12 μm, and the cysts less than 10 μm in diameter.

Entamoeba coli. This ameba, resembling, but distinguishable from *E. histolytica* is considered to be a nonpathogen.

Endolimax nana and Iodamoeba beutschlii. The organisms of these species are also considered nonpathogens.

FLAGELLATES

Chilomastix mesnili, Pentatrichomonas hominis, Enteromonas hominis,* and *Retortamonas intestinalis. These species are all nonpathogenic.

Cryptosporidiosis

Epidemiology and Life Cycle

Cryptosporidium is a genus of coccidian protozoa related to the other coccidia found in humans, including *Isospora belli, Toxoplasma gondii,* and *Sarcocystis* species. Taxonomy is uncertain because cross transmission experiments indicate a lack of host specificity. Apparently, two species affect mammals and are distinguishable by a difference in size, *C. parvum* being the smaller and *C. muris* the larger of the two. The former is thought to be a cause of diarrhea in humans and cattle, and the latter is found in the stomach of mammals.[61] Caution has been expressed about this classification, however, indicating that work on taxonomy of *Cryptosporidium* is not yet complete.[62] Cryptosporidia are found worldwide. The parasite is found in a wide range of animals, including birds, reptiles, fish, and mammals. Prior to 1981, the parasite was recognized as a cause of diarrhea in calves, goats, lambs, turkeys, and several other mammals, but infections in humans were considered rare and almost entirely confined to immunocompromised patients. After 1981, however, the infection received great attention when it was recognized that cryptosporidia are important pathogens in patients with acquired immunodeficiency syndrome (AIDS). The infection is acquired in a variety of ways. It may be acquired through contaminated water and presumably through contaminated food.[63] It can, however, be acquired directly from farm animals[61, 64] and perhaps most often by human-to-human transmission via the fecal-oral route. Outbreaks of cryptosporidiosis in day care centers and families[65] and acquisition by health-care workers[66] are examples of human-to-human transmission. Transmission in the homosexual community by the fecal-oral route is common. In one case, transmission by fomites was suspected.[63] Cryptosporidia have been found in river water and sewage and have been responsible for waterborne outbreaks.[67] They are a cause of gastroenteritis in children in developing countries and a recognized cause of traveler's diarrhea.[68] The parasite is unaffected by chlorination, 5% solution of formalin, aldehyde-based disinfectants, and 3% hypochlorite, but it can be killed by freezing, boiling, concentrated bleach, and 10% formalin.[61] The minimal infective load of cryptosporidia is not established but is believed to be small, probably less than 1000 cysts.[61]

Infection occurs with ingestion of the infective oocyst, which is 2 to 8 µm in diameter. Upon excystation, sporozoites emerge, penetrate epithelial cells of the small or large bowel, and develop into trophozoites. The trophozoites divide asexually by merogony, releasing into the lumen 6 to 8 meronts that reinvade other epithelial cells and repeat merogony. Other meronts develop intracellularly into micro- and macrogametocytes. Fertilized macro-

gametes develop into oocysts to complete the cycle. Oocysts may reinfect the same host or may be passed out to infect another host (Fig. 10–6).

Pathology

Most of our knowledge of the pathologic consequences of cryptosporidiosis comes from the study of patients with AIDS. In these patients, the parasite can be found throughout the intestinal tract from the mouth to the anus. The small and large bowel appear to be the sites most commonly involved, and which of these sites is preferentially involved is not yet clear. The developing forms of the parasite are small, being 2 to 5 µm, and are attached to the brush border (Fig. 10–7). They lie under the plasma membrane but are considered extracytoplasmic since they reside within a parasitophorous vacuole.[62] In addition, one sees blunting of the villi, infiltration of inflammatory cells into the lamina propria, and elongation of crypts.[69, 70] The few immunocompetent patients who have been studied have similar findings. In one case of AIDS, cryptosporidia were seen within the patient's blood vessels in the colonic wall, suggesting intravascular transport as a possible mechanism for spread to other parts of the body.[71] In AIDS patients, the parasite may also be found in the gallbladder and various levels of the respiratory tree. Varying degrees of malabsorption and excessive fluid loss may occur in the immunocompromised host. See also Chapters 17 and 25.

Clinical Findings

The incubation period of cryptosporidiosis varies between 2 and 14 days. In the immunocompetent host, the disease starts suddenly with diarrhea, cramps, and watery stool without blood. Low grade fever, nausea, vomiting, abdominal discomfort, and headache may also be present. A summary of many case reports indicates that the syndrome generally lasts 3 to 20 days, with diarrhea almost always being the most prominent complaint.[61] Longer duration is not uncommon, however. In one series, the median period of diarrhea was 15 days, with 75% of patients having diarrhea for 32 days.[72] Occasionally, patients may have a prolonged course, in one case lasting 4 months.[73, 74] Malnutrition in children can lead to prolongation of diarrhea.[75] A small percentage of patients require hospitalization. Oocysts may be shed for up to 50 days (mean: 12–14 d) after exposure, with the occasional patient showing a positive stool examina-

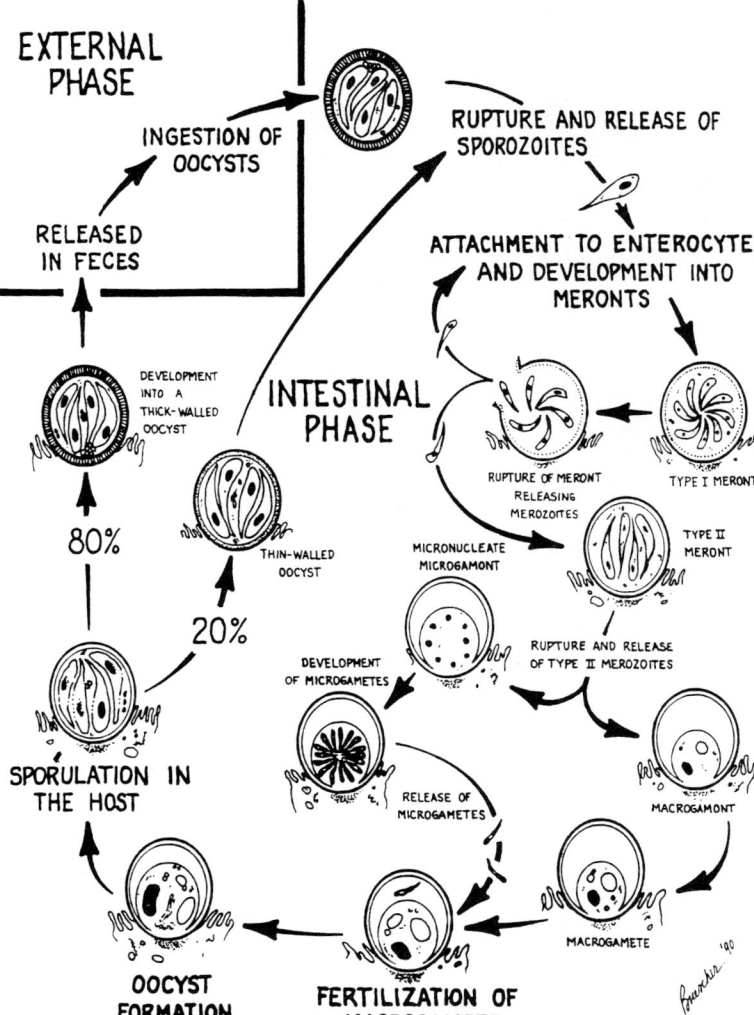

EXTERNAL PHASE

INGESTION OF OOCYSTS

RELEASED IN FECES

RUPTURE AND RELEASE OF SPOROZOITES

ATTACHMENT TO ENTEROCYTE AND DEVELOPMENT INTO MERONTS

DEVELOPMENT INTO A THICK-WALLED OOCYST

INTESTINAL PHASE

RUPTURE OF MERONT RELEASING MEROZOITES

TYPE I MERONT

80%

THIN-WALLED OOCYST

MICRONUCLEATE MICROGAMONT

TYPE II MERONT

20%

DEVELOPMENT OF MICROGAMETES

RUPTURE AND RELEASE OF TYPE II MEROZOITES

SPORULATION IN THE HOST

RELEASE OF MICROGAMETES

MACROGAMONT

OOCYST FORMATION

FERTILIZATION OF MACROGAMETE

MACROGAMETE

FIGURE 10–6.
Life cycle of *Cryptosporidium.* SOURCE: O'Ryan ML, Owen RL, Pickering LK. Cryptosporidiosis, isosporiasis and microsporidiosis. In Textbook of Pediatric Infectious Diseases. Feigin RD, Cherry JD, eds. 3rd ed. Philadelphia: WB Saunders; 1992:1941.

tion even later, after a period of negative findings in stools.[76] A chronic carrier state and documented reinfection have not been found in an immunocompetent host.

In patients with AIDS or other immunocompromising disorders, the diarrhea may be prolonged and severe, leading sometimes to severe weight loss, dehydration, electrolyte imbalance, and death. The exact cause of this profuse diarrhea is not known. Asymptomatic infection and spontaneous recovery may also occur in patients with AIDS, a fact underscoring the need for controlled studies in evaluating therapies.

The blood count is usually normal. Stool examination usually shows no blood or inflammatory cells. Malabsorption of fat, vitamin B12, and D-xylose have all been shown in patients with the chronic diarrhea syndrome. Radiographic studies in chronic cases may show motility abnormalities and flocculation consistent with malabsorption.

Diagnosis and Treatment

The diagnosis of cryptosporidiosis in both immunocompetent and immunocompromised patients is made by stool examination. The usual method is to use a modified acid-fast stain, which will color the organisms red and allow them to be identified quickly (Fig. 10–8). Not all cysts take up the stain, but the technique is reliable.[77, 78] In the case of negative findings, at least 2 stools should be examined before ruling out the diagnosis. Concentration techniques, such as Sheather's sucrose flotation, are sensitive but more laborious and not generally necessary.[69] Recently, monoclonal antibodies have been used to detect oocysts.[79] Antibodies can be detected in sera of patients by various means. Serologic tests are not helpful clinically but can be useful epidemiologic tools.

No therapy for cryptosporidiosis is known to be effective.[80] In an immunocompetent host, the infection is self-limiting, and no therapy

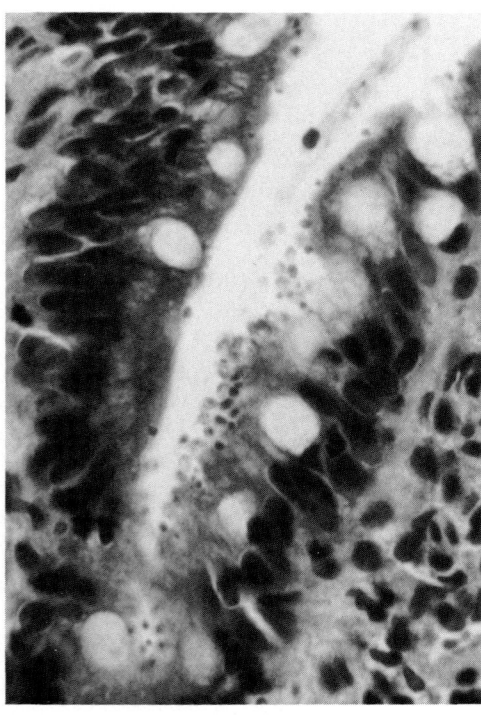

FIGURE 10–7.
Biopsy of colon, showing numerous cryptosporidia attached to epithelial cells on luminal surface. SOURCE: Courtesy of John H. Cross, PhD. Dept Preventive Medicine and Biometrics, Uniformed Services University of the Health Sciences, Bethesda MD.

other than adequate fluid replacement and symptomatic relief is needed. In AIDS patients who have persistent and severe diarrhea, the three main approaches to treatment are the use of pharmacologic agents, the use of immunomodulating agents, and supportive therapy. Initial reports of the success of spiramycin[81] were put into perspective by a placebo-controlled trial that failed to show any efficacy.[80] A similar study in infants reached the same conclusion.[82] Over 90 agents have been tried in the treatment and prevention of this disease with no clear success.[62] Diclazuril, a benzene acetonitrile derivative that is active against the related *Eimeria* species found in animals, was not effective in a small trial.[83]

Manipulation of the immune status of the patient has received attention. In cases of malnutrition, steroid usage, chemotherapy, and other immunosuppressive regimens correction or adjustment of the agents responsible for the poor immune status is indicated. Proper nutrition, reduction of steroid dosage, and temporary cessation of chemotherapy are all measures that may help the host shed this infection.[62] In AIDS patients, attempts have been made to improve local gut immunity by ingestion of antibody- or cell-containing substances. Hyperimmune bovine colostrum has given mixed results,[84, 85] and a single case report of the use of human serum immunoglobulin suggested its efficacy.[86] A double-blind crossover study of the use of transfer factor from lymphocytes of immunized and nonimmunized cows given to AIDS patients has suggested its efficacy.[87] All of these forms of treatment require further trial.

Supportive measures remain the most important ones for immunocompromised patients with chronic diarrhea. The stool volume can be enormous, with up to 17 liters daily being reported. Fluid and electrolyte replacement is essential and may be difficult to accomplish. The various antimotility drugs, such as opiates, loperamide, and diphenoxylate, may be helpful.

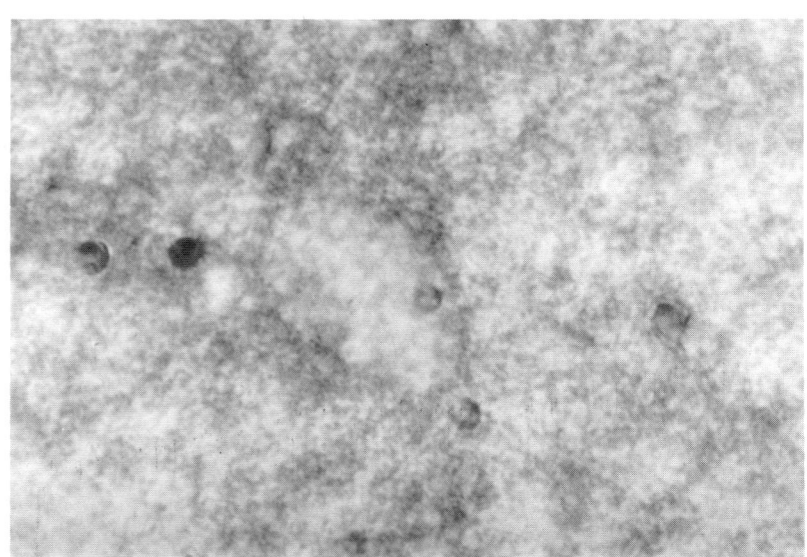

FIGURE 10–8.
Stool sample stained with modified acid-fast method, showing round cryptosporidial oocysts. SOURCE: Courtesy of John H. Cross PhD. Dept Preventive Medicine and Biometrics, Uniformed Services University of the Health Sciences, Bethesda MD. [See also Color Plate 3]

They need to be used on a trial-and-error basis. The somatostatin analog octreotide has been helpful in some cases.[88]

Prevention

Prevention of cryptosporidiosis is achieved by careful hand washing, pasteurizing or boiling water for drinking, and, in regions with poor sanitation, avoiding uncooked vegetables. Iodination and chlorination of water are not effective. Oral-anal contact should be avoided. In the hospital setting, since, as noted earlier, many disinfectants do not kill the organism, reliance must be placed on heat or gas sterilization and proper enteric and body fluid precautions. A difficult and unresolved area is the proper method for disinfecting flexible sigmoidoscopes and colonoscopes. Transmission by these instruments seems not to have been reported, but the potential for transmission by this means certainly exists. These instruments can be damaged by excessive heat and may be damaged by certain chemicals. The Centers for Disease Control has issued guidelines on this subject. Endoscopes are classified as semicritical in reference to the degree of risk of their transmitting infection. Such items should receive high-level disinfection between use on patients, including careful cleansing and wiping followed by either gas sterilization or soaking for a specified period in one of various disinfecting solutions.[89] In England, mechanical cleansing followed by immersion for 1 hour in 2% glutaraldehyde is recommended before and after use on immunocompromised patients, although the activity of the glutaraldehyde against cryptosporidia is not clear (it has been found ineffective when used for 30 minutes.)[90, 91] These or similar procedures seem reasonable for ordinary use, but gas sterilization after, and possibly before, use should be considered for immunocompromised patients.

Chagas' Disease

Organism and Epidemiology

Although we are concerned here with Chagas' disease only as it pertains to the colon, a brief review of the responsible organism and its epidemiology is useful. Chagas' disease is caused by *Trypanosoma cruzi*. The organism is found throughout Central and South America and parts of the southern United States. It parasitizes over 100 species of mammals, including domestic animals, rodents, and humans. It is transmitted by the bite of triatomid bugs. The three species responsible for most transmissions of *T. cruzi* are *Triatoma infestans*, *Panstrongylus megistus*, and *Rhodnius prolixus*. The bugs prefer to inhabit mud huts with cracked walls and thatched roofs. It follows that the infection is most common among the poorer classes, who inhabit such dwellings. Since the disease is a zoonosis, domestic animals and rodents in and near homes also play a role in bringing the infection to humans. Transmission may also occur by blood transfusion, a common event in Brazil, and congenitally. Clinically apparent Chagas' disease is most common in South America, diminishing in frequency as one moves northward. It is very rare in the United States. This geographic pattern probably results from differences in parasite strain, distribution of triatomid bugs, and standard of living. Zymodeme and DNA analyses are giving new insight into strain differences.

The life cycle of *T. cruzi* involves a reproductive phase in the host as well as in the insect vector. The flagellate form circulating in the blood is termed a trypomastigote. It is 15 to 20 μm in length and has a posterior kinetoplast. It is able to invade a variety of cells, where the organisms round up to form small (3 μm) amastigotes. These amastigotes multiply by binary fission, enlarging the cell and leading to rupture. The new circulating trypomastigotes then invade other cells, leading to a repetitive cycle. When patients infected with *T. cruzi* are bitten by a triatomid bug, trypomastigotes are aspirated and transformed in the insect gut into epimastigotes, flagellate forms with an anterior kinetoplast. The epimastigotes multiply by binary fission, then migrate to the hind gut where, changed to metacyclic trypomastigotes similar to them in appearance, they are excreted in the feces. This form is infective, and the host is infected by rubbing the triatomid bite, thus assisting the penetration of the metacyclic trypomastigotes through the skin. The organism then becomes the trypomastigote and the cycle is completed.

Pathogenesis and Pathology

At the site of penetration of the *T. cruzi* organism an inflammatory reaction often occurs, with invasion of local macrophage, muscle, and fat cells—the area being surrounded by inflammatory cells. This reaction is known as Romaña's sign (unilateral palpebral and periorbital edema) if the organisms are rubbed into the conjunctiva, or as a chagoma (an erythematous indurated area with local crust formation), if a small break in the skin is infected. The organisms migrate to local lymph nodes, reproduce intra-cellularly, and circulate through the body. They may invade almost any cell but preferentially parasitize cardiac and smooth muscle cells, neuroglia cells, and cells of the reticuloendothelial system. A chronic meningeal infection also occurs. This invasive and proliferative stage of parasite invasion is seen in the acute phase of Chagas' disease.

After a latent period that often lasts 10 or more years, a relatively small proportion of patients develop signs of chronic Chagas' disease: cardiomyopathy, megaesophagus, and megacolon. Pathologic examination of the colon shows a depletion of neuronal cells of Auerbach's plexus, with some fibrous tissue replacing this plexus, focal inflammatory lesions in the muscular layer, and hypertrophy of the muscular layer.[92, 93] The exact mechanism of the neuronal depletion is not settled. Direct invasion of neuronal cells does occur but is not thought to be extensive enough to account for such a profound loss. Autoantibodies against neurons and Schwann's cells, as well as cardiac muscle cells, have been demonstrated, and a form of auto-immunity may be operative.[94] Release of a toxic substance from the demonstrated local inflammatory sites in the adjacent muscle layer has also been postulated to explain this.[92, 93] At any rate, the result is a relatively denervated colon, particularly in the sigmoid and rectal areas. The muscle cells have an increased sensitivity to cholinergic drugs. The loss of Auerbach's plexus results in a dyskinetic rectum, which does not assist in propulsion of stool. Stasis of fecal material, subsequent dilatation of colon proximal to the rectum, and hypertrophy of the muscular layer occur. Similar changes are seen in the esophagus. These conditions lead, after a long latent period, to the megasyndromes of megacolon and megaesophagus.

Clinical Findings, Diagnosis, and Treatment

The pathogenesis just described suggests a separation of the clinical picture into three phases. In phase one, the chagomas and Romãna's sign are seen. In addition, many patients have a febrile course, with lymphadenopathy, splenomegaly, and often meningeal signs. This phase lasts up to 3 months. Approximately 10% of patients are asymptomatic throughout this phase. Next, the patient's disease enters a silent phase, during which no clinical illness is evident but the organism is quietly invading cardiac and bowel neuroglial cells. Years later, the patient may evidence a cardiomyopathy, megaesophagus, megacolon, or some combination of these.

Patients with colonic involvement complain of constipation, abdominal distention, and some degree of pain. Often, however, complaints are relatively few in spite of the enormous dilation and elongation of the colon that may exist. The colon can reach immense proportions, with a length of over 2 meters and a capacity of 30 to 40 liters.[93] Often one of the complications of megacolon brings the patient in: these include fecal impaction related to fecaloma, volvulus of the dilated sigmoid, or perforation related to ulceration at the site of fecaloma or severe torsion.[95]

The diagnosis of chagasic megacolon is made by noting the combination of enlarged colon, geographic origin of the patient, presence of other stigmata of the disease such as megaesophagus or cardiomyopathy, and a positive serologic test. Flat plate radiography of the abdomen shows the hugely dilated bowel, and the atonicity is evident on barium enema. Although the entire bowel is usually affected, the rectum is more severely involved. The amastigotes can be seen on histologic section of removed bowel wall but are usually scarce and hard to find.

If the symptoms and lack of bowel tonicity are not too severe, the patient may be treated with high fiber diet, stool softeners, and laxatives, as needed. In more severe cases the treatment is surgical. A number of procedures have been tried, with varying degrees of success. Simple partial or total colectomy with anastomosis to the remaining rectum results in dilation of the bowel above the rectum, emphasizing the important role played by the dyskinetic rectum. Operations favored today are the abdominoperineal endoanal pull-through resection with delayed colorectal anastomosis, and the Duhamel-Haddad operation. Both of these procedures depend on pulling the colon through the anus and making an anastomosis of less dilated colon to rectum just above the sphincter.[95] Drug treatment directed against the parasite is not helpful in the chronic stage. Of use only during the acute stage, nifurtimox and benznidazole are effective.

HELMINTHIC INFECTION: NEMATODES

Although a large number of helminths may infest the human intestinal tract, only a few cause pathologic conditions in the large bowel. Those of interest in this regard are known as nematodes, or round worms, and trematodes, or flukes. The nematodes causing disease of the colon and rectum are *Trichuris trichiura, Entero-bius vermicularis,* and *Stronglyoides stercoralis,* and the only trematodes are the *Schistosoma* species. Many other familiar worms, such as *Ascaris,* or hookworm, *Trichostrongylus, Clonorchis, Opisthorchis, Fasciola hepatica* and *Fasciolopsis buski,* may be diagnosed by examination of stool for ova, but they do not cause pathologic conditions of the large bowel.

Trichuris trichiura

Trichuris trichiura is a nematode that almost exclusively infests the large bowel, causing a condition known as trichuriasis. The parasite is most common in geographic areas with warm moist climates, particularly where poor sanitation is prevalent.

Life Cycle and Pathogenesis

The adult worms reside in the large intestine, though in heavy infections some may be found in the terminal ileum and the appendix. The worms have a whiplike shape with a "handle" at the posterior end and a head at the tapering anterior end. Their length ranges from 30 to 50 mm. The worms' heads are embedded in the mucosal layer of the intestine, where they obtain nutrition by sucking nutrients from the mucosal cells.

These worms produce eggs that are characteristically barrel-shaped, with a mucoid plug at each end. They are passed in the stool, and after a development period of 10 to 20 days in warm moist soil, they become infective. When reingested via contaminated food or water, they pass through the stomach and into the intestine, where the eggs hatch. The larvae attach to the small bowel temporarily while undergoing growth, then pass to the colon, where the slender head embeds itself into the crypts. The adults mate there, and the females eventually produce from 3000 to 7000 eggs daily. Three to 4 months elapse between egg ingestion and the appearance of new eggs.

Because the anterior end of the worm is embedded in the mucosal layer, secondary irritability and local inflammation in the bowel occur. In light infections, these symptoms are mild, but in heavy infections, considerable irritability, edema, and some degree of blood loss may ensue, and, in severe cases, rectal prolapse.

Clinical Findings and Diagnosis

Patients with light infections of *T. trichiura* generally do not have any symptoms. With a heavier infection, patients have varying degrees of diarrhea; some blood loss is possible, though not severe hemorrhage. Rectal prolapse occurs in heavy infections and is seen primarily in children. Continued diarrhea may lead to cachexia and protein loss.[96]

Diagnosis is generally accomplished by finding the typical barrel-shaped eggs in stool samples, either by direct smear or by one of several concentration techniques. In the case of rectal prolapse or during sigmoidoscopic examination, the worms may be visualized directly (Fig. 10–9). Sigmoidoscopic examination may also reveal edema and inflammatory changes. If the stool sample shows only a few eggs, the infection is probably light enough not to cause significant symptoms, and in such a case, significant diarrhea or other complaints should prompt investigation for other causes. Eosinophilia is not a feature of the infection.

Treatment and Prevention

The infection is best treated with 100 mg of mebendazole, given 2 times a day for 3 days. A cure rate of approximately 80% may be expected with this treatment, with a considerable reduction in worm load in those who are not totally cured.[97, 98]

The key to prevention lies in interrupting the fecal-oral transmission cycle. The provision of sufficient facilities for the deposition of human excreta and the education of the population are important measures. The avoidance of foods

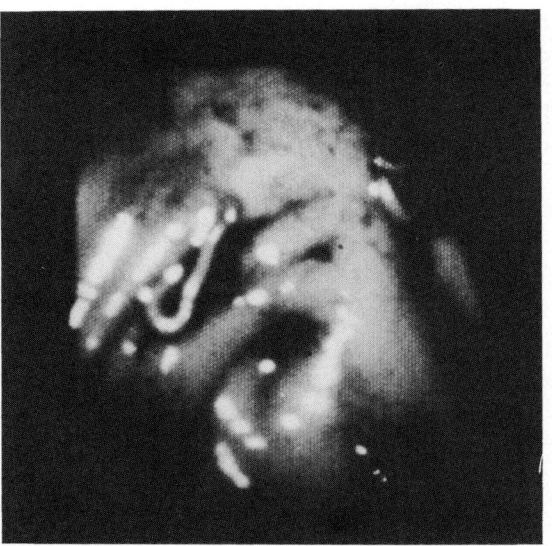

FIGURE 10–9.
A *Trichuris trichiura* worm as seen through the sigmoidoscope.

that may be contaminated, such as uncooked vegetables, lettuce, and the like and the proper preparation of these foods are effective. Eggs must incubate in soil before they become infective, and therefore direct person-to-person transmission does not occur.

Enterobius vermicularis

The disorder, known as pinworm, is due to infection by *Enterobius vermicularis*. It is primarily a disease of children, but adults may be afflicted. It has worldwide distribution, is more frequent in temperate and cold climates than in tropical areas, and affects all socioeconomic levels.

Life Cycle and Pathogeneis

The adult worms live in the cecum, appendix, and ascending colon but do not penetrate the mucosa. They are thin, white, curly and have tapered ends; the males measure from 2 to 5 mm and the females from 8 to 13 mm. The adults mate in the cecum, and the gravid female migrates down and out of the anus. The eggs are laid on the perianal skin or may be shed in large numbers if the worm dies and ruptures. The female dies and does not reenter the bowel. If the patient scratches, the eggs are lodged under the fingernails and may either be passed to another person or reintroduced into the patient's mouth, a process termed autoinfection. Eggs may survive 2 or more weeks outside the body under the favorable circumstance of humid and cool weather, may be passed through contaminated bedding and clothing, and may even be airborne. The eggs are then swallowed by the same or a different host and hatch in the intestine, and the emerging larvae migrate directly to the colon, where they mature about a month to 6 weeks after ingestion.

Clinical Findings and Diagnosis

The ova cause irritation and itching, leading to anal pruritus, the main symptom of this disease. Continued scratching in this region can lead to excoriation and weeping. The majority of patients, however, have no symptoms at all. In female children the worms may lay eggs on the vulva, producing vulvar itching and a vulvovaginitis. The worms may be found in the appendix but do not appear to be a cause of appendicitis. In rare cases, the adults may migrate to the cervix, uterus, fallopian tubes, and even the peritoneum. In the last-named case, abdom-

inal pain may be a complaint. Also in rare cases, the worms penetrate the intestine, leading to peritoneal signs, and penetrating worms may form granulomata in the anal canal.[99, 100]

The diagnosis should be suspected in patients, especially children, with anal pruritus. Conventional stool examination for ova frequently misses the diagnosis. The best method of demonstrating the eggs is by applying clear cellophane tape to the perianum, then placing it sticky side down on a microscope slide and examining it under low power for the eggs. The best time to apply the tape is early in the morning before the patient has bathed or defecated. Commercial kits are available that enable the patient to accomplish this maneuver at home. The eggs are oval, with one side flattened. They have a translucent shell, inside of which one can see the embryo, often moving. Three cellophane tape tests are sufficient for diagnosis in more than 90% of *Enterobius* infections. Also, worms are often seen directly emerging from the anus by a parent or physician. If observed at home, the worm should be collected and placed in 70% alcohol and brought in for identification. The patient's blood count is not affected unless the peritoneum is involved, in which case, changes suggestive of inflammation may be seen.

Treatment and Prevention

Asymptomatic patients need not be treated, and opinions vary on how aggressive a physician should be with patients with few or no symptoms. If the patient can be taught sufficient appropriate hygiene so as to eliminate autoinfection, the infection is self-limiting. Since appropriate drugs are quite safe, however, treatment is generally recommended. In a family setting, all members of the family are customarily treated empirically. Instruction on hygiene, especially hand washing, is important, and sheets and underwear should be washed during and immediately after treatment. A standard washing machine cycle kills the eggs.

Effective drugs for the treatment of *E. vermicularis* infection are pyrantel pamoate, given in a single dose of 11 mg/kg (to a maximum 1 g)[101] and a single dose of 100 mg of mebendazole given orally.[102] Pyrantel pamoate is ineffective against worms in the early stages of development and sometimes causes vomiting or diarrhea. Mebendazole appears to be one of the easiest treatments, with rare side effects, though it is still not recommended in patients less than 2 years of age. Pyrvinium pamoate, previously widely used, is no longer marketed in the

United States. It is frequently recommended that patients be retreated in approximately 2 weeks to eradicate worms being ingested at the time of initial treatment.

The eggs are relatively hardy, surviving up to 15 days outside the body, and can be found on skin, under fingernails, and on clothing, sheets, doorknobs, and other objects. Some are even airborne. Therefore, the key to prevention is appropriate hygienic behavior, including meticulous hand washing before eating and after defecation. Proper cutting and cleansing of fingernails, washing of affected clothing and bedding, and vacuuming in affected children's rooms all help to prevent spread within households. Families with small children are often faced with reintroduction of the parasite in spite of efforts to the contrary.

Strongyloides stercoralis

Strongyloidiasis is caused by the nematode *Strongyloides stercoralis*. This worm, in the adult form, lives in the small bowel, but through autoinfection affects the large bowel, especially in heavy infections. The parasite is found in patients of all ages, and it is more common in areas of poor sanitation but may be found throughout the world. In temperate climates, it has some predilection for institutional settings, such as mental hospitals.

Life Cycle and Pathogenesis

The life cycle of *S. stercoralis* nematodes is presented in detail in Chapter 7; only a brief outline is presented here. The adult female lives burrowed in the mucosal epithelium of the upper small bowel, where eggs are laid and hatch. The larvae, in their initial, noninfective stages known as rhabditiform larvae, transform, as a result of unknown stimuli, into infective, or filariform larvae. The filariform larvae penetrate the bowel at any part, including ileum, colon, or rectum, in a process of internal autoinfection or may penetrate the skin in the perianal area. The untransformed rhabditiform larvae pass outside in stool to complete another developmental cycle outside the body, also resulting in filariform larvae that penetrate the skin. After penetration, larvae travel via the bloodstream to the lungs, up the bronchial tree and trachea, molting en route, eventually to be swallowed. They then enter the jejunum, where they mature into female adults and renew the cycle. The penetration of the large bowel is the center of interest in this chapter.

Pathology and Clinical Findings

The pathologic condition of the large bowel in strongyloidiasis derives from autoinfection by filariform larvae. The severity and extent of the pathologic condition depend in part on the immune state of the host. Primarily, conditions that impair cellular immunoresponses predispose to syndromes of overwhelming invasive strongyloidiasis. These conditions include malnutrition, steroid administration, leukemias, lymphomas, and organ transplantation. Patients with AIDS have been described with invasive strongyloidiasis but only in small numbers. Patients with these immunodeficiencies have greater numbers of autoinfecting larvae, reduced immunoresponse, and, consequently, greater degrees of tissue invasion.

In the host with no immunodeficiency, relatively little reaction may occur at sites of larval penetration, and the filariform larvae in such a patient are seen in the colon wall almost without cellular response. Edema of the mucosal layer may be present. One may also see granulomata, however, usually with eosinophils, and sometimes focal necrosis and eosinophilic abscesses.[103, 104] These conditions are presumably responses to dead or dying larvae. Most larval penetration occurs in the cecum, appendix, and transverse colon. Areas of apparent intense penetration seen histologically coexist with nearby areas that are free of larvae.[105] In heavy infections, seen most frequently in immunocompromised patients but occasionally in apparently intact hosts, edema, hyperemia, and scattered ulcerations of the bowel may occur.[106] Granulomata are less well developed, and Langhans's giant cells, rare. The extreme end of the spectrum is characterized by diffuse ulceration, hemorrhage, and pronounced bowel wall edema. Also in heavy infections one may see gravid female worms nestled in the mucosal layer as low as the colon. Chronic fibrotic changes, leading to loss of haustral markings, may occur. The appendix is a frequent site of larval penetration, but clinical appendicitis is rare.[107] For further discussion, see Chapter 7.

Clinically, most patients with strongyloidiasis are asymptomatic. When symptoms are present they generally suggest small bowel rather than colon disease. Symptoms of mild infection include epigastric pain, dyspepsia, bloating, and diarrhea. Patients with heavier infections have more accentuated symptoms. As mentioned, clinical appendicitis is rare. Unless rectal bleeding occurs, it is hard to point to symptoms that are specifically colonic in origin.

The immunocompromised patient with invasive disease may have severe diarrhea, malabsorption, hemorrhage, fever, sepsis, evidence of pulmonary involvement, and meningitis.[108] Invasion of the large bowel undoubtedly contributes to this picture, but characteristic clinical features are seldom found.

Diagnosis and Treatment

The diagnosis of strongyloidiasis should be suspected in any patient with unexplained eosinophilia, particularly if the patient's history includes living in areas of poor sanitation. Intestinal complaints should increase suspicion. In immunocompromised patients, abdominal complaints or unexplained fever, pulmonary infiltrates, or meningitis might suggest the diagnosis. Stool examination is the most direct way to find the parasite. In normal hosts, examination of 3 stools by routine methods leads to the diagnosis approximately 75% of cases. Since the eggs hatch in the intestine, larvae are seen in the stool. The yield of identifiable organisms is improved by using the Baermann technique, a method that extracts larvae from stool using wet gauze and warm water.[109] The yield may also be improved by the use of the Entero-test and with small bowel intubation and biopsy (see Chapter 7).

With particular reference to identifying involvement of the colon, barium enema is usually normal, but may show irritability and sometimes ulcerations and decreased haustral markings, suggestive of chronic ulcerative colitis.[110, 111] A somewhat tubular-looking left colon has been described. Sigmoidoscopy and colonoscopy have been useful in making the diagnosis. With these methods one can see erythema, ulcerations, hemorrhage, and, rarely, polyps.[103, 112–114] Biopsy may show the larvae themselves or only eosinophilic granulomata and inflammatory tissue. Larvae are more concentrated in the proximal colon, and the yield of larvae on biopsy is presumably higher from that area. No data are available to evaluate whether this approach is as good as small bowel intubation and biopsy for diagnosis.

Marked peripheral eosinophilia is a common finding, though it may be absent in cases of overwhelming infection and is sometimes absent in otherwise normal hosts. Serologic tests are helpful. The Centers for Disease Control currently performs an ELISA test, which overall is approximately 85 to 90% sensitive.[115, 116] Immunocompromised patients tend to have lower positivity rates, but the sensitivity in normal hosts exceeds 90%. False-positive results can occur in cases of bancroftian filariasis and tropical eosinophilia. Use of *S. stercoralis* larvae as antigen gives optimal sensitivity and specificity. The test is also available through commercial laboratories.

Treatment of this infection is recommended. The infection is long-lasting owing to autoinfection, and severe disease is a potential risk if the patient is treated with steroids or becomes otherwise immunocompromised. Thiabendazole is the drug of choice, with albendazole and ivermectin being alternative choices, though more difficult to obtain. For details of treatment and prevention see Chapter 7.

Angiostrongylus costaricensis

Life Cycle and Pathogenesis

This nematode is found in Central and South America from Mexico to Argentina, and a case has been reported from Africa. Whether it is transmitted in the United States is not certain, but rats infected with the parasite have been found. The adult worms are small and slender, the male measuring approximately 20 mm long and the female, 33 mm. In the rat, they live in the mesenteric arterioles in the region of the terminal ileum and the ascending colon. There the female lays eggs, which are carried into the intestinal wall where they hatch. The first-stage larvae penetrate the lumen and are passed out into the stool. They are ingested by slugs and molt twice in the slug to form third-stage larvae, the infective form. The infective larvae are ingested by rats or humans who eat a slug or ingest its larvae-containing slime that has been deposited on vegetables. The ingested larvae penetrate the intestine and travel to the lymphatics and thence to the mesenteric arterioles by penetration of the vessel walls. In the rat, the cycle then proceeds as described above, but in the human, the eggs degenerate in the intestinal wall and incite a granulomatous reaction.

Pathologically, the findings are usually in the cecum, appendix, and terminal ileum. Yellow granulations of the subserosa and edema and rigidity of the intestinal wall are the most common findings. The appendix is often inflamed and may be perforated. The worms in the arterioles cause local vasculitis, which may lead to small areas of infarction. Perforation can occur. Microscopically, one sees granulomata and eosinophilic inflammatory tissue in the bowel wall, edema, and, of course, eggs and larvae. Vessel thrombosis and areas of infarction may be seen. The transverse or descending colon is occasionally involved, and worms may also be found in the liver, abdominal lymph nodes, and testes.[117] The worms may obstruct arteries in the spermatic cord.

Clinical Findings and Diagnosis

Children rather than adults are chiefly affected by this disease, especially those of school and preschool age. Right lower quadrant pain and fever are the main symptoms, but nausea, vomiting, and either diarrhea or constipation may occur. On physical examination, the abdomen is tender, usually in the right lower quadrant, and signs of peritonitis are often present. A mass may be palpated, which corresponds to the edematous bowel. Rectal examination may be painful. The resemblance of the clinical picture to appendicitis is evident. Laboratory study shows the white blood cell count to be generally in the 15,000 to 50,000 range, usually with significant eosinophilia (11–61%). If radiologic examination is carried out, it usually shows changes relating to edema and spasm confined to the area of the terminal ileum, cecum, and ascending colon.[118]

The diagnosis is often made at surgery. The combination of abdominal pain, right lower quadrant mass, and high eosinophil count in a child with an appropriate geographic history is, however, certainly suggestive of *A. costaricensis* infection. Serologic tests are available in some areas. Eggs and larvae are not found in the stool.

Treatment and Prevention

The treatment of infection by *A. costaricensis* is often surgical. In some cases, surgery is performed because of the concern over appendicitis but may be necessary in this infection because necrosis or perforation may occur. Thiabendazole and diethylcarbamazine have been used in treatment but have not been subjected to proper trial, and their efficacy is not known. In rats, the drugs appear to excite the worms rather than to kill them, and it is probably best to avoid drug therapy until further study is carried out.

The disease can be prevented by not eating uncooked vegetables and, of course, avoiding the ingestion of slugs. The parasite is not transmitted directly from rats to humans.

HELMINTHIC INFECTION: TREMATODES

Schistosoma Species

Schistosomiasis, one of the world's most prevalent diseases, is estimated to afflict about 200 million people. The genus *Schistosoma* differs from other trematodes in having no cystic metacercarial form: the adults live in blood vessels, and the eggs are not operculated. Three different species of the *Schistosoma* trematode cause the vast majority of human infections: *S. haematobium, japonicum,* and *mansoni.* To some degree, the organisms of all three may involve the large bowel, although those of *S. mansoni* are the major culprits. Other *Schistosoma* that less commonly infect man are *S. mekongi, S. intercalatum,* and *S. matthei.*

Schistosoma haematobium is found in northern and sub-Saharan Africa. Infections in the Nile Valley are especially severe. It is also found on the Arabian Peninsula and in scattered areas of the Middle East, particularly in Lebanon, Syria, Iraq, and Iran. *Schistosoma mansoni* is found throughout tropical Africa, Madagascar, Sudan, Ethiopia, Egypt, and Yemen. In the western hemisphere, *S. mansoni* is found in Brazil, Surinam, several islands in the West Indies, and Puerto Rico, and it is the only cause of schistosomiasis found in the western hemisphere. *Schistosoma japonicum* is confined to Asia, most cases being found in China, especially along river basins. The parasite is also found in scattered areas of Taiwan, the Philippines, the Mekong Valley, and the Celebes. *Schistosoma mekongi* is found along the Mekong River and adjacent parts of southeast Asia, but *S. intercalatum* is found only in West Africa and *S. matthei* in South Africa.

Life Cycle and Epidemiology

With some differences, which will be noted, all the schistosomes have a similar life cycle. Eggs are passed by urine or stool into fresh water, where they promptly hatch. Ciliated larvae, called miricidia, are released, which penetrate appropriate snails and develop into sporocysts, in each of which thousands of daughter sporocysts form. These forms emerge from the snail in 3 to 5 weeks as fork-tailed free-swimming organisms called cercariae. As many as 100,000 may develop from a single miracidium. The cercariae penetrate human skin on contact, enter the venous circulation, and terminate in various places. Larvae of *S. mansoni* terminate in the venules of the inferior mesenteric venous system, and those of *S. haematobium* in the inferior hemorrhoidal and vesicle plexuses. Larvae of *S. japonicum* reside primarily in the inferior mesenteric system, with some larval worms terminating and developing in the superior mesenteric veins.[119] The worms are slender, being 0.5 mm in diameter, and about 6 to 20 mm long. The female lies within a longitudinal body cleft of the male, and both reside within their predetermined venous system in this copulatory position (Fig. 10–10). To lay eggs, the females migrate peripherally to terminal venules over the bowel and bladder walls. The eggs subsequently laid generally move through the venules to bowel or bladder wall, but many are swept to the liver or lungs by venous drainage. The eggs work their way through bowel and bladder tissue to their respective lumens. The mechanism of this passage is incompletely understood but includes the secretion of enzymes that have lytic properties. After reaching the lumen, the eggs are passed to the outer world and the cycle is complete. Eggs are first detected some 6 to 10 weeks after cercarial penetration. Infection in humans is acquired only by contact with fresh water that is infested with cercariae. *Schistosoma japonicum* infects humans and a number of animal hosts, including water buffalo, and dogs, cattle, and several other domestic animals. *Schistosoma mansoni* has been found in rodents, baboons, and insectivores, but these animals do not seem to be involved in transmission to humans. *Schistosoma haematobium* has only rarely been seen in animals.

Pathology and Pathogenesis

Most of the pathologic conditions of schistosomiasis can be related to the eggs. The eggs release enzymes that have lytic and thus irritative properties to facilitate their movement through tissues. The enzymes and other released substances are also antigenic and sensitize the host to produce reactions, using delayed hypersensitivity and humoral pathways. Thus,

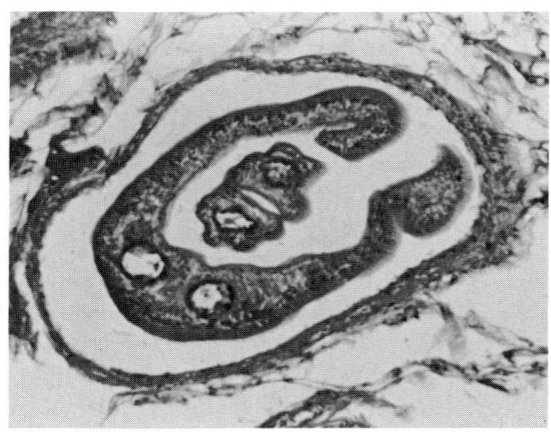

FIGURE 10–10.
A pair of *Schistosoma mansoni* worms seen within a venule. The female rests within the male. SOURCE: Courtesy Dr. Herman Zaiman: A Pictorial Presentation of Parasites, Valley City, ND.

around eggs in the bowel and bladder wall as in the portal venules of the liver, the typical lesion is a granuloma composed of lymphocytes, macrophages, eosinophils, fibroblasts, and sometimes giant cells. Younger granulomata have more neutrophils and eosinophils, and older ones show more lymphocytes, macrophages, fibroblasts, and giant cells. One often sees a degenerating egg at the center of the lesion, and this finding is diagnostic. All three species produce granulomata of similar appearance, though in *S. japonicum* the eggs are laid in bunches and a granuloma may show more necrosis around a central cluster of eggs. In *S. haematobium* and *S. mansoni* infection, granuloma formation is related primarily to cellular immune responses, whereas in *S. japonicum* infection, humoral responses are thought to play a larger role. With extensive egg production and the attendant granulomata in the portal venules, the flow of portal venous blood is obstructed, with a resultant portal hypertension (see Chapter 17).

In the colon, chronic granulomata are seen grossly as "sandy patches," collections of small yellow nodules appearing mainly on the serosa. Under microscopic examination these patches are inflammatory tissue and granulomata. Eggs are also seen throughout the bowel wall without organized granuloma formation. Hyperemia, petechiae, mucosal ulcerations, irritability, varying degrees of fibrosis, and, in severe cases, polyposis are also seen. Schistosomal polyposis, seen in its most florid form with *S. mansoni* in Egypt, is an advanced and severe form of the disease (Fig. 10–11, 10–12 A). Pathologically, the polyps show a heaping up of combined inflammatory and granulomatous tissue, masses of eggs, and a proliferative response of the overlying epithelium.[120] The polyps may range from small to quite large, may be pedunculated, and may bleed. They are most common in the distal colon and rectum. Occasionally polyps may be produced by eggs of *S. haematobium* in the rectal mucosa. Polyps of *S. japonicum* tend to be smaller but are frequently found. Chronic disease may also lead to extensive fibrotic changes that can produce ahaustral, tubular areas in the colon that are either extensive or focal, and can occasionally lead to strictures. The process may cause an overall thickening of the colonic wall. The appendix is often infected, but clinical appendicitis is rare. In addition, extracolonic masses called bilharziomas, produced by a combination of fibrotic and inflammatory tissue around eggs, may form (see Fig. 10–11). These masses are in the outer aspects of the bowel wall or may actually be extrinsic to the colon. The

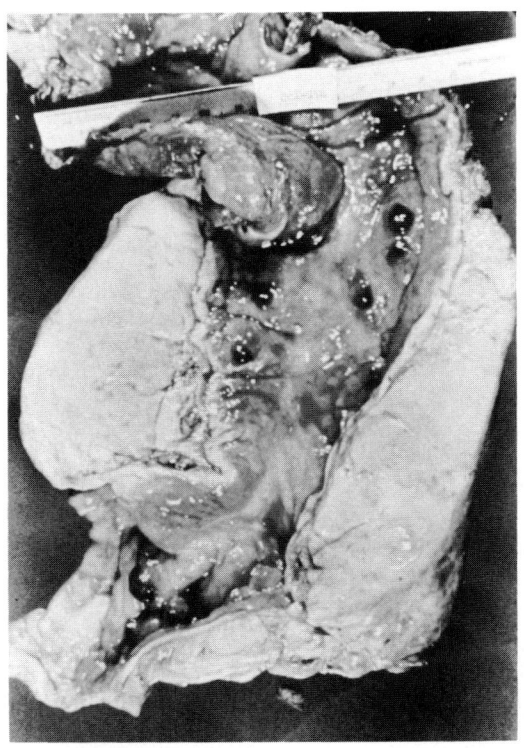

FIGURE 10–11.
Specimen from a hemicolectomy on an Egyptian patient with both *S. mansoni* and *S. haematobium*. Note the polyps, the thickened bowel wall, and the rounded white fibrotic bilharziomas exterior to the bowel on the right and left. SOURCE: Photo by Dr. AW Cheever, NIAID, NIH. Bethesda, MD, from *A Pictorial Presentation of Parasites*, edited by Herman Zaiman, Valley City, ND.

main changes due to *S. haematobium* are found in the bladder, where one also sees granulomatous inflammatory and fibrotic change, but, as mentioned, the rectal area may be involved, producing varying degrees of colitis and sometimes polyps.[121, 122]

Schistosoma mansoni and *S. haematobium* do not predispose to carcinoma of the bowel. Some clinicians speculate, however, that chronic *S. japonicum* infection may lead to this complication.[122, 123] Cellular atypia and proliferative adenomatous changes are seen and are considered to be precursors of carcinoma. Some data also indicate that patients with schistosomiasis and colon carcinoma are younger than those with carcinoma alone. The relationship of these two diseases has not yet been fully clarified.

Clinical Findings

The clinical picture of all three types of schistosomiasis can be divided into three stages: initial penetration, acute condition known as Ka-tayama fever, and chronic condition. The first two stages will be described only briefly, but the third discussed in detail in this chapter.

Stage I: Cercarial penetration is usually caused by contact with animal schistosomes but can also be caused by those infesting humans. In an unsensitized person exposed to infested fresh water, the penetration of the cercaria may cause a mild itchy or prickly sensation locally, and faint red macules may appear within 12 hours. In a person previously sensitized, exposure to cercariae leads to an erythematous papular eruption, itching, and sometimes vesicle formation. This reaction, referred to as "swimmer's itch," resolves in the course of approximately a week.

Stage II: The acute stage, named Katayama fever after a valley in Japan where this disease was endemic, generally starts 4 to 6 weeks and sometimes as late as 10 weeks or more after infection. It coincides with the initial egg production of newly acquired worms. Stage II of the disease is seldom seen clinically, however, as most infections in endemic areas are either not apparent or mild. In a nonendemic area, stage II infection might present in a tourist who has recently acquired a heavy infection. Depending on severity, it consists of varying degrees of fever, chills, weakness, sweating, anorexia, nausea, vomiting, diarrhea, abdominal pain, cough, and headache. Also frequent are urticaria and enlarged lymph nodes. The laboratory studies show eosinophilia and increased levels of immunoglobulins G and E (IgG, IgE). The syndrome usually lasts several days to weeks.

Stage III: Manifestations of the third, chronic, stage depend on the species in question and the severity of the infection. Findings pertinent to the colon are emphasized here.

Schistosoma mansoni. Infection by this species regularly produces large bowel involvement since the egg-laying worms are found in the venules of the inferior mesenteric system. Many patients in the chronic phase are asymptomatic, especially if infections are mild. In heavier infections, chronic mild diarrhea may be a symptom, sometimes with abdominal cramps. Mucus and small amounts of blood may be in the stool, but gross hemorrhage is unusual. Iron deficiency anemia can result from persistent blood loss. Mild weight loss or difficulty in maintaining weight, fatigue, and tiredness may be seen.[124] Several population-based studies, however, show no particular relation between schistosomal infection and symptoms.[125] In addition the relation of symptoms to infection in expatriates after returning home to Britain is not always clear.[126] Evaluation of complaints such as tired-

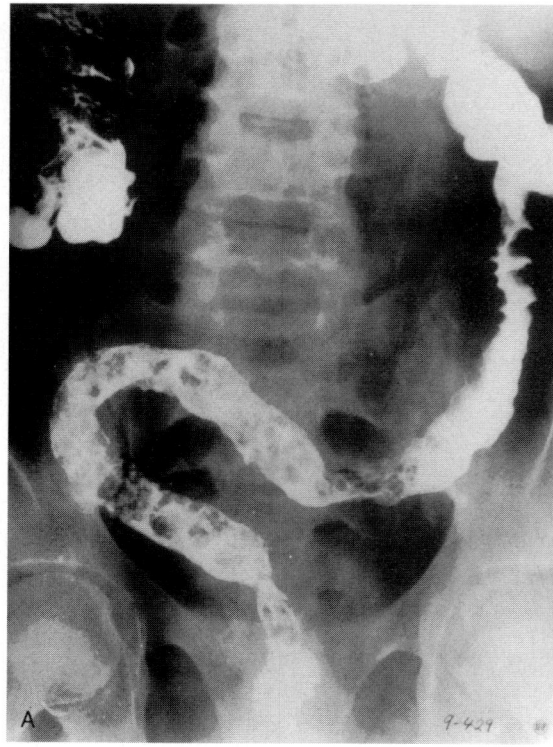
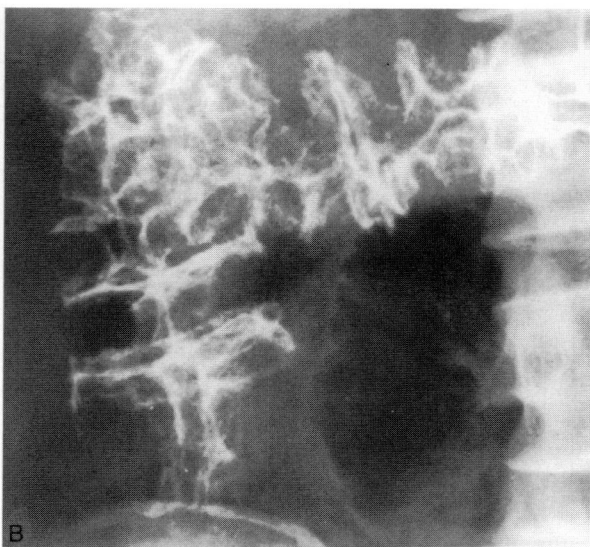

FIGURE 10–12.
A, Barium enema on a 20-year-old Egyptian man, demonstrating severe polypoid disease and generalized narrowing, with scattered areas of stricture formation. The rectosigmoid is displaced upward by a large pericolic bilharzioma. B, Close-up of hepatic flexure in a 20-year-old Puerto Rican man. Note the spasm and granular mucosal pattern due to tiny punctate mucosal ulcerations. SOURCE: Reeder MM, Palmer PES. The Radiology of Tropical Diseases with Epidemiological, Pathological and Clinical Correlation. Baltimore: Williams & Wilkins; 1981.

ness and milder intestinal dysfunction in the individual patient is therefore difficult. Improvement with treatment, if it occurs, helps to confirm an actual relationship.

A special form of *S. mansoni* infection is colonic polyposis, which is particularly frequent in Egypt, but may be seen elsewhere, though seldom in the western hemisphere. It is associated with heavy infections. Patients with multiple polyps can develop a particular syndrome, characterized by varying degrees of diarrhea, protein-losing enteropathy, hypoproteinemia, extensive blood loss, emaciation, dehydration, and electrolyte imbalance.[127]

Chronic deposition of eggs in the liver via the portal venous system leads to portal hypertension, splenomegaly, and esophageal varices. The varices may produce hematemesis, which may be fatal. Portal hypertension also opens up pathways for eggs to be shunted to the lungs, and in advanced cases cor pulmonale may result.

Examination of patients with *S. mansoni* infection may show nothing. More commonly, one finds mild degrees of splenomegaly and hepa-

tomegaly. The presence of these findings correlates roughly with worm load. The abdomen may be mildly tender, but usually local masses are not palpable. Weight loss, emaciation, and pallor, may, of course, be present, depending upon the severity of the infection. Patients with greater degrees of portal hypertension have larger spleens, sometimes extending into the pelvis, enlarged nontender livers, and dilated abdominal veins. Ascites implies either concomitant liver disease from chronic hepatitis or alcohol abuse of else a late stage of portal hypertension.

A mild eosinophilia is usually present in the range of 6 to 15% of the total leukocyte count. Mild anemia is common, and in cases of significant splenomegaly, pancytopenia may be present. The results of liver function tests are usually slightly abnormal, with modest rises in alkaline phosphatase and transaminase being the rule. Hypoproteinemia is possible. The bilirubin is usually normal. The urine is generally normal, although proteinuria may occur.

Radiographic findings vary. Flat plate radio-

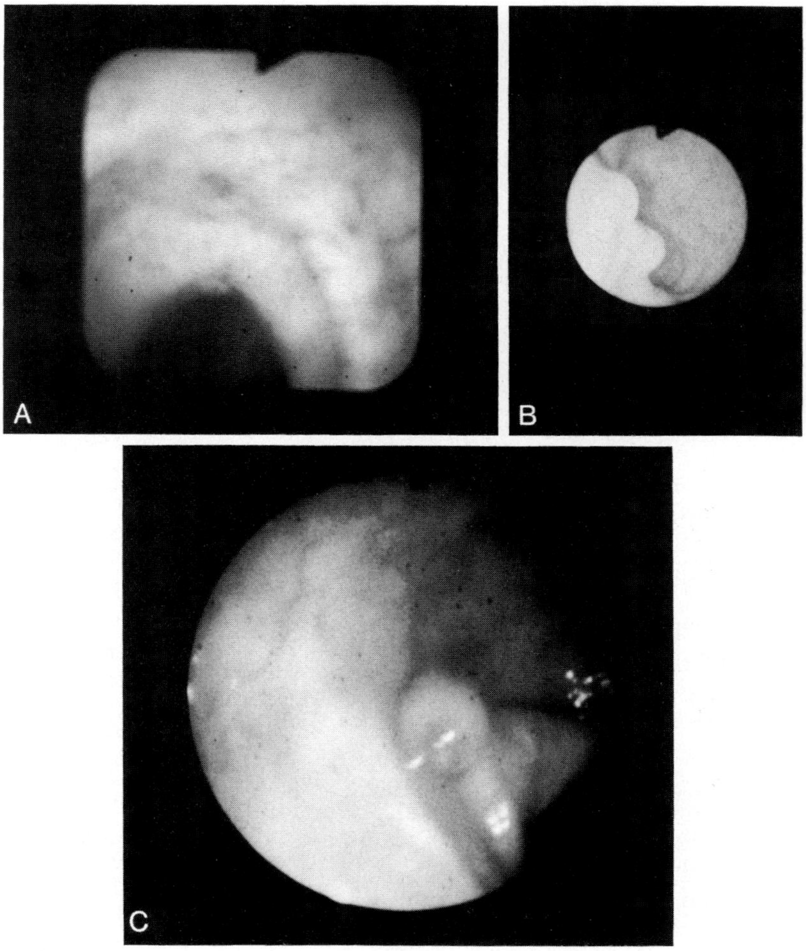

FIGURE 10–13.
Schistosomiasis mansoni as seen through the sigmoidoscope. *A,* Scattered hyperemia and petechial hemorrhages in the colon. *B,* Schistosomal rectal varices. *C,* Schistosomal colonic polyp. These patients were all examined in Saudi Arabia. SOURCE: Courtesy of Dr AE Mohamed, Riyadh Armed Forces Hospital, Riyadh, Saudi Arabia. [See also Color Plate 3]

graphs are often normal, but one may see calcification of the rectal wall in *S. mansoni* infection.[128] Barium enema findings can be normal. In *S. mansoni* infection, however, a granular pattern of the barium due to tiny mucosal ulcerations may be seen (Fig. 10–12*B*) or changes suggesting edema, spasm, and incomplete distention of the colon. These conditions tend to be relatively early signs. In more severe disease, polyps may be present, easily seen on barium enema, and more pronounced in the distal portions of the colon and rectosigmoid. They are seldom seen in *S. mansoni* infection from the western hemisphere. Later stages of disease may show loss of haustral pattern, a spiculated appearance, evidence of thickening of the wall of the colon, a tubular appearing colon, and signs of extrinsic masses due to bilharziomas (see Fig. 12*B*).[122, 129] The findings of thickening and narrowing of the colon are more common in patients in the western hemisphere. Sometimes, bilharziomas or strictures suggest malignancy on radiographic examination. Intestinal obstruction has been described, but seems to be rare.

Improvements in endoscopic techniques have allowed greater visualization of colon pathologic changes in schistosomiasis. With flexible instruments, as with the rigid sigmoidoscope, one may see irritation, spasm, small petechial lesions, small ulcerations, and, in advanced cases, varices and polyps (Fig. 10–13*A, B, C*).[130, 131] The newer flexible endoscopes show in addition that polyps are usually limited to the left colon and rectum. The colon may also look normal in the presence of schistosome eggs, in which case a paucity of inflammatory histologic changes are seen on biopsy. Polyps are smaller and less common in patients in the western hemisphere with this disease.

Schistosoma haematobium. Infection caused by *S. haematobium* infection generally presents with hematuria. More advanced stages of this disease may present with urinary tract infections and complications resulting from distorted urinary tract anatomy. Colonic involvement with *S. haematobium* is limited to the rectum. Symptoms in severe cases may include diarrhea, polyposis, and blood loss, but colonic symptoms from infection by this species are generally not pronounced. The hepatosplenic and pulmonary changes may be identical to those seen in *S. mansoni* infection. Radiographic findings are limited to irritability and signs of polyps in the rectum. Sigmoidoscopic examination may show findings similar to but less pronounced than those in *S. mansoni* infection and are limited to the lower colon.

Schistosoma japonicum. Infections by *S. japonicum* also present with a symptomatic spectrum ranging from none to varying degrees of diarrhea, hematochezia, weight loss, protein loss, abdominal discomfort, cramps, and pains. The radiographic picture less often shows polyposis, but the varying inflammatory changes of the colon may be seen as described in *S. mansoni* infection. Likewise, endoscopic examination may show a similar picture, though the polyps seem smaller than in *S. mansoni* disease.[132] The same hepatosplenic and pulmonary changes seen in *S. mansoni* infection may result from long-standing infection with *S. japonicum.*

Schistosoma mekongi. Disease due to *S. mekongi* resembles that due to *S. japonicum.* The eggs are similar to those of *S. japonicum* but are slightly smaller and rounder. The clinical presentation is similar. Many patients are asymptomatic, but some show similar lower intestinal symptoms and sigmoidoscopic findings. Enlargement of the left lobe of the liver is a common early finding. Portal hypertension may occur. Diagnosis is made by finding eggs in stool or on rectal biopsy in association with a compatible geographic history.[133]

Schistosoma intercalatum. Infection due to *S. intercalatum* is found in West Africa and the Central African Republic in scattered distribution, and the worms may hybridize with those of *S. haematobium.* The eggs resemble those of *S. haematobium* but have a slightly bent terminal spine, and they infect the entire colon. The clinical picture resembles that of schistosomiasis from *S. mansoni* but is much milder, and most patients are asymptomatic. Signs of portal hypertension have *not* been seen. Diagnosis is by stool examination or rectal biopsy.[134]

Schistosoma matthei. The *matthei* species of *Schistosoma* is an animal schistosome that also infects humans in South Africa. The eggs resemble those of *S. intercalatum* and may be found in urine or stool. The colon and liver are primarily affected, though the bowel disease is mild. In fact, most patients are asymptomatic, and the relation between symptoms and infection is obscure since co-infection with *S. mansoni* or *S. haematobium* often occurs.[135]

Diagnosis

The diagnosis of schistosomiasis is best made by finding the eggs of the parasite. Stool examination, either by direct smear or by concentration technique, is the usual method of finding eggs. The greatest sensitivity is achieved using one of the formalin-ether concentration methods. The eggs of *S. haematobium* are most often found in urine but may appear in stool. If possible, an assessment of the viability of the eggs should be made, particularly in a patient removed for some time from an endemic area or in a patient already treated. Their viability can be assessed by observing moving organelles (flame cells) of a living embryo during examination of a fresh preparation or by a hatching test, in which eggs are placed in fresh water in narrow-mouthed flasks and observed for hatching. Although most cases can be diagnosed by proper stool examination, if the diagnosis is still suspect, a still higher yield may be obtained by a biopsy of one of the transverse rectal folds. Two or 3 small biopsy samples should be obtained, and at least 1 should be crushed in the fresh state between two glass slides and examined directly (Fig. 10–14). This examination reveals the eggs and allows an assessment of viability by noting movements of the enclosed embryo. At least 1 biopsy specimen should also be sent for formal pathologic examination. *Schistosoma haematobium* infection can be diagnosed by bladder wall biopsy and sometimes by rectal biopsy. Biopsy of a polyp usually produces a positive specimen and may yield schistosomal eggs in cases in which schistosomiasis is not suspected. Liver biopsy may also reveal the eosinophilic granulomata surrounding degenerating eggs of any of the three types of schistosomiasis (see Chapter 17).

Various serologic tests are available. Some require the use of live schistosome eggs or larval forms and are not practical. Others vary in their sensitivity and specificity. The subject was reviewed in 1986.[136] Of the tests available, some bear mention. The indirect immunofluorescent (IIF) test has been found useful in screening patients in a nonendemic area, but cross-reaction with trichinella, some lack of sensitivity, and observer subjectivity exist. The ELISA is similar but quantitatively more precise and more sensitive.[136] A Falcon Assay Screening Test ELISA system (FAST-ELISA) has been developed that uses adult schistosomal microsomal antigens.[137] This test measures antibodies and is rapid, accurate, and species-specific. Another related test currently available through the Cen-

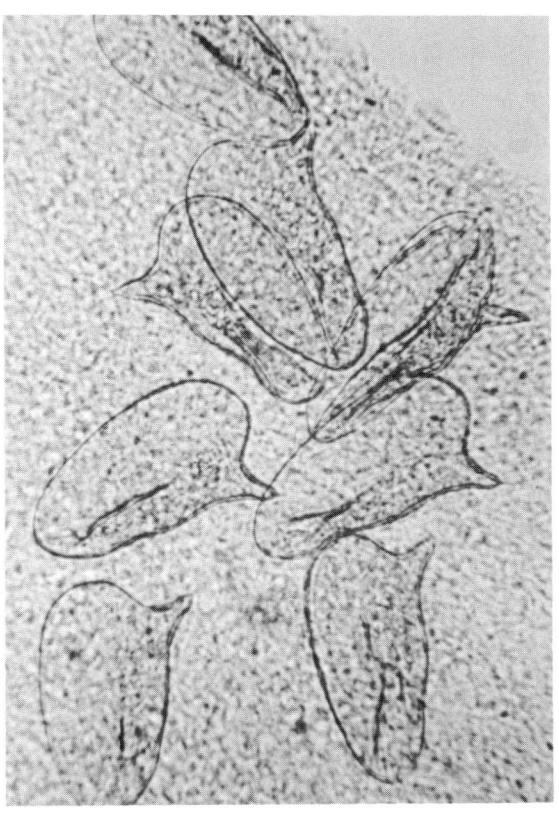

FIGURE 10–14.
Biopsy of a rectal valve crushed fresh between two glass slides. *Schistosoma mansoni* eggs are clearly visible. Larvae are absent from this specimen. SOURCE: Courtesy of Dr Herman Zaiman from A Pictorial Presentation of Parasites, Valley City, ND

ters for Disease Control is an immunoblot assay, which measures antibodies to the same antigens and is highly sensitive and species-specific.[138]

In a heavily infected patient, the diagnosis is rarely difficult since the eggs are easily found. In lightly infected individuals, however, serologic tests may be useful, in which instance a positive test would prompt further efforts to find eggs. The sensitivity of the ELISA-based tests is high enough (over 90%) to allow their use to screen individuals who have been at risk for exposure.[126] The disadvantages of the tests are that they may take weeks or months to become positive and in some cases they lack full specificity, though the newer tests have corrected this problem. It is still generally accepted that the demonstration of eggs constitutes grounds for treatment. Test results may remain positive for some time after treatment, limiting their usefulness in the assessment of recurrent or persistent infections. Serologic studies are useful, of course, for epidemiologic investigation.

Treatment

Large strides have been made in the treatment of schistosomiasis. The use of toxic agents such as antimony and even niridazol has all but disappeared. Treatment is reserved for those individuals in whom a parasitologic diagnosis, with or without serologic study, has been established. In addition, one should assess the viability of the recovered eggs, if possible, either by direct observation or by the use of a hatching test described earlier. For general purposes, however, the presence of eggs in the stool or biopsy specimen of a person known not to have received treatment and not to have been a long time away from an endemic area can usually be taken as grounds for treatment. Considering the safety of current drugs against schistosomiasis, it is generally believed that any patient who is diagnosed as having active schistosomiasis, regardless of intensity of infection, should be treated.

The most exciting of the new drugs is praziquantel.[139] It is active against all species of *Schistosoma* and has a low level of toxicity. It is efficiently absorbed and has an extensive first-pass metabolism in the liver, yielding inactive metabolites. Thus, liver disease leads to higher blood levels. Its mode of action is not completely known, but it induces a tetanic contraction in the worms and causes a blistering of the integument. For *S. haematobium* and *S. mansoni* infection, it is given as a single dose of 40 mg/kg, though in some severely infected patients, 20 mg/kg, given 3 times a day, may be advisable. Treatment of *S. japonicum* and *S. mekongi* infection is accomplished with a dosage of 20 mg/kg, given 3 times for 1 day. Side effects are generally mild but may consist of abdominal pains, nausea, vomiting, dizziness, and occasionally urticaria, slight fever, aching in the limbs, and mild increases in liver enzymes.[140-143] Diarrhea, sometimes with blood, has been noted in some studies, presumably relating to toxicity from sudden injury of large numbers of eggs.[144] Side effects may be accentuated in patients with portal hypertension. Cure rates in children infected with *S. mansoni,* particularly in the western hemisphere, may be lower, and careful follow-up is needed.[145]

Oxamniquine, a tetrahydroquinoline, effective only against *S. mansoni* infection, is also a useful drug. It is absorbed rapidly, metabolized extensively, and excreted in the urine. The mode of its action is unknown. Patients from the western hemisphere with *S. mansoni* infection are given a single dose of 15 mg/kg, but for African and Middle Eastern patients, 15 mg/kg, given 2 times a day, for 2 days is recommended. Children in the western hemisphere have a lower cure rate with conventional dosages, and should receive 20 mg/kg. Side effects include dizziness and lightheadedness. Seizures have been recorded, though usually in patients with a prior history of seizure, and the drug is contraindicated for such patients. Other side effects include headache, drowsiness, nausea, abdominal pain, and itching. These effects are usually not severe. Approximately 2 to 4 days after administration, patients often experience fever lasting 2 or 3 days.[146–148] Strains of *S. mansoni* worms resistant to oxamniquine have been found in South America.

Schistosoma haematobium may also be treated with metrifonate, a cholinesterase inhibitor. It is given in a dose of 7.5 to 10 mg/kg every 2 weeks for 3 doses. The worms are paralyzed and swept by the bloodstream to the lungs, yet pulmonary complications do not appear to result from this treatment. The drug is not available for general use in the United States, but it is obtainable from the Centers for Disease Control. Serum cholinesterase levels should be measured in patients receiving the drug.[149]

Assessing patients for cure is not always easy. Nonviable eggs may be passed for weeks or months after a successful treatment course. Examination of patients' stools 3 and 6 months after the completion of treatment is advised, and the eggs should be checked for viability. If viable eggs are being passed after 6 months, the patient is not cured, and retreatment is recommended. In many cases, particularly in young patients, regression of splenomegaly occurs. In cases of polyposis, the polyps usually have all but disappeared after a year. Surgical polypectomy is not needed. Reversal of hepatic fibrosis, and presumably prevention of portal hypertension, occurs if the fibrosis is not too old. It is therefore important to treat patients before these chronic complications occur.

Prevention

Schistosomiasis can be prevented by avoiding contact with fresh water that is contaminated with infected snails. In endemic areas, usually owing to low public health budgets, primitive living conditions, and inadequate health education, control of schistosomiasis has made poor progress. Programs that have been developed include mass chemotherapy of infected populations; snail control programs, with the use of molluscacides, biologic predators, and environmental alteration; and educational efforts directed at reducing snail contact, proper disposal of excreta, providing latrines, and the like.

Though some success has been recorded with such programs,[150] in many parts of the world, gains have been modest or nonexistent.[151] This poor result is in part due to the enormous output of cercariae, up to 100,000 by a snail infected with a single miracidium.

The use of medications to prevent clinical illness in a patient in whom infection is presumed has been inadequately studied. A vaccine is not expected in the near future. This is not surprising, since the presence of a natural infection for years does not provide total immunity.

REFERENCES

1. Salata RA, Ravdin JI. Review of the human immune mechanisms directed against *Entamoeba histolytica*. Rev Infect Dis. 1986;8:261–272.
2. Eisert J, Hannibal JE, Sanders SL. Fatal amebiasis complicating corticosteroid management of *Pemphigus vulgaris*. N Engl J Med. 1959;261:843–845.
3. Abioye AA. Fatal amoebic colitis in pregnancy and puerperium: A new clinico-pathological entity. J Trop Med Hyg. 1973;76:97–100.
4. Rode H, Davies MRQ, Cywes S. Amebic liver abscesses in infancy and childhood. S Afr J Surg. 1978;16:131–138.
5. Sargeaunt PG, Zymodemes of *Entamoeba histolytica*. In. Ravdin JI, ed. Amebiasis: Human Infection by *Entamoeba histolytica*. New York: John Wiley & Sons; 1988;370–387.
6. Krogstad DJ. Isozyme patterns and pathogenicity in amebic infection. N Engl J Med. 1986;315:390–391.
7. Tannich E, Scholze H, Nickel R, et al. Homologous cysteine proteases of pathogenic and nonpathogenic *Entamoeba histolytica*. J Biol Chem. 1991;266:4798–4803.
8. Bracha R, Diamond LS, Ackers JP, et al. Differentiation of clinical isolates of *Entamoeba histolytica* by using specific DNA probes. J Clin Microbiol. 1990;28:680–684.
9. Jackson TFHG. *Entamoeba histolytica* cyst passers: To treat or not to treat? S Afr Med J. 1987;72:657–658.
10. Ravdin JI. Pathogenesis of disease caused by *Entamoeba histolytica*: Studies of adherence, secreted toxins, and contact-dependent cytolysis. J Infect Dis. 1986;8:247–260.
11. Prathap K, Gilman R. The histopathology of acute intestinal amebiasis. Am J Pathol. 1970;60:229–239.
12. Juniper K Jr, Steele VW, Chester CL. Rectal biopsy in the diagnosis of amebic colitis. South Med J. 1958;51:545–553.
13. Perez-Tamayo R, Brandt H. Amebiasis. In: Marcial-Rojas RA, ed. Pathology of Protozoal and Helminthic Diseases. Baltimore: Williams & Wilkins; 1971;145–188.
14. Kean BH, Gilmore HR, Van Store WW. Fatal amebiasis: Report of 148 fatal cases from the Armed Forces Institute of Pathology. Ann Intern Med. 1956;44:831–843.
15. Krogstad DJ, Spencer HC Jr, Healy GR, et al. Amebiasis: Epidemiologic studies in the United States, 1971–1974. Ann Intern Med. 1978;88:89–97.
16. Garcia LS, Ash L. Diagnostic Parasitology Clinical Laboratory Manual. St. Louis. CV Mosby; 1979:384.
17. Ash LR, Orihel TC. Parasites: A Guide to Laboratory Procedures and Identification. Chicago. ASCP Press; 1987:12.
18. Healy GR. Diagnostic techniques for stool samples. In: Ravdin JI, ed. Amebiasis. Human Infection by *Enta-*

moeba histolytica. New York. John Wiley & Sons; 1988;644.

19. Baumann D, Gottstein B. A double-antibody sandwich ELISA for the detection of *Entamoeba histolytica* antigen in stool samples of humans. Trop Med Parasitol. 1987;38:81–83.

20. Samuelson J, Acuna-Soto R, Reed S, et al. DNA hybridization probe for clinical diagnosis of *Entamoeba histolytica.* J Clin Microbiol. 1989;27:671–676.

21. Gilman R, Islam M, Paschi J, et al. Comparison of conventional and immunofluorescent techniques for the detection of *Entamoeba histolytica* in rectal biopsies. Gastroenterology. 1980;78:435–439.

22. Reeder MM, Palmer PES. The Radiology of Tropical Diseases. Baltimore: Williams & Wilkins; 1981;83–156.

23. Cardoso JM, Kimura K, Stoopen M, et al. Radiology of invasive amebiasis of the colon. AJR Am J Roentgenol. 1977;128:935–941.

24. Balikian J, Uthman S, Khouri NF. Intestinal amebiasis. AJR Am J Roentgenol. 1974;122:245–256.

25. Levine SM, Stover JF, Warren JG, et al: Ameboma, the forgotten granuloma. JAMA. 1971;215:1461–1464.

26. Matsui T, Iida M, Tada S, et al. The value of double-contrast barium enema in amebic colitis. Gastrointest Radiol. 1989;14:73–78.

27. Patterson M, Healy G, Shabot JM. Serologic testing for amebiasis. Gastroenterology. 1980;78:136–141.

28. Healy GR. Serology. In. Ravdin JI, ed. Amebiasis: Human infection by *Entamoeba histolytica.* New York: John Wiley & Sons; 1988;659–660.

29. Patel AS, DeRidder PH. Amebic colitis masquerading as acute inflammatory bowel disease: The role of serology in its diagnosis. J Clin Gastroenterol. 1989;11:407–410.

30. Gilman AG, Rall TW, Nies AS, Taylor P, eds. Goodman and Gilman's The Pharmacologic Basis of Therapeutics. 8th ed. Elmsford NY: Pergamon Press; 1990;1000–1001.

31. Rosenblatt JE, Edson RS. Metronidazole. Mayo Clin Proc. 1967;62:1013–1017.

32. Klatskin G, Friedman H. Emetine toxicity in man: Studies on the nature of early toxic manifestations, their relation to the dose level, and their significance in determining safe dosage. Ann Intern Med. 1948;28:892–915.

33. Adams EB, MacLeod IN. Invasive amebiasis: I, Amebic dysentery and its complications. Medicine. 1977;56:315–323.

34. Powell SJ, Wilmot AJ, Elsdon-Dew R. Further trials of metronidazole in amebic dysentery and amebic liver abscess. Ann Trop Med Parasitol. 1967;61:511–514.

35. Ravdin JI, Petrie WA Jr. *Entameba histolytica* (amebiasis). In: Mandell GL, Douglas RG, Bennett JE, eds. Principles and Practice of Infectious Diseases. New York: Churchill Livingstone; 1990;2045.

36. Sawyer PR, Brogden RN, Pinder RM, et al. Tinidazole: A review of its antiprotozoal activity and therapeutic efficacy. Drugs. 1976;11:423–440.

37. Bakshi JS, Ghiara JM, Nanivadekar AS. How does tinidazole compare with metronidazole? Drugs. 1978; 15(suppl 1):33–42.

38. Wolf MS. Nondysenteric intestinal amebiasis. Treatment with diloxanide furoate. JAMA. 1973;224:1601–1604.

39. Woodruff AW, Bell S. Clinical trials with entamide furoate and related compounds. Trans R Soc Trop Med Hyg. 1960;54:389–395.

40. Sullam PM, Slutkin G, Gottlieb AB, et al. Paromomycin therapy of endemic amebiasis in homosexual men. Sex Transm Dis. 1986;13:151–155.

41. Wagner ED, Burnett HS. Paromomycin in the treat-

ment of amebiasis in Nyasaland. Trans R Soc Trop Med Hyg. 1961;55:428–430.

42. Powell SJ, Wilmott AJ, Elsdon-Dew R. Potentiating effect of quinolones on the action of tetracycline in amebic dysentery. Lancet. 1960;1:76–77.

43. Nanda R, Baveja U, Anand BS. *Entamoeba histolytica* cyst passers: Clinical features and outcome in untreated subjects. Lancet. 1984;2:301–303.

44. Variyam EP, Gogate P, Hassan M, et al. Nondysenteric intestinal amebiasis: Colonic morphology and search for *Entamoeba histolytica* adherence and invasion. Dig Dis Sci. 1989;34:732–740.

45. Allason-Jones E, Mindel A, Sargeaunt P, et al. *Entamoeba histolytica* as a commensal intestinal parasite in homosexual men. N Engl J Med. 1986;315:353–356.

46. Gathiram V, Jackson TFHG. A longitudinal study of asymptomatic carriers of pathogenic zymodemes of *Entamoeba histolytica.* S Afr Med J. 1987;72:669–672.

47. Mirelman D, Bracha R, Chayen A, et al. *Entamoeba histolytica:* Effect of growth conditions and bacterial associates on isoenzyme patterns and virulence. Exp Parasitol. 1986;62:142–148.

48. Ravdin JI. Intestinal disease caused by *Entamoeba histolytica.* In: Ravdin JI, ed. Amebiasis: Human Infection by *Entamoeba histolytica.* New York; John Wiley & Sons; 1988;508–509.

49. Robinson A, Levinson M. Amebic appendicitis associated with hepatic abscess. South Med J. 1984;77:1047–1048.

50. Thacker SB, Simpson S, Gordon TJ, et al. Parasitic disease control in a residential facility for the mentally retarded. Am J Public Health. 1979;69:1279–1281.

51. Salaki JS, Shirey JL, Strickland GT. Successful treatment of symptomatic *Entamoeba polecki* infection. Am J Trop Med Hyg. 1979;28:190–193.

52. Yang J, Scholten TH. *Dientamoeba fragilis:* A review with notes on its epidemiology, pathogenicity, mode of transmission, and diagnosis. Am J Trop Med Hyg. 1977;26:16–22.

53. Schein R, Gelb A. Colitis due to *Dientamoeba fragilis.* Am J Gastroenterol. 1983;78:634–636.

54. Kean BH, Malloch CL. The neglected ameba: *Dientamoeba fragilis.* Am J Dig Dis. 1966;11:735–746.

55. Swartzwelder JC. Balantidiasis. Am J Dig Dis. 1950;17:173–179.

56. Walzer PD, Judson FN, Murphy KB, et al. Balantidiasis outbreak in Truk. Am J Trop Med Hyg. 1973;22:33–41.

57. Garcia-Laverde A, De Bonilla L. Clinical trials with metronidazole in human balantidiasis. Am J Trop Med Hyg. 1975;24:781–783.

58. Zierdt CH. *Blastocystis hominis:* Past and future. Clin Microbiol Rev. 1991;4:61–79.

59. Miller RA, Minshew BH. *Blastocystis hominis:* An organism in search of a disease. Rev Infect Dis. 1988;10:930–938.

60. Markell EK, Udkow MP. *Blastocystis hominis:* Pathogen or fellow traveler? Am J Trop Med Hyg. 1986;35:1023–1026.

61. Fayer R, Ungar BLP. *Cryptosporidium* spp. and cryptosporidiosis. Microbiol Rev. 1986;50:458–483.

62. Current WL, Garcia LS. Cryptosporidiosis. Clin Microbiol Rev. 1991;4:325–358.

63. Crawford FG, Vermund SH. Human cryptosporidiosis. Crit Rev Microbiol. 1988;16:113–159.

64. Current WL, Reese NC, Ernst JV, et al. Human cryptosporidiosis in immunocompetent and immunodeficient persons: Studies of an outbreak and experimental transmission. N Engl J Med. 1983;308:1252–1257.

65. Heijbel H, Slaine K, Seigel B, et al. Outbreak of diarrhea in a day care center with spread to household members: The role of *Cryptosporidium.* Pediatr Infect Dis J. 1987;6:532–535.

66. Koch KL, Phillips DJ, Aber RC, et al. Cryptosporidiosis in hospital personnel: Evidence for person-to-person transmission. Ann Intern Med. 1985;102:593–596.
67. Rush BA, Chapman PA, Ineson RW. A probable waterborne outbreak of cryptosporidiosis in the Sheffield area. J Med Microbiol. 1990;32:239–242.
68. Soave R, Ma P. Cryptosporidiosis: Traveler's diarrhea in two families. Arch Intern Med. 1985;145:70–72.
69. Soave R, Armstrong D. Cryptosporidium and cryptosporidiosis. Rev Infect Dis. 1986;8:1012–1023.
70. Pitlik SD, Fainstein V, Garza D, et al. Human cryptosporidiosis, spectrum of disease: Report of six cases and review of the literature. Arch Intern Med. 1983;143:2269–2275.
71. Gentile G, Baldassarri L, Caprioli A, et al. Colonic vascular invasion as a possible route of extraintestinal cryptosporidiosis. Am J Med. 1987;82:574–575.
72. Wolfson JS, Richter JM, Waldron MA, et al. Cryptosporidiosis in immunocompetent patients. N Engl J Med. 1985;312:1278–1282.
73. Edelman MJ, Oldfield EC. Severe cryptosporidiosis in an immunocompetent host. Arch Intern Med. 1988;148:1873–1874.
74. Fafard J, Lalonde R. Long-standing symptomatic cryptosporidiosis in a normal man: Clinical response to spiramicin. J Clin Gastroenterol. 1990;12:190–191.
75. MacFarlane DE, Horner-Bryce J. Cryptosporidiosis in well-nourished and malnourished children. Acta Pediatr Scand. 1987;76:474–477.
76. Jokipii L, Jokipii AMM. Timing of symptoms and oocyst excretion in human cryptosporidiosis. N Engl J Med. 1986;315:1643–1647.
77. Garcia LS, Bruckner DA, Brewer TC, et al. Techniques for the recovery and identification of Cryptosporidium oocysts from stool specimens. J Clin Microbiol. 1983;18: 185–190.
78. Casemore DP, Armstrong M, Sands RL. Laboratory diagnosis of cryptosporidiosis. J Clin Pathol. 1985;38: 1337–1341.
79. Arrowood MJ, Sterling CR. Comparison of conventional staining methods and monoclonal antibody–based methods for Cryptosporidium oocyst detection. J Clin Microbiol. 1989;27:1490–1495.
80. Soave R. Treatment strategies for cryptosporidiosis. Ann N Y Acad Sci. 1990;616:442–451.
81. Portnoy D, Whiteside ME, Buckley E III, et al. Treatment of intestinal cryptosporidiosis with spiramycin. Ann Intern Med. 1984;101:202–204.
82. Wittenberg DF, Miller NM. Spiramycin is not effective in treating cryptosporidium diarrhea in infants: Results of a double-blind randomized trial. J Infect Dis. 1989;159:131–132.
83. Connolly GM, Dryden MS, Shanson DC, et al. Diclazuril in the treatment of severe cryptosporidial diarrhea in AIDS patients. AIDS. 1990;4:700–701.
84. Ungar BLP, Ward DJ, Fayer R, et al. Cessation of cryptosporidium-associated diarrhea in an acquired immunodeficiency patient after treatment with hyperimmune bovine colostrum. Gastroenterology. 1990;98: 486–489.
85. Nord J, Ma P, Dijohn D, et al. Treatment with bovine hyperimmune colostrum of cryptosporidial diarrhea in AIDS patients. AIDS. 1990;4:581–584.
86. Borowitz SM, Saulsbury FT. Treatment of chronic cryptosporidial infection with orally administered human serum immune globulin. J Pediatr. 1991;4:593–595.
87. McMeeking MW, Borkowsky W, Klesius PH, et al. A controlled trial of bovine dialyzable leukocyte extract for cryptosporidiosis in patients with AIDS. J Infect Dis. 1990;161:108–112.
88. Simon D, Weiss L, Tanowitz HB, et al. Resolution of cryptosporidium infection in an AIDS patient after improvement of nutritional and immune status with octreotide. Am J Gastroenterol. 1991;86:615–618.
89. Guideline for Handwashing and Hospital Environmental Control. Atlanta GA: Centers for Disease Control: 1885. US Dept of Commerce, National Technical Information Service publication 22161.
90. British Society of Gastroenterology. Cleaning and disinfection of equipment for gastrointestinal flexible endoscopy: Interim recommendations. Gut. 1988;29: 1134–1151.
91. Casemore DP, Blewett DA, Wright SE. British Society of Gastroenterology. Cleaning and disinfection of equipment for gastrointestinal flexible endoscopy: Interim recommendations. Gut. 1989;30:1156–1157.
92. Andrade ZA, Andrade SG, Chagas' disease (American trypanosomiasis). In: Marcial-Rojas RA, ed. Pathology of Protozoal and Helminthic Diseases. Baltimore: Williams & Wilkins; 1971:69–85.
93. Koberle F. Chagas' disease and Chagas' syndromes: The pathology of American trypanosomiasis. Adv Parasitol. 1968;6:63–116.
94. Takle GB, Hudson L. Autoimmunity and Chagas' disease. Curr Top Microbiol Immunol. 1989;145:79–92.
95. Cutait DE, Cutait R. Surgery of chagasic megacolon. World J Surg. 1991;15:188–197.
96. Gilman RH, Chong YH, et al. The adverse consequences of heavy trichuris infection. Trans Soc Trop Med Hyg. 1983;77:432–438.
97. Wolfe MS, Wershing JM, Mebendazole: Treatment of trichuriasis and ascariasis in Bahamian children. JAMA. 1974;240:1408–1411.
98. Sargent RG, Savory AM, Mina A, et al. A Clinical evaluation of mebendazole in the treatment of trichuriasis. Am J Trop Med Hyg. 1974;23:375–377.
99. Chandrasoma PT, Mendis KN. Enterobius vermicularis in ectopic sites. Am J Trop Med Hyg. 1977;26:644–649.
100. Vafai M, Mohit P. Granuloma of the anal canal due to Enterobius vermicularis: Report of a case. Dis Colon Rectum. 1983;26:349–350.
101. Bumbalo TS, Fugazzotto DJ, Wyczalek JV. Treatment of enterobiasis with pyrantel pamoate. Am J Trop Med Hyg. 1969;18:50–52.
102. Miller MJ, Krupp IM, Little MD, et al. Mebendazole: An effective anthelmintic for trichuriasis and enterobiasis. JAMA. 1974;230:1412–1414.
103. Stemmermann GN. Strongyloidiasis in migrants: Pathological and clinical considerations. Gastroenterology. 1967;53:59–70.
104. Berry AJ, Long EG, Smith JH, et al. Chronic relapsing colitis due to Strongyloides stercoralis. Am J Trop Med Hyg. 1983;32:1289–1293.
105. Genta RM, Caymmi-Gomes M. Pathology. In: Grove DA, ed. Strongyloidiasis: A Major Roundworm Infection of Man. London: Taylor & Francis; 1989:105–132.
106. Purtilo DT, Meyers WM, Connor DH. Fatal strongyloidiasis in immunosuppressed patients. Am J Med. 1974;56:488–493.
107. Shakir AA, Youngberg G, Alvarez S. Strongyloides infestation as a cause of acute appendicitis. J Tenn Med Assoc. 1986;79:543–544.
108. Scowden EB, Schnaffner W, Stone WJ. Overwhelming strongyloidiasis. Medicine (Baltimore). 1978;57:527–544.
109. Lima JP, Delgado PG. Diagnosis of strongyloidiasis: Importance of Baermann's method. Am J Dig Dis. 1961;6:899–904.
110. Dallemand S, Waxman M, Farman J. Radiological manifestations of Strongyloides stercoralis. Gastrointest Radiol. 1983;8:45–51.
111. Drasin GF, Moss JP, Cheng SH. Strongyloides stercoralis

colitis: Finding in four cases. Radiology. 1978;126:619–621.

112. Stoopack PM, Raufman J-P. Aphthoid ulceration of the colon in strongyloidiasis. Am J Gastroenterol. 1991; 86:639–642.

113. Carp NZ, Nejman JH, Kelly JJ. Strongylodiasis: An unusual cause of colonic pseudopolyposis and gastrointestinal bleeding. Surg Endosc. 1987;1:175–177.

114. Kang JY, Yap I. Colitis due to strongyloidiasis. Gastrointest endosc. 1989;35:71–72.

115. Gam AA, Neva FA, Krotoski WA. Comparative sensitivity and specificity of ELISA and IHA for serodiagnosis of strongyloidiasis with larval antigens. Am J Trop Med. 1987;37:157–161.

116. Pelletier LL, Baker CB, Gam AA, et al. Diagnosis and evaluation of treatment of chronic strongyloidiasis in ex–prisoners of war. J Infect Dis. 1988;157:573–576.

117. Morera P. Abdominal angiostrongyliasis. In: Strickland GT, ed. Hunter's Tropical Medicine. 7th ed. Philadelphia: WB Saunders, 1991:771–773.

118. Loria-Cortes R, Lobo-Sanahuja JF. Clinical abdominal angiostrongylosis: A study of 116 children with intestinal eosinophilic granuloma caused by Angiostrongylus costaricensis. Am J Trop Med Hyg. 1980;29:538–544.

119. Chen MG. Relative distribution of Schistosoma japonicum eggs in the intestine of man: A subject of inconsistency. Acta Trop (Basel). 1991;48:163–171.

120. McCully RM, Barron CN, Cheever AW. Schistosomiasis. In: Binford CH, Connor DH, eds. Pathology of Tropical and Extraordinary Diseases. Washington DC: US Armed Forces Institute of Pathology; 1976:482–508.

121. Dimmette RM, Sproat AF. Rectosigmoid polyps in schistosomiasis: I, General clinical and pathological considerations. Am J Trop Med Hyg. 1955;4:1057–1067.

122. Ming-Chai C, Chi-Yuan C, Pei-Yu C, et al. Evolution of colorectal cancer in schistosomiasis: Transitional mucosal changes adjacent to large intestinal carcinoma in colectomy specimens. Cancer. 1980;46:1661–1675.

123. Shindo K. Significance of Schistosomiasis japonica in the development of cancer of the large intestine: Report of a case and review of the literature. Dis Colon Rectum. 1976; 19:460–469.

124. Evengård B. Diagnostic and clinical aspects of schistosomiasis in 182 patients treated at a Swedish ward for tropical diseases during a ten-year period. Scand J Infect Dis. 1990;22:585–594.

125. Arap Siongok TK, Mahmoud AAF, Ouma JH, et al. Morbidity in Schistosomiasis mansoni in relation to intensity of infection: Study of a community in Machakos, Kenya. Am J Trop Med Hyg. 1976;25:273–284.

126. Harries AD, Fryatt R, Walker J, et al. Schistosomiasis in expatriates returning to Britain from the tropics: A controlled study. Lancet. 1986;1:86–88.

127. Nebel OT, el-Masry NA, Castell DO, et al. Schistosomial disease of the colon: A reversible form of polyposis. Gastroenterology. 1974;67:939–943.

128. Fataar S, et al. Radiographic spectrum of recto-colonic calcification from schistosomiasis. Bassiony H, Hamed MS, et al. Radiographic spectrum of rectocolonic calcification from schistosomiasis. AJR Am J Roentgenol. 1984;142:933–936.

129. Medina JT, Seaman WB, Guzman-Acosta C, et al. The roentgen appearance of Schistosomiasis mansoni involving the colon. Radiology. 1965;85:682–688.

130. Mohamed ARE, Karawi MA, Yasawy MI. Schistosomal colonic disease. Gut. 1990;31:439–442.

131. Radhakrishnan S, Nakib BA, Shaikh H, et al. The value of colonoscopy in schistosomal, tuberculous, and amebic colitis. Dis Colon Rectum. 1986;29:891–95.

132. Recio PM. The diagnosis and treatment of colorectal schistosomiasis. Dis Colon Rectum. 1958;1:111–115.

133. Hofstetter M, Nash TE, Cheever AW, et al. Infection with Schistosoma mekongi in Southeast Asian refugees. J Infect Dis. 1981;144:420–426.

134. Chen MG, Mott KE. Progress in assessment of morbidity due to Schistosoma intercalatum infection: A review of recent literature. Trop Dis Bull. 1989;86:R1–R18.

135. Van Wyk JA. The importance of animals in human schistosomiasis in South Africa. S Afr Med J. 1983;63:201–203.

136. Madison SE. Schistosomiasis. In: Schantz PM, Walls KW, eds. Immunodiagnosis of Parasitic Diseases. Academic Press: 1986;1:1–37.

137. Hancock K, Tsang VCW. Development and optimization of the FAST-ELISA for detecting antibodies to Schistosoma mansoni. J Immunol Methods. 1986;92:167–176.

138. Andrews J, Tsang VC, Maddison SE. Evidence of triple infections with Schistosoma japonicum, S. haematobium, and S. mansoni in two siblings. J Infect Dis. 1989;160:171–173.

139. Pearson RD, Guerrant RL. Praziquantel: A major advance in antihelminthic therapy. Ann Intern Med. 1983;99:195–198.

140. Katz N, Rocha RS, Chaves A. Preliminary trials with praziquantel in human infections due to Schistosoma mansoni. Bull WHO. 1979;57:781–785.

141. Santos AT, Blas BL, Nosenas JS, et al. Preliminary clinical trials with praziquantel in Schistosoma japonicum infections in the Philippines. Bull WHO. 1979;57:793–799.

142. Nash TE, Hofstetter M, Cheever AW, et al. Treatment of Schistosoma mekongi with praziquantel: A double-blind study. Am J Trop Med Hyg. 1982;31:977–982.

143. Andrews P, Thomas H, Pohlke R, et al. Praziquantel. Med Res Rev. 1983;3:147–200.

144. Polderman AM, Gryseels B, Gerold JL, et al. Side effects of praziquantel in the treatment of Schistosoma mansoni in Maniema, Zaire. Trans R Soc Trop Med Hyg. 1984;78:752–754.

145. deRezende GL. Survey on the clinical trial results achieved in Brazil comparing praziquantel and oxamniquine in the treatment of mansoni schistosomiasis. Rev Inst Med Trop Sao Paulo. 1985;27:328–336.

146. Lambertucci JR, Greco DB, Pedroso ERP, et al. A double blind trial with oxamniquine in chronic Schistosomiasis mansoni. Trans R Soc Trop Med Hyg. 1982;76:751–755.

147. Bassily S, Farid Z, Higashi GI, et al. Treatment of complicated Schistosomiasis mansoni with oxamniquine. Am J Trop Med Hyg. 1978;27:1284–1286.

148. Katz N, Zicker F, Pereira JP. Field trials with oxamniquine in a schistosomiasis mansoni–endemic area. Am J Trop Med Hyg. 1977;26:234–237.

149. Jewsbury JM, Cooke MJ, Weber MC. A field trial of metriphonate in treatment and prevention of schistosomiasis infection in man. Ann Trop Med Parasit. 1977;71:67–83.

150. Jordan P, Bartholomew RK, Grist E, et al. Evaluation of chemotherapy in the control of Schistosoma mansoni in Marquis Valley, Saint Lucia: I, Results in humans. Am J Trop Med Hyg. 1982;31:103–110.

151. Gryseels B. The relevance of schistosomiasis for public health. Trop Med Parasitol. 1989;40:134–142.

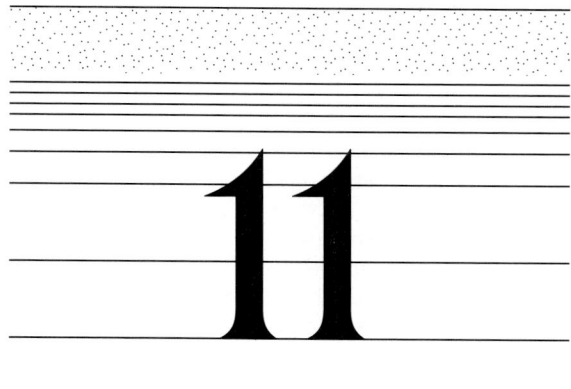

11

Anal Papillomavirus Infections

JANE M. KUYPERS, Ph.D.
NANCY B. KIVIAT, M.D.

GENITAL WARTS AND HUMAN PAPILLOMAVIRUS INFECTION

Human papillomavirus (HPV), the causative agent of genital warts, is the most common sexually transmitted viral infection in the United States.[1] Genital warts have been known since ancient times, with the term condylomata acuminata appearing in the 1800s.[2] The viral etiology of warts was established early in the twentieth century and was confirmed in 1969 by electron microscopy.[3]

Human papillomavirus usually infects the basal cells of the squamous epithelium, although it can also infect transitional and cuboidal epithelium. Infection is thought to occur after trauma to the epithelium, and it results in cellular hyperplasia of the basal cells.[4] Infectious viral particles are produced only by completely differentiated cells of the upper epithelium because cellular differentiation is necessary for the HPV growth cycle.[5] Infection with HPV can result in a clinical, subclinical, or latent infection, and in some cases it is thought to lead to the development of cancer.[6]

DETECTION OF HUMAN PAPILLOMAVIRUS

Human papillomavirus can not be cultured. At present, the only reliable way to detect and type HPV infection is by nucleic acid hybridization. A variety of nucleic acid hybridization techniques (dot blot, Southern transfer, in situ) can detect infection with HPV, differentiate between HPV types, and quantitate HPV deoxyribonucleic acid (DNA). Exfoliated epithelial cell samples or tissue biopsies, either fresh or fixed, can be analyzed. The collection, processing, and analysis of samples for dot blot, filter in situ, Southern transfer, and in situ hybridization assays have been extensively described elsewhere.[7] These assays vary considerably in sensitivity. Dot blot and Southern transfer have been shown to have equivalent sensitivity, specificity, and reproducibility for HPV DNA detection.[8] The amplification of HPV DNA prior to hybridization using a consensus primer polymerase chain reaction (PCR) technique offered increased sensitivity of detection.[9] A solution hybridization assay that can quantitate the HPV DNA in the

279

sample has become available.[10] The choice of method depends on the information desired, the expertise of the laboratory performing the test, and the turnaround time required for a result. Further studies are needed to determine the clinical significance of HPV DNA testing, including the clinical relevance of a positive HPV DNA result in the absence of a lesion, the importance of persistent HPV detection, and the significance of HPV DNA levels.

At present, we have no way of assessing past exposure to HPV. The detection of HPV antibodies in patient sera using a variety of HPV antigens has been described.[11] Currently, however, sensitive and specific serologic tests for detection of type-specific HPV are unavailable.

CLINICAL MANIFESTATIONS AND NATURAL HISTORY OF GENITAL HUMAN PAPILLOMAVIRUS INFECTION

HPV infections can result in clinically apparent and inapparent lesions. Clinically apparent lesions are raised and often papillary and are seen on physical examination on the vulva and in the perianal region. These lesions most commonly contain types of HPV not generally found in HPV-related cancers. Subclinical lesions, which are best visualized by colposcopy, are flat lesions seen on the cervix and in the internal anal canal. It is these lesions that are thought to be most closely related to cancer.[12] Perianal condylomata, the most common visible manifestations of anal HPV infection,[13] are frequently multifocal and may reach substantial size. Internal anal condylomata affect over 50% of men with external warts. Most of these are in the anal canal, but they can occur above the dentate line.

Since HPV can not be cultured and because only recently have techniques been developed allowing for sensitive and specific detection of the virus, little is known about the prevalence, development, and natural history of HPV infections. The reported incidence and prevalence of genital HPV infection are dependent on the population studied, the site or sites sampled, and the specific sampling method used. In addition, prevalence varies depending on whether HPV DNA is amplified prior to hybridization and on the number and type of HPV-specific probes used.[14–24] One 1991 study using PCR and a probe that detected a wide range of HPV types, found that in 46% of women attending a university health center, HPV was detected in vaginal or cervical specimens.[14] We have previously reported that 120 of 500 consecutive women (24%) attending a sexually transmitted disease (STD) clinic had cervical HPV DNA that was detected by using probes to 14 genital types of HPV without amplification of DNA. Few studies have focused on anal HPV. Our studies among consecutive women attending an STD clinic detected anal HPV in 53 of 1069 samples tested (5%), with HPV detected by dot blot hybridization. In contrast, among homosexual men with and without HIV infection, we found that 92% of those with, and 78% of those without, HIV infection had anal HPV DNA detected by PCR.

Genital warts, including anal warts, are thought to be very transmissible by direct sexual contact. Up to 60% of sexual partners of patients with genital warts developed genital warts themselves after an incubation period of 1 to 8 months.[25] The age at onset of genital warts parallels that of other sexually transmitted diseases. It is thought that sexual transmission of subclinical genital HPV infection may be as common as is that of condylomata. Studies have shown that the male sexual partners of females with cervical lesions were infected with mainly subclinical lesions in 43 to 77% of cases.[26–28] The average incubation period for developing genital warts after infection was 4 to 12 weeks.[25, 29] Subclinical or latent HPV infections are common and may persist for long periods.[6]

ASSOCIATION OF HUMAN PAPILLOMAVIRUS WITH GENITAL TRACT NEOPLASIA

Although the oncogenic properties of the cottontail rabbit papillomavirus (CRPV, or Shope's papillomavirus) was recognized as early as 1930, the importance of papillomaviruses in humans was not appreciated until the 1970s.[12, 30, 31] The development of recombinant DNA technology at this time allowed researchers to clone HPV DNA. On the basis of subsequent hybridization studies examining the DNA homology of HPV DNA in clinical samples, it became apparent that a large variety of types of HPV existed. Nearly 70 types of HPV have been characterized, with each type showing tropism for specific types of epithelium.[32] For example, HPV 1 is the cause of plantar warts and is rare in genital tract epithelium, whereas the so-called genital types of HPV, such as HPV 16, are generally found only in genital tract epithelium. Some genital HPVs are also found in the upper respiratory tract and are responsible for laryngeal papillomatosis.

The suggestion by Purola and Savia[33] and Meisels and Fortin[34] that changes seen in cervical cancer precursor lesions are related to genital wart virus infection led to studies of HPV in genital tract neoplasia. The ability to detect HPV in clinical samples by nucleic acid hybridization techniques enabled researchers to show that most genital warts as well as squamous cell cancers and precancerous lesions of the cervix and vulva contained specific types of HPV DNA.[35, 36] Genital types of HPV are often referred to as high-, intermediate-, or low-risk viruses on the basis of the frequency with which they are found in invasive cervical cancer.[37] The most common high-risk types are HPV 16, 18, 45, and 56. Intermediate-risk HPV viruses are 31, 33, 35, 39, 51, and 52. Those genital HPV viruses with a low oncogenic potential, most commonly found in clinically apparent vulvar and anal warts, include 6, 11, 42, 43, and 44.

A number of large case-control and cohort studies of the epidemiology of cervical cancer and the development of cervical intraepithelial neoplasia (CIN) have been carried out since the early 1970s that implicate HPV as the principal infectious agent.[38, 39] These studies along with extensive laboratory studies characterizing the oncogenic potential of specific types of HPV[40] have provided compelling evidence that specific types of HPV are the causal agent of most genital tract squamous cell cancers. Using what is now considered to be a relatively insensitive method for detection of HPV, a case-control study in Latin America among 759 women with invasive cervical cancer and 1467 randomly selected age-matched controls,[41] found HPV 16 or 18 in 471 of the patients (62%) and in 469 of the controls (32%), with a dose–response relationship observed with the strength of the hybridization reaction to HPV 16 or 18, after adjustment for age at first intercourse, number of sexual partners, parity, and Papanicolaou (Pap) smear history. Human papillomavirus 6 or 11 was also associated with cancer even in the absence of HPV 16 or 18 infection, but this is explained by their being surrogate markers of exposure to oncogenic types of HPV. A hospital-based, case-control study in China, with 101 cases and 146 controls selected from among women attending gynecology clinics and using the more sensitive PCR method, detected HPV 16 in 32 of 92 women (35%) with squamous cell carcinoma (but not in women with adenocarcinoma) and in 1% of 146 control women (odds ratio = 32.9 adjusted for age, age at first marriage, and age when starting smoking, 95%

confidence intervals = 7.7, 141.1).[42] Human papillomavirus 33 was detected in 2 cases of squamous cell carcinoma, 1 case of adenocarcinoma, and 0 of the control cases. Munoz and colleagues used three detection methods (ViraPap, Southern blot, and PCR with a consensus primer and generic and type-specific probes) in two population-based studies of invasive cervical cancer conducted in Colombia and Spain.[43] They reported that detection of HPV was strongly associated with cancer, with odds ratios greater than 10, adjusted for age, education, age at first coitus, and number of partners; that is, cancer patients were more than 10 times as likely to have HPV detected than were patients without cancer. The magnitude of associations between detection of DNA and cancer was higher when HPV DNA was detected by ViraPap or Southern blot compared with detection of HPV DNA by PCR.

Our understanding of the molecular biology of oncogenic types of HPV has increased considerably since the early 1990s. It is now thought that inactivation of two regulatory proteins by HPV proteins may be the mechanism important in cellular transformation.[40] It has been shown that HPV E6 and E7 proteins bind to, and inactivate, cellular proteins p53 and Rb105, respectively, which normally function as tumor suppressor proteins. The specificity of certain HPV types for development of cancer is demonstrated by the fact that primary cell lines have been transformed in vitro when infected with the E6 and E7 genes from HPV 16 or 18 but not with E6 or E7 genes from HPV 6 or 11, HPV types that are not often detected in genital cancer.

HUMAN PAPILLOMAVIRUS AND INVASIVE ANAL SQUAMOUS CELL CANCER

As with genital tract squamous epithelial neoplasias, HPV is thought to be involved in the pathogenesis of anal cancer and anal squamous intraepithelial lesions (ASIL). Squamous cell cancer of the anus has been shown to be strongly associated with a clinical history of genital or anal warts or both, and a high percentage of anal cancers have been found to contain the same HPV types (types 16, 18, and 31) found in cervical cancers.[44–52] Beckmann and colleagues, in a population-based, case-control study of anal cancer, found HPV DNA using in situ hybridization in 23 of 70 patients (33%) with anal squamous cell cancer (11 were types 16 or 18) and in 0 of 110 patients with adenocarcinoma of the colon.[53] Daling and colleagues, in a larger series of cases from the same population-based registry, found HPV using PCR in 89 of 129 cases (69%) of anal cancer.[54] Wolber and colleagues detected HPV DNA in 14 of 21 squamous cell tumors (67%) (12 were types 16 or 18) and in 0 of 14 cloacogenic carcinomas.[55] Scholefield and colleagues, using PCR to detect HPV DNA, found HPV type 16 in 50 of 173 anal squamous cell carcinomas (29%) taken from India, South Africa, Switzerland, Poland, Brazil, and the United Kingdom.[56]

ROLE OF COFACTORS IN DEVELOPMENT OF HUMAN PAPILLOMAVIRUS–RELATED MALIGNANCIES

Infection with specific HPV types is thought to be necessary, but not sufficient, for development of cancer. The development of malignancy also appears to depend on additional cofactors such as other sexually transmitted diseases or chemical cocarcinogens such as tobacco.[54, 57]

It is well established that iatrogenically immunosuppressed patients are at increased risk for HPV-related neoplasia, presumably as the result of decreased immunosurveillence of HPV.[58, 59] Human papillomavirus–related squamous cell cancers have been reported to be from 14 to 100 times higher in renal transplant patients than in women with a normal immune response. Not surprisingly, HIV-infected men and women, especially those with marked immunosuppression, also appear to be at increased risk for precancerous lesions, with reported odds ratios relating human immunodeficiency virus type 1(HIV 1) to squamous intraepithelial lesion (SIL) ranging from 3.3 to 14.7 times the likelihood of having SIL as HIV-negative persons.[60–69] We have reported that anal HPV DNA and anal cancer precursor lesions (high-grade ASIL) were significantly more common among HIV-seropositive men than among HIV-seronegative men.[70] Case reports of invasive cervical cancer among young HIV 1–infected women have also appeared.

NATURAL HISTORY OF ANAL HUMAN PAPILLOMA VIRUS INFECTION, ANAL INTRAEPITHELIAL LESIONS, AND INVASIVE ANAL CANCER

Although the relationship between CIN and invasive cervical cancer is well established,[71] un-til recently the relationship between what are presumed to be anal cancer precursor lesions, termed anal intraepithelial neoplasia 2-3 (AIN 2-3), and invasive anal cancer has not been closely examined. In part, this is due to the fact that although studies have demonstrated that cytologic detection of AIN lesions is possible with a sensitivity and specificity similar to that seen with cytologic examination of the cervix, there is no routine screening for AIN 2-3 among the population at risk, and detection of such lesions before the appearance of invasive cancer is rare. There are many reasons to believe that the relationship between AIN 2-3 and invasive anal cancer is similar to that between CIN 2-3 and invasive cervical cancer. First, AIN-2-3 and CIN 2-3 are thought to give rise to cancers that are remarkably similar, in regard to both their probable causal agent and their microscopic appearance.[72] Likewise, CIN and AIN appear to be closely related. They are histologically indistinguishable, and CIN 3, previously called carcinoma in situ, is frequently found adjacent to areas of invasive cervical cancer. In a review of 450 cases of anal cancer from a population-based study of anal cancer in Washington State and British Columbia, high-grade AIN was found adjacent to invasive tumor in more than 70% of cases. Furthermore, preliminary analysis of data from a continuing natural history study in Seattle shows that data for the development of AIN 2-3 as well as risk factors for progression to AIN 2-3 among HIV-seronegative men are similar to data previously reported by the Seattle group among HIV-seronegative women in regard to CIN 2-3. In summary, AIN 2-3 is likely to be a premalignant lesion, and some percentage of patients with this lesion, if untreated, are likely to develop invasive cancer.

ANAL NEOPLASIA IN HOMOSEXUAL MEN

Although anal cancer is rare in the general population, with an incidence among all men of 1.1 in 100,000, even before the acquired immunodeficiency syndrome (AIDS) epidemic, it was recognized as being from 25 to 50 times more common among homosexual men.[73] In 1980, prior to AIDS, Daling and colleagues estimated that the annual incidence of anal cancer among homosexual men was 12 to 36 in 100,000,[73] a rate approaching the annual incidence of cervical cancer in the United States (42/100,000) in 1947 before the establishment of Pap screening. Our own studies have demonstrated ASIL by anal cytology in 12% of homosexual men presenting to a community-based clinic for HIV testing and counseling, a rate similar to that of cervical squamous intraepithelial lesions (CSIL) among high-risk women attending an STD clinic.[70] The association between anal cancer and homosexual activity is presumably the result of receptive anal intercourse, with increased exposure of the anal epithelium to oncogenic HPV types. Anal intercourse has also been identified as a risk factor for anal cancer in women.[57] The increased risk of anal cancer among homosexual men has become of even greater importance since the advent of HIV. In our studies of homosexual men with and without HIV infection, we found that HPV DNA was detected by PCR among 92% of men with, and 78% of men without, HIV infection (OR = 4.7, 95% CI = 2.4, 9.1). Furthermore ASIL was noted in 24% of HIV-seropositive men and in 4.5% of seronegative men (OR = 9.1, 95% CI = 4.0, 21.4). High-grade SIL was noted only in men with HIV infection (2%). Among HIV-infected men, ASIL, detection of each anal HPV type studied, and detection of high levels of anal HPV DNA (i.e., levels of HPV DNA detectable by both Southern blot and PCR) were all associated with immunosuppression. Given these data, screening for AIN 2-3 among high-risk populations using anal cytologic smears may prove to be of considerable importance.

TREATMENT

Since fewer than 50% of patients infected with high-risk HPV types are thought to develop cancer subsequently, treatment of HPV-related lesions is based on the morphology, and not on the type, of HPV DNA present in the lesion. Furthermore, since there is no way of treating the viral infection, the aim of treatment is to eradicate the lesion, not to eliminate the virus. Local destructive treatment by means of surgery (including excision, CO_2 laser, electrocautery, cryotherapy) or of drugs (including cytotoxic agents, such as podophyllin, 5-fluorouracil, and trichloroacetic acid, and immune modulating agents such as interferon) have been described.[74, 75] There is no one method that has been considered superior to all others. Although intralesional interferon was previously shown to be effective in the treatment of condylomata acuminata, systemic interferon was of no benefit for cervical HPV disease in a placebo-controlled trial.[76]

Frequent follow-up visits are recommended after therapy because the rate of recurrence of HPV infection is high, ranging from 10 to 65%.[32] Since the virus may persist in normal adjacent tissue after treatment,[77, 78] recurrence may result from the reactivation of a latent infection. There is no therapy for latent or subclinical infection. Since it is not known if infection with HPV confers protection against subsequent reinfection with the same type and since no vaccine against HPV infection is available, recurrence may result from exogenous reinfection. It is difficult to distinguish between exogenous reinfection and the reactivation of latent infection. Prevention of reinfection through the examination and treatment of partners or the use of condoms has been suggested.[74]

REFERENCES

1. Stone KM. Epidemiologic aspects of genital HPV infection. Clin Obstet Gynecol. 1989;32:112–116.
2. Baefverstedt B. Condylomata acuminata—past and present. Acta Dermatol Venereol. 1967;47:376–381.
3. Krebs HB. Milestones in HPV research. Clin Obstet Gynecol. 1989;32:107–111.
4. Taichman LB, LaPorta RF. The expression of papillomaviruses in epithelial cells. In: Salzman NP, Howley PM, eds. The Papoviridiae. New York: Plenum Press; 1987;2:109.
5. Broker TR. Structure and genetic expression of papillomaviruses. Obstet Gynecol Clin North Am. 1987;14:329–348.
6. Syrjanen KJ. Epidemiology of human papillomavirus infections and their association with genital squamous cell cancer. APMIS. 1989;97:957–970.
7. Lorincz AT. Human papillomavirus detection tests. In: Holmes KK, Mardh PA, Sparling PF, et al. Sexually Transmitted Diseases. 2nd ed. New York: McGraw-Hill; 1990;953–959.
8. Kiviat NB, Koutsky LA, Critchlow CW, et al. Comparison of Southern transfer hybridization and dot filter hybridization for detection of cervical human papillomavirus infection with types 6, 11, 16, 18, 31, 33, and 35. Am J Clin Pathol. 1990;94:561–565.
9. Bauer HM, Greer CE, Manos MM. Detection of genital HPV infection using PCR. In: Herrington C, McGee J, eds. Diagnostic Molecular Pathology: A practical approach. Oxford: Oxford University Press; 1992;131–152.
10. Garcia M, Impraim C, Schiffman M, et al. Quantitative detection of HPV DNA with a sensitive chemiluminescence-based assay reveals a positive association between higher amounts of DNA and prevalent cervical disease. 11th International Papillomavirus Workshop. University of Edinburgh and Lothian Health Board, Edinburgh, Scotland, 1992; Abstract 297.
11. Galloway DA. Serological assays for the detection of HPV antibodies. In: Munoz N, Bosch FX, Shah KV, Meheus A, eds. The epidemiology of human papillomavirus and cervical cancer. IARC Sci Publ. 1992;119:147–161.
12. Laverty CR, Russell P, Hills E, et al. The significance of noncondylomatous wart virus infections of the cervical transformation zone. Acta Cytol. 1978;22:195–201.
13. Palefsky J. Human papillomavirus infection among HIV-infected individuals: Implications for development of

malignant tumors. Hematol Oncol Clin North Am. 1991;5:357–370.

14. Bauer HM, Ting Y, Greer CE, et al. Genital human papillomavirus infection in female university students as determined by a PCR-based method. JAMA. 1991;265:472–477.

15. Burmer GC, Parker JD, Bates J, et al. Comparative analysis of human papillomavirus detection by polymerase chain reaction and Virapap/Viratype kits. Am J Clin Pathol. 1990;94:554–560.

16. Gravitt PE, Hakenwerth A, Stoerker J. A direct comparison of methods proposed for use in widespread screening of human papillomavirus infections. Mol Cell Probes. 1991;5:65–72.

17. Hallum N, Green J, Gibson P, et al. Prevalence of HPV cervical infection in a family planning clinic determined by polymerase chain reaction and dot blot hybridization. J Med Virol. 1991;4:154–158.

18. Melchers W, van den Brule A, Walboomers J, et al. Increased detection rate of human papillomavirus in cervical scrapes by the polymerase chain reaction as compared to modified FISH and southern-blot analysis. J Med Virol. 1989;27:329–335.

19. Morris BJ, Rose BR, Flanagan JL, et al. Automated polymerase chain reaction for papillomavirus screening of cervicovaginal lavages: Comparison with dot-blot hybridization in a sexually transmitted diseases clinic population. J Med Virol. 1990;32:22–30.

20. Morrison EAB, Ho GYF, Vermund SH, et al. Human papillomavirus infection and other risk factors for cervical neoplasia: A case-control study. Int J Cancer. 1991;49:6–13.

21. Schiffman MH, Bauer HM, Lorincz AT, et al. Comparison of Southern blot hybridization and polymerase chain reaction for the detection of human papillomavirus DNA. J Clin Microbiol. 1991;29:573–577.

22. Tham KM, Chow VTK, Singh P, et al. Diagnostic sensitivity of polymerase chain reaction and Southern blot hybridization for the detection of human papillomavirus DNA in biopsy specimens from cervical lesions. Am J Clin Pathol. 1991;95:638–646.

23. Guerrero E, Daniel RW, Bosch FX, et al. Comparison of ViraPap, Southern hybridization and polymerase chain reaction methods for human papillomavirus identification in an epidemiological investigation of cervical cancer. J Clin Microbiol. 1992;30:2951–2959.

24. Kuypers J, Critchlow CW, Gravitt PE, et al. Comparison of detection of anal human papillomavirus infection by dot filter hybridization, Southern transfer hybridization and polymerase chain reaction amplification. J Clin Microbiol. 1993;31:1003–1006.

25. Oriel JD. Natural history of genital warts. Br J Vener Dis. 1971;47:1–13.

26. Schiffman MH. Recent progress in defining the epidemiology of human papillomavirus infection and cervical neoplasia. J Natl Cancer Inst. 1992;84:394–398.

27. Barrasso R, DeBrux J, Croissant O, et al. High prevalence of papillomavirus-associated penile intraepithelial neoplasia in sexual partners of women with cervical intraepithelial neoplasia. N Engl J Med. 1987;317:916–923.

28. Schneider A, Kirchmayr R, DeVilliers EM, et al. Subclinical human papillomavirus infections in male sexual partners of female carriers. J Urol. 1988;140:1431–1434.

29. Barrett TJ, Silbar JD, McGinley JP. Genital warts—a venereal disease. JAMA. 1954;54:333–334.

30. Kessler II. Human cervical cancer as a venereal disease. Cancer Res. 1976;36:783–791.

31. zur Hausen H. Human papillomaviruses and their possible role in squamous cell carcinomas. Curr Top Microbiol Immunol. 1977;78:1–30.

32. von Krogh G. Genital papillomavirus infection: Diagnostic and therapeutic objectives in the light of current epidemiological observations. Int J STD AIDS. 1991;2:391–404.

33. Purola E, Savia E. Cytology of gynecologic condyloma acuminatum. Acta Cytol. 1977;21:26–31.

34. Meisels A, Fortin R. Condylomatous lesions of the cervix and vagina: I, Cytologic patterns. Acta Cytol. 1976;20:505–509.

35. zur Hausen H, Schneider A. The role of papillomaviruses in human anogenital cancer. In: Howley PM, Salzman NP, eds. The Papillomaviruses. New York: Plenum; 1987;2:245–263.

36. Riou G, Favre M, Jeannel D, et al. Association between poor prognosis in early-stage invasive cervical carcinomas and non-detection of HPV DNA. Lancet. 1991;335:1171–1174.

37. Lorincz AT, Reid R, Jenson AB, et al. Human papillomavirus infection of the cervix: Relative risk association of 15 common anogenital types. Obstet Gynecol. 1992;79:328–337.

38. Munoz N, Bosch FX. HPV and cervical cancer: Review of case-control and cohort studies. In: Munoz N, Bosch FX, Shah KV, Meheus A, eds. The epidemiology of human papillomavirus and cervical cancer. IARC Sci Pub. (Lyon) 1992;119:251–261.

39. zur Hausen H. The role of papillomaviruses in anogenital cancer. Scand J Infect Dis. 1990;69:107–111.

40. Howley PM. Role of the human papillomaviruses in human cancer. Cancer Res. 1991;51(suppl):S5019–S5022.

41. Reeves WC, Brinton LA, Garcia M, et al. Human papillomavirus infection and cervical cancer in Latin America. N Engl J Med. 1989;320:1437–1441.

42. Peng HQ, Liu SL, Mann V, et al. Human papillomavirus types 16 and 33, herpes simplex virus type 2 and other risk factors for cervical cancer in Sichuan Province, China. Int J Cancer. 1991;47:711–716.

43. Munoz N, Bosch RX, Sanjose S, et al. The causal link between human papillomavirus and invasive cervical cancer: A population-based case-control study in Colombia and Spain. Int J Cancer. 1992;52:743–749.

44. Hill SA, Coghill SB. Human papillomavirus in squamous carcinoma of anus. Lancet. 1986;2:1333.

45. Duggan MA, Boras VF, Inoue M, et al. Human papillomavirus DNA determination of anal condylomata, dysplasias, and squamous carcinomas with in situ hybridization. Am J Clin Pathol. 1989;92:16–21.

46. Gal AA, Saul SH, Stoler MH. In situ hybridization analysis of human papillomavirus in anal squamous cell carcinoma. Mod Pathol. 1989;2:439–443.

47. Kiyabu MT, Shibata D, Arnheim N, et al. Detection of human papillomavirus in formalin-fixed, invasive squamous carcinomas using the polymerase chain reaction. Am J Surg Pathol. 1989;13:221–224.

48. Kulski JK, Demeter T, Mutavdzic S, et al. Survey of histologic specimens of human cancer for human papillomavirus types 6/11/16/18 by filter in situ hybridization. Am J Clin Pathol. 1990;94:566–570.

49. Scholefield JM, Sonnex C, Talbot IC, et al. Anal and cervical intraepithelial neoplasia: Possible parallel. Lancet. 1989;12:765–769.

50. Palefsky J, Holly EA, Gonzales J, et al. Detection of human papillomavirus DNA in anal intraepithelial neoplasia and anal cancer. Cancer Res. 1991;51:1014–1019.

51. Scholefield JH, McIntyre P, Palmer JG, et al. DNA hybridization of routinely processed tissue for detecting HPV DNA in anal squamous cell carcinomas over 40 years. J Clin Pathol. 1990;43:133–136.

52. Palmer JG, Scholefield JH, Coates PJ, et al. Anal cancer and human papillomaviruses. Dis Colon Rectum. 1989;32:1016–1022.

53. Beckmann AM, Daling JR, Sherman KJ, et al. Human papillomavirus infection and anal cancer. Int J Cancer. 1989;43:1042–1049.

54. Daling JR, Sherman KJ, Hislop TG, et al. Cigarette smoking and the risk of anogenital cancer. Am J Epidemiol. 1992;135:180–189.

55. Wolber R, Dupuis B, Thiyagaratnam P, et al. Anal cloacogenic and squamous carcinomas: Comparative histologic analysis using in situ hybridization for human papillomavirus DNA. Am J Surg Pathol. 1990;14:176–182.

56. Scholefield JH, Kerr IB, Shepherd NA, et al. Human papillomavirus type 16 DNA in anal cancers from six different countries. Gut. 1991;32:674–676.

57. Daling JR, Weiss NS, Hislop TG, et al. Sexual practices, sexually transmitted diseases, and the incidence of anal cancer. N Engl J Med. 1987;317:973–977.

58. Penn I. Cancers of the anogenital region in renal transplant recipients. Cancer. 1986;58:611–615.

59. Sillman FH, Sedlis A. Anogenital papillomavirus infection and neoplasia in immunodeficient women. Obstet Gynecol Clin North Am. 1987;15:537–558.

60. Byrne MA, Taylor-Robinson D, Munday PE, et al. The common occurrence of human papillomavirus infection and intraepithelial neoplasia in women infected by HIV. AIDS. 1989;3:379–382.

61. Caussy D, Goedert JJ, Palefsky J, et al. Interaction of human immunodeficiency and papilloma viruses: Association with anal epithelial abnormality in homosexual men. Int J Cancer. 1990;46:214–219.

62. Feingold AR, Vermund SH, Burk RD, et al. Cervical cytologic abnormalities and papillomavirus in women infected with human immunodeficiency virus. J Acquir Immune Defic Syndr. 1990;3:896–903.

63. Frazer IH, Medly G, Crapper RM, et al. Association between anorectal dysplasia, human papillomavirus, and human immunodeficiency virus infection in homosexual men. Lancet. 1986;2:657–660.

64. Henry MJ, Stanley MW, Cruikshank S, et al. Association of human immunodeficiency virus–induced immunosuppression with human papillomavirus infection and cervical intraepithelial neoplasia. Am J Obstet Gynecol. 1989;160:352–353.

65. Laga M, Icenogle JP, Marsella R, et al. Genital papillomavirus infection and cervical dysplasia: opportunistic complications of HIV infection. Int J Cancer. 1992;50:45–48.

66. Melbye M, Palefsky J, Gonzales J, et al. Immune status as a determinant of human papillomavirus detection and its association with anal epithelial abnormalities. Int J Cancer. 1990;46:203–206.

67. Palefsky JM, Gonzales J, Greenblatt R, et al. Anal intraepithelial neoplasia and anal papillomavirus infection among homosexual males with group IV HIV disease. JAMA. 1990;263:2911–2916.

68. Schafer A, Friedmann W, Mielke M, et al. The increased frequency of cervical dysplasia–neoplasia in women infected with the human immunodeficiency virus is related to the degree of immunosuppression. Am J Obstet Gynecol. 1991;164:593–599.

69. Vermund SH, Kelley KF, Klein RS, et al. High risk of human papillomavirus infection and cervical squamous intraepithelial lesions among women with symptomatic human immunodeficiency virus infection. Am J Obstet Gynecol. 1991;165:392–400.

70. Kiviat NB, Critchlow CW, Holmes KK, et al. Association of anal dysplasia and human papillomavirus with immunosuppression and HIV infection among homosexual men. AIDS. 1993;7:43–49.

71. Kiviat NB, Critchlow CW, Kurman RJ. Reassessment of the morphological continuum of cervical intraepithelial lesions: Does it reflect different stages in the progression to cervical carcinoma? In: Munoz N, Bosch FX, Shah KV, Meheus A, eds. The epidemiology of human papillomavirus and cervical cancer. IARC Sci Pub. (Lyon, France) 1992;119:59–66.

72. Melbye M, Sprogel P. Aetiological parallel between anal cancer and cervical cancer. Lancet. 1991;338:657–659.

73. Daling JR, Weiss NS, Klopfenstein LL, et al. Correlates of homosexual behavior and the incidence of anal cancer. JAMA 1982;247:1988–1990.

74. Koutsky LA, Pal WH. Genital papillomavirus infections: Current knowledge and future prospects. Sex Transm Dis. 1989;16:541–564.

75. Kraus SJ, Stone KM. Management of genital infection caused by human papillomavirus. Rev Infect Dis. 1990;12(suppl):S620–S632.

76. Gall SA, Hughes CE, Trofatter K. Interferon for the therapy of condylomata acuminata. Am J Obstet Gynecol. 1985;153:157.

77. Ferenczy A, Mitao M, Nagai N, et al. Latent papillomavirus and recurring genital warts. N Engl J Med. 1985;313:784–788.

78. MacNab CM, Walkinshaw SA, Cordiner JW, et al. Human papillomavirus in clinically and histologically normal tissue of patients with genital cancer. N Engl J Med. 1986;315:1052–1058.

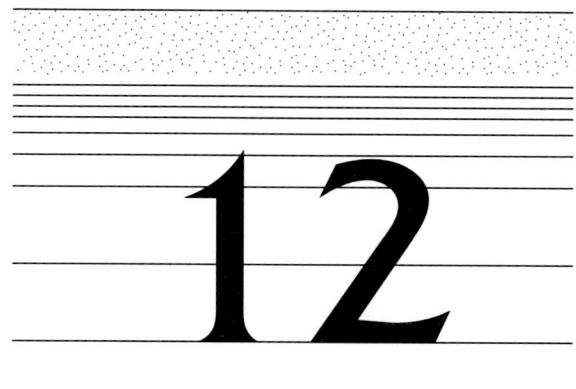

Colorectal Spirochetosis

CHRISTINA M. SURAWICZ, M.D.

In 1967 when Harland and Lee described intestinal spirochetes on the mucosal surface of a rectal biopsy from a man with chronic diarrhea,[1] they revived interest in spirochetes, which had been recognized in the intestinal flora with the advent of microscopy more than a century earlier. Numerous reports have detailed the presence of nontreponemal spirochetes in the bowel and in stool specimens since Harland and Lee's report, but it is still not clear whether these organisms are pathogens or, as is more likely, commensal flora. The term intestinal spirochetosis is misleading, however, because these organisms are found only in the colon, rectum, and appendix and not in the small intestine or more proximal locations. For this reason, the term colorectal spirochetosis is preferable.

HISTORICAL ASPECTS

Van Leeuwen first observed motile spirochete organisms in human stools, and Escherich first detailed human colorectal spirochetosis in a report published in 1884.[2] By 1923, more than 50 articles had described the presence of these organisms in patients with various intestinal conditions, including dysentery and cholera as well as nondiarrheal diseases.[3] Two reviews of colorectal spirochetosis were published in 1989 and 1990,[4, 5] one of which presents a table of the

results of early surveys of spirochetes in the stools, documenting a much higher rate than that seen today.[5] The differences may be due to differences in the populations examined or to an actual change in prevalence.

In the patient studied by Harland and Lee,[1] a 64-year-old man with chronic diarrhea, electron microscopy was used to visualize the organisms, which were described as penetrating a short distance into the epithelial cells, with occasional vacuoles around the organisms at the tip of infected colonic epithelial cells. When 100 colon biopsies were reviewed, spirochetosis was present in 10 patients, all of whom had intestinal symptoms.[6] The term intestinal spirochetosis was used. The morphology resembled the *Spirochaeta eurygyrata* described by Hogue in 1922.[7]

These organisms are present in monkeys as well as humans.[8–10] In monkeys, they were present in 14% of controls. The prevalence of spirochetosis in the human colon varies from between 1.9 and 6.9% in unselected populations[5] to between 30 and 36% in homosexual men.[11, 12]

Spirochetosis is present in 2.1 to 7.6% of normal appendices, 0.7 to 44% of inflamed appendices, and 9.8 to 12.6% of normal appendices that have been removed for symptoms of appendicitis.[13]

It is difficult to know the true prevalence of spirochetosis, since colon biopsies are usually taken only if symptoms are present, and this infestation, detected by biopsy, is not associated with gross changes in the colonic mucosa. The organisms have also been cultured.[14]

DIAGNOSIS: PATHOLOGY AND MICROBIOLOGY

When present, spirochetes can be detected by careful microscopic examination of the luminal surface of colonic biopsies (Figs. 12–1, 12–2). Standard hematoxylin and eosin (H & E) stains reveal a thickened (3 μm) blue band that coats the surface of the epithelial and goblet cells and extends a short distance into the crypts. Under higher power, individual spiral organisms can be detected. The organisms are gram-negative, stain strongly with periodic acid-Schiff (PAS) and weakly with alcian blue. Occasionally, when the mucus layer stains similarly, the diagnosis can be confused with spirochetosis,[15] but this confusion can be avoided by using silver stains. Silver stains, such as Steiner or Dieterle's stains, make diagnosis of spirochetosis easier. In a study of spirochetosis in rectal biopsies in homosexual men, silver stains increased the detection by 100% (Fig. 12–3).[12] The surface epithelium is normal, and there is no inflammation in the lamina propria. It is easy to miss this somewhat subtle finding, which can appear patchy by light microscopy but usually appears widespread by electron microscopy.[16]

The organism attaches diffusely to the surface of the mucosa, both to absorptive and to goblet cells (Figs. 12–4, 12–5). In some instances, organisms are present in vacuoles and lysosomes in the apical cytoplasm of the absorptive cells and in macrophages in the lamina propria. By immunohistochemical analysis, some have found an increase in immunoglobulin E–(IgE)–containing plasma cells in the lamina propria.[17] Cystlike associated structures have been seen in epithelial cells and in mucosal macrophages,[18] suggesting that the organism may act like a parasite in certain circumstances.

By electron microscopy, some spirochetes have a wave length of 2 μm, a width of 0.2 μm, and a length of 1.7 to 6.0 μm, and there are usually four flagella at each end. Some variants, however, may be wider or have six flagella. Spirochetes attach to the end of microvilli or between them, and the microvilli may be more sparse than is normal (see Fig. 13–4).

There are at least two different types of spirochetes. The larger *Spirochaeta eurygyrata*, has the characteristics of 4 to 10 μm length, 0.2 to 0.5 μm diameter, and irregular coils. It is a strict anaerobe and is now classified in the genus *Treponema*. The smaller organism is a regularly coiled spirochete up to 6 μm in length and 0.2 μm in diameter, with differences in morphology and growth characteristics that distinguish it from other treponemes. The original organisms described by Harland and Lee were smaller than treponemes and were considered to be in the *Borrelia* genus. Isolation of organisms by Danish[19, 20] and Italian[21] investigators has led to suggestions of a new genus of the family Treponemataceae, with proposed names *Brachyspira aalborgi* and Treponeae D 60. With the advent of culture methods,[14] the organisms have been isolated from stool specimens from people in Italy, Belgium, and Rwanda. The organisms isolated in 1986 from homosexual men were believed to be different from *B. aalborgii* because they were less fastidious, grew faster, and were culturable at 39° and 42° C.[22, 23] They are strict anaerobes. They are classified as *Treponema* species, because they resemble nonpathogenic commensal treponemes from pig intestine. It appears that there are at least two, a smaller and a larger organism, as noted in 1974.[24]

CLINICAL SIGNIFICANCE

Spirochetosis has been found in individuals from widely separated regions, including the United States, United Kingdom, Denmark, Belgium, Italy, and Africa, suggesting that spirochetes are present worldwide.

After their initial case report, Harland and Lee surveyed rectal biopsies and appendiceal specimens. In a Scottish population, they found a prevalence of 6.9%, although in none of the 14 cases found was there any relationship of spirochetosis to clinical symptoms.[6] Symptoms were usually due to underlying disease, although the cause of symptoms in two middle-aged men with diarrhea could not be established since they were lost to follow-up. In a survey of rectal biopsies from 300 consecutive patients in Denmark who were referred for sigmoidoscopy for a variety of reasons, spirochetosis was present in 15 (5%). In all cases, the colonic mucosa was normal both grossly and histologically. The persistence of symptoms in patients whose treatment with neomycin and bacitracin eliminated the spirochetes argues against pathogenesis of symptoms by spirochetes.[19]

Although most of the larger surveys suggest no pathogenic role for these organisms, individual case reports suggest that they may occasionally cause symptoms. Individual patients with

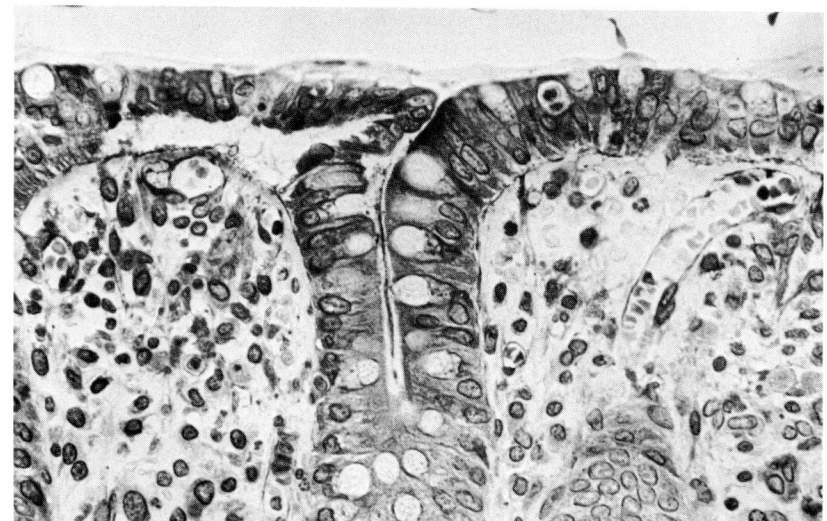

FIGURE 12–1.
Rectal biopsy specimen without spirochetosis.

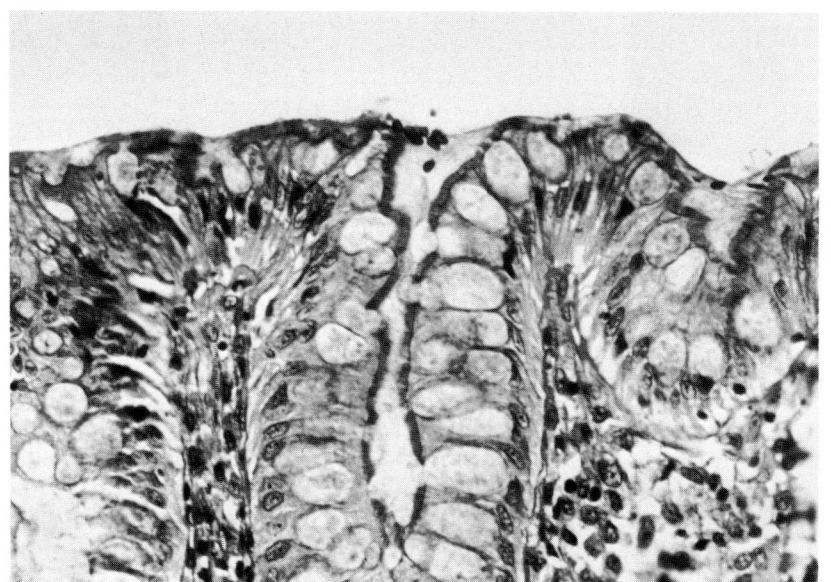

FIGURE 12–2.
An otherwise normal rectal biopsy specimen from a homosexual man shows a thickened band of spirochetes along the surface of the sample. The organisms often extend a short distance into the top of crypts. (hematoxylin-eosin, alcian blue, × 1000) SOURCE: Surawicz CM, Goodell SE, Quinn TC, et al. Spectrum of rectal biopsy abnormalities in homosexual men with intestinal symptoms. Gastroenterology. 1986;91:651–659.

FIGURE 12–3.
The spirochetes stain darkly with silver and are even more apparent along the surface of the rectal biopsy specimen (Warthin-Starry, × 550) SOURCE: Surawicz CM, Roberts PL, Rompalo A, et al. Intestinal spirochetosis in homosexual men. Am J Med. 1987;82:587–592.

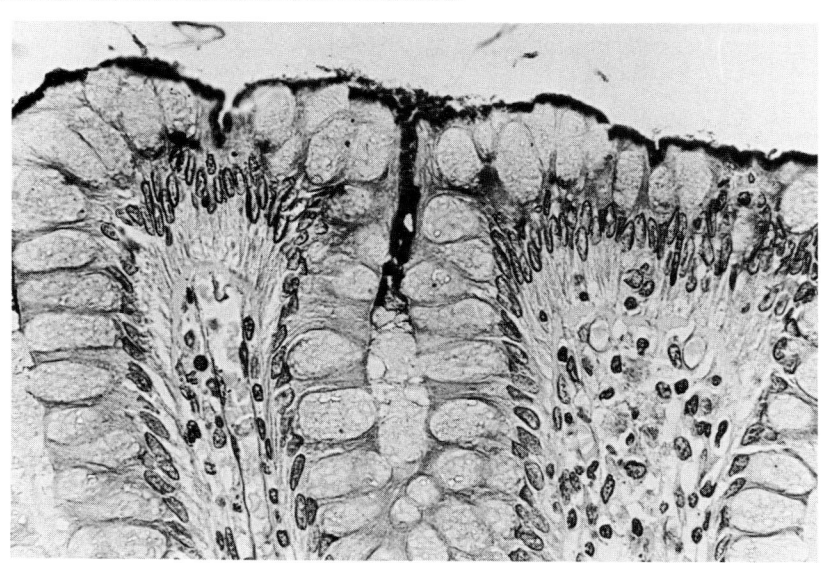

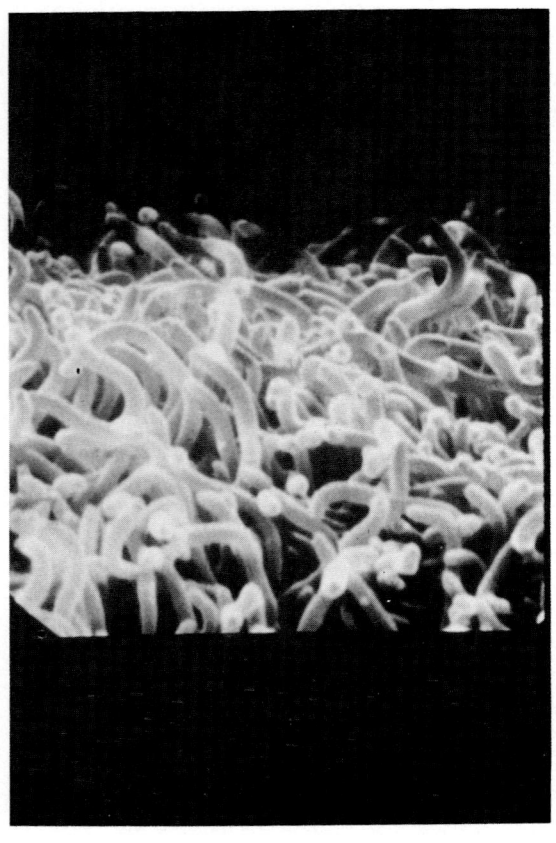

FIGURE 12–4.
Scanning electron microscopy shows spirochetes coating the mucosal surface of the rectum. SOURCE: Courtesy of Mr Ben O Spurlock, BA, Medical College of Georgia, Augusta, GA.

spirochetosis have had resolution of symptoms after metronidazole therapy.[25] For example, one patient with ulcerative colitis and adenomatous polyps had a heavy infestation and responded to treatment,[16] and the author has had a similar experience with another young man with ulcerative colitis and spirochetosis. In this setting, however, it is hard to know whether the symptoms were due to the organism or to the underlying bowel disease. It is possible that the alteration in bowel flora due to the ulcerative colitis or its treatment permits an overgrowth of spirochetes. Similarly, the occurrence of spirochetosis in a 16-year-old female who developed chronic

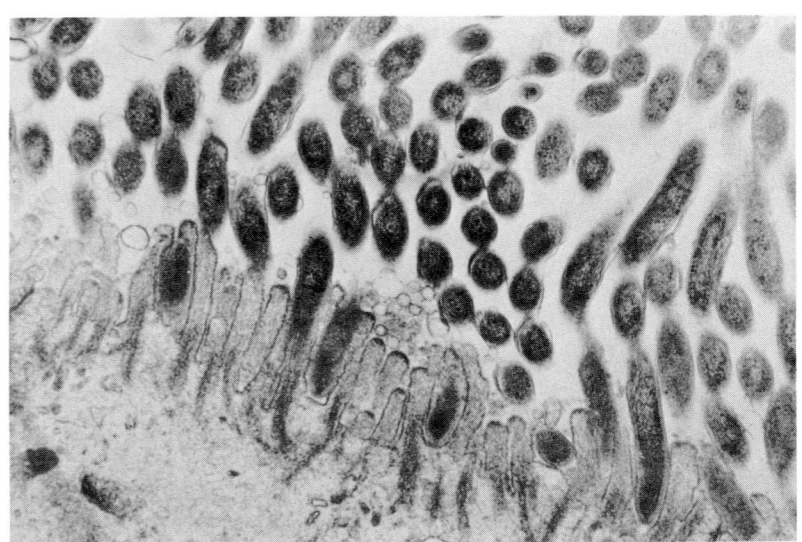

FIGURE 12–5.
Transmission electron microscopy shows spirochetes coating the mucosal surface of the rectum. Note spiral-shaped spirochetes attached longitudinally between the microvilli. Stained with uranyl acetate and lead citrate. SOURCE: Courtesy of Dr. Kenneth F Grant, MD, Blodgett Memorial Hospital, Grand Rapids, MI.

diarrhea after a course of amoxicillin raises the possibility that the bowel flora altered by antibiotics allowed colonization with the spirochetes. This patient had a spontaneous resolution of spirochetosis after she used metronidazole suppositories for only 2 days; interestingly, she experienced a relapse and was found to be reinfected with spirochetes and was retreated.[26]

With the advent of methods for culture, populations can be screened by analysis of stool specimens or rectal swab. Tompkins, in a 1986 evaluation of rectal swabs or stool analysis in 1527 people, detected 23 (1.5%) with spirochetosis, all of whom were either Asian (especially East Indian) or homosexual.[22] These individuals were screened from two different cities in England: Bradford, where there was a large immigrant population, and Leeds. In Bradford, spirochetosis was detected in 11.6% of those screened, all of whom were Asians and only one of whom had diarrhea. Of the Leeds group, only homosexuals tested positive (20%), and none of them had any intestinal symptoms.

A survey from Greece found spirochetosis in 24 of 145 cases (17%),[27] and in a Gulf Arab population it was present in 11.4% of hospitalized patients but also in 26.7% of 292 healthy controls. There was no association with gastrointestinal symptoms or other abnormalities in the stool.[28] In this study, the spirochetes were cultured from stool specimens and were found to be morphologically identical to the larger *Spirochaeta eurygyrata*. The higher prevalence in this study is probably due to many factors, which may include the methods used as well as the population studied.

In summary, individual case reports suggest occasional cure of intestinal symptoms with eradication of spirochetosis, but most larger surveys show no association. Geographic variation suggests that different populations have differing prevalence of spirochetosis, possibly reflecting differences in intestinal microflora.

APPENDICITIS

Spirochetosis had been seen in 9.6% of appendices removed for appendicitis-like symptoms in the 1930s.[29] One of the patients with spirochetosis noted in Harland and Lee's 1967 paper had attacks of abdominal pain that led to appendectomy, and spirochetes were found in the resected appendix.[1] In a later survey of surgically excised appendices, spirochetosis was found in 9.8% of appendices resected for appendicitis-like symptoms and 4.4% of appendices from patients with appendicitis.[6] An exten-

sive study from Denmark evaluated 671 appendectomy specimens. Of the 564 patients with suspected acute appendicitis, 414 actually had histologically confirmed appendicitis, but only 3 of these (0.7%) had spirochetosis. In contrast, 13 (12.6%) of the 106 patients without histologic appendicitis had spirochetosis. None of 44 patients with other pathologic conditions had spirochetosis, yet 2 (1.9%) of 107 incidentally removed appendices showed spirochetosis.[13] This paper suggests an increase in spirochetosis in patients who clinically presented with appendicitis, but in whom the appendix was normal. The prevalence of spirochetosis in the two studies is shown in Table 12–1.

SPIROCHETOSIS IN HOMOSEXUAL MEN

Since the 1970s, there has been recognition that the incidence of spirochetosis is increased in homosexual men. In 1979 a 36-year-old homosexual man with an 18-month history of anal discharge was found to have spirochetosis; the man's symptoms cleared after treatment with penicillin.[30] The two largest surveys of spirochetosis in homosexual men come from Glasgow[11] and Seattle.[12] In the Glasgow study, spirochetosis was present in 36% of men attending a genitourinary clinic. In the Seattle study of sexually transmitted colitis, 136 homosexual men were evaluated, most of whom (92%) had intestinal symptoms. Spirochetosis was present in biopsies from 30% of homosexual men and absent in all heterosexual controls. Most of the colonic biopsies were otherwise normal, although there was an association with rectal gonorrhea.

Ruane found spirochetosis in 33 patients at the West Los Angeles Veterans Administration Medical Center and was able to do clinical follow-up.[5] All 33 were men, reflecting their patient population; the average age was 44 (25–75 years old); 18 were homosexual, and 10 of these

TABLE 12–1. ASSOCIATION OF SPIROCHETOSIS AND APPENDECTOMY SPECIMENS

	LEE	HENRIK-NIELSEN
Appendicitis	4.4	0.7%
Negative appendectomy	9.8	12.6
Incidental appendectomy	3.8	1.9

REFERENCE: Lee FD, Kraszewski A, Gordon J, et al. Intestinal spirochetosis. Gut. 1971; 12:126–133.
Henrik-Nielsen R, Lundbeck FA, Teglbjaerg PS, et al. Intestinal spirochetosis of the vermiform appendix. Gastroenterology. 1985;88:971–977.

had HIV infection. Five men had other gastrointestinal illnesses (Crohn's disease, irritable bowel syndrome, and peptic ulcer disease), and 10 had other intestinal pathogens. Two men had no diarrhea. Of the seven men with diarrhea, five had resolution after treatment and two did not. Diarrhea had resolved spontaneously in an additional three men who were not treated.[5]

Treatment results in homosexual populations have been variable, with individual men who have responded to treatment with penicillin or metronidazole. In this population, however, multiple infections are frequent,[31] as evidenced by the association with gonorrhea. It is possible that the antibiotics are actually eradicating another pathogen that was not detected. Similarly, the presence of spirochetosis may indicate an overall alteration in the bowel flora associated with anal sexual contact. One gay man with 6 weeks of abdominal pain, nausea, diarrhea, and malaise had threadworms in his stool and spirochetosis by biopsy. He was treated with both metronidazole and mebendazole. He was reported as a treatment success attributed to metronidazole because the threadworm was thought unlikely to have caused his symptoms.[32] As these authors point out, spirochetosis is associated with normal rectal mucosa, and therefore its presence is often underestimated, as biopsies are less likely to be taken. Other individual cases suggest occasional pathogenicity.[33]

A few cases of spirochetosis are reported in patients with AIDS, but there is no clear or convincing evidence that the organism is a pathogen in this immunosuppressed population. Three persons with AIDS and chronic diarrhea had resolution of chronic diarrhea and eradication of spirochetes after a course of metronidazole.[34, 35] There is no certainty that this resolution was a treatment response, since there are many causes for diarrhea in persons with AIDS.

Thus, the evidence for pathogenicity relies on individual case reports of diarrhea. In a series of 15 patients who were treated with neomycin and bacitracin, there was no change in symptoms.[12]

SUMMARY

Colorectal spirochetosis probably has worldwide distribution. In selected populations, it has been found in 1.9 to 16.5% of persons when rectal biopsies have been evaluated. It has been found in up to 10% of appendectomy specimens.

The organism can be present when there are no gastrointestinal symptoms[36] or when other abnormalities, such as colon cancer, are present.[1] In some cases, symptoms resolve with therapy.[37] The organism can be eradicated with metronidazole, but symptoms may persist.[19] In other cases, spirochetosis or gastrointestinal symptoms or both may resolve spontaneously.[34]

In homosexual men, the prevalence of spirochetosis is high: 30 to 36%. In such patients, symptoms of diarrhea, bleeding, or purulent discharge have been attributed to spirochetosis. Two men with proctitis noted resolution of symptoms after metronidazole therapy. It is possible, however, that their symptoms were due to one or more of the many other pathogens that are present in such populations.[31] These studies, done before the recognition of the AIDS epidemic, showed frequent spirochetosis and frequent intestinal pathogens. There is evidence that sexually transmitted colitis has decreased markedly, probably owing to changes in sexual practice. Whether spirochetosis has decreased is not known, but the 1989 survey in Los Angeles suggests that it is still a common finding.[5] Not surprisingly, spirochetosis has been found in men with HIV infection but has not been demonstrated to be a pathogen.

There is no evidence that the organism is invasive, and there is no convincing evidence for pathogenicity. Most likely, the finding of spirochetosis indicates altered gut microecology, but spirochetes may be pathogens in occasional cases.

REFERENCES

1. Harland WA, Lee FD. Intestinal spirochetosis. Br Med J. 1967;3:718–719.
2. Escherich T. Klinisch-therapeutische Beobachtungen aus der Cholera Epidemie in Neapel. Munchener Medizinische Wochenschrift. 1884;31:561–564.
3. Parr LW. Intestinal spirochetes. J Infect Dis. 1923;33: 369–383.
4. Teglbjaerg PS. Intestinal spirochaetosis. Curr Top Pathol. 1990;81:247–256.
5. Ruane PJ, Nakata MM, Reinhardt JF, George WL. Spirochete-like organisms in the human gastrointestinal tract. Rev Infect Dis. 1989;11:184–196.
6. Lee FD, Kraszewski A, Gordon J, et al. Intestinal spirochetosis. Gut. 1971;12:126–133.
7. Hogue MJ. *Spirochaeta eurygyrata*. A note on its life history and cultivation. J Exp Med. 1922;36:617–626.
8. Takeuchi A, Zeller JA. Ultrastructural identification of spirochetes and flagellated microbes at the brush border of the large intestinal epithelium of the rhesus monkey. Infect Immun. 1972;6:1008–1018.
9. Takeuchi A, Jervis HR, Nakazawa H, et al. Spiral-shaped organisms on the surface colonic epithelium of the monkey and man. Am J Clin Nutr. 1974;27:1287–1296.
10. Takeuchi A, Zeller JA. Scanning electron microscopic observations on the surface of the normal and spiro-

chete-infested colonic mucosa of the rhesus monkey. J Ultrastruct Res. 1972;40:313–324.

11. McMillan A, Lee FD. Sigmoidoscopic and microscopic appearance of the rectal mucosa in homosexual men. Gut. 1981;22:1035–1041.

12. Surawicz CM, Roberts PL, Rompalo A, et al. Intestinal spirochetosis in homosexual men. Am J Med. 1987;82:587–592.

13. Henrik-Nielsen R, Lundbeck FA, Teglbjaerg PS, et al. Intestinal spirochetosis of the vermiform appendix. Gastroenterology. 1985;88:971–977.

14. Tompkins DS, Waugh MA, Cooke EM. Isolation of intestinal spirochaetes from homosexuals. J Clin Pathol. 1981;34:1385–1387.

15. Roberts KM, Cotton DWK, Shortland JR. Electron microscopy to differentiate intestinal spirochetosis from other conditions. Genitourin Med. 1989;65:200. Letter.

16. Willen R, Carlen B, Cronstedt J, et al. Intestinal spirochaetosis of the colon diagnosed with colono-ileoscopy and multiple biopsies. Endoscopy. 1985;17:86–88.

17. Gebbers JO, Ferguson DJP, Mason C, et al. Spirochaetosis of the human rectum associated with an intraepithelial mast cell and IgE plasma cell response. Gut. 1987;28:588–593.

18. Gebbers JO, Marder HP. Unusual in vitro formation of cyst-like structures associated with human intestinal spirochaetosis. Eur J Clin Microbiol Infect Dis. 1989;8:302–306.

19. Nielsen RH, Orholm M, Pedersen JO, et al. Colorectal spirochetosis: Clinical significance of the infestation. Gastroenterology. 1983;85:62–67.

20. Hovind-Hougen K, Birch-Andersen A, Henrik-Nielsen R, et al. Intestinal spirochetosis: Morphological characterization and cultivation of the spirochete *Brachyspira aalborgi* gen. nov., sp. nov. J Clin Microbiol. 1982;16:1127–1136.

21. Sanna A, Dettori G, Grillo R, et al. Isolation and propagation of a strain of treponema from the human digestive tract: Preliminary report. L'Igiene Moderna. 1982;77:287–297.

22. Tompkins DS, Foulkes SJ, Godwin PG, et al. Isolation and characterisation of intestinal spirochaetes. J Clin Pathol. 1986;39:535–541.

23. Cooper C, Cotton DWK, Hudson MJ, et al. Rectal spirochaetosis in homosexual men: Characterisation of the organism and pathophysiology. Genitourin Med. 1986;62:47–52.

24. Harris DL, Kinuon JM. Significance of anaerobic spirochetes in the intestines of animals. Am J Clin Nutr. 1974;27:1297–1304.

25. Cotton DWK, Kirkham N, Hicks DA. Rectal spirochaetosis. Br J Vener Dis. 1984;60:106–109.

26. Rodgers FG, Rodgers C, Shelton AP, et al. Proposed pathogenic mechanism for the diarrhea associated with human intestinal spirochetes. Am J Clin Pathol. 1986;86:679–682.

27. Delladetsima K, Markaki S, Papadimitriou K. Intestinal spirochaetosis: Light and electron microscopic study. Pathol Res Pract. 1987;182:780–782.

28. Barrett SP. Intestinal spirochaetes in a Gulf Arab population. Epidemiol Infect. 1990;104:261–266.

29. Mazza S. Espiroquetosis apendiculares. Prensa Med Argent. 1930;17:464–468.

30. Kaplan LR, Takeuchi A. Purulent rectal discharge associated with nontreponemal spirochete. JAMA. 1979;241:52–53.

31. Quinn TC, Stamm WE, Goodell SE, et al. The polymicrobial origin of intestinal infections in homosexual men. N Engl J Med. 1983;309:576–582.

32. Burns DG, Hayes MM. Rectal spirochetosis. Symptomatic response to metronidazole and mebendazole, a case report. S Afr Med J. 1985;68:335–336.

33. Douglas JG, Crucioli V. Spirochaetosis: A remediable cause of diarrhoea and rectal bleeding? Br Med J. 1981;283:1362.

34. Nathwani D, McWhinney PHM, Green ST, et al. Intestinal spirochaetosis in a man with the acquired immune deficiency syndrome (AIDS). J Infect. 1990;21:318–319.

35. Lafeuillade A, Quilichini R, Benderitter T, et al. Intestinal spirochaetosis in HIV infected homosexual men. Postgrad Med J. 1990;66:253–254. Letter.

36. Mooney EE, Casey M, Dervan PA. Intestinal spirochaetosis: Pathological entity of no clinical significance. Ir J Med Sci. 1988;157:324–325.

37. Crucioli V, Busuttil A. Human intestinal spirochaetosis. Scand J Gastroenterol. 1981;16(suppl 70):177–179.

4

Hepatobiliary Disorders

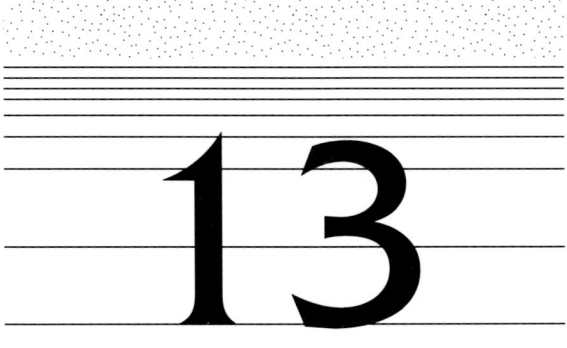

13

Diagnosis of Viral Hepatitis

RAYMOND S. KOFF, M.D.

Viral hepatitis is a major cause of acute and chronic liver disease throughout the world. Rates of infection by the various responsible agents vary from region to region and may even differ importantly among populations within a specific region. Increasing appreciation of the multiplicity of hepatitis viruses, the spectrum of the acute illness, and the wide range of sequelae of viral hepatitis, coupled with dramatic advances in strategies for the prevention of viral hepatitis and treatment of chronic viral hepatitis, support the necessity for accurate diagnosis of the responsible causal form. In addition, the practitioner must recognize and understand the clinical and epidemiologic context in which viral hepatitis has occurred, the influence of that context on the natural history of the disease, and the prevention of transmission. Gauging the immunocompetency of the affected patient is also an important issue because this information may prove prognostically and therapeutically critical in management.

Fortunately, for many of the forms of viral hepatitis now recognized, specific serologic tests are widely available and batteries of hepatitis markers can be routinely measured. Nonetheless, appropriate interpretation of these tests requires an understanding of the common and atypical patterns of appearance and disappearance of specific antigens and antibodies (for some agents specific viral nucleic acid can also

be measured) and the specificity, sensitivity, and limitations of the individual tests. Because knowledge of the virology and serology of viral hepatitis is incomplete and some serologic test procedures are investigational and restricted to a few research sites, many unresolved questions remain. In this chapter, current knowledge of the responsible agents, their epidemiologic features, natural history, and serologic diagnosis are reviewed. The influence of immunocompetency and immunodeficiency on diagnosis, course, and sequelae of viral hepatitis is presented. Where gaps in information and understanding exist, they are identified throughout the text.

ETIOLOGY OF VIRAL HEPATITIS

Responsible Agents

The major agents of viral hepatitis and their tentative classification into virus families are listed in Table 13–1. None of the known agents, with the exception of hepatitis B virus (HBV) and the HBV mutants is genetically related to any other. Hence, their shared association with hepatic necrosis and inflammation (Fig. 13–1) leads to their grouping here. Reported cases, studies of underreporting rates, and estimates of anicteric to icteric ratios and asymptomatic

TABLE 13–1. THE HUMAN HEPATITIS VIRUSES

VIRUS	GENOME	GENOME SIZE (In KB)	ENVELOPED	CLASSIFICATION	CYTOPATHIC IN VIVO
HAV	RNA	7.5	No	Picornavirus	No
HEV	RNA	7.5	No	?Calicivirus	?
HBV	DNA	3.2	Yes (HBsAg)	Hepadnavirus	No
HBV mutants	DNA	3.2	Yes (HBsAg)	Hepadnavirus	?No
HDV	RNA	1.7	Yes (HBsAg)	?Plant satellite	?
HCV	RNA	10.0	Yes	?Pestivirus	?

KEY: KB = Kilobase (1000 base pairs).

to symptomatic cases suggest that in excess of 600,000 new cases of viral hepatitis occur annually in the United States. Approximately 45 to 50% of these cases may be attributable to HBV infection, 25% are due to hepatitis A virus (HAV), and 25% to hepatitis C virus (HCV). Hepatitis D (delta virus) (HDV) infections probably account for less than 5% of cases; fewer than 100 cases of hepatitis E virus (HEV) are likely to be encountered in the United States.

Hepatitis A Virus

Hepatitis A virus, a small, 27 nm in diameter, nonenveloped RNA virus with a genome length of about 7470 nucleotides, has been classified as a member of the picornavirus family, presumably, but not definitively, in a new heparnavirus genus. HAV appears to be the only picornavirus that replicates in hepatocytes and is associated with hepatic injury. HAV has three incompletely characterized capsid proteins and a single copy of plus-stranded ribonucleic acid (RNA) with a

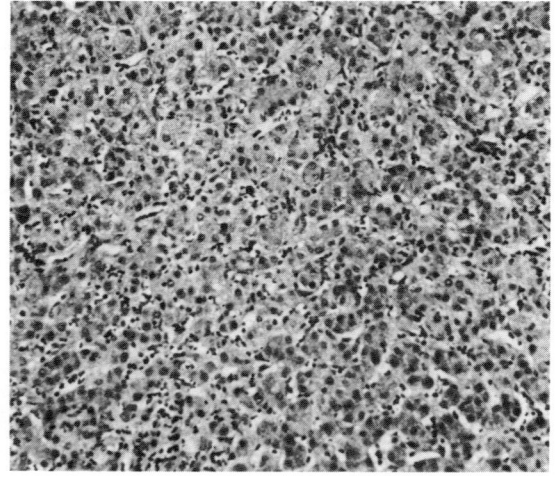

FIGURE 13–1.
Acute viral hepatitis, demonstrating hepatocyte degeneration, lobular disarray, and extensive lymphocytic infiltration of the hepatic parenchyma. Hematoxylin and eosin, × 120.

3'polyadenylated noncoding end and a 5' noncoding end that is covalently bound to protein. HAV is a hardy agent, demonstrating remarkable stability on exposure to acid, heat, or conventional agents of chemical inactivation. HAV can survive in water for prolonged periods lasting months and in the dried state, for as long as a week.

Distinct strains of HAV have been identified, based on the heterogeneity of HAV RNA nucleotides in sequenced isolates, but only one serotype is recognized. All HAV isolates appear to have one major immunodominant neutralization epitope on the surface of the capsid. The mechanism of HAV attachment to hepatocytes is uncertain. In vitro, HAV has been shown to attach to a wide range of cultured cells. This observation suggests that a specific receptor may not be present. Attachment is enhanced by calcium but not by magnesium, is greater at 4°C than at 37°C, and may be inhibited by some serum glycoproteins.[1] HAV can replicate, slowly, with a low virus yield, and without cytopathic effect, in human and monkey cell lines. In these cell cultures, HAV appears to be predominantly cell-associated and possesses some of the characteristics of a virus capable of producing persistent infection. Persistent HAV infection in vivo is thought to be extraordinarily rare.[2] HAV variants that replicate more rapidly and produce cytopathic effects have been isolated, but their biologic importance remains uncertain.

Replication of HAV in hepatocytes in vivo is generally noncytolytic. Hence, hepatic injury in HAV infection appears to be mediated through immunologic mechanisms. HAV-specific human leukocyte antigen (HLA) class I restricted cytotoxic T lymphocytes and possibly nonspecific natural killer cells are believed to be responsible for necrosis of infected hepatocytes. By mechanisms still poorly understood, HAV is released from infected hepatocytes, enters bile, and transits through the intestine. HAV appears in stool during the late incubation period, the 2 weeks before the onset of symptoms, usually peaking just before or on the day symptoms begin. HAV concentration in stool may exceed 10^8 HAV/ml. HAV may also be present in other body fluids, such as blood, saliva, and throat secretions, but usually at considerably lower levels. In patients with relapsing HAV infection, an uncommon clinical form, HAV may reappear in stool. Although yet to be confirmed, the persistence of intermittent fecal HAV excretion for months in infected neonates has been suggested by tests for HAV RNA with the polymerase chain reaction (PCR).[3] For older children and infected adults, fecal shedding sought by less sensitive techniques cannot be detected with any consistency 1 to 2 weeks after the onset of illness; no epidemiologic evidence of persistent HAV excretion exists (Table 13–2).

Hepatitis E Virus

Hepatitis E virus is a small spherical nonenveloped RNA-containing viruslike particle with a mean diameter of about 32 nm. The presence of spikes and indentations on the surface of HEV has led to the suggestion that HEV may belong to the calicivirus family. These agents are known to induce diarrheal disease in human beings. Only one serologic strain of HEV has been identified, and HEV is believed to be the major and perhaps the only agent of enterically transmitted non-HAV hepatitis.

HEV has been cloned; it is a single-stranded, positive-sense, polyadenylated RNA virus with a genome size of about 7500 nucleotides. A single open reading frame appears to encode RNA-dependent RNA polymerase and the HEV antigen, a protein that appears on the surface of the HEV particle and has been identified in the cytoplasm of infected hepatocytes. HEV has not been propagated in tissue culture, and evidence of a cytopathic effect is absent. The mechanism of HEV replication is not known for certain. The presence of HEV in the bile and feces of infected nonhuman primates is consistent with the notion that HEV replication occurs in the liver. Whether other tissues also support HEV replication is uncertain.

Hepatitis B Virus

Hepatitis B virus belongs to a small family of mammalian and avian deoxyribonucleic acid (DNA)-containing agents labeled hepadnaviruses. In addition to human wild-type HBV, HBV mutants have been identified. The human HBV is a double-shelled spherical particle with a diameter of 42 nm. The outer shell, or envelope, of HBV is composed of the hepatitis B surface antigen (HBsAg), which comprises three related proteins, the large, middle, and major (or small) HBsAg proteins. The three HbsAg proteins share a common C-terminal 226 amino acid sequence but differ in their N-terminal extensions. The large protein, with a 174 amino acid extension, may serve as a binding site for a putative hepatocyte receptor. In addition to its presence on the HBV particle, HBsAg is present in the form of 20 to 22 nm spherical and tubular particles that circulate in the blood of infected individuals. The core of HBV contains a nucleocapsid antigen, the hepatitis B core antigen (HBcAg). A nonstructural, soluble antigen, the hepatitis B e antigen (HBeAg) is also present in the nucleocapsid. In contrast to HBcAg, which is rarely detected as a free particle in serum, HBeAg is detected with some regularity in patients in whom HBV replication is active.

HBV DNA, also localized to the core of the virus particle, is a circular, partially double-stranded molecule with a genome length of close to 3200 nucleotides. The genome has a single-stranded region of variable length. Four open reading frames have been identified: the pre-S and S region, the pre-core and C region, the HBV DNA polymerase (reverse transcriptase) coding region, and the X region, which codes for a transcriptional, transactivating factor, the x antigen. Although this protein has been shown to transactivate viral and cellular

TABLE 13–2. PERSISTENT INFECTION AND SEQUELAE OF HEPATITIS VIRUS INFECTION

VIRUS	PERSISTENT INFECTION	CHRONIC HEPATITIS	HEPATOCELLULAR CARCINOMA
HAV	No	No	No
HEV	No (?)	No	No
HBV	Age-dependent, immune-mediated	Yes	Yes
HBV Mutants	Yes	Yes	?
HDV	Linked with HBV (superinfection)	Yes	Indirectly
HCV	Yes	Yes	Yes

genes, its role, if any, in the replication of the HBV genome remains uncertain. In addition to the four identified open reading frames, promoters associated with the S, C, and X regions, a glucocorticosteroid response element and enhancer elements embedded in the reverse transcriptase and X genes have been described. Their precise roles in HBV genomic replication have yet to be completely defined.

HBV replication occurs in the liver and in extrahepatic tissues, as, for example, in circulating lymphocytes and monocytes in the spleen and possibly in other organs in which the HBV genome is transcriptionally and translationally active. HBV genomic replication strategy appears analogous to that of the RNA-containing retroviruses: The 3200-nucleotide long, negative DNA strand of HBV DNA is generated by reverse transcription of a HBV-specific RNA pregenomic intermediate, which is longer than genome length, through the action of HBV-specific reverse transcriptase. The positive DNA strand is then synthesized, using the negative DNA strand as a template. Integration of the HBV genome into host hepatocyte DNA is not a requisite step in the HBV replicative cycle but may occur nonetheless. This integration of HBV DNA sequences may play a role in the development of hepatocellular carcinoma in individuals with persistent HBV infection (see Table 13–2).

Mutant Hepatitis B Viruses

Because it employs a retrovirus-like reverse transcription genomic replication strategy, HBV is believed to have a mutation rate consistently greater than that of other DNA viruses. Multiple mutants of HBV have been reported, with mutations in single or multiple sites. Although some mutants of HBV are capable of replicating in vivo and in vitro,[4] others are incapable of producing intact viral particles.[5] Many HBV mutants have yet to be fully characterized, and their biologic properties and clinical importance are under study. Mutations affecting the pre-core region of HBV have been implicated in the pathogenesis of fulminant hepatitis and may be responsible for clinically severe exacerbations of chronic hepatitis associated with HBV infection (see Table 13–2).[6, 7] Whether HBV mutants play a role in the development of hepatocellular carcinoma in patients with chronic HBV infection remains to be established.[8]

Hepatitis D Virus

Hepatitis D virus (36 nm in diameter) is a defective RNA virus that resembles satellite RNAs and satellite RNA plant viruses. HDV is believed to require a helping hepadnavirus (HBV in the case of human beings) for its entry into hepatocytes, its expression, and its release from hepatocytes.

HDV is encapsulated within an envelope supplied by its helper hepadnavirus. In human beings, the envelope is the HBsAg of the helper HBV. No definite nucleocapsid structure has been identified for HDV. Disruption of HDV particles with removal of the HBsAg envelope releases HDV RNA and HDV antigen. The HDV genome is a circular, single-stranded RNA molecule with a length of about 1700 nucleotides. Cloned, full-length HDV complementary DNA (cDNA) has been used successfully to transfect chimpanzees. HDV RNA can fold itself into an unbranched rodlike structure by base-pairing. Genomic and antigenomic HDV RNA have been shown to be capable of self-cleavage and self-ligation, suggesting that HDV has the properties of a ribozyme class of agents. Both genomic and antigenomic RNA are produced by RNA-directed RNA synthesis. The HDV antigen is believed to be a phosphoprotein capable of binding to at least three sites on both genomic and antigenomic HDV RNA.[9] HDV antigen exists in the form of two proteins: one with 195 and the other with 214 amino acids. HDV antigen appears to play a role in the replication of HDV by transporting HDV RNA from the cytoplasm to the nucleus, the site of HDV replication.[10]

HDV does not appear to require HBV for the replication of its genomic or antigenomic RNA or for the expression of the HDV antigen. HDV replication is believed to occur through a rolling circle mechanism, but the precise steps have not been fully elaborated. Nucleotide heterogeneity of about 10% has been found in comparisons of HDV isolates. Whether these HDV mutants are responsible for highly virulent or avirulent infections remains to be determined.

HDV appears to be strictly hepatotrophic. No evidence of HDV, HDV antigen, or HDV replicative intermediates has been found in extrahepatic tissue. HDV may be present in sera in concentrations as high as 10^{12} genomes/ml.[11] Circulating HDV RNA can be detected in infected individuals. Levels of HDV RNA appear to fluctuate with changes in the rate of HDV and HBV replication.

Hepatitis C Virus

Hepatitis C virus, the predominant and possibly the sole agent of bloodborne non-A, non-B hepatitis, is a lipid-enveloped, chloroform-sensitive agent. The genome of this RNA-containing virus, which is believed to be genetically related in a distant manner to the pestiviruses, comprises a single-stranded, positive-sense RNA molecule with a length of about 10,000 nucleotides. A single, large, open reading frame that can encode a polyprotein of 3000 amino acids has been identified. A 5' terminal noncoding, highly conserved region of about 330 nucleotides may play a regulatory role in HCV replication. The 5' terminal noncoding region is followed by a nucleocapsid core region, a region coding for envelope proteins and glycoproteins, and then four nonstructural regions. Nonstructural region 3 codes for a helicase, a double-stranded RNA unwinding enzyme, and a protease; nonstructural region 5 appears to code for a RNA-dependent RNA polymerase.

HCV had been estimated by membrane filtration studies to have a diameter of between 30 and 38 nm.[12] Visualization of a rare 55 nm HCV particle in serum or liver tissue by electron microscopy, however, has not confirmed this estimate. Low levels of viremia and low tissue concentrations of HCV may be responsible for difficulties in visualizing the agent. HCV RNA may be present in extrahepatic tissues such as lymphocytes, but evidence of replication outside the liver has not yet been established. The mechanism of HCV replication is not yet known. Limited but growing data based on differences in HCV genome nucleotide sequences in the region coding for envelope proteins support the notion that distinct HCV genotypes exist. Two, and possibly three, strains have been partially characterized. In addition to the existence of distinct HCV genotypes and a substantial natural mutation rate, little evidence exists to suggest that HCV infection confers immunity to reinfection by the homologous strain. Thus, it is possible that HCV infections may be recurrent. The host range of HCV infections may be limited to human beings and nonhuman primates such as chimpanzees. Propagation of HCV in tissue culture has yet to be reported.

The PCR method has been used to detect HCV RNA in both serum and liver. A wide range of serum HCV RNA concentrations has been found in infected patients: 10^5 to 10^6 copies of HCV RNA/ml of serum in one study[13] and 10^2 to 5×10^7 HCV virions/ml of plasma in another.[14] HCV RNA has been detected by PCR in patients with both chronic hepatitis C and in some patients with biochemically resolved disease.[15] These observations suggest that an asymptomatic viremic HCV carrier state may persist in the absence of biochemical abnormalities.

Viral Interference

When simultaneously present, the hepatitis viruses may interfere with the expression or replication of one another. The underlying mechanisms are ill defined but may involve the induction and release of interferon or other lymphokines, or they may involve other factors, such as the necrosis of hepatocytes that harbor persistently replicating virus or the monopolization of the macromolecular biosynthetic apparatus of the hepatocyte by the superimposed acute virus infection. Examples of viral interference have been reported in patients infected by HAV and HCV, HDV and HBV, HAV and HBV, and HBV and HCV. In one noteworthy report, evidence of HBV replication diminished or became undetectable in patients with chronic HBV infection superinfected by HAV.[16] Since simultaneous infections are unusual, with the exception of HDV/HBV co-infection or HDV superinfection of HBV carriers, the fact that the interaction of HDV and HBV has been more carefully assessed than other interactions is not surprising. These studies indicate that HDV co-infection or superinfection may partially inhibit the replication of HBV.[17] The clinical importance of this inhibition is uncertain, and, furthermore, inhibition is not an invariable feature of dual infection.[18, 19] Thus, the response to one hepatitis virus infection may or may not interfere with the response to the other agent. The interactions of nonhepatitis viruses, such as human immunodeficiency virus (HIV), with HBV, HDV, and HCV require further study.

Hepatic Injury Produced by Other Viral Agents

In immunocompetent individuals, cytomegalovirus (CMV) and Epstein-Barr virus (EBV) infections are often associated with a clinically silent or mild hepatitis and may be serologically confirmed by specific antibody studies. Recognized CMV hepatitis may be relatively more common in immunocompromised than in immunocompetent patients. It may be detected by identification of histopathologic features compatible with CMV infection (e.g., the presence of intracellular viral inclusion bodies) or the presence of CMV antigens in liver tissue or of CMV DNA detected by hybridization probes in hepatocytes. In immunocompromised patients, hepatic CMV infection may be accompanied by extensive hepatocyte damage with a relatively scant inflammatory infiltration.[20] In this setting, the disease may be clinically severe and present as fulminant hepatic failure. In EBV-induced infectious mononucleosis in immunocompetent individuals, although serum aminotransferase elevations are an almost inevitable finding, jaundice is present in no more than 5%. Infectious mononucleosis hepatitis without features of mononucleosis occurs but must be uncommon. In addition to the relatively common infections, mild hepatitis-like illnesses may accompany infection by a large number of diverse viral agents, including herpes simplex, rubella, varicella, adenovirus, reovirus, and enteric cytopathogenic human orphan (ECHO) viruses. Other responsible agents include Marburg and Ebola viruses and Rift Valley fever and Lassa fever viruses. In most, but not all, instances, involvement of other organ systems is more prominent than is hepatic involvement. As a consequence, the hepatitis may be ignored in cases of extensive extrahepatic injury.

An unusual form of sporadic acute or chronic hepatitis has been linked with paramyxovirus infection.[21] Affected individuals presented with subacute hepatic failure or evidence of chronic hepatitis, often associated with serologic features of autoimmune disease. Syncytial multinucleated giant cells that replaced hepatocyte cords were accompanied by necrosis, ballooning, and dropout of hepatocytes, cholestasis, and round cell inflammation resembling typical viral hepatitis. Electron microscopic examination revealed the presence within giant cells of viruslike structures that resembled paramyxovirus nucleocapsids in 8 of the 10 liver specimens examined. Serologic evidence of a specific paramyxovirus infection was not found. The finding of syncytial giant cells in the liver biopsy of a patient with hepatitis in whom serologic or epidemiologic features of typical viral hepatitis are absent must raise the question of paramyxovirus infection. Unfortunately, with the exception of hepatic transplantation, no treatment for this severe disease is available.

EPIDEMIOLOGY AND NATURAL HISTORY

Immunocompetent Hosts

Hepatitis A Virus

Epidemiologic patterns of HAV are consistent with the predominance of fecal-oral spread by direct person-to-person contact. HAV transmission in households, daycare centers for pre–toilet-trained children, institutions for the men-

tally disabled, neonatal intensive care units, international travelers, and military forces is well known. Although the prevalence of HAV infection does not appear to be increased in homosexual men, the risk of HAV infection in homosexual men probably increases as the number of sexual partners increases. Furthermore, active oral-anal sexual behavior is likely to enhance the efficiency of HAV transmission among sexual partners.

Common-source outbreaks of infection have been attributed to the contamination of food during collection or by HAV-infected foodhandlers and the contamination of water supplies via cross-connections or flooding. Ingestion of undercooked or raw bivalve mollusks such as clams, oysters, or mussels (the predominant vehicles) that have been harvested from contaminated waters has been implicated in both large and small outbreaks. Bloodborne transmission of HAV is unusual. In fact, transfusion-associated HAV infection is a rare event. Mini-outbreaks of HAV among parenteral drug users who share tissue penetration equipment and those who are exposed to HAV-contaminated drugs are, however, no longer uncommon. The exposure to drugs contaminated by HAV may reflect the use of the gastrointestinal tract to carry and hide illicit drugs when crossing national borders.

The major sources of HAV infection include personal contact with an acutely infected individual, attendance in daycare centers or personal contact with a daycare-associated case, parenteral drug use, international travel, and ingestion of contaminated food or water in the setting of a recognized outbreak or an unrecognized mini-outbreak. No risk factors can be identified in approximately one third of cases.

HAV infection is invariably self-limited, but uncommonly relapses and prolonged cholestatic forms may be seen. The overall case fatality rate is no higher than 0.4% but climbs in individuals over 40 years of age to just more than 1.1%.[22] Convincing evidence for persistent HAV infection and chronic hepatitis is not available (see Table 13–2). Rarely, acute HAV infection appears to trigger autoimmune chronic active hepatitis in susceptible individuals.[23]

Hepatitis E Virus

Enteric transmission involving the fecal-oral route is the predominant and possibly the sole mode of spread of HEV infection. Although the disease has been recognized in epidemic form in the Indian subcontinent, Asia, Africa, some former Soviet republics, and Mexico, endemic zones with high sporadic HEV infection rates seem likely in developing regions. The majority of recognized outbreaks have been attributed to waterborne transmission. Secondary infection rates among household contacts as measured by the development of clinical illness are surprisingly low for an infection that is enterically transmitted. Whether this reflects a relative instability of HEV, a low frequency of clinical disease among infected individuals, or other poorly defined factors is not known. Vehicles of infection such as fecally contaminated food or bivalve mollusks may also play a role, but their epidemiologic importance remains uncertain. HEV infection of domestic pigs[24] and nonhuman primates[25] has been suggested, but it has not yet been established whether these animals serve as a reservoir of infection for human beings.

Age-specific attack rates of clinically apparent HEV infection reveal that young adults are the most frequently affected. These observations are consistent with the notion that most HEV infections, like other enteric infections, probably occur in children and are anicteric and subclinical. If this notion is correct, however, the high attack rate in young adults may reflect reinfections in individuals in whom immunity to HEV infection has been lost over time. HEV infections in the United States have been limited to imported cases in individuals returning from endemic zones. Secondary spread of infection from these travelers has not yet been reported and seems unlikely. Whether a proportion of HEV-infected individuals become intestinal carriers of HEV remains uncertain.

Although most cases of HEV infection are self-limited and chronic liver disease is not a reported sequel (see Table 13–2), as many as 20% of pregnant women infected in the third trimester appear to be at risk for fulminant hepatitis.

Hepatitis B Virus

Hepatitis B virus is present in a variety of body fluids and secretions. Concentrations are highest in blood, lower in semen, and then, in descending order, in saliva, vaginal secretions, breast milk, urine, tears, and cerebrospinal fluid (CSF). Given the high levels of viremia found in acute HBV infection and in HBV carriers with high levels of HBV replication, that HBV is readily spread by the sharing of equipment for the injection of illicit drugs is not surprising. HBV is also spread through accidental needlesticks or contact of mucosal surfaces or broken skin with contaminated blood or body secretions by health-care workers or other individuals likely to be exposed, such as first-responders, emergency medical technicians, paramedics, and police and firefighters. HBV infection must also be considered a sexually transmitted disease, since both homosexual and heterosexual contact has been linked with spread of infection and sexual transmission appears to be a highly efficient means of spread.

Maternal-neonatal transmission of HBV from pregnant carriers or from pregnant women with acute HBV infection is also a well-known and important route of spread. Its importance is a consequence of the fact that infection early in life, particularly in the first year, is closely associated with the development of persistent infection in the infant. The precise mechanisms underlying maternal-neonatal transmission remain to be fully defined. Although the risk of infection is greatest when the mother is highly viremic, as reflected by the detection of HBeAg and HBV DNA in maternal serum, maternal-neonatal infection and even fulminant HBV infection have been observed in the offspring of women who test HBsAg-positive, HBeAg-negative who do not have detectable HBV DNA in serum as measured by the highly sensitive PCR technique.[26] In a few such instances, maternal mononuclear cells, which can traverse the placenta intact and circulate in the newborn, have been shown to carry HBV DNA by PCR.[26] The specific role of mononuclear cells in spreading HBV infection in this and other settings, including sexual contact, requires further investigation.

The natural history of HBV infection is dependent on both virus and host factors. As previously indicated, a growing body of evidence supports a role for virulent HBV mutants in the pathogenesis of fulminant HBV infection, an event observed in about 1% of acutely infected adults. Host factors appear to play a critical role in the development of persistent HBV infection associated with chronic hepatitis. The major host factors that have been unequivocally linked to persistent HBV infection are age at the time of infection and immunocompetency. The risk of persistent infection is inversely related to age at the time of infection. Newborns have the highest risk, approaching 80 to 90%, infants a risk of about 50%, children a risk of about 20%, and in most healthy adults the risk falls to significantly less than 2%. By contrast, the risk of persistent HBV infection in immunocompromised adults may exceed 10%. Rough estimates of the HBV carrier rate on every continent based on incomplete population statistics indicate that the number of HBV carriers throughout the world may approach 300 million.

The spectrum of hepatic disease associated with persistent HBV infection, as indicated by the prolonged presence of HBsAg in serum, is quite broad. In some individuals, only nonspecific histopathologic findings are present; in others, the lesions of chronic persistent or chronic active hepatitis (Fig. 13–2) may be found. Although chronic active hepatitis has long been linked with the development of cirrhosis, progression to cirrhosis may also occur in an uncertain number of patients with chronic persistent hepatitis. Prolonged HBV infection, particularly when initiated early in life and when accompanied by the development of cirrhosis, appears to be a precursor of primary hepatocellular carcinoma (see Table 13–2), a major form of malignancy throughout the world.

Extrahepatic manifestations of persistent HBV infection include HBV-associated polyarteritis nodosa, membranoproliferative glomerulonephritis, and cryoglobulinemia.

Hepatitis D Virus

Although the modes of HBV and HDV transmission are identical, the prevalence of HDV is not directly correlated with the prevalence of HBV. In fact, although the distribution of HDV overlaps that of HBV, the prevalence of HDV infection varies widely from area to area. Estimates suggest that as many as 15 million persons may be carriers of HDV throughout the world. Since HDV infection can repress the expression of HBsAg to levels below the sensitivity of most current commercial assays and because antibody to HDV (anti-HDV) might not be measured in HBsAg-negative patients, the frequency of infection may have been underestimated.

Nonetheless, HDV endemicity appears low in the United States, and HDV infection is most often identified in parenteral drug abusers and their sexual contacts. Sexual transmission of HDV infection appears to be less efficient than sexual transmission of HBV infection, even among homosexual populations. Maternal-neonatal transmission is a relatively uncommon mode, presumably because most HDV-infected women may have relatively low levels of HBV replication. This low level of HBV replication favors infrequent transmission of HBV to the newborn, and, in the absence of HBV transmission, HDV infection is unlikely to be established in the newborn. Other modes of transmission that may play a critical role in HDV-endemic areas include spread by inapparent permucosal or percutaneous transfer of contaminated secretions or entry of virus through open skin lesions.

Two forms of HDV infection have been identified. In HDV/HBV co-infections, exposure to both agents usually leads to a self-limited or biphasic acute hepatitis that is indistinguishable from acute HBV infection alone. In a small proportion of patients, co-infection leads to fulminant hepatitis. In contrast to the generally benign course of co-infection, HDV superinfection of an individual with preexisting persistent HBV infection may lead to fulminant disease or rapid progression to severe chronic hepatitis, cirrhosis, and hepatic failure. No evidence directly links HDV infection to hepatocellular carcinoma. Because HDV infection can lead to the rapid development of cirrhosis, a lesion likely to promote the development of hepatocellular carcinoma (see Table 13–2), HDV may serve as an indirect promoter of malignant transformation.[27]

Hepatitis C Virus

Hepatitis C virus appears to be a bloodborne pathogen, and parenteral transmission is a well-established route of its spread. Observations in chimpanzees suggest the likelihood that HCV viremia occurs within days of exposure and persists through much, if not all, of the acute phase

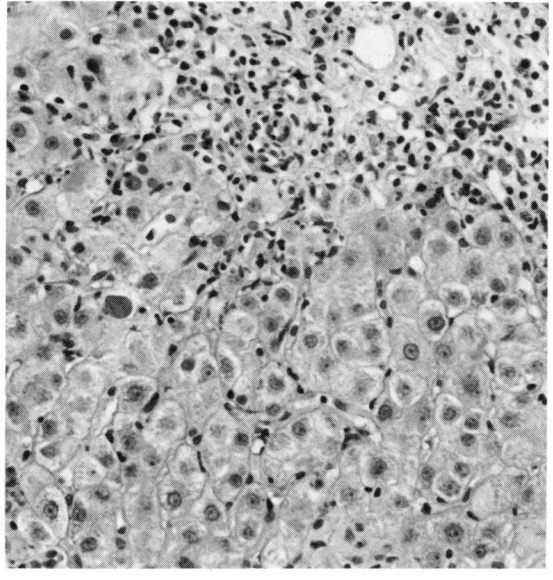

FIGURE 13–2.
Chronic active hepatitis, demonstrating piecemeal necrosis and portal lymphocytic inflammation extending across the limiting plate into the parenchyma. Hematoxylin and eosin, × 250.

of infection.[28] HCV has been transmitted through blood transfusion, through accidental needle-sticks in health-care workers, and through equipment shared by parenteral drug users. Evidence suggests that the HCV carrier rate may be lower than the HBV carrier rate, but direct estimates of the frequency of HCV viremia in the general population have yet to be undertaken.

Whether HCV is also present in body fluids and secretions remains uncertain. Although preliminary reports of the presence of HCV RNA in peripheral blood mononuclear cells and saliva suggest that transmission may occur through these vehicles, convincing evidence for such transmission is scanty. Nonetheless, epidemiologic data indicate that sexual contact with an infected individual and multiple sexual contacts are risk factors favoring HCV infection. The actual risk appears to be small. Testing of sexual and household contacts of HCV-infected individuals has infrequently revealed first-generation antibody markers of HCV infection. Limited testing of contacts for HCV RNA has also failed to support frequent transmission by person-to-person contact. Thus, although some epidemiologic data support the possibility of sexual transmission, such transmission is likely to be relatively inefficient and therefore uncommon. Similarly, transmission of HCV from infected mothers to their newborn infants may occur but appears to be an uncommon event. Hence, sexual and maternal-neonatal transmission appear to be less important in the epidemiology of HCV than in HBV. Co-infection with HIV may, however, facilitate HCV transmission through a number of routes.

Because circulating HCV RNA may persist for prolonged periods after clinical and biochemical recovery, even after loss of antibody to HCV (anti-HCV), the low frequency of person-to-person transmission cannot be due to a limited viremic period. A low level of viremia, and therefore a reduced HCV concentration in body fluids, is a more likely explanation for the relative inefficiency of contact transmission.

The natural history of HCV infection is incompletely defined. A large body of evidence indicates that approximately 50% of HCV infections, regardless of route of transmission, become persistent as determined by the presence of persistent elevations or fluctuating levels of serum aminotransferases for more than 6 months after infection is first identified. Liver biopsy of individuals with persistent aminotransferase elevations reveal features of chronic active or chronic persistent hepatitis in most cases. On prolonged follow-up, as many as 20% of patients may develop cirrhosis, although in most instances the progression to cirrhosis is clinically silent and features of portal hypertension or hepatic failure appear to be uncommon. Nonetheless, studies have linked HCV-induced cirrhosis to the development of primary hepatocellular carcinoma (see Table 13–2).

In addition to chronic hepatitis, extrahepatic organ involvement may occur in rare patients. The precise frequency of leukocytoclastic vasculitis, glomerulonephritis, and cryoglobulinemia as sequelae of persistent HCV infection is uncertain, but it must be very low.

Immunocompromised Hosts

Hepatitis A Virus

Hepatitis A virus infection has not been identified as a distinctly different disease in either homosexual men or immunosuppressed patients. Furthermore, because the prevalence of HAV infection is not dramatically increased in homosexual men or immunodeficient populations, these groups are not currently considered as candidates for HAV vaccine when that product becomes available. An HAV superinfection appears to be associated with an increased case-fatality rate in patients with underlying chronic liver disease. For this reason and because homosexual men and immunosuppressed patients may be at increased risk for chronic viral hepatitis due to the other agents, namely HBV, HBV/HDV, and HCV, it is likely that HAV is a more severe disease in these groups than in other groups.

Hepatitis E Virus

Although extensive studies have yet to be undertaken, HEV RNA, detected by PCR, is likely to be present concurrently for relatively short periods in serum and bile.[29] Whether viremia and intestinal shedding of HEV are of longer duration in immunocompromised patients remains to be determined. In fact, patterns of viremia in uncomplicated or fulminant HEV infection remain to be identified. Whether HEV infection is clinically more severe in immunocompromised patients is also not yet known. The peculiar susceptibility of pregnant women in the third trimester to HEV-induced fulminant hepatitis is enigmatic. Since only HEV and not HAV, HBV, HDV, or HCV has been linked to this devastating complication, the phenomenon is likely to be virus-specific rather than host-related.

Hepatitis B Virus

The serologic response to HBV and the natural history of infection appear to be conditioned by the immunoresponsiveness of the host. In immunocompromised individuals, HBV infection may lead to extensive replication of the virus, with the appearance of relatively large amounts of HBV DNA in the circulation and the delayed appearance of antibody directed to HBcAg of the immunoglobulin M class (IgM anti-HBc).[30] Titers of IgM anti-HBc may remain low, and loss of both anti-HBc and antibody directed to HBsAg (anti-HBs) may be accelerated in the immunodeficient. HBV replication in extrahepatic sites may also be enhanced in immunosuppressed patients. The evidence to suggest that immunocompromised patients are considerably more likely to develop persistent infection than are immunocompetent individuals is abundant. The HBV carrier state, as determined by the persistence of HBsAg for more than 6 to 12 months after acute infection, is probably 5 to 10 times more common in the immunocompromised. HBV carrier rates between 5 and 15% have been reported in homosexual men, HIV-infected individuals, individuals with Down's syndrome residing in large institutions, patients with lepromatous leprosy, and those in similar immunodeficiency states.

Although a spectrum of chronic hepatitis may be seen in immunocompromised HBV carriers, in many individuals the disease is clinically mild, reflecting the importance of the host immunologic response in the cytolytic destruction of infected hepatocytes. HBV infection of new liver grafts in patients with chronic HBV infection who undergo hepatic transplantation and are immunosuppressed by drug therapy is a common complication. In many patients, the new HBV infection is a typical acute hepatitis but has a high risk of progression to chronic hepatitis. In some patients, intracellular HBV antigens accumulate in the graft, and this feature is associated with graft dysfunction and only minimal inflammatory change in the liver. This disorder has been termed fibrosing, cholestatic hepatitis.[31]

Hepatitis D Virus

In immunocompromised patients, HDV antigen may be readily detected in serum and, in contrast to the pattern seen in immunocompetent hosts, anti-HDV may not appear. In HIV-positive patients in whom HDV and HBV infection are present, the suppression of HBV replication by HDV may be less and the anti-HDV response may be absent or blunted. The influence of HIV infection and immunosuppression remains incompletely defined. Both IgM and immunoglobulin G (IgG) anti-HDV may be undetectable or present in low titer, but serum HDV RNA appears to be unaffected by the presence of HIV infection.[32] Since commercial laboratory assays for HDV RNA are not yet available, measurement of HDV RNA provides the only direct means of assessing HDV replication. This method appears to be more sensitive than the detection of an isolated IgM anti-HDV response in acute infection.[33]

Although the increased virulence of chronic HDV infection has received considerable attention, that some chronic HDV infections may be asymptomatic and liver tests may be within normal limits is abundantly clear. Such observations suggest that host, immunologic, and viral factors may influence the pathogenicity of HDV infection. In anti-HIV–positive patients, HDV infection does not appear to run a different course. Anti-HIV–positive patients with chronic hepatitis D may demonstrate enhanced HBV and HDV replication, but evidence of an increased severity of the liver disease is not present.[34] Hepatitis D viremia may be aggravated and HDV may be more virulent in certain patients with active HBV replication, but no major role for HBV mutants in this increased severity has been established. The helper function for HDV may be greater for the wild-type HBV that expresses HBeAg than for the pre-core, HBeAg-negative HBV mutant. Thus, in patients in the last mentioned group, HDV infection is less virulent, producing a more slowly progressing and milder disease.

Hepatitis C Virus

The impact of host immunologic status on the epidemiologic, virologic, clinical, and immune responses to HCV infection is poorly understood. Limited studies of HCV infection in HIV-infected individuals have suggested that HCV can be transmitted more efficiently in the presence of HIV.[35] In a study of female sexual contacts of multiply transfused men with hemophilia, the frequency of HCV transmission to sexual contacts was 5 times higher when HIV was also transmitted.[35] Further support for an interaction between immunologic status, HIV, and HCV comes from a report indicating that maternal-neonatal transmission of HCV is greatly enhanced in the presence of coexisting HIV infection.[36] Whether these observations reflect an impaired immunologic mechanism for the clearance of HCV or enhanced HCV replication through another mechanism is unknown. Rapid progression of acute HCV infection to severe chronic hepatitis may occur in some patients with HIV co-infection, but the frequency of this phenomenon is unknown.

In contrast to this interaction of HCV with HIV, in patients with concurrent HCV and HBV infection, as, for example, in parenteral drug abusers, HBV replication may be inhibited. The mechanism responsible for this phenomenon is not understood. (See the discussion of viral interference earlier in this chapter.) In immunosuppressed patients who develop chronic hepatitis after liver transplantation for other disorders, HCV RNA may be detected in the serum and liver, but anti-HCV reactivity, as measured with the first-generation enzyme-linked immunosorbent assay (ELISA), may be absent.

SEROLOGIC DIAGNOSIS

Diagnostic Tests and Patterns

Hepatitis A Virus

Testing for HAV or for HAV RNA in blood or stool by hybridization or PCR techniques is not routinely performed. Serologic diagnosis of HAV requires detection of IgM antibody to HAV (anti-HAV). The test is highly sensitive and specific, with rare false-positive results. IgM anti-HAV–positivity in a patient with acute viral hepatitis is diagnostic of acute HAV infection. IgM anti-HAV is invariably present by the time symptoms develop. Hence, the absence of IgM anti-HAV in a symptomatic patient is strong evidence against the diagnosis of HAV infection. Commercially available assays have been designed so that in the majority of patients the IgM anti-HAV has disappeared by 3 to 6 months after the onset of illness. The persistence of IgM anti-HAV for many months after the acute phase of illness has been identified in a small proportion of patients, generally less than 10%. In rare patients, IgM anti-HAV may persist for years. Asymptomatic patients may have IgM anti-HAV for a significantly shorter period than do symptomatic patients, and males may have lower titers and remain positive for a shorter period than females.[37]

Although assays utilizing monoclonal antibodies promise an even greater sensitivity than is currently available with polyclonal reagents, none has become available commercially. Microparticle enzyme immunoassays for anti-HAV have been developed. These tests can detect both IgM and IgG antibodies and appear to be more sensitive but equal in specificity to the currently available radioimmunoassays and enzyme immunoassays.[38]

IgG anti-HAV develops more gradually than does IgM anti-HAV and reaches high levels during the convalescent phase of illness. IgG anti-HAV persists for many years after acute infection, and its presence indicates resistance to reinfection.

Hepatitis E Virus

Hepatitis E virus infection should be suspected in travelers returning to the United States with viral hepatitis or in those developing hepatitis within 2 to 7 weeks of travel in the developing world. Although most such instances are likely to be HAV infection, HEV should be considered in those patients in whom testing for IgM anti-HAV proves negative.

The presence of antibody to HEV (anti-HEV) in the sera of infected patients was initially shown by immune aggregation of HEV particles through immune-electron microscopy. Subsequently, anti-HEV was identified by immunofluorescent techniques.[39] Fluorescent antibody blocking assays have been developed at the Federal Centers for Disease Control in Atlanta, but they remain a research tool. Cloning of HEV cDNA has permitted the expression of encoded recombinant HEV proteins in *Escherichia coli*.[40] Expressed HEV proteins were shown to react serologically when incubated with sera from HEV-infected patients. Most of the detected antibodies were IgG, but some IgM antibodies were also detected. No commercial assay for anti-HEV is available; western blot and enzyme immunoassays are under development.

Hepatitis B Virus

Hepatitis B virus DNA may be the first detectable serologic marker of HBV infection. With the highly sensitive PCR technique, HBV DNA has been identified in experimentally infected chimpanzees 2 to 3 weeks before the appearance of HBsAg and for as long as 2 weeks after the appearance of anti-HBs.[41] Analyses with PCR also demonstrate that, regardless of HBeAg status, most HBsAg-positive acutely or chronically infected patients do have circulating HBV DNA. The exact duration of circulating HBV DNA and the serum concentration of HBV DNA in acute, self-limited HBV infection has yet to be established. Low-level replication of HBV may persist for prolonged periods, however, even after loss of HBsAg in chronic hepatitis B in some patients.[41] Although these observations suggest that HBV DNA may be detected weeks before other markers in patients with acute HBV infection, PCR studies for HBV DNA are not widely available.

The first conventionally measured and readily detected serologic marker of HBV infection is HBsAg. Serum pre-S antigens also appear early in the course of HBV infection, approximately at the same time as HBsAg becomes detectable, but assays for these antigens are not widely available. HBsAg is present in blood 1 to 10 weeks after exposure to HBV and several weeks before the onset of symptoms or biochemical evidence of liver injury. HBsAg, measured by conventional assays, is present for a variable but generally short period of a few weeks during the acute phase of the illness; measured by monoclonal radioimmunoassays, HBsAg may be seen to persist for several months before clearance. HBeAg may be detected in the sera of acutely infected individuals, concomitantly, just after, or within a week or so of the appearance of HBsAg. HBeAg usually disappears within 2 weeks, often before clearance of HBsAg.

IgM anti-HBc is usually the first antibody detected in acute HBV infection. It may be the sole identifiable marker of HBV infection in the interval between the disappearance of HBsAg and the appearance of anti-HBs. Available data indicate that about 10% of IgM anti-HBc–positive patients with acute HBV infection are HBsAg-negative within 1 week after the onset of clinical illness. Hence, measurement of HBsAg alone would have missed these cases and possibly resulted in misclassification and misdiagnosis. IgM anti-HBc persists throughout the acute phase of illness but then declines and ultimately disappears. It is replaced by an IgG anti-HBc that develops during the convalescent phase and persists, usually for decades, in decreasing titers. Antibody to HBeAg (anti-HBe) appears after anti-HBc and may also persist for years.

The last antibody to be regularly detected during HBV infection, Anti-HBs, is usually detected during the late convalescent phase. Anti-HBs may be synthesized earlier in the course of acute HBV infection but may not be detectable as free antibody because HBsAg is present in excess, forming HBsAg–anti-HBs immune complexes. Anti-HBs is the neutralizing, protective antibody that indicates the development of immunity. The presence of anti-HBs generally marks clearance of HBsAg and recovery from infection. In 10 to 40% of HBV carriers, low-titer heterotypic anti-HBs may be detected but has no clinical meaning; these carriers cannot be distinguished from those without detectable anti-HBs.

The appearance of anti-HBs without preceding HBsAg or anti-HBc is the classic immunogenic response to HBV vaccines containing HBsAg. In natural HBV infection, anti–pre-S IgM and IgG antibodies have been detected concomitantly with anti-HBs; they appear to be relatively short lived, persisting in serum for several weeks only. They are not routinely measured.

Hepatitis D Virus

Serologic detection of HDV in HDV/HBV co-infection may not be sought since the clinical disease may be indistinguishable from acute HBV infection and HDV may not be considered. Even when considered, either because an outbreak is suspected or exposure to HDV infection is thought likely, detection may not be attempted since current serologic techniques for diagnosis are imperfect. HDV antigen may be present in serum prior to or at the onset of illness but may disappear shortly thereafter, except in immunocompromised hosts. Detection of HDV antigen by immunoblot assay, however, may prove useful in diagnosis.[42] Similarly, HDV RNA detected by slot blot hybridization, is present in serum in about 40% of HDV infected individuals at onset but has been cleared 1 month later. Although HDV antigen can persist within hepatocytes for a longer period, liver biopsy to detect antigen is not a practical tool for diagnosis of the acute illness.

In immunocompetent patients in whom HDV/HBV co-infection occurs, and in whom HBsAg and IgM anti-HBc are identified, anti-HDV is present in only 15% of patients at the time of clinical presentation.[43] By 1 month after onset, more than 90% will have anti-HDV. IgM anti-HDV, with or without the subsequent appearance of IgG anti-HDV, may be identified.[43] In some patients, IgG anti-HDV may appear late and in isolation. An immunoglobulin A (IgA) anti-HDV has been detected in patients with chronic HDV infection,[44] but its utility in diagnosis has yet to be studied.

Measurement of all known HDV markers (HDV antigen, HDV RNA, anti-HDV) at presentation may permit diagnosis of co-infection in about 55 to 70% of infected patients. Repeated measurement of anti-HDV one or more months later seems likely to provide a valid diagnosis in most, but not all, infected patients.

Anti-HDV may be short-lived and may not persist after resolution of HDV/HBV co-infection. Hence, no serologic evidence of past infection may be present. HBV carriers superinfected by HDV are distinguished from patients with co-infection by the absence of IgM anti-HBc in superinfections. In patients with HDV superinfection, anti-HDV tends to persist for indefinite periods, and prolonged persistence of IgM anti-HDV has been correlated with prolonged HDV replication. No known protective antibodies against HDV have been identified.

Hepatitis C Virus

Serologic diagnosis of HCV infection remains in an early phase of development, but important innovations in assays are expected. Although measurement of HCV RNA by PCR may be used to identify viremia and viremic carriers, a test procedure is not available commercially and, even if available, probably would not prove useful in identifying infections that were not associated with prolonged viremia. Hence, serologic assays for antibodies to HCV antigens should prove more helpful. The first widely available assay, a first-generation capture assay for IgG anti-HCV was developed through the fusion of a recombinant HCV nonstructural antigen, termed C100, composing no more than 10% of the HCV polyprotein, to the polypeptide of human superoxide dismutase to form a fusion polypeptide termed C100-3. In addition to the ELISA, which uses the recombinant C100-3 antigen on a solid phase, a recombinant immunoblot assay (RIBA) has been developed. The first RIBA employed two antigens; a four-antigen assay has also been developed.

The first-generation enzyme immunoassays have been plagued by the occurrence of both false-positive and false-negative results. False-positives have been observed in patients with autoimmune chronic active hepatitis, rheumatoid factor, high serum globulin levels, and, inexplicably, in others in whom past exposure to HCV is unlikely. Prolonged storage of serum and repeated freezing and thawing may also increase the frequency of false-positives. False-negatives indicate that the current first-generation immunoassay for anti-HCV has limited sensitivity; blood donors who have repeatedly tested negative for anti-HCV have nonetheless been implicated in the transmission of HCV to transfusion recipients.[45]

Additional antigenic components have been incorporated into second-generation assays. These assays initially served as supplementary anti-HCV tests to distinguish between true-positive and false-positive test results on first-generation assays. The second-generation assays have replaced the initial test procedures because of their heightened sensitivity and specificity. Even some of the second-generation assays for anti-HCV may, however, fail to identify patients with acute or chronic hepatitis in whom HCV RNA can be detected in serum.

Current evidence indicates that the anti-HCV antibodies detected by enzyme immunoassay are neither neutralizing nor protective antibodies. HCV RNA may be detected by PCR in the plasma and liver of anti-HCV–positive patients[46]; thus this IgG anti-HCV appears to be a marker of past or present HCV replication. It appears slowly over a variable time after the onset of HCV infection. Seroconversion may occur as early as 15 days after onset of recognized hepatitis in about one third of patients. Seroconversion occurs by 3 months in 60% and at the end of 9 months in 85%. In a small number of patients, seroconversion may take 12 or more months.[47] In one early analysis, anti-HCV seroconversion occurred at a mean interval of nearly 4 months after the onset of clinical transfusion-associated hepatitis.[48] Seroconversion is detectable sooner when second generation assays are used: as many as 60% of patients may have positive tests during the acute phase of infection.

Anti-HCV may persist for prolonged periods after acute infection. When HCV infection appears to be self-limited, that is, when serum aminotransferases return to normal, approximately 50 to 80% of patients may lose anti-HCV within a 10-year period. In patients in whom evidence of persistent HCV infection develops, only 5 to 20% lose anti-HCV.

Unusual Serologic Patterns

Detection of HBsAg without Other HBV Markers

Patients with fulminant HBV infection may test HBsAg-negative on presentation. Even if HBsAg-positive, they typically test HBeAg-negative and HBV DNA-negative by spot or dot blot hybridization techniques. Whether they would also test HBV DNA-negative by the more sensitive PCR remains to be established. Rapid clearance of HBV associated with massive destruction of infected hepatocytes is believed to be responsible, but other mechanisms may play a role. For example, the pre-core HBV variant, which is unable to produce HBeAg because of a novel translational stop codon, has also been linked to fulminant HBV infection. This HBV variant may breed true when transmitted between individuals, but its spontaneous emergence during

TABLE 13–3. SEROLOGIC DIAGNOSIS OF ACUTE VIRAL HEPATITIS

IgM Anti-HAV	IgM Anti-HBc	HBsAg	Anti-HDV	IgG Anti-HCV	DIAGNOSIS
+	−	−	−	−	Acute HAV infection
−	+	+	−	−	Acute HBV infection
−	+	−	−	−	Acute HBV infection
−	+	+	+	−	HBV/HDV co-infection
−	−	+	+	−	HDV superinfection of HBV carrier
−	−	+	−	−	HBV reactivation or HBeAg seroconversion
−	−	−	−	+	Acute HCV infection
−	−	−	−	−	Acute HCV infection with delayed anti-HCV response or acute HEV infection

the course of infection with the wild-type HBV is also possible.[49]

In patients with nonfulminant HBV infection, HBsAg may be seen during the incubation period prior to the appearance of IgM anti-HBc. Should IgM anti-HBc not appear after an observation period of several weeks to months, the likelihood of a false-positive test result looms large. Such false-positives may be identified by specificity testing with an anti-HBs blocking test. Although believed to be rare in the United States, HBsAg confirmed by anti-HBs blocking or inhibition testing has been detected without other markers of HBV infection in Senegalese infants.[50] This unusual HBV serologic pattern has been attributed to a HBV mutant. The responsible agent has been termed HBV2.

Detection of Anti-HBc without Other HBV Marker

Anti-HBc reactivity, in the absence of other markers, may reflect false-positive test results, but these findings occur in only a small fraction of patients in whom isolated anti-HBc is found.[51] Passive acquisition of anti-HBc by the newborn infants of HBV-infected mothers accounts for the presence of anti-HBc in these infants. In other individuals in whom anti-HBc is found, fractionation reveals the presence of IgM anti-HBc. That some of these individuals have had clinically silent HBV infection and have lost circulating HBsAg seems likely. Follow-up of these individuals reveals the replacement of IgM anti-HBc by IgG anti-HBc and the development of anti-HBs. Under unusual circumstances that remain poorly understood, anti-HBs does not reach detectable levels or else declines more rapidly than anti-HBc. In this circumstance, the presence of anti-HBc reflects past infection and recovery. Considerable evidence also exists to support the notion that some patients with isolated anti-HBc are HBV carriers in whom circulating HBsAg levels are just below the threshold for detection with current assays.

Detection of Anti-HBs without Other HBV Markers

The presence of anti-HBs alone may indicate successful immunization with HBV vaccine or passive acquisition of the antibody through transfusion of blood, blood products, or hepatitis B immune globulin. In each of these passive acquisition settings, anti-HBs disappears on follow-up, with a half-life identical to that of immunoglobulins. Although uncommon, in some individuals who have recovered from HBV infection and developed both anti-HBs and anti-HBc, the anti-HBc disappears well before the anti-HBs. Rarely, a circulating IgM anti-HBs of uncertain significance may be detected.[52] This IgM reactivity does not indicate resistance to HBV infection.

Initial Serologic Diagnosis in Acute Viral Hepatitis

For initial serologic diagnosis of acute viral hepatitis, the following combination of tests should be undertaken: IgM anti-HAV, IgM anti-HBc, HBsAg, and IgG anti-HCV (Table 13–3). The presence of a positive result for IgM anti-HAV provides a diagnosis of acute HAV infection. A positive test for IgM anti-HBc, with or without HBsAg, indicates the presence of acute HBV infection. If IgM anti-HBc and HBsAg are both positive, and HDV infection is suspected on epidemiologic grounds, further testing for anti-HDV should be considered. The presence of IgM anti-HBc and HBsAg, together with positive findings for anti-HDV strongly supports a diagnosis of HDV/HBV co-infection. In some instances, HBsAg may not be detected despite the presence of HDV/HBV co-infection. In

HBsAg-positive patients with acute hepatitis in whom IgM anti-HBc is not detected but IgG anti-HBc is present, testing for anti-HDV should be undertaken. Positive findings for anti-HDV in this setting suggest the presence of HDV superinfection of an HBV carrier. An acute hepatitis may be seen in some persistently HBsAg-positive patients without HDV infection in whom HBV reactivation occurs with the reappearance of HBeAg and HBV DNA, indicating enhanced HBV replication. In others, an acute hepatitis may be associated with HBeAg seroconversion.

The presence of anti-HCV in the absence of the other serologic markers supports the diagnosis of acute HCV infection. If anti-HCV is also absent at presentation, follow-up testing should be undertaken, since the appearance of anti-HCV is often delayed for several months. Serologic testing for HEV infection is not available. The diagnosis can be suspected if the other markers of hepatitis are absent and the epidemiologic circumstances are consistent with possible exposure.

Serologic Diagnosis of Chronic Viral Hepatitis

Since the only etiologic forms of viral hepatitis associated with chronic viral hepatitis are HBV, HDV, and HCV infections, testing for HAV and, in the future, HEV is unnecessary in the evaluation of patients with chronic viral hepatitis. Since chronic HBV infection is almost invariably associated with the persistence of HBsAg, HBsAg testing should be undertaken. HBsAg-positive patients should be further tested for the presence of HBeAg and HBV DNA to assess the level of HBV replication and the response to treatment with antiviral or immunomodulatory drugs. Testing for anti-HDV should also be performed in HBsAg-positive patients with chronic hepatitis, particularly when chronic HDV is suspected because of epidemiologic features. The detection of anti-HDV in an HBsAg-positive patient with chronic hepatitis suggests that chronic HDV infection is also present. Positive findings on second-generation tests for anti-HCV support a diagnosis of chronic HCV infection in the patient with chronic hepatitis. It seems possible that testing for HCV RNA will become available in the near future and that these tests will be used to assess the level of HCV replication and the response to treatment with antiviral or immunomodulatory drugs.

REFERENCES

1. Zajac AJ, Amphlett EM, Rowlands DJ, et al. Parameters influencing the attachment of hepatitis A virus to a variety of continuous cell lines. J Gen Virol. 1991;72:1667–1675.
2. Fagan E, Yousef G, Brahm J, et al. Persistence of hepatitis A virus in fulminant hepatitis and after liver transplantation. J Med Virol. 1990;30:131–136.
3. Rosenblum LS, Villarino ME, Nainan OV, et al. Hepatitis A outbreak in a neonatal intensive care unit: Risk factors for transmission and evidence of prolonged viral excretion among preterm infants. J Infect Dis. 1991;164:476–482.
4. Tong S, Diot C, Gripon P, et al. In vitro replication competence of a cloned hepatitis B virus variant with a nonsense mutation in the distal pre-C region. Virology. 1991;181:733–773.
5. Blum HE, Galun E, Liang TJ, et al. Naturally occurring missense mutation in the polymerase gene terminating hepatitis B virus replication. J Virol. 1991;65:1836–1842.
6. Omata M, Ehata T, Yokosuka O, et al. Mutations in the precore region of hepatitis B virus DNA in patients with fulminant and severe hepatitis. N Engl J Med. 1991;324:1699–1704.
7. Liang TJ, Hasegawa K, Rimon N, et al. A hepatitis B virus mutant associated with an epidemic of fulminant hepatitis. N Engl J Med. 1991;324:1705–1709.
8. Blum HE, Liang J, Galun E, et al. Persistence of hepatitis B viral DNA after serological recovery from hepatitis B virus infection. Hepatology. 1991;14:56–62.
9. Chao M, Hsieh SY, Taylor J. The antigen of hepatitis delta virus: Examination of in vitro RNA-binding specificity. J Virol. 1991;65:4057–4062.
10. MacNaughton TB, Gowans EJ, McNamara SP, et al. Hepatitis delta antigen is necessary for access of hepatitis delta virus RNA to the cell transcriptional machinery but is not part of the transcriptional complex. Virology. 1991;184:387–390.
11. Ponzetto A, Hoyer BH, Popper H, et al. Titration of the infectivity of the hepatitis D virus in chimpanzees. J Infect Dis. 1987;155:72–78.
12. Yuasa T, Ishikawa G, Manabe S, et al. The particle size of hepatitis C virus estimated by filtration through microporous regenerated cellulose fibre. J Gen Virol. 1991;72:2021–2024.
13. Simmonds P, Zhang LQ, Watson HG, et al. Hepatitis C quantification and sequencing in blood products, haemophiliacs, and drug users. Lancet. 1990;336:1469–1472.
14. Ulrich PP, Romeo JM, Lane PK, et al. Detection, semiquantitation, and genetic variation in hepatitis C virus sequences amplified from the plasma of blood donors with elevated alanine aminotransferase. J Clin Invest. 1990;86:1609–1614.
15. Shibata M, Morishima T, Kudo T, et al. Serum hepatitis C virus sequences in posttransfusion non-A, non-B hepatitis. Blood. 1991;77:1157–1160.
16. Davis GL, Hoofnagle JH, Waggoner JG. Acute type A hepatitis during chronic hepatitis B virus infection: Association of depressed hepatitis B virus replication with appearance of endogenous alpha interferon. J Med Virol. 1984;14:141–147.
17. Lopez Morante A, de la Cruz F, de Lope CR, et al. Hepatitis B virus replication in hepatitis B and D coinfection. Liver. 1989;9:65–70.
18. Bas C, Bartolome J, La-Banda F, et al. Assessment of hepatitis B virus DNA levels in chronic HBsAg carriers with or without hepatitis delta virus superinfection. J Hepatol. 1988;6:208–213.

19. Farci P, Karayiannis P, Lai ME, et al. Acute and chronic hepatitis delta virus infection: Direct or indirect effect on hepatitis B virus replication. J Med Virol. 1988;26: 279–288.
20. Ten Napel HH, Houthoff HJ, The TH. Cytomegalovirus hepatitis in normal and immune compromised hosts. Liver. 1984;4:184–194.
21. Phillips MJ, Blendis LM, Poucell S, et al. Syncytial giant-cell hepatitis: Sporadic hepatitis with distinctive pathological features, a severe clinical course, and paramyxoviral features. N Engl J Med. 1991;324:455–460.
22. CDC. Hepatitis Surveillance Report No. 53, 1990:23.
23. Vento S, Garofano T, Di Perri G, et al. Identification of hepatitis A virus as a trigger for autoimmune chronic hepatitis type 1 in susceptible individuals. Lancet. 1991;337:1183–1187.
24. Balayan MS, Usmanov RK, Zamyatine NA, et al. Brief Report: Experimental hepatitis E infection in domestic pigs. J Med Virol. 1990;32:58–59.
25. Balayan MS. HEV infection: Historical perspectives, global epidemiology, and clinical features. In: Hollinger FB, Lemon SM, Margolis HS, eds. Viral Hepatitis and Liver Disease. Baltimore: Williams & Wilkins; 1991:498–500.
26. Shimizu H, Mitsuda T, Fujita S, et al. Perinatal hepatitis B virus infection caused by antihepatitis Be positive maternal mononuclear cells. Arch Dis Child. 1991;66:718–721.
27. Verme G, Brunetto MR, Oliveri F, et al. Role of hepatitis delta virus infection in hepatocellular carcinoma. Dig Dis Sci. 1991;36:1134–1136.
28. Shimizu YK, Weiner AJ, Rosenblatt J, et al. Early events in hepatitis C virus infection of chimpanzees. Proc Natl Acad Sci USA. 1990;87:6441–6444.
29. Uchida T, Suzuki K, Iida F, et al. Virulence of hepatitis E virus with serial passage to cynomolgus monkeys and identification of viremia. In: Viral Hepatitis and Liver Disease. Hollinger FB, Lemon SM, Margolis HS, eds. Baltimore: Williams & Wilkins; 1991:526–527.
30. Gerlich WH, Uy A, Lambrecht F, et al. Cutoff levels of immunoglobulin M antibody against viral core antigen for differentiation of acute, chronic, and past hepatitis B virus infections. J Clin Microbiol. 1986;24:288–293.
31. Davies SE, Portman B, Smith HM, et al. Unique pattern of tissue damage with recurrent HBV post-orthoptic liver transplantation. Hepatology. 1991;13:150–157.
32. Cassidy WM, Govindarajan S, Gupta S, et al. Influence of HIV on chronic hepatitis B and D infection. Hepatology. 1989;10:690.
33. Gupta S, Govindarajan S, Cassidy WM, et al. Acute delta hepatitis: Serological diagnosis with particular reference to hepatitis delta virus RNA. Am J Gastroenterol. 1991;89:1227–1231.
34. Buti M, Esteban R, Espanol MT, et al. Influence of human immunodeficiency virus infection on cell-mediated immunity in chronic D hepatitis. J Infect Dis. 1991;163:1351–1353.
35. Eyster ME, Alter HJ, Aledort LM, et al. Heterosexual cotransmission of hepatitis C virus (HCV) and human immunodeficiency virus (HIV). Ann Intern Med. 1991;115:764–768.
36. Giovannini M, Tagger A, Ribero ML, et al. Maternal-infant transmission of hepatitis C virus and HIV infections: A possible interaction. Lancet. 1990;335:1166.
37. Hatzakis A, Hadziyannis S. Sex-related differences in immunoglobulin M and in total antibody response to hepatitis A virus observed in two epidemics of hepatitis A. Am J Epidemiol. 1984;120:936–942.
38. Robbins DJ, Krater J, Kiang W, et al. Detection of total antibody against hepatitis A virus by an automated microparticle enzyme immunoassay. J Virol Methods. 1991;32:255–263.
39. Krawczynski K, Bradley DW. Enterically transmitted non-A, non-B hepatitis: Identification of virus-associated antigen in experimentally infected cynomolgus macaques. J Infect Dis. 1989;159:1042–1049.
40. Ichikawa M, Araki M, Rikihisa T, et al. Cloning and expression of cDNAs from enterically transmitted non-A, non-B hepatitis virus. Microbiol Immunol. 1991;35:535–543.
41. Kaneko S, Kobayashi K, Miller RH. Detection of hepatitis B virus DNA using the polymerase chain reaction technique. J Clin Lab Anal. 1990;4:479–482.
42. Buti M, Esteban R, Jardi R, et al. Chronic delta hepatitis: Detection of hepatitis delta virus antigen in serum by immunoblot and correlation with other markers of delta viral replication. Hepatology. 1989;10:907–910.
43. Chaggar K, McFarlane IG, Smith HM, et al. An enzyme immunoassay for detection of IgA class antibodies against hepatitis delta virus. J Virol Methods. 1991;32: 193–199.
44. Salassa B, Daziano E, Bonino F, et al. Serological diagnosis of hepatitis B and delta virus (HBV/HDV) coinfection. J Hepatol. 1991;12:10–13.
45. Esteban JI, Gonzalez A, Hernandez JM, et al. Evaluation of antibodies to hepatitis C virus in a study of transfusion-associated hepatitis. N Engl J Med. 1990;323:1107–1112.
46. Weiner AJ, Kuo G, Bradley DW, et al. Detection of hepatitis C viral sequences in non-A, non-B hepatitis. Lancet. 1990;335:1–3.
47. Tremolada F, Casarin C, Tagger A, et al. Antibody to hepatitis C virus in post-transfusion hepatitis. Ann Intern Med. 1991;114:277–281.
48. Alter HJ, Purcell RH, Shih JW, et al. Detection of antibody to hepatitis C virus in prospectively followed transfusion recipients with acute and chronic non-A, non-B hepatitis. N Engl J Med. 1989;321:1494–1500.
49. Carman WF, Fagan EA, Hadziyannis S, et al. Association of a precore genomic variant of hepatitis B virus with fulminant hepatitis. Hepatology. 1991;14:219–222.
50. Coursaget P, Yvonnet B, Bourdil C, et al. HBsAg positive reactivity in man not due to hepatitis B virus. Lancet. 1987;2:1354–1358.
51. Koff RS. Difficult serologic diagnoses in viral hepatitis. In: Hollinger FB, Lemon SM, Margolis HS, eds. Viral Hepatitis and Liver Disease. Baltimore: Williams & Wilkins, 1991:790–791.
52. Swenson PD, Escobar MR, Carrithers RL Jr, et al. Failure of pre-existing antibody against hepatitis B surface antigen to prevent subsequent hepatitis B infection. J Clin Microbiol. 1983;18:305–309.

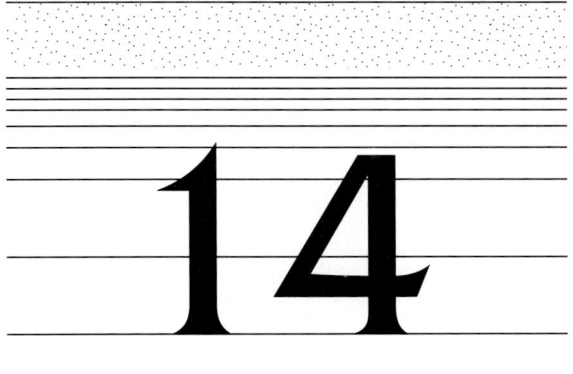

14

Treatment of Chronic Viral Hepatitis

RICHARD A. WILLSON, M.D.

CHRONIC HEPATITIS

Chronic hepatitis comprises a group of disorders with inflammation of the liver that has been present for more than 6 months.[1-3] Such a time frame is required in order to exclude slowly resolving acute hepatitis. The majority of patients with acute hepatitis resolve their infection within 3 months, and therefore the possibility of an acute hepatitis evolving into a chronic hepatitis becomes an issue at approximately 4 to 6 months. This evolution of acute hepatitis to chronic hepatitis is not, however, commonly observed in practice. The majority of patients with chronic hepatitis are diagnosed by serum aminotransferase elevations, a finding often obtained incidentally as part of a biochemical screen for an unrelated problem. Since these patients commonly have no recall of an episode of acute hepatitis, the beginning of the hepatitis cannot be dated. In this setting, both the finding of an elevated level of serum aminotransferase must be validated and its persistence documented during an arbitrary period of at least 6 months. Having done both, the physician has established the diagnosis of chronic hepatitis.

Etiologic Spectrum

Chronic hepatitis has a number of causes (Table 14–1) that either may be considered simultaneously with the above establishment of chronicity or must be determined after the establishment of chronicity.[4] The most common cause is chronic viral hepatitis related to viral hepatitis B, C, or D. The relative prevalence of these three viruses varies considerably from one area or population studied to another, but in general their frequency in decreasing order is hepatitis C virus (HCV), hepatitis B virus (HBV), and hepatitis D virus (HDV). These three viruses can be distinguished by serologic testing.[5] The next most common cause of chronic hepatitis is the idiopathic or so-called autoimmune type of hepatitis.[6] This form of chronic hepatitis may be associated with other autoimmune disorders, can often be distinguished by specific testing for serum autoantibodies, and is usually responsive to treatment with corticosteroids and other immunosuppressive drugs.[7] Drug-induced hepatitis is not a common cause of chronic hepatitis, but it is essential to exclude it from a differential diagnosis, since discontinuation of the offending drug resolves

313

TABLE 14–1. ESTABLISHED ETIOLOGY OF CHRONIC HEPATITIS

Viral hepatitis
B
C
D
Idiopathic autoimmune
Drug therapy
Metabolic disorders
Wilson's disease
α_1-Antitrypsin deficiency

TABLE 14–2. OCCASIONALLY MAY BE CONFUSED WITH CHRONIC HEPATITIS

Primary biliary cirrhosis
Primary sclerosing cholangitis
Alcohol-induced liver disease
Steatonecrosis (nonalcoholic)
Hemochromatosis

the chronic hepatitis in the majority of instances. Drug-induced liver injury can mimic virtually all naturally occurring liver diseases,[8] and, therefore, a careful, and often a repeated, drug history is mandatory. Isoniazid, methyldopa, and nitrofurantoin have, on occasion, been associated with chronic hepatitis, but other drugs have been incriminated as well.[9, 10] The metabolic disorders associated with chronic hepatitis are the least common causes. Wilson's disease, in young individuals, presents as chronic hepatitis, often in the absence of neurologic abnormalities.[11, 12] Wilson's disease is uncommon but has a known specific treatment; copper chelating agents specifically prevent the progression of the disease. Alpha$_1$-antitrypsin deficiency in adults may present with features suggesting chronic hepatitis and with no evidence of pulmonary disease.[13]

On occasion, other chronic liver diseases, since they are not conventionally considered in the differential diagnosis of chronic hepatitis, may cause confusion in the initial evaluation of a patient with chronic inflammation of the liver (Table 14–2).[4] Primary biliary cirrhosis, although typically a cholestatic condition, may in its early stages appear similar to the idiopathic autoimmune form of chronic hepatitis.[14] Another typically cholestatic condition, primary sclerosing cholangitis, in its early stages may have features that are indistinguishable from those of chronic hepatitis. The presence of inflammatory bowel disease may be a clue, and cholangiography may be required to confirm the diagnosis.[15] Alcohol-induced liver injury may cause confusion, albeit uncommonly.[16] One needs to be aware of any superimposition of a chronic viral hepatitis, whether B or C, or both, in a patient with alcohol-induced liver injury.[17–20] Many alcoholics have risk factors for acquiring the various forms of viral hepatitis. Steatonecrosis (non–alcohol-related) is an entity that is incompletely defined,[21–23] but it presents with elevated serum aminotransferase levels. Its histologic features usually distinguish it from classic chronic hepatitis. Hemochromatosis may present with elevated serum aminotransferase levels and therefore initially appear as a chronic hepatic inflammatory disorder. Serum ferritin levels, percent transferrin saturation, and iron that has been determined on liver histopathologic analysis confirm the diagnosis.[24]

Histopathology

Essential to the evaluation of chronic hepatitis is a liver biopsy (Table 14–3). The liver biopsy may provide a specific diagnosis by means of immunocytochemical assessment for specific viruses, quantitative iron and copper determinations, detection of α_1-antitrypsin globules, and the presence of specific features of cholestatic liver conditions, alcohol-induced liver disease, and steatonecrosis. Moreover, the liver biopsy provides evidence for both the extent and severity of the underlying liver injury. Indeed, the findings on liver biopsy are the basis for the pathologic classification of chronic hepatitis.[1–3]

The widely accepted histologic classification of chronic hepatitis is summarized in Table 14–4.[4] Chronic persistent hepatitis (CPH) is characterized by mild inflammation confined to the portal tract (Fig. 14–1) without fibrosis, and it is usually considered a benign or nonprogressive process. Chronic lobular hepatitis (CLH) is

TABLE 14–3. VALUE OF LIVER BIOPSY IN CHRONIC HEPATITIS

Diagnose specific cause
Pattern recognition
Immunocytochemical
Examination for specific viruses
α_1-Antitrypsin
Globules
Copper determination
Identify or exclude other liver diseases
Cholestatic
Alcohol-induced
Nonalcoholic steatonecrosis
Hemochromatosis
Determine extent and severity of liver injury
Assess natural history or effects of specific therapies
Detect hepatocellular carcinoma

TABLE 14–4. HISTOLOGIC CLASSIFICATION OF CHRONIC HEPATITIS

CHRONIC PERSISTENT HEPATITIS (CPH)
The inflammation is confined to the portal tract, and the limiting plate of hepatocytes surrounding the portal tract is intact.
Fibrosis is minimal.
Occasional mild focal inflammation may be present within the hepatic lobule.

CHRONIC LOBULAR HEPATITIS (CLH)
The inflammation is predominantly found within the hepatic lobule.
Periportal and portal inflammation are minimal, as is fibrosis.

CHRONIC ACTIVE HEPATITIS (CAH)
The inflammation and fibrosis may be severe.
Extensive portal and periportal inflammation (piecemeal necrosis) is present, and the limiting plate is disrupted.
Bridging hepatic necrosis between portal tracts and central veins may be present.
Multiple hepatic lobules may be involved, with extensive necrosis.

CIRRHOSIS (C)
The inflammation, acute or chronic, is variable.
Regenerative nodules and extensive fibrosis are the histologic hallmarks of cirrhosis.

characterized by focal lobular inflammation with minimal portal or periportal inflammation and no bridging necrosis or fibrosis (Fig. 14–2). Most patients with CLH have a chronic viral hepatitis. Little evidence exists to suggest progression to either chronic active hepatitis or cirrhosis. Chronic active hepatitis (CAH) is characterized by more severe inflammation of the portal tracts with extension outside of the portal areas into the lobule, often manifesting as piecemeal necrosis (Fig. 14–3). Extensive fibrosis and bridging hepatic necrosis may be present. Chronic active hepatitis is considered a variably progressive process that eventually leads to cirrhosis. Cirrhosis is the recognized end stage of chronic hepatitis and is characterized by varia-

ble degrees of acute and chronic inflammation, nodular regeneration, and extensive fibrosis (Fig. 14–4). Cirrhosis may be latent clinically or manifested with decompensated liver disease in such signs as ascites, edema, variceal bleeding, and encephalopathy. Hepatocellular carcinoma (HCC) is a recognized complication of cirrhosis.

These histologic classifications of chronic hepatitis are useful only in the broad sense, and their etiologic or clinical application is limited. Indeed, the categories CPH, CLH, and CAH are likely to be replaced by morphologic terms that describe portal and lobular necroinflammation, with and without fibrosis, and grade the severity of disease from mild to moderate to severe.[25–27] Although the severity of liver injury can be quantified,[28] the method is of limited value in practice, and its major application is in clinical trials, in which it is used to assess the efficacy of various therapeutic agents.

Diagnosis: Immunocytochemistry and in Situ Hybridization

In the future as our diagnostic means become more precise, the pathologic classification of chronic hepatitis will be made by specific causal agent (see Table 14–1). For example, in the differential diagnosis of chronic viral hepatitis, the detection of the specific virus in the liver would be very helpful clinically. Although serologic or serum hybridization assays are essential for diagnosis, they are an indirect measure of virologic events that are occurring in the liver in chronic viral hepatitis. Examining these virologic events directly in the liver biopsy can be accomplished with current molecular biologic techniques. Such an examination provides in-

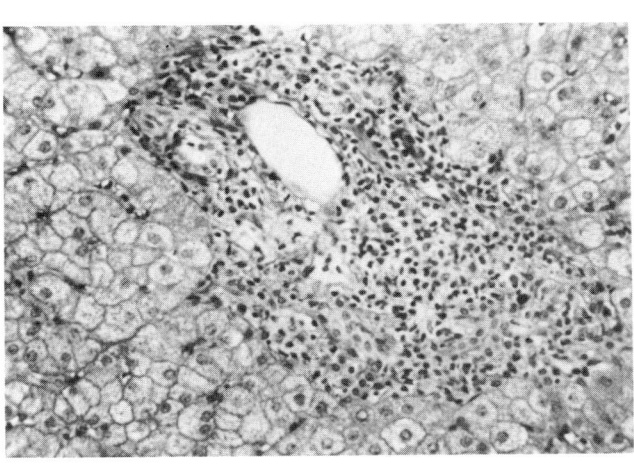

FIGURE 14–1.
Chronic persistent hepatitis. Mild portal inflammation with absence of piecemeal necrosis and no fibrosis. (Hematoxylin and eosin × 100)

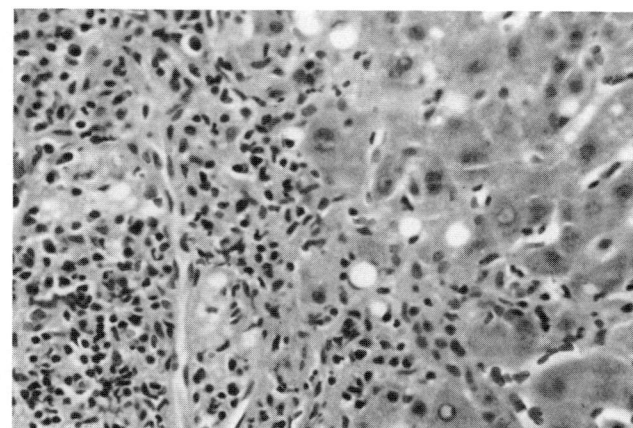

FIGURE 14–2.
Chronic lobular hepatitis. Hepatocellular necrosis within the hepatic lobule, but with minimal portal and periportal inflammation. (Hematoxylin and eosin × 100)

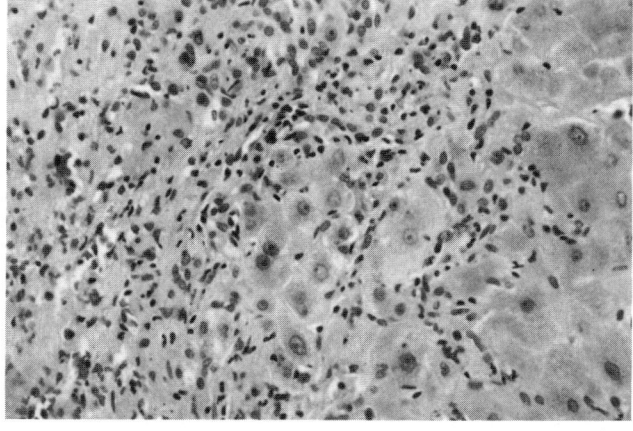

FIGURE 14–3.
Chronic active hepatitis. Prominent portal and periportal inflammation with disruption of the limiting plate and the presence of piecemeal necrosis. (Hematoxylin and eosin × 100)

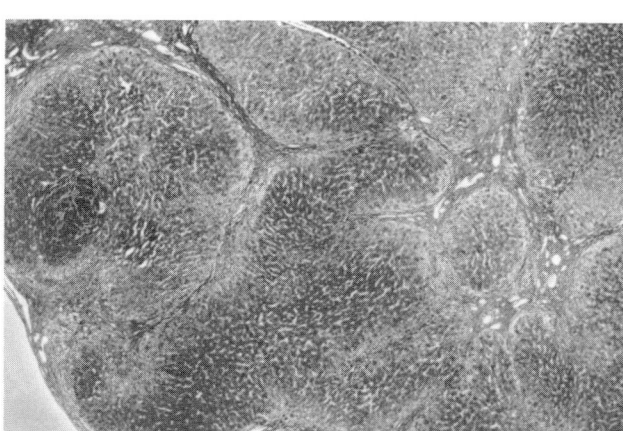

FIGURE 14–4.
Cirrhosis. Mild chronic inflammatory infiltrate, extensive fibrosis, and regenerative nodules. (Hematoxylin and eosin × 100)

creased understanding of viral replication in the liver and its role in the pathogenesis of chronic viral hepatitis. The presence of viral antigens and nucleic acids in liver biopsy specimens may be detected either by assaying a homogenized liver biopsy sample or by directly assaying the tissue sample. From the homogenized sample, the molecular weight of the viral products as well as information about viral integration can be obtained. The assay methods include Southern blot, which examines deoxyribonucleic acid (DNA); Northern blot, which examines ribonucleic acid (RNA); and immunoblot, which tests for antigens. In situ hybridization of DNA and RNA and immunocytochemical testing for antigens in tissue sections are able to provide information about the distribution of infected cells, intracellular location of virus products, types of liver cells infected, correlation between different viral antigens and nucleic acid, and the relation of all these factors to the activity and extent of the underlying chronic viral hepatitis in the given liver biopsy sample. Most of the studies on in situ hybridization and immunocytochemical analysis have been carried out to investigate aspects of chronic infection with HBV or HDV.[29] Preliminary reports on in situ hybridization[30] and immunocytochemistry[31, 32] indicate that such techniques are promising for the investigation of chronic hepatitis C.

In immunocytochemical analysis, commercial reagents are available for immunostaining for hepatitis B surface antigen (HB$_s$Ag), hepatitis B core antigen (HB$_c$Ag), and hepatitis D antigen (HDAg). Frozen liver sections are more sensitive for detecting these antigens than are formalin-fixed paraffin-embedded liver samples. Indeed, the stains for HB$_s$Ag on formalin-fixed tissue are recognized to be unreliable in confirming the diagnosis of hepatitis B. Stains for HB$_c$Ag on formalin-fixed tissue are more reliable and therefore more useful clinically.[33, 34] Nevertheless, these stains do not commonly show the HB$_c$Ag in the cytoplasm, which indicates the replicative cycle of the HBV, nor do they show the HB$_c$Ag on the plasma membrane of the hepatocyte, which is believed to be the important form of HB$_c$Ag involved in the immunologic response to HBV. In summary, 95% of patients with chronic hepatitis B demonstrate HB$_c$Ag located in the nucleus of infected hepatocytes on liver sections fixed in formalin. So-called healthy, inactive carriers of HB$_s$Ag produce negative results on HB$_c$Ag immunostaining of their liver biopsy. Thus, immunostaining can be very helpful in distinguishing a patient with chronic hepatitis B from a patient who is an apparently healthy, or inactive, carrier.[33] In

chronic hepatitis D, immunocytochemical staining for HDAg in formalin-fixed tissue is reliable. Indeed, immunostaining for HDAg is the current gold standard for the diagnosis of chronic hepatitis D. The HDAg is usually detected in the nuclei of infected hepatocytes, but on occasion it may be within the cytoplasm. Large amounts of HDAg are produced within hepatocytes during chronic hepatitis D infection, and this allows ready detection of the HDAg by immunostaining.

In situ hybridization also allows study of hepatitis viruses in liver tissue. For maximum sensitivity, the use of ^{125}I-labeled probes and frozen liver sections is advisable. In situ hybridization of liver sections shows the presence of replicative intermediates of HBV DNA in the cytoplasm of infected hepatocytes in patients with chronic hepatitis B, but not in inactive carriers. Nevertheless, low levels of HBV DNA can still be detected in their livers by polymerase chain reaction (PCR) analysis.[35, 36]

Compared with its use in chronic hepatitis B, the use of in situ hybridization for the detection of HDV RNA in liver samples from patients with chronic hepatitis D has been limited. Nevertheless, the in situ hybridization studies have confirmed that the nucleus of the hepatocytes is the intracellular location of HDV RNA replication and showed that HDAg and HDV RNA are present in the same cells. Thus, HDAg appears to be a good marker for HDV replication.

Since the technique is available to most pathology laboratories, immunocytochemistry will continue to provide useful information on the expression of viral antigens and the relationship of those antigens to hepatocellular injury. By contrast, in situ hybridization is a more difficult technique, and all pathology laboratories may not be able to provide this service. Nevertheless, kits for in situ hybridization are becoming increasingly available commercially, and therefore more diagnostic laboratories will employ this method.

Clinical Features and Management

The clinical features of chronic hepatitis are protean; they range from an asymptomatic disease detected by incidental biochemical screening to a rapidly progressive disease leading to hepatic decompensation.[4] In general, the silent nature of chronic hepatitis, particularly the forms caused by chronic viral hepatitis, is not widely appreciated. Even when present in the early stages of chronic hepatitis, however, the symptoms are relatively nonspecific but include fatigue, malaise, anorexia, depression, and right upper quadrant discomfort. In chronic hepatitis, the correlation between clinical symptoms and the extent of the biochemical abnormality or the severity of the underlying histopathologic condition is recognized to be poor. For example, asymptomatic patients with mild serum aminotransferase elevations may have severe underlying liver disease. This absence of correlation emphasizes the need for liver biopsy in the proper evaluation of patients with presumed chronic hepatitis.

No effective treatments are available for most of the disabling symptoms of chronic hepatitis, especially the marked fatigue that is commonly a dominant symptom. Nevertheless, supportive care, including patient education about chronic hepatitis, use of alcohol or other drugs, proper diets, efficacy of vitamins, and the role of exercise, may prove to be very helpful to the patient.[4] In more severe disease, in which fluid retention and hepatic encephalopathy are manifested, salt restriction and protein restriction are dietary maneuvers that have proved their clinical efficacy, but no other dietary changes have been proved to be of value. Supplemental vitamins do not appear beneficial, but most patients take multivitamins regardless. Patients should be forewarned of the potentially harmful effects to the liver and other organs of excessive dosages of certain vitamins. Patients with significant cholestasis and jaundice may require supplementary fat-soluble vitamins A, D, and K. A regular exercise program is recommended for most patients, and prolonged bed rest is to be discouraged. Except for drugs that have been associated with causing chronic hepatitis, patients with mild to moderately severe chronic hepatitis can tolerate most medications. No evidence suggests that patients with chronic hepatitis are more likely than patients without liver disease to develop an idiosyncratic drug reaction. Unless the patient has advanced chronic hepatitis or cirrhosis, most therapeutic drugs can be administered safely, but dosage adjustments may be required. Small amounts of alcohol are not harmful to patients with chronic hepatitis, and they frequently inquire about its use. Excessive alcohol intake is not to be allowed, and evidence of such abuse must be sought in evaluating some patients with marked depression or other confounding symptoms or behavior.[4]

CHRONIC VIRAL HEPATITIS

Human viral hepatitis occurs in both acute and chronic forms.[37] At least five different clinical hepatitis diseases caused by five distinct viruses are known. These viruses include the hepatitis A virus (HAV), HBV, HCV, HDV, and the hepatitis E virus (HEV). Additional viruses are likely to be found to play a role in human viral hepatitis. For example, in the posttransfusion hepatitis setting, reasonable evidence suggests that another virus may be responsible for a small number of cases (approximately 10%) that appear to be unrelated to HCV.[38] Moreover, a new viral hepatitis syndrome was described in the early 1990s that is associated with the paramyxovirus.[39] Although all of the five viruses mentioned cause acute hepatitis, only HBV, HCV, and HDV are associated with persistent infection and chronic viral hepatitis. A comparison of the three types of viruses associated with chronic viral hepatitis in humans is outlined in Table 14–5. The clinically important points in Table 14–5 are that all three viruses are commonly transmitted by parenteral routes and that the frequency of evolving into chronic hepatitis varies considerably among the three viruses.

TABLE 14–5. COMPARISON OF THREE TYPES OF VIRUSES ASSOCIATED WITH CHRONIC VIRAL HEPATITIS IN HUMANS

FEATURES	HEPATITIS B	HEPATITIS C	HEPATITIS D
Virus	HBV	HCV	HDV
Virus class	Hepadnavirus	?Flavivirus or pestivirus	Satellite virus
Virus size	42 nm	30–60 nm	40 nm
Genome	ds DNA	ss RNA(+)	ss RNA(−)
Antigens	HB_sAg	HCAg	HDAg
	HB_cAg		
	HB_eAg		
	HB_xAg		
Transmission	Parenteral and sexual	Largely parenteral	Largely parenteral
Frequency of chronicity	3–10%	40–70%	2–70%*

*Higher rate of chronicity when HDV occurs as a superinfection
SOURCE: Adapted from: Hoofnagle JH, et al. Antiviral Agents and Viral Diseases of Man. Raven Press;1990:416.

Since chronic viral hepatitis is more likely to follow a mild subclinical acute illness than a severe, icteric acute viral hepatitis, the progression from acute to chronic disease often goes undetected clinically.[37] Most patients with chronic viral hepatitis do not remember an acute episode of viral hepatitis, and many patients are, in fact, relatively asymptomatic. Estimates suggest that 0.5–1.0% of the United States population has chronic hepatitis B, 1–2% has chronic hepatitis C, and less than 0.05% has chronic hepatitis D.[37] Cirrhosis and HCC are the major serious sequelae of chronic viral hepatitis, and they contribute to its recognized high rates of morbidity and mortality. Serologic testing facilitates the identification of the specific agent in chronic viral hepatitis.[5] On occasion, however, the interpretation of the serologic tests may be complex, and in certain settings several viruses may be present simultaneously, particularly in those individuals who are frequently exposed, such as drug addicts.[40] The treatment of chronic viral hepatitis is directed at inhibiting viral replication, eliminating the virus, resolving hepatic inflammation, improving the underlying histopathologic condition, and preventing cirrhosis and the development of HCC.

Chronic Hepatitis B

The HBV (see Table 14–5), a member of the hepadna group, is a double-stranded DNA virus that replicates by reverse transcription. The HBV has multiple antigens that, although leading to a complex serologic picture, are essential for diagnosis, staging, and assessment of treatment. This virus is endemic in the human population and hyperendemic in certain regions of the world, including Southeast Asia and Southern Africa. Natural hepadnavirus infections occur in woodchucks, ground squirrels, and the Peking duck. These animal models will be helpful in enhancing our understanding of the natural history of HBV infection as well as in providing insights into potential antiviral treatments.

Hepatitis B Epidemiology

Worldwide, chronic HBV infection is a major cause of chronic hepatitis, cirrhosis, and primary HCC.[41] In those areas where hepatitis B is highly endemic, such as China and Africa, chronic HBV infection is primarily an infection of infants and children. In areas of low rates of infection, such as the United States and Western Europe, transmission during infancy and childhood is uncommon, and parenteral routes or sexual transmission are very important in the spread of hepatitis B. The HBV infection occurs primarily in young adults with certain behavioral, occupational, or lifestyle risk factors.[42] Sexual activity—commonly promiscuous, both homosexual and heterosexual—is a frequently cited risk factor for HBV infection.[43, 44] Since 1985, the number of cases of hepatitis B in homosexual men has declined by 65%. This decrease is related almost entirely to a reduction in high-risk sexual activity in response to the acquired immunodeficiency syndrome (AIDS) epidemic. With the decline of hepatitis B in homosexual males, however, the incidence of hepatitis B in heterosexual men and women has increased, strikingly, by 40%.[45] Heterosexual activity is now the mode of transmission in at least 25% of cases of HBV infection. Intravenous drug abuse is commonly associated with HBV infection, and needlestick exposure is an occupational hazard also associated with HBV infection.[42] Underlining the potential for occupational exposure to parenterally transmitted viruses, a 1992 report from an inner city emergency room in the United States indicated that HBV, HCV, and human immunodeficiency virus (HIV) are all highly prevalent among such workers: 5% have HBV, 18% have HCV, and 6% have HIV.[46] Because of the availability of sensitive serologic assays, HBV infection related to administered blood products is now very uncommon.

Natural History of Hepatitis B

Some patients with acute hepatitis B do not recover completely and go on to develop chronic hepatitis B. Determinants that are recognized to be important in the development of chronic hepatitis B include age at acquisition, gender, and immune status. Vertical transmission from mother to child at birth is almost always (90–100% of cases) associated with chronic hepatitis B, whereas the frequency of chronic hepatitis B decreases to 25% in children and to only 5% in adults. Chronic hepatitis B is more prevalent in males and in those who have chronic diseases with an altered immune status, such as renal failure. The clinical course of chronic hepatitis B is extremely variable, and its activity and severity can wax and wane over time.[47–50] In some patients, the disease is rapidly progressive, and cirrhosis may evolve within several years after the onset of the disease. In others, the disease progresses more slowly and episodically, and cirrhosis may develop many years later. In a small proportion, the disease is rather mild, and ultimately a spontaneous remission occurs. A spontaneous loss of 2% of HB$_s$Ag per year in patients with chronic hepatitis B is recognized.

The clinical, biochemical, and serologic course of a typical case of chronic HBV infection is shown in Figure 14–5. After 5 years of chronic hepatitis, hepatitis B e antigen (HB$_e$Ag) and HBV DNA are spontaneously lost and serum aminotransferase decreases into the normal range. The loss of HB$_e$Ag from the serum is the most sensitive and reliable serologic marker for eradication of viral replication, and patients who lose HB$_e$Ag from serum usually manifest a clinical and biochemical mitigation of their disease activity, despite the continued presence of HB$_s$Ag.[51] The chronic HBV infection can, however, undergo spontaneous reactivation.[52, 53] The frequency of a spontaneous reactivation has not been accurately determined, but in one report it occurred in 30% of the patients followed long term.[52] These episodes of reactivation may be relatively more common in male homosexuals than in heterosexuals and in Asian patients or patients with advanced liver disease. Reactivation invariably occurs within 1 year of HB$_e$Ag seroconversion and may be severe. Thus, HB$_e$Ag seroconversion to antibody to hepatitis B$_e$ (anti-

HB$_e$) is not necessarily an indicator of a permanent remission of the chronic hepatitis B, and the subsequent spontaneous reactivation may be an important cause of progression of liver injury. Nevertheless, the seroconversion of the HB$_e$Ag to anti-HB$_e$ is commonly used as the end point of successful antiviral therapy.[37]

In chronic hepatitis B, clinical symptoms are an unreliable guide to either the presence or the severity of chronic hepatic injury. The majority of patients with chronic viral hepatitis have no symptoms or have complaints only of mild to moderate degrees of fatigue. For this reason, chronic viral hepatitis is often a silent disease, and the absence of symptoms does not allow accurate differentiation between clinically unimportant underlying liver disease and severe progressive liver injury. In chronic HBV infection, chronic hepatitis B must be distinguished from the so-called healthy HB$_s$Ag carrier state.[33]

In the patient with persistent HB$_s$Ag in the serum, the serum aminotransferases are often tested to determine presence or absence of underlying chronic liver disease. These biochemical tests are more reliable than are symptoms in identifying patients who have chronic hepatitis. The magnitude of the elevation in the aminotransferases does not, however, accurately reflect the severity of the underlying liver disease.

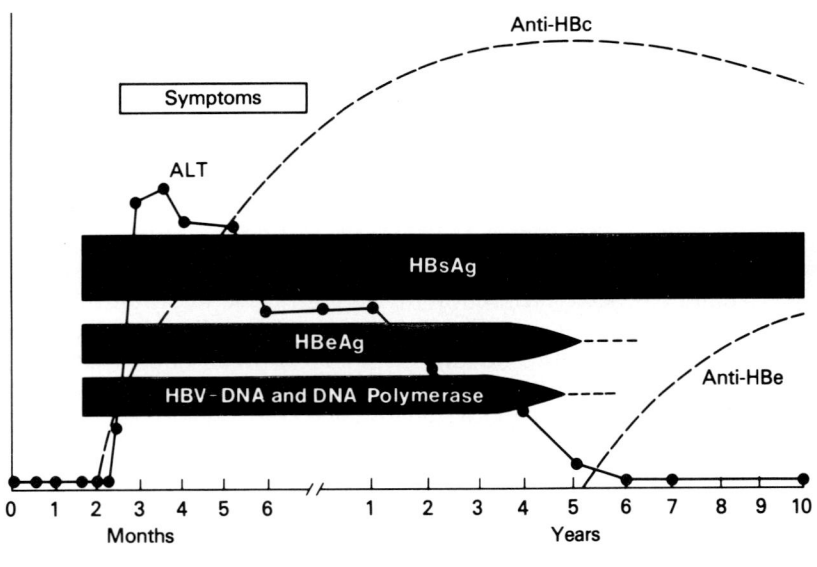

FIGURE 14–5.
The clinical, serum biochemical, and serologic course of a typical case of chronic hepatitis B. A 5-year period of chronic hepatitis is followed by a spontaneous improvement in the disease, with the fall of serum aminotransferase activities into the normal range and the loss of serum markers of HBV replication despite the continued presence of HB$_s$Ag. KEY: ALT = alanine aminotransferase, anti-HB$_c$ = antibody to hepatitis B core antigen, anti-HB$_e$ = antibody to hepatitis B e antigen, DNA-p = deoxyribonucleic acid polymerase activity, HB$_e$Ag = hepatitis B e antigen, HB$_s$Ag = hepatitis B surface antigen, HBV = hepatitis B virus. SOURCE: Hoofnagle JH, DiBisceglie AM. Antiviral therapy of viral hepatitis. In: Galasso GJ, Whitley RJ, Merigan TC, eds. Antiviral Agents and Viral Diseases of Man. 3rd ed. New York: Raven Press;1990:428.

In inactive cirrhosis, the serum aminotransferases are often only slightly elevated. During some periods, moreover, the serum aminotransferases are normal in patients with chronic viral hepatitis. Thus, the serum aminotransferases are not always reliable in distinguishing the patient with chronic viral hepatitis B from the patient in the healthy carrier state.[33]

Clinically available serologic tests may distinguish more accurately those patients with chronic hepatitis B from the so-called healthy carrier. Patients with chronic hepatitis B usually have HB_eAg and HBV DNA in their serum, whereas healthy carriers usually have no or low levels of HBV DNA in their serum and are anti-HB_e–positive. These two forms may represent two different phases or stages of chronic HBV infection: One may be an early replicative form and the other a later nonreplicative form.[33] The most practical and readily available test for measuring the state of viral activity assesses the serum HB_eAg. Most patients with active viral replication have HB_eAg in their serum, whereas those without active viral replication do not have HB_eAg in their serum and test positive for the HB_e antibody. Thus, most patients with chronic hepatitis B test HB_eAg-positive, and the healthy carrier tests negative for HB_eAg. This generalization has, however, many exceptions. Indeed, the level of HBV replication, as measured by serum HB_eAg, DNA polymerase activity, or HBV DNA testing does not correlate well with severity of underlying chronic liver disease.

Consequently, liver biopsy has been the standard means of distinguishing the patient with significant liver disease from the so-called healthy carrier.[33] The healthy carrier should have either normal liver histologic findings or only minimal abnormalities. The cytoplasm of healthy carriers frequently has large numbers of hepatocytes with abundant HB_sAg, which appear histologically as ground-glass hepatocytes. The liver biopsy is not invariably accurate, however, in distinguishing these two types of infection because liver histologic study does not indicate the state of viral replication. Immunocytochemical stains for HB_sAg and HB_cAg allow more accurate assessment of the chronic hepatitis B. These immunocytochemical techniques demonstrate that patients with chronic hepatitis B and active viral replication almost always have HB_cAg detectable in the liver, whereas the healthy carrier does not; HB_sAg can be found in both and may be more prominent in the healthy carrier. The research techniques for determining HBV DNA in liver tissue may eventually become the tests of choice in defining the state of HBV infection in the liver.[29]

In summary, an accurate assessment of whether a patient has chronic hepatitis B or is in a healthy carrier state requires a combination of clinical, biochemical, serologic, and histologic study (Table 14–6). The healthy carrier is usually asymptomatic with no signs of chronic liver disease, has normal levels of serum aminotransferases, serologically tests negative for HB_eAg, DNA polymerase activity, and HBV DNA, and has an essentially normal liver biopsy, with evidence for HB_sAg but not HB_cAg, by immunocytochemical analysis. The patient with chronic hepatitis B may not have symptoms or signs of chronic liver disease but usually has elevated serum aminotransferases, has serologic evidence of HB_eAg, DNA polymerase activity, or HBV DNA; evidence shows on liver biopsy of chronic hepatitis; and demonstrates by immunocytochemical study both HB_sAg and HB_cAg.[33, 34]

This proposed distinction between chronic hepatitis B and the healthy carrier does not apply to all patients, however, since some patients do not fall into either category. This observation is especially true if HB_eAg is used as the only serologic marker for active HBV replication. Many patients with HB_sAg-positive liver disease are negative for HB_eAg, and the question arises whether their underlying liver disease is secondary to another process or cause or merely another variation in the spectrum of chronic HBV infection. In the clinical setting, when an HB_sAg-positive, HB_eAg-negative patient continues to demonstrate active liver disease, certain factors must be considered (Table 14–7). An HBV mutant has been described that clinically presents with serious chronic liver disease but is HB_eAg-negative and anti-HB_e–positive.[54, 55] The coexistence of HDV or HCV infection needs to be excluded as well as drug-induced liver injury. Other unrelated liver diseases must also be considered as the cause for progressive liver disease.

Because of advances in molecular biologic techniques, the standard division of chronic

TABLE 14–6. DIAGNOSIS OF CHRONIC HEPATITIS B

Elevated (persistent or fluctuating) serum aminotransferase levels for at least 6 months or longer
HB_sAg-positive serum for at least 6 months or longer
Liver biopsy evidence of chronic hepatitis (mild, moderate, severe) with or without cirrhosis
Evidence of HBV replication:
  HB_eAg-positive serum
  HBV DNA in serum
  HB_cAg in liver

KEY: DNA = deoxyribonucleic acid, HB_cAg = hepatitis B core antigen, HB_eAg = hepatitis B e antigen, HB_sAg = hepatitis B surface antigen, HBV = hepatitis B virus.

TABLE 14–7. CHRONIC HEPATITIS B

HB$_s$Ag-positive, HB$_e$Ag-negative, anti-HB$_e$–positive case with evidence for active liver disease. Consider:

HBV mutant with continued HBV replication as evidenced by serum HBV DNA
Coexistence of hepatitis D or hepatitis C
Drug-induced liver disease
Unrelated liver disease

hepatitis B into an early replicative phase and a later nonreplicative phase is undergoing some modification.[56] A 1991 report indicates that after HB$_e$Ag seroconversion and loss of HBV DNA in serum, as measured by a soluble hybridization assay, serum HBV DNA actually persists at a low level, as measured by the more sensitive PCR technique.[35] This report demonstrates that HBV DNA, as measured by PCR, disappears from the serum only after HB$_s$Ag seroconversion. A preliminary report has indicated, moreover, that low levels of HBV DNA still exist in the liver of patients with chronic hepatitis B who have undergone HB$_e$Ag and HB$_s$Ag seroconversion and normalized their serum aminotransferase levels yet still show mild residual hepatitis on liver biopsy.[36] Both of these observations have been confirmed by other investigators.[57] Consequently, the nonreplicative phase might better be changed to a low-replicative, or latent, phase.[56]

Treatment: Interferons as Antiviral Agents

The interferons are a family of proteins that are produced in response to viral and other stimuli and are one of the body's natural defenses against viral infections. In addition, interferons have antiproliferative and immunomodulatory effects. Although interferon was discovered more than 30 years ago, the therapeutic potential as well as the mechanisms for actions of interferons remain actively investigated.[58–61]

Three families of interferons are recognized. Alpha-interferon is produced by B lymphocytes and monocytes. Approximately 17 different human alpha-interferon subtypes are known. Beta-interferon is produced by fibroblasts, one interferon-β gene exists. Gamma-interferon is produced by helper, or inducer, T lymphocytes, and only one interferon-γ gene exists.

Interferons are generally grouped with the intercellular signaling proteins, that is, the hormones, lymphokines, and cytokines. Interferons activate their target cells by first binding to specific receptors on the cell surface to induce synthesis of various intracellular proteins. These in-

tracellular proteins mediate the varied actions of interferon. For example, one antiviral effect of interferon is believed to be the intracellular activation of the enzyme 2′,5′-oligoadenylate synthetase, which in turn activates ribonucleases that destroy viral messenger ribonucleic acid (mRNA) within infected cells. Another intracellular protein system that is activated by interferon is the protein kinase system, which mediates its antiviral effect by inhibiting the translation of viral proteins. Interferons may also inhibit viral entry and other viral replicative events within the cell. In addition, the immunoregulatory effects of interferon on the expression of major histocompatibility antigens, the activation of macrophages, the modulation of natural killer and cytotoxic T cells, and the induction of cytokines would be likely to influence viral replication and spread.

The interferon system is active during acute viral hepatitis, regardless of its cause. Although interferon may not be measurable in the systemic circulation, its local introduction is sufficient to induce recognized effects. In chronic viral hepatitis, however, local interferon production appears to be deficient since the markers of interferon induction are not present. This process has been investigated mainly in chronic HBV disease.[59, 62, 63] The finding of the suboptimal response by the interferon system in chronic hepatitis B stimulated the therapeutic application of interferon in that setting. Indeed, early studies of alpha-interferon treatment for chronic hepatitis B were encouraging since rapid lowering of the hepatitis B virus level in serum was demonstrated.[37] The lack of sufficient amounts of alpha-interferon, however, restricted its early therapeutic clinical application. These preliminary and uncontrolled pilot studies nevertheless provided valuable information on dosage and duration of interferon therapy. For example, lower dosages of 5 to 10 million units (mU) per day were as effective as very high dosages of greater than 30 mU per day in inhibiting viral replication and were tolerated better.[37] The optimal duration of therapy was 3 to 4 months. Moreover, a delayed response or transient flare in the activity of the underlying chronic hepatitis seen in approximately two-thirds of patients appeared to be necessary for a lasting therapeutic response. This clinical exacerbation of disease activity suggested that alpha-interferon was active not only by inhibiting viral replication but also by strengthening the patient's immune response to the HBV. This combined effect of viral inhibition and immune stimulation was necessary for both serologic and clinical response.

With the advent of the recombinant interferons, controlled studies have been carried out in the treatment of chronic hepatitis B, C, and D in an attempt to define better the role of interferon in the treatment of chronic viral hepatitis. These controlled studies are discussed more thoroughly in sections dealing with antiviral therapy of chronic hepatitis B, C, and D.

Adverse Effects. Alpha-interferon therapy is frequently associated with mild to moderate systemic side effects characterized by a flulike illness that begins several hours after the injection of interferon (Table 14–8).[64] These systemic side effects consist of mild fever, chills, headache, arthralgias, and myalgias. These effects are dose-related, but they are experienced initially by most patients given 3 to 5 MU of interferon. These side effects are commonly responsive to acetaminophen. Patients, if forewarned, usually tolerate these side effects well. More serious side effects (see Table 14–8), however, particularly neuropsychiatric, may encompass mild confusion, difficulty with concentrating ability, general irritability, abusive behavior, or frank depression. A history of serious antecedent depression is probably a contraindication to interferon therapy. In our experience, and as noted by others,[65] neuropsychiatric side effects are the most common reason for discontinuing interferon therapy. Other associated toxicities include a decrease in the leukocyte and platelet counts. These decreases may temporarily require either dosage reduction or dose-skipping for their management. These hematologic toxicities usually occur within the first 4 weeks of therapy, and therefore patients require weekly monitoring of blood count for the first month. Patients with evidence of prominent hypersple-

nism require extra attention, and the hematologic toxicities may be the limiting factor in the tolerance of alpha-interferon therapy.

Slight serum aminotransferase elevations have been reported in association with alpha-interferon therapy.[66] Reports of 1990 and 1991 suggest, however, that alpha-interferon therapy may induce serious liver injury.[67–70] In one report, since no antecedent liver disease was present and other potential causes for acute liver injury were not found, the serious liver injury was attributed to interferon-induced toxicity.[69]

The induction of autoimmune disease by interferon therapy is well recognized.[66, 71, 72] Thyroid disease, both hyper- and hypothyrodism, hemolytic anemia, and thrombocytopenia are among the more common disorders reported.[64, 66, 72, 73] Autoantibodies occur in these induced disorders as well as in the interferon treatment setting in general.[74] The significance of the circulating autoantibodies in the setting of interferon treatment remains unclear. Alpha-interferon therapy may worsen the course of chronic autoimmune hepatitis when it is erroneously diagnosed as chronic hepatitis C.[75] Autoimmune disease or a predisposition to it may, however, occur in association with chronic hepatitis C.[70, 76, 77] The induction of autoimmune phenomena is also important when interferon therapy is applied after the transplantation of liver, bone marrow, or kidney, as they may be associated with an increased incidence of organ rejection.[60]

Some patients under treatment with alpha-interferon develop neutralizing antibodies to the given interferon preparation. The incidence of these antibodies depends on both the particular alpha-interferon preparation and the assay system used for detection.[78] The biologic significance of the antibodies and their role in the clinical efficacy of alpha-interferon are under investigation.[79] Several reports indicate that the level of the interferon antibody titer may relate to a lower efficacy in treatment of chronic hepatitis B[80] and chronic hepatitis C.[81] This phenomenon may be related to the type of interferon used.[82] The neutralizing antibodies to a subspecies of recombinant alpha-interferon do not appear, however, to affect the antiviral activity of the multiple subspecies of natural or lymphoblastoid interferon.[60]

ALPHA-INTERFERON ANTIVIRAL TREATMENT OF CHRONIC HEPATITIS B

The early studies of antiviral therapy for chronic HBV infection showed that three re-

TABLE 14–8. ADVERSE EFFECTS OF ALPHA-INTERFERON THERAPY

Mild to moderate side effects that usually do not require change in the administration of alpha-interferon
    Fatigue
    Fever
    Chills
    Myalgia
    Arthralgias
    Anorexia
    Nausea
    Insomnia
    Difficulty with concentration

More severe side effects that may require a change in the administration of alpha interferon
    Bone marrow suppression of platelets, neutrophils
    Infections
    Autoimmune disorders
    Psychiatric disturbance

sponses can occur; these responses are summarized in Table 14–9.[37] The most common of the three responses is transient. Some patients (30–40%), however, have a partial response. The clinical, biochemical, and serologic course of a typical patient with chronic HBV infection who had a partial response to recombinant alpha-interferon treatment is shown in Figure 14–6. The partial response is indicated by the disappearance of detectable serum HBV, as measured by serum HBV DNA, by DNA polymerase activity in association with clearance of serum HB$_e$Ag and by biochemical improvement of the liver disease, as measured by serum aminotransferase level, but persistence of serum HB$_s$Ag. The majority of patients (65%) who have a response to alpha-interferon therapy demonstrate a flare in their disease activity, or an increase in serum aminotransferase level, while on therapy. This flare in disease activity usually occurs after 1 to 3 months of therapy and coincides with the disappearance of HBV DNA and HB$_e$Ag from serum. After these events, the liver disease abates, despite the presence of HB$_s$Ag, as as-

TABLE 14–9. THREE RESPONSES OF CHRONIC HEPATITIS B TO ALPHA-INTERFERON THERAPY

Transient response
  A lowering of HBV replication as indicated by decreasing levels of either serum DNA polymerase activity or HBV DNA. These are not sustained when therapy is stopped.
Partial response
  A disappearance of either measurable serum DNA polymerase activity or HBV DNA, along with seroconversion of HB$_e$Ag, improvement in biochemical and histologic findings, but persistence of serum HB$_s$Ag.
Complete response
  A loss of serum HBV DNA, DNA polymerase activity, HB$_e$Ag, and HB$_s$Ag as well as biochemical and histologic improvement.

sessed on follow-up liver biopsy.[83–87] This remission in disease activity is usually sustained and represents a transition from chronic hepatitis B to a healthy carrier state. The continued presence of HB$_s$Ag in serum appears to be explained by integrated molecules of HBV DNA

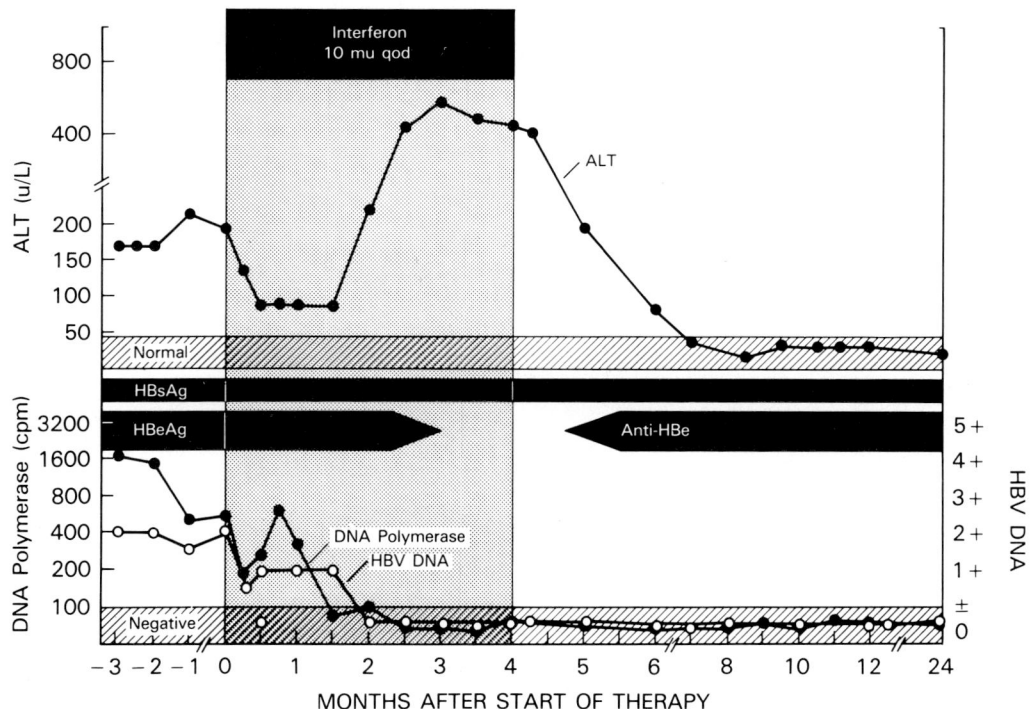

FIGURE 14–6.
The clinical, serum biochemical, and serologic progression of a patient with chronic hepatitis B, who partially responded to treatment with recombinant human interferon-α. During therapy, HBV DNA and DNA polymerase fell to undetectable levels and HB$_e$Ag disappeared and was followed by the development of anti-HB$_e$. This patient remained positive for HB$_s$Ag but had a clinical remission of the disease with serum ALT levels falling to normal. Four years later, this patient was still an HB$_s$Ag carrier but had no symptoms of liver disease and had normal serum aminotransferase levels. KEY: ALT = alanine aminotransferase, anti-HB$_e$ = antibody to hepatitis B e antigen, HB$_e$Ag = hepatitis B e antigen, HB$_s$Ag = hepatitis B surface antigen, HBV = hepatitis B virus. SOURCE: Hoofnagle JH, DiBisceglie AM. Antiviral therapy of viral hepatitis. In: Galasso GJ, Whitley RJ, Merigan TC, eds. Antiviral Agents and Viral Diseases of Man. 3rd ed. New York: Raven Press;1990:432.

in the hepatocytes, which retain an intact S gene but do not produce intact virions.

A complete response to alpha-interferon therapy is optimal but uncommon, occurring in only 10 to 15% of patients. Some patients, both those with a partial and those with a complete response to alpha-interferon therapy, are left with an inactive cirrhosis secondary to their chronic hepatitis B and may yet suffer from the consequences of portal hypertension or HCC or both.

A large number of alpha-interferon studies have been reported since the 1980s, but most of the more recent studies have not been controlled or involve a small number of patients or both. In addition, comparison between these studies is often difficult because of differences in dosages, administration regimens, source and type of interferon used, length of treatment, and heterogeneity of patient characteristics.[88] A summary of selected controlled trials of recombinant alpha-interferon therapy for chronic hepatitis B in adults is given in Table 14–10.[81, 84–86, 89–91]

Although the dose, duration, and type of alpha-interferon varied among the studies carried out on white subjects, approximately 40 to 45% of patients with chronic hepatitis B responded with loss of their serum HB_eAg, and approximately 15% of patients also lost their serum HB_sAg. By contrast, the response rate in controls was approximately 10% and less than 1%, respectively. The relapse rate in white subjects is approximately 10% or less, and most studies indicated an improvement in histologic findings on follow-up liver biopsy. In Asian patients, the response rate for seroconversion of both HB_eAg and HB_sAg was considerably lower than in whites, and, in addition, their relapse rate was high.[91, 92]

An updated report from Hong Kong confirms that alpha-interferon therapy in adult Chinese patients with chronic hepatitis B is not efficacious in patients with normal serum aminotransferse levels.[82] The response rate was significantly better, however, in patients with elevated serum aminotransferses, and was, in fact, similar to the response rates noted in whites. The rate of relapse was not given.

The dosage of interferon varied considerably in the trials and ranged from 1 to 20 MU, given daily, every other day, or thrice weekly. The higher dosages were associated with more side effects but also with higher positive response rates. In a United States multicenter trial of alpha-interferon treatment for chronic hepatitis B, the greater efficacy of the 5 MU per day regimen compared with the 1 MU per day regimen is shown in Figure 14–7. After treatment, the loss of both serum HBV DNA and HB_eAg was significantly greater in patients on the 5 MU per day regimen compared with that of both the control group and patients on the 1 MU per day regimen.[83]

The duration of alpha-interferon therapy varied among the trials. The serologic response to interferon therapy usually does not occur until after 2 to 3 months of therapy, and therefore the continuation of interferon therapy for at least 3 to 4 months is recommended. Continuation of alpha-interferon for longer than 4 to 6 months has not consistently increased the response rate to therapy. The trials carried out in the United States examined a 4-month course of therapy.[83, 84, 90]

The accumulated experience with alpha-interferon treatment for chronic hepatitis B suggests that a number of clinical factors appear to predict a favorable response in adults with chronic hepatitis B; these factors are listed in Table 14–11. In the multicenter study carried out in the United States and reported in 1990,

TABLE 14–10. CONTROLLED TRIALS OF RECOMBINANT ALPHA-INTERFERON THERAPY FOR CHRONIC HEPATITIS B IN ADULTS

				% RESPONSE*					
				WHITE		ASIAN			
REFERENCE	N	DOSAGE/ DURATION†	TYPE	Interferon	Control	Interferon	Control	% RELAPSE	HISTOLOGIC IMPROVEMENT
Alexander (1987)[89]	46	20/6	L	26 (14)	0 (0)			NE	Yes
Hoofnagle (1988)[84]	45	5–10/4	2B	32 (7)	7 (0)			10	Yes
Lok (1988)[91]	18	5/6	2A			17 (0)	0 (0)	47	NC
	18	10/6	2A			28 (0)	0 (0)		
Brook (1989)[85]	37	20/6	2A	43 (18)	0 (0)			NE	Yes
Saracco (1989)[86]	64	10/6	L	70 (24)	39 (3)			0	Yes
Perrillo (1990)[83]	41	5/4	2B	37 (12)	7 (0)			2	Yes
DiBisceglie (1991)[90]	47	10/4	2B	42 (15)	5 (0)			NE	NE

*Response = loss of HB_eAg (in parenthesis, loss of HB_sAg) in serum.

†Dosage in million units (mU) of interferon daily (some studies qod or 3 × week); duration in months of treatment.

KEY: 2A = recombinant interferon-α-2A; 2B = recombinant interferon-α-2B; L = lymphoblastoid; NC = no change; NE = not evaluated.

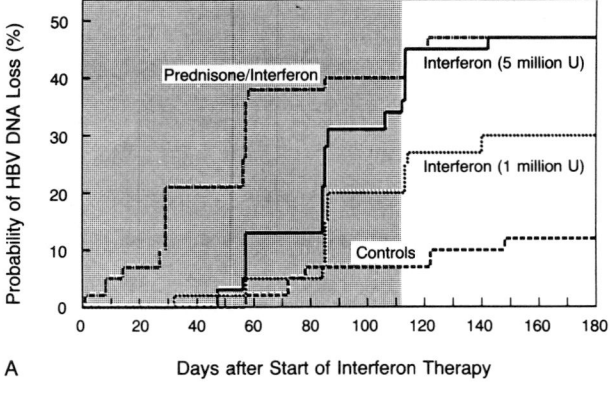

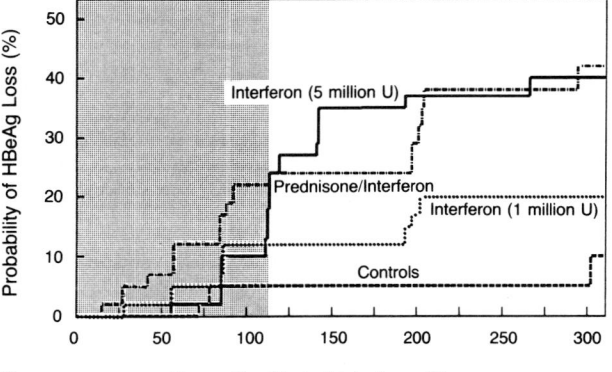

FIGURE 14–7.
Actuarial curves of loss of HBV DNA (*A*) and HB$_e$Ag (*B*) in treated patients and untreated controls. *A*, the differences between the treated patients and the controls were as follows: P=0.06 for the group that received 1 million units of interferon, P=0.0017 for the group that received 5 million units of interferon, and P=0.0001 for the group that was treated with prednisone. *B*, the differences between treated patients and controls were as follows: P was not significant for the 1-MU interferon group, P=0.0007 for the 5-MU interferon group, and P=0.0006 for the prednisone-treated group. The shaded areas indicate the period of interferon treatment. KEY: HB$_e$Ag = hepatitis B e antigen, HBV = hepatitis B virus. SOURCE: Perillo RP, Schiff ER, Davis GL, et al. A randomized controlled trial of interferon-α-2B alone and after prednisone withdrawal for the treatment of chronic hepatitis B. N Engl J Med. 1990;323:298.

lower levels of HBV DNA at entry, higher levels of serum aminotransferases, heterosexual orientation, and shorter duration of chronic hepatitis B were associated with a higher response rate to treatment.[83] A 1991 preliminary report confirmed the predictive value of higher serum aminotransferase levels but did not find that HBV DNA level or histologic scoring was of predictive value.[90] Women responded more frequently than men, but the difference was not statistically significant. The disease is rare in women, and men accounted for 80 to 90% of the patients with chronic hepatitis B. Asians are generally nonresponsive to alpha-interferon therapy[82, 93] and patients from the Mediterra-

nean area may have higher rates of response for reasons that remain unclear.[37] Some studies have suggested that male homosexuals, with or without HIV positivity, were less likely to respond to antiviral therapy, but not all studies have supported this finding.[94] Although the evidence is conflicting, male homosexuals should not be excluded from antiviral treatment even though the presence of HIV infection may reduce their response to treatment. Patients with evidence for hepatic decompensation or those who are taking immunosuppressive treatments, as, for example, those undergoing solid organ transplant or cancer chemotherapy, have generally been considered to be poor candidates for interferon therapy, as is discussed later in this chapter.

The mechanisms involved in the efficacy of alpha-interferon treatment for chronic hepatitis B are not known. Evidence suggests that the hepatitis associated with chronic HBV infection is mediated by immune lysis of infected hepatocytes.[95] Natural killer (NK) and cytotoxic T cells compose the inflammatory infiltrate in chronic hepatitis B. Alpha-interferon stimulates the differentiation of NK cells, increases the expression of class I major histocompatibility com-

TABLE 14–11. FACTORS THAT PREDICT RESPONSE OF ADULTS WITH CHRONIC HEPATITIS B TO ALPHA-INTERFERON THERAPY

Increased disease activity (higher serum aminotransferase levels)
Lower levels of serum HBV DNA
Non-Asian ethnic background
Female gender
Absence of other diseases (AIDS, renal disease, and other immunocompromised states).
Heterosexual orientation

plexes on the surface of hepatocytes, and activates cellular enzymes (2', 5'-oligoadenylate synthetase and protein kinase) that inhibit viral protein synthesis.[60] These changes, if induced by alpha-interferon, would produce an antiviral state in uninfected regenerating hepatocytes. The viral antigens HB$_c$Ag and HB$_e$Ag present on the surface of infected hepatocytes in association with class I major histocompatibility complexes induced by alpha interferon make the infected hepatocytes a target for cytotoxic T-cell lysis.[95]

In chronic hepatitis B studies, a clinical, biochemical, and serologic evaluation 1 year after the alpha-interferon therapy has been standard. This 1-year follow-up period may be too short, however, to evaluate accurately either histologic changes[87] or loss of serologic markers of hepatitis B infection.[96] For example, the report by Korenman and colleagues indicates that the biochemical and serologic remissions induced by alpha-interferon treatment are of long duration and are followed in time by the eventual loss of HB$_s$Ag and all evidence of residual virus replication.[96] The serologic and biochemical findings in 20 patients who had a long-term response to alpha-interferon therapy are shown in Figure 14–8. The likelihood of their serum becoming negative for HBV DNA, by PCR analysis

and of their HB$_s$Ag becoming negative increased to approximately 75% over the 5-year period of observation. In this report, 20 of the 23 patients (87%) who lost serum HB$_s$Ag after treatment with alpha-interferon sustained a remission of 3 to 7 years in their disease. The 3 patients who relapsed did so within 1 year of treatment. All 3 of these patients possessed factors (Asian ethnicity, advanced cirrhosis, and HIV infection) that have been reported as predisposing factors to reactivation of HBV infection.[52, 53, 97] This report demonstrates that approximately two thirds of the patients who responded to alpha-interferon treatment initially lost their serum HB$_s$Ag months to years after HB$_e$Ag seroconversion. Untreated patients with a spontaneous seroconversion of HB$_e$Ag also had a high rate of loss of serum HB$_s$Ag, but the loss was significantly slower for these patients than for the alpha-interferon–treated group. Thus, the overall frequency of serum HB$_s$Ag loss may be the same in the untreated and the alpha-interferon–treated groups, but the rate of loss appears to be faster in the alpha-interferon–treated groups. Although the predictive factors for loss of HB$_s$Ag were not apparent, the treatment group was composed of patients who were adult Caucasians with well-compensated chronic hepatitis B acquired in

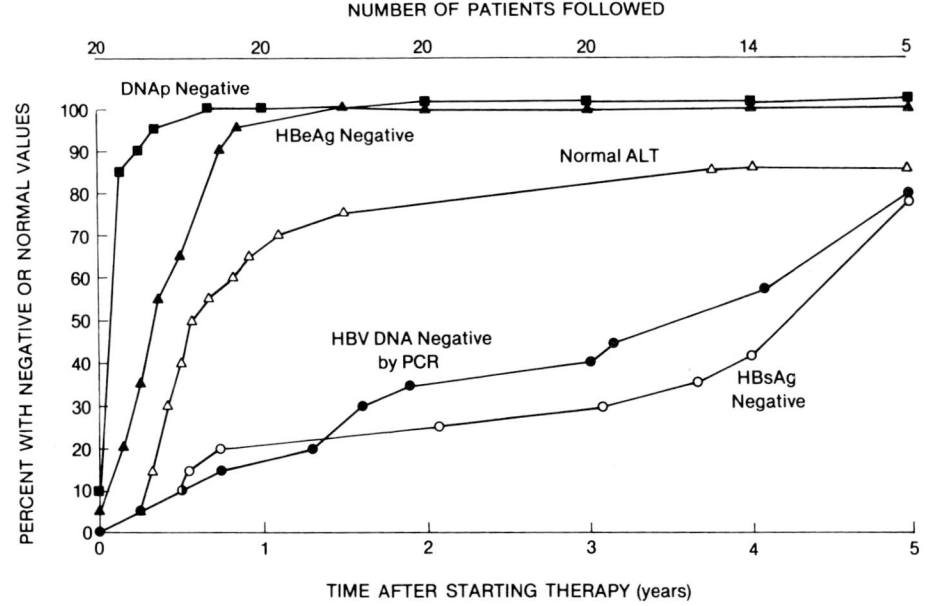

FIGURE 14–8.
Life-table analysis. Percentage of 20 patients who had negative or normal values for serologic and biochemical assays of response to long-term therapy with interferon-α. The duration of treatment was 4 months for most patients, with the exception noted in the text. KEY: ALT = alanine aminotransferase, DNA-p = deoxyribonucleic acid polymerase activity, HB$_e$Ag = hepatitis B e antigen, HB$_s$Ag = hepatitis B surface antigen, HBV = hepatitis B virus, PCR = polymerase chain reaction, time O = time of start of interferon therapy. SOURCE: Korenman J, Baker B, Waggoner J, et al. Long-term remission of chronic hepatitis B after alpha-interferon therapy. Ann Intern Med. 1991;114:630.

adulthood. Consequently, patients with childhood-acquired chronic hepatitis B and those with advanced decompensated liver disease may not demonstrate the favorable rates of loss of HB_sAg, as described by Korenman and colleagues.[96] The seroconversion of HB_sAg was usually accompanied by the loss of serum HBV DNA, as measured by both the slot blot hybridization technique and PCR.[96] This evidence indicates that with HB_eAg seroconversion, low levels of HBV replication persist and that when HB_sAg seroconversion occurs, HBV replication ceases. These observations suggest that alpha-interferon–treated patients who lose their serum HB_eAg but persist with serum HB_sAg may benefit from additional alpha-interferon therapy, especially those with persistent elevation of serum aminotransferases. A report from Spain suggests, however, a somewhat less optimistic long-term outcome.[98] The differences in outcome of the Spanish study, as compared with the findings of Korenman and colleagues,[96] were thought to be related to the characteristics of the patients included in the Spanish study.

Children. A summary of the controlled trials of recombinant alpha-interferon therapy for chronic hepatitis B in children is shown in Table 14–12.[99–101] Fewer studies have been carried out in children than in adults. Approximately 40% of white children respond with loss of serum HB_eAg, which is similar to the response in white adults. None of the children lost serum HB_sAg over the time period that these studies were carried out, however, and this response is considerably less than that found in white adults (see Table 14–10). Disappointingly, Asian children did not appear to respond at all to alpha-interferon therapy.[93, 101]

COMBINATION OF PREDNISONE AND ALPHA-INTERFERON

In an attempt to discover a way to enhance the response rate to alpha-interferon therapy, several combination therapies have been evaluated. Preliminary reports indicated that in patients with chronic hepatitis B, when corticosteroid therapy was withdrawn, an associated clinical flare of the hepatitis with an immunologic rebound occurred and was followed by a decline in the serum markers of HBV replication.[102, 103] With this preliminary information, a randomized controlled study was carried out to evaluate the efficacy of a short course of corticosteroids given prior to alpha-interferon therapy.[104] In this study, prednisone was given and withdrawn during a 6-week period: an initial dosage of 60 mg per day was decreased by 20 mg daily every 2 weeks. This 6-week course of prednisone was followed by 2 weeks of no treatment and then by 3 months of alpha-interferon therapy. HB_eAg seroconversion occurred in 44% of patients, and serum HB_sAg disappeared in 22%. Ninety percent of the HB_eAg seroconverters maintained their seronegative status for an interval of from 2 to 5 years. Owing to the encouraging results of this study, a large multicenter study was carried out in the United States that evaluated the outcome of corticosteroid pretreatment prior to alpha-interferon therapy.[83] As shown in Figure 14–7, the response rates in patients with chronic hepatitis B of both the loss of serum HBV DNA and the loss of serum HB_eAg were similar in those treated with prednisone and interferon and in those treated with 5 MU of interferon alone. This study indicates that the higher response rate associated with combination therapy is restricted to patients with lower baseline serum aminotransferase levels (<100 U/L).[83] By contrast, in Asian patients, pretreatment with prednisone appeared to have only a marginal benefit in those with elevated serum aminotransferases and no benefit in those with normal serum aminotransferases.[82] Consequently, the precise role of prednisone pretreatment remains unclear. Some risk is associated with this combination

TABLE 14–12. CONTROLLED TRIALS OF RECOMBINANT ALPHA-INTERFERON THERAPY FOR CHRONIC HEPATITIS B IN CHILDREN

				% RESPONSE*			
				WHITE		ASIAN	
REFERENCE	N	DOSAGE/ DURATION†	TYPE	Interferon	Control	Interferon	Control
Lai (1987)[101]	24	20/3	2A			0 (0)	0 (0)
Ruiz-Moreno (1991)[99]	12	10/6	2B	42 (0)	17 (0)		
	12	20/6		58 (0)			
Utili (1991)[100]	20	3/12	2A	20 (0)	10 (0)		

*Response = loss of HB_eAg (in parentheses, loss of HB_sAg) in serum.
†Dosage in million units (MU) of interferon daily (some studies qod or 3 × week); duration in months of treatment.
KEY: 2A = recombinant interferon-α-2A; 2B = recombinant interferon-α-2B.

therapy for patients who have active cirrhosis or who are marginally compensated. The clinical flare of the hepatitis that they experience after prednisone withdrawal may be fatal.[105]

COMBINATIONS OF DIFFERENT INTERFERONS

In further attempts to increase the response rate of interferon therapy, combinations of different interferons (alpha, beta, and gamma) have been evaluated in pilot clinical studies in patients with chronic hepatitis B.[106, 107] The clinical rationale for their use in combination was based on the speculation that their antiviral and immunomodulatory actions may be different and that when used in combination in vitro they appear to have a synergistic antiviral effect.[108] In one study in which a combination of beta- and gamma-interferon was evaluated, the findings suggested that early therapy with this combination may be effective since both inhibition of HBV replication and biochemical and histologic remission were demonstrated in treated patients as compared with controls.[106] Although these authors did not evaluate either beta- or gamma-interferon treatment alone in a controlled manner, neither interferon appears to have significant benefit alone in the treatment of chronic hepatitis B.[109] Additional studies of this combination of beta- and gamma-interferon for the treatment of chronic hepatitis B appear warranted. In another study, a combination of alpha- and gamma-interferon therapy was evaluated. This report demonstrated that the combination of these two interferons showed no additive or synergistic effects on HBV replication.[107] Gamma-interferon alone had a minimal effect on HBV viral replication, moreover, and was associated with more troublesome side effects. Thus, the addition of gamma-interferon to an alpha-interferon regimen does not offer any additional antiviral effects but contributes significantly to side effects.

INTERFERON TREATMENT OF CHRONIC HEPATITIS B PATIENTS WITH VARIOUS CHARACTERISTICS

HB_eAg-Negative Patients. In general, seroconversion from HB_eAg to anti-HB_e signals the loss of viremia and mitigation of the underlying chronic hepatitis.[33] In some cases, however, evidence for ongoing viral replication persists, as does the chronic hepatitis.[54, 55, 110, 111] Early in the 1990s, this clinical situation was shown to be related to an HBV mutant, or variant.[112] In this mutant strain of HBV, a genetic alteration in the sequencing of the HB_eAg protein prevents the secretion of the HB_eAg from the hepatocyte

into the blood.[111] Whether this situation occurs owing to an initial infection with the HBV variant or the variant evolves later in the course of a wild-type HBV infection remains unknown.

It is known, however, that the natural history of this anti-HB_e–positive form of chronic hepatitis B is more aggressive than is the HB_eAg-positive form and rapidly progresses to cirrhosis.[110] Therefore, an efficacious treatment for this form of chronic hepatitis B would be welcomed. A 1992 report indicates that a 6-month course of 10 MU of lymphoblastoid interferon, given 3 times per week, provided only a transient antiviral effect, having a relapse rate of 89% in patients with anti-HB_e–positive chronic hepatitis B.[113] This report supports previous experiences with alpha-interferon therapy in this setting, in which high relapse rates have been observed.[114, 115] By contrast, another 1992 report, using the same lymphoblastoid interferon and dosing schedule, indicates that the interferon therapy provided a complete response in 50% of patients and that their relapse rate was only 27%.[116] The relative youth and lower frequency of cirrhosis in the patients studied may account for the difference in treatment response from that of previous reports.[113–115, 117] Thus, alpha-interferon therapy at an early stage of disease may be efficacious in anti-HB_e, HBV-DNA–positive chronic HBV infection. Future therapeutic studies should focus on earlier stages of disease in anti-HB_e–positive patients and longer periods of antiviral treatment.

Decompensated Patients. Most of the previously described studies in which alpha-interferon therapy of chronic hepatitis B was evaluated were of patients with relatively mild disease, many of whom were asymptomatic. Patients with more severe disease were excluded, although they would clearly be in need of some form of effective treatment. A report of 18 patients with decompensated chronic hepatitis B found that some patients may benefit from alpha-interferon treatment but that lower dosages than usual may be required since these patients do not tolerate alpha-interferon well.[118] Serious complications are common, moreover, and may necessitate the drug's being discontinued. Consequently, if treated, these patients should be treated in a center that has experience with alpha-interferon therapy.[119]

Patients with Extrahepatic Manifestations. Glomerulonephritis associated with chronic hepatitis B, particularly in children, is recognized.[120–124] Neither the mechanism of renal injury nor the natural history of this HBV-related renal disease is clearly defined. Early case reports suggested that alpha-interferon therapy might mitigate the renal disease after the clearance of serum markers of HBV replication.[125-127] An interesting report evaluated 7 adults with HBV-related glomerulonephritis and the nephrotic syndrome.[128] These patients were treated with 5 MU of alpha-interferon daily for 4 months. In 5 patients, serum markers of HBV replication disappeared in association with marked improvement in their nephrotic symptoms. This study suggests that alpha-interferon therapy in this setting may result in a long-term mitigation of the nephrotic syndrome in those patients who have clearance of HBV replication.

The association of chronic HBV infection with a necrotizing vasculitis has been recognized for a long time.[129-131] It is a multisystem illness with a high mortality. Most patients have the angiographic findings of polyarteritis nodosa.[132] Immunosuppressive therapy, with corticosteroids or cyclophosphamide, is thought to improve survival rate.[132] The role of alpha-interferon therapy in this setting has not been evaluated.

Immunocompromised Patients. Chronic HBV infection frequently occurs in immunosuppressed patients. These patients commonly include those who are undergoing hemodialysis for chronic renal failure, cancer chemotherapy, and immunosuppressive therapy after organ transplantation.[94] In these immunosuppressed patients, the HBV replicates without any interference from the host's immune system. Consequently, the levels of circulating markers of HBV replication are often very high, although evidence for chronic hepatitis, either histologic or biochemical, is often not very apparent. The treatment of the chronic hepatitis B in these immunosuppressed patients presents a problem. For example, the use of alpha-interferon after organ transplantation has been of concern because of both interferon-induced toxicity and the potential for interference with graft function. A preliminary report suggests, however, that alpha-interferon therapy for liver transplant patients with chronic hepatitis B is tolerated well.[133] Whether it is efficacious in this setting remains to be shown. Previous experience with alpha-interferon treatment in patients with chronic hepatitis B has shown that those patients with high levels of viral replication and low serum ALT levels, such as is the case in immunosuppressed patients, are unlikely to respond to this treatment.[83] Indeed, early reports suggest that alpha-interferon does not appear efficacious in preventing chronic hepatitis B reinfection of the graft after liver transplantation.[134-136]

HIV-Infected Patients. Evidence increasingly suggests that interactions between HIV and HBV at the molecular level alter the pathogenesis and clinical manifestations both of the diseases they cause and of the responses to therapy.[137] Serologic evidence for combined HBV and HIV infection is common in high-risk groups such as male homosexuals, intravenous drug abusers, and hemophiliacs. The course of the chronic HBV infection changes, however, during the evolution of the HIV infection.[138, 139] For example, patients with chronic hepatitis B and AIDS usually have only mild hepatocellular injury, despite high levels of HBV replication in serum and liver. As in immunosuppressed patients in general, AIDS patients with chronic hepatitis B would not be likely to respond to alpha-interferon treatment, and a number of reports indicate that HIV-positive homosexual patients are less responsive to alpha-interferon treatment than are heterosexuals or HIV-antibody–negative homosexuals.[94] Thus, alpha-interferon treatment appears to be ineffective in HIV-antibody–positive patients with chronic hepatitis B, and this ineffective response is most likely related to diminished immunocompetency. Whether other antiviral agents will be more effective in this setting remains to be determined.

OTHER ANTIVIRAL THERAPIES FOR CHRONIC HEPATITIS B

Antiviral drug development in chronic hepatitis B has been enhanced by several in vitro and in vivo models of chronic hepatitis B. The evaluation of appropriate antiviral drugs or of their combinations can be conducted with selected animal models, addressing mechanisms of viral inhibition as well as effects on the course of chronic hepatitis B, including the development of HCC. Several antiviral agents, including thymosin, foscarnet, suramin, zidovudine, *Phyllanthus amarus*, and dideoxyadenosides, have been tested with either an in vitro or an in vivo chronic hepatitis B model system, and these agents may have therapeutic application.[140-145] In addition, some antiviral agents, including levamisole, transfer factor, ribavirin, thymosin, and interleukin-2 have been reported in pilot clinical studies and may have potential use in chronic hepatitis B.[146-152] As a single agent, acyclovir or any of its derivatives is not useful in the treatment of chronic hepatitis B.[95] Although a pilot study suggested that the combination of acyclovir and alpha-interferon might be more efficacious than either agent alone,[95] the results from a later multicenter controlled trial indicated that such a combination is not efficacious.[153]

ADENINE ARABINOSIDE AND ADENINE ARABINOSIDE MONOPHOSPHATE

Adenine arabinoside (ara-a) has been shown to inhibit HBV replication in duck HBV chronic infection,[154] and its clinical application has demonstrated inhibition of HBV replication.[155] Its clinical usefulness has been limited, however, by its poor solubility and its consequent need to be administered intravenously. Most reports have been based on the more water-soluble form, adenine arabinoside monophosphate (ara-AMP), which is administered intramuscularly. The use of ara-AMP has been evaluated clinically in the treatment of chronic hepatitis B both alone[156–159] and in combination with alpha-interferon.[160] The response rate to ara-AMP therapy has been variable, and the widely different rates of response may have been related to differences in the populations studied.[158] Nevertheless, the major drawback of ara-AMP therapy is the associated severe neurotoxicity,[161] which has limited its use, and therapeutic studies in the United States have stopped. A 1991 study involving the model of woodchuck chronic hepatitis B indicated that the dosage of ara-AMP required to inhibit HBV replication can be strikingly reduced by coupling the drug with a carrier human serum albumin.[162] These results suggest that such selective drug-conjugate vectors may inhibit HBV replication with reduced side effects. An uncontrolled pilot study of ara-AMP conjugated with lactosaminated albumin has documented HB_eAg seroconversion with limited side effects.[163] Further studies are required to evaluate this novel therapeutic approach.

Summary of Antiviral Treatment of Chronic Hepatitis B

Antiviral therapy for chronic hepatitis B continues to be experimental. Studies indicate that a 4- to 6-month course of alpha-interferon at dosages of 5 to 10 MU 3 times a week results in clinical, biochemical, and serologic improvement in 30 to 40% of patients with chronic hepatitis B. Clinical features that indicate the likelihood of a positive response to therapy include a high initial serum aminotransferase level and low levels of HBV DNA in the serum. Asian patients, both adults and children, are generally unlikely to respond well to alpha-interferon treatment. Pretreatment of patients with high-dosage corticosteroids may help to increase the response rate to alpha-interferon therapy alone, but this effect is seen mainly in patients who have mild disease, as indicated by lower levels of serum aminotransferases and less active chronic hepatitis on liver biopsy. Such pretreatment may best be left to those patients with mild disease or to patients who have failed to respond to alpha-interferon alone. The treatment of patients with decompensated hepatic disease remains uncertain, as does the treatment of recurrent HBV after liver transplantation. The somewhat limited efficacy and the side effects of alpha-interferon therapy should be considered in the decision whether to treat patients with chronic hepatitis B. Future therapeutic trials should focus on newer antiviral agents with or without alpha-interferon.

Hepatitis B Vaccine

The recombinant form of the hepatitis B vaccine has been shown to be stable, safe, highly immunogenic, and effective in individuals at high risk,[164, 165] and it is free from serious adverse effects.[166] Immunization with the HBV vaccine is the most effective means for preventing HBV infection and its consequences. Since the routes of transmission of HBV and HDV are similar, preventing acute and chronic HBV infection of susceptible persons also prevents HDV infection. In the United States, since most HBV infections occur in adults and adolescents, the original strategy recommended for the prevention of hepatitis B was the selective vaccination of adults with identified risk factors.[167] This strategy has not, however, lowered the incidence of HBV infections. From studies carried out in areas where HBV infection is endemic, childhood immunization programs have demonstrated that the rate of acute hepatitis B decreased by more than 90%.[168] Consequently, immunization during early childhood is now considered the most effective way to eliminate the transmission of HBV infection and ultimately to reduce the incidence of acute and chronic hepatitis B in the United States. Accordingly, the recommendations for implementing this strategy include making hepatitis vaccine a part of routine vaccination schedules for infants.[169] Such a program should result in the ultimate control of hepatitis B, but it might take 15 to 20 years before the effects of such an immunization program would be seen. The cost of a universal vaccine policy remains a concern, but the cost of immunization for hepatitis B in children is marginal compared with the cost of adult immunization since the amount of vaccine required in children is only one quarter of that required in adults. A cost-benefit analysis has shown that the cost of the vaccine program is significantly less than the cost to society of the consequences of HBV infection. The Immunization Advisory Committee of the Federal Centers for Disease Control (CDC) in Atlanta also urges continued efforts to immunize those adults at high risk for acquiring hepatitis B. In addition, the committee recommends continued evaluation of the long-term efficacy of the HBV vaccine in order to determine if and when booster doses may be needed.[165, 170]

Chronic Hepatitis C

Although the recently cloned HCV appears to be a novel virus, some evidence suggests that it may be a distant relative of the human flaviviruses (yellow fever, dengue, Japanese encephalitis) and animal pestiviruses (bovine viral diarrhea, hog cholera), which are now all considered members of the same Flaviviridae family.[171] Variations in hepatitis C virus genes exist, and four types have been characterized on the basis of differences in nucleotide sequences.[172] The distribution patterns of these genotypes vary from country to country. This genomic variation of the hepatitis C virus may be important both in the clinical manifestations of chronic hepatitis C[173, 174] and in its response to alpha-interferon therapy.[175, 176] This observed heterogeneity among the different isolates of HCV deserves close attention with respect to interactions between virus and host, evolution of chronic disease, response to antiviral treatment, potential induction by antiviral therapy, and vaccine development.[171, 177] One of the unique features of the HCV is that its molecular biology has largely preceded knowledge of its virology, immunology, and biology.

HCV contains a positive-stranded RNA genome that does not replicate through a DNA intermediate (see Table 14–5). Therefore, the chronicity of HCV in comparison with HBV cannot be explained as the latency of the virus through integration of the viral genome into the host genome.[171] Moreover, the strong association between HCV infection and development of HCC cannot be explained in terms of chromosomal genome integration as it can be for HBV. Thus, the presence of cirrhosis in most cases of HCV-associated HCC may indicate an indirect role for HCV in carcinogenesis.[178–180]

By the use of molecular biologic techniques, the nucleotide sequence of the entire HCV genome has been determined.[181] The genome consists of a 5' noncoding region, followed by core (nucleocapsid) and envelope structural regions, and then by five nonstructural regions (Figure 14–9). The entire genome is approximately 10 kilobases (kb), which code for approximately 3000 amino acids. The original clone, the 5-1-1 antigen, was derived from the nonstructural region NS4, and the larger clone, the c100-3 antigen, was derived from polypeptide sequences in both the NS3 and the NS4 regions. New antigens are being established that will be incorporated into the second generation assays, a c33c antigen from the nonstructural region NS3 and a c22 antigen from the nucleocapsid region (see Fig. 14–9).

Serologic Testing for Chronic Hepatitis C

The cloning of HCV has led to the development of an antibody assay that, although imperfect, is extremely useful in the differential diagnosis of acute and chronic hepatitis and in the screening of blood donors. With the advent of the serologic assay, it was documented that the majority (90%) of post-transfusion non-A, non-

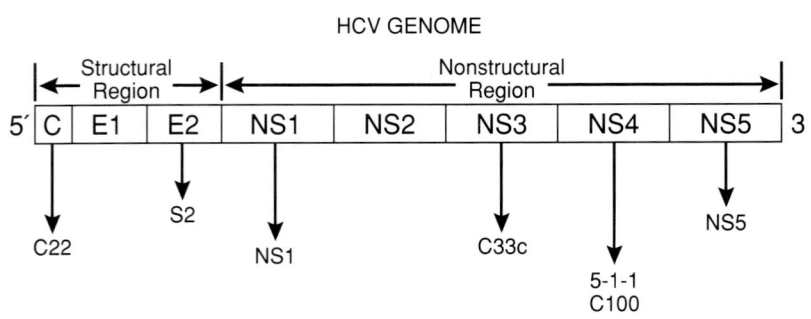

FIGURE 14–9.
The proposed genomic organization of the hepatitis C virus. The structural and nonstructural regions are shown. The structural region consists of the nucleocapsid (core) sequences and the envelope sequences. The nonstructural region is composed of five domains (NS1 to NS5). These domains have various postulated functions. The immunoreactive proteins, which are used in the current and newer generation of diagnostic assay for HCV, are indicated by arrows. KEY: C = core, E = envelope, HCV = hepatitis C virus, S = structural, NS = nonstructural.

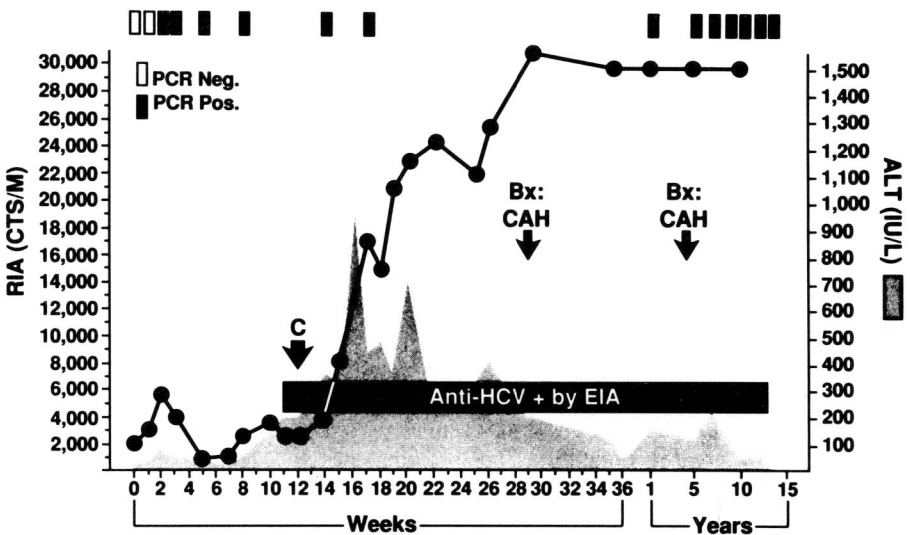

FIGURE 14–10.
Sequence of events in a patient with posttransfusion hepatitis C virus infection. The patient had the transfusion at time zero. The gray area indicates the ALT level (upper limit of normal, 44 U/L; onset of hepatitis, week 9); the solid circles indicate the onset and duration of anti-HCV as measured by RIA; the horizontal bar indicates the onset and duration of anti-HCV as measured by EIA. PCR was noted 2 weeks after exposure and 9 weeks before the first appearance of anti-HCV. KEY: ALT = alanine aminotransferase, anti-HCV = antibody to hepatitis C virus, bx = biopsy, C = infectivity established by chimp innoculation, CAH = chronic active hepatitis, EIA = enzyme immunoassay, PCR = polymerase chain reaction, RIA = radioimmunoassay. SOURCE: Atter HJ. Descartes before the horse: I clone, therefore I am: the hepatitis C virus in current perspective. Ann Intern Med. 1991;115:647.

B hepatitis was hepatitis C. The current assay is an enzyme-linked immunosorbent assay (ELISA) antibody test using the recombinant nonstructural polypeptide c100-3 coded for by the genome of HCV.[182] Using this ELISA assay in a well-defined setting of posttransfusion hepatitis, the antibody to the hepatitis C virus (anti-HCV) becomes detectable on average about 6 months after the onset of the posttransfusion hepatitis and may be delayed as long as 1 year.[183] Sixty percent of these well-defined posttransfusion hepatitis patients developed antibody within 15 weeks of exposure, and 90% within 6 months. None of these patients developed anti-HCV in less than 10 weeks. This antibody test may be negative in about 20% of patients whose clinical diagnosis of posttransfusion non-A, non-B hepatitis has been firmly established, indicating either a lack of sensitivity or the possible presence of other viruses in this setting or both. The anti-HCV assay has a fairly large window of seronegativity between exposure to HCV and the first appearance of the anti-HCV. The biochemical and serologic events in a typical patient with posttransfusion HCV infection are shown in Figure 14–10. The patient's serum becomes positive for HCV RNA, as measured by PCR, 2 weeks after the blood transfusion, referred to as time

zero, and 9 weeks before the appearance of the anti-HCV. After approximately 7 months, CAH was demonstrated on liver biopsy. Once formed, the antibody tends to persist throughout the course of chronic hepatitis C, and antibody persistence for at least 15 years has been documented.[38] The anti-HCV generally disappears in patients whose disease has resolved, but it does so at a very variable rate. Occasionally, the anti-HCV and the HCV RNA, as measured by PCR, may reappear after apparent clearance. Nevertheless, the persistence or the loss of the anti-HCV is a useful serologic marker of persistent infection or of recovery, respectively. As indicated, the assay lacks sensitivity both in the early period of infections with HCV and in chronic HCV infection.

Although the issue of assay sensitivity is very important clinically, the specificity of the antibody test is also of concern. The lack of specificity has been noted in the screening of blood donors and other low-risk populations as well as in patients with some forms of chronic liver disease such as autoimmune CAH and alcohol-induced liver disease. In most nonimplicated blood donors, only 30 to 50% of those who test positive with the current anti-HCV assay have true-positive results, as determined by supplemental testing with either a neutralization assay or the recombinant immunoblot assay (RIBA).

Several additional research assays have been developed to improve the accuracy of the current anti-HCV assay. These assays include the RIBA, a neutralization assay, and PCR. The first-generation RIBA (RIBA I) measured antibodies to two recombinant polypeptide antigens from the HCV genome, the c100-3 and the 5-1-1, and to the antigen superoxide dismutase, an enzyme used to enhance the expression of the HCV proteins in yeast. Early reports analyzing the RIBA I indicated that it was more sensitive and more specific than the first generation ELISA as well as a good indicator of infectivity. A second-generation RIBA (RIBA II) has been evaluated.[184, 185] The RIBA II has two additional recombinant polypeptide antigens from the HCV genome: c33c (from the nonstructural NS3 region) and c22 (from the capsid region) (see Fig. 14–9). A positive RIBA II is defined as reactivity with two or more of the HCV antigens c100-3, 5-1-1, c33, and c22, and an indeterminant RIBA II is defined as reactivity to only one of these HCV antigens. The validity of RIBA II has been confirmed by PCR. Two recent reports demonstrate the enhanced sensitivity of the RIBA II. One report involved patients with clinically presumed non-A, non-B chronic hepatitis, and 70% of these patients tested anti-HCV–positive by the first-generation ELISA, whereas, when their sera were tested by the RIBA II, 96 to 98% of the patients tested positive for HCV.[186] This enhanced sensitivity appeared to be due mainly to the addition of the c33c and c22 epitopes to the RIBA II assay. The second report involved the testing of blood donors; approximately half the blood donors who had tested positive by the second-generation ELISA tested negative by RIBA II, and about a quarter each were either RIBA II–positive or RIBA II–indeterminate.[187] The positive RIBA II samples were further analyzed by PCR, and the majority (46 of 49, 94%) tested positive for HCV RNA. The indeterminate RIBA II samples were also analyzed by PCR, and 76% were negative for HCV RNA. This report suggests that almost all RIBA II–positive blood donors have chronic HCV infection, and that RIBA II–indeterminate samples should be tested by PCR analysis to allow definitive identification of chronic HCV infection. Many blood banks use the RIBA II or a neutralization test as supplemental or so-called confirmatory tests of the anti-HCV ELISA results. Studies have indicated that screening blood donors with combined anti-HCV and RIBA reduces the incidence of transfusion-associated hepatitis by at least 70 to 80%.[188] Moreover, in a report from

Spain, almost three quarters (70%) of blood donors who were found to be positive for anti-HCV by both ELISA and RIBA II were documented to have substantial underlying liver disease, with 21% having CPH, 45% having CAH, and 7% having cirrhosis.[189] Similar findings have been reported from Italy.[190] In summary, supplemental testing is very important in these low-risk populations, and results of the supplemental testing must be checked before notifying the blood donors of their reactive antibody screening test for HCV. Supplemental testing is also important in some forms of chronic liver disease to clarify the diagnosis and arrange for appropriate therapy.[191, 192]

The application of the PCR technique permits a very sensitive assay for viral RNA circulating in the bloodstream and in tissue biopsy specimens. This detection of HCV RNA in serum and liver tissue aids in the diagnosis of HCV infections in many ways. For example, data obtained using the PCR assay have indicated that hepatitis C viremia can be detected within several days of exposure to the virus, which is many weeks before elevations of the serum aminotransferases occur and months before circulating viral antibodies are detectable.[184] The PCR assay allows the determination of the viremic status of patients who test positive to anti-HCV but have normal liver function tests, the so-called carrier state.[193, 194] In addition, the PCR assay provides a valuable tool to monitor therapeutic efficacy; a decrease of HCV RNA level after alpha-interferon therapy has been described.[195, 196] The PCR assay can be used to diagnose HCV infection in chronic non-A, non-B hepatitis patients who may be anti-HCV–negative by current serologic testing or, because of their immune status, may not be able to marshal an antibody response. To perform the general PCR assay for HCV RNA, primers specific for the 5′ terminus, the so-called 5′-untranslated region (see Fig. 14–9), should be used since this region is highly conserved among all isolates studied to date.[171, 197, 198] As is the case in serologic tests in general, the development of RNA assays specific for the different groups and types of HCV is desirable, and it is readily achievable by the appropriate selection of specific primers and probes.[171, 176]

In summary, although the current anti-HCV assay has been a major advance in defining chronic hepatitis C as well as in its potential prevention, the assay has serious limitations in both sensitivity and specificity. The presence of the c100-3 antibody in the serum does not allow differentiation among active HCV infection, recovery from a prior HCV infection, and a false-positive reaction. For the future, the addition of further polypeptide antigens from the HCV genome may well allow even more accurate and earlier diagnosis of infection with HCV.[199] A 1992 editorial, summarizing the advantages of the second-generation assays over the first-generation assays,[200] included better sensitivity and specificity as well as earlier detection of acute hepatitis C. A comparison of first-generation and second-generation assays, both ELISA and RIBA, and PCR has been reported as well and indicates that better assays remain to be developed.[201] Accordingly, the development of type-specific assays is of importance, particularly if the different variants of HCV exhibit different clinical outcomes and degrees of liver injury or therapeutic sensitivities and if co-infection with multiple variants of HCV influences disease development.[171]

Hepatitis C Epidemiology and Clinical Course

The estimated prevalence of anti-HCV from various areas around the world is as follows: 0.3% in Canada and northern Europe, 0.6% in the United States and central Europe, and 1.2 to 1.5% in southern Europe (Spain, Italy, Greece) and Japan.[202] Chronic hepatitis C is clearly a major cause of morbidity and mortality from liver disease in the United States. For example, chronic hepatitis C accounts for 10 to 20% of patients with end-stage liver disease who undergo liver transplantation.[203] Inasmuch as the current serologic assay lacks sensitivity, the magnitude of chronic hepatitis C may be greatly underestimated. Persistent infection and chronic hepatitis are the hallmarks of HCV infection.

Two forms of chronic hepatitis C are described: parenteral and nonparenteral.[204, 205] In the parenteral form, the high-risk associations include blood and plasma products, intravenous drug abuse, hemodialysis, and occupational exposure.[202-210] The relative frequencies of these associations are 5 to 6%, 45%, 15%, and 2 to 3%, respectively. Parenteral modes of transmission account for approximately two thirds of all cases of chronic hepatitis C.[202] Posttransfusion-associated hepatitis is the most commonly recognized and best-characterized form of chronic hepatitis C.[183, 184, 211] Indeed, hepatitis C virus is the cause of 80 to 90% of posttransfusion non-A, non-B hepatitis. The natural history of posttransfusion non-A, non-B hepatitis has been evaluated in several reports,[212, 213] and 50% or more of acute posttransfusion hepatitis has been found to progress to chronic hepatitis (Table 14–13).

TABLE 14–13. HISTOPATHOLOGY OF POSTTRANSFUSION CHRONIC HEPATITIS

CHRONIC HEPATITIS	% OF POSTTRANSFUSION PATIENTS
Chronic active hepatitis	25
Chronic persistent hepatitis	15
Cirrhosis	10
Total	50

A histologic evaluation of patients with chronic hepatitis led to the estimate that 30% have CPH, 50% CAH, and 20% cirrhosis.[212] The evolution to cirrhosis may be very rapid in some patients, whereas in others it is slow. Factors that might predict the development of cirrhosis have not been identified.[214] Both viral factors, such as initial viral load and strain of virus, and host factors, such as age, immune status, co-infections with other viruses such as HBV and HIV, and excess alcohol consumption, may play an important role in disease severity and rate of progression.[205] Earlier studies have suggested that the natural history of posttransfusion non-A, non-B hepatitis only infrequently resulted in clinically apparent liver disease, even though liver biopsy commonly documented cirrhosis.[212] A 1991 report suggested that patients with chronic hepatitis C may improve spontaneously over time, as demonstrated by a progressive decline in their serum aminotransferase levels, and most patients were asymptomatic after 10 years of follow-up.[214] Consequently, prolonged follow-up is required to assess fully the natural history of posttransfusion chronic hepatitis C. A preliminary report, which evaluated mortality and morbidity in chronic posttransfusion non-A, non-B hepatitis over an 18-year period, demonstrated that no significant difference existed in all-cause mortality in the chronic non-A, non-B hepatitis group as compared with control groups. Liver-related deaths were, however, more common in the chronic hepatitis group.[215] This liver-related mortality appeared to be related to alcoholism. Cirrhosis and HCC rates were similar in the chronic hepatitis C and the control groups.

In the posttransfusion chronic hepatitis setting, the clinical spectrum of the chronic hepatitis may be different in anti-HCV–positive cases from that of the anti-HCV–negative cases.[202] The anti-HCV–positive patients are more likely to have severe disease, as measured by serum aminotransferase or serum bilirubin levels, and are more likely to progress to severe chronic hepatitis. This difference may arise either because two distinct viruses may be associated with posttransfusion non-A, non-B hepatitis, or because the anti-HCV–negative group may be a misclassification of hepatitis in the complex setting of the postoperative state. The reasons for this difference may eventually be clarified with the newer generation of anti-HCV assays. In addition, application of PCR may in the future allow detection of HCV RNA in serum and liver tissue, HCV antigens (HCAg) may be detected in liver tissue by immunofluorescence, and in situ hybridization may allow more critical separation of the so-called non-A, non-B, non-C hepatitis, perhaps to be known as hepatitis F.

In the nonparenteral, that is, sporadic or community-acquired, form of chronic hepatitis C, the proposed associations include perinatal (vertical, from mother to newborn), sexual, and household transmission.[202, 205] Approximately 40% of cases of chronic hepatitis C are believed to be nonparenteral. The relative frequency of the proposed routes of transmission is not known, but evidence suggests low frequencies for all three.[202] Therefore, the mode of transmission of nonparenteral cases of chronic hepatitis C is largely unknown. Evidence indicates that vertical transmission from mother to infant rarely occurs unless the mother is co-infected with both HCV and HIV.[216, 217] The frequency of sexual transmission of hepatitis C is controversial,[44, 207, 218–221] but it is apparently of low frequency, particularly when compared with the transmission of HBV and HIV by sexual contact. This low frequency of sexual transmission may relate to the recognized low levels of viremia in most chronic hepatitis C carriers.[207] Sexual transmission of HCV may be enhanced in individuals with combined HIV infection since their immune deficiency may allow the HCV to reach higher titers, thereby facilitating transmission.[222] The spread of hepatitis C through household contact appears to be low as well.[219, 223] In summary, the modes of transmission of the nonparenteral or sporadic form of chronic hepatitis C remain unsettled. Indeed, the major transmission factors in community-acquired HCV infection may be but variations on known risk factors such as intravenous drug abuse, blood transfusion, or inapparent percutaneous exposure.[224] Two studies have indicated that body fluids such as saliva and semen of patients with chronic hepatitis C are rarely, if ever, contaminated with the hepatitis C virus,[223, 225] but this finding remains controversial.[224, 226–228] Although the HCV has similarities with the flaviviruses, which are arthropod-borne and spread, such transmission of HCV does not appear likely in view of its currently recognized epidemiologic features.

The natural history of the nonparenteral sporadic form of chronic hepatitis C is not known. Serologic testing with the anti-HCV assay indicates that 50 to 70% of patients with sporadic acute non-A, non-B hepatitis test positive for the antibody.[229] Moreover, in the long-term follow-up of posttransfusion and sporadic chronic hepatitis non-A, non B, a frequency of circulating anti-HCV of approximately 75% has been reported for both forms.[230] Early studies of sporadic or nonparenteral non-A, non-B hepatitis suggested that its clinical course was more benign than that of posttransfusion non-A, non-B hepatitis.[231] Fewer of the sporadic cases progressed to chronic hepatitis, but when they did, the hepatitis was more likely to be CPH than the more serious CAH. Several more recent reports, however, have suggested a more serious outcome for the sporadic form than originally thought, and its long-term course now appears to be similar to that of posttransfusion hepatitis.[232, 233] More sensitive serologic testing, including PCR, will be required to define better the heterogeneous nonparenteral form and natural history of chronic hepatitis C.

A very important epidemiologic observation is the strong association between HCC and the presence of the anti-HCV. In Japan, 70 to 80% of patients with HCC are anti-HCV–positive without evidence for HBV and ethanol.[234] Similar observations have been reported from Italy[178] and Spain.[206] A more recent report from Italy suggests that HCV infection is an independent risk factor for HCC, both because it induces cirrhosis and because it increases the risk in patients with cirrhosis.[235] A 1990 report from Japan demonstrated the close association between the presence of chronic hepatitis, cirrhosis, or HCC and the presence of anti-HCV. The report also demonstrated the long interval between viral exposure, in this case by blood transfusion, and clinical recognition of the chronic hepatitis, cirrhosis, or HCC, the mean intervals being 10 years, 20 years, and 30 years, respectively.[236] This study, along with others, suggests that hepatitis C evolves slowly and often silently from an anicteric acute hepatitis to chronic hepatitis after blood-transfusion exposure. The long interval between blood transfusion and the development of clinically apparent disease may be the reason why blood transfusion is not always considered to be causally associated with a chronic liver disease. When the chronic liver disease occurs so long after blood transfusion, the history of the transfusion may not be obtained or may not be considered relevant. This strong epidemiologic association suggests a causal role for HCV in the development of primary HCC, a role that has also been demonstrated for HBV. It is unknown whether either of these hepatitis viruses is directly oncogenic or whether the cirrhosis they eventually cause is the important factor in the development of HCC. The hepatocellular replication and regeneration that occurs in chronic inflammatory conditions of the liver may result in a mutation that causes malignant transformation.

The establishment of the diagnosis of chronic hepatitis C is outlined in Table 14–14. Because the test for anti-HCV lacks specificity, liver biopsy is required to make an accurate diagnosis of chronic hepatitis C. For example, liver biopsy is essential in excluding the other diagnoses listed in Tables 14–1 and 14–2. On occasion, the most difficult diagnosis to exclude is autoimmune CAH, and the liver biopsy does not help here. The anti-HCV test is frequently falsely positive in autoimmune chronic hepatitis.[192, 237, 238] Autoantibodies (e.g., anti-nuclear antibodies, anti–smooth muscle autoantibodies) in higher titer may help to establish a diagnosis of autoimmune chronic hepatitis, but low titers of these autoantibodies are relatively common in chronic hepatitis B and C.[239, 240] Therefore, supplemental serologic testing or the determination of HCV RNA by PCR may be required in this difficult diagnostic situation to determine which disease is present. If supplemental testing or PCR is not available, a therapeutic trial of corticosteroids has been recommended,[191] but the interpretation of a therapeutic response may be complex. Because of the possibility of a serious reaction from alpha-interferon therapy for autoimmune CAH,[75] a definitive distinction is imperative, hence the need for either the supplemental testing or the PCR assay.

Treatment

ALPHA-INTERFERON ANTIVIRAL TREATMENT OF CHRONIC HEPATITIS C

A preliminary report in 1986 indicated that alpha-interferon therapy may be efficacious in chronic non-A, non-B hepatitis.[241] Since the publication of that report, a number of therapeutic trials have been carried out. The clinical and biochemical course of a typical patient with chronic posttransfusion non-A, non-B hepatitis who was treated for 1 year with alpha-interferon is shown in Figure 14–11. The serum aminotransferase level decreased to normal after 2 months of therapy and persisted in the normal range after therapy was stopped. The liver biopsy reverted from the demonstration of CAH before treatment to nonspecific reactive changes at the end of therapy.

TABLE 14–14. DIAGNOSIS OF CHRONIC HEPATITIS C

Elevated (persistent or fluctuating) serum aminotransferase levels for at least 6 months or longer
Positive anti-HCV in serum by ELISA I or II
Liver biopsy evidence of chronic hepatitis (mild, moderate, severe) with or without cirrhosis
Specific histologic changes include: bile duct damage, lymphoid aggregates or follicles, macrovesicular fat, Mallory's bodies
Evidence of HCV replication: HCV RNA in serum or liver, by PCR

KEY: Anti-HCV = antibody to hepatitis C virus, ELISA I or II = first- or second-generation enzyme-linked immunosorbent assay, HCV = hepatitis C virus, PCR = polymerase chain reaction, RNA = ribonucleic acid.

A summary of selected controlled trials of recombinant alpha-interferon therapy for chronic hepatitis C in adults is outlined in Table 14–15. Eleven reports have been collated.[242–252] Although the dosage, duration, and type of alpha-interferon varied among the studies, approximately 45 to 50% of these patients with chronic hepatitis C had a biochemical response demonstrated by the normalization of serum aminotransferase levels, whereas the control patients had a spontaneous biochemical response rate of approximately 4%. Disappointingly, the biochemical relapse rate in the responding patients was approximately 50 to 60%. The majority of reports indicated histologic improvement in the liver biopsy done after the course of alpha-interferon treatment.

In a United States multicenter trial of alpha-interferon treatment for patients with chronic hepatitis C,[242] the response rates of 2 dosages, 3 MU and 1 MU, of alpha-interferon were evaluated, and the different response rates are given in Figure 14–12. Approximately 45% of the patients responded to the 3-MU dosage during the 24 weeks of treatment, and this response was significantly better than the response in the 1-MU dosage group or the control group. In this multicenter trial, however, approximately 50% of the patients who had responded to alpha-interferon treatment relapsed in the follow-up period (Fig. 14–13). The relapse rate was similar in the two groups, whether the patients had been treated with a 3-MU or a 1-MU dosage of alpha-interferon.

A controlled study of alpha-interferon therapy for chronic hepatitis C, carried out at the National Institutes of Health,[243] compared liver biopsy scores before and after alpha-interferon treatment; the extent of injury was less in the interferon-treated group after therapy than before therapy (Fig. 14–14). By contrast, no difference in the liver biopsy scores before and after therapy was seen in the placebo group.

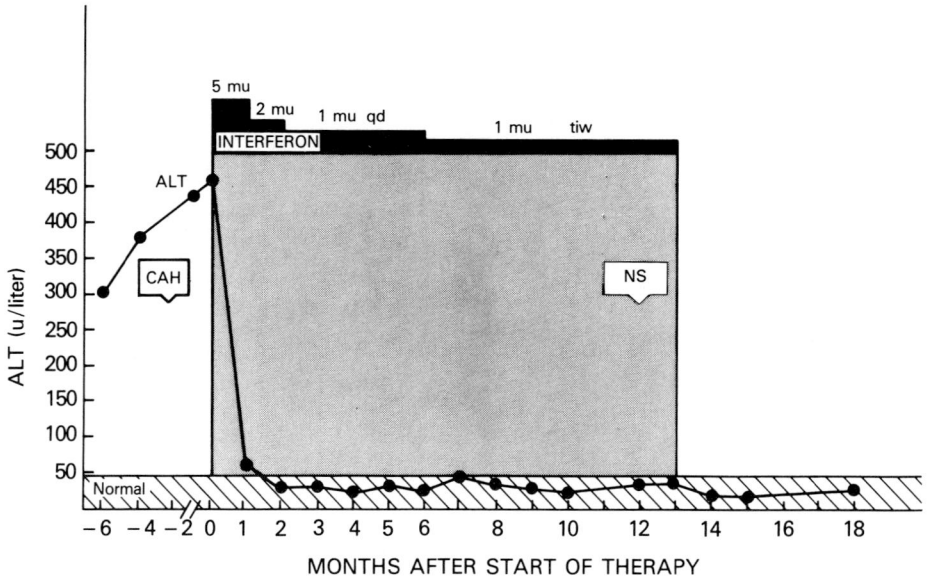

FIGURE 14–11.

The clinical, serum biochemical, and serologic course of a patient with chronic posttransfusion non-A, non-B hepatitis who was treated with interferon-α for 1 year and sustained a clinical and serum biochemical remission of disease. Serum ALT levels fell to normal within 2 months of the start of therapy. Despite a decrease in the dosage of interferon, the liver disease remained in remission, and liver biopsy, which revealed CAH before therapy, showed nonspecific reactive changes at the end of therapy. This patient had normal ALT levels and no symptoms of liver disease 2 years after the conclusion of therapy. KEY: ALT = alanine aminotransferase, CAH = chronic active hepatitis, NS = nonstructural. SOURCE: Hoofnagle JH, DiBisceglie AM. Antiviral therapy of viral hepatitis. In: Galasso GJ, Whitley RJ, Merigan TC, eds. Antiviral Agents and Viral Diseases of Man. 3rd ed. New York: Raven Press;1990:452.

TABLE 14–15. CONTROLLED TRIALS OF RECOMBINANT ALPHA-INTERFERON THERAPY FOR CHRONIC HEPATITIS C IN ADULTS

REFERENCE	N	DOSAGE/ DURATION†	TYPE	% BIOCHEMICAL RESPONSE* INTERFERON	CONTROL	% BIOCHEMICAL RELAPSE‡	HISTOLOGIC IMPROVEMENT
Davis (1989)[242]	109	3/6	2B	38 (22/58)	4 (2/51)	50 (11/22)	Yes
DiBisceglie (1989)[243]	41	2/6	2B	48 (10/21)	5 (1/20)	80 (8/10)	Yes
Jacyna (1989)[250]	14	3/4	L	71 (5/7)	0 (0/7)	NE	NE
Weiland (1989)[246]	33	3/9	2B	52 (11/21)	0 (0/12)	64 (7/11)	Yes
Gomez-Rubio (1990)[252]	30	5/18#	2B	40 (6/15)	7 (1/14)	33 (2/6)	Yes
Realdi (1990)[251]	60	6/12¶	2A	70 (21/30)	0 (0/30)	62 (13/21)	Yes
Saracco (1990)[245]	71	3/6	2B	46 (12/26)	0 (0/25)	50 (6/12)	Yes
Causse (1991)[248]	90	3/6	2B	43 (13/30)	7 (2/30)	87 (9/13)	Yes
Omata (1991)[249]	49	3/6	2A	29 (7/24)	4 (1/25)	85 (6/7)	Yes
Marcellin (1991)[244]	36	3/6	2B	39 (7/18)	0 (0/18)	28 (2/7)	Yes
Saez-Royuela (1991)[247]	20	5/12§	2C	50 (5/10)	10 (1/10)	40 (2/5)	Yes

*Response = normal transaminase levels.
†Dosage in million units (mU) of interferon 3 × week; duration in months of treatment.
‡Relapse = persistent increased transaminase levels.
§Initial dosage 15 mU for 3 months, then 10 mU for 3 months, then 5 mU for 6 months.
¶Initial dosage 6 mU for 1 month, then 3 mU for 3 months, then 1 mU for 8 months.
#Initial dosage 5 mU for 2 months, then 1.5 mU for 16 months.
KEY: 2A = recombinant interferon-α-2A, 2B = recombinant interferon-α-2B, 2C = recombinant interferon-α-2C, L = lymphoblastoid, NE = not evaluated.

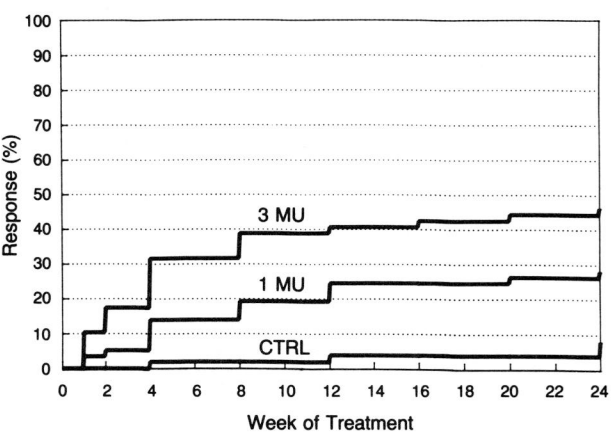

FIGURE 14–12.
Probability of complete or nearly complete response during treatment with recombinant interferon-α in patients with chronic hepatitis C. $P<0.0001$ for the difference between the 3-MU-group and the untreated group, $P<0.05$ for the difference between the two treatment groups, and $P<0.02$ for the difference between the 1-MU-group and the untreated group. KEY: 3 MU = 3 million units of interferon administered 3 times a week, 1 MU = 1 million units of interferon administered 3 times a week, CTRL = untreated control group. SOURCE: Davis GL, Balart LA, Schiff ER, et al. Treatment of chronic hepatitis C with recombinant interferon-α. N Engl J Med. 1989;321:1503.

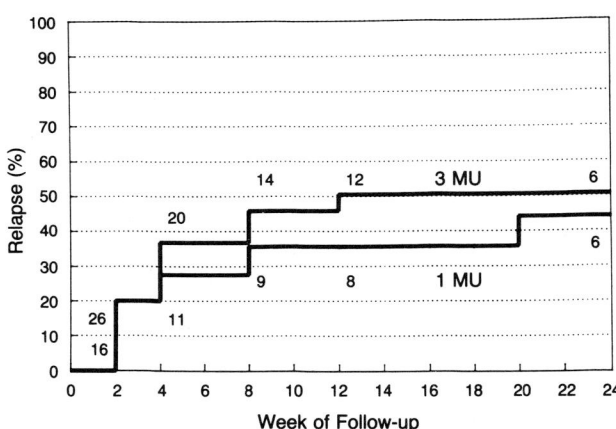

FIGURE 14–13.
Probability of relapse after discontinuation of treatment with recombinant interferon-α in patients with chronic hepatitis C. The number of patients studied at each time is shown for each group. The probability of relapse in each group was similar. KEY: 3 MU = 3 million units of interferon administered 3 times a week, 1 MU = 1 million units of interferon administered 3 times a week, CTRL = untreated control group. SOURCE: Davis GL, Balart LA, Schiff ER, et al. Treatment of chronic hepatitis C with recombinant interferon-α. N Engl J Med. 1989;521:1504.

FIGURE 14–14.
Changes in ranking of current hepatic injury on histologic examination in patients with chronic hepatitis C before and after receiving interferon or placebo. Injury including portal inflammation, piecemeal necrosis, and lobular injury was measured. The open circles indicate the ± SEM values at each time for each group. SOURCE: DiBisceglie AM, Martin P, Kassianides C, et al. Recombinant interferon-α therapy for chronic hepatitis C. N Engl J Med. 1989;321:1509.

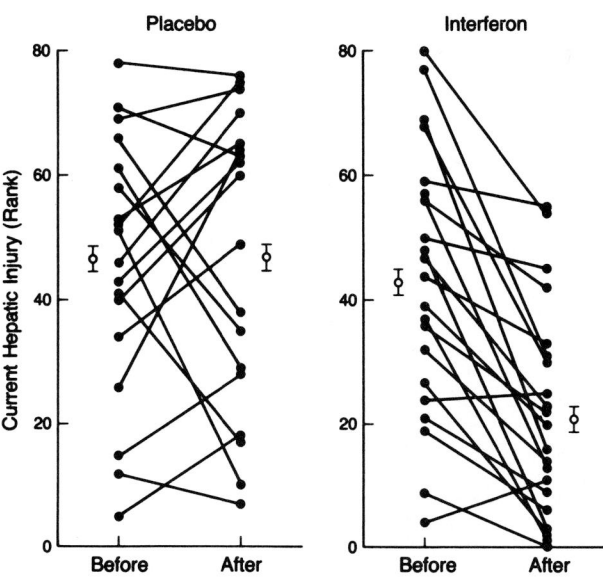

Higher dosages of alpha-interferon and more prolonged periods of treatment are under investigation. In the few full reports of these studies published, neither higher dosages nor longer periods of treatment has had a dramatic effect upon either the initial response rate or the rate of relapse.[247, 252] Certainly, side effects of alpha-interferon increase concomitantly with increases in dosage schedules. These issues of dosage and duration of therapy remain under intense investigation, and preliminary reports indicate that escalating the dosages from 1.5 to 10 MU of alpha-interferon does not appear to improve either the response rate or the relapse rate, as measured by initial response of the aminotransferase level,[253–255] and that extending the period of treatment from 6 months to 1 year brought either a modest improvement in efficacy[256, 257] or no apparent improvement in efficacy.[258, 259]

A 1991 meta-analysis evaluated 17 randomized controlled trials of either lymphoblastoid or recombinant alpha-interferon treatment for chronic non-A, non-B hepatitis.[260] Seven of these trials had been published as full reports and 10 as abstracts; in total, 916 patients were enrolled. Anti-HCV testing was carried out in 12 studies only and positive findings ranged from 55 to 100%. The response to alpha-interferon treatment, indicated by a normalization of ALT, and the rate of relapse both during and after treatment were measured. Overall, a 50% positive response rate was demonstrated. Twenty-five to 80% of patients (median 57%) relapsed after the cessation of therapy. The analysis of short-term treatment of 6 months versus long-term treatment of 9 to 18 months showed no difference in either response or relapse rate.

Several studies have suggested that lower grades of histologic severity of CPH respond better to alpha-interferon therapy than do the more severe grades of CAH with cirrhosis. Other studies have suggested that women and patients with higher initial serum aminotransferase levels may respond better to treatment with alpha-interferon. These suggested predictors of response need to be confirmed in controlled studies with larger number of patients. From the United States multicenter study, no predictors of response[261] or of relapse[262] (other than dosage) could be identified.

The mechanism behind the beneficial effects of alpha-interferon in chronic hepatitis C is unknown, but presumably interferon inhibits replication of HCV, which in turn results in mitigation of the disease. Although earlier studies that examined alpha-interferon therapy in chronic hepatitis C used normalization of the serum aminotransferase level as a measure of treatment response, HCV RNA can now be measured directly in both serum and liver by PCR.[195] This report examined the effect of alpha-interferon therapy on the inhibition or eradication of HCV and demonstrated that serum levels of HCV RNA decreased in all patients who had responded to alpha-interferon therapy with improvements in serum aminotransferase levels. The effect of interferon therapy on serum HCV RNA is shown in Figure 14–15. After 6 months of alpha-interferon treatment, the HCV RNA became negative and remained negative during the 8 months of follow-up. In patients treated with placebo, the HCV RNA remained detectable by PCR. In the 61% of the initial responders who relapsed after the treatment ended, HCV RNA reappeared in the serum.

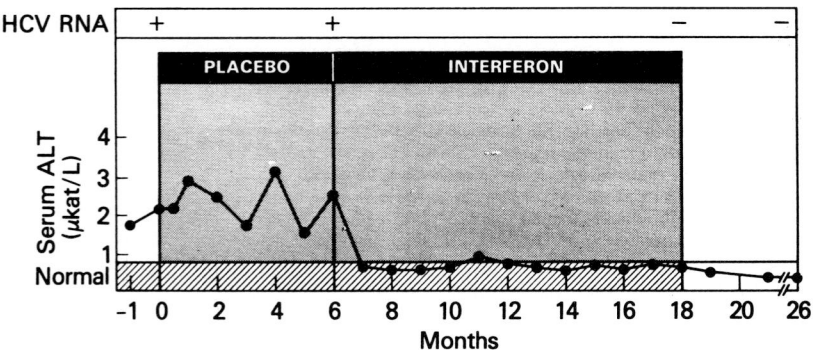

FIGURE 14–15.
Hepatitis C viral RNA levels during and after alpha-interferon treatment. Course of a patient who had a sustained response to interferon-α therapy after a 6-month period of placebo treatment. Hepatitis C viral RNA, which was detected during the placebo treatment, was not detectable during and after interferon therapy. KEY: ALT = alanine aminotransferase, HCV = hepatitis C virus. SOURCE: Shindo M, DiBisceglie AM, Cheung L, et al. Disease in serum hepatitis C viral RNA during alpha-interferon therapy for chronic hepatitis C. Ann Intern Med. 1991;115:703.

These findings indicate that the serum biochemical response to alpha-interferon therapy in chronic hepatitis C is associated with loss of detectable HCV genome from the serum. Although measurement of HCV RNA in serum is helpful in determining a virologic response to therapy, disappearance of detectable HCV RNA in serum does not provide absolute evidence of long-term clearance of the virus.[263] Testing for HCV RNA in liver tissue may ultimately provide the virologic marker necessary to identify clearance of HCV and to predict long-term remission in chronic hepatitis C.[195]

A long-term follow-up of the original pilot study of interferon therapy for chronic non-A, non-B hepatitis was reported in 1992.[264] During a follow-up of 3 to 6 years, HCV RNA remained undetectable in 6 of 8 patients who had initially responded, as indicated by normalization of aminotransferase levels, to interferon therapy. All 6 patients had persistently normal serum aminotransferase levels during the period of observation. Thus, those patients who have prolonged normalization of serum aminotransferases after interferon therapy also have an associated sustained loss of HCV RNA from serum, and a long-term beneficial response to therapy.

SUMMARY OF ALPHA-INTERFERON TREATMENT OF CHRONIC HEPATITIS C

Alpha-interferon therapy given in dosages from 1 to 10 MU, usually 3 times a week for 6 months to 1 year with or without escalating dosages or dosage titration, results in a 35 to 60% complete response rate in patients with chronic hepatitis C. An additional 10 to 20% of patients have an incomplete response, defined as greater than 50% decrease in pretreatment ALT level. These response rates are contrasted with 5 to 10% spontaneous improvement in serum aminotransferase level in control patients. Relapse rates are high, from 50 to 90%, but retreatment of patients who relapse results uniformly in a similar response to treatment. Although most studies of alpha-interferon therapy for chronic hepatitis C have involved patients with the parenterally transmitted form of the disease, the community-acquired form also appears to respond to alpha-interferon.[265] Several multicenter studies are being carried out to define further the therapeutic response of community-acquired chronic hepatitis C to interferon. Prolonged treatment, dosage escalation, and dosage titration regimens have not shown consistent improvement in either the initial response rate or the rate of relapse. No definite predictors of response or relapse have been identified. Monitoring HCV RNA by means of PCR seems increasingly likely to be required to identify the response to interferon therapy. For example, one report indicates that hepatitis C viremia can persist in chronic hepatitis C patients despite the absence of the anti-HCV; that normalization of the serum aminotransferase level does not predict loss of hepatitis C viremia; that loss of HCV RNA, as measured by PCR, does not predict a long-term loss of the HCV infection; and that the spontaneous elimination of HCV RNA in patients with chronic hepatitis C appears to be a rare event in its natural history.[202, 263]

More readily available measures of treatment response are needed. Measuring or monitoring the biologic activity of interferon treatment, as demonstrated by $2',5'$-oligoadenylate synthetase activity, may be helpful in determining dosage adjustments. Monitoring measures indicative of hepatic fibrosis might be useful. For example, serum procollagen III peptide levels have been reported to decrease in response to alpha-interferon therapy in patients with chronic hepatitis C.[266] In addition, a recent report suggests that adjuvant therapy with a nonsteroidal anti-inflammatory drug (NSAID) might enhance the therapeutic response to alpha-interferon.[267] Measuring anti-HCV titers, either by standard or newer tests, does not appear to be helpful in evaluating interferon therapy. Nevertheless, newer epitopes may come to light that might prove to be helpful in this regard. An evaluation of an immunoglobulin M (IgM) antibody to HCV c100-3 antigen in acute and chronic hepatitis C has been carried out.[268] This report demonstrated that 65% of acute hepatitis C patients tested positive for the IgM antibody and 57% for the immunoglobulin G (IgG) antibody. The IgM antibody disappeared in self-limited cases but persisted in cases of chronic infection. The IgG antibody was not helpful since it persisted in both circumstances. The presence of the IgM antibody did not, however, correlate with disease severity or progression. Nevertheless, a more recent report suggested that the presence of the IgM anti-HCV directed to the c100-3 antigen correlates with the biochemical evidence of active hepatitis C and that its disappearance from serum correlates with normalization of serum aminotransferase levels after alpha-interferon therapy.[269] Thus, if these observations are confirmed, the disappearance of the IgM anti-HCV directed to c100-3 antigen may be a serologic predictor of a sustained response to alpha-interferon treatment. A preliminary report suggests that quantification of the circulating viral load may be useful in predicting response to alpha-interferon therapy,[270] as it is to chronic hepatitis B.

Alpha-interferon therapy in chronic hepatitis C is clearly beneficial for some patients. Studies currently under way should clarify the appropriate dosage and duration of treatment. The long-term effect of alpha-interferon treatment of chronic hepatitis C is not well established, but two reports suggest that the long-term prognosis for persistent responders to alpha-interferon therapy is optimistic.[264, 271] Future studies must evaluate alternative approaches for those patients who do not respond to alpha-interferon therapy, approximately 50% of patients, as well as for those who relapse after the discontinuation of the drug.

OTHER ANTIVIRAL THERAPIES FOR CHRONIC HEPATITIS C

Ribavirin. Ribavirin, a synthetic triazole nucleoside, has antiviral activity, in that it inhibits viral synthesis, against DNA and RNA viruses in vitro and in vivo.[272] Although ribavirin, a noninterferon-inducing nucleoside analog, is most often used to treat respiratory syncytial virus infection, its therapeutic efficacy has been examined in patients infected with HIV, HBV, and Lassa fever virus. Two pilot studies evaluated its therapeutic efficacy in patients with chronic hepatitis C.[273, 274] In one study, 10 patients with anti-HCV–positive chronic hepatitis were treated with oral ribavirin, given in dosages of 1000 to 1200 mg per day for 3 months.[273] The serum aminotransferase level in these patients decreased significantly by the end of the treatment period, but their aminotransferase level increased to pretreatment levels almost immediately after treatment was stopped. Patients were not evaluated histologically pre- and post-treatment. A decrease in the mean serum hemoglobin was noted during ribavirin therapy, and this level had returned to normal by 6 weeks after therapy. A mild hemolytic anemia is a recognized adverse effect of ribavirin therapy at dosages of 1000 mg or greater. Other adverse reactions were reported to be mild and fully reversible; 6 of 10 patients had no side effects. The other pilot study, reported in preliminary form, also demonstrated efficacy for ribavirin therapy.[274] In this study, 13 patients with chronic hepatitis C were treated with oral ribavirin, given in increasing dosages from 600 mg to 1000 mg to 1200 mg per day. Of the 10 patients who completed 6 months of treatment, all had decreases in their serum ALT levels, and in 4 patients the levels returned to normal. In all

patients, however, serum ALT levels returned to pretreatment values after ribavirin therapy was stopped. HCV RNA titers, as determined by PCR, decreased slightly but did not become negative. A comparison of pretreatment and post-treatment liver biopsies showed no significant improvement in liver histologic appearance. Ribavirin was generally tolerated well, and the major side effect was a dose-dependent, rapidly reversible hemolytic anemia. Both of these preliminary studies indicate that ribavirin appears to have at least a short-term antiviral effect against hepatitis C. Ribavirin is the first drug to offer potentially effective oral therapy for chronic hepatitis C. These observations are preliminary, however, and further controlled studies are required to define better the role of ribavirin, whether alone or in combination with alpha-interferon, in the treatment of chronic hepatitis C. For those patients who do not respond to alpha-interferon therapy or who cannot tolerate its side effects, ribavirin offers a potential alternative.

Acyclovir and Gamma-Interferon. A pilot study of the efficacy of acyclovir treatment for chronic non-A, non-B hepatitis reported that at least a short, 10-day course of acyclovir does not appear to have a beneficial effect on the course of chronic non-A, non-B hepatitis.[275] One report examining gamma-interferon therapy for chronic hepatitis C indicated limited efficacy.[247]

Inosine Pranobex. A 1991 preliminary report suggested that an immunomodulatory drug, inosine pranobex, was associated with biochemical improvement in a patient with chronic hepatitis C as well as seroconversion from positive to negative HCV RNA, assessed by PCR.[276] Additional studies are necessary to confirm this potentially important observation.

Bile Acid Therapy. Ursodeoxycholic acid (UDCA) has been observed to reduce serum aminotransferase levels in some patients with chronic hepatitis.[277–279] In a recent double-blind placebo-controlled study, UDCA treatment was associated with significant improvement in serum aminotransferase levels in patients with chronic hepatitis; (17 of 24 subjects (71%) were anti-HCV–positive and 4 of 24 subjects (17%) were HB$_s$Ag-positive).[280] From the same center, a UDCA dose-response study also indicated efficacy in patients with chronic hepatitis, with 13 of 18 subjects (72%) being anti-HCV–positive.[281] A 1991 preliminary report further supports the potential therapeutic efficacy of UDCA in patients with chronic hepatitis C.[282] The mechanism of action of the UDCA in this therapeutic setting remains unclear, but possibilities include the displacement of more hydrophobic and toxic bile acids in the liver, membrane stabilizing effects, and immunomodulatory effects.[283] Collectively, these studies suggest that long-term controlled studies are needed to establish whether improvements in serum aminotransferase levels in patients with chronic hepatitis C treated with UDCA are clinically important. The relationships among the serum aminotransferase levels, liver histologic changes, and clinical events need to be determined. A preliminary report indicates that a combination of alpha-interferon and UDCA is more efficacious in the treatment of chronic hepatitis C than is alpha-interferon therapy alone.[284] Future studies should be designed to document further the value of UDCA therapy in combination with alpha-interferon treatment of chronic viral hepatitis C.

ANTIVIRAL TREATMENT OF ACUTE AND CHRONIC HEPATITIS C PATIENTS WITH VARIOUS CHARACTERISTICS

Patients with Acute non-A, non-B Hepatitis. Since the chronicity rate is very high after acute non-A, non-B hepatitis, the use of antiviral therapy during the acute illness is a reasonable course to consider. What effect does interferon treatment of acute non-A, non-B hepatitis have on the natural history of the disease? Preliminary reports, using both alpha-interferon[285, 286] and beta-interferon,[287] suggest that interferon therapy prevents the progression of acute non-A, non-B hepatitis to chronicity by eradicating HCV, as measured by PCR. In another report from a randomized controlled trial of alpha-interferon in acute posttransfusion hepatitis C, evidence indicated that a course of 3 MU of alpha-interferon administered for 3 months in patients with acute hepatitis C was associated with a shorter course of hepatitis.[288] The relapse rate however, was high after the discontinuation of therapy, and after a mean of 44 weeks follow-up, no difference from the control group was demonstrated. The study also indicated that the seroconversion rate to anti-HCV may be lower and that the liver biopsy histologic findings may be less abnormal in the alpha-interferon–treated group. These preliminary observations are potentially important, but further studies are needed to confirm these findings. The lack of an accurate serologic assay in acute hepatitis C hampers these studies. As reported in 1992, an IgM anti-HCV response to a capsid antigen may prove to be a useful serologic marker for acute viral infection.[289]

Children. The prevalence and course of chronic hepatitis C in children is not well defined, but one report indicates that it may be more common than currently thought.[290, 291] The rate of progression to chronicity may be less in children.[292] The vertical transmission from a chronic HCV-infected mother to a child has been reported,[216] and although the frequency of this form of transmission is thought to be low,[202] it appears to be particularly enhanced when the mother has a combined infection of HCV with HIV.[217] A preliminary report suggests that alpha-interferon therapy is efficacious in children with chronic hepatitis C.[293]

Immunocompromised Patients. Since the sensitivity of the current serologic assay for hepatitis C in immunocompromised patients is incompletely defined, the actual prevalence and course of chronic hepatitis C in this setting are unknown. In patients with combined HCV and HIV infection, a recent report indicates that chronic hepatitis C may be more rapidly progressive in HIV-positive patients.[294] A 1989 report suggests that the response to alpha-interferon therapy for chronic hepatitis C with and without HIV infection is similar.[295] Antiviral therapy in this setting remains to be defined but will be likely to require a combination of antiviral agents.

Chronic hepatitis C has been reported after solid organ transplantation. It may play a significant role in the morbidity and mortality in the renal posttransplantation setting,[296] and its role in the hepatic posttransplantation setting is being established.[135, 297–299] Persistent HCV infection is almost universal in patients with pretransplant infection.[300] Peritransplant acquisition of hepatitis C in patients without previous HCV infection is high (35%).[300] Studies suggest that apart from rejection and cytomegalovirus infection, HCV infection is the most frequent cause of hepatic dysfunction in liver transplant patients, and it has the potential to evolve into more serious liver disease.[301] As with chronic hepatitis B in the organ posttransplantation setting, the role of antiviral therapy is problematic, and future studies are needed to assess the efficacy of alpha-interferon and other antiviral agents in treating chronic hepatitis C in immunosuppressed patients.[302]

Patients with Extrahepatic Manifestations. With the availability of HCV serologic testing, chronic hepatitis C has been reported in association with several extrahepatic manifestations. Although many of these reports are preliminary, the manifestations include mixed cryoglobulinemia,[303, 304] polyarteritis nodosa,[305] a sicca-like syndrome,[306] and a membranoproliferative glomerulonephritis.[307] Alpha-interferon therapy has been reported to be beneficial in chronic hepatitis C infection and cryoglobulinemia,[308, 309] and two preliminary reports suggest that alpha-interferon therapy may mitigate the membranoproliferative glomerulonephritis.[307, 310] Both the association of these extrahepatic manifestations in chronic hepatitis C and their response to alpha-interferon therapy need to be more extensively documented by future reports, but the evidence indicates that HCV infection, like HBV infection, has diverse extrahepatic manifestations and that alpha-interferon therapy may prove efficacious. Detection of the minus strand of HCV RNA in tissue implies viral replication in the tissue.[311–313] Whether HCV replicates in tissue outside of the liver is controversial.[312–314] Although non-A, non-B hepatitis has been associated with aplastic anemia, evidence suggests that HCV infection is not the causal agent in this setting.[315]

Hepatitis C Vaccine

Recent progress in vaccine approaches to the related flaviviruses and pestiviruses is cause for optimism that a recombinant vaccine for HCV is feasible,[171] but HCV vaccine development is still at an early stage. To date, a neutralizing antibody has not been identified, and the considerable heterogeneity among the HCV isolates has been recognized, making vaccine development a difficult problem.[316] Two 1992 reports suggest that immunity in hepatitis C infections is relatively weak.[317, 318] This evidence comes from multiple cross-challenges with HCV in chimpanzees. HCV does not appear to confer either homologous or heterologous immunity.[318] Whether a sufficiently conserved region exists in the HCV genome that could code for an antigen capable of eliciting broad-base immunity remains unknown.[202] For the future, in vitro systems for growing the hepatitis C viruses need to be developed to allow investigations into potential specific antiviral agents and to facilitate vaccine development.

Chronic Hepatitis D (Delta)

The HDV is an unusual single-stranded circular RNA virus with some similarities to certain plant viroids (see Table 14–5). This virus requires hepadna virus helper functions for its propagation in hepatocytes. Thus, hepatitis D occurs only in individuals who are currently infected with hepatitis B, and it increases the severity of acute and chronic hepatitis B.[319] Hepatitis D is found endemically in some areas of the world, particularly in the Middle East and parts of South America, but in most areas it is found mainly in high-risk groups, including intravenous drug abusers and recipients of multiple plasma products such as hemophiliacs. Hepatitis D is clinically recognized to occur in two forms. A known chronic carrier of hepatitis B can be infected with HDV in what is called superinfection. Alternatively, HDV can be transmitted simultaneously with HBV in what is called a co-infection. These two forms of HDV infection need to be distinguished because of differences in their clinical course and prognosis.[319] The diagnosis of acute hepatitis D can be made in the setting of clinical features of acute hepatitis, and both HBsAg and anti-HDV are found in the patient's serum.[4, 320] The acute hepatitis D can be assumed to be a co-infection if IgM anti-HBc is present, since this marker suggests acute hepatitis B. The acute hepatitis D can be assumed to be a superinfection if IgM anti-HBc is absent, since this finding suggests an underlying chronic hepatitis B or HBsAg carrier state. The diagnosis of chronic hepatitis D can be assumed in the clinical setting of chronic hepatitis with a duration greater than 6 months to 1 year and both HBsAg and anti-HDV present in the serum (Table 14–16). It can be confirmed by assaying for HDV RNA or HDAg in serum or liver tissue. Both co-infection and superinfection can result in fulminant hepatitis, but it is more common with superinfection. Co-infection usually resolves without sequelae and rarely results in chronic infection. Superinfection, by contrast, usually leads to chronic hepatitis D (see Table 14–5). Chronic hepatitis D is often severe and leads to cirrhosis in the majority of patients.[319] Because of the recognized severity of chronic hepatitis D, attempts have been made at treatment with antiviral agents.

Antiviral Treatment for Chronic Hepatitis D

The treatment of chronic hepatitis D remains problematic. Pilot studies assessing the efficacy

TABLE 14–16. DIAGNOSIS OF CHRONIC HEPATITIS D

Elevated (persistent or fluctuating) serum aminotransferase levels for at least 6 months or longer
HBsAg-positive serum
Anti-HDV in serum at high titer
Liver biopsy evidence of chronic hepatitis (mild, moderate, severe), with or without cirrhosis
Evidence of HDV replication:
  HDAg in liver, by immunocytochemistry
  HDAg in serum, by immunoblot
  HDV RNA in serum, by hybridization

KEY: Anti-HDV = antibody to hepatitis D virus, HBsAg = hepatitis B surface antigen, HDAg = hepatitis D antigen, HDV = hepatitis D virus, RNA = ribonucleic acid.

TABLE 14-17. CONTROLLED TRIALS OF RECOMBINANT ALPHA-INTERFERON THERAPY FOR CHRONIC HEPATITIS D IN ADULTS

| REFERENCE | N | DOSAGE/ DURATION† | TYPE | % BIOCHEMICAL RESPONSE* | | % BIOCHEMICAL RELAPSE | HISTOLOGIC IMPROVEMENT |
				INTERFERON	CONTROL		
Porres (1989)[324]	20	20/6	2C	20 (2/10)	0 (0/10)	100 (2/2)	NC
Rosina (1991)[325]	61	10/12‡	2B	26 (8/31)	0 (0/30)	87 (7/8)	NC

*Response = normalization or 50% reduction of serum transaminase.
†Dosage in million units (mU) of interferon 2-3 × weeks; duration in months of treatment.
‡10 mU for 4 months, then 6 mU for 8 months.
KEY: 2B = recombinant interferon-α-2B, 2C = recombinant inferon-α-2C, NC = no change, relapse = persistent increased transaminase level.

of alpha-interferon treatment of chronic hepatitis D suggested that such treatment may be associated with diminished HDV replication and improvement of serum aminotransferase levels,[321-323] but that once the drug was stopped, relapse was common. A summary of selected controlled trials of recombinant alpha-interferon therapy for chronic hepatitis D in adults is given in Table 14-17.[324, 325] A biochemical response, defined as normalization or 50% or greater decrease in the serum aminotransferase level, was observed in approximately 25% of patients with chronic hepatitis D. None of the control patients experienced a biochemical response. Of those patients who responded, a biochemical relapse was very common, approximately 85%. Histologic improvement was not apparent.

A 1991 meta-analysis of five randomized, controlled trials indicated that, whereas alpha-interferon therapy had a statistically significant effect on normalization of serum aminotransferase values during the treatment period, this therapy, even when carried out for 1 year, had no statistically significant effect on serum aminotransferase activity after therapy was stopped.[326] In addition, this analysis revealed no correlation between the decrease in serum aminotransferase activity and the inhibition of HDV replication. Studies suggest that the best alpha-interferon dosage schedule for chronic HDV infection appears to be 5 MU daily or 9 MU 3 times a week for at least 1 year. Unlike in chronic hepatitis B, no factors have been identified that predict the outcome of interferon treatment of chronic HDV. The response to interferon treatment, as measured by decrease in serum aminotransferase activity, usually occurs within 3 months, and termination of treatment is recommended if no decrease in serum aminotransferase activity occurs after 3 months. Alternatives to alpha-interferon have been evaluated in some pilot studies. Although both

acyclovir and ribavirin have an effect on HDV replication in vitro, neither agent appears promising in clinical studies.[326] The effect of a combination of alpha-interferon and other interferons has not been reported.

In summary, the lack of an effective therapy for chronic hepatitis D is disappointing. Even with prolonged treatment with alpha-interferon, the effect on disease activity and on HDV replication is not impressive. The availability of animal models of HDV infection and in vitro HDV culture systems offers the opportunity to test newer antiviral agents and offers hope for the discovery of an effective treatment for chronic HDV infection. Perhaps the most reasonable approach to the treatment of chronic hepatitis D is to initiate therapy with 5 MU of alpha-interferon daily. If no biochemical response has occurred in 2 to 3 months, therapy should be discontinued. If a beneficial response is noted, however, then therapy may be considered for as long as 2 to 3 years.[327]

REFERENCES

1. DeGroote J, Desmet VJ, Gedigk P, et al. A classification of chronic hepatitis. Lancet. 1968;2:626–628.
2. Bianchi L, DeGroote J, Desmet VJ, et al. Acute and chronic hepatitis revised. Lancet. 1977;2:914–919.
3. Sherlock S. Classifying chronic hepatitis. Lancet. 1989;2:1168–1170.
4. Maddrey WC. Chronic hepatitis. In: Zakim D, Boyer TD, eds. 2nd ed. Hepatology: A Textbook of Liver Disease. Philadelphia: WB Saunders; 1990;1025–1061.
5. Hoofnagle JH, Di Bisceglie AM. Serologic diagnosis of acute and chronic viral hepatitis. Semin Liver Dis. 1991;11:73–83.
6. Johnson PJ, McFarlane IG, Eddleston ALWF. The natural course and heterogeneity of autoimmune-type chronic active hepatitis. Semin Liver Dis. 1991;11:187–196.
7. Czaja AJ, Beaver SJ, Shields MT. Sustained remission after corticosteroid therapy of severe hepatitis B surface antigen–negative chronic active hepatitis. Gastroenterology. 1987;92:215–219.

8. Willson RA. The liver: Its role in drug biotransformation and as a target of immunologic injury. Immunol Allergy Clin North Am. 1991;11:555–574.

9. Kaplowitz N, Aw TY, Simon FR, et al. Drug-induced hepatotoxicity. Ann Intern Med. 1986;104:826–839.

10. Lewis JH, Zimmerman HJ. Drug-induced liver disease. Med Clin North Am. 1989;73:775–792.

11. Sternlieb I. Perspectives on Wilson's disease. Hepatology. 1990;12:1234–1239.

12. Stremmel W, Meyerrose KW, Niederau C, et al. Wilson disease: Clinical presentation, treatment, and survival. Ann Intern Med. 1991;115:720–726.

13. Perlmuller DH. The cellular basis for liver injury in alfa-1-antitrypsin deficiency. Hepatology. 1991;13:172–185.

14. Kaplan M. Primary biliary cirrhosis. N Engl J Med. 1987;316:521–528.

15. Porayko MK, LaRusso NF, Wiesner RH. Primary sclerosing cholangitis: A progressive disease? Semin Liver Dis. 1991;11:18–25.

16. Takase S, Takada N, Enomoto N, et al. Different types of chronic hepatitis in alcoholic patients: Does chronic hepatitis induced by alcohol exist? Hepatology. 1991;13:876–881.

17. Wands JR, Blum HE. Hepatitis B and C virus and alcohol-induced liver injury. Hepatology. 1991;14:730–733.

18. Caldwell SH, Jeffers LJ, Ditomaso A, et al. Antibody to hepatitis C is common among patients with alcoholic liver disease with and without risk factors. Am J Gastroenterol. 1991;86:1219–1223.

19. Mendenhall CL, Seeff L, Diehl AM, et al. Antibodies to hepatitis B virus and hepatitis C virus in alcoholic hepatitis and cirrhosis: Their prevalance and clinical significance. Hepatology. 1991;14:581–589.

20. Pares A, Barrera JM, Caballeria J, et al. Hepatitis C virus antibodies in chronic alcoholic patients: Association with severity of disease. Hepatology. 1990;12:1295–1299.

21. Hay JE, Czaja AJ, Rakela J, Ludwig J. The nature of unexplained chronic aminotransferase elevations of a mild to moderate degree in asymptomatic patients. Hepatology. 1989;9:193–197.

22. Diehl AM, Goodman Z, Ishak KG. Alcohol-like liver disease in non-alcoholics. Gastroenterology. 1988;95:1056–1062.

23. Powell EE, Cooksley GE, Hanson R, et al. The natural history of non-alcoholic steatohepatitis: A follow-up study of forty-two patients for up to 21 years. Hepatology. 1990;11:74–80.

24. Adams PC, Halliday JW, Powell LW. Early diagnosis and treatment of hemochromatosis. Adv Intern Med. 1989;34:111–126.

25. Scheuer PJ. Classification of chronic viral hepatitis: A need for reassessment. J Hepatol. 1991;13:372–374.

26. Scheuer PJ, Ashrafzadeh P, Sherlock S, et al. The pathology of hepatitis C. Hepatology. 1992;15:567–571.

27. Gerber MA. Chronic hepatitis C: The beginning of the end of a time-honored nomenclature? Hepatology. 1992;15:733–734.

28. Knodell RG, Ishak KG, Black WC, et al. Formulation and application of numerical scoring system for assessing histological activity in asymptomatic chronic active hepatitis. Hepatology. 1981;1:431–435.

29. Gowans EJ, Jilbert AR, Burrell CJ. The detection of specific DNA and RNA sequences by in situ hybridization. In: Symons RH, ed. Nucleic Acid Probes. Orlando: CRC Press; 1989;139–158.

30. Negro F, Pacchioni D, Shimizu Y, et al. Detection of intrahepatic replication of hepatitis C virus RNA by in situ hybridization and comparison with histopathology. Proc Natl Acad Sci U S A. 1992;89:2247–2251.

31. Krawczynski K, Beach MJ, Bradley DW, et al. Hepatitis C virus antigen in hepatocytes: Immunomorphologic detection and identification. Gastroenterology. 1992;103:622–629.

32. Hiramatsu N, Hayashi N, Haruna Y, et al. Immunohistochemical detection of hepatitis C virus–infected hepatocytes in chronic liver disease with monoclonal antibodies to core, envelope and NS3 regions of the hepatitis C virus genome. Hepatology. 1992;16:306–311.

33. Hoofnagle JH, Shafritz DA, Popper H. Chronic type B hepatitis and the "healthy" HBsAg carrier state. Hepatology. 1987;7:758–763.

34. Naoumov NV, Portmann BC, Tedder RS, et al. Detection of hepatitis B virus antigens in liver tissue: A relation to viral replication and histology in chronic hepatitis B infection. Gastroenterology. 1990;99:1248–1253.

35. Baker BL, DiBisceglie AM, Kaneko S, et al. Determination of hepatitis B virus DNA in serum using the polymerase chain reaction. Hepatology. 1991;14:632–636.

36. Fong TL, DiBisceglie AM, Feinstone SM, et al. Persistent hepatic HBV-DNA after clearance of HBsAg from serum of patients with chronic hepatitis B. Hepatology. 1991;14:130A.

37. Hoofnagle JH, DiBisceglie AM. Antiviral therapy of viral hepatitis. In: Galasso GJ, Whitley RJ, Merigan TC, eds. 3rd ed. Antiviral Agents and Viral Diseases of Man. New York: Raven Press; 1990;415–459.

38. Farci P, Alter HJ, Wong D, et al. A long-term study of hepatitis C virus replication in non-A, non-B hepatitis. N Engl J Med. 1991;325:98–104.

39. Phillips MJ, Blendis LM, Poucell S, et al. Syncytial giant cell hepatitis: Sporadic hepatitis with distinctive pathological features, a severe clinical course, and paramyxoviral features. N Engl J Med. 1991;324:455–460.

40. Fong TL, DiBisceglie AM, Waggoner JC, et al. The significance of antibody to hepatitis C virus in patients with chronic hepatitis B. Hepatology. 1991;14:64–67.

41. Hoofnagle JH. Chronic hepatitis B. N Engl J Med. 1990;323:337–339.

42. Margolis HS, Alter MJ, Hadler SC. Hepatitis B: Evolving epidemiology and implications for control. Semin Liver Dis. 1991;11:84–92.

43. Alter MJ, Ahtone J, Weisfuse I, et al. Hepatitis B virus transmission between heterosexuals. JAMA. 1988;256:1307–1310.

44. Alter MJ, Coleman PJ, Alexander WJ, et al. Importance of heterosexual activity in the transmission of hepatitis B and non-A, non-B hepatitis. JAMA. 1989;262:1201–1205.

45. Alter MJ, Hadler SC, Margolis HS, et al. The changing epidemiology of hepatitis B in the United States: Need for alternative vaccination strategies. JAMA. 1990;263:1218–1222.

46. Kelen G, Green GB, Purcell RH, et al. Hepatitis B and hepatitis C in emergency department patients. N Engl J Med. 1992;326:1399–1404.

47. Fattovich G, Rugge M, Brollo L, et al. Clinical, virologic and histologic outcome following seroconversion from HBeAg to anti-HBe in chronic hepatitis type B. Hepatology. 1986; 6:167–172.

48. Fattovich G, Brollo L, Alberti A, et al. Long-term follow up of anti HBe-positive chronic active hepatitis B. Hepatology. 1988;8:1651–1654.

49. Bortolotti F, Cadrobbi P, Crivellaro C, et al. Long-term outcome of chronic type B hepatitis in patients who acquire hepatitis B virus infection in childhood. Gastroenterology. 1990;99:805–810.

50. Fattovich G, Brollo L, Giustina G, et al. Natural history and prognostic factors for chronic hepatitis B. Gut. 1991;32:294–298.

51. Hadziyannis SJ, Lieberman HM, Karvountzis GG, et al. Analysis of liver disease, nuclear HB$_c$Ag, viral replication and hepatitis B virus DNA in liver and serum of HB$_e$Ag versus antiHB$_e$ positive carriers of hepatitis B virus. Hepatology. 1983;3:656–662.

52. Davis GL, Hoofnagle JH, Waggoner JG. Spontaneous reactivation of chronic hepatitis B virus infection. Gastroenterology. 1984;86:230–235.

53. Perrillo RP, Campbell CR, Sanders GE, et al. Spontaneous clearance and reactivation of hepatitis B virus infection among male homosexuals with chronic type B hepatitis. Ann Intern Med. 1984;100:43–46.

54. Carmen WF, Jacyna MR, Hadziyannis S, et al. Mutation preventing formation of hepatitis B e antigen in patients with chronic hepatitis B infection. Lancet. 1989;2:588–590.

55. Brown JL, Carman WF, Thomas HC. The clinical significance of molecular variation within the hepatitis B virus genome. Hepatology. 1992;15:144–148.

56. Davis GL. Loss of HB$_s$Ag after interferon treatment: Cure of chronic hepatitis B virus? Hepatology. 1991;14:953–954.

57. Loriot MA, Marcellin P, Bismuth E, et al. Demonstration of hepatitis B virus DNA by polymerase chain reaction in the serum and the liver after spontaneous or therapeutically induced HB$_e$Ag to anti-HB$_e$ or HB$_s$Ag to anti-HB$_s$ seroconversion in patients with chronic hepatitis B. Hepatology. 1992;15:32–36.

58. Peters M. Mechanisms of action of interferons. Semin Liver Dis. 1990;9:235–239.

59. Peters M, Davis GL, Dooley JS, et al. The interferon system in acute and chronic viral interferon system in acute and chronic viral hepatitis. In: Popper H, Schaffner F, eds. Progress in Liver Disease. Philadelphia: WB Saunders; 1986;8:453–468.

60. Baron S, Tyring SK, Fleischmann WR, et al. The interferons: Mechanisms of action and clinical applications. JAMA. 1991;266:1375–1383.

61. Sen GC, Lengyel P. The interferon system. A bird's eye view of its biochemistry. J Biol Chem. 1992;267:5017–5020.

62. Pirovino M, Aguet M, Huber M, et al. Absence of detectable serum interferon in acute and chronic viral hepatitis. Hepatology. 1986;6:645–649.

63. Davis GL, Hoofnagle JH. Interferon in viral hepatitis: Role in pathogenesis and treatment. Hepatology. 1986;6:1038–1041.

64. Renault PF, Hoofnagle JH. Side effects of alpha interferon. Semin Liver Dis. 1989;9:273–277.

65. Renault PF, Hoofnagle JH, Park Y, et al. Psychiatric complications of long-term interferon alfa therapy. Arch Intern Med. 1987;147:1577–1580.

66. Quesada JR, Talpaz M, Rios A, et al. Clinical toxicity of interferons in cancer patients: A review. J Clin Oncol. 1986;4:234–243.

67. Silva MO, Reddy KR, Jeffer LJ, et al. Interferon-induced chronic active hepatitis? Gastroenterology. 1991;101:840–842.

68. Marcellin P, Colin JF, Boyer N, et al. Fatal exacerbation of chronic hepatitis B induced by recombinant alpha-interferon. Lancet. 1991;338:828.

69. Durand JM, Kaplanski G, Portal I, et al. Liver failure due to recombinant alfa interferon. Lancet 1991;338:1268–1269.

70. Shindo M, DiBisceglie AM, Hoofnagle JH. Acute exacerbation of liver disease during interferon alfa therapy for chronic hepatitis C. Gastroenterology. 1992;102:1406–1408.

71. Schattner A. Review: Interferons and autoimmunity. Am J Med Sci. 1988;295:532–544.

72. Conlon KG, Urba WJ, Smith JW, et al. Exacerbation of symptoms of autoimmune disease in patients receiving alpha-interferon therapy. Cancer. 1990;65:2237–2242.

73. Lisker-Melman M, DiBisceglie AM, Usala SJ, et al. Development of thyroid disease during therapy of chronic viral hepatitis with interferon alfa. Gastroenterology. 1992;102:2155–2160.

74. Mayet WJ, Hess G, Gerken G, et al. Treatment of chronic type B hepatitis with recombinant alpha interferon induces autoantibodies not specific for autoimmune chronic hepatitis. Hepatology. 1989;10:24–28.

75. Papo T, Marcellin P, Bernnan J, et al. Autoimmune chronic hepatitis exacerbated by alpha-interferon. Ann Intern Med. 1992;116:51–53.

76. Lee WM. Where is the dividing line between autoimmune hepatitis and hepatitis C? Gastroenterology. 1992;102:1814–1815.

77. Friedman LS, Patel KP, Munoz SJ. Hepatitis C virus and autoimmune chronic active hepatitis: Closing the ring. Gastroenterology. 1992;102:1436–1438.

78. Antonelli G, Currenti M, Turriziani O, et al. Neutralizing antibodies to interferon alfa: Relative frequency in patients treated with different interferon preparations. J Infect Dis. 1991;163:882–885.

79. Steis RG, Smith JW, Urba WJ, et al. Resistance to recombinant interferon alpha-2A in hairy cell leukemia associated with neutralizing anti-interferon antibodies. N Engl J Med. 1988;318:1409–1413.

80. Lok ASF, Lai CL, Leung EKY. Interferon antibodies may negate the antiviral effects of recombinant alfa interferon treatment in patients with chronic hepatitis B virus infections. Hepatology. 1990;12:1266–1270.

81. Douglas DD, Rakela J, Douglas ML, et al. Do antiinterferon antibodies effect the clinical response to recombinant alfa-2a interferon? Gastroenterology. 1992;102:A802.

82. Lok ASF, Pui-chee WU, Ching-Lung L, et al. A controlled trial of interferon with or without prednisone priming for chronic hepatitis B. Gastroenterology. 1992;102:2091–2097.

83. Perrillo RP, Schiff ER, Davis GL, et al. A randomized controlled trial of interferon alfa-2b alone and after prednisone withdrawal for the treatment of chronic hepatitis B. N Engl J Med. 1990;323:295–301.

84. Hoofnagle JH, Peters M, Mullen KD, et al. Randomized controlled trial of recombinant human alpha-interferon in patients with chronic hepatitis B. Gastroenterology. 1988;95:1318–1325.

85. Brook MG, McDonald JA, Karayiannis P, et al. Randomized controlled trial of interferon alfa 2a for the treatment of chronic hepatitis B virus infection: Factors that influence response. Gut. 1989;30:1116–1122.

86. Saracco G, Mazzella G, Rosina F, et al. A controlled trial of human lymphoblastoid interferon in chronic hepatitis B in Italy. Hepatology. 1989;10:336–341.

87. Perrillo RP, Brunt EM. Hepatic histologic and immunohistochemical changes in chronic hepatitis B after prolonged clearance of hepatitis B e antigen. Ann Intern Med. 1991;115:113–115.

88. Perrillo RP. Treatment of chronic hepatitis B with interferon: Experience in western countries. Semin Liver Dis. 1989;9:240–248.

89. Alexander GJM, Brahm J, Fagan EA, et al. Loss of HB$_s$Ag with interferon therapy in chronic hepatitis B virus infection. Lancet. 1987;2:66–69.

90. DiBisceglie AM, Bergasa NV, Fong TL, et al. A randomized controlled trial of recombinant alfa interferon therapy for chronic hepatitis B. Hepatology. 1991;14:70A.

91. Lok ASF, Lai CL, Wu PC, et al. Long-term follow-up in a randomized controlled trial of recombinant alfa-2a

interferon in Chinese patients with chronic hepatitis B infection. Lancet. 1988;2:298–302.

92. Lok ASF, Lai CL. Acute exacerbations in Chinese patients with chronic hepatitis B virus (HBV) infection: Incidence, predisposing factors and etiology. J Hepatol. 1990;10:29–34.

93. Lok ASF, Lai CL, Wu PC, et al. Treatment of chronic hepatitis B with interferon: Experience in Asian patients. Semin Liver Dis. 1989;9:249–253.

94. Davis G. Interferon treatment of viral hepatitis in immunocompromised patients. Semin Liver Dis. 1989;9:267–272.

95. Schalm SW, Thomas HC, Hadziyannis SJ. Chronic hepatitis B. In: Popper H, Schaffner F, eds. Progress in Liver Disease. Philadelphia: WB Saunders; 1990;9:443–462.

96. Korenman J, Baker B, Waggoner J, et al. Long-term remission of chronic hepatitis B after alpha-interferon therapy. Ann Intern Med. 1991;114:629–634.

97. Lok AS, Lai CL, Wu PC, et al. Spontaneous hepatitis B e antigen to antibody seroconversion and reversion in Chinese patients with chronic hepatitis B virus infection. Gastroenterology. 1987;92:1839–1843.

98. Carreno V, Castillo I, Molina J, et al. Long-term follow-up of hepatitis B chronic carriers who responded to interferon therapy. J Hepatol. 1992;15:102–106.

99. Ruiz-Moreno M, Rua MJ, Molina J, et al. Prospective randomized controlled trial of interferon in children with chronic hepatitis B. Hepatology. 1991;13:1035–1039.

100. Utili R, Sagnelli E, Galanti B, et al. Prolonged treatment of children with chronic hepatitis B with recombinant alfa-2a interferon: A controlled, randomized study. Am J Gastroenterol. 1991;86:327–330.

101. Lai CL, Lok ASF, Lin HJ, et al. Placebo controlled trial of recombinant interferon alfa 2a in Chinese HB$_s$Ag-carrier children. Lancet. 1987;2:877–880.

102. Rakela J, Redeker AG, Weliky B. Effect of short term prednisone therapy on aminotransferase levels and hepatitis B virus markers in chronic type B hepatitis. Gastroenterology. 1983;84:956–960.

103. Nair PV, Tong MJ, Stevenson D, et al. A pilot study on the effects of prednisone withdrawal on serum hepatitis B virus DNA and HB$_e$Ag in chronic active hepatitis B. Hepatology. 1986;6:1319–1324.

104. Perrillo RP, Regenstein FG, Peters MG, et al. Prednisone withdrawal followed by recombinant alpha interferon in the treatment of chronic type B hepatitis. A randomized, controlled trial. Ann Intern Med. 1988;109:95–100.

105. Katkov WN, Dienstag JL. Prevention and therapy of viral hepatitis. Semin Liver Dis. 1991;11:165–174.

106. Caselmann WH, Eisenburg J, Hofschneider PH, et al. Beta and gamma interferon in chronic active hepatitis B: A pilot trial of short-term combination therapy. Gastroenterology. 1989;96:449–455.

107. DiBisceglie AM, Rustgi VK, Kassianides C, et al. Therapy of chronic hepatitis B with recombinant alpha and gamma interferon. Hepatology. 1990;11:266–270.

108. Czarniecki CW, Fennie CW, Poers DB, et al. Synergistic antiviral and antiproliferative activities of *E. coli*–derived human alfa, beta and gamma interferons. J Virol. 1984;49:490–496.

109. Bissett J, Eisenberg M, Gregory P, et al. Recombinant fibroblast interferon and immune interferon for treating chronic hepatitis B virus infection: Patients' tolerance and the effect on viral markers. J Infect Dis. 1988;157:1076–1080.

110. Brunetto MR, Stemler M, Bonino F, et al. A new hepatitis B virus strain in patients with severe anti-HB$_e$ positive chronic hepatitis B. J Hepatol. 1990;10:258–261.

111. Bonino F, Brunetto MR, Rizzetto M, et al. Hepatitis B virus unable to secrete e antigen. Gastroenterology. 1991;100:1138–1141.

112. Foster GR, Carman WF, Thomas HC. Replication of hepatitis B and delta viruses: Appearance of viral mutants. Semin Liver Dis. 1991;11:121–127.

113. Pastore G, Santantonio T, Milella M, et al. Anti-HB$_e$–positive chronic hepatitis B with HBV-DNA in the serum response to a 6-month course of lymphoblastoid interferon. J Hepatol. 1992;14:221–225.

114. Brunetto MR, Oliveri F, Rocca G, et al. Natural course and response to interferon of chronic hepatitis B accompanied by antibody to hepatitis B e antigen. Hepatology. 1989;10:198–202.

115. Hadziyannis S, Bramou T, Makris A, et al. Interferon alfa-2b treatment of HB$_e$ Ag negative/serum HBV-DNA positive chronic active hepatitis B. J Hepatol. 1990;11(suppl):S133–S136.

116. Fattovich G, Farci P, Rugge M, et al. A randomized controlled trial of lymphoblastoid interferon-alfa in patients with chronic hepatitis B lacking HB$_e$Ag. Hepatology. 1992;15:584–589.

117. Brunetto MR, Oliveri F, DeMartini A, et al. Treatment with interferon of chronic hepatitis B associated with antibody to hepatitis B e antigen. J Hepatol. 1991;13(suppl 1):S8–S11.

118. Hoofnagle JH, DiBisceglie AM, Waggoner JG, et al. Interferon alfa for patients with clinically apparent cirrhosis due to chronic hepatitis B. Gastroenterology. 1993;104:1116–1121.

119. DiBisceglie AM. Interferon therapy of complicated hepatitis B virus infection. Semin Liver Dis. 1989;9:254–258.

120. Johnson RJ, Couser WG. Hepatitis B infection and renal disease: Clinical, immunopathogenetic and therapeutic considerations. Kidney Int. 1990;37:663–676.

121. Lai KN, Li PKT, Lui SF, et al. Membranous nephropathy related to hepatitis B virus in adults. N Engl J Med. 1991;324:1457–1463.

122. Lai KN, Lai FM. Clinical features and the natural course of hepatitis B virus–related glomerulopathy in adults. Kidney Int. 1991;40(suppl 35):S40–S45.

123. Levy M, Chen N. Worldwide perspective of hepatitis B–associated glomerulonephritis in the 80s. Kidney Int. 1991;40(suppl 35):S24–S33.

124. Venkataseshan VS, Lieberman K, Kim DU, et al. Hepatitis B–associated glomerulonephritis: Pathology, pathogenesis, and clinical course. Medicine. 1990;60:200–216.

125. Garcia G, Scullard G, Smith C, et al. Preliminary observation of hepatitis B–associated membranous glomerulonephritis treated with leukocyte interferon. Hepatology. 1985;5:317–320.

126. Mizushima N, Kanai K, Matsuda H. Improvement of proteinuria in a case of hepatitis B associated glomerulonephritis after treatment with interferon. Gastroenterology. 1987;95:524–526.

127. deMan RA, Schalm SW, vander Heijden AJ, et al. Improvement of hepatitis B–associated glomerulonephritis after anti-viral combination therapy. J Hepatol. 1989;8:367–372.

128. Lisker-Melman M, Webb D, DiBisceglie AM, et al. Glomerulonephritis caused by chronic hepatitis B virus infection: Treatment with recombinant human alpha-interferon. Ann Intern Med. 1989;111:479–483.

129. Sergent JS, Lockshin ML, Christian CL, et al. Vasculitis with hepatitis B antigenemia. Medicine. 1976;55:1–18.

130. Duffy J, Lidksy MD, Sharp JT, et al. Polyarthritis, polyarteritis and hepatitis B. Medicine. 1976;55:19–37.

131. Shusterman N, London WT. Hepatitis B and immune complex disease. N Engl J Med. 1984;310:43–46.

132. McMahon BJ, Heyward WL, Templin DW, et al. Hepatitis B associated polyarteritis nodosa in Alaskan Eskimos: Clinical and epidemiologic features and long-term follow-up. Hepatology. 1989;9:97–101.

133. Wright HI, Cavaler JS, Todo S, et al. Interferon alfa 2b therapy of viral hepatitis following liver transplantation. Hepatology. 1991;14:71A.

134. Lake JR. Liver transplantation for patients with hepatitis B: What have we learned from our results? Hepatology. 1991;13:796–799.

135. Martin P, Munoz SJ, Friedman LS. Liver transplantation for viral hepatitis: Current status. Am J Gastroenterol. 1992;87:409–418.

136. O'Grady JG, Smith HM, Davies SE, et al. Hepatitis B virus reinfection after orthotopic liver transplantation: Serologic and clinical implications. J Hepatol. 1992;14:104–111.

137. Housset C, Pol S, Carnot F, et al. Interactions between human immunodeficiency virus-1, hepatitis delta virus and hepatitis B virus infections in 260 chronic carriers of hepatitis B virus. Hepatology. 1992;15:578–583.

138. Pomerantz RJ, Friedman LS. Hepatitis B and human immunodeficiency virus: Double trouble. Gastroenterology. 1991;101:862–863.

139. Hadler SC, Judson FN, O'Malley PM, et al. Outcome of hepatitis B virus infection in homosexual men and its relation to prior human immunodeficiency virus infection. J Infect Dis. 1991;163:454–459.

140. Korba BE, Tennant BC, Cote PJ, et al. Treatment of chronic woodchuck hepatitis virus infection with thymosin alpha-1. Hepatology. 1990;12:880.

141. Sherlar AH, Hirota K, Omata M, et al. Foscarnet decreases serum and liver duck hepatitis B virus DNA in chronically infected ducks. Gastroenterology. 1986;91:818–824.

142. Petcu DJ, Aldrich CE, Coates L, et al. Suramin inhibits in vitro infection by duck hepatitis B virus, Rous sarcoma virus, and hepatitis delta virus. Virology. 1988;167:385–392.

143. Tsiquaye K, Collins P, Zuckerman AJ. Screening of antiviral drugs for treatment of hepatitis B. J Hepatol. 1986;3:545–548.

144. Venkateswaran PS, Millman I, Blumberg BS. Effects of an extract from *Phyllanthus niruir* on hepatitis B and woodchuck hepatitis viruses: In vitro and in vivo studies. Proc Natl Acad Sci U S A. 1987;84:274–278.

145. Kassianides C, Hoofnagle JH, Miller RH, et al. Effects of 2′, 3′-dideoxycytidine on duck hepatitis B virus. Gastroenterology. 1988;94:A552.

146. Chadwick RG, Jain S, Cohen BJ, et al. Levamisole therapy for chronic HB$_s$Ag-positive chronic liver disease. Scand J Gastroenterol. 1980;15:973–978.

147. Fattovich G, Brollo L, Pontisso P, et al. Levamisole therapy in chronic type B hepatitis: Results of a double blind randomized trial. Gastroenterology. 1986;91:692–696.

148. Jain S, Thomas HC, Sherlock S. Transfer factor in the attempted treatment of patients with HB$_s$Ag-positive chronic liver disease. Clin Exp Immunol. 1977;30:10–15.

149. Jain S, Thomas HC, Oxford JS, et al. Trial of ribavirin for treatment of HB$_s$Ag-positive chronic liver disease. J Antimicrob Chemother. 1978;4:367–373.

150. Fried MW, Fong TL, Swain MG, et al. Hepatitis B virus DNA suppression during long term therapy with ribavirin. Gastroenterology. 1992;102:A808.

151. Mutchnick MG, Appelman HD, Chung HT, et al. Thymosin treatment of chronic hepatitis B: A placebo-controlled pilot study. Hepatology 1991;14:409–415.

152. Kakumu S, Fuji A, Yoshioka K, et al. Pilot study of recombinant human interleukin 2 for chronic type B hepatitis. Hepatology. 1987;8:487–492.

153. Berk L, Schalm SW, deMan RA, et al. Failure of acyclovir to enhance the antiviral effect of alfa lymphoblastoid interferon on HB$_e$-seroconversion in chronic Hepatitis B: A multicentre randomized controlled trial. J Hepatol. 1992;14:305–309.

154. Hirota K, Sherkes AH, Omata M, et al. Effects of adenine arabinoside on serum and intrahepatic replicative forms of duck hepatitis B virus in chronic type B hepatitis. Hepatology. 1987;8:487–492.

155. Bassendine MF, Chadwick RG, Salmeron J, et al. Adenine arabinoside therapy in HB$_s$Ag-positive chronic liver disease: A controlled study. Gastroenterology. 1981;80:1016–1021.

156. Hoofnagle JH, Hanson RG, Minuk GY, et al. Randomized controlled trial of adenine arabinoside monophosphate for chronic type B hepatitis. Gastroenterology. 1984;86:150–157.

157. Weller IVD, Lok ASF, Mindel A, et al. Randomized controlled trial of adenine arabinoside 5′-monophosphate (ara-AMP) in chronic hepatitis B virus infection. Gut. 1985;26:745–751.

158. Marcellin P, Ouzan, Degos F, et al. Randomized controlled trial of adenine arabinoside 5′-monophosphate in chronic active hepatitis B: Comparison of the efficacy in heterosexual and homosexual patients. Hepatology. 1989;10:328–331.

159. Perrillo RP, Regenstein FG, Bodicky CJ, et al. Comparative efficacy of adenine arabinoside 5′-monophosphate in the treatment of chronic active hepatitis B. Gastroenterology. 1985;88:780–786.

160. Garcia G, Smith CI, Weissberg JI, et al. Adenine arabinoside monophosphate in combination with human leukocyte interferon in the treatment of chronic hepatitis B: A randomized, double-blind, placebo-controlled trial. Ann Intern Med. 1987;107:278–285.

161. Lok ASF, Wilson LA, Thomas HC. Neurotoxicity associated with adenine arabinoside monophosphate in the treatment of chronic hepatitis B virus infection. J Antimicrob Chemother. 1984;14:93–99.

162. Ponzetto A, Forzani B, Song SY, et al. Adenosine arabinoside monophosphate and acyclovir monophosphate coupled to lactosaminated albumin reduce woodchuck hepatitis virus viremia at doses lower than do the unconjugated drugs. Hepatology. 1991;14:16–24.

163. Finne L, Cerenzia MRT, Bonino F, et al. Inhibition of hepatitis B virus replication by vidarabine monophosphate conjugated with lactosaminated serum albumin. Lancet. 1987;2:13–15.

164. Troisi CL, Hollinger FB. Hepatitis B vaccines. In: Popper H, Schaffner F, eds. Progress in Liver Disease. Philadelphia: WB Saunders; 1990;9:405–442.

165. Catterall AP, Murray-Lyon IM. Strategies for hepatitis B immunization. Gut. 1992;33:576–579.

166. McMahon BJ, Helminiak C, Wainwright RB, et al. Frequency of adverse reactions to hepatitis B vaccine in 43,618 patients. Am J Med. 1992;92:254–256.

167. Protection against viral hepatitis: Recommendations of the immunization practices advisory committee (ACIP). MMWR Morbid Mortal Wkly Rep. 1990;39(RR-2):1–26.

168. Wainwright RB, McMahon BJ, Bulkow LR, et al. Duration of immunogenicity and efficacy of hepatitis B vaccine in a Yupik Eskimo population. JAMA. 1989;261:2362–2366.

169. Hepatitis B virus: A comprehensive strategy for eliminating transmission in the United States through universal childhood vaccination: Recommendations of the

Immunization Practices Advisory Committee (ACIP). MMWR Morbid Mortal Wkly Rep. 1991;40(RR-13):1–25.

170. Coursaset P, Yvonnet B, Gilles WR, et al. Scheduling of revaccination against hepatitis B virus. Lancet. 1991; 337:1180–1183.

171. Houghton M, Weiner A, Han J, et al. Molecular biology of the hepatitis C viruses: Implications for diagnosis, development and control of viral disease. Hepatology. 1991;14:381–388.

172. Takada N, Takase S, Takada A, et al. HCV genotypes in different countries. Lancet. 1992;339:808.

173. Takada N, Takase S, Enomoto N, et al. Clinical background of the patients having different types of hepatitis C virus genomes. J Hepatol. 1992;14:35–40.

174. Davis GL. Genomic variation of hepatitis C virus: Clues to clinical variation? Gastroenterology. 1992;103:344–346.

175. Kanai K, Kako M, Okamoto H. HCV genotypes in chronic hepatitis C and response to interferon. Lancet. 1992;339:1543.

176. Yoshioka K, Kayumu S, Wakita T, et al. Detection of hepatitis C virus by polymerase chain reaction and response to interferon alfa therapy: Relationship to genotypes of hepatitis C virus. Hepatology. 1992;16:293–299.

177. Weiner AJ, Geysen M, Christopherson C, et al. Evidence for immune selection of hepatitis C virus (HCV) putative envelope glycoprotein variants: Potential role in chronic HCV infections. Proc Natl Acad Sci U S A. 1992;89:3468–3472.

178. Colombo M, DeFranchis R, Del Ninno E, et al. Hepatocellular carcinoma in Italian patients with cirrhosis. N Engl J Med. 1991;325:675–680.

179. Wands JR, Blum HE. Primary hepatocellular carcinoma. N Engl J Med. 1991;325:729–731.

180. DiBisceglie AM, Order SE, Klein JL, et al. The role of chronic viral hepatitis in hepatocellular carcinoma in the United States. Am J Gastroenterol. 1991;86:335–338.

181. Choo QL, Kuo G, Weiner AJ, et al. Isolation of a cDNA clone derived from a blood borne non-A, non-B viral hepatitis genome. Science. 1989;244:359–361.

182. Kuo G, Choo QL, Alter HJ, et al. An assay for circulating antibodies to a major etiologic virus of human non-A, non-B hepatitis. Science. 1989;244:362–364.

183. Alter HJ, Purcell RH, Shih JW, et al. Detection of antibody to hepatitis C virus in prospectively followed transfusion recipients with acute and chronic non-A, non-B hepatitis. N Engl J Med. 1989;321:1494–1500.

184. Widdell A, Mansson AS, Sundstrom G, et al. Hepatitis C virus RNA in blood donors' sera detected by the polymerase chain reaction: Comparison with supplementary hepatitis C antibody assays. J Med Virol. 1991;35:253–258.

185. Van Der Poel CL, Cuypers HTM, Ressink HW, et al. Confirmation of hepatitis C virus infection by new four-antigen recombinant immunoblot assay. Lancet. 1991;337:317–320.

186. Marcellin P, Martinot-Peignoux M, Boyer N, et al. Second generation (RIBA) test in diagnosis of chronic hepatitis C. Lancet. 1991;337:551–552.

187. Follett EAC, Dow BC, McOmish F, et al. HCV confirmatory testing of blood donors. Lancet. 1991;338:1024.

188. Barrera JM, Bruguera M, Ercilla G, et al. Incidence of non-A, non-B hepatitis after screening blood donors for antibodies to hepatitis C virus and surrogate markers. Ann Intern Med. 1991;115:596–600.

189. Esteban JI, Lopez-Talavera JC, Genesca J, et al. High rate of infectivity and liver disease in blood donors with antibodies to hepatitis C virus. Ann Intern Med. 1991;115:443–449.

190. Alberti A, Chemello L, Cavalletto D, et al. Antibody to hepatitis C virus and liver disease in volunteer blood donors. Ann Intern Med. 1991;114:1010–1012.

191. Black M, Peters M. Alpha-interferon treatment of chronic hepatitis C: Need for accurate diagnosis in selecting patients. Ann Intern Med. 1992;116:86–88.

192. Nishiguchi S, Kuroki T, Ueda T, et al. Detection of hepatitis C virus antibody in the absence of viral RNA in patients with autoimmune hepatitis. Ann Intern Med. 1992;116:21–25.

193. Kato N, Yokosuka O, Omata M, et al. Detection of hepatitis C virus ribonucleic acid in the serum by amplification with polymerase chain reaction. J Clin Invest. 1990;86:1764–1767.

194. Ulrich PP, Romeo JM, Lane PK, et al. Detection, semi-quantitation, and genetic variation in hepatitis C virus sequences amplified from the plasma of blood donors with elevated alanine aminotransferase. J Clin Invest. 1990;86:1609–1617.

195. Shindo M, DiBisceglie AM, Cheung L, et al. Decrease in serum hepatitis C viral RNA during alfa-interferon therapy for chronic hepatitis C. Ann Intern Med. 1991;115:700–704.

196. Hagiwara H, Hayashi N, Mita E, et al. Detection of hepatitis C virus RNA in serum of patients with chronic hepatitis C treated with interferon alfa. Hepatology. 1992;15:37–41.

197. Inchaupse G, Abe K, Zebedee S, et al. Use of conserved sequences from hepatitis C virus for the detection of viral RNA in infected sera by polymerase chain reaction. Hepatology. 1991;14:595–600.

198. Cristiano E, DiBisceglie AM, Hoofnagle JH, et al. Hepatitis C viral RNA in serum of patients with chronic nonA, nonB hepatitis: Detection by the polymerase chain reaction using multiple primer sets. Hepatology. 1991;14:51–55.

199. McHutchison JG, Person JL, Govindarajan S, et al. Improved detection of hepatitis C virus antibodies in high risk populations. Hepatology. 1992;15:19–25.

200. Alter HJ. New kit on the block: Evaluation of second-generation assays for detection of antibody to the hepatitis C virus. Hepatology. 1992;15:350–353.

201. Nakatsuji Y, Matsumoto A, Tanaka E, et al. Detection of chronic hepatitis C virus infection by four diagnostic systems: First-generation and second-generation enzyme-linked immunosorbent assay, second-generation immunoblot assay and nested polymerase chain reaction analysis. Hepatology. 1992;16:300–305.

202. Alter HJ. Descartes before the horse: I clone, therefore I am; The hepatitis C virus in current perspective. Ann Intern Med. 1991;115:644–649.

203. Read AE, Donegan E, Lake J, et al. Hepatitis C in patients undergoing liver transplantation. Ann Intern Med. 1991;114:282–284.

204. Dewar TN. Non-A, non-B hepatitis. West J Med. 1990;153:173–179.

205. Genesca J, Esteban JI, Alter HJ. Blood-borne non-A, non-B hepatitis: Hepatitis C. Semin Liver Dis. 1991;11:147–164.

206. Esteban JI, Viladomiu L, Gonzalez A, et al. Hepatitis C virus antibodies among risk groups in Spain. Lancet. 1989;2:294–296.

207. Alter MJ, Hadler SC, Judson FN, et al. Risk factors for acute non-A, non-B hepatitis in the United States and association with hepatitis C virus infection. JAMA. 1990;264:2231–2235.

208. Kiyosawa K, Sodeyama T, Tanaka E, et al. Hepatitis C in hospital employees with needle stick injuries. Ann Intern Med. 1991;115:367–369.

209. Seeff LB. Hepatitis C from needlestick. Ann Intern Med. 1991;115:411.
210. Klein RS, Freeman K, Taylor PE, et al. Occupational risk for hepatitis C virus infection among New York City dentists. Lancet. 1991;338:1539–1542.
211. Estaban JI, Gonzalez A, Hernandez JM, et al. Evaluation of antibodies to hepatitis C virus in a study of transfusion associated hepatitis. N Engl J Med. 1990;323:1107–1112.
212. Berman M, Alter HJ, Ishak KG, et al. The chronic sequelae of non-A, non-B hepatitis. Ann Intern Med. 1979;91:1–6.
213. Dienstag JL. Non-A, non-B hepatitis: Recognition, epidemiology, and clinical features. Gastroenterology. 1983;85:439–462.
214. DiBisceglie AM, Goodman ZD, Ishak KG, et al. Long-term clinical and histopathological follow-up of chronic post transfusion hepatitis. Hepatology. 1991;14:969–974.
215. Seef LB, et al. Mortality of non-A, non-B transfusion-associated hepatitis in the U.S. 18 years after infection. Hepatology. 1991;14:90A.
216. Thaler MM, Park GK, Landers DV, et al. Vertical transmission of hepatitis C virus. Lancet. 1991;338:17–18.
217. Wejstal R, Hermodsson S, Iwarson S, et al. Mother to infant transmission of hepatitis C virus infection. J Med Virol. 1990;30:178–180.
218. Hess G, Massing A, Rossol S, et al. Hepatitis C virus and sexual transmission. Lancet. 1989;2:987.
219. Everhart JE, DiBisceglie AM, Murrey LM, et al. Risk for non-A, non-B (type C) hepatitis through sexual or household contact with chronic carriers. Ann Intern Med. 1990;112:544–545.
220. Melbye M, Biggar RJ, Wantzin P, et al. Sexual transmission of hepatitis C virus: Cohort study (1981) among European homosexual men. Br Med J. 1990;301:210–212.
221. Silva M, Findor A, Roach K, et al. Prevalence of HVC infection in stable sexual partners of patients with chronic hepatitis C. Gastroenterology. 1991;100:A797.
222. Eyster ME, Alter HJ, Aledort LM, et al. Heterosexual co-transmission of hepatitis C virus (HCV) and human immunodeficiency virus (HIV). Ann Intern Med. 1991;115:764–768.
223. Hsu HH, Wright TL, Luba D, et al. Failure to detect hepatitis C virus genome in human secretions with the polymerase chain reaction. Hepatology. 1991;14:763–767.
224. Hollinger FB, Lin HJ. Community-acquired hepatitis C virus infection. Gastroenterology. 1992;102:1426–1429.
225. Fried MW, Shindo M, Fong TL, et al. Absence of hepatitis C viral RNA from saliva and semen of patients with chronic hepatitis C. Gastroenterology. 1992;102:1306–1308.
226. Akahane Y, Aikawa T, Sugai Y, et al. Transmission of HCV between spouses. Lancet. 1992;339:1059–1060.
227. Kotwal G, Rustgi VK, Baroudy BM. Detection of hepatitis C virus–specific antigens in semen from non-A, non-B hepatitis patients. Dig Dis Sci. 1992;37:641–644.
228. Liou TC, Chang TT, Young KC, et al. Detection of HCV RNA in saliva, urine, seminal fluid, and ascites. J Med Virol. 1992;37:197–202.
229. Bortolotti F, Tagger A, Cadrobbi P, et al. Antibodies to hepatitis C virus in community-acquired acute non-A, non-B hepatitis. J Hepatol. 1991;12:176–180.
230. Hopf U, Moller B, Kuther D, et al. Longterm follow-up of post transfusion and sporadic chronic hepatitis non-A, non-B and frequency of circulating antibodies to hepatitis C virus (HCV). J Hepatol. 1990;10:69–76.
231. Mathieson RD, Sampliner RE, Latham PS, et al. Chronic liver disease following community-acquired

non-A, non-B hepatitis. Am J Clin Pathol. 1986;85:353–356.
232. Wejstal R, Lindberg J, Lundin P, et al. Chronic non-A, non-B hepatitis: A long-term follow-up study in 49 patients. Scand J Gastroenterol. 1987;22:1115–1122.
233. Mattsson L, Weiland O, Glaumann H. Chronic non-A, non-B hepatitis developed after transfusions, illicit self-injections or sporadically: Outcome during long-term follow-up, a comparison. Liver. 1989;9:120–127.
234. Nishioka K, Watanabe J, Furuta S, et al. A high prevalence of antibody to the hepatitis virus in patients with hepatocellular carcinoma in Japan. Cancer. 1991;67:429–433.
235. Simonetti RG, Camma C, Fiorello F, et al. Hepatitis C virus infection as a risk factor for hepatocellular carcinoma in patients with cirrhosis: A case control study. Ann Intern Med. 1992;116:97–102.
236. Kiyosawa K, Sodeyama T, Tanaka E, et al. Interrelationship of blood transfusion, non-A, non-B hepatitis and hepatocellular carcinoma: Analysis by detection of antibody to hepatitis C virus. Hepatology. 1990;12:671–675.
237. McFarlane IG, Smith HM, Johnson PJ, et al. Hepatitis C virus antibodies in chronic active hepatitis: Pathogenetic factor or false-positive result? Lancet. 1990;335:754–757.
238. Czaja AJ, Taswell HT, Rakela J, et al. Frequency and significance of antibody to hepatitis C virus in severe corticosteroid-treated cryptogenic chronic active hepatitis. Mayo Clin Proc. 1990;65:1303–1313.
239. Czaja AJ, Manns M, Homburger HA. Specificity of antibodies to liver/kidney microsome type 1 for type 2 auto-immune chronic active hepatitis: Evidence against overlapping syndromes and hepatitis B and C viruses as important immunogenic stimuli. Hepatology. 1991;14:134A.
240. Sterneck M, Ferrell L, Lake J, et al. Liver disease of undefined etiology: Relative roles of hepatitis C, autoimmune disease and cryptogenic cirrhosis. Hepatology. 1991;14:60A.
241. Hoofnagle JH, Mullen KD, Jones DB, et al. Treatment of chronic non-A, non-B hepatitis with recombinant human alpha interferon. N Engl J Med. 1986;315:1575–1578.
242. Davis GL, Balart LA, Schiff ER, et al. Treatment of chronic hepatitis C with recombinant interferon alfa. N Engl J Med. 1989;321:1501–1505.
243. DiBisceglie AM, Martin P, Kassianides C, et al. Recombinant interferon alfa therapy for chronic hepatitis C. N Engl J Med. 1989;321:1506–1510.
244. Marcellin P, Boyer N, Giostra E, et al. Recombinant human alfa interferon in patients with chronic non-A, non-B hepatitis: A multicenter randomized controlled trial from France. Hepatology. 1991;13:393–397.
245. Saracco G, Rosina F, Torrani Cerenzia MR, et al. A randomized controlled trial of interferon alfa-2b as therapy for chronic non-A, non-B hepatitis. J Hepatol. 1990;11(suppl):S43–S49.
246. Weiland O, Schvarcz R, Wejstal R, et al. Interferon alpha-2b treatment of chronic post transfusion non-A, non-B hepatitis: Interim results of a randomized controlled open study. Scand J Infect Dis. 1989;21:127–132.
247. Saez-Royuela F, Porres JC, Moreno A, et al. High doses of recombinant alfa-interferon or gamma-interferon for chronic hepatitis C: A randomized controlled trial. Hepatology. 1991;13:327–331.
248. Causse X, Godinot H, Chevallier M, et al. Comparison of 1 or 3 MU of interferon alfa-2b and placebo in patients with chronic non-A, non-B hepatitis. Gastroenterology. 1991;101:497–502.

249. Omata M, Ito Y, Yokosuka O, et al. Randomized, double-blind, placebo-controlled trial of eight-week course of recombinant alfa interferon for chronic non-A, non-B hepatitis. Dig Dis Sci. 1991;36:1217–1222.

250. Jacyna MR, Brooks MG, Loke RHT, et al. Randomized controlled trial of interferon alpha (lymphoblastoid interferon) in chronic non-A, non-B hepatitis. Br Med J. 1989;298:80–82.

251. Realdi G, Didati G, Bonetti P, et al. Recombinant human interferon alfa-2a in community acquired non-A, non-B chronic active hepatitis. Preliminary results of a randomized, controlled trial. J Hepatol. 1990;11:S68–S71.

252. Gomez-Rubio M, Porres JC, Castillo I, et al. Prolonged treatment (18 months) of chronic hepatitis C with recombinant alfa-interferon in comparison with a control group. J Hepatol. 1990;11:S63–S67.

253. Marcellin P, Pouteau M, Boyers N, et al. Absence of efficacy of an increasing dosage schedule on the response rate during and after recombinant alfa interferon therapy in chronic hepatitis C. Hepatology. 1991;14:71A.

254. Feinman SV, Willems B, Minuk G, et al. Treatment of chronic non-A, non-B hepatitis, blood related and sporadic, with recombinant interferon alfa: A controlled randomized multicenter study from Canada. Hepatology. 1991;14:71A.

255. Bosch O, Tapia L, Marriott E, et al. Evaluation of the effect of a dose escalating interferon treatment of chronic hepatitis C. Hepatology. 1991;14:72A.

256. Cerini R, Gozzolino G, Morante R, et al. Relatively high dose for 12 months recombinant alfa interferon treatment in chronic hepatitis C: A randomized controlled study. Hepatology. 1991;14:70A.

257. Colombo M, Rumi MG, Marcelli R, et al. Randomized controlled trial of recombinant interferon alfa in patients with chronic hepatitis C. Hepatology. 1991; 14:73A.

258. Metreau JM, Calmus Y, Poupon R, et al. Twelve month treatment, compared to 6 month treatment, does not improve the efficacy of alfa interferon in non-A, non-B chronic active hepatitis. Hepatology. 1991;14:72A.

259. Ferenci P, Vogel W, Hentschel E, et al. One year interferon alfa treatment of chronic hepatitis non-A, non-B. Hepatology. 1991;14:72A.

260. Tine F, Magrin S, Craxi A, Pagliaro L. Interferon for non-A, non-B chronic hepatitis. A meta-analysis of randomized clinical trials. J Hepatol. 1991;13:192–199.

261. Davis GL, Lindsay K, Albrecht J, et al. Predictors of response to recombinant alpha interferon treatment of patients with chronic hepatitis C. Hepatology. 1990;12:905.

262. Lindsay KL, Davis GL, Bodenheimer HC, et al. Predictors of relapse and response to retreatment in patients with an initial response to recombinant alpha interferon therapy for chronic hepatitis C. Hepatology. 1990;12:847.

263. Garson JA, Brillanti S, Ring C, et al. Hepatitis C viremia rebound after "successful" interferon therapy in patients with chronic non-A, non-B Hepatitis. J Med Virol. 1992;37:210–214.

264. Shindo M, DiBisceglie AM, Hoofnagle JH. Long-term follow up of patients with chronic hepatitis C treated with alfa-interferon. Hepatology. 1992;15:1013–1016.

265. Brillanti S, Garson JA, Tuke PW, et al. Effect of alfa-interferon therapy on hepatitis C viremia in community acquired chronic non-A, non-B Hepatitis: A quantitative polymerase chain reaction study. J Med Virol. 1991;34:136–141.

266. Yargas CA, Jeffers L, Civantos F, et al. Serum procollagen-III peptide in chronic viral C hepatitis and its correlation with aminotransferase levels and liver histology in the assessment of disease activity and cirrhosis. Gastroenterology. 1992;102:A905.

267. Hannigan GE, Williams BRG. Signal transduction by interferon alfa through arachidonic metabolism. Science. 1991;251:204–207.

268. Quiroga JA, Campillo ML, Catillo I, et al. IgM antibody to hepatitis C virus in acute and chronic hepatitis C. Hepatology. 1991;14:38–43.

269. Brillanti S, Masci C, Ricci P, et al. Significance of IgM antibody to hepatitis C virus in patients with chronic Hepatitis C. Hepatology. 1992;15:998–1001.

270. Wilber JC, Detmer J, Jeffers L, et al. Monitoring for the effect of alfa interferon with a new quantitative method for measurement of HCV-RNA in serum of patients with chronic hepatitis C. Gastroenterology. 1992;102:A910.

271. Silva M, Kuhns M, Laverne J, et al. Long-term remission of chronic hepatitis C after interferon therapy: Virologic, histologic and biochemical features. Gastroenterology. 1992;102:A888.

272. Patterson JL, Fernandez-Larson R. Molecular action of ribavirin. Rev Infect Dis. 1990;12:1132–1146.

273. Reichard O, Andersson J, Schvarcz R, et al. Ribavirin treatment for chronic hepatitis C. Lancet. 1991;337:1058–1061.

274. DiBisceglie AM, Shindo M, Fong TL, et al. A pilot study of ribavirin therapy for chronic hepatitis C. Hepatology. 1992;16:649–654.

275. Pappas SC, Hoofnagle JH, Young N, et al. Treatment of chronic non-A, non-B hepatitis with acyclovir: Pilot study. J Med Virol. 1985;15:1–9.

276. Prohaska W, Kleesiek K. Treatment of chronic hepatitis C with inosine pranobex. Lancet. 1991;338:390–391.

277. Leushcner U, Leushcner M, Sieratzki J, et al. Gallstone dissolution with ursodeoxycholic acid in patients with chronic active hepatitis and two year follow up: A pilot study. Dig Dis Sci. 1985;30:642–649.

278. Osuga T, Tanaka N, Matsuzaki Y, et al. Effect of ursodeoxycholic acid in chronic hepatitis and primary biliary cirrhosis. Dig Dis Sci. 1989;34(suppl):S49–S51.

279. Bellentani S, Tabarroni G, Barchi T, et al. Effect of ursodeoxycholic acid treatment on alanine aminotransferase and gamma-glutamyltranspeptidase serum levels in patients with hypertransaminasemia: Results from a double-blind controlled trial. J Hepatol. 1989;8:7–12.

280. Podda M, Ghezzi C, Battezzati PM, et al. Effects of ursodeoxycholic acid and taurine on serum liver enzymes and bile acids in chronic hepatitis. Gastroenterology. 1990;98:1044–1050.

281. Grosignani H, Battezzati PM, Setchell KDR, et al. Effects of ursodeoxycholic acid on serum liver enzymes and bile acid metabolism in chronic active hepatitis: A dose-response study. Hepatology. 1991;13:339–344.

282. Kiso S, Kawata S, Imai Y, et al. Prominent effect of ursodeoxycholic acid on serum gamma-glutamyl-transpeptidase in patients with chronic type C hepatitis. Hepatology. 1991;14:82A.

283. DeCaestecker JS, Jazrawi RP, Petroni ML, et al. Ursodeoxycholic acid in chronic liver disease. Gut. 1991, 32:1061–1065.

284. Angelico M, Gandin C, Goffredo F, et al. A combination of interferon-alfa and ursodeoxycholic acid is more effective than interferon-alfa alone in anti-HCV positive chronic hepatitis: A randomized histology-controlled clinical trial. Gastroenterology. 1992;102:A775.

285. Ohnishi K, Nomura F, Iida S. Treatment of post transfusion non-A, non-B acute and chronic hepatitis with human fibroblast beta-interferon. Am J Gastroenterol. 1989;84:596–600.

286. Ohnishi K, Nomura F, Nakano M. Interferon therapy

for acute posttransfusion non-A, non-B hepatitis: Response with respect to anti-hepatitis C virus antibody status. Am J Gastroenterol. 1991;86:1041–1049.

287. Omata M, Yokosuka O, Takano S, et al. Resolution of acute hepatitis C after therapy with natural beta interferon. Lancet. 1991;338:914–15.

288. Viladamiu L, Genesca J, Esteban JI, et al. Interferon-alfa in acute posttransfusion hepatitis C: A randomized, controlled trial. Hepatology. 1992;15:767–769.

289. Chen PJ, Wang JT, Hwang LH, et al. Transient immunoglobulin antibody response to hepatitis C virus capsid antigen in posttransfusion hepatitis C: Putative serological marker for acute viral infection. Proc Natl Acad Sci U S A. 1992;89:5971–5975.

290. al-Faleh FZ, Ayoola EA, al-Jeffry M, et al. Prevalence of antibody to hepatitis C virus among Saudi Arabian children: A community-based study. Hepatology. 1991;14:215–218.

291. Alter MJ. Inapparent transmission of hepatitis C: Foot prints in the sand. Hepatology. 1991;14:389–391.

292. Hsu SC, Chang MH, Chen DS, et al. Non-A, non-B hepatitis in children: A clinical, histologic, and serologic study. J Med Virol. 1991;35:1–6.

293. Ruiz-Moreno M, Rua MJ, Castillo I, et al. Treatment of children with chronic hepatitis C with recombinant interferon alfa: A pilot study. Hepatology. 1992;16:882–885.

294. Martin P, DiBisceglie AM, Kassinanides C, et al. Rapidly progressive non-A, non-B hepatitis in patients with human immunodeficiency virus infection. Gastroenterology. 1989;97:1559–1561.

295. Boyer N, Marcellin P, Degott C, et al. Recombinant interferon alfa for chronic hepatitis C in patients positive for antibody to human immunodeficiency virus. J Infect Dis. 1992;165:723–726.

296. Pereira BJG, Milford EL, Kirkman RL, et al. Transmission of hepatitis C virus by organ transplantation. N Engl J Med. 1991;325:454–460.

297. Poterucha JJ, Rakela J, Lumeng L, et al. Diagnosis of chronic hepatitis C after liver transplantation by detection of viral sequences with polymerase chain reaction. Hepatology. 1992;15:42–45.

298. Shah G, Demetris AJ, Gavaler JS, et al. Incidence, prevalence, and clinical course of hepatitis C following liver transplantation. Gastroenterology. 1992;103:323–329.

299. Feray C, Samuel D, Thiers V, et al. Reinfection of liver graft by hepatitis C virus after liver transplantation. J Clin Invest 1992;89:1361–1365.

300. Wright TL, Donegan E, Hsu HH, et al. Recurrent and acquired hepatitis C viral infection in liver transplant recipients. Gastroenterology. 1992;103:317–322.

301. Rakela J. Hepatitis C viral infection in liver transplant patients: How bad is it really? Gastroenterology. 1992;103:338–339.

302. Wright TL, Ferrell L, Lake J, et al. Hepatitis C viral RNA in patients on interferon alfa for post-liver transplant hepatitis. Gastroenterology. 1992;102:A911.

303. Pascual M, Perrin L, Giostra E, et al. Hepatitis C virus in patients with cryoglobulinemia type II. J Infect Dis. 1990;162:569–570.

304. Ferri C, Greco F, Longombardo G, et al. Association between hepatitis C virus and mixed cryoglobulinemia. Clin Exp Rheumatol. 1991;9:621–624.

305. Cacoub P, Lunel-Fabiani F, Du LTH. Polyarteritis nodosa and hepatitis C virus infection. Ann Intern Med. 1992;116:605–606.

306. Haddad J, Deny P, Munz-Gotheil, et al. Lymphocytic sialadentitis of Sjögren's syndrome associated with chronic hepatitis C virus liver disease. Lancet. 1992;339:321–323.

307. Hartwell P, Willson RA, Hart J, et al. Chronic hepatitis C, glomerulonephritis, and alfa interferon-2b. Gastroenterology. 1992; 102:A818.

308. Knox TA, Hillyer CD, Kaplan MA, et al. Mixed cryoglobulinemia responsive to interferon-alfa. Am J Med. 1991;91:554–555.

309. Durand JM, Kaplanski G, Lefevre P, et al. Effect of interferon-alpha 2b on cryoglobulinemia related to hepatitis C virus infection. J Infect Dis. 1992;165:778–779.

310. Pappas SC, Lewtas I, Terrault N, et al. Chronic hepatitis C associated with vasculitis, cryoglobulins and glomerulonephritis: Clinical features and response to interferon therapy. Hepatology. 1991;14:78A.

311. Fong TL, Shindo M, Feinstone SM, et al. Detection of replicative intermediates of hepatitis C viral RNA in liver and serum of patients with chronic hepatitis C. J Clin Invest. 1991;88:1058–1060.

312. Takehara T, Hayashi N, Mita E, et al. Detection of the minus strand of hepatitis C virus RNA by reverse transcription and polymerase chain reaction: Implications for hepatitis C virus replication in infected tissue. Hepatology. 1992;15:387–390.

313. Shindo M, DiBisceglie AM, Biswas R, et al. Hepatitis C virus replication during acute infection in the chimpanzee. J Infect Dis. 1992;166:424–427.

314. Shimizu YK, Iwamoto A, Hijikata M, et al. Evidence for in vitro replication of hepatitis C virus genome in a human T-cell line. Proc Natl Acad Sci U S A. 1992;89:5477–5481.

315. Hibbs JR, Frickhofen N, Rosenfeld SJ, et al. Aplastic anemia and viral hepatitis. Non-A, non-B, non-C? JAMA. 1992;267:2051–2054.

315. Daugherty D: Genetic structure and heterogeneity of hepatitis C virus: A vaccine impediment? Hepatology. 1992;15:739–741.

317. Prince AM, Brotman B, Huima T, et al. Immunity in hepatitis C infection. J Infect Dis. 1992;165:438–443.

318. Farci P, Alter HJ, Govindarajan S, et al. Lack of protective immunity against reinfection with hepatitis C virus. Science. 1992;258:135–140.

319. Hoofnagle JH: Type D (delta) hepatitis. JAMA. 1989;261:1321–1325.

320. DiBisceglie AM, Negro F. Diagnosis of hepatitis delta virus infections. Hepatology. 1989;10:1014–1016.

321. Hoofnagle JH, Mullen KD, Peters M, et al. Treatment of chronic delta hepatitis with recombinant human alfa interferon. Prog Clin Biol Res. 1987;234:291–298.

322. Thomas HC, Farci P, Shein R, et al. Inhibition of hepatitis delta virus (HDV) replication by lymphoblastoid human alpha interferon. Prog Clin Biol Res 1987; 234:277–290.

323. Rosina F, Saracco G, Lattore V, et al. Alpha 2 recombinant interferon in the treatment of chronic hepatitis delta virus (HDV) hepatitis. Prog Clin Biol Res. 1987;234:299–303.

324. Porres JC, Carreno V, Bartolome J, et al. Treatment of chronic delta infection with recombinant human interferon alfa 2c at high doses. J Hepatol. 1989;9:338–344.

325. Rosina F, Pintus C, Meschievitz C, et al. A randomized controlled trial of a 12 month course of recombinant human interferon-alfa in chronic delta (type D) hepatitis: A multicenter Italian study. Hepatology. 1991; 13:1052–1056.

326. Hadziyannis SJ. Use of alfa interferon in the treatment of chronic delta hepatitis. J Hepatol. 1991;13(suppl 1):S21–S26.

327. DiBisceglie AM, Martin P, Lisker-Melman M, et al. Therapy of chronic delta hepatitis with interferon alfa-2b. J Hepatol. 1990;11:S151–S154.

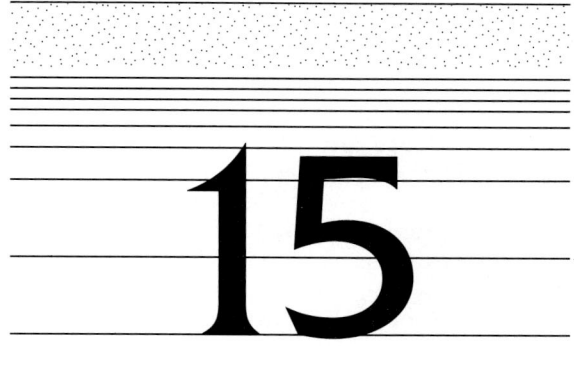

15

Bacterial Infections of the Liver and Biliary System

MARCIA IRENE F. CANTO, M.D.
ANNA MAE DIEHL, M.D.

PYOGENIC LIVER ABSCESS

Incidence

Pyogenic liver abscesses are relatively uncommon. In autopsy series, the prevalence of this condition is between 0.45 and 1.47%.[1] The incidence of liver abscesses was between 0.03 and 0.04% of hospital admissions in the early 1900s, with a female to male ratio of 2.5 to 1.0. These figures have not changed significantly since the early 1940s.[1,2]

By contrast, there has been a shift in the incidence of liver abscesses in different age groups. In the preantibiotic era, when liver abscesses were most commonly associated with pylephlebitis due to appendicitis, they occurred in patients between 10 and 40 years of age. Pyogenic abscesses are now most commonly diagnosed in patients, those in the fifth decade of life and beyond, who have associated cholangitis due to biliary obstruction. Obstruction can be due to choledocholithiasis, postsurgical strictures, and benign and malignant tumors of the biliary tree and pancreas.

Pathogenesis

Infection usually reaches the liver by contiguous spread from adjacent organs. Cholecystitis and cholangitis are the most frequently associated conditions. Liver abscesses can also arise from metastatic tumors within the liver as well as from infections extending from adjacent organs, such as in subphrenic collections, perforated peptic ulcers, pneumonia, and ascending pelvic infections.

Portal bacteremia and embolization can arise from assorted intra-abdominal diseases such as diverticulitis, peptic ulcer disease, appendicitis, pancreatitis, proctitis, and gastrointestinal (GI) tract malignancy.[1] However, liver abscesses only rarely complicate inflammatory bowel disease, despite frequent portal bacteremia. Portal bacteremia by itself is not uncommon or harmful. It may, however, lead to liver parenchymal infection when small areas of hepatic infarction related to intrahepatic thromboembolism or necrotic tumor provide a nidus for infection.[2] Hepatic arterial bacteremia due to sepsis from infections such as osteomyelitis, endocarditis, or distant purulent abscesses leads to liver abscesses less frequently than does portal venous seeding. Direct blunt trauma and penetrating liver injuries are also associated with liver abscesses. Other reported but rare risk factors are liver biopsy, congenital polycystic disease, and therapeutic hepatic artery ligation.[3, 4]

Host factors also play a role. Infants and children develop pyogenic abscesses due to umbilical infection or sepsis. Others can have associated immune defense abnormalities, such as leukemia and chronic granulomatous disease. There is also an increased incidence in diabetics and patients with metastatic cancer.[5] Five to forty-five percent of cases have no identifiable route or source of infection.[6] These are the so-called cryptogenic liver abscesses. If the biliary and GI tracts are carefully examined, the incidence of cryptogenic abscesses of the liver decreases to 10% (Table 15–1).[7]

Clinical Features

The clinical and laboratory features of pyogenic liver abscesses are variable and nonspecific. Patients most commonly present with fever, chills, weakness, sweats, and anorexia. Most patients have abdominal pain. This usually is located in the right upper quadrant but may occur in the left upper quadrant (as in left hepatic lobe lesions) or diffusely, when peritonitis occurs. Many patients have diarrhea and significant weight loss. Other patients may complain of cough, pleuritic chest pain, or right shoulder pain (Table 15–2).

Most patients have an enlarged liver. Right

TABLE 15–1. FREQUENCY OF DISEASES UNDERLYING PYOGENIC LIVER ABSCESS

CONDITION	FREQUENCY (%)
BILIARY	19–51
Ascending cholangitis	
Malignant obstruction	
Iatrogenic stricture	
Parasites	
CRYPTOGENIC	19–36
GASTROINTESTINAL (PORTAL)	14–26
Appendicitis	
Diverticulitis	
Colitis	
Perforated ulcer	
Chronic pancreatitis	
Crohn's disease	
HEMATOGENOUS	10–19
DIRECT EXTENSION	10–11

SOURCE: Data from reference nos. 4, 9, 11, 16, 18, 19.

TABLE 15–2. SYMPTOMS ASSOCIATED WITH LIVER ABSCESS

SYMPTOM	PATIENTS (%)
Fever	78–100
Anorexia	38–80
Abdominal pain	48–80
Weakness, malaise	30–96
Chills	38–88
Weight loss	25–68
Nausea, vomiting	28–53
Diarrhea	17–48
Cough	11–28
Jaundice	15–21
Pleuritic pain	9–24
Dyspnea	7
Abdominal mass	4
Hiccups	3

SOURCE: Adapted from: Brandborg LL, Goldman IS. Bacterial and miscellaneous infections of the liver. In: Zakim D, Boyer TD, eds. Hepatology 2nd ed. Philadelphia PA: WB Saunders; 1990:1087, Table 40–1.
Additional data from reference nos. 4, 11, 16, 17, 23, 24.

upper quadrant tenderness is found in about 40 to 70% of cases. Other signs, such as a palpable liver mass, splenomegaly, and chest findings (rales, friction rub, or dullness), occur in only 20% of patients or fewer. Jaundice is infrequent and may be due to underlying biliary obstruction or sepsis (Table 15–3). The majority of patients have elevated leukocyte counts and anemia. The serum alkaline phosphatase is high in most cases, although aminotransferases may be normal or mildly elevated. Prothrombin time is usually prolonged. Serum albumin may be normal or low. Bilirubinemia is variable (Table 15–4).

Diagnosis

Clinical Features

Patients may be symptomatic for varying lengths of time. Most are symptomatic for at

TABLE 15–3. SIGNS ASSOCIATED WITH PYOGENIC LIVER ABSCESS

SIGN	PATIENTS (%)
Hepatomegaly	51–92
Right upper quadrant tenderness	41–72
Jaundice	23–43
Chest signs	11–48
Splenomegaly	21–24
Abdominal mass	17–18

SOURCE: Adapted from: Brandborg LL, Goldman IS. Bacterial and miscellaneous infections of the liver. In: Zakim D, Boyer TD, eds. Hepatology 2nd ed. Philadelphia PA: WB Saunders; 1990:1087, Table 40–2.

TABLE 15–4. LABORATORY FINDINGS
ASSOCIATED WITH PYOGENIC LIVER ABSCESS

LABORATORY FINDING	PATIENTS (%)
Elevated alkaline phosphatase	84–100
Leukocytosis	73–96
Prolonged prothrombin time	71–87
Anemia	50–80
Decreased albumin	33–87
Elevated AST or ALT	48–60
Elevated bilirubin	28–73

SOURCE: Adapted from: Brandborg LL, Goldman IS. Bacterial and miscellaneous infections of the liver. In: Zakim D, Boyer TD, eds. Hepatology 2nd ed. Philadelphia PA: WB Saunders; 1990:1087, Table 40–3.

Additional data from reference nos. 4, 11, 16, 18, 24.

least 2 or more weeks before diagnosis. Delays in diagnosis may result from the nonspecific presenting symptoms and signs. Mistaken initial diagnoses have included pneumonia, cholangitis, pancreatitis, arterial occlusion, perforated viscus, tumor, and fever of unknown origin. Delay in diagnosis may also be due to previous antibiotic use.

Findings of routine blood cultures are often negative. Systemic bacteremia is documented by blood cultures in only one fourth to one half of cases. Thus, percutaneous aspiration should always be attempted for proper identification of causal organisms. Abscess cavity aspirates are more accurate than are blood cultures in identifying the bacteria involved, particularly since other organisms may be present in the abscess that may not be present in the blood.

Imaging Studies

A chest radiograph can frequently show abnormalities.[1, 4] An elevated right hemidiaphragm, atelectasis, and pleural effusion are associated findings. Rarely, there may be an air-fluid level present in the right upper quadrant. Ultrasound is highly recommended as the preferred initial diagnostic test because of its accuracy, sensitivity, and ability to identify associated abnormalities of the biliary tract. It can detect lesions as small as 1 cm. Even if accuracy is operator dependent, it is said to be as high as 97%.[8] In addition, ultrasound is helpful in distinguishing pyogenic from amebic abscesses. The latter are homogeneous, well circumscribed, and oval or round, whereas the former appear hypoechoic with irregular margins (Fig. 15–1).[9] Computed tomography (CT) is said to be more sensitive than ultrasound, but it is more expensive. It also helps identify other underlying intra-abdominal diseases.

Differential Diagnosis

Amebic abscesses may mimic pyogenic abscesses in clinical and radiographic presentation. Amebiasis should be excluded, particularly in areas with Hispanic or immigrant populations. This may be difficult, but differentiation is crucial because spillage and resulting peritonitis can occur in amebic liver abscesses after attempted drainage. Hydatid disease should be excluded by either an indirect hemagglutination or a complement fixation test for antibodies to *Echinococcus* (see Chapter 17). Findings from these tests may be positive in at least 80% of cases.[10]

Bacteriology

Blood cultures produce positive findings for bacteria in 33 to 64% of cases.[4, 5, 11] Multiple abscesses are more likely to be associated with positive findings on blood cultures than are solitary ones.[11]

The bacteriology of pyogenic liver abscesses has changed considerably over the years. In the past, as many as 50% of abscesses were sterile.[1] This was due to the inability to transport and culture specimens for anaerobic organisms properly. Currently, bacteria can be recovered in about 86 to 100% of aspirates.[11] With strict anaerobic techniques, about half of bacterial liver abscesses may be found to be due to anaerobic organisms, either alone or in combination with aerobic organisms.[11] Cultures from aspirates of liver abscesses are frequently polymicrobial.[11, 12] The isolated organisms vary, but anaerobic and facultative gram-negative enteric bacilli and microaerophilic streptococci are the most common (Table 15–5).

Pathology

Most series report about an equal frequency of solitary and multiple abscesses in the liver. The majority of abscesses originating from the biliary tract are multiple, whereas most abscesses related to portal system bacteremia are single and in the right lobe. Multiple abscesses occur in both lobes. Liver abscesses may be microscopic or macroscopic. Most microscopic abscesses are multiple and more difficult to diagnose.

Complications

Complications of pyogenic liver abscesses are due to local extension into surrounding tissues

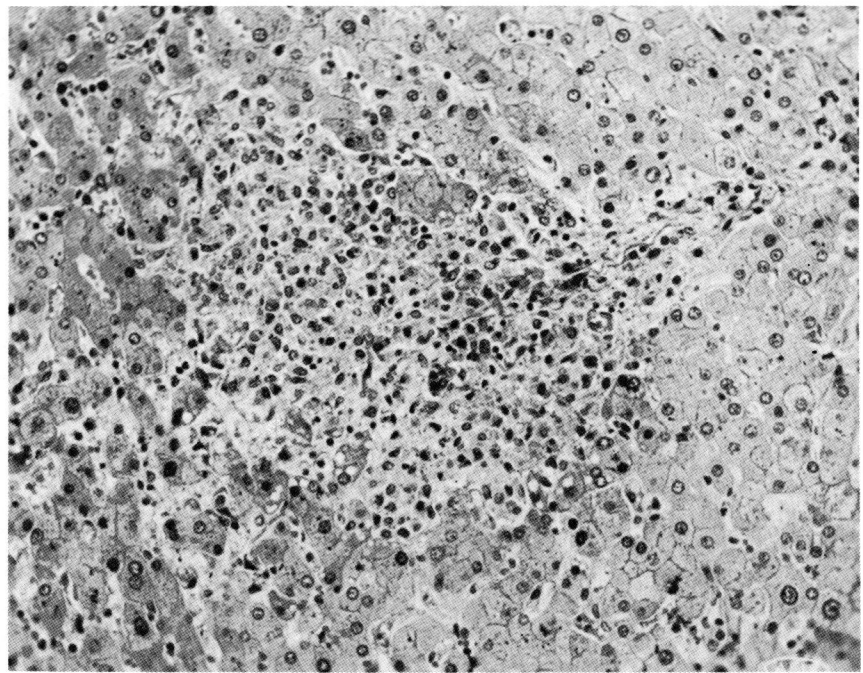

FIGURE 15–1.
Typhoid nodule. Section from a necropsy liver showing a focus of necrosis with "granulomatoid" appearance. (H & E, ×195) (Courtesy of Dr. Kamal G. Ishak, Armed Forces Institute of Pathology.)

or free rupture (Table 15–6). In a series of 73 patients with liver abscesses, rupture occurred in 15.1% of patients but did not result in any death.[13] Rupture of an abscess into the abdomen presents as acute abdominal pain and leads to peritonitis. Pleuropulmonary complications are the most common complications and are usually due to transdiaphragmatic extension or embolization. Subphrenic abscesses occur in about 2 to 5% of cases.

Rupture of rapidly enlarging liver abscesses through the diaphragm leads to empyema.

Slowly growing abscesses cause pleurisy, adhesions, and obliteration of the pleural space.[10] This, in turn, can result in direct rupture of pus into the lung and to abscess formation. Subsequently, these abscesses can involve the pericardial space, hepatic veins, or inferior vena cava. Liver abscesses can also, but more rarely, rupture into the abdominal wall or thoracic ducts.

Mortality

Death is almost certain with untreated pyogenic liver abscesses, and even with therapy, the mortality is high. In 1938, the overall mortality was 77%.[1] From the 1950s through the 1970s, despite the use of intravenous (IV) antibiotics and surgical drainage, the death rate was still 31% for solitary abscesses and 88% for multiple abscesses, with an overall mortality of 65%.[14]

Most reviews since the late 1980s have reported improved but significant death rates.[15–17] With advances in radiologic imaging tests and the development of potent antimicrobial agents, the mortality from pyogenic abscesses of the liver has decreased. Since the early 1970s, mortality figures have ranged between 11 and

TABLE 15–5. ORGANISMS ISOLATED FROM PYOGENIC LIVER ABSCESSES

AEROBIC	ANAEROBIC
Escherichia coli	Anaerobic streptococci
Klebsiella	Microaerophilic streptococci
Enterococcus	Bacteroides
Proteus	Fusobacterium
Citrobacter	Clostridium
Pseudomonas aeruginosa	Actinomyces
Serratia	
Enterobacter	
Staphylococcus aureus	
Streptococcus pneumoniae	
Listeria	
Yersinia	

SOURCE: Data from reference nos. 4, 11, 16, 24, 28.

TABLE 15–6. COMPLICATIONS IN PATIENTS WITH PYOGENIC LIVER ABSCESS

Rupture into abdomen, peritonitis
Rupture into pleural space
  Empyema
  Pleuritis, adhesions
Lung abscess
Rupture into abdominal wall, pericardium, thoracic duct,
  hepatic vein

SOURCE: Data from reference nos. 4, 18.

32%, which coincides with the increased use of CT scans to aid in diagnosis as well as therapy.

Factors Associated with Increased Mortality

Several factors are associated with increased mortality from pyogenic liver abscesses (Table 15–7).

LABORATORY TESTS

Pitt and Zuidema described 80 patients over a 20-year period and found that elevations of bilirubin and aspartate aminotransferase (AST) levels, hypoalbuminemia (<3 g/dl), and polymorphonuclear (PMN) leukocyte count of more than 80% were associated with a significantly increased death rate.[18]

Lee and colleagues from Taiwan analyzed 73 patients with pyogenic liver abscesses seen from 1978 to 1988.[17] They found that the overall mortality was 19%. A multivariate stepwise logistic regression analysis detected three factors that independently predicted increased mortality from a liver abscess. These were marked leukocytosis (>20,000/mm³), hypoalbuminemia (<2.5 g/dl), and the presence of pleural effusion. In fact, the risk of death was 9 times greater in patients with pleural effusions than in those without. This study emphasizes the association of liver abscess with pleural effusion and the importance of aggressive diagnostic imaging of the liver in febrile patients with right-sided pleural effusions of unknown origin. It also underscores the role of a chest radiograph as an essential initial study in the diagnosis of a liver abscess.

NUMBER OF ABSCESSES

Multiple abscesses carry a much worse prognosis than does a solitary liver abscess (mortality of 88% vs 31%).[18]

BACTERIOLOGY

Patients who have polymicrobial infections have a higher mortality rate (75%) than do those with infections from a single organism (54%). In one series, all 14 patients who had multiple organisms isolated from the blood died.[18] Furthermore, the type of bacterial infection (e.g., aerobic versus anaerobic) appeared to influence mortality. There was a significantly lower death rate in those patients with pure anaerobic or mixed aerobic and anaerobic infections compared with those with pure aerobic infections. However, patients with pure or mixed anaerobic infections were more likely to have a solitary liver abscess compared to those with pure aerobic infections (68% versus 37%, respectively). This might at least account for the lower mortality rate in the former group.

AGE

The influence of age on mortality is controversial. Some authors have reported higher mortality rates in patients older than 60 or 70 years.[18, 19] Others have reported no significant difference in mortality between different age groups.[17]

Treatment

Choice of Antibiotic

When a hepatic abscess is suspected, parenteral broad-spectrum antibiotics should be administered. Preferably these drugs are started after an imaging test confirms the diagnosis and material is obtained for culture and sensitivity studies. Antibiotics should be directed against both aerobic and anaerobic gram-negative and gram-positive organisms, usually those of enteric origin. Most infections are found to be polymicrobial when pus from the liver is cultured, even if blood cultures are positive for only one organism. The most commonly used antibiotics are a combination of an aminoglycoside, ampicillin

TABLE 15–7. FACTORS ASSOCIATED WITH INCREASED MORTALITY FROM PYOGENIC LIVER ABSCESSES

VARIABLE	MORTALITY RATE (%)
Polymicrobial	88
Multiple abscesses	43–75
Marked leukocytosis >20,000/mm³	38
Elevated ALT, AST	26–37
Jaundice	29–36
Pleural effusion	31
Hypoalbuminemia	22–37

KEY: ALT = alanine aminotransferase, AST = aspartate aminotransferase.
SOURCE: Data from reference nos. 9, 18.

TABLE 15–8. MORBIDITY AND MORTALITY OF SURGICAL- AND PCD-TREATED GROUPS

	PERCUTANEOUS DRAINAGE (%)	SURGICAL DRAINAGE (%)
Morbidity	69	48
Mortality	13	17

KEY: PCD = percutaneous catheter drainage.
SOURCE: Bertel CK, VanHeerden JA, Sheedy PF. Treatment of pyogenic hepatic abscess: Surgical vs. percutaneous drainage. Arch Surg. 1986; 121:554.

or penicillin, and metronidazole. The last named has the added benefit of treating amebiasis as well as anaerobic infection.

As soon as blood and abscess culture results are available, the antibiotic regimen should be modified according to their findings. Intravenous antibiotics are given until at least 48 hours after fever disappears and symptoms and leukocytosis abate. Most patients are treated with oral antibiotics for at least 2 to 4 weeks. In patients with renal failure, third-generation cephalosporins or imipenem can be used.

Surgery versus Percutaneous Drainage

Despite the use of appropriate therapy, the mortality from pyogenic hepatic abscesses is still high and ranges from 11 to 58%.[16–21] Treatment of liver abscesses has evolved over the years. Open drainage plus antibiotics has been regarded as the treatment of choice. During the operation, the infection can be localized and drained and the underlying intra-abdominal condition can be identified and possibly corrected. However, multiple liver abscesses can make surgical drainage technically problematic. Despite proper therapy, the mortality can be as high as 71%.[18]

Percutaneous drainage is now an accepted alternative to open drainage. This technique is not new. As early as 1898, Surgeon-Colonel W.F. Stevenson treated 150 patients with liver abscesses and advocated diagnostic aspiration before surgery. Therapeutic drainage was first successfully performed in combination with antibiotics in 1953, when 13 of 14 patients were cured.[22] It took at least 2 decades before it became widely accepted. With the advent of CT scanning and increased use of percutaneous drainage, many series have shown that antibiotic therapy alone or in combination with percutaneous drainage can treat most patients with liver abscesses. This is particularly true of solitary lesions, which can be localized accurately and adequately drained. Moreover, other authors have described equal success with multiple abscesses,[11] although most failures occur in this group.

In a retrospective review of 54 cases treated in Los Angeles, Stain and colleagues reported that 22 of 29 patients (79%) were cured with diagnostic percutaneous aspiration and antibiotics alone.[11] Nineteen of 23 patients (83%) recovered completely with therapeutic drainage. Four patients were treated successfully with antibiotics alone and without diagnostic aspiration. Only 1 patient died after failed aspiration, catheter, and surgical drainage. Bertel and colleagues at the Mayo Clinic studied 39 patients (treated between 1977 and 1984) and in 1986 reported the morbidity and mortality of patients treated surgically or with percutaneous drainage in addition to antibiotics (Table 15–8).[19] The rate of morbidity was high for both treatment groups. They recommended that surgery be reserved for patients who have failed percutaneous drainage or for those with concurrent disease requiring laparotomy. In 1991, Cheng and colleagues compared the results of 162 patients of similar age and sex distribution who were treated over a span of 8 years with medical treatment, percutaneous catheter drainage (PCD), or surgical drainage.[23] All three groups were similar in the proportion of underlying conditions such as diabetes, malignancy, cirrhosis, biliary tract disease, and peptic ulcer. The surgical group had a higher fraction of patients with gallstone disease compared with the medical and PCD groups (42% vs 24% and 19%, P = .033). The 57 patients in the medical treatment group received only antibiotics, with or without diagnostic needle aspiration. The 62 patients in the PCD group received antibiotics in addition to sonogram-guided drainage. The surgical group consisted of 43 patients operated on electively. Only 60% of the medically treated patients were cured, compared with 84% and 90% of patients in the surgical and PCD groups, respectively. There was a significant difference in success rate between patients treated with drainage (surgical or percutaneous) versus those treated only with antibiotics and diagnostic aspiration (Table 15–9).

Percutaneous drainage can spare the patient the morbidity of major abdominal surgery, the attendant perioperative risks, and intra-abdomi-

TABLE 15–9. RESULTS OF PERCUTANEOUS DRAINAGE

STUDY	METHOD	NO. PATIENTS	SUCCESS %
Bertel et al. (1986)[19]	Retrospective	39	81
Cheng et al. (1990)[23]	Retrospective	162	90
Stain et al. (1991)[11]	Retrospective	54	79–83

nal spread of infection. Rapid responses are common, with a mitigation of fever and leukocytosis. Perforation of other abdominal organs, pneumothorax, bleeding, and intraperitoneal leakage of pus are reported but unusual complications of transperitoneal drainage.

Among the reported complications of pyogenic liver abscesses is rupture of undrained abscesses treated only with antibiotics.[23] Patients can also develop septic emboli in various organs. Third-generation cephalosporins are useful in patients who develop endophthalmitis because of penetration of the blood-brain barrier.

Major bleeding diathesis and ascites have been cited as relative contraindications to percutaneous aspiration or drainage.[16] Because of excellent results and minimal complications, these procedures are now advocated for most patients with a single abscess. Open surgical drainage tends to be reserved for patients who have failed percutaneous aspiration or catheter drainage or who have other coexisting abdominal conditions requiring surgery.

Approach to Therapy

For patients who have a suspected pyogenic liver abscess with no coexistent intra-abdominal condition requiring emergency laparotomy the following are recommended:

1. Exclusion of amebiasis with an amebic hemagglutination test
2. Immediate ultrasound or CT scan to confirm the diagnosis
3. Concurrent diagnostic aspiration of abscess for Gram stain, culture, and sensitivity testing
4. Parenteral antibiotic therapy, initially broad-spectrum treatment (such as metronidazole, penicillin, and an aminoglycoside) to cover anaerobes and aerobes, with later modifications according to results of bacteriologic cultures
5. Repeat radiologic imaging and aspiration to obtain additional material for culture and sensitivity testing and to perform catheter drainage for persistent sepsis after 7 to 10 days of antibiotic therapy

6. Open surgical drainage for patients with coexistent intra-abdominal abnormality or failures of PCD

OTHER INFECTIONS INVOLVING THE LIVER

Yersinia enterocolitica

Yersinia enterocolitica infection in humans presents as ileocolitis in children and terminal ileitis and mesenteric adenitis in adults. Arthritis, cellulitis, erythema nodosum, and septicemia are reported complications.[24] Most patients have an underlying disease such as diabetes, cirrhosis, or hemochromatosis. Excess iron has been implicated as a factor predisposing to infection with this organism.

The septicemic form mimics malaria or typhoid fever. Abscesses in the liver and spleen characterize the localized subacute form of this disease. These abscesses were multiple and diffusely distributed in the liver of 16 of the 21 patients reported in the literature.

Treatment with antibiotics is problematic. Beta-lactamase production renders the organism resistant to ampicillin. Trimethoprim-sulfamethoxazole or an aminoglycoside or both appears to be the most effective treatment but penicillin and metronidazole have been used with varying success. The subacute form has a poor prognosis, and most cases have been diagnosed at autopsy. Overall mortality is 48%. One report described the successful treatment of 1 patient with CT-guided drainage and antibiotics.[25]

Listeria monocytogenes

The propensity of *Listeria monocytogenes* to invade the liver is well documented in animal and human neonatal infections.[24] There are a few reports in the literature of hepatic involvement in the course of adult infections with *L. monocytogenes*. One report described a solitary culture-negative liver abscess successfully treated with percutaneous drainage and penicillin.[26] Another report described 3 cases of disseminated listeriosis presenting as acute hepatitis.[27]

Almost all the cases had some underlying liver abnormality, such as cirrhosis, hemochromatosis, chronic active hepatitis, Felty's syndrome, or a hematologic malignancy. The degree of liver enzyme elevation may be moderate or severe, mimicking an acute viral hepatitis. Blood cultures have usually led to the correct diagnosis. Liver histopathology was remarkable for multiple abscesses or granulomatas.

Typhoid Fever

Salmonella typhi is a gram-negative bacillus that causes typhoid fever. Enteric fever is a systemic infection that involves the liver. Some patients may actually present with a viral hepatitis–like illness, including fever, hepatomegaly, and liver tenderness. Cholecystitis and liver abscess are well-known complications. Hepatomegaly is found in 13 to 65% of patients.[28] As many as 43% of patients develop splenomegaly.[29] Although a minority of patients (4–16%) are jaundiced, mildly elevated bilirubin levels are present in almost 25% of cases. The serum aminotransferase levels are abnormal in about 50% of cases.[29] Many patients with normal-sized livers have abnormal findings on liver function tests.

Liver involvement appears to be related to endotoxin. Although intact *Salmonella* organisms can be found in liver tissue, an endotoxin may be present that produces focal cell necrosis, mononuclear infiltration, and hyperplastic Kupffer cells with debris.[28] These changes are similar to those seen in sepsis. Histologic examination of the liver can show mononuclear cell infiltration, marked Kupffer cell hyperplasia, and focal necrosis.[28, 30] Typhoid nodules are characteristic of typhoid fever and may be seen distributed throughout the liver (see Fig. 15–1).[31] They are composed of marked hypertrophy and proliferation of Kupffer cells. Biochemical and clinical abnormalities resolve within 2 to 3 weeks after therapy. Chronic carrier states are due to persistence of infection in the gallbladder and liver.

Paratyphoid Fever

Salmonella paratyphi A and B are the most common causal organisms of paratyphoid fever. Elevated findings on liver function tests, with or without hepatomegaly, may be seen, as in typhoid fever. Elevation of AST is the most common abnormality (82%) of patients, with occa-sional slight serum alkaline phosphatase (39%) and bilirubin elevations (18%).[32] In epidemics of *Salmonella* infection, severe jaundice can be due to paratyphoid fever, suppurative cholangitis (SC), or co-infection with hepatitis virus.[28]

Shigella Hepatitis

Shigellosis is a common enteric infection. Jaundice that occurs in epidemics is most often due to concomitant hepatitis A virus infection. Hepatomegaly has been reported.[33] A few case reports describe a cholestatic hepatitis.[33, 34] Hepatic histopathologic findings include focal portal and periportal polymorphonuclear inflammation and necrosis, prominent cholestasis, and bile ductule involvement.

Melioidosis

Melioidosis is an infection endemic to Southeast Asia caused by *Pseudomonas pseudomallei*. The organism is found in soil and water. The incubation period may range from a few days to several weeks. Clinical disease may range from asymptomatic infection to a severe fulminant septicemia, with GI tract, lung, and liver involvement.[28] On histologic examination, focal hepatic necrosis, inflammatory infiltrates, and multiple small liver abscesses may be seen. Giemsa stains can demonstrate organisms on liver biopsy specimens.[35] In chronic disease, granulomatous inflammation may be seen in the liver.

Tularemia

Francisella tularensis is a gram-negative coccobacillus that causes tularemia. Although elevated levels of liver enzymes are fairly common, overt hepatitis is rare and liver injury is usually mild. In disseminated disease, however, jaundice, hepatomegaly, ascites, and peritonitis have been described.[28]

Gonococcal Infections

About 50% of patients with gonococcal bacteremia have abnormal findings on liver function tests.[28] Almost all these patients have ele-vated serum alkaline phosphatase levels, ar the AST level is abnormal in about 30 to 4C Jaundice occurs in fewer than 10% of patier

Curtis in 1930 first called attention to the "violin-string" adhesions between the liver and anterior abdominal wall as well as the association with gonococcal pelvic inflammatory disease. Fitz-Hugh described gonococcal perihepatitis and the name Fitz-Hugh–Curtis was given to the syndrome.[37] Perihepatitis is thought to occur through direct spread of infection from the pelvic organs, although there have been cases reported in men, which suggests that the liver is involved during bacteremia.[37]

The Fitz-Hugh–Curtis syndrome is the most common liver complication of gonococcal infection.[36, 37] Most patients are young women. They complain of the sudden onset of sharp right upper quadrant pain, which can be mistaken for acute cholecystitis, pleurisy, pyelonephritis, or cholelithiasis. Oral cholecystograms may demonstrate nonvisualization of the gallbladder, which has led to operations for cholecystectomy.[38] In retrospect, most patients have had a prior history of pelvic inflammatory disease. On examination, there may be liver tenderness or a friction rub. Diagnosis is readily made by vaginal swab cultures for gonococcus. Prognosis is not affected by liver involvement.

Bartonellosis

Bartonellosis is caused by *Bartonella bacilliformis,* a small, gram-negative coccobacillus. The disease is endemic to Colombia, Ecuador, and Peru. It usually presents as an acute febrile illness, with jaundice, hemolysis, hepatosplenomegaly, and lymphadenopathy.[28] Splenic infarction and centrilobular necrosis may also occur. As many as 40% of patients die from sepsis or acute hemolysis. Treatment with chloramphenicol or tetracycline is usually effective.

Clostridium perfringens

As many as 20% of patients with gas gangrene due to *Clostridium perfringens* may be jaundiced.[28] Most of the hyperbilirubinemia is due to hemolysis caused by the exotoxin released by the bacteria. Many cases are also associated with cholecystitis or biliary tract obstruction. The mortality from clostridial infections is high and unrelated to primary liver dysfunction.

Legionnaire's Disease

Legionnaire's disease is caused by a fastidious gram-negative bacterium called *Legionella pneu-*

mophila, Epidemiologic evidence indicates that this disease is acquired from environmental sources. Profound weakness, dry cough, malaise, anorexia, and watery diarrhea are common symptoms. Although pulmonary disease usually dominates the clinical presentation, abnormalities in the findings of liver function tests can occur. These consist of elevated serum aminotransferases (50%), total bilirubin (20%), and serum alkaline phosphatase (45%).[39] Jaundice is usually mild, and bilirubin is usually less than 5 mg/dl. Liver involvement is of no consequence in the outcome of this disease.

Histologic changes in the liver include microvesicular fat and focal necrosis. *Legionella pneumophila* has been seen on liver biopsies. The diagnosis is usually made by serologic testing (direct fluorescent antibody) or by testing postmortem tissue by Dieterle's staining or by both. Serologic evaluation is important only in retrospective confirmation of suspected cases because of the time required for seroconversion. The treatment of choice is the administration of erythromycin for at least 3 weeks.

Syphilis

The liver is involved in congenital syphilis, secondary syphilis, and late syphilis. There was a marked decrease in the incidence of early syphilis after World War II and the advent of effective antibiotic therapy. In the 1970s, numerous cases of syphilitic hepatitis were reported that mimicked viral hepatitis.

Secondary Syphilis

Hepatic involvement in secondary syphilis has been recognized for four hundred years, but it has been thought to be uncommon.[40, 41] In 1943, Hahn found only 80 patients with hepatomegaly in 33,825 cases of secondary syphilis.[41a] The incidence of syphilitic hepatitis may be as low as 1%,[28] but in a series of 175 patients with secondary syphilis, 10% of patients had "clinical, biochemical, and immunological" evidence of liver damage.[42] In another series, 9 of 18 patients with secondary syphilis had abnormal findings on liver function tests.[41]

The most common presenting symptoms of syphilitic hepatitis are anorexia, weight loss, malaise, fever, and a rash.[28, 42, 43] Jaundice, hepatomegaly, and hepatic tenderness are not consistently present. Many patients do not have a previous history of primary chancre. Concomitant rectal syphilis may produce diarrhea, bleeding, or pain on defecation. The clearest sign of secondary syphilis is the well-described rash that is often present when the liver is involved. It is a diffuse and symmetric and pink, dark red, or coppery macular rash, located on the ribs and trunk, that later spreads to the rest of the body. It develops into a generalized pruritic papular rash that characteristically affects the palms and soles. Almost all patients have generalized lymphadenopathy, including the epitrochlear nodes.[28] Biochemical abnormalities include slight to moderate elevations of AST, alanine aminotransferase (ALT), bilirubin, and lactate dehydrogenase as well as a disproportionate increase in serum alkaline phosphatase.[43] Sometimes, only the last named may be abnormal, and it remains so for several weeks after appropriate treatment.

Characteristic histologic abnormalities in syphilitic hepatitis include focal liver necrosis, particularly in the periportal areas and around the central vein. There are inflammatory cells composed of neutrophils, eosinophils, mast cells, plasma cells, and lymphocytes.[41–45] There may also be Kupffer cell hyperplasia and thickening of central vein branches. There is little or no damage to bile ductules and no bile stasis. Spirochetes have been seen with the use of silver stains in the livers of about half of patients with secondary syphilis.[44] They can be found in the inflammatory necrotic foci, in sinus endothelial cells, in the space of Disse, or in intrahepatic bile capillaries (Fig. 15–2).[42]

Late Syphilis

The hepatic lesions in tertiary syphilis are well described but have been uncommonly encountered since the advent of the antibiotic era. Most patients are asymptomatic. Some complain of abdominal pain, weight loss, anorexia, or fever. Others may have a large, nodular, tender liver similar to that seen in metastatic malignancy.[28] Ascites, jaundice, and portal hypertension have also been reported.[45] The classic lesion is the syphilitic gumma. Gummata are focal, single, or multiple lesions with central necrosis and surrounding granulation tissue. There may be plasma cells and lymphocytes, fibrosis, and endarteritis surrounding the gummata. Scarring is common upon healing.

Granulomatous Hepatitis

Mycobacteria

Tuberculosis (TB) is the second most common single cause of hepatic granulomatas and

accounts for 10 to 54% of cases in several series.[46] Tuberculosis is the most common infectious cause of granulomatous hepatitis (Table 15–10). The clinical presentation of hepatic granulomata may mimic other diseases that cause granulomatous hepatitis. Fever (82% of patients), weight loss (60%), abdominal pain (35%), and pulmonary symptoms (60%) are present along with liver enlargement (67%) and, less frequently, splenomegaly (19%), ascites (21%), lymphadenopathy (16%), and jaundice (10%).[47] About 50% patients are anemic and about 67% are hypoalbuminemic. Liver function tests frequently demonstrate abnormalities. An abnormal chest radiograph may be an important clue, since about 40% of patients show findings consistent with miliary TB. Table 15–11 presents a comparison of clinical findings in patients with hepatic granulomata.

Hepatic TB can be classified as follows: primary acute pulmonary TB with liver involvement, miliary TB, primary TB of the liver, tuberculoma (abscess), chronic pulmonary TB with liver involvement, and tuberculous cholangitis.[48]

Primary acute TB often affects the liver. Klatskin reported that as many as 64% of patients with primary TB had some liver involvement, which is often asymptomatic.[45] Primary macronodular hepatic TB with tubercles ranging from 1 to 3 cm and minimal involvement of other organs (e.g., spleen) is rare in the western world (Fig. 15–3).[49] Patients with chronic pulmonary TB may have hepatic granulomata in 0 to 79% of liver biopsy and 50 to 100% in autopsy specimens.[50] Miliary TB may affect the liver, with reported incidence rates of 25 to 97% in several series.[51] Because of this, some authors consider liver biopsy to be the most sensitive test to diagnose miliary TB (Tables 15–12 and 15–13). Tuberculous cholangitis is a rare infection of the biliary tree.

The tuberculoma is an aggregation of granulomata with caseation necrosis in which TB bacilli can be seen through specific stains. Some granulomata may be noncaseating. There may be a particularly dense cuff of lymphocytes surrounding the lesion.[52] The organisms are identified by visual examination in 0 to 35% of granulomatas. Tuberculosis is cultured in only 0 to 10% of cases.[51] The highest premortem diagnostic yield is from biopsy-obtained granulomata in patients with miliary TB, from whom 43 to 60% of cultures or smears are positive for the organism.[52, 53]

Brucellosis

Brucellosis is an infection found in individuals who work with pigs, cattle, goats, or sheep.

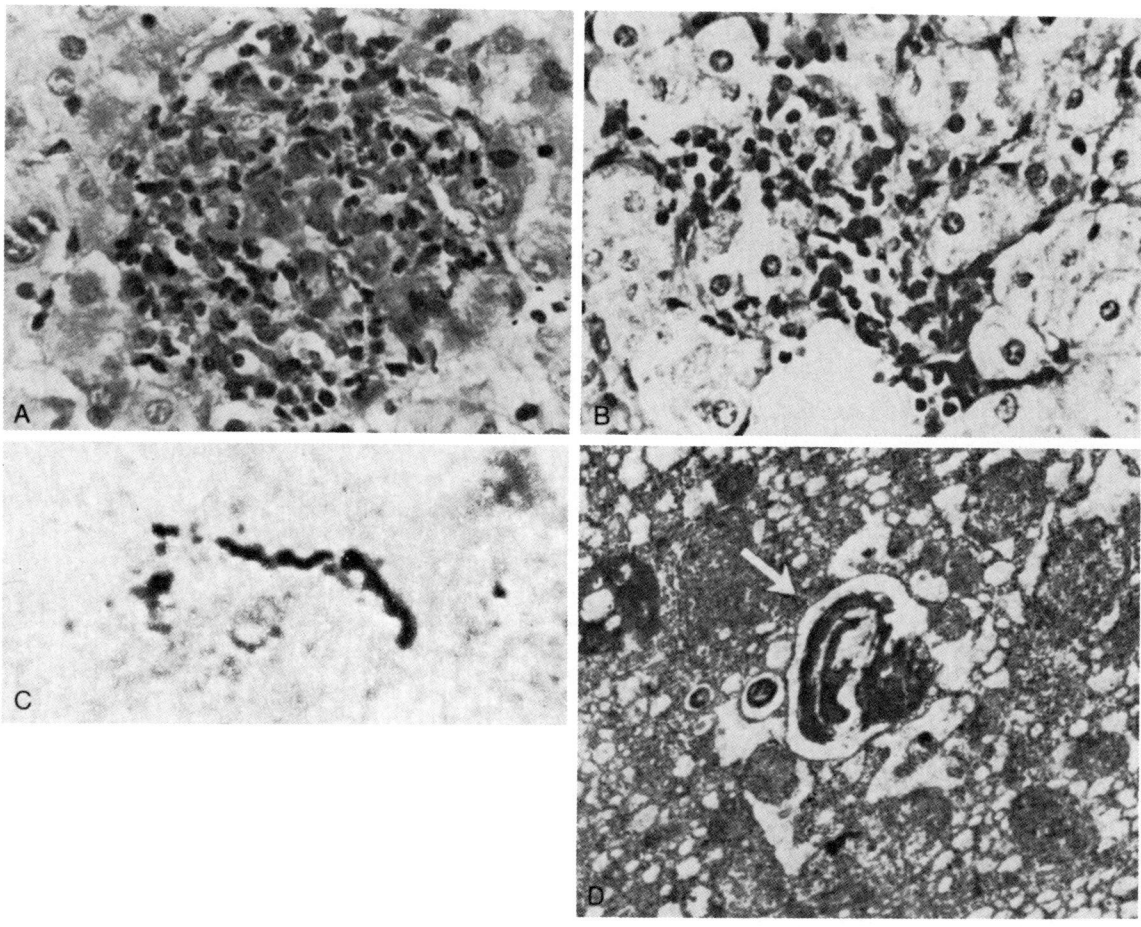

FIGURE 15–2.
Early syphilitic hepatitis. *A*, Light micrograph of liver tissue from patient with early syphilis showing focal inflammatory reaction. (H & E, reduced to ⅔ from ×400) *B*, Light micrograph of liver tissue from patient with early syphilis showing lymphocytic infiltration of region around central vein. (H & E, reduced to ⅔ from ×400) *C*, Light micrograph of liver tissue from patient with early syphilis showing treponeme (Warthin-Starry, ×1000) *D*, Electron micrograph of liver cell showing tubularization of endoplasmic reticulum and intracellular treponeme. (×9200) SOURCE: Feher J, Somogyi T, Timmer M, et al. Early syphilitic hepatitis. Lancet. 1978;2:896–899.

Hepatic noncaseating granulomata are the most frequent histologic findings. There may also be nonspecific focal accumulation of lymphocytes in the portal tracts or lobules.[45] Liver function tests often show abnormalities, and jaundice may be present in severe cases. Diagnosis is confirmed by isolation of the organism from liver tissue culture, although the yield is low. The history of animal exposure is of vital importance. Serologic testing using counterimmunoelectrophoresis or the rose bengal test is reliable.[53]

BACTERIAL INFECTION IN PATIENTS WITH LIVER DISEASE

Despite the use of broad-spectrum antibiotics, bacterial infection is responsible for as many as 25% of deaths in patients with liver disease. The most susceptible seem to be those with alcoholic cirrhosis, especially when complicated by GI tract bleeding. Rimola and colleagues reviewed 187 patients with alcoholic cirrhosis admitted to the hospital and found that bacterial infection was present in 46%.[54]

By contrast, patients with chronic active hepatitis or primary biliary cirrhosis (PBC) do not appear to be so susceptible to infection. This is also true of patients with acute viral hepatitis or drug-induced liver disease, unless complicated by fulminant or subacute hepatic failure.[55] Death results directly from infection or from precipitation of encephalopathy, bleeding, or renal failure. Diagnosis may be difficult in the absence of fever, chills, leukocytosis, or hypotension. Deterioration of mental status or renal

TABLE 15–10. INFECTIOUS CAUSES OF HEPATIC GRANULOMAS

BACTERIAL INFECTIONS	PARASITIC INFECTIONS
Mycobacterial diseases	Schistosomiasis
Tuberculosis	Visceral larva migrans
Atypical mycobacteriosis	Fascioliasis
BCG immunization	Capillariasis
Leprosy	Strongyloidiasis
Brucellosis	Ascariasis
Tularemia	Ancylostomiasis
Granuloma inguinale	Amebiasis
Melioidosis	Toxoplasmosis
Listeriosis	Malaria
Nocardiosis	Tongue-worm
Actinomycosis	**VIRAL INFECTIONS**
Typhoid fever	Cytomegalovirus
Paratyphoid B	Infectious mononucleosis
FUNGAL INFECTIONS	Acute viral hepatitis
Histoplasmosis	Influenza B
Cryptococcosis	**OTHER INFECTIONS**
Coccidioidomycosis	Q-fever
Blastomycosis	Mediterranean fever (Olmer's disease)
Candidiasis	Syphilis
Torulopsosis	Lymphogranuloma venereum
Aspergillosis	Psittacosis
	Whipple's disease (?)

KEY: BCG = bacille Calmette-Guérin.
SOURCE: Harrington PT, Gutierrez JJ, Ramirez-Ronda CH, et al. Granulomatous hepatitis. Rev Infect Dis. 1982;4:638–655.

dysfunction may be the only sign. Infections are usually due to gram-negative enteric organisms (particularly *Escherichia coli*) and to pneumococci. Infection with anaerobes is unusual.

Types of Infection

Bacteremia

Urinary tract infection, bacteremia, and pneumonia are the most common types of infection, aside from spontaneous bacterial peritonitis. Bacteremia is present in 7 to 20% of patients admitted to the hospital with cirrhosis. It is present in as many as 36% of patients in coma from fulminant hepatic failure, irrespective of the cause.[55] The likelihood of bacteremia increases after the second day of coma. Typically, infection may precipitate the initial encephalopathy or be present as a recurrence of coma during the recovery phase. The mortality for bacteremia in decompensated alcoholic cirrhotics is about 70% compared with that of patients with compensated liver disease.

Although urinary tract or respiratory tract in-

TABLE 15–11. CLINICAL FINDINGS IN PATIENTS WITH HEPATIC GRANULOMATA

GROUP OR FINDING	TUBERCULOSIS (%)	SARCOIDOSIS (%)	FUNGAL INFECTIONS (%)	OTHER DISEASES (%)*	UNDETERMINED ETIOLOGY (%)	TOTAL (%)
Male	54	32	78	69	49	52.4
Female	46	68	22	31	51	47.6
Fever	87	47	89	44	68	69.4
Fever of unknown origin	62	21	78	31	36	44.4
Hepatomegaly	49	58	56	63	44	50.8
Splenomegaly	26	42	22	31	24	28.2
Hyperbilirubinemia	37	18	0	47	21	26
Increased alkaline phosphatase	52	47	25	57	51	48.9
Increased aminotransferase	47	50	25	57	51	48.9
Increased gammaglobulins	68	83	86	86	74	76.5
Abnormal cholesterol	33	0	17	45	23	26.7
Increased BSP retention	73	80	56	90	60	68.1
Total no. of patients	39	19	9	16	41	124

*Lymphoma, 6 cases; cirrhosis, 4; postnecrotic cirrhosis, 3; Wegener's granulomatosis, 1; brucellosis, 1; and leprosy, 1.
KEY: BSP = bromosulfophthalein.
SOURCE: Gilinsky NH, Campbell JAH, Kirsch RE. The clinical spectrum of hepatic granuloma. S Afr Med J. 1981;60:691–694.

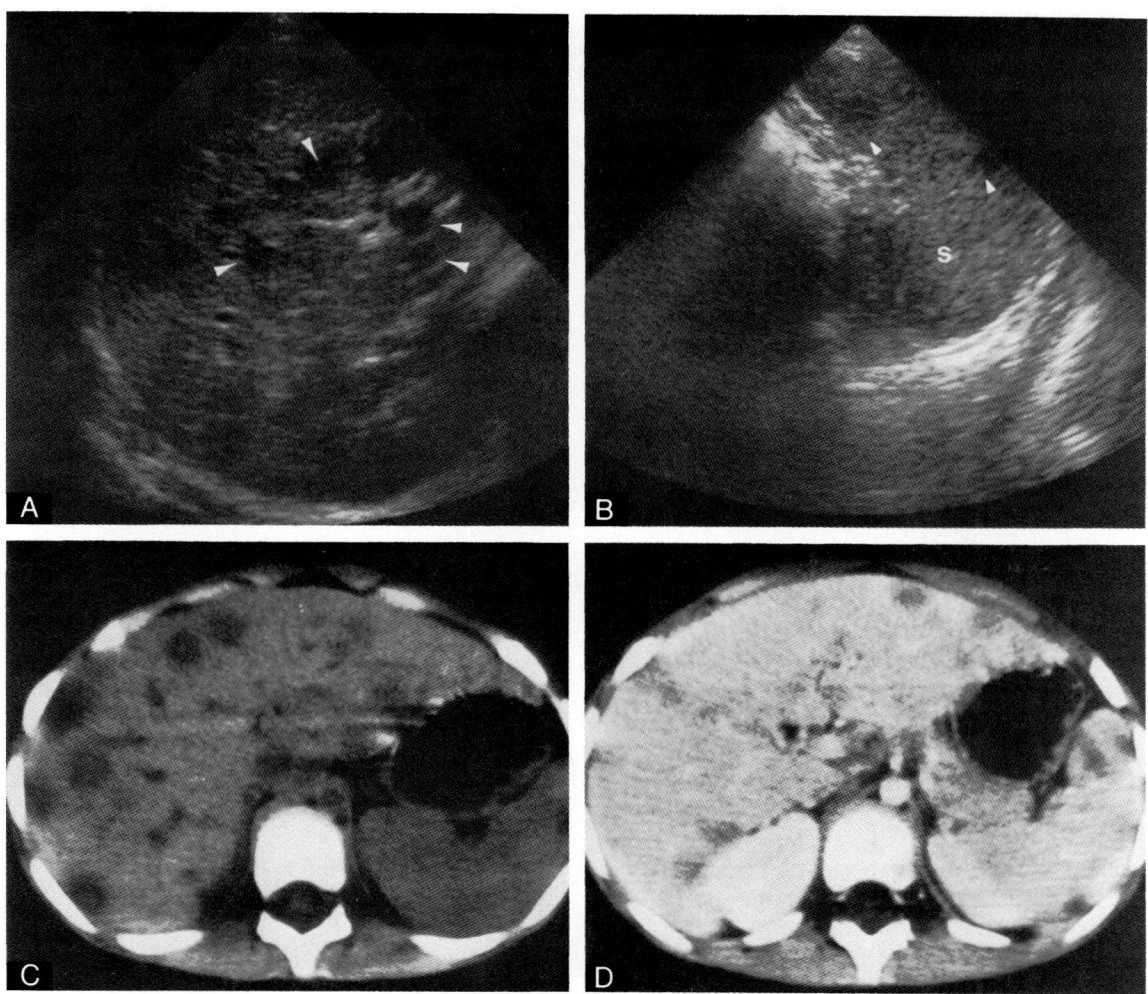

FIGURE 15–3.
Macronodular hepatic tuberculosis. Ultrasound of the abdomen shows multiple, rounded, hypo- and anechoic areas scattered diffusely throughout the liver (*A*) and spleen (*B*). *C*, Precontrast computed tomography (CT) scan of the upper abdomen shows multiple, rounded hypodense lesions scattered throughout the liver parenchyma. *D*, Contrast-enhanced CT scan of the midabdomen shows some rim enhancement of the nodules within the liver and spleen. SOURCE: Levine C. Primary macronodular hepatic tuberculosis: US and CT appearances. Gastrointest Radiol. 1990;15:307–309.

TABLE 15–12. DIAGNOSTIC PROCEDURES YIELDING HEPATIC GRANULOMATA

PROCEDURE	NO. OF PATIENTS
Needle biopsy of the liver	94
Peritoneoscopy	6
Laparotomy	
Diagnostic	4
Staging	6
Nonhepatic reason	6
Total	116

SOURCE: Gilinsky NH, Campbell JAH, Kirsch RE. The clinical spectrum of hepatic granuloma. S Afr Med J. 1981;60:691–694.

fections are responsible for half of the cases of bacteremia, the source of infection is found less often in patients with decompensated liver disease.[55] The frequent isolation of enteric organisms suggests that the GI tract is an important source of infection. Furthermore, bacteremia and endotoxemia are reduced in cirrhotic patients who are treated with gut sterilization.[54]

Pneumonia

Death caused by pneumonia is more common in alcoholics than in age- and sex-matched con-

TABLE 15–13. DIAGNOSTIC YIELD OF BIOPSY OF LIVER GRANULOMATA IN 116 PATIENTS

DIAGNOSIS	NO. OF CASES
Tuberculosis	
Organism	7
Caseation	10
Culture	2
Leprosy	1
Schistosomiasis	1
Parasite	1
Drugs	3
Hepatobiliary disease	3
Amyloidosis	1
Carcinoma	1
Polyarteritis nodosa	1
Total	31 (27%)

SOURCE: Gilinsky NH, Campbell JAH, Kirsch RE. The clinical spectrum of hepatic granuloma. S Afr Med J. 1981;60:691–694.

trols.[55] Pneumonia is also more common in these patients because of their recumbency from ascites and bleeding from esophageal varices, especially if managed by Sengstaken-Blakemore tubes or sclerotherapy. Furthermore, female alcoholics and patients with hepatomegaly have a higher mortality rate.[56] Complications of infections are also more common in alcoholics. There is increased fever and consolidation and increased incidence of abscesses, empyema, and atelectasis. Pneumonia in alcoholic cirrhotics is associated with a death rate of about 30%.[56] This contrasts with the 5% mortality rate from pneumonia in patients with PBC.

Certain organisms cause pneumonia more frequently in alcoholic patients. Approximately half of all patients with primary *Klebsiella* pneumonia, and of adult patients with *Haemophilus influenzae* or pneumonia from gram-negative or pneumococcal bacteremia are alcoholics.[57]

Urinary Tract Infections

Urinary tract infections occur in as many as 40% of cirrhotic patients who are hospitalized, regardless of the cause. They occur in 50% of all patients with decompensated cirrhosis. Bacteriuria occurs more than twice as often in women with PBC (19%) compared with those with other types of chronic liver disease (7%) or age-matched controls.[58] Although 50% of the episodes are asymptomatic, 50% of the patients develop recurrent attacks during a 2-year follow-up. However, only a small fraction of patients with PBC develop acute pyelonephritis. The most common organism is *E. coli*, which is responsible for 70% of episodes. The reason for the increased susceptibility to bacteriuria is not understood but appears not to be related to structural abnormalities of the urinary tract or to the degree of cholestasis.

Bacterial Endocarditis

Bacterial endocarditis is rare in patients with liver disease but affects mainly alcoholic cirrhotics. In fact, pneumococcal endocarditis occurs almost exclusively in patients who are either alcoholic or cirrhotic.[59] It may accompany pneumococcal pneumonia or meningitis.

Meningitis

Bacterial meningitis is also rare in patients with chronic liver disease.[55] Alcoholism, however, was present in 25% of patients with pneumococcal meningitis, 19% of patients with *Listeria* meningitis, and 6% of those with meningococcal meningitis.[55] The diagnosis can be easily overlooked, especially in alcoholics who are confused or encephalopathic or who have head injuries.

Pathobiology of Bacterial Infection

Predisposing Conditions

Certain events appear to predispose patients with liver disease to the development of bacterial infection. The most common is GI tract hemorrhage, especially from esophageal varices. A major source of infection is the bowel, and gut sterilization has been shown to decrease the incidence of infections after GI hemorrhage.[54]

DEFECTS OF HOST DEFENSES

The high incidence of infections with encapsulated organisms in patients with liver disease suggests defects in humoral responses and polymorphonuclear function. In hepatic failure, the severe complement deficiency causes impairment of opsonization. This can be improved by transfusion of fresh frozen plasma and humoral responses return to normal within a week of recovery from coma.[60, 61] Furthermore, neutrophils of most patients with fulminant hepatic failure and of 60% of patients with alcoholic liver disease have defective chemoattractant activity and adherence.

Patients with decompensated alcoholic cirrhosis have impaired Kupffer cell phagocytosis.[55] This has been associated with a poor prognosis and an increased susceptibility to infection. Plasma fibronectin, which is an opsonin for Kupffer cells, is frequently reduced in patients with liver disease. Furthermore, monocytes have been shown to exhibit abnormal chemotactic function. By contrast, patients with chronic liver disease (especially those with PBC), do not usually have problems with opsonization.

EFFECT OF ALCOHOL ON HOST DEFENSES

Animal studies have shown that alcohol intoxication causes impaired glottic closure, macrophage migration and white blood cell mobilization, phagocytosis, and bacterial killing.[62] Humans given alcohol into the bloodstream showed reversible depression of serum bactericidal activity from certain bacteria, and this may have been due to abnormal complement synthesis. Acute alcohol abuse also has a direct toxic effect on bone marrow and can depress the white blood cell count.[55]

Hepatic Dysfunction during Infection

Jaundice

Extrahepatic and systemic infections can often lead to jaundice and other biochemical changes suggestive of a primary hepatic or biliary tract disease. Hepatic dysfunction during systemic infection can result in errors in diagnosis and treatment that could be serious if a systemic bacterial infection were the cause of icterus. In infants, gram-negative sepsis is a well-recognized cause of cholestatic jaundice.[28] In adults, this syndrome is less common and is usually mild, unless it occurs in the setting of pregnancy or severe sepsis.

In neonates, blood tests during gram-negative infection demonstrate a predominantly conjugated form of hyperbilirubinemia, minimal to moderately elevated aminotransferases, and widely varying change in alkaline phosphatase level.[31] In adults, there is a wider range of associated changes in findings on liver function tests in the setting of infection. Jaundice in an adult due to bacterial sepsis is well described. It has been associated with several organisms (Table 15–14), including aerobic and anaerobic gram-negative and gram-positive organisms. It has occurred with different sources of infection, although in many cases bacteremia was suspected but not proved.

Pirovino and colleagues described 5 adult patients with jaundice from severe extrahepatic infection who were studied prospectively with liver function tests.[63] Intraperitoneal infection was found to be a major risk factor for the develop-

ment of jaundice. Pneumonia is one infection well known to be associated with clinical jaundice. It was first described in 1836 by Garvin.[64] Since then, numerous authors have described this entity. Many reports list *Streptococcus pneumoniae* as the infecting organism (reported incidence is between 3.0 and 67.7%). *Klebsiella pneumoniae* and other forms of bacterial pneumonia may also present with jaundice.[65]

For reasons unknown, jaundice complicates pneumonia, particularly in black male patients.[31] The male to female ratio of patients who develop jaundice with pneumococcal pneumonia is 10 to 1. Although malnutrition and hemolysis due to glucose-6-phosphate dehydrogenase (G6PD) deficiency were listed as contributory factors, other researchers have disputed these theories. Bacteremic jaundice is frequently cholestatic in nature and appears early in the course of bacteremia, usually within a few days. Hepatomegaly occurs in about 50% of patients. The serum bilirubin is usually between 5 and 10 mg/dl but may be as high as 30 to 50 mg/dl.[31] Most (75–80%) of the bilirubin is conjugated. The serum aminotransferases are normal or mildly elevated. Albumin levels may be low but are similar to levels in nonjaundiced patients with sepsis. The prothrombin time is normal or correctable with vitamin K therapy. Serum alkaline phosphatase is elevated in almost half of patients, but usually only 2 to 3 times normal (Fig. 15–4). Marked elevation in serum alkaline phosphatase activity compared with bilirubin may also be a manifestation of systemic infection.[66] This may mimic extrahepatic biliary obstruction. There are reports of disproportionate increases of liver alkaline phosphatase levels in infections from shigellosis,[33] legionnaire's disease,[39] and in anaerobic bacteria.[66]

The diagnosis of bacteremic jaundice should be strongly considered in a patient who becomes acutely jaundiced and febrile but whose serum enzymes are normal or near normal. The major differential diagnosis is cholangitis or liver abscess, but there may be other causes of jaundice in the same patient. These include multiple blood transfusions, shock or anoxia, and use of hepatotoxic drugs. Neale and colleagues reported that jaundice due to intrahepatic infection can be differentiated from that due to extrahepatic infection by serum B$_{12}$ levels.[67] In all 6 patients with bacteremic jaundice they studied, the serum B$_{12}$ levels were normal. This contrasted with 4 patients with either liver abscess or cholangitis who had elevated levels. The distinction between a hepatic and a sys-

TABLE 15–14. NONHEPATIC BACTERIAL INFECTIONS THAT CAN LEAD TO JAUNDICE

REFERENCE*	CASES M/F	CASES AGE	BILIRUBIN TOT/DIR (mg/dl)	LIVER HISTOLOGY	AGENT OF INFECTION	DEATHS
Bernstein & Brown (1962)	8/1	2 wk–2 mo	12–22/5–8†	Bile stasis Mild toxic changes	*Escherichia coli* (6) Paracolon (2) *Pseudomonas aeruginosa* (1)	9
Hamilton & Sass-Kortsak (1963)	13/11	1d–3 mo	3–31/1–15†	Bile stasis No necrosis	*E. coli* (11) *Aerobacter* (4)	11
Fahrlander et al. (1964)	5/3	44–80 yr	3–16	Intrahepatic cholestasis Electron microscopy bile canalicular dilation with loss of microvilli	*E. coli* (3) *P. aeruginosa*	1
Eley et al. (1965)	2/3	35–54	3–23/3–15†	Intrahepatic cholestasis	*E. coli* *Proteus* *Bacteroides*	1
Danks et al. (1965)	16/9	1 wk–4 wk	10–30		*E. coli* (13) Enterobacteriaceae (11) *Staphylococcus aureus*	2
Kenny et al. (1966)	11/0	2 wk–8 wk	2–39/2–38†	Intrahepatic cholestasis	*E. coli* (11)	4
Arthur & Wilson (1967)	2/2	3 wk–8 wk 12 yr	3–6		*E. coli* (3)	0
Miller & Irvine (1969)	9	Adults	1.5–2.5†		*E. coli* (8)	0
Seeler & Hahn (1969)	10/1	1 wk–8 wk	6–48/2–24†		*E. coli* Paracolon *Aerobacter*	0
Vermillon et al. (1969)	4/3	18 yr–72 yr	5–24/4–16†	Intrahepatic cholestasis Mild focal cell necrosis Kupffer cell hyperplasia	*E. coli* (3) *P. aeruginosa* (2) Anaerobic streptococcus	6
Rooney et al. (1971)	22	1 wk–3 wk	6–50/1–37†		*E. coli* (13) *Proteus* Paracolon	0
Ng & Rawstron (1971)	6/0	2 wk–8 wk	7–30/5–20†		*E. coli* (5) Paracolon	0
Borges et al. (1972)	8/5	2 mo–10 mo	3–30/2–14†	Intrahepatic cholestasis Kupffer cell hyperplasia	*E. coli* *Proteus*	0
Miller et al. (1976)	15/15	15 yr–27 yr	2–20† mean 8.7 (mean 6.8)	Intrahepatic cholestasis Kupffer cell hyperplasia	*E. coli* *P. aeruginosa* *S. aureus* Paracolon *Klebsiella*	13

*References cited by source publication.
†Range.
SOURCE: Zimmerman HJ, Fang M, Utili R, et al. Jaundice due to bacterial infection. Gastroenterology. 1979;77:362–374.

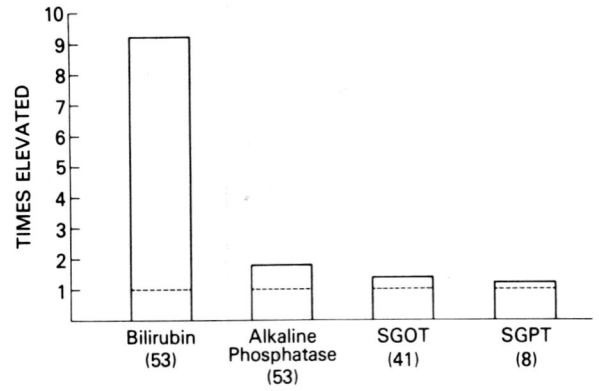

FIGURE 15–4.
Mean height of serum bilirubin, alkaline phosphatase, serum glutamic-oxaloacetic transaminase (SGOT, now AST), and serum glutamic pyruvate transaminase (SGPT, now ALT) in 53 cases of jaundice associated with sepsis from six reports. SOURCE: Jaundice due to bacterial infection (clinical conference). Gastroenterology. 1979;77(2):362–374.

temic infection is arbitrary unless the chief threat is to the liver, and the systemic manifestations are only of secondary importance.

POSTULATED MECHANISMS FOR JAUNDICE DURING INFECTION

Most investigators currently think that the jaundice that occurs with pneumonia is mainly hepatocellular and cholestatic. This correlates well with findings on liver biopsy that show cloudy hepatocyte swelling, patchy necrosis, hepatocellular bile deposits, and dilated bile canaliculi.

Endotoxin. The mechanism of liver involvement in sepsis and nonhepatic bacterial infections may be related to functional or structural changes caused by circulating toxins or to invasion of the liver by bacterial organisms. Similarities in manifestations during different gram-negative infections and the presence of a cholestatic syndrome despite the absence of actual biliary obstruction suggest a role for circulating endotoxin.

Endotoxin is a complex lipopolysaccharide from the outer membrane of the bacterial cell wall. The lipid moiety, called lipid A, has a similar biochemical structure among gram-negative bacteria of the Enterobacteriaceae and is responsible for the toxicity of the lipopolysaccharide.[68] In experimental animals, endotoxin from E. coli[69] and Salmonella enteritidis[70] causes dose-dependent decreases in bile flow and excretion of organic anions. Specifically, the bile salt–independent fraction of bile is affected by both endotoxins through the inhibition of Na^+ and K^+-ATPase activity.[31] This may partly account for the cholestatic effect of the lipopolysaccharide. It is amplified in neonates who have a lower synthetic rate for, and circulating pool of, bile salts, and thus, selective inhibition of the bile salt–independent fraction would aggravate the already low bile salt–dependent bile flow.

Decreased Hepatic Perfusion. Because some of the histologic changes seen in the liver after trauma or sepsis are similar to those seen after hepatic ischemia, a decrease in nutrient blood flow to the liver may cause hepatocyte dysfunction.[71] However, both human and animal studies show that during the early hyperdynamic phase of sepsis, hepatic blood flow and oxygen consumption are increased.[72] It is therefore not clear if changes in hepatic nutrient supply are the cause of liver dysfunction or if they are important only during the terminal stages of septic shock.

Liver Injury. By contrast, certain bacterial infections such as typhoid fever have been shown not only to cause jaundice but also to induce liver injury. Typhoid hepatitis is characterized by hyperbilirubinemia (usually below 10 mg/dl) and a moderate elevation of serum alkaline phosphatase and aminotransferases.[31] The latter are usually elevated less than 5 times normal but may be markedly abnormal. In contrast to patients with E. coli–related cholestasis who have almost normal hepatic parenchyma, the liver histologic findings of patients with typhoid fever shows focal cell necrosis with mononuclear cell infiltration and marked Kupffer cell hyperplasia with mild cholestasis. These changes completely resolve on follow-up liver biopsies after therapy. When Salmonella endotoxin was injected into rabbits, the liver showed similar changes.[73] However, because bacteremia is well documented in typhoid fever, the role of blood-borne bacteria in producing hepatocellular injury cannot be disregarded. Direct invasion of hepatic parenchyma by bacteria is unlikely to be responsible for liver abnormalities because bacteria are rarely isolated from the liver, even in the presence of specific lesions such as granulomata.

Another mechanism for hepatic injury during infection was suggested by Holman and Saba.[74] They studied the idea that the vascular entrance of both bacterial and nonbacterial particulate material could lead to hepatic parenchymal cell injury, due either to postphagocytic Kupffer cell activity or to the margination of activated leukocytes in the liver. They injected denatured, collagen-coated particles as well as heat-killed Pseudomonas aeruginosa bacteria to serve as particulate challenges. They then measured plasma AST and ornithine carbamoyltransferase enzyme levels for 3 to 72 hours. The AST and ornithine carbamoyltransferase levels were elevated 350 to 400% after injection of the nonbacterial particles and the IV injection of the heat-killed Pseudomonas after either laparotomy plus cecal ligation (for mild sepsis) or laparotomy. Furthermore, the authors found that activated PMNs (exposed to dead bacteria) but not Kupffer cells induced a significant (P <0.05) release of ornithine carbamoyltransferase from cultured liver parenchymal cells. They concluded that the transient hepatic parenchymal cell injury with postoperative sepsis may be mediated by the margination of activated PMNs in the liver.

The mechanism for the disproportionate increase in serum alkaline phosphatase in some patients with mild jaundice is unknown. One postulated theory is a blockage of reticuloendothelial system function by circulating bacteria or products of metabolism, causing prolonged half-life of endogenous alkaline phosphatase.

Hemolysis. Hemolysis may contribute to the jaundice in patients with infection. *Clostridium* exotoxin induces hemolysis. Shurin and colleagues studied the capsular polysaccharide of *H. influenzae* type B, polyribosyl ribitol phosphate (PRP), which is released from growing organisms during human infection and can be found in body fluids.[75] It binds to untreated erythrocytes and appears to induce intravascular, complement-mediated hemolysis as well as extravascular hemolysis. Patients with invasive infection therefore develop hemolysis when circulating PRP and antibody to PRP are present simultaneously. The hemolytic anemia that occurs during human infection with *H. influenzae* type B may be due to binding of PRP to red blood cells and immune destruction of sensitized erythrocytes.

LIVER HISTOLOGY

Microscopic sections of the liver in patients with jaundice associated with sepsis show prominent intrahepatic cholestasis, with little or no focal hepatic necrosis. Less frequently, there may also be a slight increase in portal lymphocytes, Kupffer cell hyperplasia, and mild fatty vacuolization. Electron microscopic examination of liver biopsies also shows marked dilatation of bile canaliculi, flattened and reduced microvilli, and abnormal mitochondria.

Caruana and colleagues examined the histopathologic findings of the liver of 19 patients who died of clinical sepsis, and they attempted to relate certain features of the illness or treatment to the observed histopathologic changes.[76] The most striking finding was midzonal and peripheral necrosis of a moderate to marked degree in 11 of the 19 patients. Other important changes were acute inflammation and cholestasis. The severity of hepatocellular necrosis did not appear to be influenced by the circulating pathogen, the nutritional support administered, or the arterial blood pressure. They suggested that hepatocellular necrosis is characteristic of sepsis and may be caused by loss of specific factors that normally maintain liver function and structure.

CLINICAL OUTCOME

Is jaundice a marker of poorer prognosis in patients with severe bacterial infection? Published series report a mortality rate as high as 90%.[77] However, the hepatic injury appears to contribute little to the morbidity or mortality due to the infection and requires no therapy. Jaundiced patients with infections die from their underlying diseases and not from liver failure. The mortality also does not correlate with level or duration of hyperbilirubinemia. However, an improved mortality rate of about 10% has been reported in patients who are not jaundiced but have minor abnormalities of alkaline phosphatase, AST, or ALT.

Hepatocyte Dysfunction During Sepsis

A number of metabolic abnormalities occur during sepsis. These are hypermetabolism, increased gluconeogenesis, accelerated ureagenesis, and increased urinary nitrogen excretion. Glucose intolerance is common with hyperglucagonemia and elevated cortisol, growth hormone, and catecholamine levels inducing gluconeogenesis. The major metabolic change during sepsis is increased protein catabolism.[78] During sepsis, amino acids are released from muscle 3 to 5 times faster than during fasting state to support gluconeogenesis. There is accelerated amino acid uptake by the liver. Some skeletal muscle amino acid release and liver uptake support acute phase protein synthesis.[79] These proteins are linked to the host's response to inflammation. At the same time, there is a depression of liver synthesis of less important carrier proteins such as albumin and transferrin.[78, 79] As such, the liver is central to the host's response to infection.

In addition to hormonal stimulation, control of protein metabolism may be related to macrophage-derived interleukin-1 and its cleaveage product proteolysis inducing factor. These induce muscle proteolysis by activating muscle prostaglandin production and lysosome proteases in muscle cells.[80, 81]

BACTERIAL INFECTIONS OF THE BILIARY SYSTEM

Acute Cholecystitis

Acute cholecystitis is defined as acute inflammation of the gallbladder. It is a clinical entity that complicates about 10 to 20% of symptomatic gallstones. Since more than 20 million Americans harbor gallstones, it is a significant cause of morbidity and an inestimable economic loss related to health care costs, disability, and loss of productivity. The overall mortality rate from acute cholecystitis is 5%. This figure increases in diabetics and elderly patients to about 6.5 to 7.9% and 10%, respectively.[82-84]

Pathogenesis

Although acute cholecystitis is a common disease, the cause is not clear-cut. It can result from ischemia or bacterial infection. More than 90% of cases are related to cholelithiasis and cystic duct occlusion. Obstruction may be due to actual stone impaction or inflammation and edema in the duct. Not all cases of cystic duct obstruction progress to the acute clinical syndrome. Experimental ligation of the cystic duct does not itself produce cholecystitis.[85] Similarly, acute cholecystitis can develop even in the absence of gallstones or apparent cystic duct obstruction. This entity, called acute acalculous cholecystitis, is uncommon and occurs in about 5 to 15% of patients.[86] Symptoms may not correlate with the severity of gallbladder pathologic findings, especially in elderly and diabetic patients. They may develop gangrene and perforation with few symptoms.

Pellegrini and Way proposed a sequence of events. The combination of cystic duct occlusion and saturated bile leads to activation of inflammatory mediators, such as the prostaglandins, in the wall of the gallbladder. Prostaglandin E_1, in particular, causes mucosal secretion but not absorption, which may explain gallbladder distention in this disease.[101] Further indirect support for this hypothesis comes from a study by Thornell and colleagues, which showed that inhibition of prostaglandin synthesis with indomethacin can relieve biliary pain in acute cholecystitis.[87] After a stone becomes impacted in the cystic duct, venous and lymphatic outflow obstruction produces gallbladder wall edema. The subsequent development of ischemia or secondary bacterial infection determines the course of events.

Components of bile have been implicated in the pathogenesis of acute cholecystitis. Cholesterol crystals in lithogenic bile may injure gallbladder mucosa directly.[88] Bile acids in high concentrations decrease the transepithelial transport of water.[89] Bile acids have also been shown to disrupt membranes and cause inflammation, an action that is normally inhibited by lecithin in normal bile. Furthermore, phospholipase A_2 may be released from injured gallbladder epithelium, resulting in conversion of lecithin into lysolecithin. Lysolecithin, in turn, experimentally causes disruption of cell membranes, derangement of the mucosa lining, and increased gallbladder permeability.[90–91] Phospholipase A_2 may also react with arachidonic acid to form prostaglandin E_2 and other potential mediators of inflammation. Other lysosomal enzymes in gallbladder mucosa may cause epithelial cell autolysis.[92]

Gallbladder wall ischemia can progress to frank gangrene and perforation. It seems to result from distention and increased intraluminal pressure related to the inflammatory response and stimulated secretory state. The increased luminal pressure correlates well with decreased gallbladder blood flow.[93] Small-vessel thromboses can also occur[94] and may partially explain why diabetics with preexisting microangiopathy are prone to gallbladder perforation.

Bacterial infection does not appear to be the initiating factor in acute cholecystitis. Organisms have been cultured from gallbladder bile in only 50% of cases.[95] If the impacted stone does not lead to gangrene or infection, bile pigments are absorbed and hydrops of the gallbladder develops. When cystic duct obstruction persists, secondary infection of gallbladder contents leads to suppurative cholecystitis or gallbladder empyema.

Clinical Manifestations

Acute cholecystitis can be diagnosed clinically by the presence of upper abdominal pain, fever, and nausea accompanied by right upper quadrant tenderness. Most patients give a history of one or more preceding episodes of biliary colic. Acute cholecystitis may mimic angina or myocardial infarction and even induce classic ischemic changes on an electrocardiogram.[96] Pain may localize to the right upper quadrant and become pleuritic in nature owing to local peritoneal irritation. Physical examination may reveal tenderness, guarding, low-grade fever, and local peritoneal signs. The presence of high fever and rigors is associated with complications such as gallbladder perforation, empyema, and cholangitis.[84] Murphy's sign (inspiratory arrest and pain with deep palpation of the right subcostal region) is highly suggestive of acute cholecystitis. In 20 to 30% of patients, a palpable, tender gallbladder is pathognomonic of acute cholecystitis when accompanied by typical symptoms.

Screening laboratory tests are nonspecific. The white blood cell count may be normal or slightly elevated. Higher counts are associated with suppurative complications of acute cholecystitis. Abnormalities in liver function tests such as slight elevations of alkaline phosphatase or aminotransferases may be present even in the absence of common duct stones. These are due to extension of the inflammatory process to the common bile duct or hepatic parenchyma. Mild jaundice (total bilirubin <5 mg/dl) is unusual but appreciable in 10 to 20% of patients without

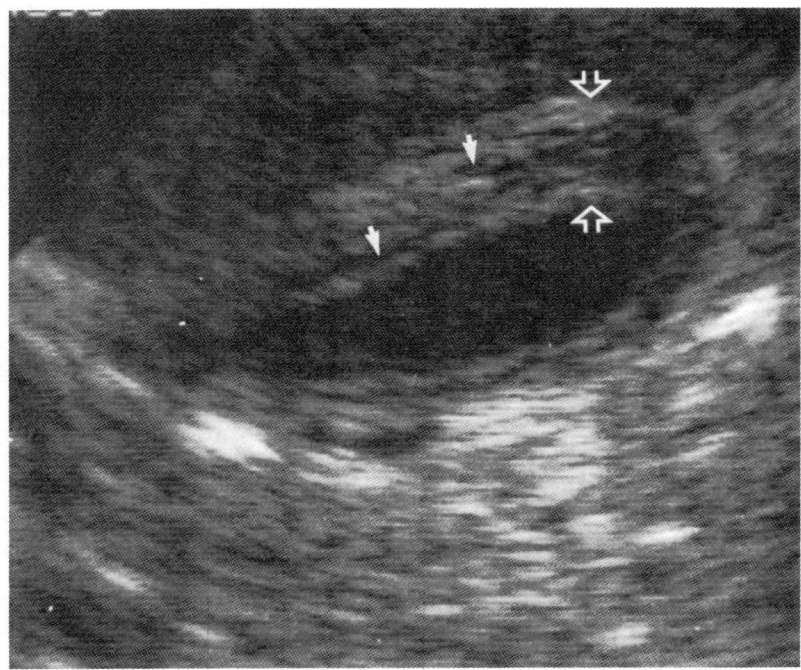

FIGURE 15–5.
Sonographic changes in acute cholecystitis. A longitudinal scan demonstrates a markedly thickened gallbladder wall (open arrows) with multiple striated lucencies (arrows) consistent with surgically proved acute cholecystitis. SOURCE: Carroll BA. Preferred imaging techniques for the diagnosis of cholecystitis and cholelithiasis. Ann Surg. 1989;210:1–12.

choledocholithiasis. Serum amylase may be normal or slightly elevated.

Differential Diagnosis

The diagnosis of acute cholecystitis is made clinically. The differential diagnosis should include acute pancreatitis, especially in patients with coexistent gallstones. Other conditions that can present with upper abdominal pain or an acute abdomen include acute hepatitis, liver abscess, primary or metastatic liver tumors, perforated peptic ulcers, kidney or ureteral stones, and acute appendicitis. Markedly obese and pregnant patients have presented atypically with retrocecal appendicitis in the right upper quadrant.[84] Fitz-Hugh–Curtis syndrome should be considered, particularly in young women. Herpes zoster infection may present with unilateral pain before the typical rash. An inferior wall myocardial infarction may be difficult to distinguish clinically. Acute bacterial cholangitis should be considered, especially in an ill, jaundiced patient.

Plain films of the abdomen are useful only if the clinical picture suggests ureteral stone, small bowel obstruction, chronic constipation, or ruptured viscus as a cause.[84] Rarely, air in the gall-bladder (emphysematous cholecystitis) or biliary tree (cholecystenteric fistula) can be diagnostic.

Supportive evidence for the diagnosis of acute cholecystitis may be provided by nuclear hepatobiliary imaging or ultrasound. These tests have replaced oral cholecystography and intravenous cholangiography (IVC) as initial procedures in the evaluation of suspected gallbladder disease. Sonographic changes include thickening of the gallbladder wall (Fig. 15–5), gallbladder distention, and a rounded (rather than oval), sonolucent area within the wall (representing subserosal edema), pericholecystic fluid (representing perforation and local abscess formation), and a sonographic Murphy's sign (focal tenderness elicited by pressure of the transducer over the gallbladder).[97] Gallbladder stones can rarely be seen impacted in the cystic duct.

Ultrasonography may, however, provide falsely negative results. Furthermore, its accuracy is operator dependent. However, ultrasonography is capable of visualizing other structures in the right upper quadrant, such as common bile duct, liver, and pancreas, which may be the source of abdominal pain. It is also superior to cholescintigraphy in diagnosing complications of acute cholecystitis such as perforation and abscess formation. It does not expose the patient to ionizing radiation and is the procedure of choice in children and pregnant women (Table 15–15).

The accuracy of ultrasound is high, but cholescintigraphy with technetium-99 iminodiacetic acid (DISIDA) compounds is considered by most to be the diagnostic test of choice. A nuclear scan can reliably diagnose cystic duct obstruction and acute cholecystitis at least 90 to 100% of the time.[98] It is also highly sensitive in the 5 to 10% of acute acalculous cholecystitis that is characterized by functional, rather than anatomic, obstruction. Adequate biliary visualization is possible, even with serum bilirubin levels as high as 20 to 30 mg/dl.[99] False-positive results (i.e., nonvisualization of the gallbladder on late scans) occur in only 4 to 5% of patients.[100] This happens after a prolonged fast, when the gallbladder is distended, or after a recent meal, owing to gallbladder contraction. It can also occur in patients who are on total parenteral nutrition and in those with congenital absence of the gallbladder. Since chronic cholecystitis and partial cystic duct obstruction can also cause delayed gallbladder visualization, images should be obtained at 4 hours and as long as 24 hours after injection.[45] By contrast, gallbladder visualization excludes the diagnosis of acute cholecystitis 98 to 100% of the time (Fig. 15–6).[97]

Complications

EMPYEMA

Suppurative cholecystitis is a complication similar to any intra-abdominal abscess. It is more common in diabetic patients.[101]

INFARCTION AND PERFORATION

Gangrene of the gallbladder wall results from progressive edema and small-vessel thrombosis. Torsion of the gallbladder has also been reported.[102] Infarction can rapidly lead to gallbladder perforation, which occurs in approximately 10% of cases.[103] Perforation can result in diffuse peritonitis or local abscess formation in the subhepatic space. A few gangrenous gallbladders can perforate into the liver parenchyma and cause a liver abscess. The overall mortality rate in patients with perforated gallbladders is 15 to 20%. However, when diffuse peritonitis develops in 30 to 35% of cases, the death rate increases to 40%. The difficulty and delay in establishing this diagnosis account for most of the mortality.

BILIARY-ENTERIC FISTULAE

About 15 to 20% of patients with gallbladder perforation develop biliary-enteric fistulae. The

TABLE 15–15. COMPARISON OF ULTRASOUND AND HEPATOBILIARY SCINTIGRAPHY

ULTRASOUND	HEPATOBILIARY SCINTIGRAPHY
CLINICAL FEATURES	CLINICAL FEATURES
Best study of anatomy	Best study of function
Visualizes other RUQ structures; detects gallstones; cannot visualize cystic duct	Visualizes cystic duct; cannot visualize gallstones or other RUQ structures
Less sensitive and specific for AC	Most sensitive and specific for AC
Diagnosis of AC rests on ancillary signs	Diagnosis of AC made on pathophysiologic basis; can distinguish acute from chronic disease
Reproduction of "sonographic Murphy's sign" may be required for diagnosis of AC	Painful manipulation of abdomen not required for diagnosis of AC
Detects complications of AC; can suggest need for common bile duct exploration	Poor anatomic resolution; cannot detect complications of AC
TECHNICAL FEATURES	TECHNICAL FEATURES
Safe, no known complications	Safe, no known complications
Rapid, readily available	Relatively rapid (may rule out AC in 1 h); may take up to 24 h to perform
Can be done as bedside exam	Cannot be done as bedside exam
Noninvasive	Minimally invasive
No ionizing radiation	Involves ionizing radiation
Inexpensive	More expensive
Does not require fasting state	Requires 24-h fast
Independent of hepatic function	Poor visualization with severe hepatic dysfunction
Technically more difficult to perform	Technically simple to perform
Operator-dependent	Not operator-dependent
Artifact with bowel gas, obesity, overlying ribs	False-positives with alcoholism, TPN, severe intercurrent illnesses

KEY: AC = acute cholecystitis, RUQ = right upper quadrant, TPN = total parenteral nutrition.
SOURCE: Cox GR, Browne BJ. Acute cholecystitis in the emergency department. J Emerg Med. 1989; 7:501–511.

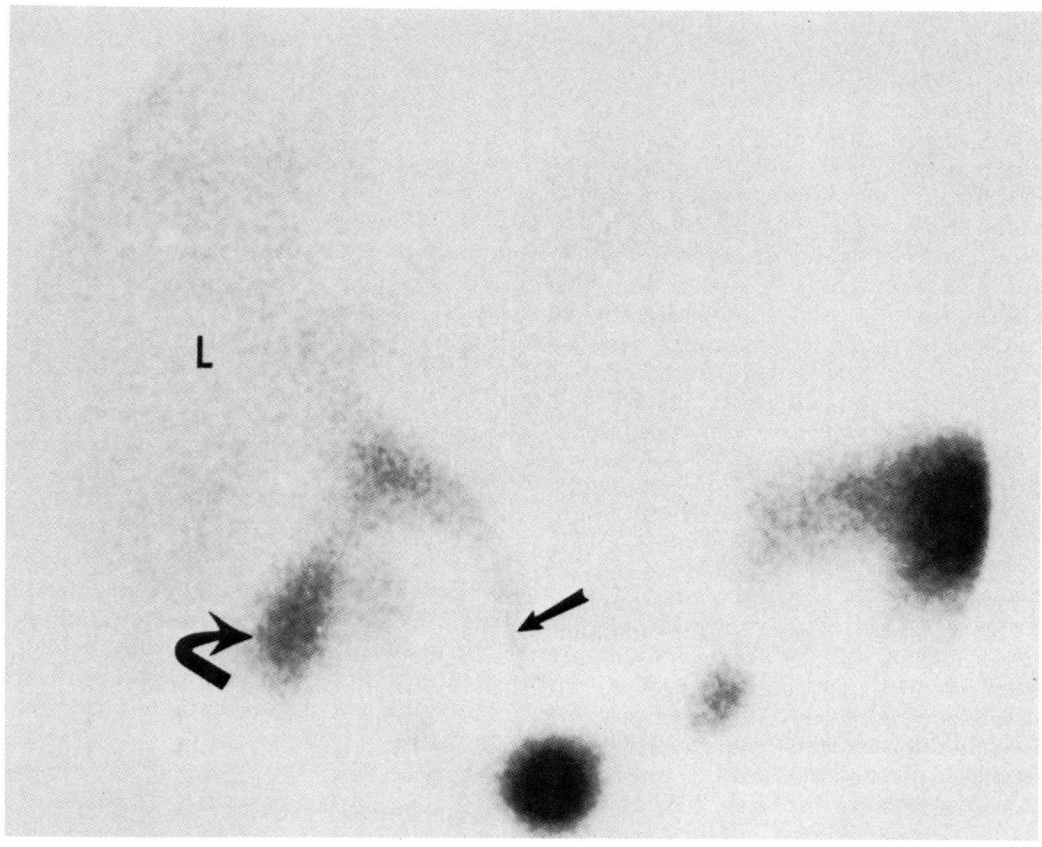

FIGURE 15–6.
Normal hepatobiliary scan. A normal hepato-iminodiacetic acid (HIDA) scan at 1 hour shows visualization of the gallbladder (curved arrow), common bile duct (arrow), and bowel. KEY: L = liver. SOURCE: Carroll BA. Preferred imaging techniques for the diagnosis of cholecystitis and cholelithiasis. Ann Surg. 1989;210:1–12.

incidence of biliary fistulae is 0.9%, with a male to female ratio of 2.3 to 1.0.[104] Gallstones cause more than 90% of cases.[105, 106] Fistulae develop after repeated attacks of cholecystitis and inflammation, which result in gallbladder adherence to an adjacent viscus. Ischemia and perforation of the gallbladder lead to erosion of the stone into the intestinal lumen. The most common fistulae are cholecystoduodenal (75% of patients).[107] Cholecystogastric (5%) and cholecystocolic (15%) fistulae also occur. Choledochoenteric fistulae are more common in Asia, where common duct pigment stones predominate. About 15% of Asian patients with choledocholithiasis develop choledochoduodenal fistulae.[108] Patients in western countries, however, develop choledochoduodenal fistulae from penetrating posterior duodenal ulcers in 80% of cases.[109]

Most biliary-enteric fistulae are diagnosed at surgery. They should be considered when a patient with acute cholecystitis develops intestinal obstruction, hyponatremia, or dehydration due to significant loss of bile. If these conditions go uncorrected, prerenal azotemia and metabolic acidosis ensue. Cholecystocolic fistulae can give rise to cholangitis and diarrhea. The latter arises from the profound secretory effect of bile that has bypassed ileal reabsorption.

Gallstone ileus can be the presenting sign of a biliary-enteric fistula in about 15% of patients. The location of obstruction is usually the small-caliber terminal ileum. Jejunal and gastric outlet obstruction (known as Bouveret's syndrome) has been reported as well.[110] The diagnosis of intestinal obstruction may be difficult to make, since gallstones moving along the intestine cause intermittent and nonspecific symptoms. Plain supine and upright films of the abdomen may show dilated small bowel loops and air-fluid levels or branching lucency in the right upper quadrant (pneumobilia). These findings are considered pathognomonic of gallstone ileus. Fistulae between the gallbladder and common bile duct can result from an impacted gallstone. This can lead to obstructive jaundice (Mirizzi's syndrome) as well.[111]

Management of Acute Cholecystitis

SUPPORTIVE THERAPY

When the diagnosis of acute cholecystitis is considered, the patient should be admitted to the hospital. Intravenous fluids are administered and a nasogastric tube placed to decompress the upper GI tract. Morphine should be avoided because it causes contraction of the sphincter of Oddi. Intravenous antibiotics should be given even before diagnostic tests are complete. Coliforms predominate among pathogens, and first- or second-generation cephalosporins (e.g., cefoxitin, cefamandole, or cefotetan) may suffice for empirical coverage. Broad-spectrum antibiotics are needed in elderly, diabetic, or toxic patients to cover enterococci, *Pseudomonas* organisms, and anaerobes. A penicillin and an aminoglycoside can be used. Single therapy with piperacillin has been shown to be as effective as combined therapy with ampicillin and tobramycin for acute cholecystitis.[112]

OPERATIVE THERAPY

Open Cholecystectomy. After supportive therapy has been initiated, the timing of cholecystectomy can be determined. This has been performed within 48 hours of the onset of acute cholecystitis or between 6 and 8 weeks after successful management. Data from four prospective randomized trials in the late 1970s and early 1980s showed that early surgery is preferable. Early surgery decreased total time of hospital stay but did not increase mortality or common duct injuries.[113–116] Furthermore, dissection was made easier during early surgery because edema delineated tissue planes. Delayed surgery was associated with almost 20% noncompliance after recovery from the initial attack. Therefore, surgery should be scheduled for within 48 hours of onset of acute cholecystitis if not contraindicated by concomitant illness. Patients with empyema should undergo cholecystectomy as soon as possible. Current mortality rate for open cholecystectomy for uncomplicated acute cholecystitis is only about 1%.[117]

The most common reason for delaying surgery is if a patient without clinical signs of suppuration presents with symptoms of more than 2 days' duration. An interval operation may be safer to perform because established inflammation may obscure the planes of dissection. Furthermore, at least two thirds of these patients may respond to initial medical therapy. The remaining one third need early surgery owing to progressive fever, pain, leukocytosis, or systemic toxicity.

Open surgery for acute cholecystitis is similar to that for chronic disease, with a few exceptions. Aspiration of the gallbladder is performed to provide specimens for bacterial cultures. Operative cholangiograms are more often performed because of the increased prevalence of common duct stones (15–20%) in acute cholecystitis. Cholangiograms facilitate dissection as well.

Laparoscopic Cholecystectomy. Laparoscopic cholecystectomy has rapidly become more popular than open cholecystectomy. Many consider this to be the procedure of choice for surgical removal of the gallbladder because of its proven advantages over open cholecystectomy. The short operative time (90–150 min), minimal morbidity (1–9.5%), high degree of success (94–99%), and no reported mortality make laparoscopic cholecystectomy more desirable than open cholecystectomy. Furthermore, the short hospital stay, reduced postoperative pain, and abbreviated recovery period have made this procedure popular with patients, physicians, and third-party payers (Table 15–16).[118–124] Conversion to open cholecystectomy occurs in 1–7% of cases, usually owing to acute inflammation, significant bleeding, and extensive adhesions. Uncommon but potential complications include bleeding, injury to the common bile duct, trocar injury to the bowel, and spillage of bile or stones or both.[120] The major contraindications to laparoscopic cholecystectomy are acute cholangitis, peritonitis, abdominal sepsis, major bleeding diathesis, and pregnancy.

Laparoscopic cholecystectomy can be performed to treat acute as well as chronic cholecystitis. In large series that have studied the use of laparoscopic cholecystectomy specifically in acute cholecystitis, even patients with severe acute disease were operated on. Approximately 6% of laparoscopic cholecystectomies for acute cholecystitis were converted to open cholecystectomy, which is comparable to the rate for elective laparoscopic surgery. When patients had severe acute cholecystitis, this rate increased to 30%, but acute disease was still not believed to be a contraindication to surgery by a well-trained laparoscopic surgeon.[125]

The optimal management of choledocholithiasis in relation to laparoscopic cholecystectomy is less well defined. When noninvasive imaging tests identify common bile duct stones preoperatively or when patients develop obstructive

TABLE 15–16. RESULTS OF LAPAROSCOPIC CHOLECYSTECTOMY

REFERENCE	NO. OF PATIENTS	MORBIDITY (%)	MORTALITY (%)	MEAN PROCEDURE LENGTH (MIN)	RATE OF CONVERSION TO OPEN CHOLECYSTECTOMY (%)	LENGTH OF HOSPITAL STAY (D)	LENGTH OF POSTOP RECOVERY (WK)
Dunn (1992)[118]	77	0	0	100	1.3	1.5	1
Smith (1991)[119]	190	9.5	0	74	3	2	1.8
Cohen (1992)[121]	140	1.4	0	106	5.7	1.6	1
Sigman (1992)[122]	500	0.6	0	88	5	1	1
Larson (1992)[123]	644	6.3	0	*	4.5	2	1
Ruers (1991)[124]	100	7.9	0	150	7	4	*

*Data not available.

jaundice or pancreatitis postoperatively, endoscopic retrograde cholangiopancreatography (ERCP) with sphincterotomy can be performed. Preoperative ERCP is often performed to avoid complications related to the small but significant presence of coexistent common bile duct stones. Approximately 3 to 15% of preoperative ERCPs may diagnose choledocholithiasis, enabling definitive papillotomy before cholecystectomy.[123, 126]

Intraoperative laparoscopic cholangiography can be done but has not yet become routine. When choledocholithiasis is unexpectedly diagnosed during a laparoscopic cholecystectomy, stone extraction can be accomplished intraoperatively by using a basket and a 9.4F flexible uteroscope through the cystic duct into the common bile duct (choledochoscopy).[127] Laparoscopic common bile duct exploration can be done but is difficult to perform because of the lack of adequate instrumentation and limited experience with this procedure.[128] Although it cannot yet be performed widely, some authors believe that it will eventually replace many open common bile duct explorations.

In 1991, British authors studied the utility of the intravenous cholangiogram to identify patients with common bile duct stones.[129] Of 100 consecutive patients with symptomatic gallstones who have undergone laparoscopic IVC, one had false-positive findings. These IVC data were compared with data from 52 patients who also had operative cholangiograms performed. One stone was detected on operative cholangiographic examination that was not identified on IVC. No additional information was gained from operative cholangiography. These data suggest that preoperative IVC is adequate for the detection of duct stones in patients considered for laparoscopic cholecystectomy.

Cholecystostomy. Cholecystectomy is successful in 85 to 97% of cases, but sometimes cholecystostomy is necessary. The latter may be performed because dissection may be too difficult and unsafe. Open cholecystostomy may be the procedure of choice in unstable, elderly patients who are poor surgical risks. The operative mortality rate for urgent cholecystostomy is approximately 15%. This high figure is due to both the severity of illness and the inadequacy of biliary drainage in the presence of cholangitis. When cholangitis is a strong consideration, choledochotomy and T-tube placement should be performed. In selected patients with acalculous cholecystitis, ultrasound-guided percutaneous cholecystostomy is performed.[130]

About 1 week after surgery, a cholangiogram is repeated to exclude the presence of retained common duct stones. If a cholecystostomy was performed, elective cholecystectomy is scheduled for about 6 weeks later. Earlier operation may be necessary since symptoms can recur in half of patients with gallbladders in situ.

Repair of Complications. The operative procedure for biliary-enteric fistulae is more controversial. When intestinal obstruction from gallstones occurs, surgery should be performed early because spontaneous passage beyond the point of obstruction rarely occurs. Patients are often unstable, and the operation should aim at relieving the obstruction without dealing with the biliary tract disease. In this case, a simple enterotomy with stone extraction suffices. Complete examination of the intestine is necessary because at least 10% of patients have passed more than one stone into the GI tract. Although gallstone ileus can recur if simultaneous cholecystectomy is not performed, this happens in only about 4% of cases. Furthermore, simultaneous cholecystectomy may actually cause greater morbidity and mortality than that caused by gallstone ileus.[131] Elective surgery for a biliary fistula should include choledochal decompression because of concomitant common

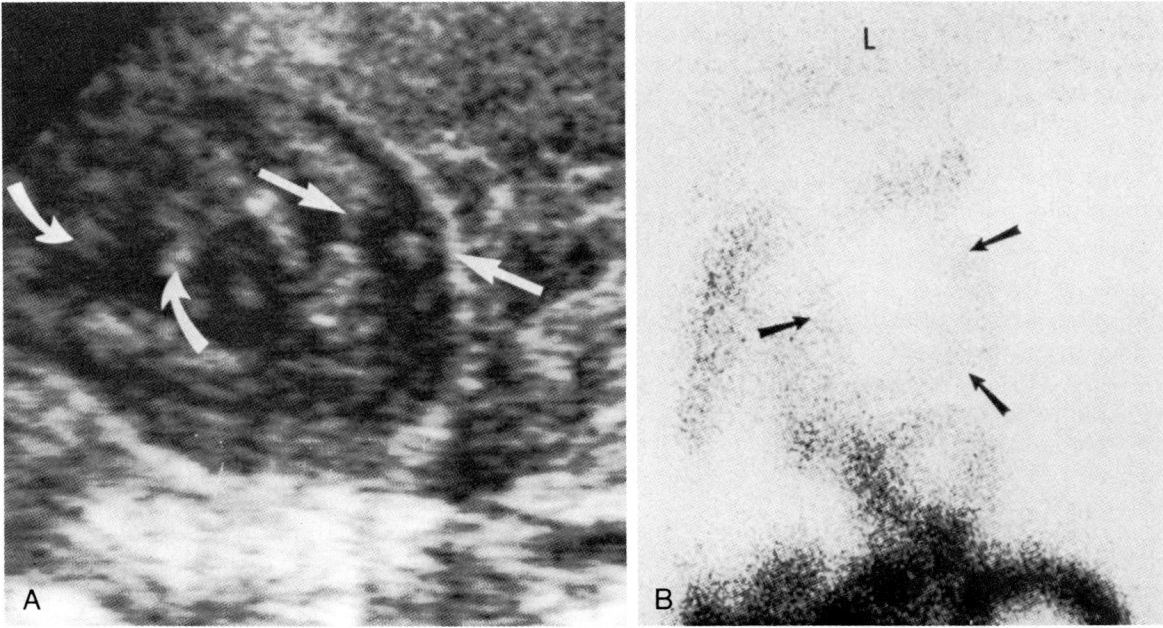

FIGURE 15–7.
Hemorrhagic, gangrenous acalculous cholecystitis. *A,* A transverse ultrasound scan shows the hemorrhagic, gangrenous gall-bladder in a patient with acalculous cholecystitis. Multiple irregular echoes consistent with hemorrhage (curved arrows) fill the lumen, and the wall shows irregular thickening (arrows). *B,* A 2-hour anterior projection technetium-DISIDA (o-diisopropyl iminodiacetic acid) radionuclide scan in this patient shows a "rim sign" of abnormal isotope (arrows) around a nonvisualized gallbladder. This is consistent with inflammation around and in the gallbladder wall. KEY: L = liver. SOURCE: Carroll BA. Preferred imaging techniques for the diagnosis of cholecystitis and cholelithiasis. Ann Surg. 1989;210:1–12.

duct stones. The repair of a biliary fistula usually includes dissection of the fistula, closure of the intestinal opening, cholecystectomy, and common duct exploration.[28] Alternatively, cholecystostomy and T-tube placement may be preferred in high-risk patients or those in whom dissection is difficult. Cholecystocolic fistulae need urgent repair because of the high frequency of cholangitis.

Acute Acalculous Cholecystitis

Acute acalculous cholecystitis (AAC) deserves special mention because the mortality rate is generally much higher (30–50%) than in acute calculous cholecystitis.[132] Diagnosis may be difficult, but certain groups of patients appear to be predisposed. Although AAC is more common in adults, about half of all children with acute cholecystitis have no gallbladder stones.[133] Adults who have burns, recent major surgery, severe

trauma, prolonged hyperalimentation, vasculitis, sepsis, coma, or diabetes or those who are on narcotics are also at high risk.[134, 135] Patients with the acquired immunodeficiency syndrome (AIDS) secondary to cryptosporidial or cytomegaloviral infection of the biliary tree have developed AAC.[136] Patients on hemodialysis who develop spontaneous intracholecystic hemorrhage have been diagnosed with acute acalculous cholecystitis (Fig. 15–7).[137]

The pathogenesis of this disease is still unclear. As in calculous cholecystitis, bile stasis and increased lysolecithin production may contribute. Impaired gallbladder emptying and bile stasis can result in a functional cystic duct obstruction. Some authors have suggested that obstruction is due to small stones that are passed or undetectable. In experimental animals, circulating coagulation factors have been associated.[138] Since gangrene is seen in about 50% of cases,[139] systemic hypotension and gallbladder hypoperfusion have also been implicated as causal agents. Other factors, such as sympathetic stimulation leading to vascular smooth muscle spasm and ischemia and the effect of positive pressure ventilation on bile flow, have been implicated. Primary infection may cause emphysematous cholecystitis, in which gas bubbles are seen in the wall of the gallbladder. Males and diabetics are preferentially affected. At least 33% of all these cases are acalculous. The causal agent is *E. coli* in 33% of cases and *Clostridium* in 45%. Anaerobes may occasionally be isolated.

The diagnosis of AAC is suggested by the presence of right upper quadrant pain and a palpable mass in the high-risk patients. This is the exception rather than the rule. Part of the high mortality rate may be due to difficulty in making the diagnosis in critically ill patients. A sign such as sepsis, insulin resistance, unexplained fever, or thrombocytopenia may be the only clue. Jaundice or abnormal alkaline phosphatase levels may also be present. It is important to remember that cholestasis may be due to drug toxicity, fatty liver from hyperalimentation, or concomitant sepsis.

Noninvasive imaging studies may help. Hepatobiliary scintigraphy (DISIDA) scans may detect acalculous cholecystitis in only 40% of cases.[140] Ultrasonographic changes include gallbladder wall thickness and pericholecystic fluid in the absence of stones. Sonographic examination may be more readily performed at the bedside in the critically ill patient.

Once the diagnosis is established, cholecystectomy should be performed emergently. Rapid progression to empyema, perforation, or gangrene is more common than in calculous disease, and more than half of all patients have at least one complication.

Acute Bacterial Cholangitis

Definition and Etiology

Acute cholangitis is a clinical syndrome with fever, right upper quadrant pain, and jaundice. Bacterial infection is the most common cause. The systemic toxicity that occurs in acute obstructive cholangitis results when biliary tree obstruction is significant enough to cause entry of bacteria or endotoxin into the blood. It is assumed that infection arises from bacteria that reach the biliary system from the duodenum by direct ascension, hence the term "ascending cholangitis." This term usually denotes the mildest form of cholangitis, which manifests as the classic triad of pain, jaundice, and fever and

chills originally described by Charcot.[141] A distinction is made between suppurative cholangitis and nonsuppurative cholangitis, which lie at opposite ends of a spectrum. The latter term has been used to describe a less severe form of biliary infection, whereas the former entity is defined by the presence of pus in the biliary tree and was described by Reynolds and Dargan in 1959.[142] They added abnormal mental status and shock to Charcot's original triad to describe the entity defined as Reynold's pentad. Although there is overlap in the clinical appearance and course of cholangitis, the term acute suppurative cholangitis usually denotes a rapidly progressive, lethal form of cholangitis.

Stones are the most common cause of biliary obstruction and may cause cholangitis even with partial occlusion of the common bile duct. Choledocholithiasis is found in approximately 9 to 15% of patients operated on for chronic cholecystitis.[143, 144] It is usually due to stones that have migrated from the gallbladder, although stones can form de novo in the common bile duct. Common duct stones can present clinically from several days to several decades after a cholecystectomy, when they are most likely due to de novo formation. Age over 60 years increases the incidence of common duct stones.[145]

Obstruction of the biliary tree due to malignancy is the next most common cause of cholangitis.[146] The most frequently diagnosed neoplasms are carcinomas of the bile ducts, pancreas, and ampulla of Vater. Infections arise less frequently from neoplasms than from stones, even if obstruction is total. Invasive diagnostic procedures such as cholangiography can often lead to cholangitis in patients with malignant obstruction.

Other causes of biliary obstruction are choledochal cysts and common duct strictures related to surgical injury. Biliary-enteric anastomoses such as transduodenal sphincteroplasty can lead to reflux of GI tract contents into the biliary tree and presumably cause cholangitis. Infection is rare, however, and is usually associated with concomitant biliary obstruction.[28]

Pathogenesis

Bile is normally sterile, and attempts to infect nonstagnant bile have been unsuccessful. The incidence of positive biliary tract cultures is higher in patients with common bile duct disease than in those with chronic gallbladder disease without common duct disease. Although gallbladder bile from patients with cholecystitis is culture-positive in as many as half of cases,[147] bile from patients with choledocholithiasis is more often infected (approximately 90% of cases).[148] Obstruction of the biliary tree is believed to cause stasis and bacterial overgrowth. This has been shown in experiments that demonstrate a temporal relationship between bile duct ligation and infection.[149] However, it is probably not only increased intraductal pressure that predisposes to infection, since complete obstruction of the common bile duct due to malignancies rarely leads to cholangitis.[150] How bacteria actually reach the biliary tree is not well established. Among the possible routes are hepatic arterial or portal blood circulation, biliary or intestinal lymphatics spread, and direct spread from the duodenum or gallbladder. Evidence for the portal pathway was provided by Dineen, who showed that a significant amount of bacteria can be cultured from portal blood and bile, particularly during biliary obstruction.[151] Systemic bacteremia is less common than portal bacteremia during acute cholangitis. Direct ascension of bacteria from the duodenum is indirectly supported as a route of infection by occasional episodes of cholangitis in patients with surgically altered biliary drainage. Furthermore, descent of bacteria from infected gallbladders is suggested by the growth of the same organism from cultures of common duct and gallbladder bile.[152]

Bacteriology

The most commonly encountered organisms in biliary sepsis arise from the GI tract. Biliary infections are often polymicrobial (48–61%), although blood cultures are usually positive for only one organism.[28, 139] Bacteremia is present in about 25 to 40% of cases, even if 92 to 100% of bile cultures are positive.[153]

Causal organisms include *E. coli*, which is the most common (recovered in about 60% of cases), *Klebsiella* (recovered in about 40% of cases), *Pseudomonas*, *Enterobacter*, and *Proteus*. Together, *E. coli* and *Klebsiella* are responsible for about 70% of positive findings of bile cultures and 85% of blood cultures. *Enterococcus* and anaerobic bacteria are cultured less frequently. Enterococcal cultures account for about 30% of positive bile cultures. Anaerobic bacteria including *Bacteroides fragilis* and *Clostridium* species are becoming more frequently recognized as pathogenic organisms and may be isolated in up to 10% of cases.

Histopathologic Features

O'Connor and colleagues studied liver biopsies obtained percutaneously or at autopsy from patients with acute cholangitis.[150] They described "acute pericholangitis" (portal acute inflammatory cell infiltrate), "microscopic acute cholangitis" (few neutrophils within bile duct lumens), and frank microabscesses in ducts and liver parenchyma. They failed to find significant differences in the histopathologic changes in the liver of patients who lived and of those who died.

Clinical Manifestations

Acute cholangitis is thought to be a continuum of diseases with a wide spectrum of clinical findings and outcome.[154] Patients can present with only mild pain and low-grade fever. Charcot's triad is present in 50 to 70% of cases.[155] Jaundice may be absent in 20% of patients. This may make diagnosis difficult because abdominal pain, fever, and chills are nonspecific. The differential diagnosis of acute cholangitis must include acute cholecystitis, pyogenic liver abscess, acute hepatitis, and acute pancreatitis. Although some patients with acute cholecystitis may be mildly jaundiced, total bilirubin levels higher than 5 mg/dl[156] are more common in patients with acute cholangitis.

O'Connor and colleagues retrospectively analyzed 65 patients with biliary sepsis and mechanical biliary obstruction and found no significant distinguishing features between suppurative cholangitis and nonsuppurative cholangitis.[154] No differences in mean temperature, presence of shock, mental status changes, peritoneal signs, white blood cell count, hemoglobin blood urea nitrogen, or liver function tests were evident in patients with or without pus within the common bile duct. Furthermore, both groups of patients had similar incidences of systemic medical illnesses (such as diabetes, liver disease, or cardiopulmonary disease) and postoperative complications. Thus, in the two largest series of patients, the two forms of cholangitis could not be distinguished before examination of the common bile duct.[155]

Diagnosis

Plain radiographs of the abdomen may show nonspecific changes such as ileus. Hepatobiliary scans have been used to diagnose biliary obstruction but are unable to define precisely biliary anatomy. There has been increasing interest in these scans, but data have been analyzed only in a retrospective manner. For example, Kaplun and colleagues and Miller and colleagues studied patients with jaundice, abdominal pain, and absence of biliary flow on cholescintigraphy.

They found that 40 to 70% of those evaluated preoperatively had normal-sized common bile ducts, as determined by ultrasound, and suggested that cholescintigraphic scans may be able to detect early acute obstruction before sonography.[156, 157]

Ultrasound has been effective in accurately differentiating extrahepatic obstruction from intrahepatic cholestasis in jaundiced patients. The reported accurancy rate is 96% in patients with dilated biliary trees.[158] However, in a study by Beinart and colleagues of 150 patients with calculi, neoplasms, or strictures, 9% of patients with ductal obstruction demonstrated by transhepatic cholangiographic examination had normal findings on ultrasound examination.[159] In a 1983 prospective study of 87 consecutive patients, ultrasound detected only 13% of patients with surgically proven choledocholithiasis. Thirty-six percent of the patients studied had a normal common bile duct caliber but had stones detected at operation.[160] Although CT scan may be more accurate at diagnosing common duct stones,[161] ultrasound is considered the reasonable initial diagnostic test of choice because of its portability, low cost, lack of ionizing radiation, and accuracy in most patients.

More invasive tests, such as percutaneous transhepatic cholangiography and ERCP, have the advantage of higher diagnostic accuracy. Moreover, they may provide better evaluation of the cause and level of biliary obstruction and a therapeutic option to decompress nonoperatively. The choice of one method over the other depends on anatomic considerations as well as the availability of technical expertise. The presence of massive ascites may make transhepatic cholangiography unfavorable. A duodenal diverticulum or history of upper intestinal tract bypass surgery may make ERCP less likely to be successful.

Therapy

SURGICAL THERAPY

In the past, standard therapy for cholangitis consisted of broad-spectrum IV antibiotic coverage, IV fluids, and operative decompression. Surgical literature has stressed the need for laparotomy, although many of the studies are retrospective. The need for early decompression of the biliary tree is clear. Even patients with poor prognostic factors, such as advanced age and sepsis, may respond to adequate drainage of the biliary tree.

The most common types of surgical procedures are common duct exploration or cholecystectomy with T-tube drainage, or both, and biliary-enteric anastomosis. Operative mortality for emergency operations ranges from 1 to 40%.[155, 162] Complications include retained common bile duct stones, duodenal fistulae or leaks, postoperative sepsis, and wound infections. Dramatic improvement in survival (i.e., as little as 3% mortality) results from elective rather than emergency operation.

NONOPERATIVE THERAPY

Nonoperative biliary decompression seems logical as either an initial or a sole therapeutic procedure. Percutaneous transhepatic decompression, endoscopic nasobiliary drainage, sphincterotomy, stone extraction, or stent placement can improve survival, particularly in high-risk elderly patients with multiple medical problems.

It is unclear whether cholecystectomy is truly necessary after successful endoscopic removal of common duct stones. Martin and Tweedle reported a 99% success rate of endoscopic sphincterotomy in 81 consecutive patients with intact gallbladders and symptomatic choledocholithiasis.[162a] The complication rate was 7%, with 1 reported death. Common duct stones were removed in 86% of patients, but only 9 patients had cholecystectomy afterwards. Short-term follow-up (mean of 24 mo) of the remaining 61 patients with gallbladders in situ showed no deaths attributable to biliary tract disease.

Percutaneous transhepatic drainage is useful for preoperative biliary decompression as well as palliation of patients with malignant obstruction. Catheter placement is successful in about 90% of cases, but complication and mortality rates are variable. The main complication is catheter-related sepsis, which increases in frequency with prolonged manipulation or drainage. Bleeding can occur in as many as 15% of patients. Death rates as high as 8.6% have been reported.[163]

Endoscopic retrograde cholangiopancreatography with endoscopic sphincterotomy (ERCP/ES) is the procedure of choice in the initial management of common duct stones. In 1985, Carr-Locke and colleagues reported 394 consecutive patients who underwent ERCP/ES.[164] Sphincterotomy was successful in 98% of cases, and common duct stones were removed in 93%. Early complications, mostly due to bleeding, were noted in 10% of patients, and the 30-day mortality rate was 3.3%. Of these deaths, 0.8% were directly related to the endoscopic sphincterotomy.

Most studies on ERCP/ES in acute cholangitis

have been retrospective (Table 15–17). In 1982, Cotton and colleagues successfully managed 12 of 14 patients with cholangitis with ERCP, sphincterotomy, stone extraction, or nasobiliary drainage.[165] Carr-Locke's group compared results from surgical and endoscopic decompression. Of 82 patients studied, 39% had surgical drainage and 61% had endoscopic drainage, with stone clearance successful in 70% of the endoscopic sphincterotomy group. The surgical group had a 30-day mortality of 21.4%, which is significantly higher than the 4.7% death rate in the endoscopically treated group. Despite greater age and its concomitant medical problems that theoretically made the endoscopic group at higher risk, fewer complications (28%, due to hemorrhage) occurred in this group than in the surgically treated group (57%, from bleeding, wound infection, multiple organ failure).[164a]

Prognosis

In the early 1980s, retrospective studies demonstrated that survival was much lower in patients treated medically, regardless of the presence or absence of biliary pus. Death in cholangitis was due to biliary sepsis in 67% of cases.[154] Surgical decompression of the biliary tree resulted in 50% survival in the suppurative cholangitis group versus 78% in the nonsuppurative cholangitis group. Nonsurvivors were more likely to have had cancer (55% vs 17%) and suppuration (41% vs 19%) than were survivors. Mean bilirubin, white blood cell count, hemoglobin, and blood urea nitrogen levels were also significantly different between the two groups.

The outcome of patients with acute bacterial cholangitis ranges from intermittent mild episodes to shock and death. Published survival rates in surgical literature from the 1960s and 1970s range from 0 to 88% (Table 15–18).[154] The presence of hypotension, advanced age, acute renal failure, and inadequate antibiotic coverage has also been associated with lower survival.[146, 164] Failure to undergo surgical decompression of the biliary tree was associated

with the higher mortality rates (58% in patients given medical therapy alone), although some patients with mild cholangitis responded to antibiotics alone.[166] Pus is not universally present in bile ducts of patients who are extremely toxic or who die. However, it is clear from multiple studies in the literature that patients with suppurative cholangitis have a worse prognosis, with a cumulative mortality of about 44% compared with 18% in patients with nonsuppurative cholangitis.

With the advent of ERCP and sphincterotomy, survival rates improved. Short-term death rates can range from 3.3 to 8% in patients with choledocholithiasis and cholangitis, even in high-risk elderly patients.[154, 155, 167, 168] Mortality is increased significantly to about 27% in patients with malignant obstruction and cholangitis.[162]

Approach to Therapy

Because of the lack of clinical trials and the wide spectrum of severity in acute cholangitis, treatment should be individualized. A brief period of about 12 to 24 hours with IV antibiotics and close observation is reasonable because a number of a patients do improve under this therapy.[146, 162] Empirical antibiotics should include coverage for enteric gram-negative bacteria, enterococci, and anaerobes. Traditional regimens have used penicillin and an aminoglycoside, and this treatment was effective in as many as 90% of patients.[169] The addition of clindamycin or metronidazole is appropriate to cover possible anaerobic infection.

Although third-generation cephalosporins have been used, particularly in elderly patients with abnormal renal function, these antibiotics are not adequate for biliary sepsis. They are not effective against enterococci and have poor activity against *Bacteroides* species.

The newer broad-spectrum acylureidopenicillins such as piperacillin have excellent activity against coliforms, anaerobes, and enterococci. These drugs may be administered in combination with an aminoglycoside for synergism against enterococci and enteric gram-negative bacteria.

TABLE 15–17. SURGICAL VERSUS ENDOSCOPIC BILIARY DECOMPRESSION IN 82 PATIENTS WITH ACUTE CHOLANGITIS*

	SURGICAL GROUP (N = 32)	ENDOSCOPIC GROUP (N = 50)
30-day mortality	21.4%	4.7%
Morbidity	57%	28%

*NOTE: Eleven patients had neither surgery nor endoscopic treatment.
SOURCE: Leese T, Neoptolemos JP, Baker AR, Carr-Locke DL. Management of acute cholangitis and the impact of endoscopic sphincterotomy. Br J Surg 1986;73:988–992.

TABLE 15–18. SURVIVAL RATES IN ACUTE BACTERIAL CHOLANGITIS

REFERENCE, YR*	NO. OF PATIENTS	OPERATIVE THERAPY		NONOPERATIVE THERAPY		SC		NSC		OVERALL MORTALITY
		NO.	MORTALITY, %	NO.	MORTALITY, %	NO.	MORTALITY, %	NO.	MORTALITY, %	
Grant, 1945	3	3	0	0	...	3	0	0	...	0
Cole, 1945	6	5	15	...	...	5	15	...	...	15
Reynolds & Dargan, 1957	5	4	25	1	100	5	40	0	...	40
Glenn and Moody, 1960	8	5	0	3	100	8	38	0	...	38
Haupert et al, 1965	15	12	33	3	100	15	47	0	...	47
Ostermiller et al, 1965	8	8	88	0	...	8	88	0	...	88
Waddell, 1966	6	3	0	3	100	6	50	0	...	50
Dow and Lindenaur, 1967	10	8	50	2	100	10	60	0	...	60
Hinchey & Cooper, 1968	24	22	27	2	100	24	33	0	...	33
Welch & Donaldson, 1970	20	16	25	4	100	20	40	0	...	40
Saharia & Cameron, 1975	78	64?‡	...	14?†	...	11	18	67	13	14
Boey & Way, 1976	99	86	17	13	23	14‡	36	72‡	10	17
Present study, 1980	65	50	32	15	87	19	70	46	36	45
Total	347	222	25	46	58	148	44	185	18	30

*Dates refer to publication year of original references cited in source.
†Excluded from total due to insufficient data.
‡Thirteen of the cases in this study could not be classified as SC or NSC.
SOURCE: O'Connor MJ, Schwartz ML, McQuarrie DG, et al. Acute bacterial cholangitis: An analysis of clinical manifestation. Arch Surg. 1982; 117:437–441.

Data on newer broad-spectrum agents such as imipenem are not yet available. This medication has the potential for effective use as a single-agent therapy for cholangitis. Antibiotics are generally given for 10 to 14 days intravenously. Any diagnostic or therapeutic manipulation of the biliary tree needs additional antibiotic coverage if performed beyond this time period.

If the patient does not respond, biliary decompression should be performed. This should be done preferably by percutaneous transhepatic cholangiography or ERCP; both provide accurate imaging of the biliary tree and can precisely define the location and nature of the obstruction. ERCP with sphincterotomy may be the preferred treatment for acute bacterial cholangitis because of its distinct advantages over percutaneous drainage and emergency operation. In experienced hands, the technique is easily performed with minimal sedation. This eliminates the risk from general anesthesia. The procedure generally is shorter than percutaneous transhepatic drainage, which requires establishing an adequate tract and internal drainage. It also avoids complications such as catheter-related sepsis, bile leakage, and the formation of a cholangiovenous fistula, favoring bacteremia. It also allows urgent decompression in stone-related cholangitis, which may be followed by elective cholecystectomy. Complication rates and 30-day mortality are lower compared with surgical decompression and sometimes percutaneous transhepatic drainage. If ERCP/ES is unsuccessful and obstruction persists, then a nasobiliary catheter should be placed. If this fails, percutaneous transhepatic drainage should be considered and operative decompression performed. A surgeon should be actively participating in the care of the patient with cholangitis because of possible need for operation, either electively or emergently if nonoperative procedures fail.

Recurrent Pyogenic Cholangitis

Recurrent pyogenic cholangitis was reported by Cook and colleagues in 1954.[170] It is also known as Oriental cholangiohepatitis because of the high prevalence of the disease in natives of and immigrants from Asia. This disease occurs when stones, usually the "pigment" type, form primarily in the intrahepatic bile ducts. Thus, the term "hepatolithiasis" has also been used. The stones can cause local obstruction or migrate distally or both and result in common bile duct occlusion. Biliary strictures from recurrent transmural ductal inflammation affect all parts of the biliary tree. The intrahepatic ducts develop patchy dilatation and stenosis. The extrahepatic ducts are also dilated and fibrotic. Recurrent cholangitis ensues, resulting in biliary sepsis and cholangitic liver abscesses.[171] With time, liver parenchymal destruction and secondary biliary cirrhosis may develop.[172]

The pathogenesis of recurrent pyogenic cholangitis has been linked to parasitic infestation of the biliary tree with *Ascaris lumbricoides* or *Opisthorchis sinensis*. These worms have been found in stones[173] but are not consistently present. Bacterial colonization of bile with *E. coli* may be another contributing factor. These bacteria contain an enzyme called β-glucuronidase that deconjugates bilirubin glucuronides to form free bilirubin and glucuronic acid.[174] Cetta reported 2 cases that support the hypothesis of infection as an initial event in the formation of brown-pigmented biliary stones. He prospectively studied 600 patients who underwent cholecystectomy, sphincterotomy, and T-tube drainage for gallstones.[175] Bile culture produced negative findings, and stones were absent before and immediately after the first operation in 2 patients. A previous sphincterotomy become stenotic. At a second operation, which occurred after *E. coli* was cultured from T-tube bile, typical pigment stones were found in the common bile duct. Another possible causative factor in recurrent pyogenic cholangitis is a low-protein diet. This reportedly results in decreased amounts of glucaro-1,4-lactone, an endogenous inhibitor of β-glucuronidase.[28] Both infection and diet are believed to result in increased stone precipitation.

Oriental cholangiohepatitis begins with transient mild attacks characterized by low-grade fever and minimal jaundice. Later on, the attacks increase in number and severity. Signs and symptoms of suppurative cholangitis finally present. Jaundice and leukocytosis are not so severe as in cholangitis. There may also be other signs of portal hypertension, such as hepatosplenomegaly.

Contrast CT scans of the liver may show ductal enhancement, liver abscesses, or parenchymal atrophy. Endoscopic retrograde cholangiopancreatography or percutaneous transhepatic cholangiography may be helpful in establishing biliary anatomy and sites of obstruction, and ERCP may show intrahepatic duct pruning, cholangiectasia, with or without stones.

Complications can include portal vein thrombosis, liver abscesses, pancreatitis (12%), peritonitis from gallbladder perforation, biliary-enteric fistulae, and gram-negative sepsis. Treatment is directed toward operative biliary decompression in addition to antibiotic coverage and supportive measures. Pathogenic organisms in recurrent pyogenic cholangitis are similar to those in ascending cholangitis. Choledochotomy and drainage are performed. Cholecystostomy or cholecystectomy is necessary for treatment of gallbladder perforation, empyema, or presence of gallstones. Choledochoscopy or cholangiography are helpful in evaluating the presence of residual intrahepatic stones. Transduodenal sphincteroplasty is performed if the common bile duct dilatation reaches the ampulla. This may actually render as many as 85% of patients asymptomatic if there are no intrahepatic stones or strictures.[146] Roux-en-Y choledochojejunostomy is indicated if the common duct is dilated proximal to the duodenum.

In 25% of patients, retained intrahepatic stones need special management. These stones are usually confined to the left hepatic lobe and may eventually require left hepatic lobectomy. A transhepatic approach to the right ductal system may be necessary to reach retained stones. Fan and colleagues retrospectively studied 88 patients with acute cholangitis due to hepatolithiasis.[171] Thirty percent required emergency operation owing to shock, peritonitis, or fever. Many of these patients had concomitant extrahepatic ductal obstruction due to strictures or impacted common duct stones. The overall operative mortality was 20 to 40%, which was attributed mostly to delay in diagnosis and therapeutic intervention.

REFERENCES

1. Ochsner A, DeBakey M, Murray S. Pyogenic abscess of the liver. Am J Surg. 1938;40:292–319.
2. Greenstein AJ, Lowenthal D, Hammer GS, et al. Continuing changing patterns of disease in pyogenic liver abscess: A study of 38 patients. Am J Gastroenterol. 1984;79:217–226.
3. Land MA, Moinuddin M, Bisno AL. Pyogenic liver abscess: Changing epidemiology and prognosis. South Med J. 1985;78:1426–1430.
4. Srivastava ED, Mayberry JF. Pyogenic liver abscess: A review of aetiology, diagnosis and intervention. Dig Dis. 1990;8:287–293.
5. Neoptolemos JP, Macpherson DS. Pyogenic liver abscess. Br J Hosp Med. 1981;26:47–55.
6. Klein B, Lewinski UH, Cohen AM, et al. Liver abscess as a late complication of percutaneous liver biopsy. Arch Surg. 1980;115:1233–1234.

7. Jochimsen PR, Zike WL, Shirazi SS, et al. Iatrogenic liver abscess: A complication of hepatic artery ligation for tumor. Arch Surg. 1978;113:141–144.

8. Barnes PF, DeCock KM, Reynolds TN, et al. A comparison of amebic and pyogenic abscesses of the liver. Medicine. 1987;66:472–483.

9. Lee FS, Block GE. The changing pattern of hepatic abscesses. Arch Surg. 1972;104:465–470.

10. Cohen JL, Martin FM, Rossie RL, et al. Liver abscess: The need for complete gastrointestinal evaluation. Arch Surg. 1989;124:561–564.

11. Stain SC, Yellin AE, Donovan AJ, Brien HW. Pyogenic liver abscess: Modern treatment. Arch Surg. 1991;126: 991–996.

12. Taylor KJW, deGraff C, Wasson JFM, et al. Accuracy of grey-scale ultrasound diagnosis of abdominal and pelvic abscesses in 220 patients. Lancet. 1978;8:83–84.

13. Ralls PW, Barnes PF, Radin DR, et al. Sonographic features of amebic and pyogenic liver abscesses: A blinded comparison. Am J Rad. 1987;149:499–501.

14. Barros JL. Hydatid disease of the liver. Am J Surg. 1978;135:597–600.

15. Sabbaj J, Sutter VL, Finegold SM. Anaerobic pyogenic liver abscesses. Ann Intern Med. 1972;77:629–638.

16. McDonald MI, Corey GR, Gallis HA, et al. Single and multiple pyogenic liver abscesses; natural history, diagnosis and treatment, with emphasis on percutaneous drainage. Medicine. 1984;63:291–302.

17. Lee KT, Sheen PC, Chen JS, Ker CG. Pyogenic liver abscess: Multivariate analysis of risk factors. World J Surg. 1991;15(3):372–376.

18. Pitt HA, Zuidema GD. Factors influencing mortality in the treatment of pyogenic hepatic abscess. Surg Gynecol Obstet. 1975;140:228–234.

19. Bertel CK, Van Heerden JA, Sheedy PF. Treatment of pyogenic hepatic abscess. Arch Surg. 1986;121:554–558.

20. Klatchko BA, Schwartz SI. Diagnostic and therapeutic approaches to pyogenic abscess of the liver. Surg Gynecol Obstet. 1989;168:332–336.

21. Gyorffy EJ, Frey CF, Silva J. Pyogenic liver abscess: Diagnostic and therapeutic strategies. Ann Surg. 1987; 206:699–705.

22. McFadzean AJS, Chang KPS, Wong CC. Solitary pyogenic abscess of the liver treated by closed aspiration and antibiotics. Br J Surg. 1953;41:141–152.

23. Cheng DL, Liu YC, Yen MY, et al. Pyogenic liver abscess: Clinical manifestations and value of percutaneous catheter drainage treatment. J Formos Med Assoc. 1990;89(7):571–576.

24. Khanna R, Levendoglu H. Liver abscess due to *Yersinia enterocolitica:* Case report and review of the literature. Dig Dis Sci. 1989;34(4):636–639.

25. Gray ML, Killinger AH. *Listeria monocytogenes* and listeric infections. Bacteriol Rev. 1966;30:309–382.

26. Al-Dajani O, Khatib R. Cryptogenic liver abscess due to *Listeria monocytogenes.* J Infect Dis. 1983;147(5):961.

27. Yu VL, Miller WP, Wing EJ, et al. Disseminated listeriosis presenting as acute hepatitis. Am J Med. 1982;73:773–777.

28. Brandborg LL, Goldman IS. Bacterial and miscellaneous infections of the liver. In: Zakim DS, Boyer TD, eds. Hepatology. 2nd ed. Philadelphia: WB Saunders, 1990:1086–1098.

29. Nasrallah SM, Nassar VH. Enteric fever: A clinicopathologic study of 104 cases. Am J Gastroenterol. 1978;69(1):63–69.

30. Khosla SN, Singh R, Singh GP, Trehan VK. The spectrum of hepatic injury in enteric fever. Am J Gastroenterol. 1988;83(4):413–416.

31. Zimmerman HJ, Fang M, Utili R, et al. Jaundice due to bacterial infection. Gastroenterology. 1979;77(2):362–374.

32. Meals RA. Paratyphoid fever. A report of 62 cases with several unusual findings and review of the literature. Arch Intern Med. 1976;136:1422–1428.

33. Horney JT, Schwartzmann SW, Galambos JT. *Shigella* hepatitis. Am J Gastroenterol. 1976;66:146–149.

34. Stern MS, Gitnick GL. *Shigella* hepatitis. JAMA. 1976;235(24):2628–2629.

35. Greenawald KA, Nash G, Foley FD. Acute systemic melioidosis. Autopsy findings in four patients. Am J Clin Pathol. 1969;52:188–198.

36. Holmes KK, Counts GW, Beaty HN. Disseminated gonococcal infection. Ann Intern Med. 1971;74:979–993.

37. Vickers FN, Maloney PJ. Gonococcal perihepatitis. Arch Intern Med. 1964;114:120–123.

38. Lightfoot RW Jr, Gotschlich E. Gonococcal disease. Am J Med. 1974;56:327–356.

39. Kirby BD, Snyder KM, Meyer RD, Finegold SM. Legionnaire's disease: Clinical features of 24 cases. Ann Intern Med. 1978;89(3):297–309.

40. Wile UJ, Karshner RC. Icterus gravis syphiliticus: Its relationship to acute yellow atrophy. JAMA. 1917;68: 1311–1314.

41. Pareek SS. Liver involvement in secondary syphilis. Dig Dis Sci. 1979;24:41–43.

41a. Hahn RD. Syphilis of the liver. Am J Syph. 1943; 27:529–562.

42. Feher J, Somogyi T, Timmer M, et al. Early syphilitic hepatitis. Lancet. 1978;2:896–899.

43. Sobel HJ, Wolfe EH. Liver involvement in early syphilis. Arch Pathol. 1972;93:565–568.

44. Baker A, Kaplan M, Wolfe H, et al. Liver disease associated with early syphilis. N Engl J Med. 1971;284(25): 1422–1425.

45. Klatskin G. Hepatitis associated with systemic infections. In: Schiff L, ed. Diseases of the Liver. 4th ed. Philadelphia: JB Lippincott, 1975:711–754.

46. Harrington PT, Gutierrez JJ, Ramirez-Ronda CH, et al. Granulomatous hepatitis. Rev Infect Dis. 1982;4(3): 638–655.

47. Gilinsky NH, Campbell JAH, Kirsch RE. The clinical spectrum of hepatic granuloma. S Afr Med J. 1981; 60:691–694.

48. Vainrub B. Bacterial infections of the liver and biliary tract: Laboratory studies to determine etiology. In: Becker S, ed. Diagnostic Procedures in the Evaluation of Hepatic Diseases. Laboratory and Research Methods in Biology and Medicine. New York: Alan R, Liss; 1983;7:119–128.

49. Levine C. Primary macronodular hepatic tuberculosis: US and CT appearances. Gastrointest Radiol. 1990; 15:307–309.

50. Guckian JC, Perry JE. Granulomatous hepatitis: An analysis of 63 cases and review of the literature. Ann Intern Med. 1963;65:400–412.

51. Cucin RL, Coleman M, Eckardt J, et al. The diagnosis of miliary tuberculosis: Utility of peripheral blood abnormalities, bone marrow, and liver needle biopsy. J Chronic Dis. 1973;26:355–361.

52. Korn RJ, Kellow WF, Heller P, et al. Hepatic involvement in extrapulmonary tuberculosis—Histologic and functional characteristics. Am J Med. 1959;27:60–71.

53. Fauci AS. Granulomatous hepatitis. In: Mandel GL, Douglas RG, Bennett JE, eds. Principles and Practice of Infectious Diseases. New York: John Wiley 1979: 1070–1075.

54. Rimola A, Bory F, Teres J, et al. Oral nonabsorbable antibiotics prevent infection in cirrhotics with gastrointestinal hemorrhage. Hepatology. 1985;5:463–467.

55. Wyke RJ. Problems of bacterial infection in patients with liver disease. Gut. 1987;28:623–641.

56. Schmidt W, Lint J. Causes of death in alcoholics. J Stud Alcohol. 1972;33:171–185.

57. Tillotson JR, Lerner AM. Pneumonias caused by gram-negative bacilli. Medicine. 1966;45:65–76.

58. Burroughs AK, Rosenstein IJ, Epstein O, et al. Bacteriuria and primary biliary cirrhosis. Gut. 1984;25:133–137.

59. Buchbinder NA, Roberts WC. Alcoholism: An important but unemphasized factor predisposing to infective endocarditis. Arch Intern Med. 1973;132:689–692.

60. Wyke RJ, Rajkovic IA, Eddleston ALWF, et al. Defective opsonization and complement deficiency in serum from patients with fulminant hepatic failure. Gut. 1980;21:643–649.

61. Larcher VF, Wyke RJ, Mowat AP, et al. Mechanism of yeast opsonization defect in children with fulminant hepatic failure. Clin Exp Immunol. 1981;46:406–411.

62. Johnson WD Jr. Impaired defense mechanism associated with acute alcoholism. Ann N Y Acad Sci. 1975; 252:343–347.

63. Pirovino M, Meister F, Rubli E, Karlaganis G. Preserved cytosolic and synthetic liver function in jaundice of severe extrahepatic infection. Gastroenterology. 1989; 96(6):1589–1595.

64. Garvin IP. Remarks on pneumosa biliosa. South Med Surg. 1836;1:382–387.

65. Miller DJ, Keeton GR, Webber BL, Saunders BJ. Jaundice in severe bacterial infection. Gastroenterology. 1976;71:94–97.

66. Fang MH, Ginsberg AL, Dobbins WO. Marked elevation in serum alkaline phosphatase activity as a manifestation of systemic infection. Gastroenterology. 1980; 78(3):592–597.

67. Neale G, Caughey DE, Mollin DL, Booth CC. Effects of intrahepatic and extrahepatic infection on liver function. Br Med J. 1966;1:382–387.

68. Luderitz O, Galanos C, Lehmann V, et al. Lipid A: Chemical structure and biologic activity. J Infect Dis. 1973;128(Suppl):17–29.

69. Utili R, Abernathy CO, Zimmerman HJ. Cholestatic effects of *Escherichia coli* endotoxin on the isolated perfused rat liver. Gastroenterology. 1976;70:248–253.

70. Utili R, Abernathy CO, Zimmerman HJ. Effects of *Salmonella enteritidis* endotoxin on the excretory function of the isolated perfused rat liver. Proc Soc Exp Biol Med. 1977;155:184–188.

71. Gimson AE. Hepatic dysfunction during bacterial sepsis. Intensive Care Med. 1987;13:162–166.

72. Imamura M, Clowes G. Hepatic blood flow and oxygen consumption in starvation, sepsis, and septic shock. Surg Gynecol Obstet. 1975;141(1):27–34.

73. Morgan HR. Pathological changes produced by rabbits by a toxic sometic antigen derived from *Eberthella typhosa*. Am J Pathol. 1943;19:135–145.

74. Holman JM Jr, Saba TM. Hepatocyte injury during post-operative sepsis: Activated neutrophils as potential mediators. J Leukoc Biol. 1988;43(3):193–203.

75. Shurin SB, Anderson P, Zollinger J, Rathbun RK. Pathophysiology of hemolysis in infections with *Hemophilus influenzae* type B. J Clin Invest. 1986; 77(4):1340–1348.

76. Caruana JA Jr, Montes M, Camara DS, et al. Functional and histopathologic changes in the liver during sepsis. Surg Gynecol Obstet. 1982;1545(5):653–656.

77. Vermillon SE, Gregg JA, Baggenstoss AH, et al. Jaundice associated with bacteremia. Arch Intern Med. 1969;124:611–618.

78. Bernuau D, Rogier E, Feldmann G. Decreased albumin and increased fibrinogen secretion by single hepatocytes from rats with acute inflammatory reaction. Hepatology. 1983;3:29–33.

79. Sganga G, Siegel J, Brown G, et al. Reprioritization of hepatic plasma protein release in trauma and sepsis. Arch Surg. 1986;120(2):187–189.

80. Clowes G, George B, Villee C, et al. Muscle proteolysis induced by a circulating peptide in patients with sepsis and trauma. N Engl J Med. 1983;308:545–552.

81. Baracos V, Rodemann HP, Dinarello C, et al. Stimulation of muscle protein degradation and prostaglandin E2 release by leukocytic pyrogen (interleukin-1): A mechanism for the increased degradation of muscle proteins during fever. N Engl J Med. 1983;308(10): 553–558.

82. Ransohoff DF, Miller GL, Forsythe SB, et al. Outcome of acute cholecystitis in patients with diabetes mellitus. Ann Intern Med. 1987;106:829–832.

83. Sandler RS, Maule W, Baltus ME. Factors associated with postoperative complications in diabetics after biliary tract surgery. Gastroenterology. 1986;91:157–162.

84. Glenn F. Surgical management of acute cholecystitis in patients 65 years of age and older. Ann Surg. 1981;193(1):56–59.

85. Matolo NM, LaMorte WW, Wolfe BM. Acute and chronic cholecystitis. Surg Clin North Am. 1981;61: 875–883.

86. Cox GR, Browne BJ. Acute cholecystitis in the emergency department. J Emerg Med. 1989;7:501–511.

87. Thornell E, Kral JG, Jansson R, et al. Inhibition of prostaglandin synthesis as treatment for biliary pain. Lancet. 1979;1(8116):584.

88. Roslyn JJ, DenBesten L, Thompson JE Jr, Silverman BF. Roles of lithogenic bile and cystic duct occlusion in the pathogenesis of acute cholecystitis. Am J Surg. 1980;140(1):126–130.

89. Thomas CG Jr, Womack NA. Acute cholecystitis, its pathogenesis and repair. Arch Surg. 1952;64:590–600.

90. Sjodahl R, Wetterfors J. Lysolecithin and lecithin in the gallbladder and bile: Their possible roles in the pathogenesis of acute cholecystitis. Scand J Gastroenterol. 1974;9(6):519–525.

91. Sjodahl R, Tagesson C, Wetterfors J. On the pathogenesis of acute cholecystitis. Surg Gynecol Obstet. 1978;146:199–202.

92. Sjodahl R, Tagesson C. On the development of primary acute cholecystitis. Scand J Gastroenterol. 1983;18: 577–579.

93. Csendes A, Sepulveda A. Intraluminal gallbladder pressure measurements in patients with chronic or acute cholecystitis. Am J Surg. 1980;139(3):383–384.

94. Rosch J, Grolman JH Jr, Steckel RJ. Arteriography in the diagnosis of gallbladder disease. Radiology. 1969; 92(7):1485–1491.

95. Claesson B, Holmlund D, Matzsch T. Biliary microflora in acute cholecystitis and the clinical implications. Acta Chir Scand. 1984;150:229–237.

96. Krasna MJ, Flancbaum L. Electrocardiographic changes in cardiac patients with acute gallbladder disease. Am Surg. 1986;52:541–543.

97. Carroll BA. Preferred imaging techniques for the diagnosis of cholecystitis and cholelithiasis. Ann Surg. 1989;210(1):1–12.

98. Fink-Benett D, Freitas JE, Ripley SD, et al. The sensitivity of hepatobiliary imaging and real time ultrasonography in the detection of acute cholecystitis. Arch Surg. 1985;120:904–906.

99. Ashley SW, Cheung LY. New diagnostic techniques in hepatobiliary disease. Surg Annu. 1985;17:41–67.

100. Weissmann HS, Berkowitz D, Fox MS, et al. The role of technetium-99m iminodiacetic acid (IDA) cholescintigraphy in acute acalculous cholecystitis. Radiology. 1983;146(1):177–178.

101. Pellegrini CA, Way LW. Acute cholangitis. In: Way LW,

Pellegrini CA, eds. Surgery of the Gallbladder and Bile Ducts. Philadelphia: WB Saunders, 1987:251.

102. Wetstein L, Attkiss M, Aufses AH Jr. Acute torsion of the gallbladder: Review of the literature and report of a case. Am Surg. 1976;42(2):138–141.

103. Strohl EL, Diffenbaugh WG, Baker JH, et al. Gangrene and perforation of the gallbladder. Inst Abstr Surg. 1962;114:1.

104. Glenn F, Reed C, Grafe WR. Biliary enteric fistula. Surg Gynecol Obstet. 1981;153(4):527–531.

105. Piedad OH, Wels PB. Spontaneous internal biliary fistula: Obstructive and nonobstructive types. Twenty-year review of 55 cases. Ann Surg. 1972;175(1):75–80.

106. LeBlanc KA, Barr LH, Rush BM. Spontaneous biliary enteric fistulas. South Med J. 1983;76:1249–1252.

107. Alberti-Flor JJ, Hernandez M, Dunn GGD, et al. Cholecystoduodenal fistula. Am J Gastroenterol. 1985; 80(8):655–657.

108. Urakami Y, Kishi S. Endoscopic fistulotomy for parapapillary choledochoduodenal fistula. Endoscopy. 1978;10(4):289–294.

109. Hoppenstein JM, Mendoza CB, Watke AL. Choledochoduodenal fistula due to perforating duodenal ulcer disease. Am Surg. 1971;173(1):145–147.

110. Cooper SG, Sherman SB, Steinhardt JE, et al. Bouveret's syndrome. Diagnostic considerations. JAMA. 1987; 258(2):226–228.

111. Starling JR, Matallana RH. Benign mechanical obstruction of the common hepatic duct (Mirizzi syndrome). Surgery. 1980;88(5):737–740.

112. Muller EL, Pitt HA, Thompson JE Jr, et al. Antibiotics in infections of the biliary tract. Surg Gynecol Obstet. 1987;165(4):285–292.

113. Jarvinen JH, Hastbacka J. Early cholecystectomy for acute cholecystitis. A prospective randomized study. Ann Surg. 1980;191(4):501–505.

114. Lahtinen J, Alhava EM, Aukee S. Acute cholecystitis treated by early and delayed surgery. A controlled clinical trial. Scan J Gastroenterol. 1978;13(6):673–678.

115. McArthur P, Cuschieri A, Sells RA, Shields R. Controlled clinical trial comparing early with interval cholecystectomy for acute cholecystitis. Br J Surg. 1975;62(10):850–852.

116. van der Linden W, Sunzel H. Early versus delayed operation for acute cholecystitis: A controlled clinical trial. Am J Surg. 1970;120(1):7–13.

117. Bateson MC. Gallstone disease—Present and future. Lancet. 1986;2:1265–1267.

118. Dunn JP. Laparoscopic cholecystectomy: Initial New Zealand experience. N Z Med J. 1992;105(928):47–49.

119. Smith JF, Boysen D, Tschirhart J, Williams T. Risks and benefits of laparoscopic cholecystectomy in the community hospital setting. J Laparoscop Surg. 1991; 1(6):325–32.

120. Talamini MA, Gadacz TR. Laparoscopic approach to cholecystectomy. Adv Surg. 1992;25:1–20.

121. Cohen MM. Initial experience with laparoscopic cholecystectomy in a teaching hospital. Can J Surg. 1992;35(1):59–63.

122. Sigman HH, Fried GM, Hinchey EJ, et al. Role of the teaching hospital in the development of a laparoscopic cholecystectomy program. Can J Surg. 1992;35(1):49–54.

123. Larson GM, Vitale GC, Casey J, et al. Multipractice analysis of laparoscopic cholecystectomy in 1,983 patients. Am J Surg. 1992;163(2):221–226.

124. Ruers TJ, Jakimowicz JJ. Laparoscopic cholecystectomy: A new trend in the management of gallstone disease. Scand J Gastroenterol Suppl. 1991;188:8–12.

125. Jacobs M, Verdeja JC, Goldstein HS. Laparoscopic cholecystectomy in acute cholecystitis. J Laparoendosc Surg. 1991;1(3):175–177.

126. Cronin KJ, Kerin MJ, Williams NN, et al. Endoscopic management of common duct stones with laparoscopic cholecystectomy. Ir J Med Sci. 1991;160(9):265–267.

127. Smith PC, Clayman RV, Soper NJ. Laparoscopic cholecystectomy and choledochoscopy for the treatment of cholelithiasis and choledocholithiasis. Surgery. 1992; 111(2):230–233.

128. Dion YM, Morin J, Dionne G, Dejoie C. Laparoscopic cholecystectomy and choledocholithiasis. Can J Surg. 1992;35(1):67–74.

129. Joyce WP, Keane R, Burke GJ, Daly M, et al. Identification of bile duct stones in patients undergoing laparoscopic cholecystectomy. Br J Surg. 1991;78(10):1174–1176.

130. Eggermont AM, Lameris JS, Jeekel J. Ultrasound-guided percutaneous transhepatic cholecystostomy for acute acalculous cholecystitis. Arch Surg. 1985; 120(12):1354–1356.

131. Kasahara Y, Umemura H, Shiraha S. Gallstone ileus. Review of 112 patients in the Japanese literature. Am J Surg. 1980;140(3):437–440.

132. Ullman M, Hasselgren PO, Tveit E. Posttraumatic and postoperative acute acalculous cholecystitis. Acta Chir Scand. 1984;150(6):507–509.

133. Pieretti R, Auldist AW, Stephens CA. Acute cholecystitis in children. Surg Gynecol Obstet. 1975;140(1):16–18.

134. Petersen SR, Sheldon GF. Acute acalculous cholecystitis. A complication of hyperalimentation. Am J Surg. 1979;138:814–817.

135. Glenn F, Becker CG. Acute acalculous cholecystitis. An increasing entity. Ann Surg. 1982;195(2):131–136.

136. Margulis SJ, Honig CL, Soave R, et al. Biliary tract obstruction in the acquired immunodeficiency syndrome. Ann Intern Med. 1986;105:207–210.

137. McFadden DW, Smith GW. Hemodialysis-associated hemorrhagic cholecystitis. Am J Gastroenterol. 1987; 82:1081–1083.

138. Becker CG, Dubin T, Glenn F. Induction of acute cholecystitis by activation of factor XII. J Exp Med. 1980;151(1):81–90.

139. Howard RJ. Acute acalculous cholecystitis. Am J Surg. 1982;141:194–198.

140. Mirvis SE, Vainright JR, Nelson AW, et al. The diagnosis of acute acalculous cholecystitis: A comparison of sonography, scintigraphy, and CT. AJR Am J Roentgenol. 1986;147(6):1171–1175.

141. Charcot JM. Leçons sur les maladies du fore des voies filares et des reins. Thesis. Paris, 1877.

142. Reynolds BM, Dargan EL. Acute obstructive cholangitis. Ann Surg. 1959;150:299–303.

143. Pitluk HC, Beal JM. Choledocholithiasis associated with acute cholecystitis. Arch Surg. 1979;114(8):887–888.

144. Stubbs RS, McLoy RF, Blumgart LH. Cholelithiasis and cholecystitis: Surgical treatment. Clin Gastroenterol. 1983;12:179–201.

145. Vennes JA. Management of calculi in the common duct. Semin Liver Dis. 1983;3:162–171.

146. Sievert W, Vakil NB. Emergencies of the biliary tract. Gastroenterol Clin North Am. 1988;17(2):245–264.

147. Flemma RJ, Flint IM, Osterhout S, et al. Bacteriologic studies of biliary tract infection. Ann Surg. 1967; 166(4):563–572.

148. Nielsen ML, Justsen T. Anaerobic and aerobic bacteriological studies in biliary tract disease. Scand J Gastroenterol. 1976;11(5):437–446.

149. Huang T, Bass JA, Williams RD. The significance of biliary pressure in cholangitis. Arch Surg. 1969; 98(5):629–632.

150. O'Connor MJ, Schwartz ML, McQuarrie DG, et al. Cholangitis due to malignant obstruction of biliary flow. Ann Surg. 1980;193:341–345.

151. Dineen P. The importance of the route of infection in experimental biliary obstruction. Surg Gynecol Obstet. 1964;119:1001–1012.

152. Scott AJ, Kahn GA. Origin of bacteria in common duct bile. Lancet. 1967;2(520):790–792.

153. Thompson JE, Tompkins RD, Longmire WP. Factors in management of acute cholangitis. Ann Surg. 1981; 195:25–26.

154. O'Connor MJ, Schwartz ML, McQuarrie DG, et al. Acute bacterial cholangitis: An analysis of clinical manifestation. Arch Surg. 1982;117:437–441.

155. Saharia PC, Cameron JL. Clinical management of cholangitis. Surg Gynecol Obstet. 1976;142(3):369–372.

156. Kaplun L, Weissmann HS, Rosenblatt RR, et al. The early diagnosis of common bile duct obstruction using cholescintigraphy. JAMA. 1985;254(17):2431–2434.

157. Miller DR, Egbert RM, Braunstein P. Comparison of ultrasound and hepatobiliary imaging in the early detection of acute total common bile duct obstruction. Arch Surg. 1984;119:1233–1237.

158. Taylor KJW, Rosenfield AT, Spiro HM. Diagnostic accurancy of gray scale ultrasonography for the jaundiced patient. Arch Intern Med. 1979;139:60–63.

159. Beinart C, Efremedis S, Cohen B, et al. Obstruction without dilatation: Importance in evaluating jaundice. JAMA. 1981;245:353–356.

160. Cronan JJ, Mueller PR, Simeone JF, et al. Prospective diagnosis of choledocholithiasis. Radiology. 1983;146: 467–469.

161. Baron RL. Common bile duct stones: Reassessment of criteria for CT diagnosis. Radiology. 1987;162:419–424.

162. Chock E, Wolfe BM, Matolo NM. Acute suppurative cholangitis. Surg Clin North Am. 1981;61:885–892.

162a. Martin DF, Tweedle DE. Endoscopic management of common duct stones without cholecystectomy. Br J Surg. 1987;74(3):209–211.

163. Joseph PK, Bizer LS, Sprayregen SS, et al. Percutaneous transhepatic biliary drainage, results and complications in 81 patients. JAMA. 1986;255(20):2763–2767.

164. Leese T, Neoptolemos JP, Carr-Locke DL. Success, failure, early complications and their management following endoscopic sphincterotomy: Results in 394 consecutive patients from a single center. Br J Surg. 1986;72(3):215–219.

164a. Leese T, Neoptolemos JP, Baker AR, Carr-Locke DL. Management of acute cholangitis and the impact of endoscopic sphincterotomy. Br J Surg 1986;73:988–992.

165. Vallon AG, Shorvon PJ, Cotton PB. Duodenoscopic treatment of acute cholangitis. Gut. 1982;23:A915.

166. Haupert AP, Carey LC, Evans WE, et al. Acute suppurative cholangitis: Experience with 15 consecutive cases. Arch Surg. 1967;94:460–468.

167. Boey JH, Way LW. Acute cholangitis. Ann Surg. 1980;191:264–270.

168. Classen M. Endoscopic papillotomy—New indications, short and long term results. Clin Gastroenterol. 1986;15:446–457.

169. Pitt HA, Postier RG, Cameron JL. Consequences of preoperative cholangitis and its treatment on the outcome of surgery for choledocholithiasis. Surgery. 1983;94(3):447–452.

170. Cook J, Hou PC, Ho HC, et al. Recurrent pyogenic cholangitis. Br J Surg. 1954;42:188–203.

171. Fan ST, Lae EC, Mok FP, et al. Acute cholangitis secondary to hepatolithiasis. Arch Surg. 1991;126(8):1027–1031.

172. Chou ST, Chan CW. Recurrent pyogenic cholangitis: A necropsy study. Pathology. 1980;12(3):415–428.

173. Teoh TB. A study of gallstones and included worms in recurrent pyogenic cholangitis. J Pathol Bacteriol. 1963;86:123–129.

174. Tabata M, Nakayama F. Bacteria and gallstones—Etiological significance. Dig Dis Sci. 1981;26(3):218–224.

175. Cetta FM. Bile infection documented as initial event in the pathogenesis of brown pigment biliary stones. Hepatology. 1986;6(3):482–489.

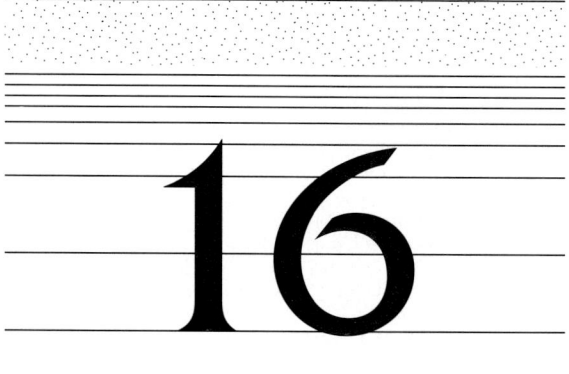

16

Hepatobiliary Infections in AIDS

SCOTT L. FRIEDMAN, M.D.

The liver and biliary tree are frequently sites of opportunistic infection in the patient with human immunodeficiency virus (HIV) infection (Table 16–1). These infections may occur at any stage of HIV disease, from the otherwise asymptomatic state to end-stage immunodeficiency. The involvement of the liver or biliary tract by opportunistic infection is not an unusual criterion to establish the diagnosis of acquired immunodeficiency syndrome (AIDS) in an HIV-infected individual[1] (Table 16–2).

Infections of liver and biliary system may be due to bacteria (including acid-fast bacilli), fungi, viruses—even HIV itself—or protozoa (see Table 16–1). Which of these opportunistic infections is most likely in a given patient is in part determined by the stage of HIV infection. For example, diseases due to most bacteria, including *Mycobacterium tuberculosis*, may be seen at early or intermediate stages of immunocompromise, when CD4 lymphocyte count is 200–750 per mm³. By contrast, infections by protozoa, fungi, and other bacteria, especially *Mycobacterium avium-intracellulare*, tend to occur with advanced immunocompromise, when CD4 counts are severely depressed ($<200/mm^3$). Infections due to the hepatotrophic viruses, hepatitis B virus (HBV), hepatitis C virus (HCV), and hepatitis D virus, or hepatitis delta virus (HDV), do not appear to be stage-specific in that liver

---

TABLE 16–1. HEPATOBILIARY INFECTIONS IN PATIENTS INFECTED WITH HIV

BACTERIA, MYCOBACTERIA	**VIRUSES**
Mycobacterium avium-intracellulare	Cytomegalovirus
Mycobacterium kansasii	Herpes simplex
Mycobacterium tuberculosis	Adenovirus
Rochalimaea henselae	Human immunodeficiency virus
Rochalimaea quintana	Hepatitis B, C, D (delta)
? *Salmonella, Shigella* sp.	
PROTOZOA	**FUNGI**
Pneumocystis carinii	*Histoplasma capsulatum*
Microsporidia (*Enterocytozoon bieneusi, Encephalitozoon cuniculi*)	*Cryptococcus neoformans*
Cryptosporidium parvum	*Coccidioides immitis*
Leishmania donovani	
Toxoplasma gondii	
Dicrocoelium dendriticum	

391

TABLE 16–2. HEPATOBILIARY INFECTIONS THAT ESTABLISH A DIAGNOSIS OF AIDS

WITHOUT LABORATORY EVIDENCE OF HIV INFECTION
Assume no other causes of immunosuppression
DEFINITE EVIDENCE OF
   Cryptosporidiosis > 1 mo
   Cytomegalovirus > 1 mo
   Herpes infection > 1 mo
   Mycobacterium avium or *Mycobacterium kansasii,*
     disseminated
WITH LABORATORY EVIDENCE OF HIV INFECTION
DEFINITE EVIDENCE OF
   Disseminated mycobacteria, non-TB
   Extrapulmonary TB
   Recurrent *Salmonella* bacteremia
   Disseminated coccidioidomycosis
   Disseminated histoplasmosis
PRESUMPTIVE EVIDENCE OF
   Mycobacterial disease, disseminated

disease due to these agents may occur during any stage of co-infection with HIV.

In addition to specific infections, a large number of so-called nonspecific pathologic conditions are frequently seen.[2] With increasing awareness of the spectrum of diseases in HIV-infected individuals has come the recognition that some formerly thought nonspecific findings are, in fact, specific manifestations of newly recognized pathogens as, for one clear example, is the case in the association of peliosis hepatis with a newly characterized bacterium.

With the exception of hepatotrophic viruses, most infections of the liver or biliary tree in HIV infection or AIDS are usually part of a systemic infection and are thus frequently identified in blood or lymph node culture prior to their isolation from liver. In particular, mycobacterial infection with *M. avium* and *M. tuberculosis,* infections with cytomegalovirus (CMV), and most fungal infections are identified in this way.

This chapter reviews hepatobiliary infections from two perspectives. First, characteristics of infections grouped according to their class are reviewed along with general guidelines for therapy. Second, practical aspects of evaluating abnormal liver chemistries and hepatobiliary symptoms are offered, emphasizing the role of imaging studies and liver biopsy.

CHARACTERISTICS OF HEPATOBILIARY INFECTIONS IN AIDS

Bacterial Infections

Mycobacterium

Mycobacterium avium-intracellulare is consistently the most frequent specific hepatic finding

in AIDS, occurring in 19 to 70% of patients.[3, 4] The pathologic hallmark of the infection is the presence of poorly formed granulomata containing large numbers of acid-fast bacilli within foamy histiocytes.[5] Organisms are less commonly seen outside of granulomata but may be cultured from liver biopsy in the absence of infected histiocytes.[6] Acid-fast smear of infected tissue typically reveals organisms that cannot be distinguished from *M. tuberculosis* until further typed by culturing. The sensitivity of acid-fast bacillus smear in diagnosing hepatic disease is not established, but the infection may be inapparent histologically and diagnosed subsequently by tissue culture.[7] In children with AIDS, *M. avium* has been reported primarily as a postmortem finding, with some unique histopathologic features, including a pseudosarcomatous variant and multinucleated giant cells.[8]

As indicated, *M. avium* infection of the liver is virtually always part of a systemic infection. It is associated with fever, night sweats, lymphadenopathy, and, occasionally, diarrhea. Bone marrow infiltration is common, and pulmonary disease is occasionally seen.[9] Large intra-abdominal adenopathy seen on imaging studies raises the suspicion of *M. avium*; directed skinny needle biopsy of such nodes may reveal the organism and obviate liver biopsy in some cases.[10] Typically, liver involvement is associated with marked elevations of serum alkaline phosphatase and with only modest elevations of bilirubin aspartate aminotransferase (AST) and alanine aminotransferase (ALT).[2] More than 25 isolates have been identified, with no single type predominating in liver.[9]

Treatment of *M. avium* in AIDS is not completely satisfactory in that some reduction in bacterial load is seen, often in association with subjective symptomatic improvement, but complete eradication of the organism is unusual. In symptomatic patients, multidrug regimes are employed; commonly used combinations may include rifampin, amikacin, ciprofloxacin, streptomycin, and azithromycin.[11, 12]

Mycobacterium tuberculosis infections, in contrast to those of *M. avium-intracellulare,* may occur before patients are profoundly immunocompromised.[13] Symptoms are those commonly associated with tuberculosis (TB) in immunocompetent patients: fever, cough, night sweats, and, occasionally, lymphadenopathy. Hepatobiliary disease may also be heralded by abdominal pain, jaundice, or hepatosplenomegaly. Extrapulmonary diseases including those of the liver are common in HIV-infected patients (25–70%),[14] and may present independent of, or in association with, pulmonary involvement.[15] Other

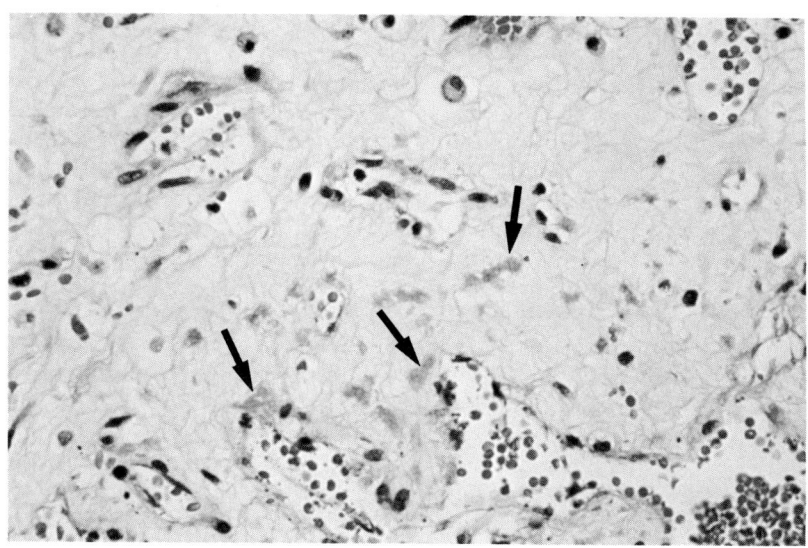

FIGURE 16–1.
Microscopic appearance of bacillary peliosis hepatis. Photomicrograph of liver biopsy specimen revealing dilated vascular spaces containing red blood cells. Dark clusters *(arrows)* within the stroma or adjacent to vascular lakes are clumps of bacteria. (hematoxylin and eosin, ×500) SOURCE: Courtesy of Dr Linda Ferrell, UCSF Department of Pathology, San Francisco, CA. [See also Color Plate 4]

manifestations, including tuberculous abscesses[16, 17] and bile duct tuberculomas[13] are rarely seen. Hepatic *M. tuberculosis* is usually diagnosed by culturing acid-fast bacilli from liver tissue obtained by percutaneous or laparoscopic biopsy; this is the most sensitive diagnostic test and may produce positive findings in the absence of overt granulomata or positive acid-fast stain. Treatment should include three-drug therapy initially (isoniazid, rifampin, and either pyrazinamide or ethambutol) followed by isoniazid and rifampin for 6 to 12 months.[14, 15, 18]

Rarer atypical mycobacteria, including *Mycobacterium kansasii* and *Mycobacterium xenopi,*[19–21] are occasionally seen in patients infected with HIV, although the prevalence of extrapulmonary disease in this small number of patients cannot be estimated accurately. Manifestations of these atypical mycobacteria in liver are similar to those of other mycobacterial diseases in AIDS.

Rochalimaea and Bacillary Peliosis Hepatis

Bacillary peliosis hepatis is a recently recognized hepatic manifestation of systemic infection by either *Rochalimaea henselae* or *Rochalimaea quintana,* two newly characterized bacteria closely related to *Bartonella* species (order Rickettsiales).[22–25] In liver, infection is associated with dilated vascular lakes typical of peliosis hepatis; non-HIV–related peliosis hepatis is not associated with these bacteria.[22, 26] HIV-associated peliotic lesions may be massive or small, single or multiple. The infection is more commonly observed in those HIV-infected patients with CD4 counts <200 per mm³, and is associated with a number of prominent extrahepatic man-

ifestations. These manifestations include cutaneous angiomatous lesions typical of cat-scratch disease (the infections are associated with either ownership or contact with cats)[27] and lytic bone lesions.[28]

Symptoms in infected patients may include fever, chills, sweats, bone pain, cutaneous angiomatous lesions, and abdominal or right upper quadrant pain; larger clinical series are awaited before the frequency and full range of symptoms can be accurately reported. A patient has been described in whom anemia was attributed to sequestration of red cells within vascular lakes.[29]

The diagnosis of bacillary peliosis hepatis may be established by blood culture in which lysis centrifugation tubes are used, by tissue culture on chocolate agar or by immunofluorescence, immunoblot, or polymerase chain reaction studies.[22] Polymerase chain reaction has proved an especially useful technique in classifying newly identified organisms that may be difficult to isolate by more conventional means.[23]

Several pathologic features are characteristic of bacillary peliosis hepatis. A hallmark of the disease is the presence of the dilated vascular lakes, which are associated with proliferation of sinusoidal endothelial cells, extravasation of red blood cells, blebbing of hepatocyte membranes, and dilation of Disse's spaces.[29] Tissue examined with Warthin-Starry silver stain reveals clumps of purple bacteria within a myxoid stroma (Fig. 16–1); bacteria can be most readily identified either with high-power light microscopy or with electron microscopy.[26, 29]

Recommendations for therapy of bacillary peliosis hepatis are evolving but include prolonged treatment for a minimum of 2 to 4

months with either erythromycin or doxycycline. Responses to antimycobacterials,[28] cephalosporins, and ampicillin with sublactams have
also been observed.[26, 29] Clinical improvement in
most cases is the rule, including resolution of
even large peliotic spaces.[29] Because the infection is relatively chronic and indolent, lifelong
antibiotic therapy may ultimately prove essential
if recurrences are frequently noted. Interestingly, earlier reports of histologic features in
liver during HIV infection identified peliosis hepatis as a common nonspecific finding.[30, 31] The
recognition that this finding is a manifestation
of a specific infection raises the question of
whether other nonspecific lesions, including
Kupffer cell hyperplasia and culture-negative
granulomata (Fig. 16–2), may also be ascribed
eventually to as yet uncharacterized microorganisms.

Low-grade hepatic persistence of enteric bacterial pathogens, particularly *Salmonella* and *Shigella* species, may explain the high rate of recurrent bacteremia from these and related
organisms in patients with HIV infection.[32, 33]
Failure to clear or kill bacteria in portal blood
may be one consequence of hepatic macrophage infection by HIV.

Viral Infections

Cytomegalovirus

Cytomegalovirus is the most frequent infectious pathogen in AIDS, and the liver is found
to be involved in 5 to 25% of liver biopsies.[7, 30]
As with most infections of liver, CMV hepatitis
is always part of systemic CMV infection; it is
uncommonly a major source of symptoms independent of other sites of CMV infection such as
retina, colon, and esophagus. Clinical findings
may include fevers and right upper quadrant
pain in association with nonspecific elevations
of liver chemistries. Typical viral inclusions that
create an owl's eye appearance are usually identified in Kupffer cells but can sometimes be
seen in hepatocytes or sinusoidal endothelial
cells (Fig. 16–3)[7, 34, 35] or in association with
granulomata.[3, 36, 37] Mononuclear cell infiltration
and microabscesses with neutrophils are common findings.[35] Monoclonal antibody staining,[38]
in situ hybridization, and viral culture of liver
tissue can be used to support the diagnosis of
hepatic CMV.[35] Rarely does it happen that treatment of CMV is required solely because of hepatic involvement, but in such cases ganciclovir
or foscarnet is likely to be effective.[39]

Biliary involvement with CMV is frequently
seen in patients with progressive ductal changes
termed HIV-associated cholangiopathy. First described in 1983 by Pitlik and colleagues[40] and
Guarda and colleagues,[41] the syndrome has
been characterized as consisting of intra- or extrahepatic ductal narrowing similar, but not
identical, to sclerosing cholangitis.[42–44] Ampullary biopsies may reveal typical CMV-like intranuclear inclusions in epithelial cells in association with positive cultures for CMV. In many
cases *Cryptosporidium* has been identified instead
of, or in addition to, CMV. The incidence of the
syndrome may be higher than originally suspected; in some patients with CMV viremia, cholestatic changes have been identified in asymptomatic individuals.[45] An etiologic role for CMV

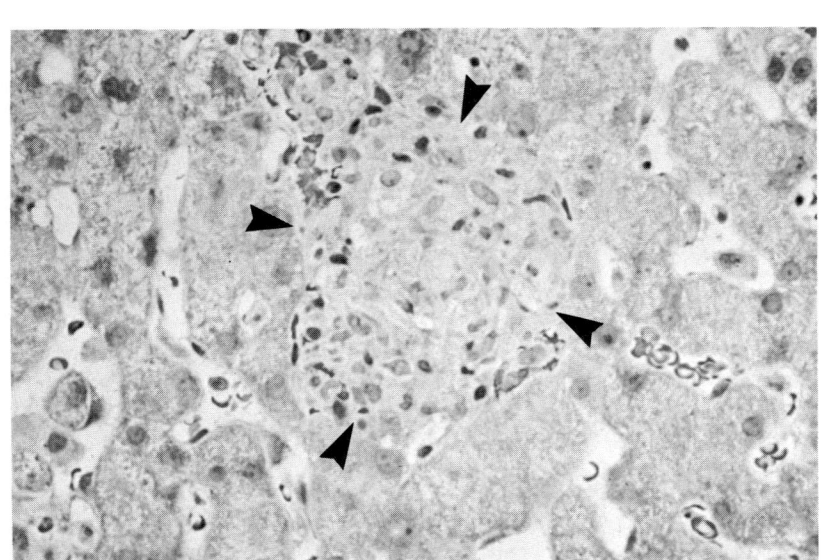

FIGURE 16–2.
Hepatic granuloma in AIDS. Liver
biopsy from a patient with AIDS
demonstrating a granuloma *(arrowheads)*, without associated microorganisms. Granulomata are frequently identified as a nonspecific
finding in patients with AIDS. (hematoxylin and eosin, ×325)
SOURCE: Courtesy of Dr Linda Ferrell, UCSF Department of Pathology, San Francisco, CA. [See also
Color Plate 4]

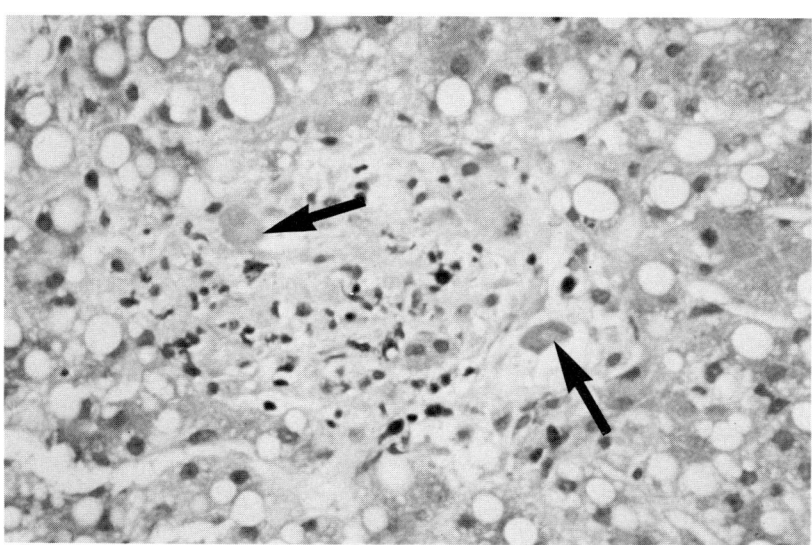

FIGURE 16–3.
Hepatic cytomegalovirus infection. Liver biopsy specimen demonstrating cytomegalic cells *(arrows)* with variable staining of the cytoplasm, which may contain inclusions of viral particles typical of hepatic CMV disease. (hematoxylin and eosin, ×250) SOURCE: Courtesy of Dr Linda Ferrell, UCSF Department of Pathology, San Francisco, CA. [See also Color Plate 4]

or *Cryptosporidium* in this syndrome has not been established, however, because not all patients have evidence of infection. Also arguing against an etiologic role for CMV has been the lack of response to ganciclovir, an agent with efficacy against CMV in other sites. One possibility is that all patients have CMV, but the virus is not detected in some. Alternatively, a subset of patients may have a unique immunologic response of the biliary system to some unidentified antigen,[43] as has been proposed for sclerosing cholangitis associated with inflammatory bowel disease.[46]

Cytomegalovirus-related acalculous cholecystitis has also been described in AIDS patients[47–50] and presents with severe abdominal pain and occasionally peritonitis. Cytomegalovirus cholecystitis does not appear to be part of the HIV-cholangiopathy syndrome since the two rarely coexist in the same patient.

Herpesvirus and Adenovirus

Like CMV, herpesvirus involvement of liver may on rare occasion be clinically important, with hepatic necrosis and hemorrhage[35, 51] in association with Cowdry-type inclusions. Increased rates of viral replication for all herpesviruses (including CMV) have been reported in patients co-infected with HIV, and direct interaction of the two viruses in co-infected cells may even contribute to enhanced expression of HIV.[52–54] Hepatic herpesvirus disease is usually seen in association with disseminated infection and viral culture of liver biopsy material may identify the organism.[55] Herpes may be a more common cause of liver disease in pediatric than in adult AIDS; a number of children with

chronic active hepatitis have been reported.[56–58] Although no reports citing treatment have been published, acyclovir would be appropriate for use in well-documented cases. A single case of adenovirus hepatitis and necrosis has been reported in an HIV-positive patient with disseminated adenovirus infection.[59]

Human Immunodeficiency Virus

Strong evidence exists for the direct infection of liver by HIV.[60] Immunohistochemical stains of human liver tissue using monoclonal antibodies to the HIV p24 antigen have demonstrated viral antigen within Kupffer cells (hepatic macrophages).[61–64] Its presence may account for the frequent nonspecific findings of Kupffer cell hyperplasia and giant cell formation reported in earlier series.[6] More recently, infection by HIV of human Kupffer cells has been achieved in culture[66, 67] and may be mediated by CD4 receptors.[67] Sinusoidal endothelial cells also express CD4 receptors, which allows for low-level infection of cultured sinusoidal endothelial cells.[60] By contrast, infection of hepatocytes has not been consistently observed in vivo or in culture.[60]

The identification of HIV in Kupffer cells is not surprising given the propensity of the virus to infect macrophages.[68] This finding has at least two important implications: 1) Any therapeutic strategies to clear the virus must account for the liver as a significant viral reservoir; 2) HIV infection of Kupffer cells is likely to result in impairment of macrophage function.[69] This impaired reticuloendothelial cell function may account, for example, for the high incidence of enteric bacteremia in patients with HIV infection. Elucidation of the role of liver cell populations in HIV infection and replication of the virus will probably be further advanced by the use of feline and primate models of the disease.[60]

Hepatitis B Virus

The prevalence of positive serologic tests indicating past or present infection with HBV is high in AIDS patients but no different from that in patients without AIDS who are homosexuals or intravenous drug users. Clinical and autopsy studies in AIDS patients have reported a prevalence approaching 90% in serologic evidence for past or present HBV infection.[7]

The high likelihood of HBV infection in the male homosexual population was well recognized before the AIDS epidemic. The likelihood of its presence has been related to the duration of homosexual activity, the number of non-steady sexual partners, and the frequency of anal-genital or oral-anal contact.[70]

In patients with past or present infection with HBV, HIV infection leads to alterations of HBV antigen-antibody display, viral replication, and clinical consequences.[71] By contrast, no definitive evidence exists to demonstrate that HBV alters the behavior of HIV.[71] Several reports have described the reappearance of hepatitis B surface antigen (HBsAg) in HIV-infected patients previously thought to be immune to HBV, as indicated by the presence of antibody directed to hepatitis B surface antigen (anti-HBs).[72, 73] Recurrence of HBsAg may arise from either reinfection or reactivation.[73] In addition, the loss of naturally acquired anti-HBs is accelerated, even in those patients who remain HBsAg-negative.[74, 75] Associated with loss or reduction in immunity to HBV is increased prevalence of hepatitis B e antigen (HBeAg) expression, elevated mean levels of deoxyribonucleic acid (DNA)-polymerase, and increased titers of antibodies directed to hepatitis B core antigen (anti-HBc).[72, 76, 77] Thus, a larger proportion of patients with HIV and HBV infections are chronic carriers of HBV[78] and have highly infectious serum and body fluids compared with those who are HIV-negative. This conclusion underscores the importance of adhering closely to universal body substance precautions and of vaccinating susceptible immunocompetent individuals with HBV vaccine.

Interestingly, although HIV leads to more prevalent chronic HBV carriage, it appears to reduce the severity of clinical liver disease in most,[76, 77, 79] but not all,[80, 81] patients, as measured by mean elevation of AST and ALT. In one study, the mean ALT level correlated with CD4 lymphocyte count.[79] One interesting case cites dramatic improvement in HBV-induced liver injury after subsequent infection by HIV.[82] The mechanism for reduced HBV-related liver injury after HIV infection is not certain but has been attributed to a diminution in lymphocyte-mediated hepatocellular injury as a result of HIV effects on lymphocytes. Specifically, the capacity to generate T and B lymphocytes sensitized to HBV proteins may be impaired.[83] Despite the general observation that liver injury from HBV may be attenuated by HIV co-infection, progressive liver disease with fatal hepatic failure is still observed in patients co-infected with the two viruses.[81]

The failure of patients with HIV infection to reliably clear HBsAg has suggested that AIDS patients have a deficient systemic alpha-interferon response,[84] a suggestion that is supported by studies showing a lack of efficacy of alpha-interferon for HBV in HIV-positive patients.[85] Antiretroviral treatment with zidovudine likewise has no effect on HBV replication.[86, 87]

Not only does HIV affect the behavior of HBV, but HBV might stimulate the expression of HIV. Several studies suggest that the X gene product of HBV may enhance transcription of HIV in a process known as transactivation,[88] which involves specific soluble transcription factors.[89] Furthermore, the localization of HBV and HIV DNA sequences together in peripheral mononuclear cells[90–92] underscores the potential relevance of transactivation to the clinical courses of HIV and HBV in vivo.

The presence of HIV also reduces the efficacy of HBV vaccination in susceptible individuals. Several studies have consistently demonstrated suboptimal response to a plasma-derived vaccine in both the magnitude and the duration of antibody response.[93–95] The efficacy of recombinant vaccines has not been reported. Patients who have received one or more HBV vaccine doses prior to HIV infection have reduced peak ALT levels, HBsAg prevalence, and chronic carriage,[78] suggesting at least partial protection in those who are immunocompetent at the time of vaccination. Despite early concerns, no evidence whatsoever suggests that the plasma-derived HBV vaccine can transmit AIDS.[96]

Delta Hepatitis

The consequences of HIV infection on delta hepatitis appear similar to those of HBV, although far fewer patients with HDV have been studied. The presence of HIV does not directly affect the prevalence of delta hepatitis, which ranges in the United States from 0 to 15%[97] and is more closely correlated with geographic location, and sexual and drug use habits.[97, 98] In a small series, however, HIV co-infection was associated with enhanced delta virus replication without increased liver disease,[99] and in a single patient reactivation of delta hepatitis was ascribed to acute HIV infection.[100]

Hepatitis C

Serum assays to detect antibody for HCV (anti-HCV) have demonstrated a variable prevalence of HCV among HIV-positive individuals, from 7% in a university clinic setting[101] to 89% among intravenous drug users.[102] Although the rate for drug users is higher than those previously reported, whether this increase can be ascribed to HIV is uncertain because the false-positive rate for first-generation enzyme-linked immunosorbent assay (ELISA) may be increased in HIV-positive patients. This higher false-positive rate emphasizes the need to perform secondary tests such as radioimmunoblot assay (RIBA) in positive ELISA samples.[101] The reportedly lower titers of anti-HCV described in the largest series to date could reflect an increased prevalence of false-positive tests, or, alternatively, they may represent an accelerated loss of antibodies to HCV, as suggested in a large survey of intravenous drug users.[103] Prevalence of HCV antibodies is increased in female sexual partners of men co-infected with HIV and HCV, suggesting that HIV may be a cofactor in the sexual transmission of HCV.[104]

The impact of HIV on the clinical course of HCV infection is not yet clear. Fluctuations in AST and ALT levels and cirrhosis occur in co-infected patients but not in a pattern clearly distinguishable from that of HIV-negative patients. Case reports have described severe chronic active hepatitis[105] and fulminant hepatic failure attributable to HCV in the setting of HIV infection.[106]

Some evidence suggests that alpha-interferon is effective for treating HCV disease in HIV-positive patients, although only small numbers of patients have been reported.[105, 107] Patients who are HIV-positive have been excluded from published interferon trials for HCV, and the drug has not yet been approved by the federal Food and Drug Administration for use in HIV-seropositive patients.

Fungal Infections

Histoplasma capsulatum is an opportunistic pathogen in AIDS, and the liver can be affected in patients with disseminated disease. Infections are reported predominantly, but not exclusively, in geographic regions of high prevalence of the organism.[108, 109] Liver biopsies may reveal caseating granulomata containing fungal organisms. Infection is often initially identified in peripheral blood smears or bone marrow.[110, 111] Culture of hepatic tissue, blood, or bone marrow can confirm the diagnosis, but several weeks may be required for the organism to grow in culture. Diagnosis may be supplemented by detection of high levels of *Histoplasma* polysaccharide antigen or *Histoplasma* antibodies.[109] In patients with documented infection, pulmonary disease is present in slightly less than half of patients, implying that a normal chest radiograph does not exclude the diagnosis of extrapulmonary infection.[108, 109] Associated skin or gastrointestinal involvement may also be present.[110]

Treatment of histoplasmosis requires parenteral therapy with amphotericin B since early trials of ketoconazole have been disappointing.[108] Chronic maintenance therapy with amphotericin or fluconazole after successful induction with amphotericin may be required to prevent relapse.

Cryptococcus neoformans may infect the liver in the setting of disseminated infection involving multiple viscera.[7, 112] Typically, in liver the organism is found in the sinusoids and is associated with a poor inflammatory response. Fungal forms may be identified by Gomori's methenamine silver stain. Similarly, coccidioidomycosis[113] and blastomycosis[114] can involve the liver as part of a systemic infection, especially in geographic regions where these fungi are endemic. The organisms typically are found as spherules within fibrosing granulomata. *Candida albicans* infection of the liver is rare in contrast with its high prevalence in mucosal sites. Hepatic micro- or macroabscesses are most likely to occur if the patient is neutropenic, especially after chemotherapy for non-Hodgkin's lymphoma.[115, 116] Treatment of cryptococcal, coccidioidal, blastomycotic, and candidal infections of liver requires initial therapy with amphotericin B followed by maintenance therapy with fluconazole; ketoconazole is less effective. For cryptococcal infections, fluconazole may be adequate for induction therapy,[117] although longer term results are awaited comparing this agent with amphotericin.

Protozoal Infections

Isolated cases of *Pneumocystis carinii* pneumonia hepatitis have been described and are attributable to the use of inhaled pentamidine aerosols, which fail to protect extrapulmonic sites from *P. carinii* pneumonia.[118, 119] In addition to *P. carinii* pneumonia, the liver may be the site of infection by protozoa of the Microsporidia order *(Encephalitozoon cuniculi)*[120] and by *Dicrocoelium dendriticum.*[121] (See Chapter 17.)

As noted, *Cryptosporidium* has been identified in several cases of HIV-associated cholangiopathy as well as in acalculous cholecystitis,[47, 48] although an etiologic role for the organisms of this genus has not been established. Rare cases of biliary disease associated with microsporidia have been reported.[122, 123]

Visceral leishmaniasis, or kala-azar, due to *Leishmania donovani,* appears to be more likely in patients with HIV infection than in immunocompetent hosts and has been reported in drug abusers and homosexuals from nonendemic areas.[124–126] In some patients, *Leishmania* amastigotes may be identified by Giemsa stain or culture of liver biopsy material or in splenic, gastrointestinal tract, and bone marrow material.[126] Treatment with antimonials is not always satisfactory; anecdotal reports suggest that amphotericin B may be effective.[126]

Toxoplasma gondii is almost exclusively a central nervous system infection in patients with AIDS, although rare instances of concurrent hepatic involvement have been noted.[127]

CLINICAL ASPECTS OF HEPATOBILIARY DISEASE IN AIDS

Hepatomegaly, with or without jaundice, and abnormal liver chemistries are frequent findings in patients with HIV infection. Hepatomegaly may be present clinically in more than 50% of patients,[7] but clinical examination may underestimate its actual prevalence since it has been found in as much as 84% of patients at postmortem. Hepatomegaly is usually associated with one or more liver function test abnormalities, although significant jaundice due to parenchymal disease is uncommon.

Conditions associated with HIV infection account for the majority of cases of liver disease. No single feature or combination of findings is common to all patients with hepatic disease in AIDS.[37, 128] From a clinical perspective, hepatobiliary disease can be broadly classified as hepatic parenchymal abnormality, biliary abnormality, or a combination of the two. Parenchymal abnormalities are most often infectious, but neither neoplasms, in particular non-Hodgkin's lymphoma, nor drug-induced disease is infrequent. In addition, the clinical and histologic features of viral hepatitis may be modified by co-infection with HIV.

Biliary tract involvement in AIDS may result in marked jaundice and right upper quadrant symptoms. The syndrome of HIV-associated cholangiopathy is a prominent cause of biliary disease.[31, 42–44, 129–131] Patients develop significant upper abdominal pain in association with marked elevation of alkaline phosphatase and moderate elevations of bilirubin, AST, and ALT.

Ductal changes of HIV-associated cholangiopathy may include papillary stenosis alone, sclerosing cholangitis-like lesions alone, a combination of the two, or long, extrahepatic strictures. Abdominal ultrasound or computed tomography (CT) scan detects ductal abnormalities in 77% of those with cholangiographically proven disease, implying that a negative finding on imaging study does not definitively exclude the diagnosis.[44] For most patients with predominantly papillary stenosis, sphincterotomy results in a symptomatic improvement.[44] Alkaline phosphatase continues to rise, however, probably reflecting progression of intrahepatic disease.[44]

Other, less common types of biliary tract disease in AIDS include primary bile duct lymphoma,[132] epithelial angiomatosis,[133] lymphomatosis nodal obstruction, Kaposi's sarcoma, microsporidiosis,[123] and biloma.[134] In addition, chronic pancreatitis and choledocholithiasis may also lead to biliary obstruction, although their prevalence is not clearly increased in HIV infection.

Evaluation

The initial decision in evaluating the AIDS patient with jaundice or hepatomegaly or both is to determine whether the findings are due to intrahepatic or extrahepatic disease. Simultaneous disease in other sites as well as the liver must also be considered. A history of mild jaundice, often in association with fever and constitutional symptoms, is more consistent with intrahepatic disease, whereas symptoms of deep jaundice associated with pain of relatively acute onset suggest extrahepatic disease.

Because the clinical history and the finding of symptomatic hepatomegaly are nonspecific, further evaluation is usually necessary. Elevations of ALT, AST, or both are seen in 35 to 40% of patients, but neither the pattern nor the extent of elevation of these tests correlates with specific findings in the liver.[2, 128] By contrast, marked elevation of alkaline phosphates correlates statistically with the presence of *M. avium* infection in the liver in AIDS patients when extrahepatic obstruction is absent.[2] Nonetheless, an imaging procedure of the liver and biliary ducts is almost always indicated. Abdominal CT scan and sonogram should be employed early because they are especially useful in identifying ductal dilatation, pathologic conditions of the gallbladder, and focal hepatic lesions.[135] Liver-spleen scintigraphy may be helpful in assessing liver and spleen size or parenchymal abnormalities[136] but is less useful than CT. If focal lesions of liver are identified with imaging studies, then directed skinny needle biopsies are appropriate.

When intrahepatic disease seems likely, the indications for percutaneous nondirected liver biopsy are not well defined. In principle, biopsy is appropriate when symptomatic, treatable disease of the liver is suspected or when a specific diagnosis of hepatic disease is needed. Biopsy is most commonly undertaken in patients with unexplained fever or persistent symptomatic elevations of liver chemistries for which remediable causes have been otherwise excluded. Tissue should be routinely stained for acid-fast bacilli and cultured for fungi, viruses, and mycobacteria.

The utility of liver biopsy in patients with suspected intrahepatic disease has not been conclusively established. Biopsies reveal abnormal findings in 90 to 100% of patients with AIDS,[2, 128] yet in one careful retrospective review, liver biopsy identified a previously undiagnosed infection or neoplasm in only 2 of 26 patients (8%), suggesting that the liver is rarely the site of disease not manifest elsewhere.[2] In a more recent report by Cappell and colleagues, liver biopsy was diagnostic in 50% of patients when primary indications were fever or abnormal liver chemistries. A review by these authors of all published studies to date reported a diagnostic utility of liver biopsy ranging from 24 to 80%.[13] Even in Cappell's study, however, the primary diagnosis was most often *M. avium* infection, which might otherwise be identified by blood or bone marrow cultures. A more compelling indication for liver biopsy might be in suspected cases of TB in which other potential sites of infection have been excluded. This approach would be especially relevant in urban populations, where *M. tuberculosis* is more prevalent. Consideration in such cases might alternatively be given to skinny needle biopsy of liver, in which adequate tissue could be recovered for acid-fast stains and culture, with a reduced risk of hemorrhage.

The significance of a number of the nonspecific findings in liver are uncertain. In particular, granulomata in the absence of fungal or bacterial organisms are often seen.[2, 3, 6] Microvesicular and macrovesicular steatosis may be identified as well, possibly due to malnutrition, since the findings are similar to those seen in patients with kwashiorkor.[2]

When liver biopsies are diagnostic, specific infections or neoplasms are usually evident on tissue sections of appropriately stained biopsy material. *Mycobacterium avium* is almost always present within hepatic granulomata, although it may occasionally be detectable only on culture of biopsy material for acid-fast bacilli.[2, 5] *Cryptococcus* and *Histoplasma* are also associated with granulomata.[7, 108, 109] Cytomegalovirus nuclear inclusions can be localized within Kupffer cells or hepatocytes.[7] Kaposi's sarcoma and lymphomas are easily identified by their homogeneous neoplastic appearance.[7, 137] When lymphoma is suspected, material should be fixed in paraformaldehyde to allow for thin plastic sections to define the histologic type. Drug-induced hepatitis may be recognized on occasion by the presence of eosinophils within granulomata.[128]

Although theoretically liver biopsy poses no increased risk in AIDS patients if coagulation studies are normal, anecdotal experience[138] (SLF, unpublished data, 1993) suggests that there may be an increased rate of hemorrhagic complications even when no vascular structures are encountered. The possibility exists but is unproved that some of these episodes may have arisen from peliotic lesions, although reports to date suggest that biopsy is safe in this condition. Nonetheless, the preliminary observation that an increased risk of hemorrhagic complication is possible underscores the importance of reserving liver biopsy for those circumstances in which less invasive methods have failed to establish a diagnosis.

When an extrahepatic cause for jaundice is suggested on CT (e.g., dilated ducts), papillary stenosis associated with CMV, cryptosporidiosis, or microsporidiosis must be considered promptly. Further evaluation, when indicated, may include endoscopic retrograde cholangiopancreatographic examination (ERCP) if CT or ultrasound demonstrates dilation of extrahepatic ducts extending to the duodenum. Ampullary and biopsy specimens collected during ERCP should be examined for the presence of viruses, protozoa, or neoplastic cells and cultured for viruses, particularly CMV.

REFERENCES

1. Revision of the CDC surveillance case definition for acquired immunodeficiency syndrome. MMWR Morb Mortal Wkly Rep. 1987;36(Suppl 1):1S–15S.
2. Schneiderman DJ, Arenson DM, Cello JP, et al. Hepatic disease in patients with the acquired immune deficiency syndrome (AIDS). Hepatology. 1987;7:925–930.

3. Orenstein MS, Tavitian A, Yonk B, et al. Granulomatous involvement of the liver in patients with AIDS. Gut. 1985;26:1220–1225.

4. Kahn SA, Saltzman BR, Klein RS, et al. Hepatic disorders in the acquired immune deficiency syndrome: A clinical and pathological study. Am J Gastroenterol. 1986;81:1145–1148.

5. Greene JB, Sidhu GS, Lewin S, et al. *Mycobacterium avium-intracellulare.* A cause of disseminated life-threatening infection in homosexuals and drug abusers. Ann Intern Med. 1982;97:539–546.

6. Nakanuma Y, Liew CT, Peters RL, Govindarajan S. Pathologic features of the liver in acquired immune deficiency syndrome (AIDS). Liver. 1986;6:158–166.

7. Glasgow BJ, Anders K, Layfield LJ, et al. Clinical and pathologic findings of the liver in the acquired immunodeficiency syndrome (AIDS). Am J Clin Pathol. 1985; 83:582–588.

8. Kahn E, Greco MA, Daum F, et al. Hepatic pathology in pediatric acquired immunodeficiency syndrome. Hum Pathol. 1991;22:1111–1119.

9. Horsburgh CR, Mason UG, Farhi DC, Iseman MD. Disseminated infection with *Mycobacterium avium-intracellulare.* Medicine. 1985;64:36–48.

10. Nyberg DA, Federle MP, Jeffrey RB, et al. Abdominal CT findings of disseminated *Mycobacterium avium-intracellulare* in AIDS. AJR Am J Roentgenol. 1985;145:297–299.

11. Young LS, Wiviott L, Wu M, et al. Azithromycin for treatment of *Mycobacterium avium-intracellulare* complex infection in patients with AIDS. Lancet. 1991;338:1107–1109.

12. Hoy J, Mijch A, Sandland M, et al. Quadruple-drug therapy for *Mycobacterium avium-intracellulare* bacteremia in AIDS patients. J Infect Dis. 1990;161:801–805.

13. Cappell MS. Hepatobiliary manifestations of the acquired immune deficiency syndrome. Am J Gastroenterol. 1991;86:1–15.

14. Chaisson RE, Slutkin G. Tuberculosis and human immunodeficiency virus infection. J Infect Dis. 1989;159:96–100.

15. Small PM, Schecter GF, Goodman PC, et al. Treatment of tuberculosis in patients with advanced human immunodeficiency virus infection. N Engl J Med. 1991;324:289–294.

16. Moreno S, Pacho E, Lopez-Herce JA. *Mycobacterium* tuberculosis visceral abscesses in the acquired immunodeficiency syndrome (AIDS). Ann Intern Med. 1988; 109:437. Letter.

17. Weinberg JJ, Cohen P, Malhotra R. Primary tuberculous liver abscess associated with the human immunodeficiency virus. Tubercle. 1988;69:145–147.

18. Theuer CP, Hopewell PC, Elias D, et al. Human immunodeficiency virus infection in tuberculosis patients. J Infect Dis. 1990;162:8–12.

19. Scherer R, Sable R, Sonnenberg M. Disseminated infection with *Mycobacterium kansasii* in the acquired immunodeficiency syndrome. Ann Intern Med. 1986; 105:710–712.

20. Eng RHK, Forrester C, Smith SM, Sobel H. *Mycobacterium xenopi* infection in a patient with acquired immunodeficiency syndrome. Chest. 1984;86:145–147.

21. Fournier AM, Dickinson GM, Erdfrocht IR. Tuberculous and nontuberculous mycobacteriosis in patients with AIDS. Chest. 1988;93:772–775.

22. Slater LN, Welch DF, Min KW. *Rochalimaea henselae* causes bacillary angiomatosis and peliosis hepatis. Arch Intern Med. 1992;152:602–606.

23. Relman DA, Loutit JS, Schmidt TM, et al. The agent of bacillary angiomatosis. An approach to the identification of uncultured pathogens. N Engl J Med. 1990;323:1573–1580.

24. Regnery RL, Anderson BE, Clarridge JE 3rd, et al. Characterization of a novel *Rochalimaea* species, *R. henselae* sp. nov., isolated from blood of a febrile, human immunodeficiency virus–positive patient. J Clin Microbiol. 1992;30:265–274.

25. Slater LN, Welch DF, Hensel D, Coody DW. A newly recognized fastidious gram-negative pathogen as a cause of fever and bacteremia. N Engl J Med. 1990;323:1587–1593.

26. Perkocha LA, Geaghan SM, Yen TSB, et al. Clinical and pathological features of bacillary peliosis hepatis in association with human immunodeficiency virus infection. N Engl J Med. 1990;323:1581–1586.

27. LeBoit PE, Berger TG, Egbert BM, et al. Epithelioid haemangioma-like vascular proliferation in AIDS: Manifestation of cat scratch disease bacillus infection? Lancet. 1988;8592:960–963.

28. Koehler JE, LeBoit PE, Egbert BM, Berger TG. Cutaneous vascular lesions and disseminated cat-scratch disease in patients with the acquired immunodeficiency syndrome (AIDS) and AIDS-related complex. Ann Intern Med. 1988;109:449–455.

29. Garcia-Tsao G, Panzini L, Yoselevitz M, West AB. Bacillary peliosis hepatis as a cause of acute anemia in a patient with the acquired immunodeficiency syndrome. Gastroenterology. 1992;102:1065–1070.

30. Welch K, Finkbeiner W, Alpers CE, et al. Autopsy findings in the acquired immunodeficiency syndrome. JAMA. 1984;252:1152–1159.

31. Czapar CA, Weldon-Linne M, Moore DM, Rhone DP. Peliosis hepatis in the acquired immunodeficiency syndrome. Arch Pathol Lab Med. 1986;110:611–613.

32. Fischl MA, Dickinson GM, Sinave C, et al. *Salmonella* bacteremia as manifestation of acquired immunodeficiency syndrome. Arch Intern Med. 1986;146:113–115.

33. Smith PD, Macher AM, Bookman MA, et al. *Salmonella typhimurium* enteritis and bacteremia in the acquired immunodeficiency syndrome. Ann Intern Med. 1985;102:207–209.

34. Mobley K, Rotterdam HZ. Lerner CW, Tapper ML. Autopsy findings in the acquired immunodeficiency syndrome. Pathology. 1985;20:45–65.

35. Bach N, Theise ND, Schaffner F. Hepatic histopathology in the acquired immunodeficiency syndrome. Semin Liver Dis. 1992;12:205–212.

36. Cappell MS, Schwartz MS, Biempica L. Clinical utility of liver biopsy in patients with serum antibodies to the human immunodeficiency virus. Am J Med. 1990;88:123–130.

37. Wilkins MJ, Lindley R, Dourakis SP, Goldin RD. Surgical pathology of the liver in HIV infection. Histopathology. 1991;18:459–464.

38. Sacks SL, Freeman HJ. Cytomegalovirus hepatitis: Evidence for direct hepatic viral infection using monoclonal antibodies. Gastroenterology. 1984;86:346–350.

39. Jacobson MA, O'Donnell JJ. Approaches to the treatment of cytomegalovirus retinitis: Ganciclovir and foscarnet. J AIDS. 1991;4:S11–S15.

40. Pitlik SD, Fainstein V, Garza D, et al. Human cryptosporidioses: Spectrum of disease. Arch Intern Med. 1983;143:2269–2275.

41. Guarda LA, Stein SA, Cleary KA, Ordonez NG. Human cryptosporidiosis in AIDS. Arch Pathol Lab Med. 1983;107:562.

42. Schneiderman DJ, Cello JP, Laing FC. Papillary stenosis and sclerosing cholangitis in patients with the acquired immune deficiency syndrome (AIDS). Ann Intern Med. 1987;106:546.

43. Cello JP. Human immunodeficiency virus–associated biliary tract disease. Semin Liver Dis. 1992;12:213–218.

44. Cello JP. Acquired immunodeficiency syndrome cho-

langiopathy: Spectrum of disease. Am J Med. 1989; 86:539–546.

45. Jacobson MA, Cello JP, Sande MA. Cholestasis and disseminated cytomegalovirus disease in patients with the acquired immunodeficiency syndrome. Am J Med. 1988;84:218–224.

46. Prochazka EJ, Terasaki PI, Park MS, et al. Association of primary sclerosing cholangitis with HLA-DRw52a. N Engl J Med. 1990;322:1842–1844.

47. Blumberg RS, Kelsey P, Perrone T, et al. Cytomegalovirus- and *Cryptosporidium*-associated acalculous gangrenous cholecystitis. Am J Med. 1984;76:1118–1123.

48. Kavin H, Jonas RB, Chowdhury L, Kabins S. Acalculous cholecystitis and cytomegalovirus infection in the acquired immunodeficiency syndrome. Ann Intern Med. 1986;104:53–54.

49. Agha FP, Nostrant TT, Abrams GD, et al. Cytomegalovirus cholangitis in a homosexual man with acquired immune deficiency syndrome. Am J Gastroenterol. 1986;81:1068–1072.

50. Kahn DG, Garfinkle JM, Klonoff DC, et al. Cryptosporidial and cytomegaloviral hepatitis and cholecystitis. Arch Pathol Lab Med. 1987;111:879–881.

51. Zimmerli W, Bianchi L, Gudat F. Disseminated herpes simplex type 2 and systemic *Candida* infection in a patient with previous asymptomatic human immunodeficiency virus infection. J Infect Dis. 1988;157:597–598.

52. Webster A, Lee CA, Cook DG. Cytomegalovirus infection and progression towards AIDS in haemophiliacs with human immunodeficiency virus infection. Lancet. 1989;2:63–66.

53. Nelson JA, Reynolds-Kohler C, Oldstone MBA, Wiley CA. HIV and CMV coinfect brain cells in patients with AIDS. Virology. 1988;165:286–290.

54. Ho WZ, Harouse JM, Rando RF. Reciprocal enhancement of gene expression and viral replication between human CMV and HIV-1. J Gen Virol. 1990;71:97–103.

55. Taylor RJ, Saul SH, Dowling JN. Primary disseminated herpes simplex infection with fulminant hepatitis following renal transplantation. Arch Intern Med. 1981;141:1519–1521.

56. Beissner RS, Rappaport FS, Diaz JA. Fatal case of Epstein-Barr virus–induced lymphoproliferative disorder associated with a human immunodeficiency virus infection. Arch Pathol Lab Med. 1987;11:250–253.

57. Duffy LF, Daum F, Kahn E. Hepatitis in children with acquired immune deficiency syndrome: Histopathologic and immunocytologic features. Gastroenterology. 1986;90:173.

58. Thung SN, Gerber MA, Benkov KJ. Chronic active hepatitis in a child with HIV infection. Arch Pathol Lab Med. 1988;112:914–916.

59. Krilov LR, Rubin LB, Frogel M. Disseminated adenovirus infection with hepatic necrosis in patients with human immunodeficiency virus infection and other immunodeficiency states. Rev Infect Dis. 1990;12:303–307.

60. LaFon M-E, Kirn A. Human immunodeficiency virus infection of the liver. Semin Liver Dis. 1992;12:197–204.

61. Ward JM, O'Leary TJ, Baskin GB, et al. Immunohistochemical localization of human and simian immunodeficiency viral antigens in fixed tissue sections. Am J Pathol. 1987;127:199–205.

62. Housset C, Boucher O, Girard PM, et al. Immunohistochemical evidence for human immunodeficiency virus-1 infection of liver Kupffer cells. Hum Pathol. 1990;21:404–408.

63. Hoda SA, White JE, Gerber MA. Immunohistochemical studies of human immunodeficiency virus 1 in liver

tissues of patients with AIDS. Mod Pathol. 1991;4:578–581.

64. Li XM, Jeffers LJ, Reddy KR. Detection of HIV in liver tissue of AIDS patients by in situ hybridization (abstract). Hepatology. 1989;10:678.

65. Schmitt MP, Steffan AM, Gendrault JL, et al. Multiplication of human immunodeficiency virus in primary cultures of human Kupffer cells: Possible role of liver macrophage infection in the physiopathology of AIDS. Res Virol. 1990;141:143–152.

66. Gendrault JL, Steffan AM, Schmitt MP. Interaction of cultured human Kupffer cells with HIV-infected CEM cells: An electron microscopic study. Pathobiology. 1991;59:223–226.

67. Scoazec J-Y, Feldmann G. Both macrophages and endothelial cells of the human hepatic sinusoid express the CD4 molecule, a receptor for the human immunodeficiency virus. Hepatology. 1990;12:505–510.

68. Gendelman HE, Orenstein JM, Baca LM, et al. The macrophage in the persistence and pathogenesis of HIV infection. AIDS. 1989;3:475–495.

69. Andreesen R, Brugger W, Kunze R, et al. Defective monocyte to macrophage maturation in human immunodeficiency virus infection. Res Virol. 1990;141:217–224.

70. Schreeder MT, Thompson SE, Hadler SC. Hepatitis B in homosexual men: Prevalence of infection and factors related to transmission. J Infect Dis. 1982;146:7–15.

71. McNair ANB, Main J, Thomas HC. Interactions of the human immunodeficiency virus and the hepatotrophic viruses. Semin Liver Dis. 1992;12:188–196.

72. Lazizi Y, Grangeot-Keros L, Delfraissy J-F, et al. Reappearance of hepatitis B virus in immune patients infected with the human immunodeficiency virus type 1. J Infect Dis. 1988;158:666–667.

73. Waite J, Gilson RJC, Weller IVD, et al. Hepatitis B virus reactivation or reinfection associated with HIV-1 infection. AIDS. 1988;2:443–448.

74. Laukamm-Josten U, Muller O, Bienzle U, et al. Decline of naturally acquired antibodies to hepatitis B surface antigen in HIV-1 infected homosexual men. AIDS. 1988;2:400–401.

75. Biggar RJ, Goedert JJ, Hoofnagle J. Accelerated loss of antibody to hepatitis B surface antigen among immunodeficient homosexual men infected with HIV. N Engl J Med. 1987;316:630–631.

76. Perrillo RP, Regenstein FG, Roodman ST. Chronic hepatitis B in asymptomatic homosexual men with antibody to the human immunodeficiency virus. Ann Intern Med. 1986;105:382.

77. Krogsgaard K, Lindhardt BO, Nielsen JO, et al. The influence of HTLV-III infection on the natural history of hepatitis B virus infection in male homosexual HBsAg carriers. Hepatology. 1987;7:37–41.

78. Hadler SC, Judson FN, O'Malley PM. Outcome of hepatitis B virus infection in homosexual men and its relation to prior human immunodeficiency virus infection. J Infect Dis. 1991;163:454–459.

79. Bodsworth N, Donovan B, Nightingale BN. The effect of concurrent human immunodeficiency virus infection on chronic hepatitis B: A study of 150 homosexual men. J Infect Dis. 1989;160:577–581.

80. Rector WG, Govindarajan S, Horsburgh CR, et al. Hepatic inflammation, hepatitis B replication, and cellular immune function in homosexual males with chronic hepatitis B and antibody to human immunodeficiency virus. Am J Gastroenterol. 1988;83:262–266.

81. Housset C, Pol S, Carnot F, et al. Interactions between human immunodeficiency virus-1, hepatitis delta virus and hepatitis B virus infections in 260 chronic carriers of hepatitis B virus. Hepatology. 1992;15:578–583.

82. Pastore G, Santantonio T, Monno L. Effects of HIV superinfection on HBV replication in a chronic HBsAg carrier with liver disease. J Hepatol. 1988;7:164–168.

83. Foster GR, Thomas HC. Hepatitis and other liver disease in patients with HIV infection. HIV: Adv Ther. 1992;2:19–24.

84. Paul RG, Roodman ST, Paul DA, Perrillo RP. Elevated HLA class I antigen expression on peripheral blood mononuclear cells of HBsAg carriers with coexistent human immunodeficiency virus infection. Hepatology. 1987;7:1326–1329.

85. McDonald JA, Harris S, Waters JA, Thomas HC. Effect of human immunodeficiency virus (HIV) infection on chronic hepatitis B hepatic viral antigen display. J Hepatol. 1987;4:337–342.

86. Gilson RJC, Hawkins AE, Kelly GK, et al. No effect of zidovudine on hepatitis B virus replication in homosexual men with symptomatic HIV-1 infection. AIDS. 1991;5:217–220.

87. Marcellin P, Pialoux G, Girard PM, et al. Absence of effect of zidovudine on replication of hepatitis B virus in patients with chronic HIV and HBV infection. N Engl J Med. 1989;32:1758. Letter.

88. Twu J-S, Robinson WS. Hepatitis B virus X gene can transactivate heterologous viral sequences. Proc Natl Acad Sci U S A. 1989;86:2046–2050.

89. Seto E, Mitchell PJ, Yen TS. Transactivation by the hepatitis B virus X protein depends on AP-2 and other transcription factors. Nature. 1990;344:72–74.

90. Laure F, Zagury D, Saimot AG. Hepatitis B virus DNA sequence in lymphoid cells from patients with AIDS and AIDS-related complex. Science. 1985;229:561.

91. Noonan CA, Yoffe B, Mansell PW, et al. Extrachromosomal sequences of hepatitis B virus DNA in peripheral blood mononuclear cells of acquired immune deficiency patients. Proc Natl Acad Sci U S A. 1986; 83:5698–5702.

92. Bartolome FJ, Moraleda G, Castillo I, et al. Presence of HBV-DNA in peripheral blood mononuclear cells from anti-HIV symptomless carriers. J Hepatol. 1990;10:186–190.

93. Collier AC, Corey L, Murphy VL, Handsfield HH. Antibody to human immunodeficiency virus (HIV) and suboptimal response to hepatitis B vaccination. Ann Intern Med. 1988;109:101–105.

94. Carne CA, Weller IVD, Waite J, et al. Impaired responsiveness of homosexual men with HIV antibodies to plasma-derived hepatitis B vaccine. Br Med J. 1987;294:866–868.

95. Mannucci M, Zanetti AR, Gringeri A, et al. Long-term immunogenicity of a plasma-derived hepatitis B vaccine in HIV seropositive and HIV seronegative hemophiliacs. Arch Intern Med. 1989;149:1333–1337.

96. Centers for Disease Control. Hepatitis B vaccine: Evidence confirming lack of AIDS transmission. JAMA. 1985;253:21–22.

97. Solomon RE, Kaslow RA, Phair JP, et al. Human immunodeficiency virus and hepatitis delta virus in homosexual men. Ann Intern Med. 1988;108:51–54.

98. Novick DM, Farci P, Croxson TS, et al. Hepatitis D virus and human immunodeficiency virus antibodies in parenteral drug abusers who are hepatitis B surface antigen positive. J Infect Dis. 1988;158:795–803.

99. Buti M, Esteban R, Espanol MT, et al. Influence of human immunodeficiency virus infection on cell-mediated immunity in chronic D hepatitis. J Infect Dis. 1991;163:1351–1353.

100. Shattock AG, Finlay H, Hillary IB. Possible reactivation of hepatitis D with chronic delta antigenaemia by human immunodeficiency virus. Br Med J. 1987;294: 1656–1657.

101. Hayashi PH, Flynn N, McCurdy SA, et al. Prevalence of hepatitis C virus antibodies among patients infected with human immunodeficiency virus. J Med Virol. 1991;33:177–180.

102. Sonnerborg A, Abebe A, Strannegard O. Hepatitis C virus infection in individuals with or without human immunodeficiency virus type 1 infection. Infection. 1990;18:347–351.

103. Chamot E, Hirschel B, Wintsch J, et al. Loss of antibodies against hepatitis C virus in HIV-seropositive intravenous drug users. AIDS. 1990;4:1275–1277.

104. Eyster ME, Alter HJ, Aledort LM, et al. Heterosexual co-transmission of hepatitis C virus (HCV) and human immunodeficiency virus (HIV). Ann Intern Med. 1991;115:764–768.

105. Berk L, Schalm SW, Heijtink RA. Severe chronic active hepatitis (autoimmune type) mimicked by coinfection of hepatitis C and human immunodeficiency viruses. Gut. 1991;32:1198–1200.

106. Martin P, DiBisceglie AM, Kassianides C, et al. Non-A, non-B hepatitis leads to rapidly progressive liver disease in patients with human immunodeficiency virus infection. Gastroenterology. 1989;96:A627.

107. Boyer N, Marcellin P, Degott C, et al. Recombinant interferon-α for chronic hepatitis C in patients positive for antibody to human immunodeficiency virus. J Infect Dis. 1992;165:723–726.

108. Wheat LJ, Slama TG, Zeckel ML. Histoplasmosis in the acquired immune deficiency syndrome. Am J Med. 1985;78:203.

109. Wheat LJ, Connolly-Stringfield PA, Baker RL, et al. Disseminated histoplasmosis in the acquired immune deficiency syndrome: Clinical findings, diagnosis and treatment, and review of the literature. Medicine. 1990;69:361–374.

110. Johnson PC, Khardori N, Najjar AF, et al. Progressive disseminated histoplasmosis in patients with acquired immunodeficiency syndrome. Am J Med. 1988;85:152–158.

111. Tomita T, Chiga M. Disseminated histoplasmosis in acquired immunodeficiency syndrome: Light and electron microscopic observations. Hum Pathol. 1988;19: 438–441.

112. Bonacini M, Nussbaum J, Ahluwalia C. Gastrointestinal, hepatic, and pancreatic involvement with *Cryptococcus neoformans* in AIDS. J Clin Gastroenterol. 1990;12:295–297.

113. Bronnimann DA, Adam RD, Galgiani JN. Coccidioidomycosis in the acquired immunodeficiency syndrome. Ann Intern Med. 1987;106:372–379.

114. Pappas PG, Pottage JC, Powderly WG, et al. Blastomycosis in patients with the acquired immunodeficiency syndrome. Ann Intern Med. 1992;116:847–853.

115. Haron D, Feld D, Tuffnell P, et al. Hepatic candidiasis: An increasing problem in immunocompromised patients. Am J Med. 1987;83:17–26.

116. Thaler M, Pastakia B, Shawker TH, et al. Hepatic candidiasis in cancer patients: The evolving picture of the syndrome. Ann Intern Med. 1988;108:88–100.

117. Saag MS, Powderly WG, Cloud GA, et al. Comparison of amphotericin B with fluconazole in the treatment of acute AIDS-associated cryptococcal meningitis. N Engl J Med. 1992;326:83–89.

118. Jules-Elysee KM, Stover DE, Zaman MB, et al. Aerosolized pentamidine: Effect on diagnosis and presentation of *Pneumocystis carinii* pneumonia. Ann Intern Med. 1990;112:750–757.

119. Fistel SH, Rueda-Pedraza E, Ishak KG, Goodman ZD. A 29-year-old man with the acquired immunodeficiency syndrome and liver dysfunction. Semin Liver Dis. 1992;12:219–225.

120. Terada S, Reddy KR, Jeffers LJ, et al. Microsporidian hepatitis in the acquired immunodeficiency syndrome. Ann Intern Med. 1987;107:61–62.
121. Drabick JJ, Egan JE, Brown SL, et al. Dicrocoeliasis (lancet fluke disease) in an HIV seropositive man. JAMA. 1988;259:567–568.
122. McWhinney PHM, Nathwani D, Green ST, et al. Microsporidiosis detected in association with AIDS-related sclerosing cholangitis. AIDS. 1991;5:1394–1395.
123. Pol S, Romana C, Richard S, et al. *Enterocytozoon bieneusi* infection in acquired immunodeficiency syndrome–related sclerosing cholangitis. Gastroenterology. 1992; 102:1778–1781.
124. Falk S, Helm EB, Hubne K, Stutte HJ. Disseminated visceral leishmaniasis (kala azar) in acquired immunodeficiency syndrome (AIDS). Pathol Res Pract. 1988;183:253–255.
125. Sendino A, Barbado J, Mostaza JM, et al. Visceral leishmaniasis with malabsorption syndrome in a patient with acquired immunodeficiency syndrome. Am J Med. 1990;89:673–675.
126. Altes J, Salas A, Riera M, et al. Visceral leishmaniasis: Another HIV-associated opportunistic infection? Report of eight cases and review of the literature. AIDS. 1991;5:201–207.
127. Oksenhendler E, Cadranel J, Sarfati C. *Toxoplasma gondii* pneumonia in patients with the acquired immunodeficiency syndrome. Am J Med. 1990;88:18.
128. Lebovics E, Thung SN, Schaffner F, Radensky PW. The liver in the acquired immunodeficiency syndrome: A clinical and histologic study. Hepatology. 1985;5:293.

129. Margulis SJ, Honig CL, Soave R, et al. Biliary tract obstruction in the acquired immunodeficiency syndrome. Ann Intern Med. 1987;105:207.
130. Viteri AL, Greene JF. Bile duct abnormalities in the acquired immune deficiency syndrome. Gastroenterology. 1987;92:2014–2018.
131. Roulot D, Valla D, Brun-Vezinet F, et al. Cholangitis in the acquired immunodeficiency syndrome: Report of two cases and review of the literature. Gut. 1987; 28:1653–1660.
132. Kaplan LD, Kahn J, Jacobson M, et al. Primary bile duct lymphoma in the acquired immunodeficiency syndrome (AIDS). Ann Intern Med. 1989;110:161–162.
133. Krekorian TD, Radner AB, Alcorn JM, et al. Biliary obstruction caused by epithelioid angiomatosis in a patient with AIDS. Am J Med. 1990;89:820–822.
134. Fritz HP, Polio J, Hewitt JK. Biloma secondary to hepatocellular carcinoma in an HIV-seropositive patient. Am J Gastroenterol. 1989;84:1560–1563.
135. Jeffrey RB. Gastrointestinal imaging in AIDS-abdominal computed tomography and ultrasound. Gastroenterol Clin North Am. 1988;17:507–521.
136. Smith R. Liver-spleen scintigraphy in patients with acquired immunodeficiency syndrome. AJR Am J Roentgenol. 1985;145:1201.
137. Caccamo D, Pervez NK, Marchcusky A. Primary lymphoma of the liver in the acquired immunodeficiency syndrome. Arch Pathol Lab Med. 1986;110:553.
138. Gordon SC, Veneri RJ, McFadden RF, et al. Major hemorrhage after percutaneous liver biopsy in patients with AIDS. Gastroenterology. 1991;100:1787.

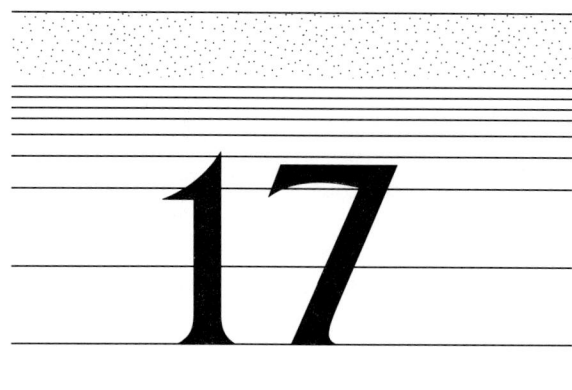

17

Parasitic Infections of the Liver and Biliary Tree

RALPH T. BRYAN, M.D.
MARCO K. MICHELSON, M.D.

For health care professionals in North America and other developed regions, parasitic infections can no longer be considered rare or unusual. We are living in an era in which the term global community is truly an accurate reflection of world affairs. Clinicians are no longer buffered from those medical conditions previously considered tropical or exotic. The reasons for this trend are quite clear; increasing immigration from developing countries, rapidly expanding tourism to exotic locales, and major military operations in the tropics are all contributing to the likelihood that the medical community in developed countries will encounter more and more patients with parasitic infections. In addition, patients with acquired immunodeficiency syndrome (AIDS) are likely to suffer from opportunistic parasitic infections. Medical professionals, therefore, have a responsibility to be prepared to deal competently with diseases in which the vast majority of them have had little or no training. In this chapter, we hope to help physicians and others fulfill that responsibility by describing the parasitic infections that affect the liver and biliary tree.

Parasites capable of causing hepatobiliary infections include both protozoa and helminths. Included among the helminths are trematodes (flukes), cestodes (tapeworms), and nematodes (roundworms). Some parasites demonstrate a predilection for hepatobiliary sites, whereas others arrive there accidentally owing to the anatomic location of the liver and biliary tree. We have organized this chapter into the two broad categories of helminthic and protozoal infections. The discussion of each of these types of infection is further divided into those conditions having major or primary hepatobiliary manifestations and those in which hepatobiliary involvement is minor, secondary, transient, or rare. Although many of these infections have multiorgan involvement, only their hepatobiliary manifestations are emphasized here.

To provide a rapid reference source for differential diagnoses, Tables 17–1 through 17–4 present the various hepatobiliary parasitic infections organized by clinical syndromes (see Tables 17–1 and 17–2), pathologic findings (see Table 17–3), and epidemiologic characteristics (see Table 17–4).

405

TABLE 17–1. CLINICAL MANIFESTATIONS OF MAJOR HEPATOBILIARY PARASITIC INFECTIONS

CLINICAL MANIFESTATION	PARASITIC INFECTION						
	SCHISTOSOMA SPECIES	*FASCIOLA* SPECIES	*CLONORCHIS/ OPISTHORCHIS*	*ECHINOCOCCUS* SPECIES	*TOXOCARA* SPECIES	*CAPILLARIA HEPATICA*	AMEBIC LIVER ABSCESS
Fever							
Acute	+	+	0	0	0	+	+
Chronic/recurrent	+	+	+	0	+	0	+
Jaundice	+	+	+	+	0	+	+
Cholecystitis and/or cholangitis	+ R	+	+	0	0	0	0
Diarrhea	+ Ac	+	+	0	0	+	+ <30%
Urticaria	+ Ac	+ Ac	0	+	+	0	0
Hepatomegaly							
Painful/tender	+ Ac	+ Ac	+	0	0	+	+
Painless	+ Cr	+ Cr	0	+	+	0	0
Hepatic mass	0	0	0	+	0	0	+
Splenomegaly	+	+ Ac	0	0	0	+	0
Ascites	+ Cr	0	+	+ *Em*	0	0	0
Lymphadenopathy	+ Ac	0	0	0	0	0	0
Leukocytosis	+	+ Ac	0	0	±	+	0
Eosinophilia	+	+	+	+ *	–	+	0
Anemia	+	+	0	0	0	+	+

KEY: + = commonly observed but not necessarily always present, 0 = never or rarely observed, R = rare, Ac = acute infection, Cr = chronic infection, *Em* = *Echinococcus multilocularis,* * = highly variable.

HELMINTHIC INFECTIONS OF THE LIVER AND BILIARY TREE

Conditions with Major Hepatobiliary Manifestations

Schistosomiasis

PARASITE LIFE CYCLE AND EPIDEMIOLOGY

Schistosomiasis is infection with digenetic trematodes of the genus *Schistosoma.* The cycle of infection begins with penetration of intact skin by free-living cercariae, the late intermediate forms of *Schistosoma* species (Fig. 17–1). After transforming into schistosomula, the young worms enter the systemic circulation and pass through the pulmonary vasculature into the portal venous system, where they reach maturity. Mated adult worms migrate to their final destinations near the intestines (*S. mansoni, S. japonicum, S. mekongi, S. intercalatum*) or ureters and bladder (*S. haematobium*). Egg deposition begins approximately 4 to 12 weeks after exposure. Egg output varies with the infecting species and ranges from 100 to 300 eggs per day for *S. mansoni,* 20 to 200 eggs per day for *S. haematobium,* and up to 3500 eggs per day for *S. japonicum.*[1–3] Nearly half of all eggs produced are retained in the tissues, where each egg may incite a vigorous granulomatous reaction, approaching 100 times the size of a single egg. Many eggs, however, migrate through the viscera into the lumen of the intestine or bladder, and from there they are expelled in the stool or urine. Ova deposited in fresh water hatch and release miracidia, early intermediate forms of this organism, which are infectious to specific snail hosts. This specificity for a given species of snail is the major determinant of the observed geographic distribution of schistosomiasis. Transformation of miracidia to cercariae within snails completes the developmental process. Released cercariae renew the cycle upon contact with another susceptible host.[1]

Infections with *Schistosoma* species affect approximately 200 million individuals in 76 countries (Fig. 17–2). An additional 600 million persons in areas with endemic schistosomiasis are believed to be at risk for acquiring this disease. Five major species account for the majority of these infections: *S. mansoni,* found in the western hemisphere, Africa, and the Middle East; *S. haematobium,* found only in Africa and the Middle East; *S. japonicum* and *S. mekongi,* found only in the Far East; and *S. intercalatum,* which has been described only from select areas on the African continent. Hepatic complications are most frequently associated with *S. mansoni, S. japonicum, S. mekongi,* and *S. intercalatum* infections.[1–3] Clinicians in developed countries are most likely to encounter patients with chronic disease among groups of immigrants or refugees, but acute disease has been reported in returning travelers.[4, 5]

CLINICAL MANIFESTATIONS

Symptoms and signs of acute schistosomiasis are thought to result from an immunologic response to the maturation of adult worms and subsequent egg deposition. Symptoms are often

TABLE 17–2. CLINICAL MANIFESTATIONS OF SELECTED RARE OR MINOR
HEPATOBILIARY PARASITIC INFECTIONS

CLINICAL MANIFESTATION	PARASITIC INFECTION						
	ASCARIS	ANGIO-STRONGYLUS	DICRO-COELIUM	CRYPTO-SPORIDIUM	ENTERO-CYTOZOON	GIARDIA	PNEUMO-CYSTIS
Fever							
Acute	0	+	0	0	0	0	0
Chronic/recurrent	0	0	0	+	+	0	0
Jaundice	0	+ R	+	+	+	0	0
Cholecystitis and/or cholangitis	+	0	0	+	+	0	0
Diarrhea	0	0	+	+	+	+	0
Urticaria	0	0	0	0	0	0	0
Hepatomegaly							
Painful/tender	0	+	0	0	0	0	0
Painless	0	0	0	0	0	0	+
Hepatic mass	0	0	0	0	0	0	0
Splenomegaly	0	0	0	0	0	0	+
Ascites	0	0	0	0	0	0	+
Lymphadenopathy	0	0	0	0	0	0	0
Leukocytosis	0	+	0	0	0	0	0
Eosinophilia	+	+	+ R	0	0	0	0
Anemia	0	0	0	0	0	0	0

NOTE: Clinical manifestations are those known to occur in patients with hepatobiliary involvement with these infections.
KEY: + = commonly observed but not necessarily always present, 0 = never, rarely observed, or unknown, R = rare.

nonspecific and may include headache, fever, chills, cough, anorexia, abdominal pain, nausea, vomiting, diarrhea, weakness, urticaria, myalgias, and arthralgias. An enlarged and tender liver, splenomegaly, lymphadenopathy, and eosinophilia frequently accompany acute intestinal infections (e.g., those caused by *S. mansoni* and *S. japonicum*) and should alert the astute clinician to this diagnosis in returning travelers and immigrants.[4, 5] Many of the acute manifestations of infection may be noted within the first 2 to 4 weeks after exposure and generally subside within 1 to 2 months.[6–8] By contrast, urinary schistosomiasis, which is caused by *S. haemato-*

bium, is less frequently associated with an acute toxemic state and is usually characterized by intermittent dysuria and hematuria.[4–9]

Hepatic involvement as a component of chronic schistosomal infections (e.g., hepatointestinal and hepatosplenic syndromes) is responsible for a large proportion of the serious morbidity seen in this disease. Periportal fibrosis, presinusoidal obstruction, and portal hypertension result from the inflammatory reaction to eggs swept into the liver by the portal circulation. Initially, patients are frequently asymptomatic. This process gradually culminates, however, in the development of ascites, peripheral

TABLE 17–3. PATHOLOGY OF HEPATOBILIARY PARASITIC INFECTIONS

PATHOLOGIC CATEGORY	PARASITIC DISEASES
HEPATOCELLULAR DISEASE	
Granulomatous hepatitis or hepatic granulomata	schistosomiasis, fascioliasis, toxocariasis, hepatic capillariasis, disseminated strongyloidiasis, angiostrongyliasis, enterobiasis, paragonimiasis, pentastomiasis
Portal fibrosis	schistosomiasis
Hepatic microabscesses or hepatocellular necrosis	paragonimiasis, amebic liver abscess, microsporidiosis, toxoplasmosis, babesiosis
Cystic liver disease	echinococcosis, amebic liver abscess
RETICULOENDOTHELIAL DISEASE	
Kupffer cell infection and/or hyperplasia	visceral leishmaniasis, toxoplasmosis, malaria (pigment deposition)
BILIARY DISEASE	
Cholangitis	fascioliasis, clonorchiasis/opisthorchiasis, ascariasis, cryptosporidiosis, microsporidiosis
Biliary hyperplasia	fascioliasis, clonorchiasis/opisthorchiasis
Cholangiocarcinoma	clonorchiasis/opisthorchiasis

TABLE 17–4. EPIDEMIOLOGIC CHARACTERISTICS OF MAJOR HEPATOBILIARY PARASITIC INFECTIONS

PARASITIC DISEASE	GEOGRAPHIC DISTRIBUTION	TRANSMISSION/INFECTION SOURCE	SPECIAL RISK GROUP
Schistosomiasis	Asia, Africa, S America, Caribbean	Cercarial larvae enter skin via contact with fresh water	Travelers, expatriates (e.g., Peace Corps)
Fascioliasis	Worldwide; cattle- or sheep-raising regions	Consumption of uncooked aquatic plants (e.g., watercress)	Consumers of wild watercress
Clonorchiasis/ opisthorchiasis	SE Asia, China, Japan, Korea, E Europe	Consumption of raw or partially cooked freshwater fish or crayfish	SE Asian immigrants
Echinococcosis	Worldwide; sheep-raising regions (*Eg*); northern latitudes of N America & Eurasia (*Em*)	Ingestion of food, water, or soil contaminated with egg-laden dog feces	Sheep herders, native Americans (*Eg*); hunters, trappers, native Alaskans (*Em*)
Toxocariasis	Worldwide	Ingestion of food, water, or soil contaminated with egg-laden feces of dogs or cats	Children <5 yr with history of pica or exposure to puppies
Hepatic capillariasis	Worldwide	Ingestion of soil contaminated with embryonated eggs	Unknown
Amebic liver abscess	Worldwide but more frequent in Africa, Asia, Mexico, S America	Person-to-person, fecal-oral	Immigrants, travelers, institutionalized persons

KEY: *Eg = Echinococcus granulosus, Em = Echinococcus multilocularis.*

edema, gastroesophageal varices, gastrointestinal bleeding, and splenomegaly. Intrahepatic shunting may also lead to the deposition of *Schistosoma* eggs in the lungs, resulting in pulmonary hypertension and cor pulmonale.[10] Urinary schistosomal infections have infrequently been associated with hepatic or splenic pathology.[11, 12] Prolonged carriage of *Salmonella* species has been noted to complicate chronic schistosomal infections and may contribute to the persistent fevers and marked splenomegaly observed in some patients. Abdominal examination reveals a palpable, nodular liver with predominant enlargement of the left lobe. The spleen is also frequently enlarged and firm, and tenderness may be noted over the descending colon. Physical signs of hepatocellular dysfunction such as jaundice, spider angiomata, palmar erythema, and encephalopathy are not usually present unless the underlying hepatic disease is very far advanced or coexists with another process such as viral hepatitis. Later stages of disease are associated with contraction of the liver, marked splenomegaly, ascites, peripheral edema, and decompensated liver function.[10]

Laboratory abnormalities include leukocytosis with eosinophilia, elevated erythrocyte sedimentation rate, anemia resulting from hypersplenism or recurrent gastrointestinal bleeding, and increased levels of circulating immunoglobulin E (IgE). Although mild elevations of serum asparate aminotransferase (AST) (previously known as serum glutamic-oxaloacetic transaminase, or SGOT) and lactate dehydrogenase (LDH) have been noted during acute infections, tests of liver function generally remain normal until the more advanced stages of the illness.[8, 10, 13]

Extrahepatic complications involving the intestinal tract (e.g., colonic polyposis), central nervous system, eyes, kidneys and genitourinary structures, and skin have also been observed either during the course of infection or as a consequence of the ectopic deposition of *Schistosoma* eggs.[7] Cholecystitis has occasionally been reported in association with chronic schistosomal infections.[14, 15]

DIAGNOSIS AND PATHOLOGY

The diagnosis of acute schistosomiasis should be considered in persons experiencing fever, gastrointestinal distress, and eosinophilia after fresh-water contact in areas affected by this disease. Stool examinations are frequently negative during the initial phases of infection. The recent development of sensitive serologic assays has facilitated earlier diagnosis before substantial egg deposition has occurred.[16, 17]

Identification of schistosome eggs in stool specimens is the most convenient and definitive method of diagnosing an active intestinal infection (Fig. 17–3). Persons with chronic infections, however, pass fewer eggs in stool and may be more reliably diagnosed by examining biopsies obtained from the rectal mucosa.[17] Needle biopsy of the liver may be useful for excluding other causes of granulomatous hepatic disease but is not sufficiently sensitive for the diagnosis of schistosomal infection.[6] Standardized ultrasonographic techniques and classification schemes

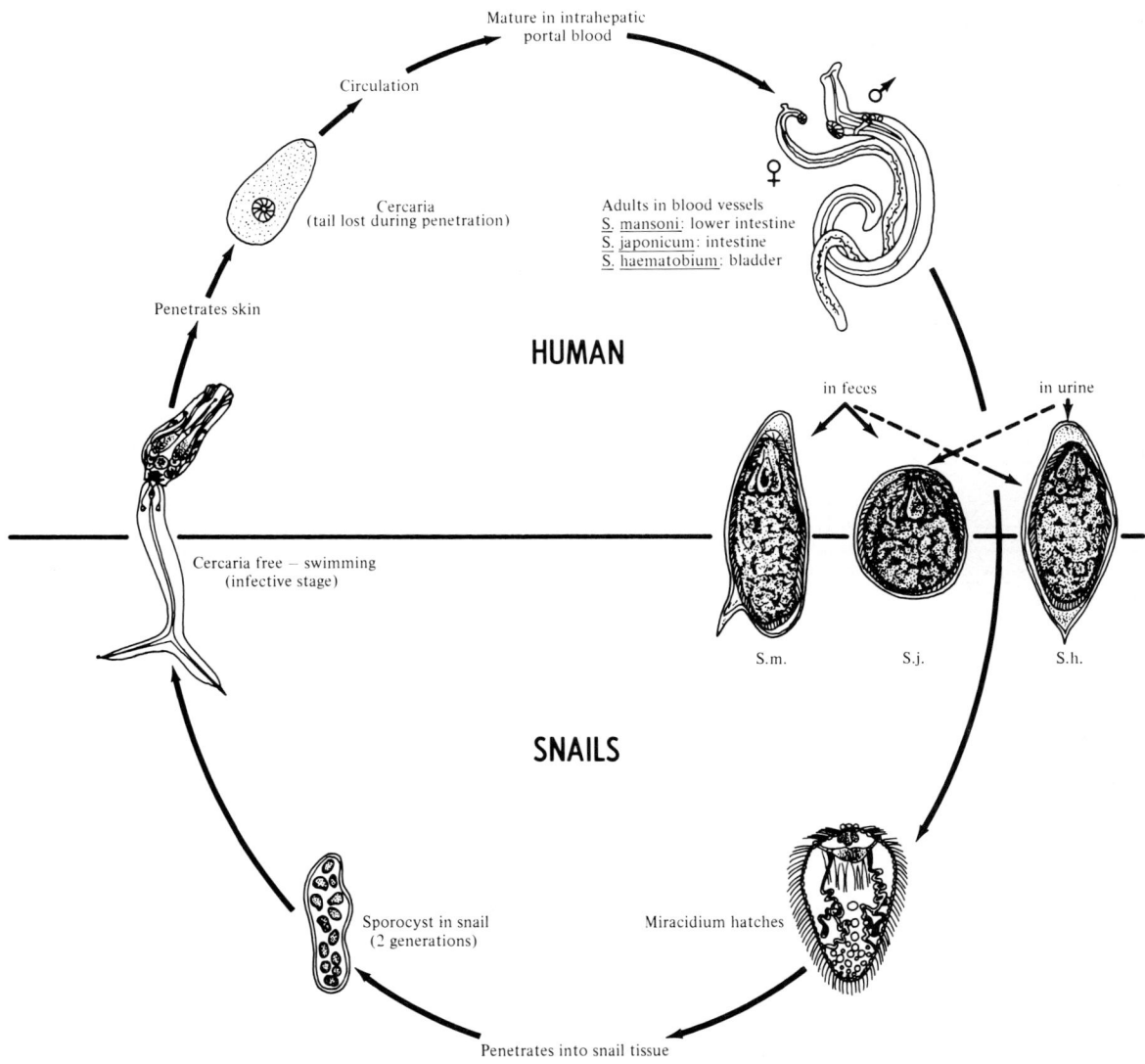

Mature in intrahepatic
portal blood

Circulation

Cercaria
(tail lost during penetration)

Adults in blood vessels
S. mansoni: lower intestine
S. japonicum: intestine
S. haematobium: bladder

Penetrates skin

HUMAN

in feces   in urine

S.m.   S.j.   S.h.

Cercaria free — swimming
(infective stage)

SNAILS

Miracidium hatches

Sporocyst in snail
(2 generations)

Penetrates into snail tissue

FIGURE 17–1.
Life cycle of schistosomes.

have also been developed to assess hepatic pathologic change noninvasively in this disease.[18, 19]

Early clinical manifestations of schistosomiasis should be distinguished from those observed in toxocariasis, trichinosis, filariasis, strongyloidiasis, and capillariasis. Hepatosplenic complications may mimic findings seen in cirrhosis, typhoid fever, visceral leishmaniasis, chronic malarial infection, leukemia, and lymphoma.[10]

TREATMENT AND PREVENTION

Praziquantel, 40 to 60 mg/kg of body weight given over one day and divided in 2 or 3 oral doses, is the treatment of choice for all species of schistosome infections. Higher dosages have

generally been reserved for the treatment of *S. japonicum* and *S. mekongi* infections or for persons heavily infected with *S. mansoni*.[20, 21] Some investigators have advocated the concurrent use of corticosteroids during the acute phase of infection to suppress immunologically mediated symptoms and to avoid adverse reactions to drug therapy.[22, 23] Short-course steroid therapy combined with furosemide and spironolactone has also been reported to offer some advantage in the management of refractory ascites complicating hepatic schistosomiasis.[24] Oxamniquine, given in oral doses of 15 to 60 mg/kg of body weight for 1 to 2 days, and metrifonate, 7.5 to 10 mg/kg of body weight given orally every other week for 3 doses, are effective alternative

WORLD DISTRIBUTION OF SCHISTOSOMIASIS

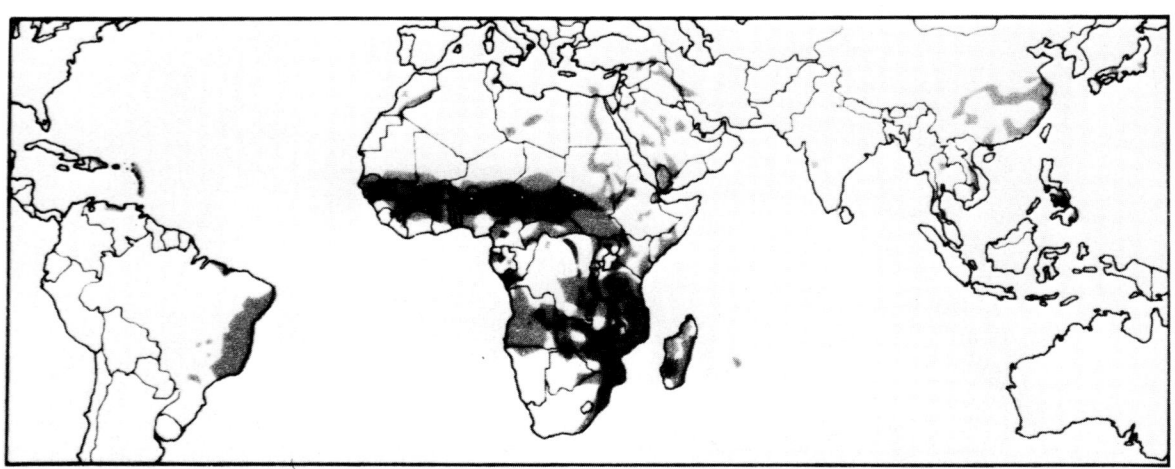

FIGURE 17–2.
Geographic distribution of schistosomiasis.

therapies for *S. mansoni* and *S. haematobium* infections, respectively, in persons who cannot tolerate praziquantel.[6, 21]

Surgical interventions, including distal splenorenal shunting, with or without splenopancreatic disconnection, and esophagogastric devascularization with splenectomy, have been reported effective in controlling recurrent variceal hemorrhage due to schistosomal liver disease.[25–28] By contrast, endoscopic sclerotherapy has not been superior to standard approaches in controlling acute variceal bleeding but is associated with a higher long-term survival than is standard therapy.[29] The role of beta-blockers in managing these complications is also being explored.[30]

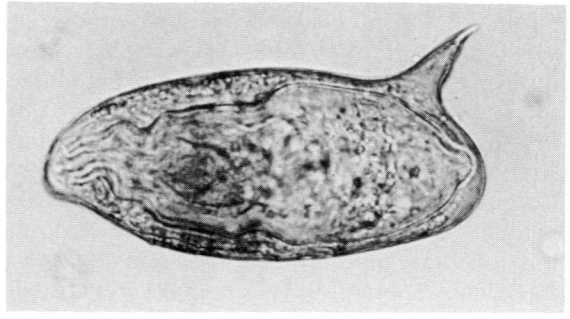

FIGURE 17–3.
Egg of *Schistosoma mansoni* in stool. SOURCE: Courtesy of ML Eberhard PhD, Centers for Disease Control and Prevention, Atlanta GA.

Prevention of infection in persons residing in areas with endemic schistosomiasis depends on the implementation of cost-effective educational and control measures directed at eliminating contamination of water sources by human waste and on instituting widespread therapy of infected individuals. Travelers to these areas should be advised of the risk of disease due to exposure to contaminated fresh water.

Fascioliasis

PARASITE LIFE CYCLE AND EPIDEMIOLOGY

Fascioliasis, or sheep liver fluke disease, is infection with *Fasciola hepatica* or *Fasciola gigantica*. Because the life cycle, pathology, and clinical manifestations of these species are similar, we will use the term *Fasciola* species to refer to both and will distinguish between the two only when discussing geographic distribution. *Fasciola* species are trematode parasites (flukes) that classically cycle between herbivorous mammals and intermediate aquatic snail hosts (Fig. 17–4). Parasite eggs, passed in the feces of infected mammals into freshwater streams or ponds, produce larval forms (miracidia) that penetrate lymnaeid snails, in which they develop into other larval stages before emerging from the snail as mobile cercariae. The cercariae seek out aquatic plants on which to attach and encyst, forming metacercariae that remain intact and infectious for long periods if not subjected to desiccation.[31–34] Definitive hosts become in-

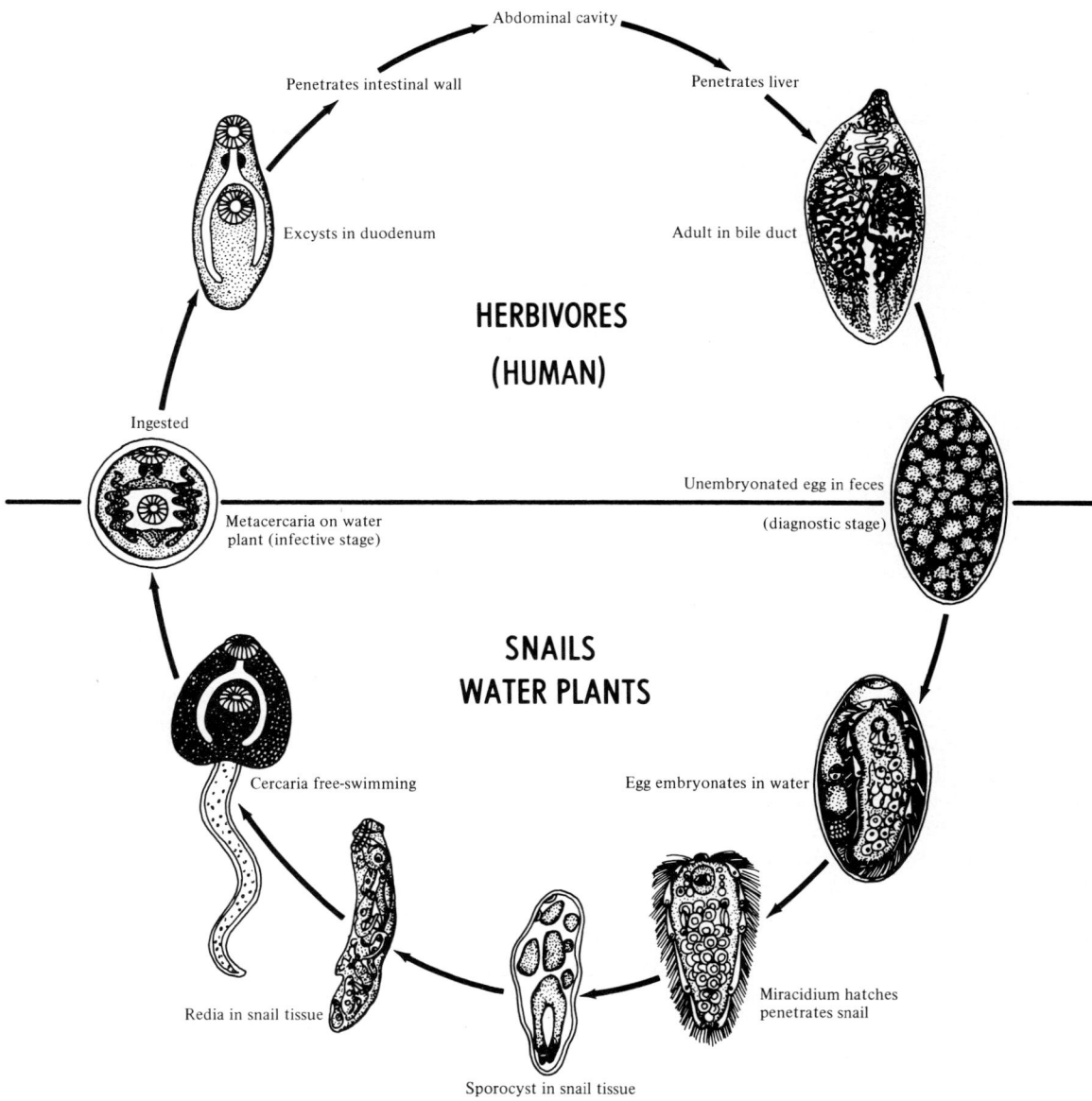

FIGURE 17–4.
Life cycle of *Fasciola hepatica*.

fected when they consume uncooked aquatic plants or water that contains encysted metacercariae. Shortly after being consumed by an appropriate host, the metacercariae excyst in the duodenum, traverse the intestinal wall, and enter the abdominal cavity. Larvae then develop into immature flukes that penetrate Glisson's capsule and migrate through the hepatic parenchyma for several weeks before settling in the bile ducts, where they eventually reach sexual maturity. Once mature, these hermaphroditic flukes produce eggs that are passed with the host's feces, thereby completing the life cycle.[31–34] Adult flukes have been reported to survive as

long as 9 to 13 years in humans. Although the prepatent period (from ingestion of metacercariae to recovery of eggs in feces) ranges from 2 to 4 months, symptoms of acute fascioliasis may occur as soon as immature flukes begin their migration through the hepatic parenchyma.[31, 34]

Human fascioliasis is classically associated with the consumption of contaminated (wild) watercress, but the ingestion of any aquatic plant or water containing viable metacercariae results in infection (Fig. 17–5). Consumption of raw *Fasciola*-infected animal liver causes "false" fascioliasis, when eggs or adult flukes contained

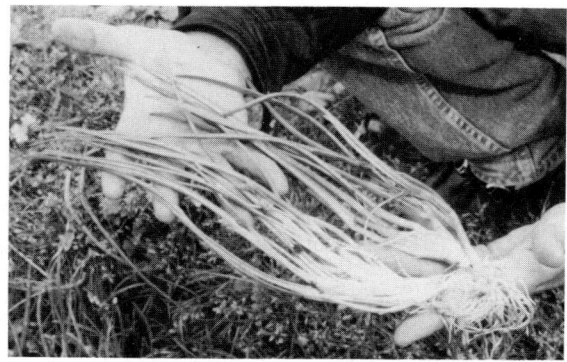

FIGURE 17–5.
Aquatic plant (kjosco) associated with *Fasciola hepatica* transmission in Bolivia.

in the ingested liver are detected in feces,[33] but it does not cause true infection as suggested in one report.[35] Unlike the cercariae of *Schistosoma* species, the metacercariae of *Fasciola* species cannot penetrate intact skin and must be consumed to initiate an infection.[31]

Fasciola gigantica, a common parasite of herbivorous mammals in Africa, Asia, and Hawaii, has been reported in humans in Zimbabwe, Uganda, Tashkent in the former Soviet Union, Iraq, and Hawaii.[32, 33] *Fasciola hepatica,* by contrast occurs throughout the world but primarily in temperate and subtropical regions where animal husbandry practices provide infected sheep, cattle, and goats with unrestricted access to aquatic vegetation (Fig. 17–6). Fascioliasis, therefore, is a zoonotic disease of primarily domestic livestock that is endemic in many regions of Europe, Latin America (including Cuba and Puerto Rico), North Africa, Asia, the Western Pacific, and various regions of the United States. Sporadic reports of human cases have been received from all these areas, and the disease may be endemic in certain human populations in Cuba, Puerto Rico, Peru, Bolivia, and Chile.[31, 36–38] Epidemics in humans, which may follow seasons of high rainfall, have occurred in France, the United Kingdom, Hungary, Egypt, Algeria, Brazil, and Bolivia.[31, 33, 38, 39] Both autochthonous and imported human cases occur in the United States but are rarely reported (CDC, unpublished data, 1992).[40]

CLINICAL MANIFESTATIONS

The incubation period of this infection in humans has been inadequately studied. Based on a few outbreaks and isolated case reports, estimates range from a few days to 3 months.[31] Such estimates have been limited, however, by the occurrence of asymptomatic acute infection and acute infections that are superimposed on chronic infections.

The clinical manifestations of fascioliasis are generally classified into three phases: acute or invasive, chronic-latent, and chronic-obstructive. A fourth category, ectopic fascioliasis, may occur during any of these three phases but is most common during the acute phase. Signs and symptoms during the invasive phase correspond to the migration of juvenile flukes through the hepatic parenchyma. Acute disease, if symptomatic, lasts from 2 to 4 months and is typically heralded by a triad of fever, abdominal pain (usually right upper quadrant), and eosinophilia. Urticaria with dermatographia occurs in up to 21% of cases, and nonspecific gastrointestinal complaints such as anorexia, nausea, and diarrhea are relatively common. Physical examination is most notable for fever and tender hepatomegaly. Splenomegaly has been noted in 12 to 25% of reported acute cases; jaundice or ascites is rarely observed. The most helpful laboratory finding is eosinophilia, which is virtually always greater than 5% and may reach as high as 83%. Leukocytosis is common, ranging from 10,000 to 43,000 cells/mm³. Mild to moderate anemia may also occur.[31] Reports of liver function abnormalities during this phase of the disease are conflicting, but several recent reports have consistently noted abnormal findings on liver function tests.[31, 40–43]

The latent phase corresponds to that period in the life cycle of *Fasciola* species when immature flukes have ceased their migration and have settled within the biliary ducts. Oviposition begins at this point, thus marking the end of the prepatent period. The chronic-latent phase may last for months or years. During this phase, the patient may be completely asymptomatic or may experience vague, nonspecific gastrointestinal symptoms. Persistent eosinophilia and intermittent fever may also occur; the former is frequently a clue to the diagnosis in asymptomatic individuals. Some patients may also exhibit recurrences of acute signs and symptoms.[31, 39]

The chronic-obstructive phase results from the biliary ductal inflammation and epithelial hyperplasia induced by the presence of adult flukes in both intra- and extrahepatic bile ducts.[31, 44] This stage of infection is often characterized by recurrent episodes of biliary colic, cholangitis, cholelithiasis, cholecystitis, and the usual laboratory and radiologic findings suggestive of biliary obstruction.[31, 33, 35, 39, 45] Hepatomegaly is common in long-standing infections.[31] Despite some published claims to the con-

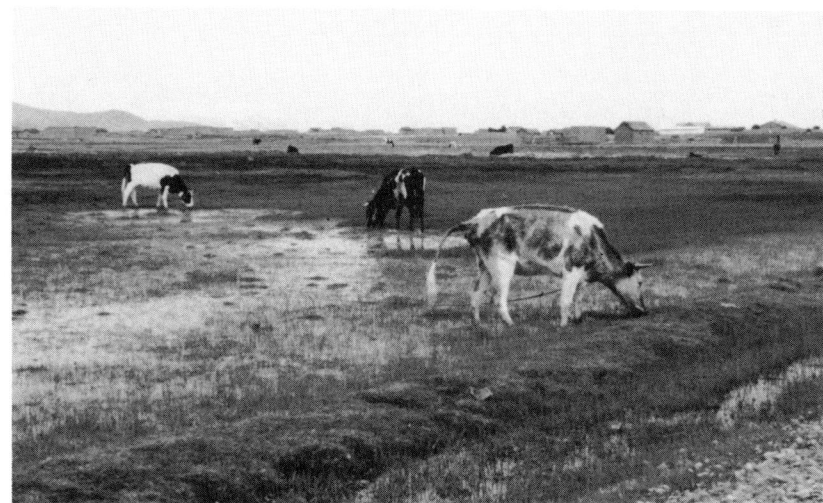

FIGURE 17–6.
Typical epidemiologic setting for endemic fascioliasis: cattle feeding on aquatic vegetation in Bolivia.

trary,[35, 40] eosinophilia may indeed be a feature during this, or any other, stage of fascioliasis and is frequently a valuable clue to the diagnosis.[31-34] Moderate to severe anemia, perhaps due to loss of blood in bile, also occurs. *Fasciola* flukes, although not true blood feeders, may ingest blood while feeding on hepatic parenchyma or ductal epithelium and may induce blood loss through epithelial injury.[33] Although not always present, abnormal findings on liver function tests, including aminotransferase, alkaline phosphatase, and bilirubin elevations, are also relatively common during this phase.[31-35, 39]

Although pericholangitis and periportal fibrosis are usually minimal, biliary cirrhosis and sclerosing cholangitis may occur in cases of prolonged heavy infection.[31] No reasonable data suggest a positive association between fascioliasis and hepatocellular carcinoma or cholangiocarcinoma.[31, 46]

Ectopic fascioliasis, which usually results from the aberrant migration of juvenile flukes, has been reported in numerous anatomic sites.[31, 32, 34, 46-50] The skin over the abdomen is the most common site of extrahepatic involvement and is sometimes associated with painful, pruritic, subcutaneous nodules.[50] In Bolivia, we have seen patients in whom ectopically migrating flukes have actually migrated to the cutaneous surface, where they are physically extracted by the patient (CDC, unpublished data, 1988).

Gastrointestinal bleeding in the form of hemobilia, an uncommon complication, has been reported as the cause of death in 3 patients.[31, 44, 47] Deaths due to fascioliasis are exceedingly rare, and only 5 other fatal cases have been reported. Hepatic subcapsular hematoma is also a rarely reported complication.[31, 50]

DIAGNOSIS AND PATHOLOGY

During the acute phase, diagnosis of fascioliasis depends on the correct observation of characteristic signs and symptoms in persons with appropriate epidemiologic histories. Because no eggs are passed during this phase, direct parasitologic confirmation of the diagnosis is unlikely to occur except in those rare cases of cutaneous ectopic migration or during laparotomy, when migrating flukes might be directly visualized. Indirect immunologic methods, however, are potentially useful.

Definitive diagnosis of fascioliasis during the latent and chronic phases is most commonly achieved by the demonstration of eggs in stool, duodenal fluid, or biliary drainage. *Fasciola* eggs are large (130–150 μm $\times$ 63–90 μm), operculated, and light yellowish brown (Fig. 17–7A). Of the numerous stool examination techniques available, sedimentation procedures appear to work best.[31, 33, 34, 51, 52] Demonstration of eggs in feces, however, may be difficult because egg excretion is often intermittent, requiring repeated stool examinations to confirm the diagnosis. Eggs of *F. hepatica* and *F. gigantica* appear identical and are difficult to distinguish from those of the intestinal fluke *Fasciolopsis buski*.[33] In areas where uncooked liver is consumed, false fascioliasis may occur but is easily ruled out by placing the patient on a liver-free diet for 3 days and repeating the stool examination.[33, 53]

In recent years, various radiologic imaging techniques have proven helpful in the evaluation of fascioliasis. Most techniques, however, yield nonspecific findings. Various case reports have commented on the use of cholangiography, endoscopic retrograde cholangiopancreatography (ERCP), radioisotope scanning, ultra-

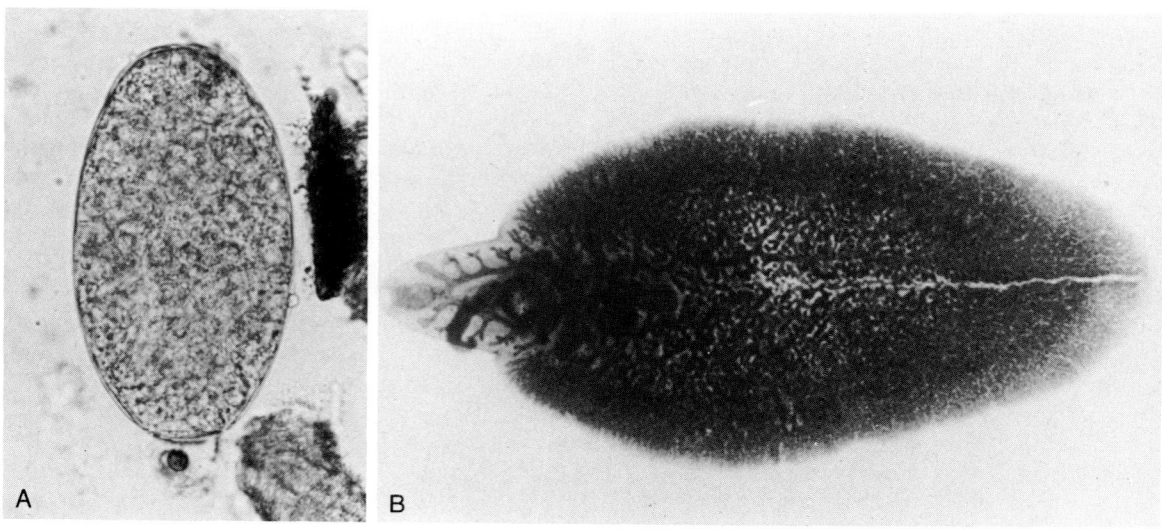

FIGURE 17–7.
(*A*), Egg of *Fasciola hepatica* in stool. (*B*), Adult fluke.

sound (US), and computed tomography (CT).[31] Published experience with magnetic resonance imaging (MRI) is too limited to warrant comment.

Oval radiolucent images consistent in size and shape with adult flukes have been visualized by intravenous cholangiography, oral cholecystography, and ERCP.[31, 45, 54, 55] Radionuclide imaging of the liver using technetium (Tc 99m) sulfur colloid may show hepatomegaly with focal defects or so-called cold lesions; imaging with gallium citrate (Ga 67) shows increased uptake, or hot spots, in the same areas.[31, 56]

Ultrasound, when used to evaluate acute disease, may produce normal results or may reveal the nonspecific findings of hepatomegaly or areas of increased hepatic echogenicity or both.[35, 45, 57] During the latent or chronic-obstructive phases, however, echogenic structures, which are sometimes motile, and consistent in size and shape with adult flukes and have been visualized in the gallbladder and common bile duct.[45, 58, 59] Other, less specific, ultrasonographic findings include biliary ductal dilatation with irregular wall thickening.[45]

Of the many radiologic imaging techniques used to evaluate fascioliasis, CT appears to be the most consistently useful, particularly during the hepatic migration phase of the disease. The findings of CT scans in patients whose disease is in the latent and chronic phases are frequently normal. A review of the literature available reveals two characteristic findings on hepatic CT. First, multiple nodular, hypodense lesions, ranging from 4 to 30 mm, may be present in the right or left hepatic lobes. These lesions, which are thought to correspond to microabscesses or areas of parenchymatous destruction, may be found both centrally and peripherally.[35, 40, 42, 45, 60] Second, peripherally located branching or tortuous lesions corresponding to the migratory tracts of the juvenile flukes may be seen with CT. Such tracts have also been seen at surgery and laparoscopy.[40, 45, 60] Both nodular, hypodense lesions and branching lesions are better visualized with contrast enhancement, and both may diminish or disappear after appropriate medical therapy.[35, 40, 42, 45, 60]

Numerous immunodiagnostic tests for infection with *F. hepatica* have been developed, but such tests vary widely in sensitivity, specificity, cost, and availability. Immunodiagnostic tests are essential during the acute prepatent stages of fascioliasis when eggs are not excreted; early diagnosis and treatment can prevent severe clinical sequelae. Excellent comprehensive reviews of immunologic tests for fascioliasis are available.[31, 53, 61] Enzyme-linked immunosorbent assays (ELISA), immunofluorescence assays (IFA), and counterelectrophoresis (CEP) appear to be the most sensitive and specific, but cross-reactions with other parasitic infections, particularly schistosomiasis, may occur. Moreover, IFA and CEP findings may not be positive during the latent and chronic-obstructive phases.[31, 34] The enzyme-linked immunoelectrotransfer blot (EITB) holds promise as a highly specific immunodiagnostic test for fascioliasis.[62] The use of CEP techniques to identify fluke antigens in stool specimens from patients with fascioliasis also pears promising.[63] Skin tests, which were once commonly used, are no longer recommended because of their low specificity.[31, 61]

Fascioliasis is sometimes diagnosed by the discovery of adult flukes in the gallbladder or bile ducts during ERCP, laparoscopy, laparotomy, or autopsy.[31, 44, 45, 47, 53, 54, 58] One report even noted flukes in postoperative biliary drainage.[64] The flukes are leaf-shaped, relatively flat, and measure up to 30 mm by 13 mm (Fig. 17–7B).[33]

During laparotomy or laparoscopy, yellowish or grayish white nodules 1 to 30 mm in diameter and ribbed or vermiform formations of similar color are often seen on the surface of the liver. Nodules have also been observed in adjacent parietal peritoneum, and hepatic capsular thickening may be present.[31, 39, 45, 65, 66] In chronic cases, the gallbladder and common bile duct are usually thickened, edematous, dilated, or all three.

Microscopically, liver lesions generally show hepatic necrosis and granulomata with Charcot-Leyden crystals and eosinophilic infiltrates. Eosinophilic abscesses and egg granulomata may also be present. Occasionally, portions of eggs or migrating flukes are seen on liver biopsy. In the bile ducts, epithelial hyperplasia and periportal fibrosis occur.[31, 33, 39, 46, 50]

TREATMENT AND PREVENTION

Although surgical intervention may be required for some of the long-term sequelae and rarer complications of fascioliasis, most patients can be treated with appropriate anthelminthic medications. Patients with parasitologically confirmed infections, whether or not they are symptomatic, should be treated without delay. For others in whom the diagnosis is unproved but strongly suspected based on appropriate clinical and epidemiologic findings, empirical therapy is reasonable, particularly if the diagnosis is supported by positive serologic results. Of the dozen or so drugs reported to have efficacy against *Fasciola* species in human trials or case reports, only four warrant discussion here. The current drug of choice is the halogenated phenol derivative bithionol. Given in an oral dosage of 50 mg/kg of body weight in 3 divided doses on alternate days for 15 days, the drug is effective in eradicating most human infections. Side effects, which are generally mild, include anorexia, nausea, vomiting, and abdominal pain.[21, 31] In the United States, bithionol is available only through the federal Centers for Disease Control and Prevention (CDC) Drug Service in Atlanta GA (404-639-3670; after hours, holidays, and weekends: 404-639-2888). A com-

parably effective alternative to bithionol is the parenterally administered alkaloid compound dehydroemetine, given intramuscularly (IM) or subcutaneously (SC) in daily doses of 1 mg/kg of body weight for 10 days. Nevertheless, dehydroemetine has been associated with more significant cardiac, hepatic, and gastrointestinal adverse reactions. This medication is also available through the CDC Drug Service.

A candidate likely soon to replace bithionol as the treatment of choice for human fascioliasis is the benzimidazole derivative triclabendazole. This compound, given in a single or split oral dose, has been effective and tolerated well in several recent case reports[42, 43, 67] and is undergoing extended clinical trials sponsored by the World Health Organization and the product manufacturer (Ciba-Geigy). Unfortunately, this drug is not commercially available in North America.

Despite comments to the contrary in some textbooks and case reports,[64] praziquantel does not appear to be consistently effective against human infection with *Fasciola* species. Several recent publications have noted its lack of efficacy.[31, 41, 43, 51, 68, 69]

The prevention of fascioliasis requires public health education and modification of animal husbandry practices. Educational efforts are directed toward potential consumers of aquatic plants, particularly wild watercress. Changes in animal husbandry practices should include measures to inspect regularly and treat livestock and to ensure separation of livestock and other potentially infected herbivores from areas where aquatic vegetation is cultivated for human consumption.

Clinicians who encounter patients with fascioliasis should inquire carefully about the circumstances of infection; other persons who may not yet be symptomatic may have been infected simultaneously. Moreover, the source of infection needs to be identified so that it may be eradicated and not pose a risk to others.[39]

Clonorchiasis and Opisthorchiasis

PARASITE LIFE CYCLE AND EPIDEMIOLOGY

The parasites that cause clonorchiasis (*Clonorchis sinensis*) and opisthorchiasis (*Opisthorchis viverrini* and *O. felineus*) are digenetic trematodes of the family Opisthorchioidea. They are liver flukes that, although taxonomically distinct, have similar life cycles and clinical manifestations. All three have low host specificity and can infect a variety of mammalian reservoir hosts, including humans. In addition, they each require two intermediate hosts: an aquatic snail and either freshwater fish or, occasionally, freshwater crayfish (Fig. 17–8). Parasite eggs are passed in the feces of infected mammals into freshwater habitats, where the eggs are consumed by an appropriate intermediate snail host and then hatch. Larvae emerge as free-swimming cercariae, which seek out and penetrate a second intermediate host, a suitable freshwater fish or crayfish, in which they encyst as metacercariae in skin or muscle. When consumed in raw or undercooked fish or crayfish by a mammalian host, the metacercariae excyst in the duodenum and migrate up the ampulla of Vater to the bile ducts, where they mature to egg-producing capability within 1 month (pre-patent period).[70–72] Adult flukes are flat, slender, and 10 to 25 mm (C. sinensis) or 8 to 12 mm (O. viverrini) in length (Fig. 17–9). They can survive in human hosts for more than 20 years.[71, 73, 74]

The Chinese or Oriental liver fluke (C. sinensis) is widespread in both humans and animals in Japan, Korea, China, Taiwan, and Vietnam. More than 20 million persons in China and 4.5 million in Korea are estimated to be infected.

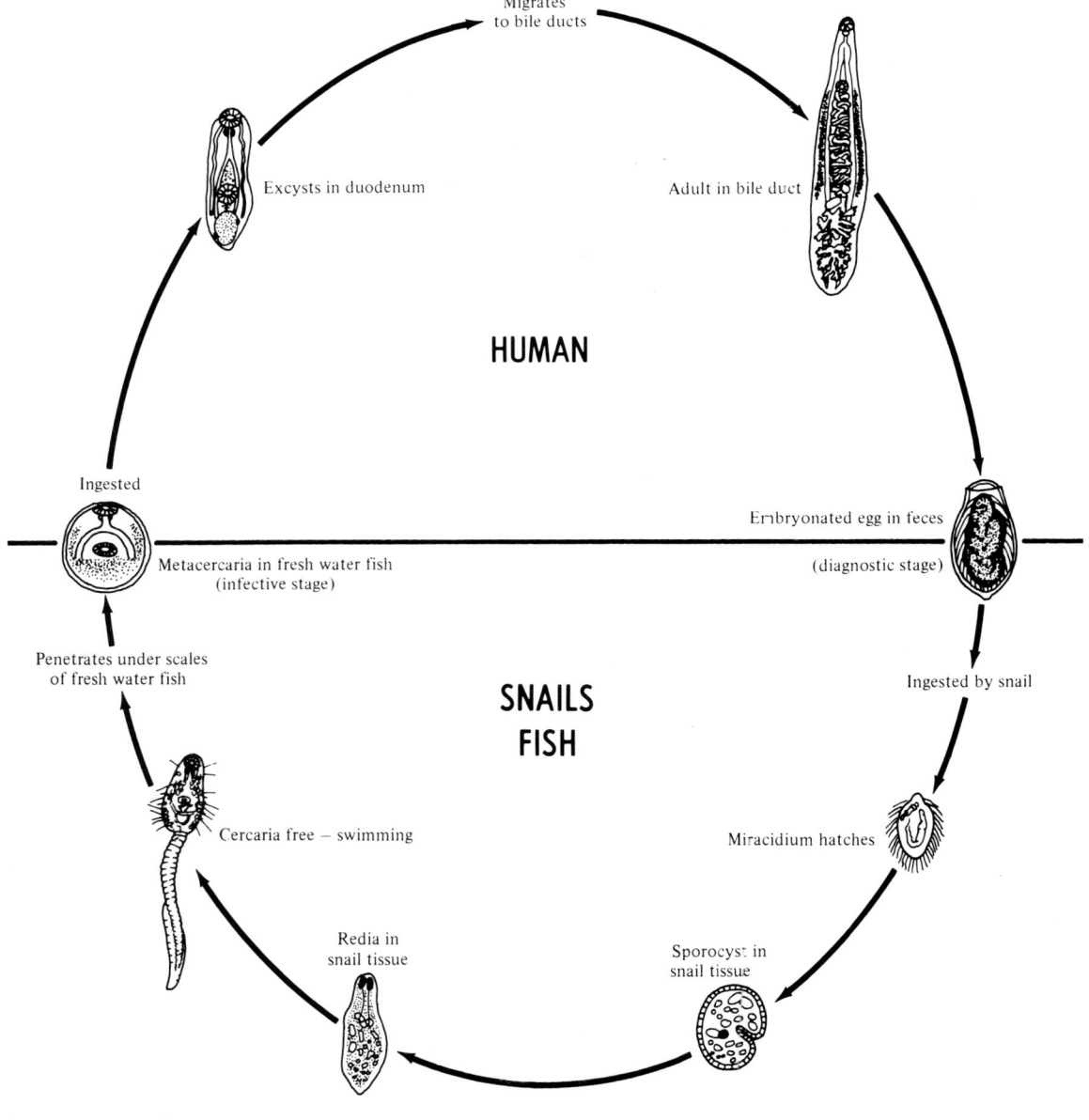

FIGURE 17–8.
Life cycle of *Clonorchis sinensis*.

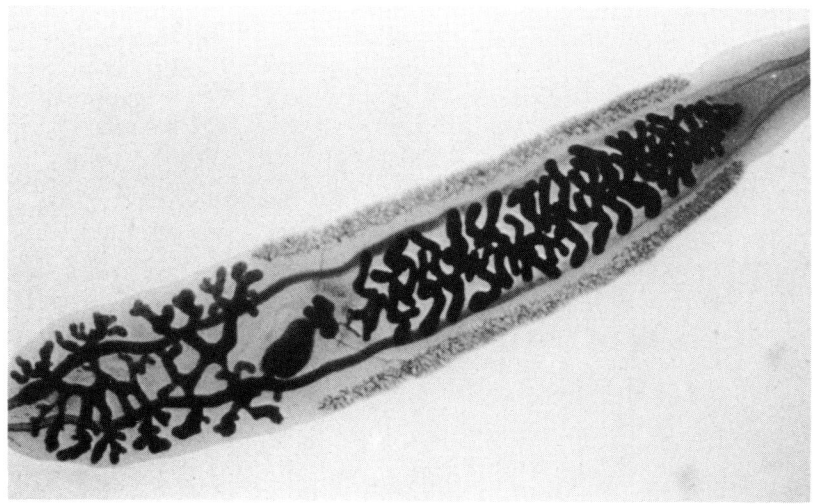

FIGURE 17–9.
Adult *Clonorchis sinensis*. SOURCE:
Courtesy of DA Schwartz, MD.
Emory University, Atlanta GA.

Its persistence in human hosts is closely linked to sociocultural factors that include dietary, animal husbandry, and agricultural practices. In South China and Hong Kong, for example, dishes such as *yue-shan* and *yue-shan chuk*, containing the raw fish known locally as "ide," are popular among adult males. In Japan, infection is often linked to the consumption of sashimi and sunomono (fish pickled in vinegar).[46, 73, 75]

Opisthorchis viverrini is also an important human parasite in Southeast Asia, where it is estimated to infect over 7 million persons in Thailand, Laos, Cambodia, Vietnam, and China.[46, 70, 73, 75, 76] Unlike clonorchiasis, *O. viverrini* opisthorchiasis is not uncommon in young age groups because *kio-pla*, a dish made from chopped raw fish, is widely consumed and often fed to infants and young children.[46, 73, 77] *Opisthorchis felineus*, the cat liver fluke, exists primarily in Eastern Europe and the former Soviet Union, where numerous domestic dogs and cats and wild mammals serve as natural reservoirs. Human infections are most commonly reported from Poland, Siberia, and Kazakhstan.[71, 72, 78]

Clonorchiasis/opisthorchiasis can be transmitted outside of areas where it is endemic through the consumption of imported raw, smoked, sun-dried, salted, or pickled freshwater fish infected with metacercariae, as has been reported among natives of Hawaii.[46, 71] In addition, hepatobiliary fluke infestations are among the most commonly identified parasitic infections in Southeast Asian immigrants entering North America.[73, 74, 78, 79]

CLINICAL MANIFESTATIONS

In the majority of persons with light infections, clonorchiasis/opisthorchiasis is asympto-

matic and is diagnosed only during routine screening for fecal parasites. Manifestations of acute infection, reported only for *C. sinensis* and *O. felineus*, are rarely observed. Such manifestations usually develop 2 to 3 weeks after the consumption of contaminated fish and include fever, abdominal pain, diarrhea, leukocytosis, and eosinophilia.[46, 73, 78, 80] Later sequelae are strongly correlated with the intensity and duration of fluke infestation.[76, 80, 81] Clinical features in symptomatic, chronically infected persons include right upper quadrant and epigastric abdominal pain, anorexia, diarrhea, low-grade fever, and tender hepatomegaly. Eosinophilia, if present, is usually less than 20%.[46, 73, 78, 80, 82] With persistent infection or increasing worm burdens, signs and symptoms of chronic or intermittent biliary obstruction develop. Cholelithiasis and cholecystitis are common; ascites, hepatic abscesses, biliary stricture, pancreatitis, and recurrent suppurative cholangitis may also develop.[46, 70, 73, 76, 78, 81, 83] These signs and symptoms are frequently accompanied by jaundice. Alkaline phosphatase and bilirubin levels are often elevated, and mild to moderate elevations of hepatic aminotransferases are common. Upper gastrointestinal bleeding with hemobilia has been reported, but this occurred in a Thai patient co-infected with *O. viverrini* and *F. hepatica*. Biliary cirrhosis has not been clearly associated with clonorchiasis/opisthorchiasis.[72, 84]

Prolonged heavy infections may lead to chronic inflammation with resultant periportal fibrosis, dilated and tortuous bile ducts, and epithelial dysplasia (Fig. 17–10).[76, 81, 83] Such dysplastic epithelium may give rise to primary hepatic malignancy in the form of cholangiocarcinoma (often mucin-secreting adenocarcinoma).[46, 83, 84, 85] Although other carcinogenic cofactors may ex-

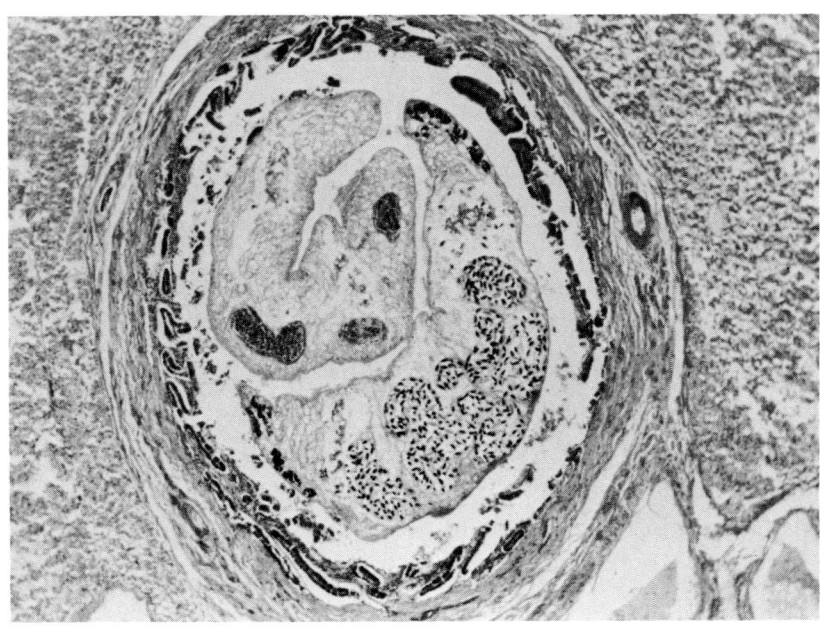

FIGURE 17–10.
Histopathology of clonorchiasis/opisthorchiasis. *Clonorchis sinensis* in a bile duct with squamous metaplasia of the epithelium and prominent periductal fibrosis. Characteristic eggs are seen in the uterus of the fluke. SOURCE: Courtesy of DA Schwartz, MD, Emory University, Atlanta GA and the Armed Forces Institute of Pathology, Washington DC; Schwartz DA. Helminths in the induction of cancer: *Opisthorchis viverrini, Clonorchis sinensis* and cholangiocarcinoma. Trop Geogr Med. 1980;32:95–109.

ert an additive or synergistic influence, the strong association and probable cause and effect relationship between clonorchiasis/opisthorchiasis and cholangiocarcinoma is well documented by clinical and epidemiologic investigations in humans and by experimental studies in animals.[46, 70, 76, 77, 84, 85] Cholangiocarcinomas are often multicentric and tend to arise in the secondary bile ducts of the hepatic hilum.[46, 85] Although most common in men older than 40 years, this condition has been found in persons as young as 23 years.[81] The signs and symptoms are nonspecific. Most patients experience involuntary, unexplained weight loss, and up to 50% of those infected have epigastric pain, abdominal mass, jaundice, and ascites.[46] Metastatic adenocarcinomas have been found in the lung, brain, gallbladder, kidney, heart, omentum, and diaphragm.[85] The vast majority of published reports relating liver fluke infections to cholangiocarcinoma refer to *C. sinensis* and *O. viverrini*, and not to *O. felineus*. Whether this means that *O. felineus* lacks this association or that *O. felineus*–associated cholangiocarcinomas are underreported is uncertain.

DIAGNOSIS AND PATHOLOGY

The diagnosis of clonorchiasis/opisthorchiasis is usually confirmed by demonstrating fluke eggs in feces. The eggs of *C. sinensis*, *O. viverrini*, and *O. felineus* are very similar and need not be distinguished for appropriate therapy to be provided. The eggs of these three species should, however, be distinguished from those of intestinal flukes. Unlike *Fasciola* species, eggs of *C. sinensis* and *Opisthorchis* species are excreted frequently and in sufficient numbers to make routine stool examination adequate for diagnostic confirmation in most uncomplicated cases. Eggs may also be found in duodenal aspirates. In patients with advanced disease and obstructive jaundice, however, eggs may not appear in feces, despite enormous worm burdens. In such cases, the diagnosis is confirmed by finding eggs or adult flukes in the biliary ducts or gallbladder at surgery or autopsy, in postoperative biliary drainage, or in biliary fluid obtained by percutaneous needle aspiration.[73, 77, 80, 81, 83, 86]

Cholangiographic studies typically reveal relatively uniform and slender filling defects within dilated intrahepatic ducts. Ducts may also show epithelial irregularities and tortuosity. Mulberry-like cystic dilatations of the intrahepatic ducts have been reported as radiographically diagnostic of biliary fluke infestation.[46, 72] Ultrasonography is usually helpful only in demonstrating the nonspecific findings of biliary obstruction; some clinicians in Thailand, however, believe that the combination of a hydrops gallbladder and dilated ducts in the absence of gallstones on ultrasound is pathognomonic for cholangio-carcinoma.[76]

Immunologic techniques have, thus far, played a relatively minor role in the diagnosis of clonorchiasis/opisthorchiasis. Immunodiagnostic tests suffer from limited availability and from poor sensitivity and specificity.[46, 73, 78] Nevertheless, recent developments in the detection of diagnostic antigens in stool specimens appear promising.[70, 87]

TREATMENT AND PREVENTION

Because of the availability of safe and effective therapy, the long life span of the parasites in human hosts, and the potentially serious sequelae of persistent infections, all patients with clonorchiasis/opisthorchiasis should be treated, regardless of whether they are symptomatic. The current treatment of choice for infections with *C. sinensis, O. viverrini,* or *O. felineus* is praziquantel, in a total dosage of 75 mg/kg of body weight given orally in 3 divided doses during 1 day.[21] In light infections, a single oral dose of 40 mg/kg may be effective. Repeated doses are occasionally required for heavier infections. Side effects, if they occur, are generally mild and transient and include headache, dizziness, and nausea. No evidence of drug resistance has been reported.[21, 70, 73, 74, 83, 86, 88–90] After treatment, dead flukes are occasionally seen in stool specimens and in postoperative biliary drainage. In successfully treated patients, eggs are undetectable in stool specimens as early as 1 week after treatment; repeating stool examinations 1 month after treatment is advisable. Clinical symptoms and radiologic signs may take several months to resolve.[73] Sphincterotomy, T-tube biliary drainage, or surgical removal of biliary stones, debris, and dead flukes may be necessary in some cases.[46]

Alternative treatment regimens might include mebendazole, given in daily doses of 30 mg/kg of body weight for 3 to 4 weeks, or albendazole, 400 mg given 2 times a day for 7 days, but either is less effective than praziquantel.[73] Chloroquine phosphate was commonly used before the availability of praziquantel.[46, 80]

Prevention depends on the thorough cooking of all freshwater fish or crayfish. Alternatively, metacercariae of *O. viverrini* are effectively destroyed by placing them in 5 to 15% saline solutions for 3 to 10 days or by freezing to −10°C for 5 days.

Echinococcosis

PARASITE LIFE CYCLE AND EPIDEMIOLOGY

Echinococcosis (hydatid disease or hydatidosis) is infection with the larval, or cystic, stage of tapeworms belonging to the genus *Echinococcus.* Adults, or cestodes, are small (5–10 mm), segmented tapeworms that reside in the small intestine of their definitive hosts, usually dogs or other canines (Fig. 17–11). The scolex, or head, attaches to the host's intestinal mucosa by means of four suckers and a double row of rostellar hooks. Eggs containing infective embryos (oncospheres) are passed with the host's feces into the external environment, where they are consumed by appropriate mammalian intermediate hosts such as sheep. Once consumed, the eggs hatch in the small intestine. Liberated oncospheres then penetrate the intestinal mucosa and migrate via venous or lymphatic vessels to distant anatomic sites. The liver is the most common site, but oncospheres may also reach lungs, kidney, spleen, brain, bone, or other tissue. In the liver (or elsewhere), the metacestode, or hydatid cyst, develops by vesiculation and production of thousands of protoscolices. The avascular cyst wall consists of three layers. The outer adventitial layer, or pericyst, is host-derived and may calcify. The intermediate, acellular laminated layer and the innermost germinal layer are both parasite-derived. A protoscolex, which consists of a scolex invaginated into a small forebody, is produced asexually within small secondary cysts (brood capsules or daughter cysts) that develop from the germinal layer. Rupture or leakage of the hydatid cyst results in the release of viable protoscolices and the subsequent development of daughter cysts in secondary anatomic sites. When consumed by a dog or other susceptible definitive host feeding on the uncooked infected viscera of an intermediate host, hundreds of thousands of protoscolices reach the definitive host's small intestine, where each protoscolex may develop into an adult tapeworm. Adults of the species *Echinococcus granulosus* can survive in dogs for up to 29 months.[91–96]

Like other intermediate hosts, humans, especially children, acquire echinococcosis by ingesting *Echinococcus* eggs. Ingestion usually occurs by hand-to-mouth transfer of eggs after contact with infected dogs but may also result from ingesting food, water, or soil contaminated by infected dog feces.[91]

Three species of *Echinococcus* cause disease in humans: *E. granulosus, E. multilocularis,* and *E. vogeli.* Epidemiology, pathogenesis, and clinical manifestations vary according to the infecting species (Table 17–5, Fig. 17–12A and B). *Echi-*

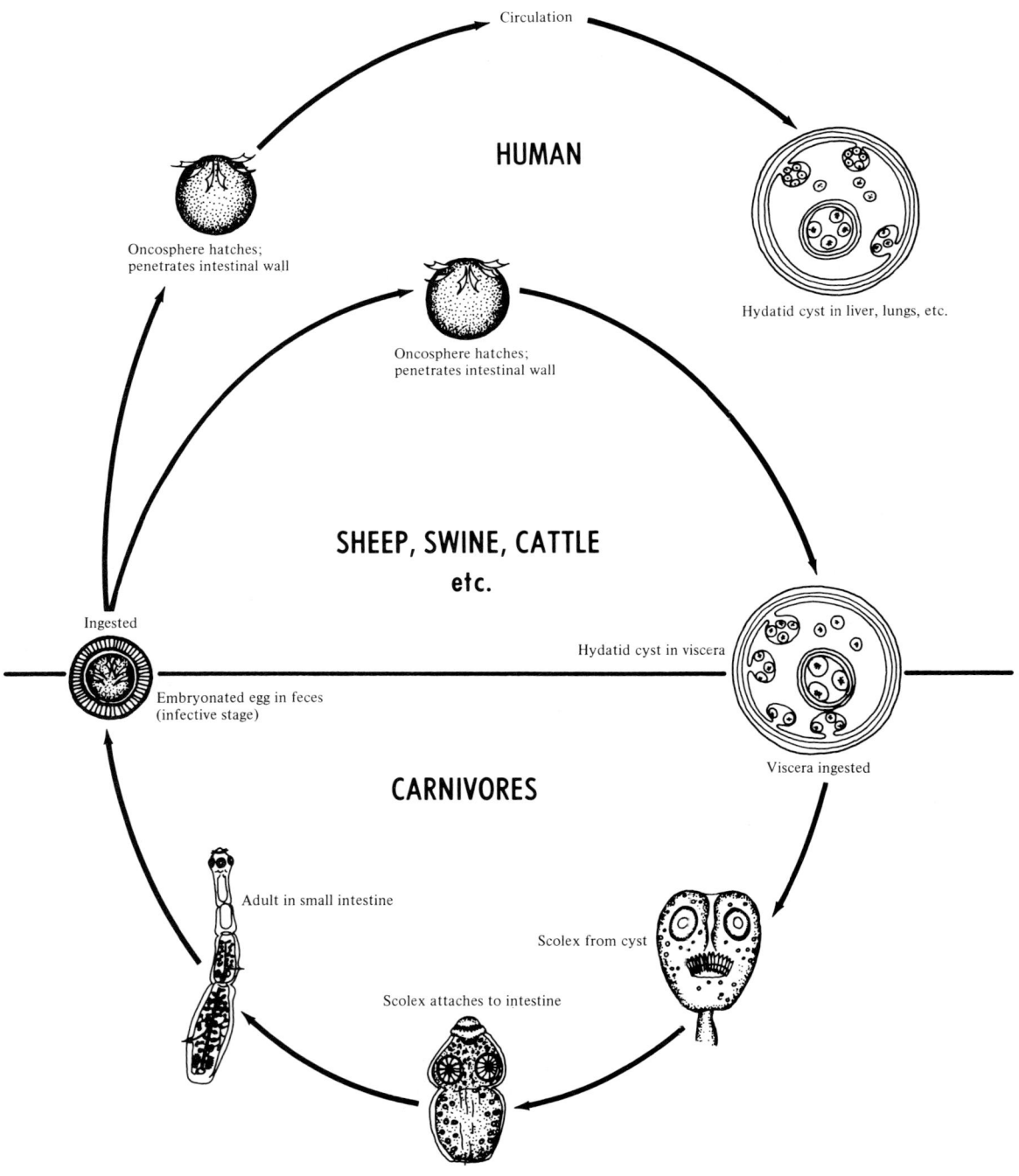

FIGURE 17–11.
Life cycle of *Echinococcus granulosus.*

nococcus granulosus, the causal agent of the cystic form of hydatid disease, is the most common and widespread species. Its usual definitive host is the domestic dog, but it also infects the wolf, coyote, jackal, and dingo. In most parts of the world, sheep are the most important intermediate hosts. In some regions, however, other domestic ungulates (e.g., goats, cattle, swine, buf-falo, horses, and camels) may serve as important reservoirs of infection. *Echinococcus granulosus* occurs worldwide and has been described on every continent except Antarctica. In regions where *E. granulosus* is endemic, infection is most common among persons who use dogs to help raise livestock. In the United States, *E. granulosus* echinococcosis is sporadically prevalent in

TABLE 17–5. ECHINOCOCCUS INFECTIONS AND HUMAN DISEASE

SPECIES	DISTRIBUTION	DEFINITIVE HOSTS	INTERMEDIATE HOSTS	HUMAN DISEASE
Echinococcus granulosus	Worldwide	Dogs, other canines	Domestic & wild ungulates: sheep, cattle, horses, pigs, goats, etc.	Cystic hydatid disease
Echinococcus multilocularis	Northern latitudes of N America & Eurasia	Foxes, dogs, other canines, cats	Rodents	Alveolar hydatid disease
Echinococcus vogeli	Central & S America	Wild & domestic canines	Rodents	Polycystic hydatid disease

sheep-raising regions of Utah, Arizona, New Mexico, and California and exists in domestic-sylvatic cycles (dog-moose or dog-caribou) in Alaska. The diagnosis is more common among native American Navajo and Zuni and in Alaskan natives than in the general population.[91, 97, 98]

The alveolar form of hydatid disease is caused by *E. multilocularis*. Definitive hosts for this species are mostly wild animals such as foxes, and intermediate hosts are usually rodents. Domestic dogs and cats can become definitive hosts, however, if allowed to feed on infected rodents such as voles. The geographic distribution of *E. multilocularis* is more restricted than that of *E. granulosus* and is most common in the northern latitudes of North America and Eurasia. Hunters, trappers, and certain indigenous populations are at highest risk for infection. In the United States, enzootic foci exist in North and South Dakota, Minnesota, Iowa, Nebraska, Montana, Wyoming, and western Alaska. Most human cases in this country have been diagnosed in Alaskan Eskimos; only 2 cases have been reported from north central states of the contiguous United States.[91, 97–100]

Echinococcus vogeli causes the polycystic form of hydatid disease, which occurs in scattered foci in Central and South America. The life cycle involves wild and domestic dogs as definitive hosts and wild rodents such as pacas, agoutis, and spiny rats as intermediate hosts.[91, 97]

CLINICAL MANIFESTATIONS

Signs and symptoms depend primarily on cyst size, location, and condition. In *E. granulosus* echinococcosis, cysts grow by endogenous proliferation of the germinal membrane and enlarge concentrically at a rate of 1 to 5 cm in diameter per year. Infections are usually acquired during childhood, and patients may remain asymptomatic for many years before the usually indolent onset of clinical manifestations. Most human infections (50–70%) involve the liver, and up to 25% of patients with hepatic cysts have concomitant pulmonary cysts. In 5 to 10% of cases, cysts are found in brain, kidney, spleen, heart, or bone. Twenty to 40% of patients have multiple cysts or multiple organ involvement. In patients with uncomplicated hepatic involvement, clinical manifestations commonly include abdominal pain, nausea, vomiting, hepatomegaly, or a palpable abdominal mass. Eosinophilia, although reported in up to 50% of cases, may not be present, even in patients with multiple large hydatid cysts. Hepatic aminotransferases and alkaline phosphatase are generally at normal levels or only mildly elevated.[92, 94–96, 100, 101]

Complications of hepatic *E. granulosus* infection are usually a result of spontaneous or traumatic cyst leakage or rupture. Allergy-like reactions to released cyst contents range from abrupt or intermittent generalized urticaria and pruritus to severe, sometimes fatal, anaphylaxis.[92, 96, 101] In addition, leakage may result in dissemination of the infection by seeding the peritoneal cavity or other locations with protoscolices capable of producing daughter cysts. Cysts rupture into the biliary tree in approximately 5% of cases, producing signs and symptoms typical of biliary obstruction, such as jaundice, nausea or vomiting, and abdominal pain. In some of these cases, daughter cysts have been recovered from the common bile duct.[86, 102, 103] Further complications of biliary involvement may include recurrent, suppurative, or sclerosing cholangitis and the development of pyogenic hepatic abscesses. The abscesses occur in up to 20% of patients with hepatic echinococcosis, and underlying echinococcal disease is reportedly the most common cause of pyogenic hepatic abscess in Greece and Spain.[86, 96, 102, 104]

Echinococcus multilocularis echinococcosis is a highly invasive and destructive disease that results in solid, tumorlike masses that are easily confused with hepatic cirrhosis or carcinoma. The name, alveolar hydatid disease, derives from the hepatic nodules or masses that, when sectioned for pathologic examination, appear as alveolus-like microvesicles.[97] Hydatid cysts of *E. multilocularis* expand into multilocular infiltrating lesions by exogenous proliferation of their

GEOGRAPHIC OCCURRENCE OF *ECHINOCOCCUS GRANULOSUS* INFECTION

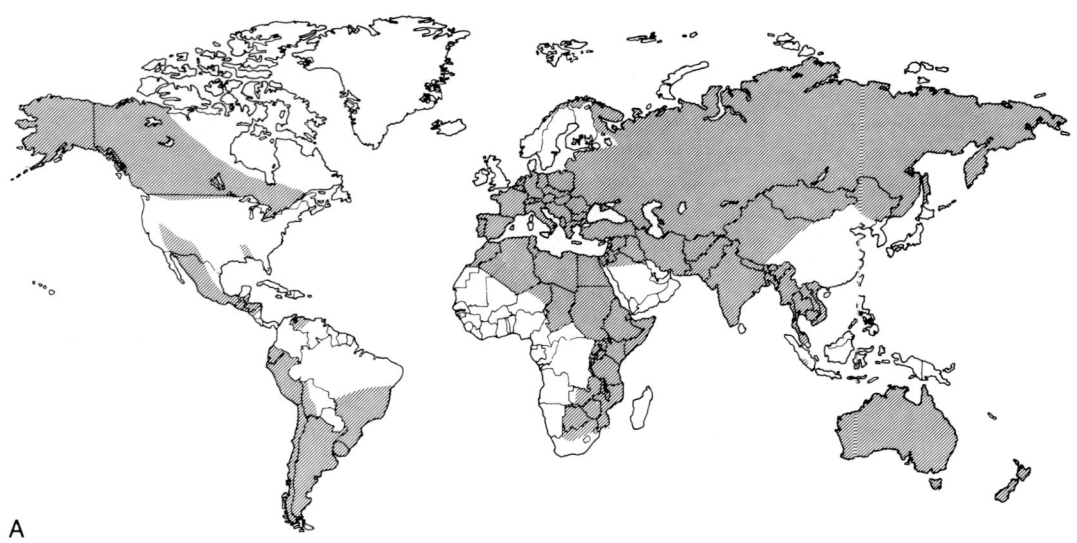

A

GEOGRAPHIC OCCURRENCE OF *ECHINOCOCCUS MULTILOCULARIS* AND *ECHINOCOCCUS VOGELI* INFECTIONS

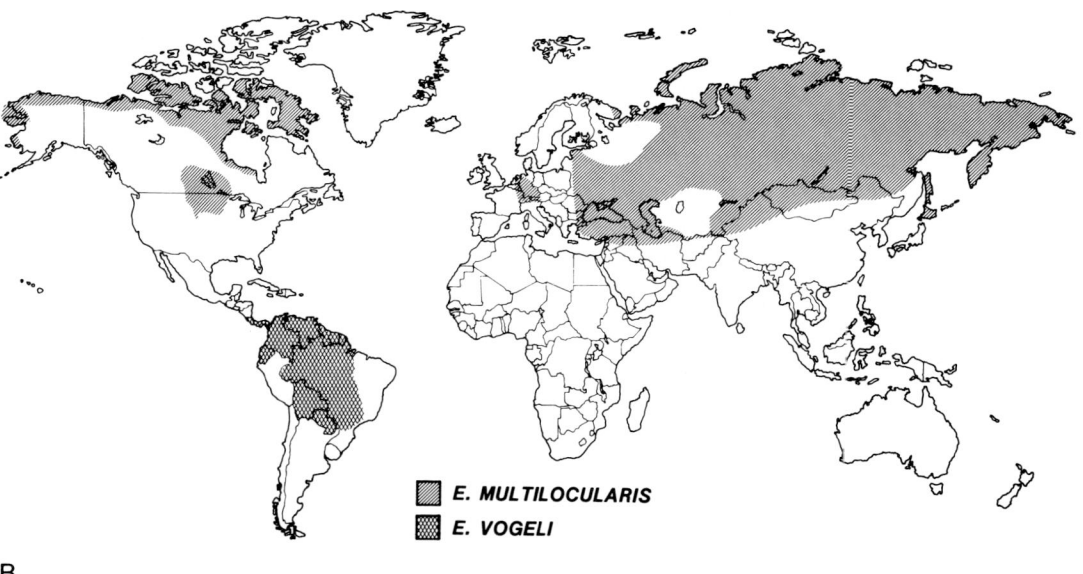

⬚ E. MULTILOCULARIS

⬚ E. VOGELI

B

FIGURE 17–12.
Geographic distribution of Echinococcosis. (*A*), *Echinococcus granulosus*. (*B*), *Echinococcus multilocularis* and *Echinococcus vogeli*. SOURCE: Courtesy of PM Schantz, VMD, PhD. Centers for Disease Control and Prevention, Atlanta GA. Schantz PM, Okelo GBA. Echinococcosis (hydatidosis). In: Warren KS, Mahmoud AAF. Tropical and Geographical Medicine. 2nd ed. New York: McGraw-Hill; 1990:505–508.

germinal membranes.[105] As with *E. granulosus* infections, patients infected during childhood may remain asymptomatic for many years before developing nonspecific manifestations such as hepatomegaly, ascites, icterus, and abdominal pain. Because of its insidious and progressive

nature, infection with *E. multilocularis* is usually not diagnosed until its lesions are inoperable owing to extensive invasion of contiguous tissues or distant metastases to lung or brain.[92, 99, 106] Although spontaneous resolution has been described in asymptomatic patients detected by

tive. The highest rates of positivity were in specimens from the southeastern United States and from Puerto Rico (Fig. 17–18).[134]

CLINICAL MANIFESTATIONS

Although the majority of infections are asymptomatic, two major syndromes related to toxocaral infections are recognized.[133, 139] Visceral larva migrans, caused by the systemic migration of larvae, is most frequently observed in young children (mean age, 5 yrs) with a history of pica. Clinical findings may include persistent and often marked eosinophilia, leukocytosis, fever, hepatomegaly, urticaria, hypergammaglobulinemia, and elevated blood group isohemagglutinins.[140–142] Pulmonary manifestations may mimic those found in asthma and pneumonitis.[143] Less frequently, neurologic involvement may result in focal or generalized seizures, encephalopathy, and behavior disorders.[142, 144] Ocular larva migrans, typically resulting from the unilateral larval invasion of an eye, is often associated with visual loss and strabismus in the absence of systemic findings. Fundoscopic findings range from a solitary posterior pole or peripheral granuloma to severe exudative endophthalmitis with retinal detachment.[145]

Occult infections with *Toxocara*, it has been suggested, may occasionally be associated with a syndrome of nonspecific symptoms including abdominal pain, anorexia, sleep and behavior disturbances, cervical adenitis, wheezing, limb pains, and fever.[146]

DIAGNOSIS AND PATHOLOGY

Visceral toxocariasis should be considered in any individual with a history of pica, exposure to dogs or cats, and persistent eosinophilia. The presence of hepatic enlargement supports the diagnosis. Clinical findings and the results of hematologic and biochemical tests are frequently inadequate for distinguishing this syndrome from other causes of eosinophilia. Although serial stool examinations are useful for excluding other gastrointestinal parasites, these techniques cannot be used to reveal the presence of *Toxocara* because these organisms do not remain in the intestinal tract and do not produce eggs in humans. By contrast, migrating worms may be identified in tissue sections (Fig. 17–19), but blind biopsies are generally low-yield procedures and are not routinely recommended.[147] Ocular toxocariasis should be considered in any patient with a unilateral raised retinal lesion. Diseases of the eye that may resemble ocular toxocaral infection include retinoblastoma and other ocular tumors, exudative retinitis, uveitis, developmental abnormalities, and trauma.[145]

Serologic tests (e.g., ELISA) using larval-stage antigens are the most reliable means of supporting the clinical diagnosis of toxocaral infection.[148] The clinical features of visceral toxocariasis should be distinguished from those of infections caused by the human hookworm, *Strongyloides stercoralis*, filaria, *Trichinella* species, and *Schistosoma* species.

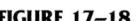

FIGURE 17–18.
Toxocariasis in the United States, 1981. Map depicting percent positive toxocaral infection by enzyme-linked immunosorbent assays submitted to state public health laboratories and the Centers for Disease Control and Prevention in 1981.

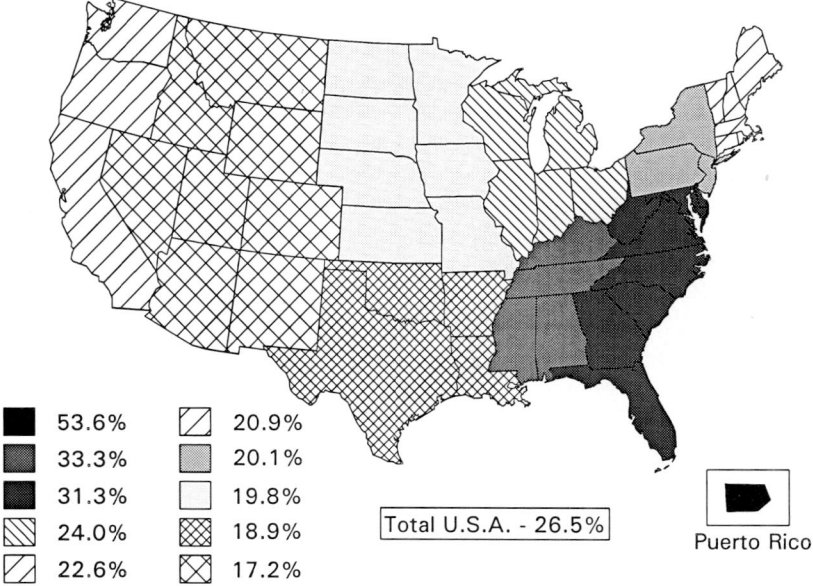

53.6%	20.9%
33.3%	20.1%
31.3%	19.8%
24.0%	18.9%
22.6%	17.2%

Total U.S.A. - 26.5%

Puerto Rico

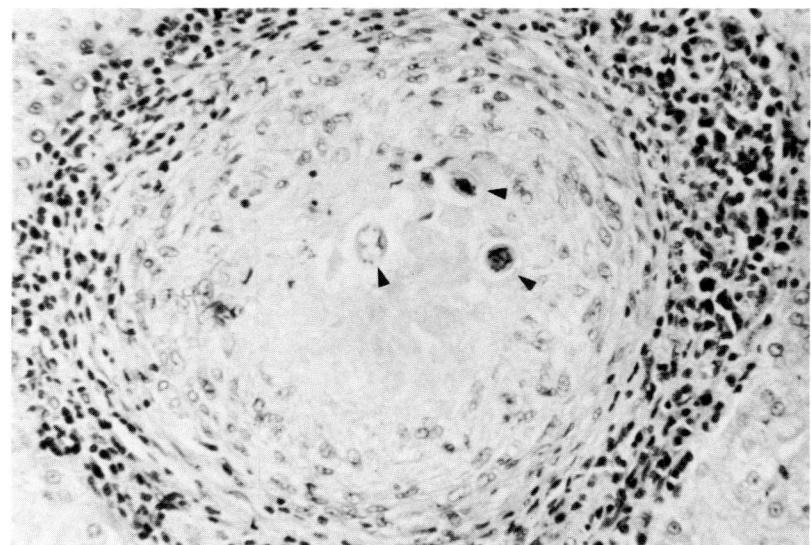

FIGURE 17–19.
Hepatic histopathology of toxocariasis. Typical hepatic granuloma surrounding *Toxocara canis* larva (arrowheads) seen in cross section. (mouse, hemotoxylin-eosin) SOURCE: Courtesy of LT Glickman, DVM, Lafayette IN.

TREATMENT AND PREVENTION

Asymptomatic visceral infections with *Toxocara* species do not require specific therapy. Eosinophilia and seropositivity often resolve spontaneously.[149]

Management of symptomatic infections is primarily supportive. Diethylcarbamazine, 50 to 150 mg given orally 3 times a day for 1 to 3 weeks, and thiabendazole, 25 to 50 mg/kg of body weight given orally daily for 1 to 3 weeks, have frequently been used with inconsistent results. Alternative preparations including mebendazole, 200 mg given orally twice a day for 5 days, and albendazole, 5 to 10 mg/kg of body weight given daily for 5 days, offer the advantage of better patient tolerance and lower toxicity.[150] Significant pulmonary, myocardial, or central nervous system complications may respond to the administration of corticosteroids. Acute ocular infections have been treated with local or systemic corticosteroids alone or in combination with anthelminthic agents or with laser photocoagulation of discernible worms. Chronic ocular infections are most effectively managed surgically.[145, 151]

Toxocaral infections can be prevented by ensuring good personal hygiene, eliminating intestinal parasites from dogs and cats, minimizing human contact with potentially contaminated environments, and encouraging pet owners to prevent their animals from fecally contaminating public areas.[152]

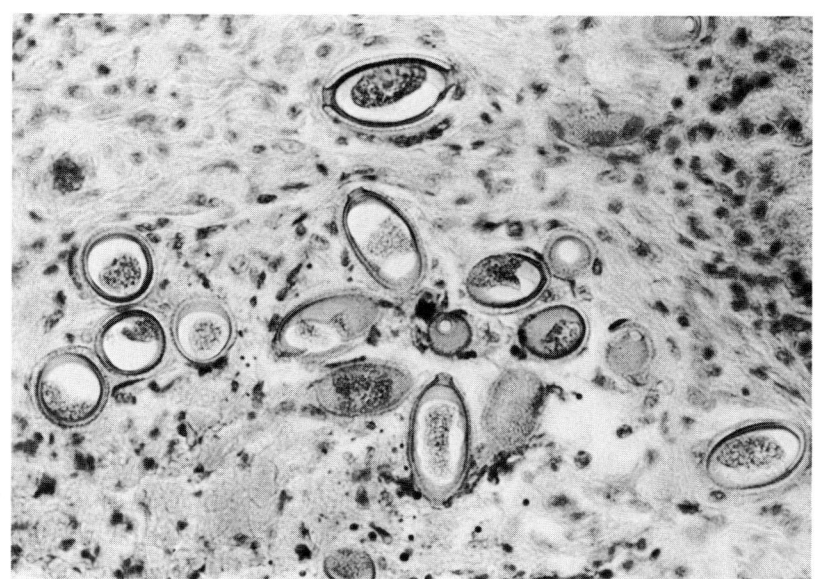

FIGURE 17–20.
Histopathology of hepatic capillariasis. Eggs of *Capillaria hepatica* with surrounding granulomata and fibrosis in liver. (green monkey, hemotoxylin-eosin) SOURCE: Courtesy of ML Eberhard, PhD. Centers for Disease Control and Prevention, Atlanta GA.

Hepatic Capillariasis

PARASITE LIFE CYCLE AND EPIDEMIOLOGY

Infection with the roundworm *Capillaria hepatica* is acquired by ingesting soil (i.e., pica) that contains embryonated eggs or soil-contaminated food or water. Larvae, released in the cecum, penetrate the intestinal mucosa. The portal venous circulation carries maturing larvae to the liver, where they ultimately become lodged. Further development into adult worms takes place during the following month. Approximately 4 weeks after infection, adult worms begin to disintegrate, releasing eggs into the hepatic parenchyma and thereby producing an intense inflammatory reaction that involves macrophages, eosinophils, and giant cells. Resolution of this process is often attended by marked fibrosis surrounding the deposits of eggs (Fig. 17–20). In nature, decomposition of an infected animal carcass allows eggs in the host tissues to embryonate in the soil. Alternatively, predation by other temporary hosts such as dogs or cats provides a means by which eggs are disseminated in the environment through the stools of these animals. The cycle is ultimately completed when the appropriate rodent host ingests mature eggs.[153]

Human infection with *C. hepatica* is a relatively rare occurrence despite its wide distribution among lower species of animals; approximately 32 cases of genuine human infestation have been described.[154-176] Humans become hosts for this parasite by inadvertently intruding upon the enzootic cycle, which typically involves rodents (e.g., rat, muskrat, squirrel, beaver, and North American prairie dog) but has included other mammals such as the peccary, pig, dog, cat, European hare, capuchin monkey, spider monkey, and chimpanzee.[175]

CLINICAL MANIFESTATIONS

Hepatic capillariasis is characterized by fever, nausea, vomiting, diarrhea or constipation, anorexia, myalgia, and arthralgia. Abdominal distention, pedal edema, and weight loss may also be seen during later stages of the illness. Physical examination may reveal tender hepatomegaly and mild splenomegaly. Laboratory abnormalities have included prominent leukocytosis with eosinophilia; mild elevations of AST, alkaline phosphatase, and serum bilirubin; anemia; and increased erythrocyte sedimentation rate. Chest radiographs may suggest pneumonitis.[154-173, 176]

DIAGNOSIS AND PATHOLOGY

Definitive diagnosis can be established only by observing the adult worms or eggs in liver biopsy or autopsy specimens, which are often associated with necrosis, granuloma formation, and fibrosis.[177]

Capillaria hepatica eggs found in stool specimens do not signify acute infection and most commonly result from the ingestion of raw or undercooked liver from an infected animal (e.g., monkey and wild boar).[178]

The clinical syndrome of fever, eosinophilia, and hepatomegaly is suggestive of this diagnosis, but *C. hepatica* infections should be distinguished from syndromes that accompany toxocariasis, trichinosis, schistosomiasis, and fascioliasis.[179] Hepatic granulomatous lesions or calcifications have also been observed after infections with other helminths (see Table 17–3).[180]

TREATMENT AND PREVENTION

Few patients have been successfully treated for this infection.[161, 168, 170, 172, 173] Agents used in these anecdotal reports have included dithiazanine iodide, sodium stibogluconate, and thiabendazole.[161, 168, 172] More recently, 2 patients appeared to respond to combinations of drugs, in one case, disophenol, pyrantel tartrate, and steroids, and, in the other case, thiabendazole, ivermectin, and steroids.[170, 173]

Prevention of infection depends on adequate rodent control and appropriate hygienic practices when preparing or eating potentially contaminated food. The ingestion of raw or undercooked liver from primary hosts should also be discouraged.

Helminthic Infections with Rare or Minor Hepatobiliary Manifestations

Ascariasis

Ascaris infections are among the most prevalent helminthic infestations encountered around the world, affecting an estimated 800 million to 1 billion persons. High worm burdens are commonly found in populations with substandard living conditions.[181] Further details regarding the life cycle, epidemiology, and usual clinical manifestations of *Ascaris lumbricoides* are presented in Chapter 7.

The majority of patients with *Ascaris* infections are either asymptomatic or mildly symptomatic during the course of larval migration, but cough, dyspnea, wheezing, rales, and substernal

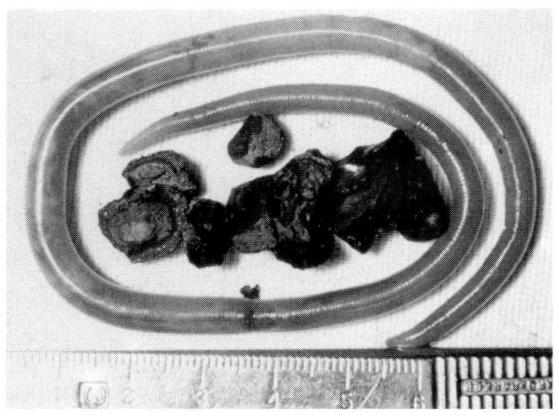

FIGURE 17–21.
Biliary ascariasis. Adult worm and gallstones extracted at autopsy from a Philippine patient with biliary ascariasis. SOURCE: Courtesy of DA Schwartz, MD, Emory University, Atlanta GA.

discomfort associated with transient pulmonary infiltrates may be observed during the first 2 weeks of infection.[182] Chronic infections are most frequently associated with vague episodic epigastric or periumbilical pain. Intestinal complications may result in serious morbidity, however, including acute obstruction, intussusception, volvulus, perforation, and appendicitis.[183–185] Although maturing worms ultimately localize in the lower portion of the small intestine, aberrant migration of adult worms through the ampulla of Vater has resulted in cholecystitis, cholangitis, hepatic abscess formation, and acute pancreatitis.[186–189] Moreover, fragments of disintegrating worms within the biliary tree can serve as a nidus for the develop-

ment of biliary calculi (Fig. 17–21).[190] Preexisting malformations of the biliary tract may facilitate worm movement into this area.[191]

A history of regurgitating a worm or passing a large worm per rectum is highly suggestive of ascariasis. In the absence of such an event, the diagnosis should be considered in any individual with an appropriate exposure history and a vague constellation of abdominal symptoms associated with mild eosinophilia. Definitive diagnosis is most easily established by identifying characteristic eggs in stool specimens. *Ascaris* larvae have also been found in sputum specimens, gastric washings, and liver (Fig. 17–22) and lung biopsy material. Persons with symptoms compatible with biliary tract or pancreatic disease may be effectively evaluated by ultrasound examination, which may identify the offending worm.[192–193] Worms may also be directly visualized and extracted by endoscopic means.[194, 195]

The vague abdominal complaints and eosinophilia associated with ascariasis should be distinguished from similar findings resulting from infection with other migrating nematodes including *Strongyloides, Trichinella, Ancylostoma* and *Necator* (hookworms), and *Toxocara*.

Asymptomatic or mildly symptomatic intestinal infections can be treated effectively with mebendazole, given in 100-mg oral doses 2 times a day for 3 days; pyrantel pamoate, given in a single oral dose of 11 mg/kg of body weight (maximum of 1 g); or piperazine citrate, given in daily doses of 75 mg/kg of body weight for 2 days (maximum of 4 g for adults or 2 g for children weighing <20 kg).[196, 197] Albendazole, given orally in a single 400-mg dose, has also been reported to be effective.[198] Intestinal or

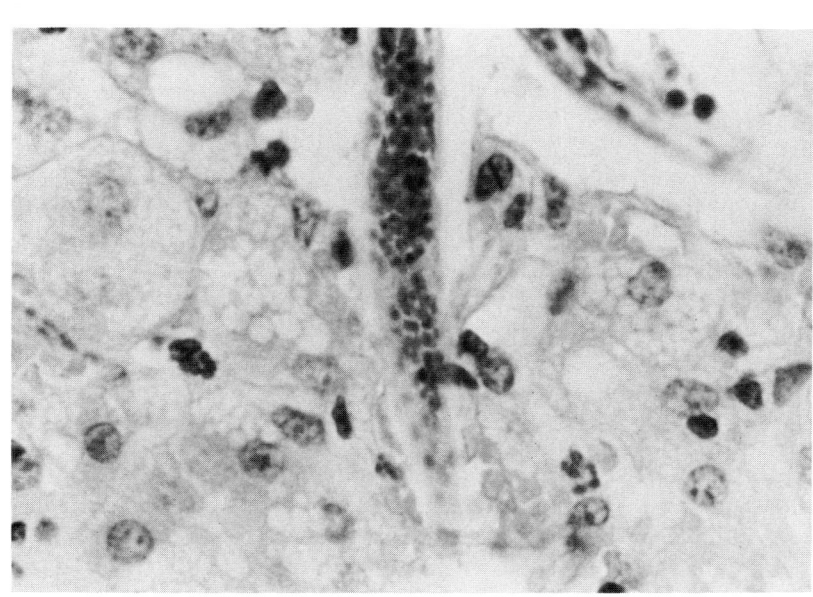

FIGURE 17–22.
Longitudinal section of an *Ascaris* larva in human liver. (hematoxylin-eosin, ×400) SOURCE: Courtesy of DA Schwartz, MD. Atlanta GA.

biliary obstruction complicating intestinal ascariasis often requires surgical intervention. In the absence of ischemic bowel, perforation, peritonitis, or established hepatic, pancreatic, or biliary ascariasis, however, conservative management may be attempted for 12 to 24 hours.[196] In addition to supportive care, piperazine syrup may be given by nasogastric tube (NGT).[199]

Prevention of *Ascaris* infections depends on careful cleaning and cooking of soil-contaminated food items and strict attention to personal hygiene, particularly in areas where proper sanitary facilities may be lacking.[200]

Strongyloidiasis

The small intestinal nematode *Strongyloides stercoralis* is discussed in further detail in Chapters 7 and 10. A discussion of strongyloidiasis is included here because hepatic manifestations may occur in immunosuppressed hosts suffering from disseminated infection with *S. stercoralis*. In transplant recipients, persons on chronic steroid therapy, persons with certain malignancies or those receiving antineoplastic medications, and, rarely, persons with AIDS, dissemination may follow the hyperinfection syndrome.[201] Hyperinfection is a result of chronic autoinfection and is an exaggeration or augmentation of the parasite's normal life cycle.[202] Dissemination, by contrast, occurs when migrating filariform larvae invade tissues that are not ordinarily part of the life cycle.

Reports documenting hepatobiliary involvement with *S. stercoralis* have appeared periodically since 1876.[202–206] Jaundice and abnormal liver function test findings suggestive of an obstructive process have been reported for disseminated strongyloidiasis, and liver biopsies or postmortem tissue specimens may reveal periportal inflammation or eosinophilic granulomatous hepatitis or both. Larvae have been observed in intrahepatic biliary canaliculi, in lymphatic vessels, and within small branches of the portal vein.[202, 203, 207]

Diagnosis of disseminated strongyloidiasis usually results from the appropriate interpretation of epidemiologic circumstances and clinical signs and symptoms (discussed in Chapters 7 and 10) rather than from sole reliance on hepatobiliary manifestations. The presence of jaundice or an obstructive condition on liver function test results in a patient with known *S. stercoralis* infection should, however, alert the clinician to the possibility of dissemination. Eosinophilia is definitely not a common finding in disseminated disease and eosinopenia may, in fact, be a poor prognostic sign.[201, 202, 206, 207] Once

it has disseminated, strongyloidiasis is difficult to treat and mortality is high (50–86%).[202, 208] Effective management, therefore, depends on prevention (i.e., screening for strongyloidiasis before giving immunosuppressive drugs) and early diagnosis and intervention in cases of intestinal disease or hyperinfection syndrome. Treatment is discussed in Chapters 7 and 10.

Angiostrongyliasis

Abdominal angiostrongyliasis due to *Angiostrongylus costaricensis* has been observed in children in Costa Rica since 1952. The disease has been reported from numerous other Latin American countries and, rarely, from Africa. Two cases presumably acquired in the United States were reported in 1992.[209] The parasite is a filariform nematode that resides in the mesenteric arteries (Fig. 17–23) of its definitive hosts, which include cotton rats, other rodents, coatis, and marmosets. Eggs pass from the arterioles to the intestinal wall, where embryonation takes place. First-stage larvae migrate to the intestinal lumen, from which they are passed in rodent feces and subsequently consumed by snail or slug intermediate hosts. The life cycle is completed when definitive hosts consume infected intermediate hosts. Humans are most commonly infected by consuming uncooked fruits and vegetables contaminated with infective larvae-laden snail or slug secretions, or by inadvertently consuming mollusk intermediate hosts.[210–212] Infections are most common in male children between the ages of 6 and 13 years; incidence tends to be highest during the wettest seasons of the year.[212]

Most clinical manifestations arise from granulomatous reactions to degenerating eggs in the ileocecal region. Common clinical signs and symptoms include abdominal pain and tenderness, fever, anorexia, palpable tumor-like masses in the right lower quadrant, vomiting, painful rectal examination, and leukocytosis with eosinophilia. Cases are frequently misdiagnosed as appendicitis. A rare but important manifestation is acute testicular pain and inflammation mimicking testicular torsion. Although liver-related symptoms are relatively uncommon, most patients with intestinal angiostrongyliasis have some degree of hepatic involvement. In those with hepatic signs and symptoms, tender hepatomegaly is the most common manifestation; jaundice is rare.[209–212] A visceral larva migrans–like syndrome due to *A. costaricensis* has also been described, and hepatic lesions in ectopic angiostrongyliasis are similar to those induced by *T. canis*.[213]

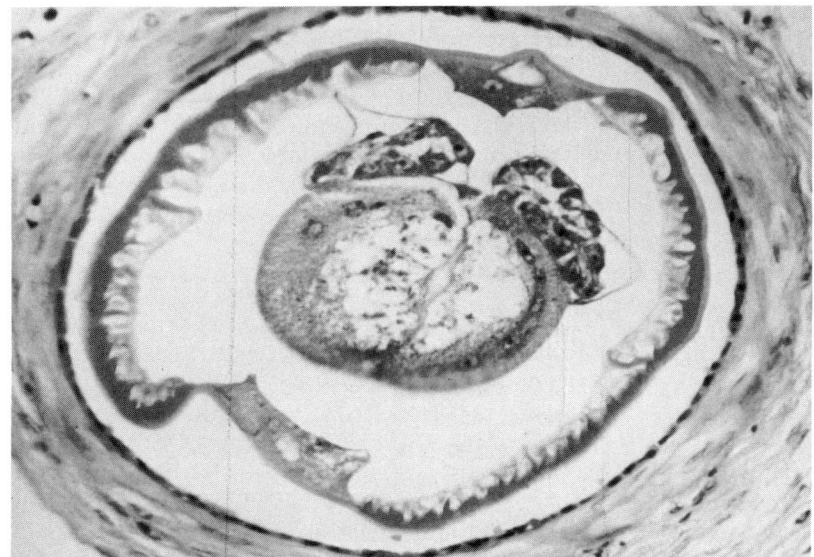

FIGURE 17–23.
Adult *Angiostrongylus costaricensis* in cross section of a mesenteric artery. (hematoxylin-eosin, ×200) SOURCE: Courtesy of LR Ash, PhD. Los Angeles CA.

Although serodiagnostic tests for abdominal angiostrongyliasis exist (latex agglutination, ELISA), they are not widely available, and hence, diagnosis usually depends on clinical manifestations and histopathologic findings. Until controlled comparative trials have been completed, treatment will probably remain supportive. Although mebendazole or thiabendazole have been recommended,[21, 209] no convincing data regarding the efficacy of various anthelminthic medications are available. Because experimental data from rats suggest that chemotherapy may actually induce erratic migrations by otherwise nonmigrating parasites, some experts advise against, rather than for, the use of chemotherapy until more information is available.[211]

Enterobiasis

Pinworm infection, or enterobiasis, is dealt with in greater detail in Chapter 10. A brief discussion is included here because of the occasional propensity of female worms to migrate to ectopic sites. The most important and widely reported ectopic sites are the appendix and the female genital tract. Such cases may be asymptomatic or associated with significant pathologic changes.[214, 215] Ectopic migration is more common in women. Hepatic granulomata due to dead worms or eggs in the liver parenchyma have been reported on several occasions, often in association with colonic malignancies.[214, 216–220] Such findings are usually incidental to the malignancy.

Paragonimiasis

Paragonimiasis is infection with *Paragonimus westermani*, the oriental lung fluke, or with any of several other *Paragonimus* species. Although most commonly associated with Southeast Asia, paragonimiasis also occurs in Japan, Korea, Africa, and Central and South America; autochthonous cases have also been reported in North America.[221, 222] The definitive hosts for *Paragonimus* species are humans and various wild or domestic mammals. The life cycle requires two intermediate hosts—first snails and then freshwater crustaceans such as crabs, crayfish, or shrimp. Infection in humans occurs when uncooked, metacercariae-infested freshwater crustaceans are consumed. Definitive hosts perpetuate the life cycle by shedding eggs in expectorated respiratory secretions or in feces that contaminate aquatic environments containing the appropriate snail and crustacean intermediate hosts.[223]

Although *P. westermani,* the most commonly reported species in humans, usually infects the lungs, ectopic localizations are not unusual. Cerebral paragonimiasis is the most severe, but almost any organ can be infected, including skin, pleura, eyes, heart, pericardium, kidney, reproductive organs, bone, intestines, pancreas, and liver. Although hepatic infections may result in abscess formation, patients are often asymptomatic or exhibit nonspecific signs and symptoms.[224–226] Biliary infections are rare and poorly documented.

Diagnosis is most often accomplished by demonstrating typical eggs in sputum, pleural fluid, cerebrospinal fluid, or feces (because egg-containing respiratory secretions are often swallowed). Immunodiagnosis can be particularly helpful in extrapulmonary cases. A sensitive and specific immunoblot assay for paragonimiasis is available at the CDC.[227] Treatment with praziquantel, given orally 3 times a day for 2 days in doses of 25 mg/kg of body weight, is safe and effective.[21]

Dicrocoeliasis and Eurytremiasis

Dicrocoelium dendriticum, the lancet fluke, is a trematode that infects the biliary tract of herbivorous mammals such as cattle and sheep. It is found in many countries of Europe, Asia, and the Middle East but has also been reported in Canada, the United States, and, rarely, in Latin America and Africa. The parasite life cycle depends on two intermediate hosts, a land snail and ants of the genus *Formica*. Definitive hosts, and occasionally humans, are infected by consuming metacercariae-containing ants on ant-infested grass, fruits, or vegetables. In addition, false parasitosis can occur when humans consume liver from infected animals and simply pass eggs in feces without actually being infected.[228, 229]

Symptoms are usually mild and include nonspecific abdominal distress, nausea, vomiting, diarrhea or constipation, flatulence, and biliary colic. Eosinophilia occurs but is relatively rare.[230] An asymptomatic case involving an HIV-positive man was recently reported, but whether he had true infection or false parasitosis was unclear.[231] Diagnosis is by identification of characteristic eggs in stool, bile, or duodenal fluid, but false parasitosis must be ruled out by a repeated stool examination. Recovery of adult flukes by biopsy or at autopsy is definitive. Praziquantel at the same dosage as for clonorchiasis is the preferred treatment, but treatment failures have occurred.[230, 232]

Eurytremiasis is infection with the pancreatic fluke, *Eurytrema pancreaticum*. This fluke commonly infests the pancreatic and, rarely, bile ducts of cattle, sheep, goats, and buffalo in Asia but has also been observed in Brazil, Venezuela, and Madagascar. The first and second intermediate hosts are land snails and grasshoppers or crickets, respectively. Human infections, occurring after inadvertent ingestion of infected insects, have been documented in Japan, Hong Kong, and China. Two cases were confirmed by the finding of adult flukes at autopsy; one of these was in a woman with gastric carcinoma. Symptoms, diagnosis, and treatment are as described for dicrocoeliasis, but it should be noted that the eggs of the two flukes are indistinguishable.[229, 232, 233]

Pentastomiasis

Pentastomiasis is infection with organisms of the class Pentastomida. Pentastomes, sometimes referred to as tongue worms, exhibit characteristics of both arthropods and annelids, and their taxonomic classification has been debated for years. Almost all human infections are due to one of two species, *Armillifer armillatus* and *Linguatula serrata*. Pentastomiasis is a parasitic zoonosis that occurs most commonly in equatorial Africa, the Middle East and Southeast Asia, but it has also been reported in Europe and the Americas, including the United States.[234-238] In definitive hosts, adult pentastomes reside in the respiratory tract of reptiles (*A. armillatus*) or the nasopharynx of carnivorous mammals (*L. serrata*). Eggs (Fig. 17–24) passed into the environment via nasal secretions, saliva, or feces are consumed by secondary hosts, usually rodents or larger herbivorous mammals such as sheep or goats. After first-stage larvae emerge in the gut, they penetrate the intestinal wall to migrate and encyst in various tissues, where they develop into second- and third-stage larvae. The life cycle is completed when a definitive host consumes the larvae-laden tissues of a secondary host.[235]

Humans may serve as temporary definitive hosts when they consume inadequately cooked liver or lymph nodes of infected sheep or goats. Third-stage larvae then migrate from the stomach to the nasopharynx, where they attach, resulting in a self-limited nasopharyngitis known as halzoun, marrara, or nasopharyngeal linguatulosis.[235, 236, 239] In the more common situation, in which humans become infected by consuming egg-contaminated food or water, humans serve as dead-end secondary hosts. First-stage larvae emerge and migrate to various visceral sites, most commonly the liver, where they usu-

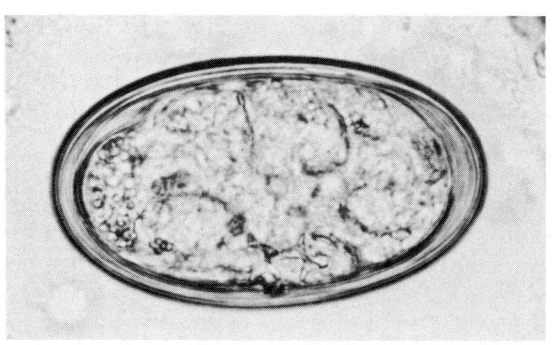

FIGURE 17–24.
Egg of *Linguatula serrata* from a dog. SOURCE: Courtesy of ML Eberhard, PhD. Centers for Disease Control and Prevention, Atlanta GA.

ally encyst, die, and calcify. Because human infections are usually asymptomatic, hepatic pentastomiasis is usually an incidental finding at autopsy or laparotomy performed for other indications. The most common lesion is a necrotic pentastomid granuloma. Plain radiographs of the abdomen may show typical C-shaped or "cashew-nut" calcifications. Eosinophilia is not a feature.[234–236] Rarely, encysted larvae may molt, with subsequent enlargement of the cyst that results in mass effects on contiguous tissues. This phenomenon has been associated with both biliary and intestinal obstruction in addition to pericarditis, pneumonitis, lung collapse, meningitis, and prostatitis. Peritonitis due to migrating third-stage larvae has also been reported.[235] Except in the rare complications noted above, when surgical intervention may be required, treatment is rarely needed. No medications have been shown to be effective.

PROTOZOAL INFECTIONS OF THE LIVER AND BILIARY TREE

Conditions with Major Hepatobiliary Manifestations

Amebic Liver Abscess

PARASITE LIFE CYCLE AND EPIDEMIOLOGY

Infection with the cosmopolitan protozoan parasite *Entamoeba histolytica* causes amebiasis. As discussed in Chapter 10, amebiasis may be an asymptomatic luminal or an invasive condition. The term invasive refers to the presence of hematophagous trophozoites in tissue and stool. The liver is the most common extraintestinal site of invasive amebiasis, and infection there results in the condition usually referred to as amebic liver abscess.[240–242] Motile, uninucleate trophozoites of invasive strains of *E. histolytica* reside in human colonic mucosa, where they either invade further or encyst. Cysts, which do not develop in tissue, are passed in the stool of infected individuals and are responsible for the ongoing transmission of the disease. With the appropriate combination of parasite traits (e.g., pathogenic zymodemes), host immune factors, and colonic bacterial flora, *E. histolytica* trophozoites are capable of lysing host intestinal epithelial and inflammatory cells and causing colonic ulceration and deep-tissue invasion.[243] Trophozoites may then spread to the liver via portal vein radicles. As hepatic colonization progresses, trophozoites are thought to disrupt sinusoidal circulation and induce periportal in-

farction. Subsequent lysis of neutrophils and hepatocytes by amebic trophozoites causes the formation of an abscess that is composed of necrotic debris and contained within a thin layer of fibrosis.[244]

Asymptomatic or luminal amebiasis occurs worldwide, but invasive disease occurs more frequently in areas such as western and southeastern Africa, Southeast Asia, Mexico, and western South America.[241] Significant numbers of cases have also been reported from India and Egypt.[245, 246] Of the estimated 500 million persons infected with *E. histolytica,* between 10 and 30% develop extracolonic sequelae.[242, 247, 248] Clinicians in developed countries are most likely to encounter amebic liver abscesses in immigrants, visitors, or travelers from amebiasis-endemic areas, persons confined to institutions for the mentally impaired, and perhaps in patients receiving immunosuppressive therapy.[242, 248–250] In areas without endemic amebiasis, isolated case reports of amebic liver abscess in immigrants are not uncommon,[251] and multiple cases in extended families have also been reported.[252] The risk for travelers appears to be relatively low, but *E. histolytica* infections leading to hepatic abscesses may occur after only brief stays abroad, may produce hepatic manifestations after years of absence from an endemic area, and may be fatal. Moreover, travelers to areas with endemic amebiasis may be more susceptible to invasive disease than are native residents.[249, 253, 254]

Although found in all age groups, amebic liver abscess is 10 times more common in adults and is seen most frequently in persons 20 to 60 years of age. For unexplained reasons, amebic liver abscess occurs much more frequently in males than in females.[241, 248] *Entamoeba histolytica* infection in male homosexuals is rarely associated with extraintestinal disease, and amebic liver abscess is not a commonly reported problem in persons with AIDS, even in areas in the tropics where amebiasis is highly endemic (Table 17–6).[242, 253, 255]

CLINICAL MANIFESTATIONS

The clinical manifestations of amebic liver abscess are typically classified as either acute or subacute (insidious).[242, 246, 248, 253] Signs and symptoms of hepatic involvement may develop within days of, or up to several years after, intestinal amebiasis. Up to 50% of patients with amebic liver abscess have no history of intestinal disease.[253, 256] Despite reports with estimates as high as 66%, concomitant diarrheal illness is usually present in less than 30% of cases.[246, 248, 256] Al-

Parasitic Infections of the Liver and Biliary Tree   **437**

TABLE 17–6. EPIDEMIOLOGIC CHARACTERISTICS OF AMEBIC LIVER ABSCESS

CHARACTERISTIC	COMMENT
Geographic distribution	Worldwide, but more common in Africa, Southeast Asia, Mexico, western South America
Age	Most common in adults 20–60 years of age
Gender	More frequent in males
High-risk populations	Residents of the tropics, patients in mental health institutions, some travelers
Populations without evidence of increased risk	Most travelers, homosexuals, persons with AIDS, women, & children

though amebic abscesses may be multiple and may occur anywhere in the liver, most patients have solitary lesions in the right lobe.[241, 246, 257]

In acute cases, those in which symptoms have been present for less than 14 days, spiking fevers, chills, hepatic tenderness, and leukocytosis are the most common initial manifestations. Point tenderness over the liver or right lower intercostal spaces is a common and helpful physical finding, particularly in the absence of hepatomegaly. Pain in the right hypochondrium may be pleuritic in nature, often with referral to the right shoulder.[241, 242, 246, 256, 257] Left-lobe abscesses are often accompanied by pain in the epigastrium, with radiation to the left shoulder. Anorexia, nausea, vomiting, and nonproductive cough are also common.[241, 246] Liver function tests are minimally elevated or normal; anemia is not a common feature in acute cases.[242, 248] There is at least one report of obstructive jaundice being more common in patients with acute manifestations.[245] Mortality and severe complications may also be more likely in such cases.[248, 258]

Patients with an insidious onset of signs and symptoms are usually older, and their initial clinical manifestations are more subtle, evolving during periods of up to 6 months. Anorexia, weight loss, hepatomegaly, and anemia (normochromic, normocytic) are common. If present, fever is usually low grade but may be either intermittent or continuous. Abdominal pain, common in acute cases, is not a consistent complaint and is absent in up to 60% of patients with insidious onset of symptoms. When present, it is often vague and nonspecific. Hepatic tenderness, however, is a common physical finding. Pulmonary manifestations such as cough and the presence of rales and rhonchi on physical examination are more common in chronic cases. Hepatic aminotransferases are usually

normal, as in acute disease, but alkaline phosphatase level is elevated in up to 90% of cases. The severity of both anemia and alkaline phosphatase elevation correlates well with the duration of symptoms. Leukocytosis is minimal or absent.[241, 242, 246, 248, 256]

Complications of amebic liver abscess are due to direct or metastatic extension.[253] Pleuropulmonary complications occur in 20 to 35% of patients and include effusions, empyema, pulmonary abscesses, and hepatobronchial fistulas. Right-sided involvement is most common.[241, 242, 246, 256] Intraperitoneal rupture, the second most common complication, may manifest as sudden perforation with acute peritonitis, gradual leak with localized abscess formation, or gradual seepage with chronic, generalized peritonitis.[248] A rarer but more severe complication is amebic pericarditis, which occurs most frequently in patients with left hepatic lobe abscesses.[256] Other uncommon complications include rupture into the gallbladder, stomach, colon, or inferior vena cava and metastasis to brain or kidney.[241, 242] Secondary bacterial infections of amebic abscesses are rare and tend to occur only after aspiration has been repeatedly attempted.[241, 242, 251] A syndrome referred to as amebic hepatitis has never been histologically confirmed, and its existence is controversial.[256, 257]

DIAGNOSIS AND PATHOLOGY

The differential diagnosis of amebic liver abscess includes pyogenic abscess, hepatic neoplasms, and echinococcosis.[241, 242, 256, 259, 260] Amebic abscesses have been mistaken for hepatic neoplasms, resulting in unnecessary surgical procedures, and malignancies have been misdiagnosed as amebic abscesses, with subsequent delay in appropriate antineoplastic therapy.[260–262] Because the onset may be insidious, with fever as the only initial manifestation, amebic liver abscess must also be considered in the differential diagnosis of fever of unknown origin.[241, 242]

The diagnosis of amebic liver abscess depends on the clinician's assessment of the clinical and epidemiologic features and on the appropriate application of serologic tests and hepatic imaging. Plain films of the abdomen or chest may reveal a characteristically elevated right hemidiaphragm. Other reliable, noninvasive imaging techniques include ultrasound, CT, MRI, and nuclear scintigraphy. Nuclear scanning techniques, although sensitive, are quite nonspecific and offer no real advantage over other hepatic imaging modalities. Published experience with MRI is limited, but its usefulness in assessing amebic liver abscess is comparable to that of

CT.[241, 253] Computer tomography scanning is superior to ultrasound in its ability to define the extent of disease. Nevertheless, it uses intravenous contrast material, delivers ionizing radiation, is expensive, and may be less effective than ultrasound in demonstrating the radiologic characteristics of amebic liver abscess.[264]

In addition to being an excellent means of assessing response to therapy, ultrasound is as effective as radionuclide scanning, CT, and MRI in determining the location, size, shape, and number of hepatic abscesses (Fig. 17–25).[246, 263] Given these characteristics, many authorities believe that ultrasound is the diagnostic imaging test of choice for this condition.[264] Characteristics of amebic liver abscesses on ultrasound include round or oval shape; absence of an abrupt transition from normal hepatic parenchyma to the abscess; internal echoes that are fine, homogeneous, low-level, and less echogenic than normal hepatic parenchyma; peripheral location within the liver; and posterior enhancement. Although all five of these sonographic traits are present in only about 30% of cases, approximately 90% of amebic liver abscesses exhibit at least three of the five.[246, 264] It should be stressed, however, that none of these findings is pathognomonic or universally present, and similar sonographic observations may occur with hepatic neoplasms and pyogenic abscesses.[246, 261, 262] Likewise, although most patients have single lesions in the right hepatic lobe, abscesses may occur anywhere in the liver, and up to 50% of persons with acute manifestations have multiple lesions.[242]

In addition to radiographic imaging techniques, serologic tests are often helpful in the diagnosis of amebic liver abscess. Commonly used serologic assays include IHA, IIF, immunodiffusion, CIEP, and ELISA. In addition, a simplified, commercially available, bicolored latex agglutination assay has recently been described.[265] Most of the commonly used assays are reliable and are positive in 85 to 98% of cases of amebic liver abscess.[266, 267] Although negative results essentially rule out the possibility of amebic liver abscess in most cases, at least 1 case with negative ELISA and positive IHA results has been reported.[251] Moreover, differences in laboratory technique and specimen handling can cause variations in antibody titers of 2- to 4-fold dilutions.[261] Explanations for such discrepancies include the use of different assays by different laboratories, the detection of different antibodies to distinct amebic antigens by various assays, and the virtual lack of standardization among amebic serodiagnostic techniques.[251, 266] Seropositivity in patients with amebic liver abscess does not distinguish between current and past infection. Indirect hemagglutination titers, for example, may remain unchanged or only slightly diminished for months or years after the resolution of an active infection.[241, 251, 261, 266, 267] Despite these drawbacks, antibody detection remains an important adjunct to the diagnosis of amebic liver abscess.

Although not yet available for routine clinical diagnosis, preliminary studies of the detection of specific antiamebic IgM and circulating immune complexes appear promising.[266-268] Antigen detection in liver abscess fluid is also possible.[266]

Diagnostic aspiration is rarely necessary but may be important in differentiating amebic from pyogenic abscesses, particularly in cases with multiple lesions. Such procedures are best

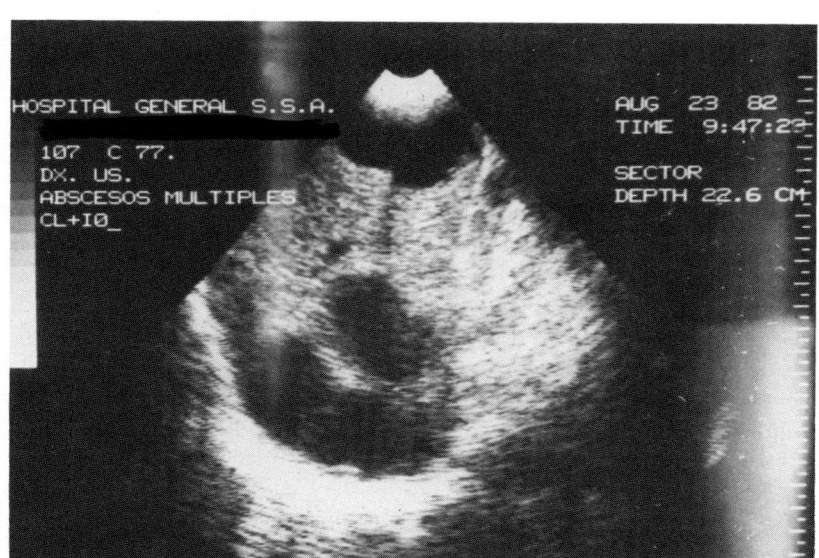

FIGURE 17–25.
Ultrasound image of multiple amebic liver abscesses. SOURCE: Courtesy of J Cross, PhD. Bethesda MD.

TABLE 17–7. SUMMARY OF MEDICATIONS USED TO TREAT AMEBIC LIVER ABSCESS

DRUG	DOSE	DURATION	COMMENT
Metronidazole	750 mg PO or IV tid	5–10 d	Oral preparation may be poorly tolerated at this dosage; often associated with disulfiram-like reactions
Tinidazole	800 mg PO tid	5 d	Better tolerated than metronidazole, but unavailable in the United States
Dehydroemetine	1.0–1.5 mg/kg/d IM (max 90 mg/d)	5 d	Adverse reactions common; available in the U.S. only through CDC Drug Service (404-639-3670)
Chloroquine phosphate	600 mg base (1 g salt) PO qd, then 300 mg base (500 mg salt) PO qd	2 d 2–3 w	Usually given immediately after, or simultaneously with, dehydroemetine

NOTE: All medications listed should always be followed by a luminal agent; see text.

carried out under ultrasound guidance and should be performed at the site of maximal tenderness or over the area of maximum dullness to percussion. Although classically described as similar to anchovy paste in character, the consistency of abscess contents ranges from thin to viscous, and its color may be white, yellow, red, gray, or brown. Abscess fluid is generally odorless and bacteriologically sterile unless it has been contaminated by previous aspirations. Microscopically, this fluid consists primarily of necrotic debris with few or no cells. Trophozoites of *E. histolytica* are rarely present in the central necrotic contents but may be found in specimens obtained from the periphery of the abscess in approximately 50% of cases. Aspirate fluid should be examined in both saline wet mounts and stained preparations. In some cases, treating the aspirate with proteolytic enzymes (e.g., streptodornase) may help in the visualization of trophozoites.[244, 251, 257, 267]

TREATMENT AND PREVENTION

Mortality in appropriately treated, uncomplicated amebic liver abscess is less than 1%; in cases with delayed diagnosis or complications, however, mortality levels may reach 13%.[242, 256, 259] The treatment of choice is parenteral or oral metronidazole, given 3 times a day in 750-mg doses for 5 to 10 days, which is effective in more than 95% of uncomplicated cases.[21, 242, 256] In patients requiring intravenous administration, 500 mg of metronidazole, given 4 times a day, may also be used.[248] Oral metronidazole has been associated with nausea, abdominal discomfort, dizziness, weakness, and mild ataxia, and patients should always be reminded of the disulfiram-like reaction that occurs with the concomitant ingestion of alcohol. Another nitroimidazole compound, tinidazole, given orally 3 times

a day in 800-mg doses for 5 days, is equally effective and tolerated better but is not available in the United States.[21, 242, 257] Although experience is relatively limited, effective single-dose therapy with these agents has also been reported.[248, 269]

Alternatives to the nitroimidazoles include emetine, dehydroemetine, chloroquine, and a dehydroemetine/chloroquine or emetine/chloroquine combination (Table 17–7). Treatment regimens using these medications are generally less preferred because of adverse side effects with emetine and dehydroemetine and higher relapse rates with chloroquine, but they are favored by some authors for use in more severe, refractory, or complicated cases.[242, 246, 248, 257, 270, 271] Because recurrent liver abscess probably results from failure to eradicate bowel-residing *E. histolytica*, whichever primary anti-amebic liver abscess regimen is used should always be followed by treatment with a luminal agent such as paromomycin, diloxanide furoate, or iodoquinol (Chapter 10).[21, 242, 248, 256, 257, 270, 272–274] This recommendation has been reemphasized in a 1992 report by Irusen and colleagues, who noted that asymptomatic intestinal colonization with pathogenic zymodemes of *E. histolytica* was present in 36 of 50 South African patients (72%) with amebic liver abscess.[269] Moreover, successful therapy for amebic liver abscess with metronidazole failed to eradicate intestinal organisms in 20 of these 36 patients (56%), 3 of whom, after not receiving luminal therapy, went on to develop recurrent invasive disease (1 with amebic liver abscess and 2 with amebic dysentery).[269] Conversely, patients with intestinal amebiasis who are treated only with luminal agents are much more likely to develop amebic liver abscess than are those who receive tissue amebicides such as metronidazole.[259]

In most patients receiving appropriate anti-amebic liver abscess chemotherapy, pain and fever are alleviated within 72 hours.[242, 246, 248] The absence of defervescence within 3 to 5 days suggests the possibility of inadequate therapy and the potential need for prescribing alternative treatment regimens or reappraising the diagnosis.[242] Resistance to metronidazole as a cause of poor clinical response, although suggested by some, has never been fully documented.[241, 248]

Patients who do not respond to initial medical therapy may sometimes require therapeutic aspiration or open surgical drainage. The therapeutic role of aspiration has been somewhat controversial. It is used routinely in some geographic areas but reserved only for selected cases in others.[242, 248, 256, 257, 263, 264, 270, 275] Percutaneous aspiration is associated with a small but increased rate of bacterial superinfection. In those areas where it is not performed routinely on all patients with suspected amebic liver abscess, indications for percutaneous aspiration include diagnostic differentiation between amebic liver abscess and pyogenic or mixed abscesses, clinical suspicion that abscess rupture is imminent, lack of response to chemotherapy within 3 to 5 days, and possibility of rupture into the pericardium by abscesses of the left hepatic lobe.[241, 242, 246, 248, 257, 264, 270] In some patients whose illness is severe, early reduction of abscess size by aspiration may be helpful in relieving patient discomfort more promptly.[270] Open surgical drainage is rarely necessary but may be required in cases in which percutaneous aspiration is unsuccessful or the abscess is inaccessible (e.g., left lobe), when abscesses have ruptured, or if bacterial superinfection has occurred.[241, 242, 248, 270]

Response to therapy is frequently monitored by ultrasound. Although often helpful, such monitoring may also lead to confusion. Images during the initial stages of therapy are highly variable and may have little, if any, correlation with actual clinical response. Early in therapy, therefore, response is best evaluated by clinical findings such as the resolution of abdominal pain and fever. Amebic liver abscesses monitored with ultrasound tend to resolve slowly and may actually increase in size during the first few weeks after successful chemotherapy. Most resolve within 6 to 7 months, but complete resolution may take up to 2 years in some cases. Residual findings include normal sonographic liver patterns, hepatic cysts that are sonographically indistinguishable from simple hepatic cysts, calcifications, and areas of increased, decreased, or heterogeneous hepatic parenchymal echogenicity. Resolution time may or may not correlate with abscess size, and abscesses that have been aspirated do not necessarily resolve faster. True amebic liver abscess recurrences are

usually within 2 months of initial therapy.[242, 257, 263, 264] Resolution time for treated amebic liver abscess is considerably longer than that for pyogenic abscesses.[275]

Prevention of amebic liver abscess depends on the prevention of intestinal amebiasis and the use of tissue amebicides in patients treated for intestinal disease. In amebiasis-endemic areas, efforts at control are directed toward environmental sanitation, detection and treatment of infected patients, and health education. No effective vaccine is available, and prophylactic medications for visitors to areas with endemic amebiasis are not recommended.

Protozoal Infections with Rare or Minor Hepatobiliary Manifestations

Cryptosporidiosis

Cryptosporidium is found in both the small intestine and colon (see Chapter 10). Microsporidia and *Giardia*, which are primarily pathogens of the small intestine, are discussed later. All three parasites, however, have been reported to have hepatobiliary manifestations. Biliary involvement with *Cryptosporidium* species (Fig. 17–26) appears to be limited to immunocompromised patients, almost exclusively those with AIDS. Acalculous cholecystitis, cholangitis (both sclerosing and nonsclerosing), and papillary stenosis have been the primary manifestations; cryptosporidial hepatitis and pancreatitis have also been reported.[276–278] Several of the reported cases of cholecystitis were co-infected with cytomegalovirus (CMV).[276, 279–281] Reported symptoms include fever, right upper quadrant abdominal pain, nausea or vomiting, and coexistent diarrhea. Jaundice may also be present, and alkaline phosphatase and bilirubin levels are almost always elevated. Abnormalities typical of cholecystitis and biliary obstruction are commonly detected with oral cholecystograms, transhepatic cholangiograms, ERCP, ultrasound, CT, and nuclear liver scans.[276, 278, 282] Definitive diagnosis may be difficult because patients with hepatobiliary involvement do not consistently shed oocysts in stool. Organisms have been detected, however, in biliary fluid, sputum, liver biopsies, surgically extracted gallbladders, and at autopsy, in both intra- and extrahepatic bile ducts.[276, 278, 283] Associated injury to biliary epithelium is often diffuse and severe.[283] Treatment options for such patients are limited, as are those for patients with only intestinal involvement, but there may be a role for endoscopic sphincterotomy when papillary stenosis is present.

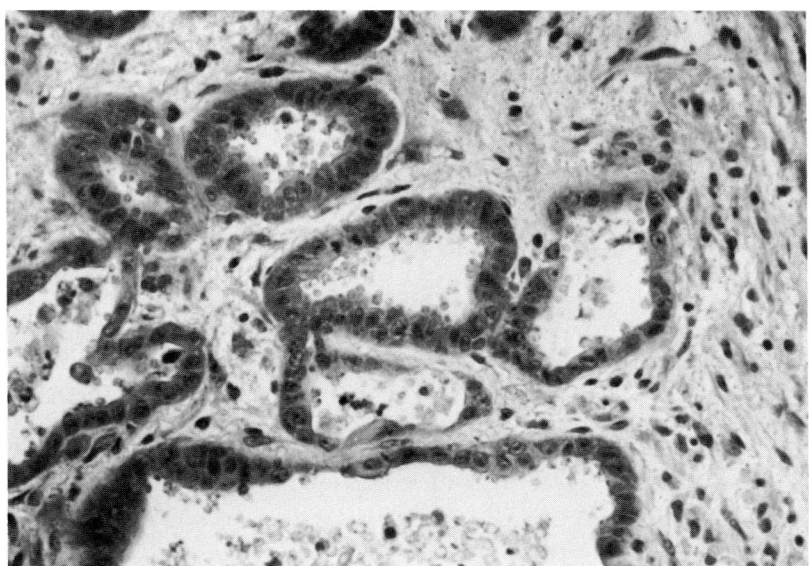

FIGURE 17–26.
Small- and medium-order intrahepatic bile ducts containing numerous *Cryptosporidium* species lining the luminal surfaces of infected cells. Oocysts are also present lying free in the biliary lumen. (hematoxylin-eosin, × 200) SOURCE: Courtesy of LR Ash, PhD. Los Angeles CA.

Microsporidiosis

Organisms of the phylum Microspora, commonly referred to as microsporidia, are noncoccidian protozoa that are taxonomically very distinct from *Cryptosporidium*.[284] Four genera of the order Microsporida (*Enterocytozoon, Septata, Encephalitozoon,* and *Nosema*) have been implicated in hepatobiliary infections, and all were in immunocompromised patients. The earliest case was that of an infant with thymic alymphoplasia who died with disseminated nosematosis (*N. connori*); an autopsy revealed focal areas of hepatocellular necrosis and intrahepatocyte organisms in addition to multiple organ involvement.[285] Microsporidia hepatitis due to *Encephalitozoon* was subsequently reported in a patient with AIDS. This patient, a 35-year-old homosexual man, died with fulminant hepatocellular necrosis after developing rapidly worsening fever, jaundice, and diarrhea. Suppurative necrosis and granulomatous changes involving primarily the portal tracts were evident at autopsy. Organisms with ultrastructural characteristics of *Encephalitozoon* were identified in hepatic tissue.[286]

Infections with *Enterocytozoon* were once thought to be limited to the intestines.[287–289] Reports in the early 1990s, however, documented biliary *Enterocytozoon* infection in patients with unexplained AIDS-related cholangitis.[290, 290a, 290b, 290c] In addition, we have identified *Enterocytozoon* spores (Fig. 17–27) in the surgically removed gallbladder of a patient with *Enterocytozoon* enteritis and presumed acute acalculous cholecystitis. As in all cases of *Enterocytozoon* infection reported so far, patients with biliary involvement are HIV-infected and severely immunosup-

pressed, usually with CD4 counts less than 200 cells/mm³. The recently described microsporidan, *Septata intestinalis*, has also been identified in biliary epithelium.[288] Because most patients

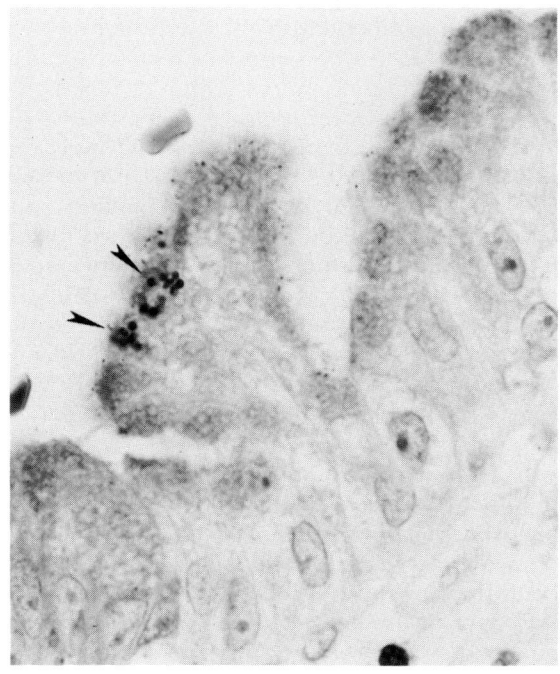

FIGURE 17–27.
Enterocytozoon bieneusi (microsporidia) in the gallbladder of a patient with intestinal microsporidiosis and AIDS. Clusters of gram-positive spores are seen (arrowheads) in the superficial biliary epithelium. SOURCE: Courtesy of L Gorelkin, MD and the Enteric Opportunistic Infections Working Group, Centers for Disease Control and Prevention and Emory University School of Medicine, Atlanta GA.

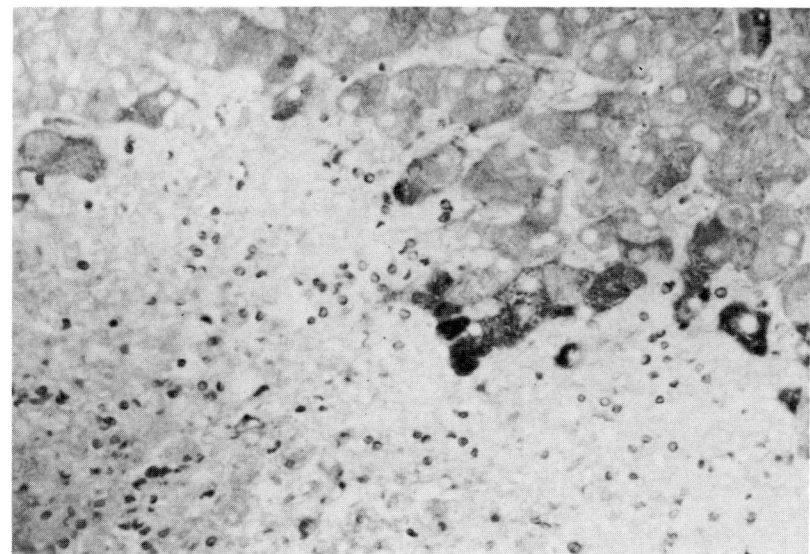

FIGURE 17–28.
Focus of *Pneumocystis carinii* in the liver of a patient with AIDS, showing characteristic cysts, many of which are partially collapsed. (Gomori's methenamine silver, × 200) SOURCE: Courtesy of LR Ash, PhD. Los Angeles CA

appear to have concomitant intestinal infections, presumptive diagnosis in patients with biliary signs and symptoms may be achieved by direct staining of stool or duodenal aspirates.[291] Until further experience is attained, treatment attempts should probably employ those agents undergoing clinical trials for intestinal infections such as albendazole.

Giardiasis

Biliary involvement with *Giardia* has been poorly documented, but colonization of the biliary tract has been reported in patients with symptomatic small bowel infections. It is uncertain how often this occurs or what, if any, symptomatic change it produces. The possibility of biliary colic and jaundice due to biliary obstruction and irritation or edema of the ampulla of Vater due to *Giardia* has been suggested.[292–296]

Pneumocystosis

Although data suggest that *Pneumocystis carinii* may soon be reclassified as a fungus,[297] it is included here because it is still thought of as a protozoan by most practicing clinicians. *P. carinii* continues to be the most common, and arguably most important, opportunistic pathogen in patients with AIDS. Known primarily for its propensity to cause serious pneumonitis in association with AIDS and other forms of immunodeficiency, extrapulmonary pneumocystosis is being reported with increasing frequency.[298–300] In 1990, the rate of extrapulmonary *P. carinii* found at autopsy in patients with AIDS ranged from 2.5 to 5.0%.[298, 299] After lymph nodes and

spleen, the liver is the third most common site of extrapulmonary *P. carinii* infection (Fig. 17–28), but hepatic infection is often seen in association with other reticuloendothelial foci. Hepatic involvement has been reported in at least 16 patients, 12 of whom had AIDS.[298–300] An additional patient has recently been identified among a cohort of HIV-infected patients in Atlanta (DA Schwartz, M.D., personal communication, 1992). Most cases of AIDS-related hepatic *P. carinii* infection have occurred in patients who were receiving prophylactic aerosolized pentamidine,[299] and most have had prior or concomitant *P. carinii* pneumonitis. Other immunosuppressive conditions associated with hepatic *P. carinii* have included hypogammaglobulinemia, postsplenectomy renal transplantation, and thymic alymphoplasia.[298, 299] Antemortem diagnosis by liver biopsy has occurred in at least 4 patients, all of whom had AIDS.[300, 302–304]

Reported clinical manifestations in patients with hepatic *P. carinii* infection are limited but have included hepatosplenomegaly, ascites, elevated hepatic aminotransferases and alkaline phosphatase levels, hypoalbuminemia, coagulopathy, and increased hepatic echogenicity on ultrasound.[298, 300, 301, 303–305] Three patients have been successfully treated with pentamidine trimethoprim-sulfamethoxazole, or trimethoprim/dapsone.[300, 303, 304]

Toxoplasmosis

Infections with *Toxoplasma gondii* are worldwide in distribution. Serologic surveys conducted in the United States suggest that approximately 20 to 40% of the population has been exposed to this parasite, and estimates of infection in pregnant women suggest that annually 1 to 2 infants of every 1000 live births are born with congenitally acquired disease.[306-309] This infection has increasingly gained attention owing to its frequent role in the generation of intracerebral mass lesions in the setting of AIDS.[310] Hepatic involvement is occasionally observed as a component of severe disseminated infections in both normal and debilitated hosts.

Toxoplasma gondii oocysts in soil or water and tissue cysts contaminating meat products are accidentally ingested and then mature within the intestinal tract of humans and other intermediate hosts, releasing infectious sporozoites. These organisms penetrate the intestinal tract, differentiating into tachyzoites, and enter the systemic circulation, through which they are widely disseminated to, and invade, somatic cells.[311, 312] Transmission to humans may also occur via transfusion of blood products, transplantation of organs containing tissue cysts, accidental inoculation of tachyzoites in the laboratory, or transplacental passage of tachyzoites from mother to infant during the course of acute infection.

The majority of infections in the immunocompetent host are asymptomatic and often undiagnosed. When present, symptoms and signs most frequently include fever, chills, headache, malaise, and lymphadenopathy. Mild elevations of serum aminotransferase levels, hepatomegaly, splenomegaly, and rash are less commonly observed.[313, 314] By contrast, infections in the immunocompromised host are associated with more severe systemic manifestations, including encephalitis, pneumonitis, myocarditis, and, rarely, hepatitis.[315, 315a] Congenital infections are evident in only 10 to 20% of affected infants but may result in hydrocephalus, hepatic and splenic enlargement, jaundice, intellectual impairment, chorioretinitis, and microcephaly.[316]

Diagnosis of *Toxoplasma* infection is most readily accomplished by identifying circulating parasite-specific IgG or IgM using any of several established serologic techniques. Negative results on a methylene blue dye test, indirect fluorescent antibody test, or enzyme immunoassay for IgG virtually excludes acute infection in an immunocompetent host. The detection of circulating IgA or IgM by capture enzyme immunoassay or immunosorbent agglutination can provide additional information regarding the recency of infection in the setting of a positive IgG assay. Specialized histopathologic staining techniques and tissue or animal culture systems are also available and can provide further diagnostic support in the appropriate clinical setting.[317, 318]

Systemic antibiotic therapy is generally reserved for severely symptomatic immunocompetent hosts, including those with chorioretinitis, and for acute infections occurring in immunocompromised patients and in the setting of pregnancy. Effective treatment typically consists of a combination of pyrimethamine, given in daily doses of 100 to 200 mg in 2 divided oral doses for 1 to 3 days and then in daily doses of 25 to 75 mg per day, for 4 weeks, with sulfadiazine (or trisulfa-pyrimidines), given in a dosage of 100 mg/kg of body weight daily, with a maximum of 6 to 8 g per day, in 4 divided oral doses for 4 to 6 weeks, and the concomitant administration of 5 to 10 mg per day of leucovorin to minimize hematologic toxicity. Higher dosages of pyrimethamine have been used in treating *Toxoplasma* infection in patients with AIDS. Spiramycin, a macrolide antibiotic not commercially available in the United States, has also shown promise in the treatment of toxoplasmosis acquired during pregnancy. Preventive measures include the adoption of sound hygienic practices when handling materials potentially contaminated with cat feces or oocysts (e.g., litter boxes, soil), thorough cooking of meat before consumption, and identification of women at risk for this infection during pregnancy.[319-321]

Leishmaniasis

Protozoa of the genus *Leishmania* have a worldwide distribution and are estimated to infect approximately 12 million persons in endemic areas.[322] Travelers to these areas are also at risk of acquiring this disease.[323-328] Recently, a more rapidly progressive form of this infection has been observed in persons with AIDS.[329-331]

Most infections with *Leishmania* species are acquired through the bite of an infected sand fly (*Lutzomyia* in the New World and *Phlebotomus* in the Old World). Rare cases of transfusion-associated infection, congenital transmission, and person-to-person transmission have also been reported.[332-335] Intracellular stages of the parasite (amastigotes) are ingested during a sand fly blood meal, change into flagellated extracellular forms (promastigotes) in the sand fly gut, and are transmitted to other hosts during subsequent feedings. Organisms ultimately invade and multiply within the reticuloendothelial system of the infected host. Primary reservoir hosts vary with geographic location and include rodents, dogs, jackals, foxes, sloths, and humans.[336]

Leishmania organisms have a complicated taxonomy and have been categorized into four species complexes based on ecologic, biochemical, and developmental characteristics, isoenzyme patterns, geographic distribution, and clinical findings most frequently associated with component organisms. Morphologic differences between species are subtle and generally inadequate for definitive species identification. The *L. tropica* complex of organisms is primarily found in the Mediterranean littoral, Africa, the Middle East, central Asia, and China (Old World) and is typically associated with cutaneous infection. New World cutaneous leishmaniasis in Central and South America, the Dominican Republic, and sporadically in the United States is caused by organisms belonging to either the *L. mexicana* complex or the *L. braziliensis* complex. The latter organism also causes mucosal disease, known as mucocutaneous leishmaniasis. Visceral leishmaniasis results from infection with organisms of the *L. donovani* complex, which are widely distributed throughout the Old World, Central America, and South America.[332, 336–339]

The clinical spectrum of *Leishmania* infections can be broadly divided into cutaneous and visceral manifestations. Only the visceral manifestations are emphasized here, although skin lesions (kala-azar dermal leishmaniasis) have been noted to appear months to years after treatment of visceral disease due to *L. donovani* species.[339–341]

Visceral infections caused by members of the *L. donovani* complex begin in a fashion similar to that of the cutaneous forms of this infection. The initial papular or ulcerative lesion at the site of inoculation (sand fly bite), however, has characteristically resolved by the time the patient presents for evaluation of possible visceral disease. The incubation period generally ranges from 2 to 6 months, although many years may elapse before the onset of clinical manifestations. Patients typically present with a gradual onset of intermittent fevers, diarrhea, weight loss, and progressive hepatic and splenic enlargement. Grayish hyperpigmentation of the skin, which gave rise to the name kala-azar, which means "black fever," is a characteristic finding in certain areas of the world (e.g., India). Frequently associated laboratory abnormalities include pancytopenia and a polyclonal hypergammaglobulinemia. Oral and nasopharyngeal nodules or ulcerations may also occur as a component of visceral infection. Uncommonly, a generalized lymphadenopathic syndrome without associated hepatosplenomegaly has been observed.[339, 342]

Chronic ulcerative or nodular skin lesions occurring in individuals who have previously resided in areas of the world where leishmaniasis is endemic should prompt an evaluation for the cutaneous form of this disease. Aspiration, scrapings, or biopsy of lesion margins for special staining (i.e., Giemsa or Leishman's stain) and culture can be diagnostic.[343, 344] Definitive diagnosis of visceral leishmaniasis requires splenic, hepatic, bone marrow, or lymph node aspirates in which amastigote-containing macrophages and noncaseating granulomata may be found.[342, 345] Serologic testing (e.g., ELISA, IFA) has been employed as an adjunct to the diagnosis of visceral leishmaniasis.[322, 341, 342] The Montenegro test (leishmanin skin test) is primarily of epidemiologic value as an indicator of recent infection with *Leishmania* species. Delayed hypersensitivity responses to intradermally inoculated promastigote antigens occur in cutaneous, mucocutaneous, and resolving visceral leishmaniasis. Skin tests are usually nonreactive in diffuse cutaneous and acute visceral leishmaniasis.[336, 340–342]

Visceral leishmaniasis should be differentiated from a number of other systemic syndromes associated with marked hepatic and splenic enlargement, including typhoid fever, brucellosis, schistosomiasis, malaria, chronic myelogenous leukemia, Hodgkin's disease, and other lymphomas.[332, 340–342]

Pentavalent antimonial compounds remain the drugs of choice for the treatment of all forms of leishmaniasis. In the United States, sodium stibogluconate (Pentostam) is available for this purpose through the CDC Drug Service. This agent is typically administered in a daily dosage of 20 mg/kg of body weight for a period ranging from 20 days in cutaneous disease to a minimum of 28 days in mucocutaneous and visceral leishmaniasis.[346, 347] Alternative agents that have been employed in patients with visceral disease who are unable to receive or are not responding to standard courses of antimony include pentamidine, amphotericin B, and combined therapy with antimony and interferon-δ.[340–342, 347–349]

Malaria

Malaria is conservatively estimated to affect 200 million individuals in over 100 countries worldwide, remaining one of the most important public health problems of Africa, Asia, and Latin America. The four major species of *Plasmodium* infecting humans include *P. falciparum*, widely distributed in Africa, Southeast Asia, South America, Haiti, New Guinea, and Oceania; *P. vivax*, occurring primarily in Central America and the Indian subcontinent but also found in South America, Southeast Asia, and Oceania; *P. ovale*, limited primarily to Africa; and *P. malariae*, which is most commonly seen in Africa.[350, 351] Imported cases in travelers as well as in immigrants and also transfusion-associated cases continue to be reported in the United States and have contributed to local outbreaks.[352–354]

Early forms of the parasite (sporozoites) are inoculated into the bloodstream by infected anopheline mosquitoes and subsequently enter hepatocytes, where they transform into exoerythrocytic forms. Further multiplication may continue, ultimately leading to cell rupture and release of merozoites infective for circulating erythrocytes. Alternatively, hepatic forms of *P. vivax* and *P. ovale* may transform into more dormant stages (hypnozoites), which cause relapsing symptoms many months or years after the initial infection. Merozoites entering red blood cells undergo further asexual reproduction, resulting in rupture of the erythrocyte membrane and liberation of additional merozoites that perpetuate the life cycle. The developmental process is completed when circulating erythrocytic forms that have differentiated into gametocytes are ingested by the appropriate mosquito host, in which sexual reproduction leads to the formation of infective sporozoites.[355]

Acute malarial infections are associated with the development of rigors, fever, malaise, anorexia, headache, nausea, vomiting, diarrhea, and myalgias typically within 30 to 60 days of exposure to an infected mosquito. Symptoms are frequently nonspecific and are attributed to an intercurrent viral syndrome. Fevers may initially be irregular in onset, although subsequent synchronization of parasite development may result in the more characteristic tertian (*P. vivax, P. ovale*) or quartan (*P. malariae*) periodicity of febrile paroxysms. Splenomegaly and tender hepatic enlargement are commonly found during acute infections and may be associated with anemia, leukopenia, thrombocytopenia, elevated aminotransferase levels, hyperbilirubinemia, and false-positive serologic tests for syphilis. Relapses are known to occur within 6 months of acute infection with *P. vivax* if a tissue schizonticide has not been employed during therapy. *Plasmodium malariae* has been reported to recur as long as 30 to 50 years after acute infection. Complications of acute infection include splenic rupture, cerebral malaria, pulmonary edema, renal insufficiency, and hemolytic anemia. Massive splenic enlargement with hepatomegaly (hyperreactive malarial syndrome, tropical splenomegaly syndrome) has also been associated with more chronic malarial infections in which

circulating immune complexes may contribute to reticuloendothelial system stimulation.[355–357]

Definitive diagnosis of acute malarial infection is dependent on the identification of trophozoites on peripheral blood smears. Initially, the limited number of the circulating parasites may preclude their detection, however, and repeated evaluation of peripheral smears should be performed if symptoms occurring in the appropriate clinical setting suggest the diagnosis. Serologic assays for the detection of malarial antigens have also been developed but remain primarily epidemiologic tools.[355, 356, 358]

Symptoms occurring during the course of acute infection should be differentiated from those observed in acute viral illnesses such as hepatitis, gastroenteritis, amebic liver disease, relapsing fever, yellow fever, typhoid, tuberculosis, brucellosis, trypanosomiasis, endocarditis, and pyelonephritis.[355]

The emergence of widespread resistance to various antimalarial preparations has significantly complicated the management of *P. falciparum* infections, although *P. vivax, P. ovale*, and *P. malariae* species remain generally susceptible to standard regimens. Thus, chloroquine salt, given orally in an initial 1000 mg dose, followed by 500 mg in 6 hours, then 500 mg a day orally for 2 consecutive days, remains the drug of choice for malaria acquired in areas in which drug resistance has not yet been observed, such as in Central America north of Panama, Mexico, Haiti, the Dominican Republic, and in the Middle East, including Egypt. *Plasmodium falciparum* infections acquired in areas known to harbor chloroquine-resistant strains can be treated with oral regimens consisting of combinations of 650 mg of quinine given 3 times a day for 3 to 7 days, and either 250 mg of tetracycline 4 times a day for 7 days, 100 mg of doxycycline 2 times a day for 7 days, or pyrimethamine/sulfadoxine (Fansidar) given in combination 75 mg/1500 mg as a single dose. Alternatively, 750 to 1250 mg of mefloquine as a single agent can be used. This agent should not be administered to individuals performing functions requiring fine-motor coordination, those with underlying neuropsychiatric disorders, pregnant women, or those persons who are receiving concurrent anti-arrhythmics, particularly beta-blockers and calcium channel blockers, or quinine. Severe infections requiring intravenous therapy can be treated with quinidine salt, given in a loading dose of 10 mg/kg of body weight to a maximum of 600 mg in normal saline administered over 1 to 2 hours and followed by a continuous infusion of 0.02 mg/kg/min for 3 consecutive days under close cardiovascular monitoring.[21, 359–361]

An oral regimen should be implemented as soon as the patient's condition stabilizes. Steroids are no longer recommended for the treatment of complications occurring during the course of acute malarial infection.[362] Primaquine, given in daily oral doses of 26.3 mg salt for 14 days, is indicated for the eradication of latent hepatic schizonts that occur during infection with either *P. vivax* or *P. ovale* if the possibility of glucose-6-phosphate dehydrogenase deficiency has been excluded. The role of newer agents including halofantrine and artemisinin in the treatment of this infection is being investigated.[363] Exchange transfusion should be considered for the treatment of high levels of parasitemia associated with *P. falciparum* infection (> 5%) in addition to the above measures.[359]

The choice of prophylactic regimens is similarly influenced by the presence or absence of chloroquine-resistance in a given area of anticipated travel. Chloroquine salt, administered weekly in an oral dose of 500 mg, beginning one week before travel and continuing for 4 weeks after departure from an endemic area, remains effective in nonresistant areas. Mefloquine, given orally in 250-mg doses weekly as outlined for chloroquine; doxycycline, given orally in 100-mg doses daily (considered investigational for this purpose); or combinations of chloroquine, given weekly in 500-mg oral doses, and either proguanil, which is not available in the United States, given orally in 200-mg doses daily for areas of sub-Saharan Africa, or pyrimethamine/sulfadoxine, taken in combination in a single dose of 75 mg/1500 mg as presumptive treatment if medical care is unavailable, are frequently employed for this purpose.[21, 363] The use of pharmacologic agents for prophylaxis should not preclude efforts to prevent direct contact with the vector mosquito by sleeping under mosquito netting, wearing appropriate clothing (long pants, and shirts with long sleeves), using insect repellents, and avoiding the use of scented lotions.[364]

REFERENCES

1. World Health Organization. The control of schistosomiasis. World Health Organ Tech Rep Ser. 1985;728.
2. World Health Organization. Parasitic diseases. Schistosomiasis, an unwelcome guest. Wkly Epidem Rec. 1987;17:122–123.
3. World Health Organization. Schistosomiasis. Wkly Epidem Rec. 1989;22:171.
4. Stuiver PC. Acute schistosomiasis in *Schistosoma haematobium* infection. In: Steffen R, Lobel HO, Haworth J, Bradley DJ. Travel Medicine. Berlin: Springer-Verlag; 1989:381–383.
5. Centers for Disease Control. Acute schistosomiasis in U.S. travelers returning from Africa. MMWR. 1990;39:141–148.
6. Nash TE, Cheever AW, Ottesen EA, Cook JA. Schistosome infections in humans: Perspectives and recent findings. Ann Intern Med. 1982;97:740–754.
7. Jordan P, Webbe G. Schistosomiasis. Epidemiology, Treatment, and Control. London: William Heinemann; 1982.
8. Hiatt RA, Sotomayor ZR, Anchez G, et al. Factors in the pathogenesis of acute schistosomiasis mansoni. J Infect Dis. 1979;139:659–666.
9. Walt F. The Katayama syndrome. S Afr Med J. 1954;28:89–93.
10. Prata A. Schistosomiasis mansoni in Brazil. In: Mahmoud AAF. Baillière's Clinical Tropical Medicine and Communicable Diseases: Schistosomiasis. London: Baillière Tindall; 1987;2:349–369.
11. Stephenson LS, Latham MC, Kinoti SN, Oduori ML. Regression of splenomegaly and hepatomegaly in children treated for *Schistosoma haematobium* infection. Am J Trop Med Hyg. 1985;34:119–123.
12. Gilles HM. Infection with *S haematobium*. In: Jordan P, Webbe G. Schistosomiasis: Epidemiology, Treatment, and Control. London: William Heinemann; 1982:79–104.
13. Watt G, Padre LP, Tuazon M, et al. Hepatic parenchymal dysfunction in *Schistosoma japonicum* infection. J Infect Dis. 1991;164:1186–1192.
14. Al-Saleem T, Al-Janabi T. Schistosomal cholecystitis: Report of six cases. Ann R Coll Surg Engl. 1989;71:366–367.
15. Marcial MA, Marcial-Rojas RA. Cholecystitis due to *Schistosoma mansoni*: Fact or fancy. Bol Asoc Med P R. 1989;81:178–179.
16. Hancock K, Tsang VCW. Development and optimization of the FAST-ELISA for detecting antibodies to *Schistosoma mansoni*. J Immunol. 1986;92:167–186.
17. Harries AD, Speare R. Rectal snips in the diagnosis of hepatosplenic schistosomiasis. Trans R Soc Trop Med Hyg. 1988;82:720.
18. Homeida M, Abdel-Gadir AF, Cheever AW, et al. Diagnosis of pathologically confirmed Symmers's periportal fibrosis by ultrasonography: A prospective blinded study. Am J Trop Med Hyg. 1988;38:86–91.
19. Doehring-Schwerdtfeger E, Mohamed-Ali G, Abdel-Rahim IM, et al. Sonomorphological abnormalities in Sudanese children with *Schistosoma mansoni* infection: A proposed staging-system for field diagnosis of periportal fibrosis. Am J Trop Med Hyg. 1989;41:63–69.
20. King CH, Mahmoud AAF. Drugs five years later: Praziquantel. Ann Intern Med. 1989;110:290–296.
21. Drugs for parasitic infections. Med Lett Drugs Ther. 1993;35:111–122.
22. Farid Z, Woody J, Kamal M. Praziquantel and acute urban schistosomiasis. Trop Geogr Med. 1989;41:172.
23. Ong ELC, Ellis ME. Acute schistosomiasis (Katayama fever): Corticosteroid as adjunct therapy. Scand J Infect Dis. 1989;21:473–474.
24. El-Zayadi A, Mohran Z, Hasseeb N, et al. Short-term course of corticosteroids in the treatment of resistant ascites complicating schistosomal liver disease. Am J Gastroenterol. 1991;86:53–56.
25. Salam AA, Ezzat FA, Abu-Elmagd KM. Selective shunt in schistosomiasis in Egypt. Am J Surg. 1990;160:90–92.
26. Abu-Elmagd KM, Ezzat FA, Fathy OM, et al. Should both schistosomal and nonschistosomal variceal bleeders be disconnected? World J Surg. 1991;15:389–398.
27. Ezzat FA, Abu-Elmagd KM, Sultan AA, et al. Schistosomal versus nonschistosomal variceal bleeders: Do they respond differently to selective shunt (DSRS)? Ann Surg. 1989;209:489–500.

28. Da Silva LC, Strauss E, Gayotto LC, et al. A randomized trial for the study of the elective surgical treatment of portal hypertension in mansonic schistosomiasis. Ann Surg. 1986;204:148–153.

29. El-Zayadi A, El-Din SS, Kabil SM. Endoscopic sclerotherapy versus medical treatment for bleeding esophageal varices in patients with schistosomal liver disease. Gastrointest Endosc. 1988;34:314–317.

30. Mies S, Pereira M de B, Orlando CD, et al. Propranolol in the prevention of recurrence of digestive hemorrhage in patients with hepatosplenic schistosomiasis. AMB Rev Assoc Med Bras. 1988;34:24–28.

31. Chen MG, Mott KE. Progress in assessment of morbidity due to *Fasciola hepatica* infection: A review of recent literature. Trop Dis Bul. 1990;87:R1–R38.

32. Bunnag D, Thanongsak B, Goldsmith R. Fascioliasis. In: Strickland GT. Hunter's Tropical Medicine. 7th ed. Philadelphia: WB Saunders; 1991;823–826.

33. Beaver PC, Jung RC, Cupp EW. Amphistomate and distomate flukes. In: Beaver PC, Jung RC. Clinical Parasitology. 9th ed. Philadelphia: Lea & Febiger; 1984:451–455.

34. Acha PN, Szyfres B. Fascioliasis. In: Zoonoses and communicable diseases common to man and animals. Pan American Health Organization; 1987;503:660–667.

35. Takeyama N, Nobuyoshi O, Sakai Y, et al. Computed tomography findings of hepatic lesions in human fascioliasis: Report of two cases. Am J Gastroenterol. 1986;81:1078–1081.

36. Bendezu P, Frame A, Hillyer G. Human fascioliasis in Corozal, Puerto Rico. J Parasitol. 1982;68:297–299.

37. Stork M, Venables G, Jennings S, et al. An investigation of endemic fascioliasis in Peruvian village children. J Trop Med Hyg. 1973;76:231–235.

38. Bjorland J, McAuley JB, Strauss W, et al. An acute outbreak of fascioliasis among Aymara Indians in the Bolivian Altiplano. Submitted for publication.

39. Jones E, Kay J, Milligan H, et al. Massive infection with *Fasciola hepatica* in man. Am J Med. 1977;63:836–842.

40. Pagola Serrano M, Vega A, Ortega E, et al. Computed tomography of hepatic fascioliasis. J Comput Assist Tomogr. 1987;11:269–272.

41. Farid Z, Trabolsi B, Boctor F, et al. Unsuccessful use of praziquantel to treat acute fascioliasis in children. J Infect Dis. 1986;154:920–921.

42. Loutan L, Bouvier M, Rojanawisut B, et al. Single treatment of invasive fascioliasis with triclabendazole. Lancet. 1989;2:383.

43. Wessely K, Reischig H, Heinerman M, et al. Human fascioliasis treated with triclabendazole (Fasinex) for the first time. Trans R Soc Trop Med Hyg. 1988;82:743–745.

44. Bannerman C, Manzur A. Fluctuating jaundice and intestinal bleeding in a 6-year-old girl with fascioliasis. Trop Geogr Med. 1986;38:429–431.

45. Beers B, Pringot J, Geubel A, et al. Hepatobiliary fascioliasis: Noninvasive imaging findings. Radiology. 1990;174:809–810.

46. Chan CW, Lam SK. Diseases caused by liver flukes and cholangiocarcinoma. Baillière's Clinical Gastroenterology 1987;1:297–318.

47. Acuna-Soto R, Braun-Roth G. Bleeding ulcer in the common bile duct due to *Fasciola hepatica*. Am J Gastroenterol. 1987;82:560–562.

48. Shazly A, Desoky I, Feky A. A case of ectopic fascioliasis in a farmer from Mansoura City, Dakahlia, Egypt. J Egypt Soc Parasitol. 1991;21:333–335.

49. Park CI, Kim H, Ro JY, et al. Human ectopic fascioliasis in the cecum. Am J Surg Pathol. 1984;8:73–77.

50. Meyers WM, Neafie RC. Fascioliasis. In: Binford CH, Connor DH. Pathology of Tropical and Extraordinary Diseases. Washington DC: Armed Forces Institute of Pathology; 1976;2:524–527.

51. Knobloch J, Delgado A, Alvarez A. Human fascioliasis in Cajamarca, Peru: I, Diagnostic methods and treatment with praziquantel. Trop Med Parasit. 1985;36:88–90.

52. Gamboa C, Biolley M, Oberg C. Distomatosis: Alternativas de diagnostico coproparasitologico. Parasitol al Dia. 1989;13:138–140.

53. Hillyer G. Fascioliasis and fasciolopsiasis. In: Balows A, Hausler WJ, Lennette EH. Laboratory Diagnosis of Infectious Diseases: Principles and Practice. New York; Springer-Verlag; 1988:855–861.

54. Campos LA, Garcia Bonilla A. *Fasciola hepatica* in the common bile duct: Presentation of a case. Rev Gastroenterol Mex. 1990;55:25–29.

55. Pandolfo I, Zimbaro G, Bartiromo G, et al. Ultrasonographic and cholecystographic findings in a case of fascioliasis of the gallbladder. JCJ J Clin Ultrasound. 1991;19:505–507.

56. Rivera JV, Bermudez RH. Radionuclide imaging of the liver in human fascioliasis. Clin Nucl Med. 1984;9:450–453.

57. Hodler J, Meier P. Infection of the liver by *Fasciola hepatica*: Sonography and CT. ROFO. 1989;151:740–741.

58. Criado MP, Mazas-Artasona L, Balmaseda C, et al. Distomatose hépatobiliaire en échographie. J Radiol. 1989;70:617–619.

59. Bassily S, Iskander M, Yousseff FG. Sonography in diagnosis of fascioliasis. Lancet. 1989;1:1270–1271.

60. Pulpeiro JR, Armesto V, Varela J, et al. Fascioliasis: Findings in 15 patients. Br J Radiol. 1991;64:798–801.

61. Hillyer GV. Fascioliasis, paragonimiasis, clonorchiasis, and opisthorchiasis. In: Walls KW, Schantz PM. Immunodiagnosis of Parasitic Diseases. Orlando, FL: Academic Press; 1986;1:40–51.

62. Hillyer GV, Soler de Galanes M. Identification of a 17-kilodalton *Fasciola hepatica* immunodiagnostic antigen by the enzyme-linked immunoelectrotransfer blot technique. J Clin Microbiol. 1988;26:2048–2053.

63. Youssef FG, Mansour NS, Aziz AG. Early diagnosis of human fascioliasis by the detection of copro-antigens using counterimmunoelectrophoresis. Trans R Soc Trop Med Hyg. 1991;85:383–384.

64. Schiappacasse RH, Mohammadi D, Christie AJ. Successful treatment of severe infection with *Fasciola hepatica* with praziquantel. J Infect Dis. 1985;152:1339–1340.

65. Uribarrena R, Borda F, Munoz M, et al. Laparoscopic findings in eight cases of liver fascioliasis. Endoscopy. 1985;17:137–138.

66. Cosme A, Alzate L, Orive V, et al. Laparoscopic findings in liver fascioliasis. Study of 13 cases. Rev Esp Enferm Dig. 1990;78:359–362.

67. Markwalder K, Koller M, Goebel N, Wolff K. Infektion mit *Fasciola hepatica*. Schweiz Med Wochenschr. 1988;118:1048–1052.

68. Sapunar J, Zenteno J. Praziquantel: Una droga inefectiva en la fascioliasis humana? Relato de cinco casos de Francaso. Parasitol al Dia. 1989;13:74–75.

69. Farid Z, Kamal M, Mansour N. Praziquantel and *Fasciola hepatica* infection. Trans R Soc Trop Med Hyg. 1989;83:813.

70. Haswell-Elkins MR, Sithithaworn P, Elkins D. *Opisthorchis viverrini* and cholangiocarcinoma in northeast Thailand. Parasitol Today. 1992;8:86–89.

71. Beaver PC, Jung RC, Cupp EW. Amphistomate and distomate flukes. In: Beaver PC, Jung RC. Clinical Parasitology. 9th ed. Philadelphia: Lea & Febiger; 1984:471–478.

72. Dooley JR, Neafie RC. Clonorchiasis and opisthor-

chiasis. In: Binford CH, Connor DH. Pathology of Tropical and Extraordinary Diseases. Washington DC: Armed Forces Institute of Pathology; 1976;2:509–516.

73. Bunnag D, Thanongsak B, Goldsmith R. Clonorchiasis. In: Strickland GT. Hunter's Tropical Medicine. 7th ed. Philadelphia: WB Saunders; 1991;822–823.

74. Jong EC, Wasserheit JN, Johnson RJ, et al: Praziquantel for the treatment of *Clonorchis/Opisthorchis* infections: Report of a double-blind, placebo-controlled trial. J Infect Dis. 1985; 152:637–640.

75. Cross JH, Murrell KD. The 33rd SEAMEO-TROPMED regional seminar on emerging problems in food-borne parasitic zoonoses: Impact on agriculture and public health. Southeast Asian J Trop Med Public Health. 1991;22:4–15.

76. Elkins DB, Haswell-Elkins MR, Mairang E, et al. A high frequency of hepatobiliary disease and suspected cholangiocarcinoma associated with heavy *Opisthorchis viverrini* infection in a small community in northeast Thailand. Trans R Soc Trop Med Hyg. 1990;84:715–719.

77. Kurathong S, Lerdverasirikul P, Wongpaitoon V, et al. *Opisthorchis viverrini* infection and cholangiocarcinoma. Gastroenterology. 1985;89:151–156.

78. Acha PN, Szyfres B. Opisthorchiasis. In: Zoonoses and Communicable Diseases Common to Man and Animals. Pan American Health Organization; 1987;503:675–678.

79. Weniger BG, Schantz PM. Praziquantel and refugee health. JAMA. 1984;251:2391–2392.

80. Cross JH. Liver and lung fluke infections. In: Spittell JA. Clinical Medicine. Philadelphia: Harper & Row; 1982;2:1–13.

81. Pungpak S, Riganti M, Bunnag D, et al. Clinical features in severe *Opisthorchis viverrini*. Southeast Asian J Trop Med Public Health. 1985;16:405–409.

82. Yue-han L, Zhong-da Q, Xiao-gen W, et al. Praziquantel in *Clonorchis sinensis*: A further evaluation of 100 cases. Chin Med J (Engl). 1982;95:89–94.

83. Hsu CCS, Kron MA. Clonorchiasis and praziquantel. Arch Intern Med. 1985;145:1002–1003.

84. Flavell DJ. Liver-fluke infection as an aetiological factor in bile-duct carcinoma of man. Trans R Soc Trop Med Hyg. 1981;75:814–824.

85. Schwartz DA. Helminths in the induction of cancer: *Opisthorchis viverrini, Clonorchis sinensis* and cholangiocarcinoma. Trop Geogr Med. 1980;32:95–109.

86. Dennis MJS, Dennison AR, Morris DL. Parasitic causes of obstructive jaundice. Ann Trop Med Parasit. 1989;83:159–161.

87. Sirisinha S, Chawengkirttikul R, Sermswan R, et al. Detection of *Opisthorchis viverrini* by monoclonal antibody-based ELISA and DNA hybridization. Am J Trop Med Hyg. 1991;44:140–145.

88. Chen CY. Clinical study of treatment and immunodiagnosis in patients with clonorchiasis. J Formosan Med Assoc. 1988;87:1170–1175.

89. Rim HJ, Lyu KS, Lee JS, et al. Clinical evaluation of the therapeutic efficacy of praziquantel (Embay 8440) against *Clonorchis sinensis* infection in man. Ann Trop Med Parasitol. 1981;75:27–33.

90. Bunnag D, Harinasuta T. Studies on the chemotherapy of human opisthorchiasis in Thailand: I. Clinical trial of praziquantel. Southeast Asian J Trop Med Public Health. 1980;11:528–531.

91. Bryan RT, Schantz PM. Zoonosis update: Echinococcosis (hydatid disease). J Am Vet Med Assoc. 1989;195:1214–1217.

92. Schantz PM, Okelo GBA. Echinococcosis (hydatidosis). In: Warren KS, Mahmoud AAF. Tropical and Geographical Medicine. 2nd ed. New York: McGraw-Hill; 1990:505–518.

93. Beaver PC, Jung RC, Cupp EW. Cyclophyllidean tapeworms. In: Beaver PC, Jung RC. Clinical Parasitology. 9th ed. Philadelphia: Lea & Febiger; 1984:527–543.

94. Schaefer JW, Khan MY. Echinococcosis (hydatid disease): Lessons from experience with 59 patients. Rev Infect Dis. 1991;13:243–247.

95. Case Records of the Massachusetts General Hospital: Case 45-1987. N Eng J Med. 1987;317:1209–1217.

96. Mathisen GE, Sokolov RT, Meyer RD: Fever, abdominal pain, and headache in an Iranian woman. Rev Infect Dis. 1990;12:529–536.

97. Schantz PM. Echinococcosis. In: Steele JH, Jacobs L, Arambulo P. CRC Handbook Series in Zoonoses. Boca Raton FL: CRC Press; 1982;1:231–277.

98. Schantz PM. Parasitic zoonoses in perspective. Int J Parasitol. 1991;21:161–170.

99. Stehr-Green JK, Stehr-Green PA, Schantz PM, et al. Risk factors for infection with *Echinococcus multilocularis* in Alaska. Am J Trop Med Hyg. 1988;38:380–385.

100. Schantz PM. Hydatid disease (echinococcosis). In: Spittell JA. Clinical Medicine. Philadelphia: Harper & Row; 1986;3:1–12.

101. Al-Kraida A, Alam MK, Qazi MS, et al. Hydatid disease of the liver in Riyadh. Ann Saudi Med. 1988;8:117–121.

102. Paone R, Mercer L, Miranda C, et al. Echinococcal disease of the extrahepatic biliary tract. Tex Med. 1989;85:36–37.

103. Kune GA, Schellenberger R. Current management of liver hydatid cysts: Results of a 10-year study. Med J Aust. 1988;149:26–30.

104. Karavias D, Panagopoulos C, Vagianos C, et al. Infected echinococcal cyst. A common cause of pyogenic hepatic abscess. Ups J Med Sci. 1988;93:289–296.

105. McGreevy PB, Nelson GS. Larval cestode infections. In: Strickland GT. Hunter's Tropical Medicine. 7th ed. Philadelphia: WB Saunders; 1991;843–846.

106. Akingolu A, Demiryurek H, Guzel C. Alveolar hydatid disease of the liver: A report on thirty-nine surgical cases in eastern Anatolia, Turkey. Am J Trop Med Hyg. 1991;45:182–189.

107. Rausch RL, Wilson JF, Schantz PM, et al. Spontaneous death of *Echinococcus multilocularis*: Cases diagnosed serologically (by Em2 ELISA) and clinical significance. Am J Trop Med Hyg. 1987;36:576–585.

108. Morel P, Robert J, Rohner A. Surgical treatment of hydatid disease of the liver: A survey of 69 patients. Surgery. 1988;104:859–862.

109. Kalovidouris A, Pissiotis C, Pontifex C, et al. CT characterization of multivesicular hydatid cysts. J Comput Assist Tomogr 1986;10:428–431.

110. Lewall DB, McCorkell SJ. Hepatic echinococcal cysts: Sonographic appearance and classification. Radiology. 1985;155:773–775.

111. Bret PM, Fond A, Bretagnolle M, et al. Percutaneous aspiration and drainage of hydatid cysts in the liver. Radiology. 1988;168:617–620.

112. Davolio Marani SA, Canossi GC, Nicoli FA, et al. Hydatid disease: MR imaging study. Radiology. 1990;175:701–706.

113. Case Records of the Massachusetts General Hospital: Case 19-1990. N Eng J Med. 1990;322:1378–1385.

114. Schantz PM. Circulating antigen and antibody in hydatid disease. N Eng J Med. 1988;318:1469. Letter.

115. Filice C, Di Perri G, Strosselli M, et al. Parasitologic findings in percutaneous drainage of human hydatid liver cysts. J Infect Dis. 1990;161:1290–1295.

116. Maddison SE, Slemenda SB, Schantz PM, et al. A specific diagnostic antigen of *Echinococcus granulosus* with an apparent molecular weight of 8 kDa. Am J Trop Med Hyg. 1989;40:377–383.

117. Hira PR, Lindberg LG, Francis I, et al. Diagnosis of

cystic hydatid disease: Role of aspiration cytology. Lancet. 1988;1:655–657.

118. Duewell VS, Marincek B, von Schulthess GK, et al. MRT und CT bei alveolärer Echinokokkose der Leber. ROFO. 1990;152:441–445.

119. Lanier AP, Trujillo DE, Schantz PM, et al. Comparison of serologic tests for the diagnosis and follow-up of alveolar hydatid disease. Am J Trop Med Hyg. 1987;37:609–615.

120. D'Alessandro A, Rausch RL, Cuello C, et al. First observation of *Echinococcus vogeli* in man, with a review of human cases of polycystic hydatid disease in Colombia and neighboring countries. Am J Trop Med Hyg. 1979;28:303–317.

121. Morris DL, Lamont G. Suction curettage in the management of hydatid cysts. Br J Surg. 1987;74:323.

122. Magistrelli P, Masetti R, Coppola R, et al. Surgical treatment of hydatid disease of the liver: A 20-year experience. Arch Surg. 1991;126:518–522.

123. Prasad J, Bellamy PR, Stubbs RS. Instillation of scolicidal agents into hepatic hydatid cysts: Can it any longer be justified? N Z Med J. 1991;104:336–337.

124. Okelo GBA. Hydatid disease: Research and control in Turkana: III, Albendazole in the treatment of inoperable hydatid disease in Kenya, a report on 12 cases. Trans R Soc Trop Med Hyg. 1986;80:193–195.

125. Morris DL, Dykes PW, Marriner S, et al. Albendazole: Objective evidence of response in human hydatid disease. JAMA. 1985;253:2053–2057.

126. Schantz PM. Effective treatment for hydatid disease? JAMA. 1985;253:2095–2097. Editorial.

127. Todorov T, Vutova K, Petkov D, et al. Albendazole treatment of human cystic echinococcosis. Trans R Soc Trop Med Hyg. 1988;82:453–459.

128. Rowley AH, Shulman ST, Donaldson JS, et al. Albendazole treatment of recurrent echinococcosis. Pediatr Infect Dis. 1988;7:666–667.

129. Morris DL. Pre-operative albendazole therapy for hydatid cyst. Br J Surg. 1987;74:805–806.

130. Morris DL, Smith PG. Albendazole in hydatid disease: Hepatocellular toxicity. Trans R Soc Trop Med Hyg. 1987;81:343–344.

131. World Health Organization. Albendazole: Fatal pancytopenia (Italy). World Health Organ Pharmaceut Newslett. 1991;4:8.

132. Berguer R, Wilson JF. Surgery in hepatic *Echinococcus multilocularis* disease. Gastroenterology. 1990;98:A–438.

133. Glickman LT, Schantz PM. Epidemiology and pathogenesis of zoonotic toxocariasis. Epidemiol Rev. 1981;3:230–250.

134. Schantz PM. *Toxocara* larva migrans now. Am J Trop Med Hyg. 1989;41:21–34.

135. Nagakura K, Tachibana H, Kaneda Y, et al. Toxocariasis possibly caused by ingesting raw chicken. J Infect Dis. 1989;160:735–736.

136. Schantz PM, Michelson MK. *Toxocara* species and other Nematodes causing larva migrans syndromes. In: Gorbach SL, Bartlett JG, Blacklow NR. Infectious Diseases. Philadelphia: WB Saunders; 1992:1343–1347.

137. Beaver PC. Zoonoses with particular reference to parasites of veterinary importance. In: Soulsby EJL. Biology of Parasites. New York: Academic Press; 1966:215–218.

138. Parsons JC. Ascarid infections of cats and dogs. Vet Clin North Am Small Anim Pract. 1987;17:1307–1339.

139. Zinkham WH. Visceral larva migrans: A review and reassessment indicating two forms of clinical expression, visceral and ocular. Am J Dis Child. 1978;132:627–633.

140. Glickman LT, Schantz PM, Cypress RH. Epidemiological characteristics and clinical findings in patients with serologically proven toxocariasis. Trans R Soc Trop Med Hyg. 1979;73:254–258.

141. Mok CH. Visceral larva migrans: A discussion based on a review of the literature. Clin Pediatr. 1968;7:565–573.

142. Huntley CC, Costas MC, Lyerly A. Visceral larva migrans syndrome: Clinical characteristics and immunologic studies in 51 patients. Pediatrics. 1965;36:523–536.

143. Beshear JR, Hendley JO. Severe pulmonary involvement in visceral larva migrans. Am J Dis Child. 1973;125:599–600.

144. Fortenberry JD, Kenney RD, Younger J. Visceral larva migrans producing static encephalopathy in an infant. Pediatr Infect Dis J. 1991;10:403–406.

145. Shields JA. Ocular toxocariasis: A review. Surv Ophthalmol. 1984;28:361–381.

146. Taylor MRH, Keane CT, O'Connor P, et al. The expanded spectrum of toxocaral disease. Lancet. 1988;1:692–694.

147. Nichols RL. The etiology of visceral larva migrans: I, Diagnostic morphology of infective second-stage *Toxocara* larvae. J Parasitol. 1956;42:349–362.

148. Glickman LT, Schantz PM, Grieve RB. Toxocariasis. In: Walls KW, Schantz PM. Immunodiagnosis of Parasitic Diseases. Orlando FL: Academic Press; 1986;1:201–231.

149. Bass JL, Mehta KA, Glickman LT, et al. Asymptomatic toxocariasis in children. Clin Pediatr. 1987;26:441–446.

150. Sturchler D, Schubarth P, Gualzata M, et al. Thiabendazole vs. albendazole in treatment of toxocariasis: A clinical trial. Ann Trop Med Parasitol. 1989;83:473–478.

151. Hagler WS, Pollard ZF, Jarrett WH, et al. Results of surgery for ocular *Toxocara canis*. Ophthalmology. 1981;88:1081–1086.

152. Schantz PM, Stehr-Green JK. Toxocaral larva migrans. J Am Vet Med Assoc. 1988;19:28–32.

153. Wright KA. Observations on the life cycle of *Capillaria hepatica* (Bancroft, 1893) with a description of the adult. Can J Zool. 1961;38:167–182.

154. McQuown AL. *Capillaria hepatica*. Report of genuine and spurious cases. Am J Trop Med. 1950;30:761–767.

155. Otto GF, Berthrong M, Appleby RE, et al. Eosinophilia and hepatomegaly due to *Capillaria hepatica*. Bull Johns Hopkins Hosp. 1954;94:319–336.

156. Turhan B, Unat EK, Yenermen M, et al. Insan Karacigerinde *Capillaria hepatica* (Bancroft, 1893) Travassos, 1915. Mikrobiol Dergisi. 1954;7:149–159.

157. Ewing GM, Tilden IL. *Capillaria hepatica*: Report of a fourth case of true human infestation. J Paediatr. 1956;48:341–348.

158. Cochrane JC, Sagorin L, Wilcocks MG. *Capillaria hepatica* infection in man. S Afr Med J. 1957;31:751–755.

159. Ward RL, Dent JH. *Capillaria hepatica* infection in a child. Bull Tulane Univ Med Fac. 1959;19:27–33.

160. Kallichurum S, Elsdon-Dew R. *Capillaria* in man: A case report. S Afr Med J. 1961;35:860–861.

161. Calle S. Parasitism by *Capillaria hepatica*. Pediatrics. 1961;27:648–655.

162. Garcia FR, Mendiola GJ, Biagi FF. Eosinofilia elevada con manifestaciones viscerales: IV, Primer caso de infeccion por *Capillaria hepatica* en Mexico. Bol Med Hosp Infant Mex. 1962;19:473–479.

163. Piazza R, Correa MO, Fleury RN. Sobre um caso de infestacao humana por *Capillaria hepatica*. Rev Inst Med Trop S Paulo. 1963;5:37–41.

164. Camain R, Dor X, Ranavo F. Hepatic infestation with *Capillaria hepatica* in an 11-month-old child. Ann Pediatr (Paris). 1965;12:559–562.

165. Cislaghi F, Radice C. Infection by *Capillaria hepatica*. First case report in Italy. Helv Paediat Acta. 1970;25:647–654.

166. Pampiglione S, Conconi C. Primo Caso di capillariosi epatica osservata nell'uomo in Italia. Parassitologia. 1970;12:125–134.

167. Slais J. The finding and identification of solitary *Capillaria hepatica* (Bancroft, 1893) in man from Europe. Folia Parasitol (Praha). 1973;20:149–161.

168. Silverman NH, Katz JS, Levin SE. *Capillaria hepatica* infestation in a child. S Afr Med J. 1973;47:219–221.

169. Vargas CG, Lopez MH, Victoria VR, et al. *Capillaria hepatica*: Report of the 2nd case found in the Mexican Republic. Bol Med Hosp Infant Mex. 1979;36:909–917.

170. Pereira VG, Franca LCM. Successful treatment of *Capillaria hepatica* infection in an acutely ill adult. Am J Trop Med Hyg. 1983;32:1272–1274.

171. Attah EB, Nagarajan S, Obineche EN, et al. Hepatic capillariasis. Am J Clin Pathol. 1983;79:127–130.

172. Berger T, Degremont A, Gebbers JO, et al. Hepatic capillariasis in a 1-year-old child. Eur J Pediatr. 1990;149:333–336.

173. Pannenbecker J, Miller TC, Muller J, et al. Severe liver involvement by *Capillaria hepatica*. Monatsschr Kinderheilkd. 1990;138:767–771.

174. McQuown AL. *Capillaria hepatica*. Am J Clin Pathol. 1954;24:448–452.

175. Beaver PC, Jung RC, Cupp EW. Aphasmid nematodes (Adenophorea). In: Beaver PC, Jung RC. Clinical Parasitology. 9th ed. Philadelphia: Lea & Febiger; 1984:245–252.

176. MacArthur WP. A case of infestation of the human liver with *Hepaticola hepatica* (Bancroft, 1893) Hall, 1916. Proc R Soc Med (Trop Dis Parasit). 1924;17:83–84.

177. Arean VM. Capillariasis. In: Marcial-Rojas RA. Pathology of Protozoal and Helminthic Diseases. Baltimore: Williams & Wilkins; 1971:666–676.

178. Acha PN, Szyfres B. Capillariasis. In: Zoonoses and Communicable Diseases Common to Man and Animals. Pan American Health Organization. 1987;503:781–786.

179. Kumar V. Hepatic *Capillaria* may simulate the syndrome of visceral larva migrans: An analysis. Ann Soc Belge Med Trop. 1985;65:101–104.

180. Marcial-Rojas RA, Ramirez-Ronda CH. Parasitic diseases of the liver. In: Schiff L, Schiff ER. Diseases of the Liver. Philadelphia: JB Lippincott; 1982:1165–1197.

181. World Health Organization. Prevention and control of intestinal parasitic infections: Report of a WHO expert committee. World Health Organ Tech Rep Ser. 1987;749.

182. Gelpi AP, Mustafa A. Seasonal pneumonitis with eosinophilia: A study of larval ascariasis in Saudi Arabia. Am J Trop Med Hyg. 1967;16:646–657.

183. Hlaing T. A Profile of ascariasis morbidity in Rangoon Children's Hospital, Burma. J Trop Med Hyg. 1987;90:165–169.

184. Blumenthal DS, Schultz MG. Incidence of intestinal obstruction in children infected with *Ascaris lumbricoides*. Am J Trop Med Hyg. 1985;24:801–805.

185. Louw JH. Abdominal complications of *Ascaris lumbricoides* infestation in children. Br J Surg. 1966;53:510–521.

186. Khuroo MS, Zargar SA, Mahajan R. Hepatobiliary and pancreatic ascariasis in India. Lancet. 1990;335:1503–1506.

187. Schulman A. Biliary ascariasis presenting in the United States. Am J Gastroenterol. 1977;68:167–170.

188. Saw HS, Somasundaram K, Kamath R. Hepatic ascariasis: A case report and review of the literature. Arch Surg. 108:733–735.

189. Parodi-Hueck LE, Wenger F, Montiel-Villasmil D. *Ascaris* hepatic abscess in children. J Pediatr Surg. 1972;7:69.

190. Schulman A. Non-western patterns of biliary stones and the role of ascariasis. Radiology. 1987;162:425–430.

191. Uflacker R, Duarte D, Silva P. Association of congenital cystic dilatation of the common bile duct and congenital diverticulum of the hepatic duct with concomitant ascariasis. Gastrointest Radiol. 1978;3:407–409.

192. Deeg KH. Sonographic diagnosis of biliary ascariasis. Eur J Paediatr. 1990;150:95–96.

193. Khuroo MS, Zargar SA, Mahajan R, et al. Sonographic appearances in biliary ascariasis. Gastroenterology. 1987;93:267–272.

194. Chen YS, Den BX, Huang BI, et al. Endoscopic diagnosis and management of *Ascaris*-induced acute pancreatitis. Endoscopy. 1986;18:127–128.

195. Manialawi MS, Khattar NY, Helmy MM, et al. Endoscopic diagnosis and extraction of biliary *Ascaris*. Endoscopy. 1986;18:204–203.

196. Cline BL. Current drug regimens for the treatment of intestinal helminth infections. Med Clin North Am. 1982;66:721–742.

197. Janssens PG. Chemotherapy of gastrointestinal nematodiasis in man. In: Bossche HV, Thienpont D, Janssens PG. Handbook of Experimental Pharmacology. Berlin: Springer-Verlag; 1985;77:183–406.

198. Ramalingam S, Sinniah B, Krishnan U. Albendazole: an effective single dose, broad-spectrum anthelminthic drug. Am J Trop Med Hyg. 1983;32:984–989.

199. Swartzwelder JC, et al. The use of piperazine for the treatment of human helminthiases. Gastroenterology. 1957;33:87–94.

200. Walsh JA, Warren KS. Selective primary health care: An interim strategy for disease control in developing countries. N Engl J Med. 1979;301:967–974.

201. Smith JW. Strongyloidiasis. Clin Microbiol Newsletter. 1991;13:33–40.

202. Scowden EB, Schaffner W, Stone WJ. Overwhelming strongyloidiasis: An unappreciated opportunistic infection. Medicine. 1978;57:527–544.

203. Marcial-Rojas RA. Strongyloidiasis. In: Marcial-Rojas RA. Pathology of Protozoal and Helminthic Diseases. Baltimore: Williams & Wilkins; 1971:711–733.

204. Meyers WM, Connor DH, Neafie RC. Strongyloidiasis. In: Binford CH, Connor DH. Pathology of Tropical and Extraordinary Diseases. Washington DC: Armed Forces Institute of Pathology; 1976;2:428–432.

205. Neefe LI, Pinilla O, Garagusi VF, et al. Disseminated strongyloidiasis with cerebral involvement: A complication of corticosteroid therapy. Am J Med. 1973;55:832–838.

206. Purtilo DT, Meyers WM, Connor DH. Fatal strongyloidiasis in immunosuppressed patients. Am J Med. 1974;56:488–492.

207. Beaver PC, Jung RC, Cupp EW. The rhabditida: *Strongyloides* and related forms. In: Beaver PC, Jung RC. Clinical Parasitology. 9th ed. Philadelphia; Lea & Febiger; 1984:253–262.

208. Pearson RD, Guerrant RL. *Strongyloides* infections. In: Strickland GT. Hunter's Tropical Medicine. 7th ed. Philadelphia: WB Saunders; 1991:706–11.

209. Hulbert TV, Larsen RA, Chandrasoma PT: Abdominal *Angiostrongylus* mimicking acute appendicitis and Meckel's diverticulum: Report of a case in the United States and review. Clin Infect Dis. 1992;14:836–840.

210. Beaver PC, Jung RC, Cupp EW. The Strongylida: Hookworms and other bursate nematodes. In: Beaver PC, Jung RC. Clinical Parasitology. 9th ed. Philadelphia: Lea & Febiger; 1984:294–296.

211. Morera P. Abdominal Angiostrongyliasis. In: Strickland GT. Hunter's Tropical Medicine. 7th ed. Philadelphia: WB Saunders; 1991:771–773.

212. Loria-Cortes R, Lobo-Sanahuja JF. Clinical abdominal angiostrongylosis: A study of 116 children with intestinal eosinophilic granuloma caused by *Angiostrongylus costaricensis*. Am J Trop Med Hyg. 1980;29:538–544.

213. Morera P, Perez F, Mora F, et al. Visceral larva migrans–like syndrome caused by *Angiostrongylus costaricensis*. Am J Trop Med Hyg. 1982;31:67–70.

214. Sun T, Schwartz NS, Sewell C, et al. *Enterobius* egg granuloma of the vulva and peritoneum: Review of the literature. Am J Trop Med Hyg. 1991;45:249–253.

215. Chandrasoma PT, Mendis KN. *Enterobius vermicularis* in ectopic sites. Am J Trop Med Hyg. 1977;26:644–649.

216. Hennequin C, Breuil J, Patey O, et al. Hepatic granuloma caused by *Enterobius vermicularis*. Bull Soc Fr Parasitol. 1988;5:205–208.

217. Slais J. A threadworm granuloma in the human liver. Helminthologia. 1963;4:479–483.

218. Little MD, Cuello CJ, D'Alessandro A. Granuloma of the liver due to *Enterobius vermicularis*. Am J Trop Med Hyg. 1973;22:567–569.

219. Mondou EN, Gnepp DR. Hepatic granuloma resulting from *Enterobius vermicularis*. J Clin Pathol 1989;91:97–100.

220. Daly JJ, Baker GF. Pinworm granuloma of the liver. Am J Trop Med Hyg. 1984;33:62–64.

221. Johnson RJ, Jong EC, Dunning SB, et al. Paragonimiasis: Diagnosis and the use of praziquantel in treatment. Rev Infect Dis. 1985;7:200–206.

222. Amunarriz M. Intermediate hosts of *Paragonimus* in the eastern Amazonic region of Ecuador. Trop Med Parasitol. 1991;42:164–166.

223. Acha PN, Szyfres B. Paragonimiasis. In: Zoonoses and Communicable Diseases Common to Man and Animals. Pan American Health Organization; 1987; 503:678–686.

224. Meyers WM, Neafie RC: Paragonimiasis. In: Binford CH, Connor DH. Pathology of Tropical and Extraordinary Diseases. Armed Forces Institute of Pathology; 1976;2:517–524.

225. Goldsmith R, Bunnag D, Bunnag T. Paragonimiasis. In Strickland GT. Hunter's Tropical Medicine. 7th ed. Philadelphia: WB Saunders; 1991;827–831.

226. Beaver PC, Jung RC, Cupp EW. Amphistome and distomate flukes. In: Beaver PC, Jung RC. Clinical Parasitology. 9th ed. Philadelphia: Lea & Febiger; 1984:464–471.

227. Slemenda SB, Maddison SE, Jong EC, et al. Diagnosis of paragonimiasis by immunoblot. Am J Trop Med Hyg. 1988;39:469–471.

228. Acha PN, Szyfres B. Dicrocoeliasis. In: Zoonoses and Communicable Diseases Common to Man and Animals. Pan American Health Organization; 1987; 503:654–657.

229. Beaver PC, Jung RC, Cupp EW. Amphistome and Distomate Flukes. In: Clinical Parasitology. 9th ed. Philadelphia; Lea & Febiger; 1984:461–463.

230. Mohamed ARE, Mummery V. Human dicrocoeliasis: Report on 208 cases from Saudi Arabia. Trop Geogr Med. 1990;42:1–7.

231. Drabick JJ, Egan JE, Brown SL, et al. Dicrocoeliasis (lancet fluke disease) in an HIV-seropositive man. JAMA. 1988;259:567–568.

232. Bunnag D, Bunnag T, Goldsmith R. Dicrocoeliasis and eurytremiasis. In: Strickland GT. Hunter's Tropical Medicine. 7th ed. Philadelphia: WB Saunders; 1991;826–827.

233. Ishii Y, Koga M, Fujino T, et al. Human infection with the pancreas fluke, *Eurytrema pancreaticum*. Am J Trop Med Hyg. 1983;32:1019–1022.

234. Gardiner CH, Dyke JW, Shirley SF. Hepatic granuloma due to a nymph of *Linguatula serrata* in a woman from Michigan: A case report and review of the literature. Am J Trop Med Hyg. 1984;33:187–189.

235. Drabick JJ. Pentastomiasis. Rev Infect Dis. 1987;9:1087–1094.

236. Meyers WM, Neafie RC, Connor DH. Pentastomiasis. In: Binford CH, Connor DH. Pathology of Tropical and Extraordinary Diseases. Armed Forces Institute of Pathology; 1976;2:546–550.

237. Haugerud RE. Evolution in the pentastomids. Parasitol Today. 1989;5:126–131.

238. Acha PN, Szyfres B. Pentastomiases. In: Zoonoses and Communicable Diseases Common to Man and Animals. Pan American Health Organization; 1987; 503:877–882.

239. Khalil GM. *Linguatula serrata* (Pentastomida) parasitizing humans and animals in Egypt, neighbouring countries, and elsewhere: A review. J Egypt Public Health Assoc. 1972;47:363–369.

240. Wanke C, Butler T, Islam M. Epidemiologic and clinical features of invasive amebiasis in Bangladesh: A case-control comparison with other diarrheal diseases and postmortem findings. Am J Trop Med Hyg. 1988;38:335–341.

241. Martinez-Palomo A, Ruiz-Palacios G. Amebiasis. In: Warren KS, Mahmoud AAF. Tropical and Geographical Medicine. 2nd ed. New York: McGraw-Hill; 1990:327–344.

242. Reed SL. Amebiasis: An update. Clin Infect Dis. 1992;14:385–393.

243. Ravdin JI. *Entamoeba histolytica*: From adherence to enteropathy. J Infect Dis. 1989;159:420–429.

244. Joyce MP, Ravdin JI. Pathology of human amebiasis. In: Ravdin JI. Amebiasis: Human Infection by *Entamoeba histolytica*. New York: John Wiley; 1988:129–146.

245. Nigam P, Gupta AK, Kapoor KK, et al. Cholestasis in amoebic liver abscess. Gut. 1985;26:140–145.

246. Ahmed L, El Rooby A, Kassem MI, et al. Ultrasonography in the diagnosis and management of 52 patients with amebic liver abscess in Cairo. Rev Infect Dis. 1990;12:330–337.

247. Walsh JA. Prevalence of *Entamoeba histolytica* infection. In: Ravdin JI. Amebiasis: Human Infection by *Entamoeba histolytica*. New York: John Wiley; 1988:93–105.

248. Reed SL, Braude AI. Extraintestinal disease: Clinical syndromes, diagnostic profile, and therapy. In: Ravdin JI. Amebiasis: Human Infection by *Entamoeba histolytica*. New York: John Wiley; 1988:511–532.

249. Pearson RD, Hewlett EL. Amebiasis in Travelers. In: Ravdin JI. Amebiasis: Human Infection by *Entamoeba histolytica*. New York: John Wiley; 1988:556–562.

250. Petri WA, Ravdin JI. Amebiasis in institutionalized populations. In: Ravdin JI. Amebiasis: Human Infection by *Entamoeba histolytica*. New York: John Wiley; 1988:576–581.

251. Case Records of the Massachusetts General Hospital: Case 7-1990. N Eng J Med. 1990;322:454–460.

252. Spencer HC, Muchnick C, Sexton DJ, et al. Endemic amebiasis in an extended family. Am J Trop Med Hyg. 1977;26:628–635.

253. Guerrant RL. Amebiasis: Introduction, current status, and research questions. Rev Infect Dis. 1986;8:218–227.

254. Weinke T, Friedrich-Janicke B, Hopp P, et al. Prevalence and clinical importance of *Entamoeba histolytica* in two high-risk groups: Travelers returning from the tropics and male homosexuals. J Infect Dis. 1990;161:1029–1031.

255. Druckman DA, Quinn TC. *Entamoeba histolytica* infections in homosexual men. In: Ravdin JI. Amebiasis: Human Infection by *Entamoeba histolytica*. New York: John Wiley; 1988:563–575.

256. Adams EB, MacLeod IN. Invasive amebiasis: II; Amebic liver abscess and its complications. Medicine. 1977; 56:324–334.

257. Wolfe MS. Amebiasis. In: Strickland GT. Hunter's Tropical Medicine. 7th ed. Philadelphia: WB Saunders; 1991:550–565.

258. Khan JA, Jafri SMW, Khan MA. Obstructive jaundice: An unusual presentation of amoebic liver abscess. J Trop Med Hyg. 1990;93:194–196.
259. Walsh JA. Problems in recognition and diagnosis of amebiasis: Estimation of the global magnitude of morbidity and mortality. Rev Infect Dis. 1986;8:228–238.
260. Case Records of the Massachusetts General Hospital: Case 19-1990. N Eng J Med. 1990;322:1378–1385.
261. LeBolt SA, Jurado R, Healy GR, et al. Hepatocellular carcinoma simulating amebic liver abscess: Report of a case and analysis of current diagnostic methods. Am J Gastroenterol. 1985;80:639–642.
262. Maharaj B, Patel A, Bhoora IG, et al. Ultrasonography and scintigraphy in liver disease in developing countries. Lancet. 1989;2:853–856.
263. Ahmed L, Salama ZA, El Rooby A, et al. Ultrasonographic resolution time for amebic liver abscess. Am J Trop Med Hyg. 1989;41:406–410.
264. Ralls PW, Colletti PM, Halls JM. Imaging in hepatic amebic abscess. In: Ravdin JI. Amebiasis: Human Infection by *Entamoeba histolytica*. New York: John Wiley; 1988:664–704.
265. Robert R, Mahaza C, Bernard C, et al. Evaluation of a new bicolored latex agglutination test for immunological diagnosis of hepatic amoebiasis. J Clin Microbiol. 1990;28:1422–1424.
266. Healy GR. Serology. In: Ravdin JI. Amebiasis: Human Infection by *Entamoeba histolytica*. New York: John Wiley; 1988:650–663.
267. Proctor EM. Laboratory diagnosis of amebiasis. Clin Lab Med. 1991;11:829–859.
268. Gandhi BM, Irshad M, Acharya SK, et al. Amebic liver abscess and circulating immune complexes of *Entamoeba histolytica* proteins. Am J Trop Med Hyg. 1988;39:440–444.
269. Irusen EM, Jackson TFHG, Simjee AE. Asymptomatic intestinal colonization by pathogenic *Entamoeba histolytica* in amebic liver abscess: Prevalence, response to therapy, and pathogenic potential. Clin Infect Dis. 1992;14:889–893.
270. Ravdin JI. *Entamoeba histolytica* (amebiasis). In: Mandell GL, Douglas RG, Bennett JE. Principles and Practice of Infectious Diseases. 3rd ed. New York: Churchill Livingstone; 1990:2036–2049.
271. Wilmot AJ, Powell SJ, Adams EB. Chloroquine compared with chloroquine and emetine combined in amebic liver abscess. Am J Trop Med Hyg. 1959;8:623–624.
272. Powell SJ, Stewart-Wynne EJ, Elsdon-Dew R. Metronidazole combined with diloxanide furoate in amoebic liver abscess. Ann Trop Med Parasitol. 1973;67:367–368.
273. McAuley JB, Juranek DD. Luminal agents in the treatment of amebiasis. Clin Infect Dis. 1992;14:1161–1162. Letter.
274. McAuley JB, Herwaldt BL, Stokes SL, et al. Diloxanide furoate for treating asymptomatic *Entamoeba histolytica* cyst passers: Fourteen years' experience in the United States. Clin Infect Dis. 1992;15:464–468.
275. Sheen IS, Chang Chien CS, Lin DY, et al. Resolution of liver abscesses: Comparison of pyogenic and amebic liver abscesses. Am J Trop Med Hyg. 1989;40:384–389.
276. Current WL, Garcia LS. Cryptosporidiosis. Clin Microbiol Rev. 1991;4:325–358.
277. Pitlik S, Fainstein V, Rios A, et al. Cryptosporidial cholecystitis. N Engl J Med. 1983;308:967.
278. Gross TL, Wheat J, Bartlett M, et al. AIDS and multiple system involvement with *Cryptosporidium*. Am J Gastroenterol. 1986;81:456–458.
279. Blumberg RS, Kelsey P, Perrone T, et al. Cytomegalovirus and *Cryptosporidium*-associated acalculous gangrenous cholecystitis. Am J Med. 1984;76:1118–1123.
280. Hinnant K, Swartz A, Rotterdam H, et al. Cytomegaloviral and cryptosporidial cholecystitis in two patients with AIDS. Am J Surg Pathol. 1989;13:57–60.
281. Kahn DG, Garfinkle JM, Klonoff DC, et al. Cryptosporidial and cytomegaloviral hepatitis and cholecystitis. Arch Pathol Lab Med. 1987;111:879–881.
282. Texidor HS, Godwin TA, Ramirez EA. Cryptosporidiosis of the biliary tract in AIDS. Radiology. 1991;180:51–56.
283. Godwin TA. Cryptosporidiosis in the acquired immunodeficiency syndrome: A study of 15 autopsy cases. Hum pathol. 1991;22:1215–1224.
284. Bryan RT, Visvesvara GS. Coccidia and microsporidia Ann Intern Med. 1991;114:343. Letter.
285. Margileth AM, Strano AJ, Chandra R, et al. Disseminated nosematosis in an immunologically compromised infant. Arch Pathol. 1973;95:145–150.
286. Terada S, Reddy R, Jeffers LJ, et al. Microsporidian hepatitis in the acquired immunodeficiency syndrome. Ann Intern Med. 1987;107:61–62.
287. Bryan RT, Cali A, Owen RL, et al. Microsporidia: Opportunistic pathogens in patients with AIDS. In: Sun T. Progress in Clinical Parasitology. Philadelphia: Field & Wood; 1991;2:1–26.
288. Bryan RT. Microsporidiosis. In: Mandell GL, Bennett JE, Dolan R, eds. Principles and Practice of Infectious Diseases. 3rd ed. New York: Churchill Livingstone; 1990:2130–2134.
289. Orenstein J, Chiang J, Steinberg W, et al. Intestinal microsporidiosis as a cause of diarrhea in AIDS. Hum Pathol. 1990;21:475–481.
290. McWhinney PHM, Nathani D, Green ST, et al. Microsporidiosis detected in association with AIDS-related sclerosing cholangitis. AIDS. 1991;5:1394.
290a. Beaugerie L, Teilhac M-F, Deluol A-M, et al. Cholangiopathy associated with microsporidia infection of the common bile duct mucosa in a patient with HIV infection. Ann Intern Med. 1992;117:401–402.
290b. Pol S, Romana C, Richard S, et al. *Enterocytozoon bieneusi* infection in acquired immunodeficiency syndrome–related sclerosing cholangitis. Gastroenterology. 1992;102:1778–1781.
290c. Pol S, Romana C, Richard S, et al. Microsporidia infection in patients with the human immunodeficiency virus and unexplained cholangitis. N Engl J Med. 1993;328:95–99.
291. Weber R, Bryan RT, Owen RL, et al. Improved light-microscopical detection of microsporidia spores in stool and duodenal aspirates. N Engl J Med. 1992;326:161–162.
292. Beaver PC, Jung RC, Cupp EW. Flagellate protozoa of the digestive and urogenital tracts. In: Beaver PC, Jung RC. Clinical Parasitology. 9th ed. Philadelphia: Lea & Febiger; 1984:44–46.
293. Wright SG. Giardiasis. In: Strickland GT. Hunter's Tropical Medicine. 7th ed. Philadelphia: WB Saunders; 1991:565–570.
294. Drew JH. Biliary giardiasis and pancreatitis. Med J Aust. 1981;1:196–197. Letter.
295. Bhattacharya AK, Mukhopadyay P. Biliary giardiasis. J Assoc Physicians India. 1982;30:223.
296. Soto JM. *Giardia lamblia*: A case presentation of chronic cholecystitis and duodenitis. Am J Gastroenterol. 1977;67:265–269.
297. Edman JC, Kovacs JA, Masur H, et al. Ribosomal RNA sequence shows *Pneumocystis carinii* to be a member of the fungi. Nature. 1988;334:519–522.
298. Telzak EE, Cote RJ, Gold JWM, et al. Extrapulmonary *Pneumocystis carinii* infections. Rev Infect Dis. 1990; 12:380–386.
299. Raviglione MC. Extrapulmonary pneumocystosis: The first 50 cases. Rev Infect Dis. 1990;12:1127–1138.

300. Poblete RB, Rodriguez K, Foust RT, et al. *Pneumocystis carinii* hepatitis in the acquired immunodeficiency syndrome (AIDS). Ann Intern Med 1989;110:737–738.

301. Radin DR, Baker EL, Klatt EC, et al. Visceral and nodal calcifications in patients with AIDS-related *Pneumocystis carinii* infection. AJR Am J Roentgenol. 1990;154:27–31.

302. Macher AM, Bardenstein DS, Zimmerman LE, et al. *Pneumocystis carinii* choroiditis in a male homosexual with AIDS and disseminated pulmonary and extrapulmonary *P carinii* infection. N Engl J Med. 1987;316:1092. Letter.

303. Sparling TG, Dong SR, Hegedus C, et al. Aerosolized pentamidine and disseminated infection with *Pneumocystis carinii*. Ann Intern Med. 1989;111:442. Letter.

304. Richie TL, Yamaguchi E, Virani NA, et al. Extrapulmonary *Pneumocystis* infection. Ann Intern Med. 1989;111:339–340. Letter.

305. Mathews WC, Bozzette SA, Harrity S, et al. *Pneumocystis carinii* peritonitis: Antemortem confirmation of disseminated pneumocystosis by cytologic examination of body fluids. Arch Intern Med.1992;152:867–869.

306. Walls KW, Kagan IG, Turner A. Studies on the prevalence of antibodies to *Toxoplasma gondii*: I, US military recruits. Am J Epidemiol. 1967;85:87–92.

307. Sever JL, Ellenberg JH, Ley AC, et al. Toxoplasmosis. Maternal and pediatric findings in 23,000 pregnancies. Pediatrics 1988;82:181–192.

308. Remington JS, Desmonts G. Toxoplasmosis. In: Remington JS, Klein JO. Infectious Diseases of the Fetus and Newborn Infant. Philadelphia: WB Saunders; 1990:89–195.

309. Wilson CB, Remington JS, Stagno S, et al. Development of adverse sequelae in children born with subclinical congenital *Toxoplasma* infections. Pediatrics. 1980;66:767–774.

310. Luft BJ, Remington JS. Toxoplasmic encephalitis in AIDS. Clin Infect Dis. 1992;15:211–222.

311. Dubey JP, Beattie CP. Toxoplasmosis of animals and man. Boca Raton FL: CRC Press; 1988.

312. Frenkel JK. Pathophysiology of toxoplasmosis. Parasitol Today. 1988;4:273–278.

313. Teutsch SM, Juranek DD, Sulzer A, et al. Epidemic toxoplasmosis associated with infected cats. N Engl J Med. 1979;300:695–699.

314. Beneson MW, Takafuji ET, Lemon SM, et al. Oocyst-transmitted toxoplasmosis associated with ingestion of contaminated water. N Engl J Med. 1982;307:666–669.

315. Ruskin J, Remington JS. Toxoplasmosis in the compromised host. Ann Intern Med. 1976;84:193–199.

315a. Kean BH, Sun T, Ellsworth RM. Color Atlas: Text of Ophthalmic Parasitology. New York: Igaku-Shoin; 1991:9–21.

316. Carter AO, Frank JW. Congenital toxoplasmosis: Epidemiologic features and control. Can Med Assoc J. 1986;135:618–623.

317. Wilson M, McAuley JB. Laboratory diagnosis of toxoplasmosis. Clinics in Lab Med. 1991;11:923–939.

318. Stepick-Biek P, Thulliez P, Araujo FG, et al. IgA antibodies for diagnosis of acute congenital and acquired toxoplasmosis. J Infect Dis. 1990;162:270–273.

319. American Academy of Pediatrics. *Toxoplasma gondii* (toxoplasmosis). In: Peter G, Lepow ML, McCracken GH, Phillips CF. Report of the committee on infectious diseases, Elk Grove Village. Am Acad Pediatr. 1991:478–480.

320. Daffos F, Forestier F, Capella-Pavlovsky M, et al. Prenatal management of 746 pregnancies at risk for congenital toxoplasmosis. N Engl J Med. 1988;318:271–275.

321. Remington JS, McLeod R. Toxoplasmosis. In: Gorbach SL, Bartlett JG, Blacklow NR. Infectious Diseases. Philadelphia: WB Saunders; 1992:1328–1343.

322. World Health Organization. Control of the leishmaniases. World Health Organ Tech Rep Ser. 1990:F93.

323. Steele NP Jr, Foshee WS, Koch F, et al. Visceral leishmaniasis acquired in Greece: Diagnosis and treatment in an American child. South Med J. 1977;70:1481–1483.

324. Geraci JE, Wilson WR, Thompson JH. Visceral leishmaniasis (kala-azar) as a cause of fever of unknown origin. Mayo Clin Proc. 1980;55:455–458.

325. Maquire JH, Gantz NM, Moscella S, et al. Leishmanial infections: A consideration in travelers returning from abroad. Am J Med Sci. 1983;285:32–40.

326. Khot AS, Thompson MH. Visceral leishmaniasis contracted in the Mediterranean area. Arch Dis Child. 1983;58:930–931.

327. Pearson RD, Sousa AQ. Leishmaniasis in travelers. Travel Med. 1985;3:2–8.

328. Case Records of the Massachusetts General Hospital: Case 7-1991. N Engl J Med. 1991;324:476–485.

329. Clauvel JP, Couderc LJ, Belmin J, et al. Visceral leishmaniasis complicating acquired immunodeficiency syndrome (AIDS). Trans R Soc Trop Med Hyg. 1986;80:1010–1011. Letter.

330. Yebra M, Segovia J, Manzano L, et al. Disseminated-to-skin kala-azar and the acquired immunodeficiency syndrome. Ann Intern Med. 1988;108:490–491.

331. Montalban C, Martinez-Fernandez R, Calleja JL, et al. Visceral leishmaniasis (kala-azar) as an opportunistic infection in patients infected with the human immunodeficiency virus in Spain. Rev Infect Dis. 1989;11:655–660.

332. Pearson RD, Sousa ADQ. Leishmania species: Visceral (kala-azar), cutaneous, and mucosal leishmaniasis. In: Mandell GL, Douglas RG, Bennett, JE. Principles and Practice of Infectious Diseases. 3rd ed. New York: Churchill Livingstone; 1990:2066–2077.

333. Low GC, Cooke WE. A congenital case of kala-azar. Lancet. 1926;2:1209–1211.

334. Symmers WStC. Leishmaniasis acquired by contagion: A case of marital infection in Britain. Lancet. 1960;1:127–132.

335. Lewis DJ, Ward RD. Transmission and vectors. In: Peters W, Killick-Kendrick R. The Leishmaniases in Biology and Medicine. London: Academic Press; 1987:235–262.

336. Chulay JD. Leishmaniasis: General principles. In: Strickland GT. Hunter's Tropical Medicine. 7th ed. Philadelphia: WB Saunders; 1991:638–642.

337. Lainson R, Shaw JJ. Evolution, classification and geographical distribution. In: Peters W, Killick-Kendrick R. The Leishmaniases in Biology and Medicine. London: Academic Press; 1987:2–120.

338. Grimaldi G, Tesh RB, McMahon-Pratt D. A review of the geographic distribution and epidemiology of leishmaniasis in the new world. Am J Trop Med Hyg. 1989;41:687–725.

339. Marsden PD, Johnson WD. Leishmania. In: Gorbach SL, Bartlett JG, Blacklow NR. Infectious Diseases. Philadelphia: WB Saunders; 1992:1978–1984.

340. Chulay JD. Cutaneous leishmaniasis of the Old World. In: Strickland GT. Hunter's Tropical Medicine. 7th ed. Philadelphia: WB Saunders; 1991:648–652.

341. Chulay JD. Cutaneous leishmaniasis of the New World. In: Strickland GT. Hunter's Tropical Medicine. 7th ed. Philadelphia: WB Saunders; 1991:652–655.

342. Oster CN, Chulay JD. Visceral leishmaniasis (kala-azar). In: Strickland GT. Hunter's Tropical Medicine. 7th ed. Philadelphia: WB Saunders; 1991:642–648.

343. Hendricks LD, Wright N. Diagnosis of cutaneous leish-

maniasis by in vitro cultivation of saline aspirates in Schneider's *Drosophila* medium. Am J Trop Med Hyg. 1979;28:962–964.

344. Navin TR, Arana FE, de Merida AM, et al. Cutaneous leishmaniasis in Guatemala: Comparison of diagnostic methods. Am J Trop Med Hyg. 1990;42:36–42.

345. Chulay JD, Bryceson ADM. Quantitation of amastigotes of *Leishmania donovani* in smears of splenic aspirates from patients with visceral leishmaniasis. Am J Trop Med Hyg. 1983;32:475–479.

346. Berman JD. Chemotherapy of leishmaniasis: Biochemical mechanisms, clinical efficacy and future strategies. Rev Infect Dis. 1988;10:560–586.

347. Herwaldt BL, Berman JD. Recommendations for treating leishmaniasis with sodium stibogluconate (Pentostam) and review of pertinent clinical studies. Am J Trop Med Hyg. 1992;46:296–306.

348. Saenz RE, Paz H, Berman JD. Efficacy of ketoconazole against *Leishmania braziliensis panamensis* cutaneous leishmaniasis. Am J Med. 1990;89:147–155.

349. Berman JD. Leishmaniasis. In: Rakel RE. Conn's Current Therapy. Philadelphia: WB Saunders; 1992:73–76.

350. Bruce-Chwatt LJ. Essential Malariology: Epidemiology of Malaria. New York: John Wiley; 1985:166–209.

351. Spencer HS. Epidemiology of malaria. In: Strickland GT. Clinics in Tropical Medicine and Communicable Diseases. Malaria. Philadelphia: WB Saunders. 1986; 1:1–28.

352. Singal M, Shaw PK, Lindsay RC, et al. An outbreak of introduced malaria in California possibly involving secondary transmission. Am J Trop Med Hyg. 1977;26: 1–9.

353. Maldonado YA, Nahlen BL, Roberts RR, et al. Transmission of *Plasmodium vivax* in San Diego County, California, 1986. Am J Trop Med Hyg. 1990;42:3–9.

354. Guerrero IC, Weniger BC, Schultz MG. Transfusion malaria in the United States, 1972–1981. Ann Intern Med. 1983;99:221–226.

355. Strickland GT. Malaria. In: Strickland GT. Hunter's Tropical Medicine. 7th ed. Philadelphia: WB Saunders; 1991:586–617.

356. Quinn TC, Strickland GT. Clinical manifestations of malaria. Clin Trop Med Comm Dis. 1986;1:127.

357. White NJ, Warrell DA, Chanthavanich P, et al. Severe hypoglycemia and hyperinsulinemia in falciparum malaria. N Engl J Med. 1983;309:61–66.

358. World Health Organization. WHO expert committee on malaria: 18th Report. World Health Organ Tech Rep Ser. World Health Organization; 1986;735.

359. Bloland PB, Campbell CC. Malaria. In: Rakel RE. Conn's Current Therapy. Philadelphia: WB Saunders; 1992:81–88.

360. White NJ. Drug treatment and prevention of malaria. Eur J Clin Pharmacol. 1988;34:1–14.

361. Phillips RE, Warrell DA, White NJ, et al. Intravenous quinidine for the treatment of severe falciparum malaria: Clinical and pharmacokinetic studies. N Engl J Med. 1985;312:1273–1278.

362. Warrell DA, Looareesuwan S, Warrell MJ, et al. Dexamethasone proves deleterious in cerebral malaria: A double blind trial in 100 comatose patients. N Engl J Med. 1982;306:313–319.

363. American Medical Association. Antiprotozoal drugs. In: Drug Evaluations Annual. 7th ed. 1991;1493–1531.

364. Advice for Travelers. Med Lett Drugs Ther. 1990; 32:33–36.

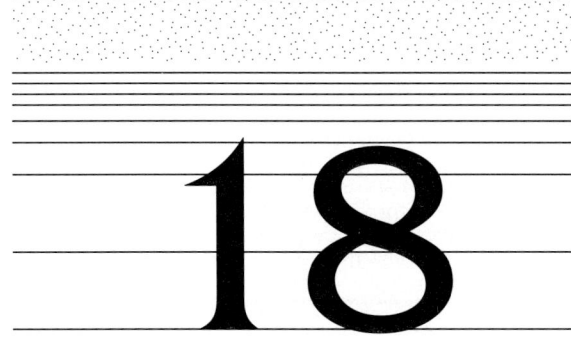

18

Spontaneous Bacterial Peritonitis

JOHN G. McHUTCHISON, M.D.
BRUCE A. RUNYON, M.D.

HISTORICAL ASPECTS

Since the recognition of infected ascites by Conn and Fessell, a large amount of information has been gathered on the entity we now refer to as spontaneous bacterial peritonitis (SBP).[1] In most instances, SBP occurs in patients with cirrhosis and ascites. Less frequently this infection can occur in individuals with acute liver diseases such as fulminant viral hepatitis or acute alcoholic hepatitis, and in rare cases, an individual with ascites that is not due to liver disease, such as the nephrotic syndrome or cardiac ascites, can also develop SBP.[2-4]

Spontaneous bacterial peritonitis or one of its variant forms is more common than previously thought and occurs in 10 to 25% of patients with ascites on hospital admission.[5-7] SBP is also frequently subclinical and accounts for up to 75% of serious infections in patients with liver disease and ascites.[8, 9] This infection carries a poor prognosis, despite adequate therapy, owing to the presence of underlying severe and often advanced liver disease.[10] Indeed, in many liver transplant centers throughout the United States, the occurrence of SBP has become an indication for considering earlier orthotopic transplantation in a patient who would for other reasons be maintained on an elective waiting

list.[10, 11] Other major advances in our knowledge of SBP include improved methods of detection and treatment, recognition of predisposing factors, and insight into the pathophysiology of infected ascites.[11] In this chapter, we have attempted to outline these advances in the hope that the practicing physician can manage this common, serious infection in a reasonable and more effective way.

DEFINITION AND CLASSIFICATION OF INFECTED ASCITES

As outlined in Table 18–1, we classify infected ascites into 5 categories.

Spontaneous Bacterial Peritonitis

Spontaneous bacterial peritonitis is defined as ascitic fluid infection when the ascitic fluid culture grows bacteria (usually a single organism) associated with an ascitic fluid polymorphonuclear neutrophil (PMN) leukocyte count of ≥250 cells per mm³, in the absence of any intra-abdominal surgical source of infection. This is the most commonly recognized type of ascitic fluid infection in the patient with liver disease

TABLE 18–1. CLASSIFICATION OF INFECTED ASCITES

TYPE OF INFECTION	PMN COUNT (per mm³)	CULTURE
Spontaneous bacterial peritonitis	≥ 250	positive (usually 1 organism)
Monomicrobial nonneutrocytic bacterascites	< 250	positive (1 organism)
Culture-negative neutrocytic ascites	≥ 250	no growth
Secondary bacterial peritonitis	≥ 250	positive (multiple organisms)
Polymicrobial bacterascites	≤ 250	positive (multiple organisms)

NOTE: Normal ascites PMN count is <250 cells/mm³.

and ascites. In a recent prospective treatment trial of 100 patients with infected ascites, two thirds were diagnosed as having this form of infection on the basis of the above criteria. The remaining one third were culture-negative.[12] SBP, as just defined, is found in 12 to 15% of hospitalized cirrhotics with ascites when the ascites is sampled by paracentesis routinely on admission.[6, 7]

Monomicrobial Nonneutrocytic Bacterascites

Monomicrobial nonneutrocytic bacterascites (MNB) is defined as ascitic fluid that grows a single organism when cultured but is associated with a normal ascitic fluid PMN count of <250 cells per mm³. The prevalence of this variant is 8% on routine admission paracentesis.[6] The significance of this form of ascitic fluid infection is discussed in a later section.

Culture-Negative Neutrocytic Ascites

Culture-negative neutrocytic ascites (CNNA) is diagnosed when the ascitic fluid PMN count is ≥250 cells per mm³ without any evident intra-abdominal surgical source of infection, yet the ascitic fluid culture does not grow pathogenic bacteria. Other causes of an elevated ascites PMN count must be excluded in order to diagnose this condition accurately, for example, the patient must not have received antibiotics and should not have pancreatitis, peritoneal carcinomatosis, tuberculous peritonitis, or hemorrhage into the ascites, all of which are known to elevate the ascites PMN count without associated infection.[13] As discussed later, many of these instances may be due to an inadequate culture technique. Depending on culture technique, the prevalence of sterile cultures among neutrocytic samples varies from 7 to 58%.[14–16]

Secondary Bacterial Peritonitis

Since secondary bacterial peritonitis is associated with a very high mortality (the authors have not seen a single patient survive without surgical intervention), it is of utmost importance to differentiate secondary bacterial peritonitis from other types of ascites infection. Secondary bacterial peritonitis is defined as an ascitic fluid PMN count of ≥250 cells per mm³ in which the culture grows bacteria (usually multiple gut organisms) and for which an intra-abdominal source of infection is evident, as for example, perforated viscus or retroperitoneal or subhepatic abscess. The signs and symptoms of secondary bacterial peritonitis resemble those of spontaneous bacterial infection, and a useful algorithm has been designed to allow the differentiation between these conditions (see Fig. 18–7). The prevalence of secondary peritonitis in cirrhotics on admission to hospital is 2%.[6]

Polymicrobial Bacterascites

Polymicrobial bacterascites results from an unintentional needlestick perforation of the gut during attempted paracentesis. The condition should be suspected when stool contents are aspirated into the syringe, when multiple organisms are seen on Gram stain (without PMNs), or when the culture reveals multiple organisms. Fortunately, this occurs only rarely and was observed in only 1 of 1000 paracenteses (0.1%) performed prospectively by one of the authors (BAR) and in 10 of 1578 paracenteses (0.6%) analyzed retrospectively.[17] Most instances (90%) of polymicrobial ascites settle spontaneously without further evidence of development of bacterial peritonitis.[17] A repeat paracentesis should be performed 6 to 12 hours after a suspected needlestick perforation of the gut to ensure that a neutrocytic response has not occurred.

PATHOGENESIS AND NATURAL HISTORY

Pathogenesis

Acute bacterial infections, including bacteremia, are common in patients with cirrhosis.[18–20] Many proposed defects in the immunologic defense mechanisms of these individuals have been documented (Table 18–2).[18, 21–24] The actual role of each of these defects in the pathogenesis of SBP has remained difficult to establish. It seems reasonable, however, that in patients with advanced liver disease (irrespective of the cause) factors including complement deficiency, defects in neutrophil and monocyte function, and impaired hepatic reticuloendothelial cell function all provide the milieu for more frequent bacteremia and perhaps for prolonged bacteremia. In keeping with this concept, cirrhotic rats with ascites have been shown to develop bacteremia after being exposed to pneumococci and have a higher mortality compared both with control rats and also with rats with cirrhosis but without ascites.[25]

How do the organisms gain entry into the ascitic fluid cavity? Hematogenous spread during episodes of spontaneous bacteremia could be responsible, and bacteremia is detected in approximately 40 to 50% of patients with bacterial peritonitis.[12] In further support of blood as a source of bacteria, some individuals with a urinary or respiratory tract infection develop SBP with the same organism cultured from a separate body fluid. Although these findings suggest that hematogenous spread of the bacteria may be the source of organisms, an alternative locus of infection and bacteremia is not found in the majority of patients with SBP. Since more than 70% of episodes of SBP are caused by gut organisms, the gut would seem to be the most likely source of infection in the majority of infected patients. An alternative mechanism to explain the source of bacteria in SBP is the translocation of gut bacteria into the ascitic fluid cavity, with the subsequent development of SBP. Gut wall mucosal edema has been demonstrated in cirrhotics with portal hypertension, and the transmural migration of radioactively labeled *Escherichia coli* from the gut lumen to the peritoneal cavity would also support such a theory.[26] Runyon and colleague have produced further evidence suggesting that translocation occurs in a rodent model of cirrhotic ascites.[27] In this study, gut flora could be successfully cultured from the mesenteric lymph nodes of 88% of cirrhotic rats with ascites but not from the control group of animals. Passage of bacteria from the gut lumen to the mesenteric lymph nodes occurs almost uniformly in a model of cirrhosis and ascites that does develop SBP. Whether this occurs in humans with cirrhosis and ascites is as yet unknown, but the permeability of the gut mucosa in cirrhotics has recently been documented to be abnormal.[28] Such a concept would certainly explain the high prevalence of gut flora observed in SBP. Whether pathogenic organisms then migrate to the ascitic fluid either directly by lymphatic rupture or indirectly via a circuitous blood-borne route is still unknown. An acceptable model of the pathogenesis of spontaneous bacterial peritonitis must take into account all the clinical data outlined here.

A proposed outline of the pathogenesis of SBP is shown in Figure 18–1. Owing to altered host defense mechanisms, organisms from the gut, or less commonly from other sources of bacteremia, would not be eradicated normally and would then be available to seed the mesenteric lymph nodes by means of translocation. The ascites could then be colonized directly via the bloodstream or potentially via the mesenteric lymph nodes. Once seeded within the ascites, a neutrophil response would occur if the host's peritoneal macrophages were not capable of destroying the organism, resulting in SBP. Further bacteremia from the infected ascitic pool could then lead to detectable bacteremia in blood, or seeding at other potential sites, including the urinary tract, or pleural effusions. Such a model explains most of the clinical data compiled to date in SBP.

Ascitic Fluid Characteristics That Predispose to Infection

Most reported episodes of SBP have been associated with portal hypertension–related ascites or the nephrotic syndrome in children.[29] One of the unifying factors of the ascites of these patients is a low protein content of ascitic fluid. By contrast, most causes of ascites that are

---

TABLE 18–2. DEFECTS IN HOST DEFENSES IN PATIENTS WITH CIRRHOSIS

↓ Hepatic reticuloendothelial phagocytic function
↓ Neutrophil phagocytosis
↓ Neutrophil degranulation
↓ Intracellular killing of bacteria by neutrophils
↓ Oxidative burst of neutrophils in response to bacteria
↓ Complement levels in serum and ascites
↓ Monocyte function

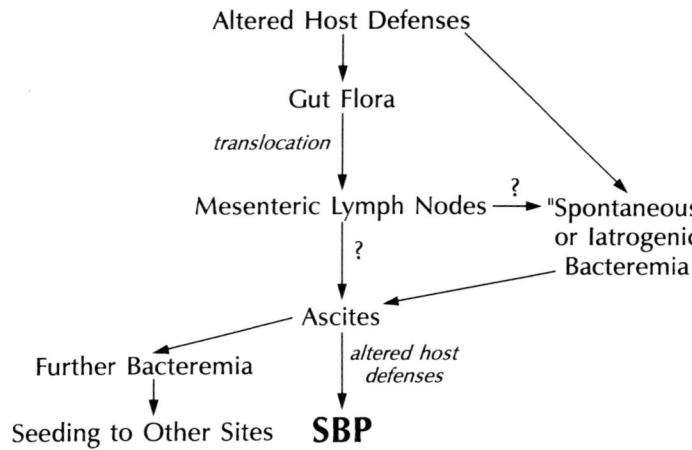

FIGURE 18–1.
Proposed pathogenesis of spontaneous bacterial peritonitis (SBP). Due to altered host defense mechanisms, gut organisms may seed mesenteric lymph nodes by translocation. Ascitic fluid is then colonized either directly or indirectly. Whether a neutrophil response then develops into SBP depends on host bacterial defense mechanisms within the ascitic fluid.

not associated with episodes of SBP are associated with a high protein content, as in ascites due to heart failure or peritoneal carcinomatosis. In keeping with these clinical observations, a retrospective analysis of data gathered in three earlier series of patients with cirrhotic ascites and SBP indicated that the ascitic fluid total protein concentration was lower when compared with fluid obtained from individuals who had cirrhotic ascites but not SBP (0.8, 1.3, and 1.6 g/dl vs. 1.8, 1.8, and 2.0 g/dl, respectively).[30–32] In a more recent prospective study, in which on admission routine abdominal paracentesis was performed on 90 cirrhotic patients with ascites, an ascitic fluid total protein concentration of ≤1 g per dl was associated with a 10-fold increased risk of developing SBP during the period of hospitalization compared with the cirrhotics whose total protein concentration was ≥1 g per dl.[5] The findings of this study suggest that the recurrence rate of SBP should be higher in individuals with lower ascitic fluid total protein concentrations. Another study aimed at investigating the recurrence of SBP and pos-

sible predictors of repeated infection verified that a low ascitic fluid total protein content is a statistically significant and independent predictor of SBP recurrence.[10]

Why does low-protein ascites predispose the patient to SBP? Presumably, the ascites is initially colonized by bacteria as outlined earlier, and whether infection supervenes to lead to SBP depends on the antimicrobial activity of the ascitic fluid. Most bacteria that are responsible for bacteremia and serious infections are resistant to activation by complement and must be engulfed and undergo phagocytosis before the microorganisms are killed.[33] For this process to occur in ascites, the bacterial cell wall must first be coated, or opsonized, with immunoglobulin G (IgG) or the third component of complement (C3) or both. The opsonic activity of ascitic fluid has been shown to correlate directly with the ascitic fluid total protein content (Fig. 18–2),[34] and in a prospective study, patients with deficient opsonic activity were found to be predisposed to the development of SBP compared with cirrhotics with a more normal opsonic ac-

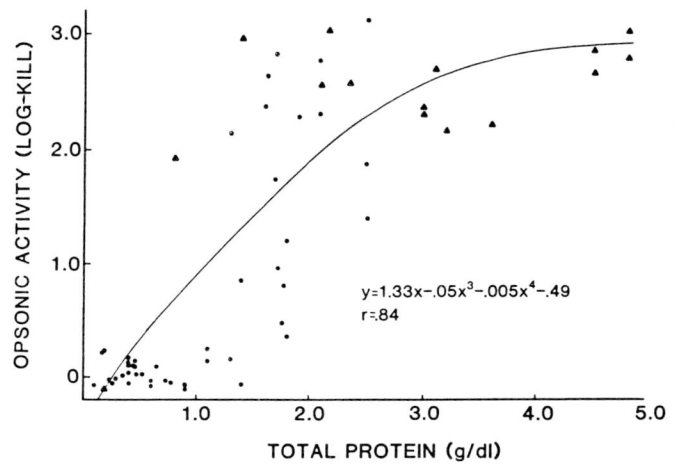

$$y = 1.33x - .05x^3 - .005x^4 - .49$$
$$r = .84$$

FIGURE 18–2.
Correlation between the opsonic activity of ascitic fluid and ascitic fluid total protein concentration. Opsonic activity is measured as the log kill of an *Escherichia coli* cultured from a patient with spontaneous bacterial peritonitis plotted against the protein concentration of the ascites. The dots represent patients with ascites due to cirrhosis and the triangles represent those with noncirrhotic ascites. SOURCE: Runyon BA, Morrissey RL, Hoefs JC, et al. Opsonic activity of human ascitic fluid: A potentially important protective mechanism against spontaneous bacterial peritonitis. Hepatology. 1985;4:634–637.

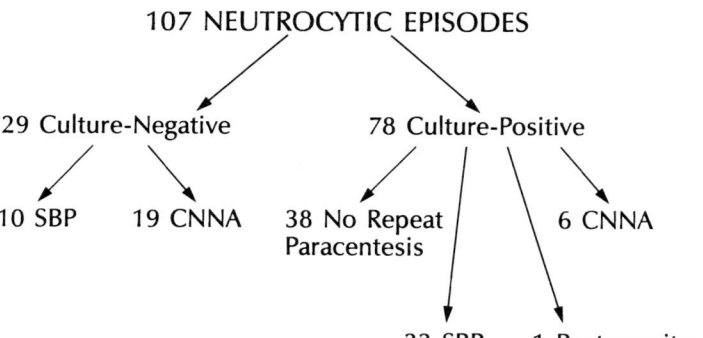

107 NEUTROCYTIC EPISODES

29 Culture-Negative   78 Culture-Positive

10 SBP   19 CNNA   38 No Repeat   6 CNNA
                       Paracentesis

33 SBP   1 Bacterascites

FIGURE 18–3.
Short-term natural history of untreated neutro-
cytic ascites in the setting of cirrhosis. KEY:
CNNA = culture-negative neutrocytic ascites,
SBP = spontaneous bacterial peritonitis.

tivity profile.[35] In keeping with the deficient bactericidal activity of patients with ascites at risk for the development of SBP, both opsonic activity and total protein levels in ascites seem to correlate with deficient levels of total hemolytic complement and C3 and C4.[34, 35] It thus seems that in patients with cirrhosis and ascites, the final event in determining whether ascites colonization results in SBP depends upon the endogenous antimicrobial activity of the ascites fluid. As the severity of the underlying liver disease advances, the protein and complement content of ascites, and therefore opsonic activity, fall. This process explains the clinical observation that SBP usually occurs in the setting of advanced liver disease.[29, 36] The sequence of events that follows colonization of ascites with bacteria probably involves the coating of bacteria with opsonins, followed by the attempted removal of the foreign particles by peritoneal macrophages, followed by the activation of complement with attraction of neutrophils into the peritoneal cavity if the peritoneal macrophages cannot eradicate the bacteria.

Short-term Natural History of Ascitic Fluid Infection

Two studies of the early 1990s attempted to characterize the natural history of MNB and have allowed us to gain insight into the dynamics of ascitic fluid infection in its early stages.[37, 38] In a 1990 prospective study of 138 episodes of ascitic fluid infection in 105 patients with liver disease, 44 episodes (32%) were due to MNB (i.e., a positive culture without a neutrocytic response).[37] A repeat paracentesis was performed in 21 of these 44 patients with MNB before the administration of antibiotics. Eight (38%) of these progressed to develop SBP, and 13 (62%) experienced spontaneous resolution. All 8 patients who later developed SBP had signs and symptoms suggestive of infection at the time of

the initial paracentesis. By comparison, 7 of the 13 patients (54%) with MNB whose ascites became sterile on repeat paracentesis were asymptomatic.

The results of this study indicate that about two thirds of patients with MNB resolve their infection without antibiotics and one third progress to SBP.[37] The only clinical feature that appears to separate these two groups is the presence or absence of clinical signs and symptoms of infection. These findings have been validated in a 1991 study of 22 patients with asymptomatic MNB.[38] Only 3 of the 22 patients (14%) had developed SBP when repeat paracentesis was performed. In both these studies, it was observed that patients with MNB have less severe liver disease, despite there being no difference detected between the two groups in ascitic fluid protein content. An important observation in one of these studies was the rapidity with which a neutrocytic response could develop in MNB. The ascitic fluid PMN count was noted to increase by a magnitude of 50- to 170-fold within 40 to 70 minutes, respectively, from the initial nonneutrocytic culture-positive specimen.[37] These data suggest that rapid entry of PMNs can occur after the initial colonization of ascites with bacteria. Also, the PMN count in infected ascites has been observed to decrease spontaneously in some patients before antibiotic therapy.[16] Whether this represents spontaneously resolving infection is unknown. To further determine the natural history of neutrocytic ascites, we have performed two paracenteses in rapid sequence before starting antibiotic therapy in patients with cirrhosis and neutrocytic ascites (Runyon BA, Antillon MR, McHutchison JG, unpublished data, 1991; Fig. 18–3). The average time interval between paracenteses was 8.4 hours. Overall, 29 of the 107 initial specimens (27%) were culture-negative and 78 specimens (73%) were culture-positive. In 19 of the initial culture-negative group (66%), the subsequent sample was also sterile, and in addition, the PMN count was lower than it had been in the initial sample in 18 of them. In the 10 remaining culture-negative patients (34%), the second specimen was culture-positive, indicating that the infection had converted from CNNA to SBP. The ascitic fluid opsonic activity was significantly higher in the specimens that remained culture-negative compared with those in which the culture became positive (0.87 ± 0.79 vs. 0.20 ± 0.50 log kill, P <0.02), suggesting that the inherent antimicrobial activity of specimens from patients with resolving infection was greater than it was in those from patients with persistent infection.

Of the 40 cases in which the findings of the initial culture were positive for SBP and a follow-up paracentesis was performed, 34 cases (85%) remained culture-positive with the same organism, but 6 patients (15%) spontaneously became culture-negative before administration of antibiotic therapy. Among those cases in which SBP persisted on repeat paracentesis, the PMN count was rising in two thirds and declining in one third. These findings suggest that most episodes of SBP progress and most CNNA episodes resolve spontaneously.

These data allow us to further understand the dynamics of ascitic fluid infection (Fig. 18–4). Episodes of spontaneous bacteremia result in occasional seeding of the ascites with bacteria, which is detected at this early stage as monomicrobial bacterascites. In certain individuals with the appropriate characteristics of host defenses, ascitic fluid protein content, opsonic activity, complement, and organism virulence, this colonization may either resolve spontaneously or progress until detected as neutrocytic ascites. At the stage of neutrocytic ascites, infection may advance, with continued positive findings on cultures and increasing neutrophil count, to SBP. In other cases, bacteria may be undergoing destruction by normal host defenses before the first paracentesis to the extent that no organisms are present or else their numbers fall below the limit of sensitivity of the culture technique, and thus the condition is diagnosed as CNNA. An additional paracentesis in this setting would reveal a decrease in the neutrophil count. Two sequential paracenteses during a phase when there is neutrophil-mediated bacterial killing may produce first a culture-positive and then a culture-negative sample. Finally, a burst in bacterial growth or exhaustion of host defenses would be expected to result in conversion of an episode of CNNA to SBP. All of these events have been observed. Obviously, the process of ascitic fluid infection represents a dynamic balance between host defense and organism virulence factors.

Long-term Natural History of Spontaneous Bacterial Peritonitis

Until the early 1990s, the recurrence rate of SBP in patients was unknown. Three prospective trials that included 134 patients have addressed this issue. The calculated rates or probabilities of recurrence of SBP at 1 year after the initial episode of ascitic fluid infection were 69% in a 1988 study,[10] 68% in a 1990 study,[39] and 47% in a study published in 1991.[40] Each of these studies included only patients with advanced liver disease of varying etiologies. Data on the effect of different causes of the liver disease and cirrhosis on SBP recurrence were presented in two of these studies.[10, 39] The cause of the cirrhosis appeared to make no difference to the probability of recurrence of SBP. The third study, from Taiwan, included only patients with cirrhosis due to hepatitis B and reported a rate of recurrence lower than but similar to the rates reported in the other two studies.[40] In the Taiwanese study, it is noteworthy that the subgroup of patients with hepatocellular carci-

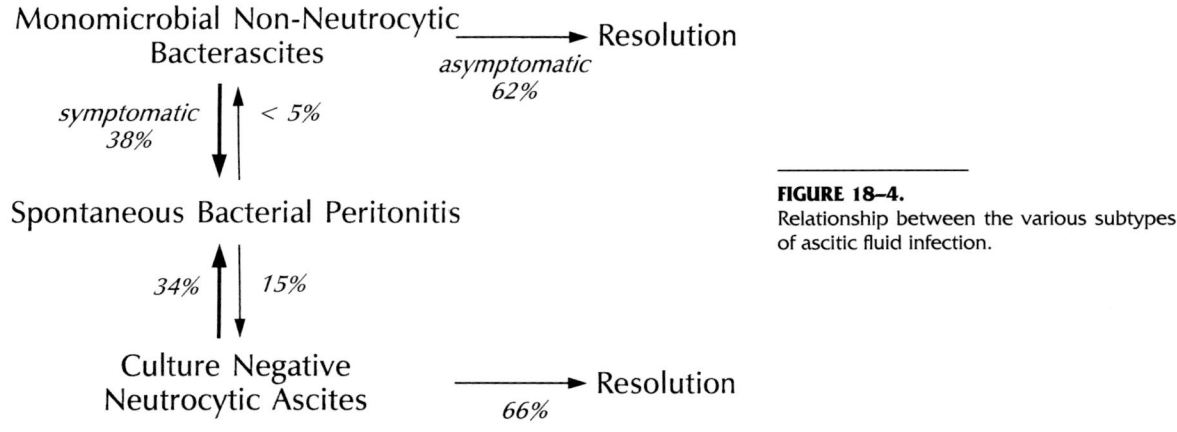

FIGURE 18–4.
Relationship between the various subtypes of ascitic fluid infection.

TABLE 18–3. IN-HOSPITAL OCCURRENCE OF SPONTANEOUS BACTERIAL PERITONITIS AND MORTALITY IN PATIENTS WITH HEPATITIS B SURFACE ANTIGEN–POSITIVE CIRRHOSIS OR HEPATOCELLULAR CARCINOMA

| | ALL CASES | IN-HOSPITAL OCCURRENCE OF SBP | |
		NO. (%) OF CASES	NO. (%) OF SBP CASES WITH MORTALITY
Cirrhosis	153	33 (22)	12 (36)*
HCC	109	8 (7)	4 (50)
Total	262	41 (16)	16 (39)

*P = 0.064 compared with 23 of 120 patients (19%) in the control group.

KEY: HCC = hepatocellular carcinoma, SBP = spontaneous bacterial peritonitis.

SOURCE: Wang SS, Tsai YT, Lee SD, et al. Spontaneous bacterial peritonitis in patients with hepatitis-B–related cirrhosis and hepatocellular carcinoma. Gastroenterology. 1991;101:1656–1662, 1659, Table 4.

noma did not have an increased incidence of recurrent SBP, as might have been expected on the grounds that they had more advanced liver disease (Table 18–3). It would thus appear that once spontaneous bacterial peritonitis occurs, for the reasons already outlined and whatever the type of underlying advanced liver disease, repeated infections occur in approximately two thirds of patients within 1 year.

CLINICAL FEATURES

Prevalence

Early retrospective studies suggested that the prevalence of SBP was of the order of 8 to 13%.[32, 41, 42] With the growing awareness that this condition is often subclinical and with fewer contraindications to perform paracentesis, a steady increase in the prevalence of SBP has been reported in the literature. In one study, a 12-fold increase in the detection of asymptomatic episodes of SBP and a 4-fold increase in detection of symptomatic cases was observed over the 6-year period 1973–1978.[31] In this same period, the number of specimens submitted for culture also increased by a factor of 7 to 8.[31] In seven more recent prospective studies, the prevalence of SBP found at the time of routine paracentesis on admission to hospital increased to between 15 and 25%.[5–7, 30, 43–45] A large series reported in 1991 confirmed these findings in 262 patients with cirrhosis and ascites. The prevalence of SBP on admission in this population was 15% and an additional 6.5% of those studied developed SBP during hospitalization, for

an overall prevalence of 21.5%.[40] This study was the first to be able to calculate the expected prevalence of SBP by prospectively following patients who had not previously been infected. The annual calculated incidence of SBP in cirrhotics with ascites was 11.3%.[40]

Signs and Symptoms and Laboratory Features

The presentation of patients with SBP has been addressed in many studies. Pooled data from 11 large studies of 489 patients with SBP are shown in Table 18–4.[6, 12, 30, 31, 36, 37, 41, 42, 46–48] As can be seen, a significant proportion of patients with SBP present with nonspecific symptoms such as altered mental status, diarrhea, or hypotension and shock. Abdominal symptoms in patients with SBP tend to be mild in comparison with those of patients without liver disease with peritonitis. The most common abdominal signs are pain and tenderness alone. Since the classic surgical sign of peritonitis, rebound tenderness, has been reported to occur in only 8 to 10% of individuals with SBP,[12, 37] it should not be relied on clinically to diagnose SBP in these patients. Apparently, the presence of ascites in SBP does not allow the contact of inflamed peritoneal surfaces that produces rebound tenderness. The signs and symptoms of SBP are thus nonspecific and mild and in general do not allow the clinician to differentiate infected from sterile ascites at the bedside.[49]

What proportion of patients with SBP are asymptomatic? In earlier studies when the threshold of indication for paracentesis was higher, only a minority of infected patients were asymptomatic.[31] More recent studies involving

TABLE 18–4. SIGNS AND SYMPTOMS OF INFECTION AT TIME OF DIAGNOSIS IN 489 PATIENTS WITH SBP*

CLINICAL FEATURE	% WITH SIGN OR SYMPTOM	NO.†
Fever	69	462
Abdominal pain	59	489
Altered mental status	54	489
Abdominal tenderness	49	462
Diarrhea	32	322
Paralytic ileus	30	413
Hypotension	21	385
Hypothermia	17	295

*Pooled data from 11 series with a total of 489 patients.[6, 12, 30, 31, 36, 37, 41, 42, 46–48]

†Number of patients (of the total 489 available in these studies) used as a base to determine the presence or absence of the clinical feature noted.

larger numbers of patients with SBP indicate, however, that the prevalence of truly asymptomatic ascitic fluid infection is as high as 10%.[12, 37] As these studies did not involve consecutive paracentesis on all patients with ascites, the true incidence of asymptomatic SBP may be underestimated in these studies. Pinzello and colleagues reported a prevalence of asymptomatic SBP of 33% (9 of 27 episodes without symptoms referable to the abdomen) in performing routine paracentesis on 234 patients with cirrhosis and ascites.[6] The true prevalence of asymptomatic SBP thus probably lies between these two estimates in patients with ascites and liver disease. Other variants of SBP such as MNB may present with a different clinical pattern. In a study comparing SBP and MNB, significantly more patients with MNB were asymptomatic (34% vs 13%, P< 0.01), and pain as an indication for paracentesis was present in only 11% of patients with MNB compared with 50% in those with SBP.[37]

Laboratory investigations of blood samples usually give no clue to the presence of SBP in a patient with cirrhosis and ascites. The disturbed laboratory parameters purely reflect the severe nature and the origin of the underlying liver disease. This is evidenced by the absence of Childs-Pugh class A patients in most published studies.[12, 47, 48] Despite the severity of the liver disease in SBP patients, individual differences among patients and among published studies make it difficult to determine if there are any distinctive laboratory features that might suggest the development of SBP. Patients with SBP and acute liver disease, those, for example, with acute alcoholic hepatitis, are more likely to have higher values for bilirubin and lower values for prothrombin activity than are patients with quiescent end-stage liver disease, in which jaundice and coagulopathy are in general not so marked. In a 1991 study of therapy in 90 patients with SBP, 0 patients had a normal prothrombin time and only 5 patients (6%) had a normal serum albumin concentration, reflecting the severity of the liver diseases in patients who develop SBP.[12] In this study only 49 individuals with SBP (54%) had a normal serum creatinine level. Elevated values of serum creatinine have also been observed in many other studies of SBP.[31, 32, 42] Renal function has been observed to return to baseline levels with successful antibiotic treatment.[48] We now consider this observation to be part of the syndrome of SBP, although the exact mechanism for the fall in glomerular filtration rate has not been established. This association has been observed so frequently that in our liver unit a rise in creatinine level in an asymptomatic patient who was not receiving diuretics would immediately lead us to perform paracentesis to exclude SBP.

Perhaps the one helpful routine laboratory test in patients with SBP is to determine the peripheral white blood cell (WBC) concentration, which is elevated in 50 to 75% of patients presenting with SBP.[31] Furthermore, it has been shown that the WBC concentration does increase in a proportion of patients who develop SBP when compared with their pre-SBP value. Of perhaps even more clinical value is our observation that SBP may be manifested by a rise in the percentage of immature PMN bands in patients who are unable to mount an actual increase in the WBC concentration (unpublished observation, B. A. Runyon, M.D., 1991). The presence of such bands in our patients with ascites and advanced liver disease is also an indication for paracentesis to exclude SBP.

Mortality and Survival

With increased awareness of SBP and improved diagnostic techniques and antibiotics, the mortality due to SBP has decreased dramatically. In the original studies in the 1970s, the reported mortality for SBP approached 100%.[36, 42] In analyzing the results from 7 studies of a total of 246 patients with SBP, the mean weighted mortality was found to be reduced to 78%.[29] This figure reflects the mortality during the hospitalization in which the index episode of SBP was recorded. Data are also available from 5 large prospective series (Table 18–5).[10, 12, 45, 47, 48] Of the 344 patients with SBP included in these studies, the mortality during the actual episode of SBP was as low as 2% in one study (mean 29%). A similar reduction in the mortality rate during the initial hospitalization (38–54%, mean 43%) was observed in these studies. Despite these improvements in short-term mortality observed in the five years bridging the 1980s and 1990s, the prognosis for these patients is still poor as reflected in the 1-year mortality figures (68–88%, mean 82%; see Table 18–5). These improved survival statistics probably reflect the increasing ability to diagnose SBP earlier, the use of improved and nonnephrotoxic antibiotics, and refinements in our medical care of the critically ill patient with severe liver disease. One could argue that the successful treatment of SBP, as reflected in this reduction in short-term mortality, is purely a reprieve from the eventual poor outcome of these patients with relatively advanced end-stage liver disease. Without treatment, however, most pa-

TABLE 18–5. MORTALITY IN PROSPECTIVE TRIALS OF SBP

| REFERENCE | NO. | MORTALITY (%) | | |
		SBP*	IN HOSPITAL†	1 YEAR‡
Ariza (1991)[48]	52	35	50	68
Runyon (1991)[12]	90	2	38	NA
Grange (1990)[47]	22	15	47	70
Tito (1988)[10]	139	46	54	88
Yang (1985)[45]	41	NA	39	72

*Mortality during the episode of SBP.
†Mortality during that hospitalization.
‡Mortality of survivors at 1 year.
KEY: NA = not available from the published data, SBP = spontaneous bacterial peritonitis.

tients with SBP die. The successful treatment of SBP allows further time for consideration of other alternatives, which include orthotopic liver transplantation in suitable patients.

What is the cause of the mortality in these patients after they have been diagnosed with SBP? In most studies a small proportion of patients die within 48 hours of the diagnosis of SBP, despite appropriate antibiotic therapy. Most of these deaths appear to be associated with hepatic and renal failure, gastrointestinal bleeding, or both.[48] These early deaths probably represent examples of overwhelming SBP complicated by multiorgan failure. A further subgroup of patients has been identified who die within 7 days of the initial diagnosis of SBP.[31] There is no doubt that many of these patients appear to have more serious underlying liver disease and often an acute superimposed component, especially acute alcoholic hepatitis. These patients tend to be deeply jaundiced with renal failure, and as few as 10% have been reported to leave hospital after they develop SBP. They probably constitute a completely separate subgroup of patients with SBP.[31]

In a review of the factors that contributed to death in SBP, infection, whether from SBP or other sources, was found to be a contributing factor in 35 of 77 patients (45%) who succumbed to an episode of SBP.[29] A more recent analysis, including studies performed between 1983 and 1991, gives slightly different results

which are presented in Table 18–6.[6, 12, 47, 48] In these studies, which were carefully designed to detect the recurrence and relapse of SBP, the major contributing factors responsible for death were either gastrointestinal bleeding, usually of variceal origin, or a combination of liver and renal failure. The infection itself, which included recurrence and relapse of SBP and superinfection, contributed to only 18% of those patients who died in hospital. As would be expected, most of these presumed causes of death relate to the severity of the underlying hepatic dysfunction. Similarly, the reported mortality in these studies at 1 year follow-up also reflects the end-stage nature of the liver disease. In the largest study, which reported 59 deaths during follow-up, liver failure itself was the main cause of death in 26 patients (44%) and recurrent SBP was the cause in 18 patients (31%).[10] Gastrointestinal hemorrhage and the development of hepatocellular carcinoma were responsible for the deaths of 12 patients (20%), with the remaining 3 deaths (5%) being associated with renal failure and other infections.

Prognostic Factors

Earlier studies attempted to define potential clinical and laboratory features that may help to predict outcome and survival in patients with SBP.[31, 41, 50] Factors that were found to predict a

TABLE 18–6. FACTORS CONTRIBUTING TO IN-HOSPITAL MORTALITY AFTER SBP

REFERENCE	NO.	INFECTION	GI BLEEDING	LIVER & RENAL FAILURE
Runyon (1991)[12]	34	2	←−−−−−−32−−−−−−→	
Ariza (1991)[48]	26	9	10	7
Grange (1990)[47]	4	1	2	1
Pinzello (1983)[6]	13	2	4	7
Total	77	14 (18%)	←−−−−−−63 (82%)−−−−−−→	

KEY: GI = gastrointestinal, SBP = spontaneous bacterial peritonitis.

poor outcome included encephalopathy, high bilirubin values ($\geq$8 mg/dl), and a low serum albumin level ($<$2.5 gm/dl), all reflecting advanced liver disease. Hoefs and colleagues analyzed two groups of patients and found that those with acute alcoholic hepatitis did poorly (10% survival) compared with those with more quiescent chronic liver disease (90% survival).[31] A further analysis of these variables revealed that the level of bilirubin and WBC concentration predicted survival through the episode of SBP, whereas survival throughout hospital stay was lowest in those who had a raised creatinine level or were older. These findings seem to make sense and verify our clinical findings: older patients and those who have more advanced disease, severe acute alcoholic hepatitis, or renal failure do not tolerate SBP well. A 1991 study of 90 cases of SBP indicated that patients with concomitant bacteremia did not have increased mortality (50% for bacteremic compared with 33% for nonbacteremic groups).[12]

Predisposing Factors and Relationship to Invasive Procedures

Apart from the importance of a low total protein content of less than 1 g per dl that has been shown to predispose to the development of SBP, other factors may be important in creating the environment for SBP. Many other sites of infection have been observed in association with SBP. These commonly include the skin, urinary tract, respiratory tract, and bowel, and infections at these sites are usually detected at the time that multiple cultures are obtained.[29] A report published in 1990 also suggested the simultaneous occurrence of spontaneous bacterial empyema and SBP in patients with cirrhotic ascites and pleural effusions.[51] This is not surprising, since 10% of patients with cirrhosis do have pleural effusions that are documented to be in communication with the ascites pool.[52] Such a communication would allow the concurrent infection of both pleural and ascitic fluid if SBP was the primary infection, or, perhaps concurrent infections are caused via hematogenous spread. In many instances, the organism cultured from these other sources is the same as that retrieved from the ascitic fluid culture.

Infections are common in cirrhotic patients. In one study, 86 of 187 consecutive patients (46%) admitted to a liver unit had documented bacterial infections at admission or during hospitalization, and in another study 35% developed proven infection.[18, 53] The high prevalence of bacterial infections and bacteremia in cirrhotic patients makes it difficult to establish cause and effect between the simultaneous occurrence of SBP and another locus of infection. No definite evidence suggests that these other loci of infection actually predispose patients to develop SBP. Concurrent infections involving the same organism in ascites and in another site may reflect either the simultaneous seeding of both sites from a spontaneous episode of bacteremia or else the seeding of other sites from the ascites via the bloodstream.

Certain invasive procedures have been reported in association with SBP. These include endoscopy, variceal sclerotherapy, percutaneous catheter placement, urinary catheters, and peritoneovenous shunts.[29, 54-56] These procedures are well documented to cause bacteremia, but a direct relationship between them and the development of SBP has not been firmly established.[57] Wang and colleagues reported that in a series of 41 patients with SBP, 4 patients (10%) had received endoscopic variceal sclerotherapy and 3 others (7%) had undergone transarterial embolization of hepatocellular carcinomas within the 3-day period before developing SBP.[40] Two reports published in 1991 finally shed some light on the risk of SBP associated with gastrointestinal hemorrhage.[54, 58] Ho and colleagues prospectively assessed the presence or absence of bacteremia in patients undergoing emergency and elective sclerotherapy. Although not all organisms isolated by blood culture were clinically significant, the overall incidence of clinically significant bacteremia probably caused by emergency sclerotherapy, and thus not present before sclerotherapy, was 5.4%.[54] The patients were not followed after the initial study, and no comment was made as to the presence of ascites, but no overt episodes of SBP were reported. Nevertheless, this study does provide us with new information; 5 to 6% of patients undergoing this procedure emergently, but not electively, have significant bacteremia that could potentially cause SBP if ascites were present. The second important 1991 study of Soriano and colleagues prospectively addressed the prevalence of SBP in cirrhotic patients with gastrointestinal hemorrhage.[58] Although no comments are made regarding the relationship of sclerotherapy, emergent or elective, to the development of SBP, the striking finding was that 17% of the patients not treated with prophylactic antibiotics developed spontaneous bacteremia or SBP or both.

These studies indicate that a significant percentage of cirrhotic patients with ascites who develop gastrointestinal bleeding or undergo endoscopy do develop bacteremia and SBP. The results further suggest that the hemorrhage and not the emergency sclerotherapy are most likely to be responsible for the bacteremia. This is not an unexpected finding. Blood loss and hypovolemia have been shown in experimental models to alter intestinal permeability to enteric organisms, which would favor translocation of bacteria, and to depress hepatic reticuloendothelial function.[59, 60] Also, the administration of salt-rich fluids to resuscitate patients with cirrhosis increases the volume of ascites, with a resultant dilution of ascitic fluid protein content that further favors the development of SBP (Runyon BA, Antillon MR, unpublished observations, 1991). For all these reasons, the patient with liver disease and gastrointestinal hemorrhage is predisposed to SBP.

A note concerning the risk of introducing infection at the time of paracentesis is pertinent. Spontaneous bacterial peritonitis very rarely develops as a result of paracentesis (0.1–0.6%).[17] We believe strongly that paracentesis should not be considered a predisposing factor for ascitic fluid infection. In our opinion, the risks of not performing paracentesis far outweigh those of performing this simple procedure.

PRINCIPLES OF EVALUATION

Because of the high prevalence of SBP of 20 to 27% detected by routine paracentesis in patients with cirrhotic ascites and because of the fact that only two thirds of patients are symptomatic, all patients with ascites should routinely undergo paracentesis on admission to hospital. Spontaneous bacterial peritonitis can be diagnosed only by paracentesis, and it is a safe procedure, even in the presence of coagulopathy. In our institutions, paracentesis is mandatory at the time of admission in all patients with ascites. We routinely repeat the paracentesis during hospitalization if the patient develops any clinical deterioration such as fever, encephalopathy, renal impairment, or deteriorating liver function without an identifiable cause.

The procedure is best performed with a 22-gauge needle in the midline between the umbilicus and symphysis pubis in the area of dullness to percussion. Areas of scarring should be avoided since they are often the site of collateral vessels, and complications (e.g., hemoperitoneum) occur when the needle is introduced through or near scars.[61] Fifty ml of fluid should be withdrawn, sent for the ascites cell count, and cultured at the bedside in blood culture bottles (Table 18–7).

TABLE 18–7. EVALUATION OF A PATIENT WITH LIVER DISEASE AND ASCITES AND SUSPECTED SBP

Always suspect SBP: 20–27% of cirrhotic patients with ascites are infected on a routine paracentesis at admission to hospital.
Coagulopathy is not a contraindication to paracentesis.
Use 22-gauge needle; withdraw 40–50 ml.
Avoid scars; this is the site of collaterals and adherent bowel.
Midline paracenteses have fewer complications.
Send ascites for cell count.
Culture 10 ml in each of 2 blood culture bottles at bedside.
Draw blood cultures.

KEY: SBP = spontaneous bacterial peritonitis.

Ascitic Fluid Analysis

The three widely accepted diagnostic criteria for SBP are an ascitic fluid PMN count of ≥ 250 cells per mm^3, a positive ascitic fluid culture, and the absence of any primary surgical source of peritonitis. Because of the serious nature and high mortality of SBP, the ideal test to confirm the diagnosis should be inexpensive and easy to perform and have a short turnaround time.

The test for ascitic fluid PMN count has met these criteria and has become the rapid presumptive diagnostic test for SBP. The test allows the initiation of treatment while awaiting culture results during the 24- to 48-hour period required. The accepted cutoff value for the ascites PMN count is ≥ 250 cells per mm.^{3} The normal ascites WBC count is 281 ± 25 cells per mm^3, of which only $27 \pm 2\%$ are PMNs.[31] The visual characteristics of the ascitic fluid are not helpful. Ascites that is cloudy is usually infected, but the appearance may be due to triglycerides, so-called opalescent ascites, and ascites with a PMN count of 250 to 300 cells per mm^3 looks essentially normal. Occasionally, a paracentesis may be traumatic. As a result, numerous red blood cells may be present in the specimen and it may appear bloody or only slightly cloudy, leading to difficulty in interpreting the cell count in this situation. As a general rule, we allow only 1 PMN per 250 red blood cells because of trauma. With this knowledge, the actual ascites PMN count can be established to determine if there is concurrent infection.[62]

Concern that the changes in ascitic fluid analysis in patients with SBP who are undergoing diuresis may result in difficulty in interpreting the PMN count also seems to be unfounded (Table 18–8). Unlike cerebrospinal, synovial, and pleural fluid, the total protein content and ascites glucose concentration do not seem to increase in SBP.[63] An increase in lactate dehydrogenase (LDH) however, seems to accom-

TABLE 18–8. COMPARISON OF CHANGES
IN ASCITIC FLUID COMPOSITION
DURING SBP AND DIURESIS

DURING SBP
↑ Ascites PMN count
↑ Ascites LDH
No change in glucose or total protein
DURING OR AFTER DIURESIS
↑ Ascites total protein (2-fold)
↑ Ascites total WBC count
No change in ascites PMN count

KEY: LDH = lactate dehydrogenase, PMN = polymorphonuclear neutrophil leukocytes, SBP = spontaneous bacterial peritonitis, WBC = white blood cell.

pany the increase in ascites PMN count and presumably represents the release of this enzyme from damaged neutrophils.[63] Fortunately, the ascitic fluid PMN count does not increase during diuresis and remains a reliable method to differentiate SBP from sterile ascites in the many patients who are receiving diuretics.[62] The contraction in the volume of ascites with diuresis does, however, result in an increase in the total ascites WBC count. During a 10 kg diuresis, for instance, the ascites WBC was observed to increase from 300 to 1200 cells per mm[3].[62] This phenomenon is probably a reflection of the short half-life of PMNs. The longer survival of monocytes and lymphocytes would allow these cell lines to remain in ascites and become concentrated. Similarly, the contraction of ascites with diuresis results in a rise in protein content of ascites.[62, 64] In these two studies, diuresis of 8 to 10 kg resulted in a 2-fold increase in the ascitic fluid total protein content.

Culture Technique

The conventional method of culturing ascites by plating out a loop of fluid on agar plates in the microbiology laboratory detects a causative organism in only 42 to 57% of cases.[15, 16, 65] In comparison, the inoculation of a larger volume of ascites into aerobic and anaerobic blood culture bottles (Fig. 18–5) at the bedside improves the sensitivity of detection of an organism to approximately 90%, a finding now verified in many studies.[11] When 10 ml of ascites is inoculated into each of the two bottles, the sensitivity of detecting an organism is superior to that produced when smaller volumes are used.[16] Larger volumes (>10 ml) do not appear to increase this sensitivity. These differences are best explained by the low concentration of organisms in SBP; the median concentration of bacteria in SBP is 1 organism per ml, and 50 to 60% of

episodes of SBP contain ≤2 organisms per ml.[16] It seems reasonable that culturing a total of 20 ml of fluid that contains a low bacteria count rather than 10 μl by loop should increase the rate of positive findings. We presume that the nutritious environment provided by the culture bottles, which contain nutrients, opsonin inhibitors, and an anticoagulant that protect bacteria from further destruction, also aids in detection.

Why culture the ascites at the bedside? In theory, a low number of organisms per ml may potentially be destroyed if left for a prolonged period of time in a hostile environment, such as in a syringe. It has been shown that a delay of 4 hours in transferring infected ascites into blood culture bottles results in a 25% reduction of the number of cultures that produce positive findings.[66] The effect of even longer delays is unknown but would be expected to be even greater.

In light of this information, the most sensitive method to culture ascites is to inoculate 10 ml of ascites into each of two blood culture bottles at the bedside as well as to perform an ascitic fluid PMN count on fluid withdrawn at the same time. Although many microbiologic laboratories routinely perform a Gram stain on most ascites specimens submitted, the low number of organisms per ml of spontaneously infected fluid in the majority of cases suggests that this would not be helpful in making a rapid diagnosis of SBP. As expected, ascites fluid that has been proved to be infected by culture has a positive Gram stain only 7% of the time.[16] If the ascitic fluid is centrifuged to concentrate the organisms, Gram stain of the sediment will still identify only 10% of patients with early SBP.[16]

Organisms Responsible

Most patients who develop SBP and in whom a positive culture is recorded have pure growth of a single organism. The pooled data from over 500 patients with SBP from several large studies show the different organisms cultured (Table 18–9).[6, 8, 12, 30, 31, 36, 40, 42, 46–48, 67] As can be seen, the majority of organisms cultured are of enteric origin, but only a small proportion are anaerobes. Although the reasons for this are unknown, a likely explanation is that the high partial pressure of oxygen in ascites fluid makes it an environment that is hostile to such organisms.[29] In 172 of the 387 patients (44%), blood cultures were also positive at the time of the initial diagnosis of SBP. In the majority of cases, the organism isolated from the blood is the same as that isolated from the ascites.

ASCITIC FLUID CULTURE TECHNIQUES

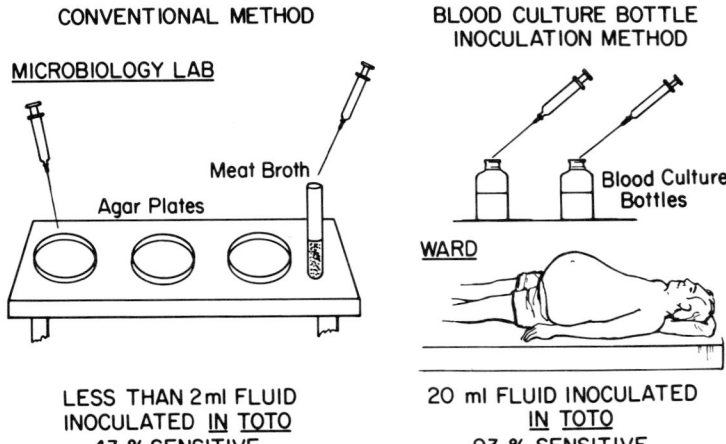

FIGURE 18–5.
Diagrammatic representation of conventional ascitic fluid culture method and blood culture bottle method. SOURCE: Runyon BA. Spontaneous bacterial peritonitis: An explosion of information. Hepatology. 1988;8: 171–175. Editorial.

Unusual organisms can occasionally cause SBP. A number of reports have identified various *Salmonella* species as the responsible organism for SBP in patients with cirrhosis.[68, 69] Of more concern, these species have also been reported to cause SBP in patients with ascites not due to liver diseases that contains a high total protein content and opsonic activity.[70] The presumption is that these virulent organisms can overcome the relatively good endogenous antimicrobial activity of high protein ascites, which is rich in opsonic activity and complement, and cause SBP in patients who would not ordinarily develop this infection.[70]

The Value of Ascitic Fluid pH and Lactate in Diagnosis

The initial interest in ascitic fluid pH and lactate levels stemmed from the idea that these two parameters might aid in the rapid diagnosis of SBP. Since the first publications in the early 1980s,[71, 72] seven further studies have been published on the utility of pH and lactate in SBP.[43–45, 73–76] The most important finding in all but one of these nine studies was that the ascitic fluid PMN count was the single most sensitive test to diagnose SBP. Unfortunately, the results of these studies are difficult to interpret and inconsistent regarding the usefulness of the pH and lactate in diagnosing SBP. Most of the earlier studies included small numbers of patients, among whom was a high proportion of patients (25–67%) with secondary peritonitis—a totally separate form of ascitic fluid infection with a completely different ascitic fluid analysis.[43–45, 73–75] Also, many of these studies did not use the optimal culture technique (see Fig. 18–5), with the result that specimens with a high PMN count and a negative culture were incorrectly interpreted as a false-positive elevated PMN count rather than as a false-negative culture, thus making the PMN count appear a less sensitive test. Other problems with these studies include differences in the classification of the variant forms of SBP and omission of important control groups with other miscellaneous causes of ascites.

Fortunately, the results of a 1991 study of over 200 ascites specimens (101 were infected) finally clarify the importance of the measurement of pH and lactate in SBP.[76] The data from this study concerning ascitic fluid pH and the sensitivities and specificities of the individual tests are shown in Figure 18–6 and Table 18–10. As can be seen, the most sensitive and accurate test was an ascitic fluid PMN count of ≥250 cells per mm³. Lactate measurements were stopped after an interim analysis during this study because

TABLE 18–9. BACTERIA ISOLATED FROM ASCITES IN 519 PATIENTS WITH SBP

ORGANISM	NO. ISOLATES	%
Escherichia coli	222	43
Klebsiella pneumoniae	55	11
Streptococcus pneumoniae	48	9
Alpha-hemolytic streptococcus	34	7
Group D streptococcus	25	5
Unclassified streptococcus	21	4
Enterobacteriaceae	21	4
Beta-hemolytic streptococcus	15	3
Staphylococcus	15	3
Pseudomonas	9	1
Miscellaneous	54	10
Total	519	100

SOURCE: Reference nos. 6, 8, 12, 30, 31, 36, 40–42, 46–48, 67.

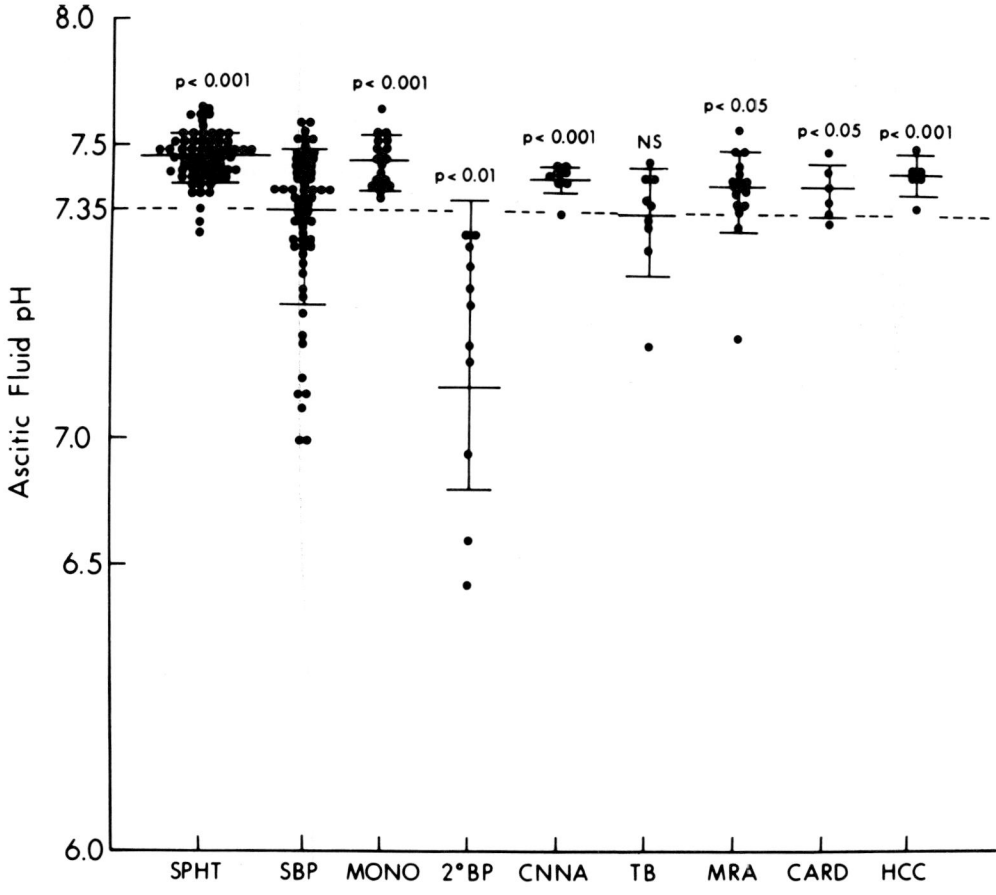

FIGURE 18–6.
Ascitic fluid pH in fluids of various types. KEY: 2° BP = secondary bacterial peritonitis, CARD = cardiac ascites, CNNA = culture-negative neutrocytic ascites, HCC = hepatocellular carcinoma, MONO = monomicrobial bacterascites, MRA = malignancy-related ascites, NS = not significant, SBP = spontaneous bacterial peritonitis, SPHT = sterile portal hypertension–related ascites, TB = tuberculous peritonitis, SOURCE: Runyon BA, Antillon MR. Ascitic fluid pH and lactate: Insensitive and nonspecific tests in detecting ascitic fluid infection. Hepatology. 1991;13:929–935.

TABLE 18–10. SENSITIVITY AND SPECIFICITY ANALYSIS OF ASCITIC FLUID TESTS IN DETECTING SBP

PARAMETER	SENSITIVITY (%)	SPECIFICITY (%)	POSITIVE PREDICTIVE VALUE (%)	NEGATIVE PREDICTIVE VALUE (%)	ACCURACY (%)
PMN ≥250 cells/mm³	100	89	69	100	91
PMN ≥500 cells/mm³	83	92	71	96	90
Lactate >3.57 mmol/L	44	93	62	87	84
pH <7.35	33	95	60	85	83
A-AF lactate >2.23 mmol/L	17	97	60	83	82
A-AF pH >0.10	28	88	36	83	76

NOTE: As can be seen, the ascitic fluid PMN count is the most sensitive and accurate test.
KEY: A-AF = arterial-ascitic fluid gradient, PMN = polymorphonuclear neutrophil leukocyte, SBP = spontaneous bacterial peritonitis.
SOURCE: Runyon BA, Antillon MR. Ascitic fluid pH and lactate: Insensitive and nonspecific tests in detecting ascitic fluid infection. Hepatology. 1991;13:929–935.

they were found to be inferior to the measurement of ascitic fluid pH. Other important findings in this study were that no specimens from patients with monomicrobial nonneutrocytic bacterascites had a pH <7.35. In this group of patients in whom the PMN count was not helpful, since by definition it was normal, the pH of the ascitic fluid was not helpful either in detecting ascitic fluid infection. In comparison with the monomicrobial nonneutrocytic bacterascites group, all other groups studied had a significantly lower ascitic fluid pH compared with sterile ascites. Since ascites that contained PMN cells was more acidic than were the sterile samples and since the samples that contained bacteria but no PMNs were not acidic, the change in pH in infected ascites was probably a reflection of the presence of PMNs rather than of bacteria. From this study it was estimated that the presence of at least 2000 PMNs is necessary before the ascitic fluid pH falls below 7.35.[76]

The results of this study are important. If one were to decide whether to treat according to the results of the pH and lactate findings alone, more than half of the documented episodes of SBP would have remained untreated.[76] The single most accurate and sensitive test to diagnose SBP rapidly is the ascitic fluid PMN count. In addition, the PMN count is the best test to detect other forms of bacterial peritonitis.

The addition of the measurement of pH and lactate to diagnose SBP requires special handling, with specimens being kept on ice and transported immediately to the laboratory, which is costly. These findings are not necessary to establish the diagnosis of SBP. We can be even more confident of the findings of Runyon's study since they have been verified in another large study of 285 ascites specimens that included 41 patients with SBP.[77]

Differentiation of Spontaneous from Secondary Peritonitis

Between 10 and 15% of patients with infected ascites are found to have secondary bacterial peritonitis.[29] The intra-abdominal source of infection in these cases may be due either to a perforated viscus (commonly a peptic ulcer, sigmoid diverticulum, or perforated gallbladder) or to so-called nonperforation secondary peritonitis (e.g., a perinephric abscess or sealed-off diverticular or appendiceal abscess).[67, 78] Clinical signs appear to be of little value in differentiating SBP from secondary peritonitis, since few patients develop classic signs of rigidity and re-

bound tenderness when a perforation occurs in the presence of ascites. It would seem prudent to diagnose patients with secondary bacterial peritonitis early, since they may not be adequately treated with antibiotics alone and may require surgical correction of a perforation or other intra-abdominal collection to survive.

Two retrospective studies indicated that peritonitis associated with perforation is characterized by an ascitic fluid protein content >1 g per dl, a glucose value <50 mg per dl, and an ascitic fluid LDH greater than normal.[30, 79] It was also found that the ascitic fluid PMN count falls exponentially in patients with SBP who are treated but continues to rise during antibiotic therapy in patients with secondary peritonitis. These findings appear to hold true in all patients with ascites, whether or not they have underlying liver disease.[30] On the basis of these findings, an algorithm has been introduced to allow the clinician to distinguish between these two conditions in the hope that earlier recognition of surgically correctable causes of peritonitis might increase survival (Fig. 18–7).[67] This algorithm does appear to be useful. A prospective study using the algorithm in 28 patients with SBP and 15 patients with secondary peritonitis indicated that it is 100% sensitive in detecting patients with secondary peritonitis due to gut perforation.[67]

Only 1 of 28 patients with SBP (3.6%) met two of the three criteria as outlined in Figure 18–7 compared with 10 of the 15 patients (67%) with secondary peritonitis. The algorithm correctly identified all 5 patients with free perforations and half of those with secondary peritonitis without a detectable perforation. Also, the PMN count at 48 hours after treatment returned to below the baseline pretreatment value in all patients with SBP compared with only a third of those with secondary peritonitis. As would be expected, in all cases of SBP in which the culture grew an organism, 89% had pure growth of a single bacteria, whereas 100% of patients with secondary peritonitis had positive cultures, and 53% of these grew multiple organisms. The mortality in the two groups of patients was similar (46% and 53%, respectively). Most episodes of SBP (86%) became sterile on repeat culture after a single dose of antibiotic, whereas most secondary cases remained culture-positive despite the use of antibiotics. Another study has identified a subgroup of patients with biliary peritonitis, which was usually due to a perforated gallbladder.[80] Perforation should be suspected when the ascitic fluid is bile-stained with an ascitic fluid bilirubin

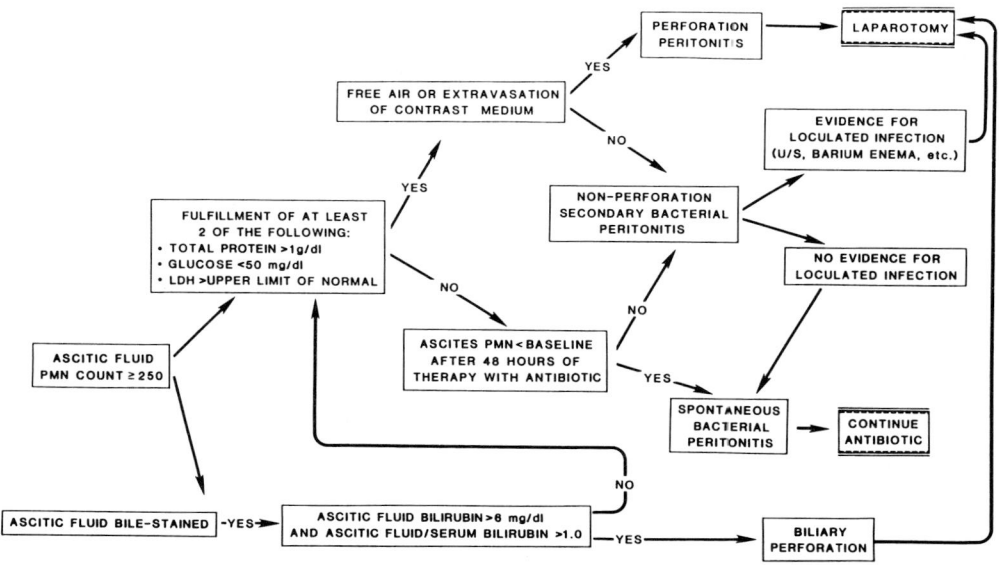

FIGURE 18–7.
Algorithm for the evaluation of patients with neutrocytic ascites (e.g., polymorphonuclear neutrophil leukocyte count ≥250 cells/mm³ in the absence of hemorrhage into ascites, tuberculosis, peritoneal carcinomatosis, or pancreatitis) in the differentiation of spontaneous bacterial peritonitis (SBP) from perforation and from nonperforation secondary peritonitis. KEY: LDH = lactate dehydrogenase, U/S = ultrasound. SOURCE: Akriviadis EA, Runyon BA. Utility of an algorithm in differentiating spontaneous from secondary peritonitis. Gastroenterology. 1990;98:127–133.

value of >6 mg per dl or an ascites to serum bilirubin ratio >1.[80]

We believe that if two of the three criteria outlined here (see Fig. 18–7) are met, secondary peritonitis should be strongly considered. Studies such as water-soluble contrast studies and ultrasound should be performed to exclude the presence of free air, perforation, and other causes of loculated pus within the abdomen. If the patient has a proven free perforation or loculated infection, surgery should be performed, since such individuals do not respond to medical therapy alone. Expectant therapy should be continued if no actual perforation can be detected. In this situation, the response of the PMN count to therapy should be monitored. A vigilant watch should be maintained, and if the PMN count does not respond and cultures remain positive despite therapy, thorough searches for an unusual intra-abdominal locus of sepsis should continue.

PRINCIPLES OF THERAPY

Treatment of Documented SBP

If the PMN count is >250 cells per mm³ or the Gram stain is positive or if the patient has

convincing signs or symptoms of peritonitis, empirical therapy should be started without waiting 48 hours for culture results. What is the most appropriate antibiotic therapy for SBP? In the past, the combination of ampicillin and gentamicin was widely recommended to cover the predominance of enteric organisms.[41] We now know that aminoglycosides such as gentamicin should not be used in patients with advanced liver disease. Apart from their narrow therapeutic window, aminoglycosides have been shown to have an unpredictable volume of distribution in cirrhosis[81] and are frequently associated with nephrotoxicity in this population in up to 73% of patients.[9, 82] In controlled trials, less toxic alternative regimens have been proved to be more effective and to have fewer side effects.[8] Also, the serum creatinine level has been shown to be an unpredictable marker of GFR in cirrhosis, making therapy with aminoglycosides even more hazardous.

Most of the flora responsible for SBP (see Table 18–9) are sensitive to either a third-generation cephalosporin or to chloramphenicol.[29] Although chloramphenicol is generally tolerated well and is inexpensive, it is only bacteriostatic for gram-negative bacteria, and fatal recurrences could arise if this drug were routinely used in SBP, as is the case in gram-negative meningitis.[83] In SBP, broader spectrum third-generation cephalosporins have been prospectively demonstrated to be as effective as the combination of ampicillin and an aminoglycoside without the related problems of nephrotoxicity.[8] A further beneficial effect of these cephalosporins is that this class of drugs has also been shown to enter ascites rapidly.[84] Most importantly, third-generation cephalosporins have been shown to cover effectively most of the organisms (94–98%) responsible for SBP in two large prospective trials.[8, 12]

Other newer agents have also been evaluated, including amoxicillin–clavulanic acid, aztreonam, ceftriaxone, and cefoperazone.[47, 48, 85, 86] It appears that most third-generation cephalosporins supply adequate coverage and are ideal for the empirical treatment of SBP. There appears to be a very low incidence of skin reactions (3%), which are not severe.[12] Unfortunately, the newer monobactam class of antibiotics (aztreonam is an example) have poor coverage against gram-positive organisms and a worrisome rate of superinfection (14% in one study).[48]

A suitable empirical regimen to start therapy when the ascites PMN count is elevated and SBP is suspected is cefotaxime or a similar cephalosporin. The dosage of cefotaxime is 2.0 g intravenously every 8 hours. As these newer antibiotics are generally more expensive, antibiotic therapy can be switched to an equally effective narrower spectrum agent when the culture and susceptibility studies have returned (usually in 48–72 h). In general, most *E. coli* bacteria are sensitive to ampicillin, and most pneumococci are sensitive to penicillin.

Response to Therapy

The ascites culture has been previously shown to become sterile in 86% of individuals with SBP after a single dose of cefotaxime.[67] A 1991 prospective large study of 90 patients verified these findings.[12] Both ascites and blood were sterilized in more than 90% of patients with SBP; the remainder had resistant flora or died before completion of therapy.[12] Also, the ascitic fluid PMN count returned to normal during therapy in 90% of the patients, and in the 10% of patients in whom it did not, there was no increased frequency of relapse or recurrences. Patients also responded clinically; 51% defervesced, and abdominal pain, when present, disappeared in 33% within 24 hours of starting treatment.[12] The rate of recurrence immediately after therapy during the hospitalization appears to be on the order of 10 to 12%.[12, 87] Most of these recurrences appear to be due to episodes of reinfection with different organisms rather than a re-

lapse with the same organism.[12] Superinfection after therapy with the third-generation cephalosporins occurs very infrequently. The long-term recurrence rate has been addressed previously.

What is the ideal length of antibiotic therapy in a patient with SBP? Prior teaching suggested 10 to 14 days of therapy in the absence of any supporting clinical data. A 1989 study suggested that empirical therapy administered until the cell count returned to normal may be equally effective, but these findings have not been prospectively confirmed.[87] Five days of therapy has now been shown to be equally effective as 10 days of therapy.[12] In this study, the cure rate, efficacy, relapse and reinfection rate, and morbidity and mortality were equal whether the patient received cefotaxime for 5 days or 10. Such short-term therapy was also shown to be cost-effective.[12] For SBP, we can now confidently recommend single-agent therapy with a third-generation cephalosporin such as cefotaxime for 5 days only. Sensitivities should be checked as soon as available to allow a further reduction in cost by switching to a narrower spectrum antibiotic, if applicable.

Prophylactic Therapy

This chapter has outlined certain factors that predispose the patient with ascites to SBP. These include an ascitic fluid total protein content >1g per dl, a prior episode of SBP (the recurrence rate at 1 year is 47–69%), and gastrointestinal hemorrhage. In view of the high recurrence rate and its associated high mortality, despite our improved methods of diagnosis and therapy, the question of whether antibiotics should be given prophylactically to these high-risk individuals is an important one. The ideal antibiotic would necessarily be nonabsorbable and would presumably act by inhibiting growth of the intestinal flora that are predominantly responsible for SBP. In 1985, a prospective trial of a prophylactic oral antibiotic regimen in cirrhotics with gastrointestinal hemorrhage showed that such treatment was effective in reducing significantly the number of episodes of spontaneous bacteremia and peritonitis.[53] Despite these results, this form of therapy did not become widely accepted because the regimen required three nonabsorbable antibiotics that were very unpalatable and were associated with significant side effects when given long-term. More recently the oral quinolone class of antibiotics has been shown to produce a selective intestinal decontamination (SID) by inhibiting aerobic gram-negative intestinal flora and preserving the anaerobic gut flora in healthy volunteers, cirrhotics, and neutropenic patients.[39, 88, 89] In neutropenic patients, one of these quinolone antibiotics, norfloxacin, decreased the incidence of gram-negative infections without producing significant side effects or overgrowth of resistant organisms.[39, 89] In two prospective trials of patients at risk for SBP because of either a low ascites protein content or a prior episode of SBP,[39, 90] norfloxacin significantly reduced the incidence of SBP in those who were treated (Fig. 18–8) from 35 to 12%[39] and from 23 to 0%.[90] Importantly, the SBP that did develop in patients treated with norfloxacin was caused by gram-positive organisms. These organisms would not be expected to be eradicated by selective intestinal decontamination. No overgrowth or infections due to resistant organisms developed, and other non-SBP infections were not increased more in these patients than in control patients. A further preliminary report has also verified these findings in cirrhotics with gastrointestinal bleeding, showing that norfloxacin

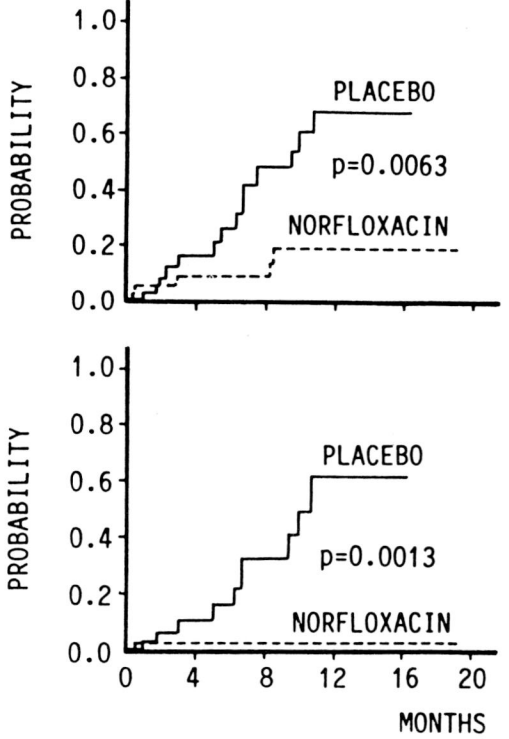

FIGURE 18–8.
Cumulative probability of spontaneous bacterial peritonitis (SBP) recurrence in patients treated with norfloxacin and placebo. The upper graph compares the recurrence rate of all episodes of SBP, whereas the lower graph indicates recurrence due only to aerobic gram-negative bacilli. SOURCE: Gines P, Rimola A, Planas R, et al. Norfloxacin prevents spontaneous bacterial peritonitis in cirrhosis: Results of a double-blind placebo-controlled trial. Hepatology. 1990;12:716–724.

reduced the incidence of SBP and bacteremia to 3% from the 17% observed in controls.[58] It has been demonstrated in another report that short-term norfloxacin therapy led to an increase in serum and ascitic fluid C3 levels,[91] a potentially beneficial effect, since low C3 levels have been directly related to SBP.[34] A further potential benefit may be obtained by treating the patient who has cirrhosis and ascites with diuretics rather than by repeated large-volume paracentesis, since diuresis has been shown to increase the opsonic activity of ascitic fluid.[64]

We thus routinely recommend long-term prophylactic therapy for patients with a documented episode of SBP because of the high rate of its recurrence. Whether patients with low ascitic fluid total protein (<1 g/dl) should always receive prophylactic therapy has not yet been proved. It does seem reasonable, however, to offer such therapy to patients who are in a high-risk situation and to those who are awaiting orthotopic liver transplantation. With the more recent evidence on gastrointestinal hemorrhage and emergency variceal sclerotherapy, we now also recommend that these patients be given norfloxacin as soon as possible after the hemorrhage begins, and this therapy should be continued empirically for at least 1 week. The role of prophylactic antibiotic therapy in other situations is at present unknown, and recommendations cannot as yet be made confidently on the basis of any published data. Only one randomized trial addressing the usage of prophylactic antibiotics in patients undergoing chronic sclerotherapy has been published.[92] There was no apparent benefit in the group receiving antibiotics compared with the placebo group. We do, however, use diuretics as the first line of therapy to treat ascites and reserve large-volume paracentesis for patients who are refractory to diuretics or who have respiratory embarrassment. Our rationale is that this may theoretically aid in further protecting these patients from SBP by increasing ascitic fluid opsonic activity.

FUTURE DIRECTIONS

A rodent model that develops cirrhosis and ascites was described in 1991.[93] Approximately 50% of these animals develop SBP. The SBP in these rats is impressively similar to that observed in humans in that the ascitic fluid PMN count rises and cultures become positive; *E. coli* is the most common organism, and bacterascites resolves spontaneously, as it does in humans. This model should allow a unique opportunity to study further both the pathogenesis of SBP and the potential benefit of important therapeutic modalities. Insight into the relationship between gastrointestinal hemorrhage and SBP and studies on the effect and importance of complement, the translocation of enteric organisms, the effect of prophylactic antibiotic therapy on survival and stool flora, and the utility of other strategies should be possible with this model and will provide important information that we hope will allow us to improve the outlook for patients with SBP and advanced liver disease.

REFERENCES

1. Conn HO. Spontaneous peritonitis with bacteremia in Laënnec's cirrhosis caused by enteric organisms. Ann Intern Med. 1964;60:568–580.
2. Thomas FB, Fromkes JJ. Spontaneous bacterial peritonitis associated with acute viral hepatitis. J Clin Gastroenterol. 1982;4:259–262.
3. Barness LA, Moll GH, Janeway CA. Nephrotic syndrome: I, Natural history of the disease. Pediatrics. 1950;5:486–503.
4. Runyon BA. Spontaneous bacterial peritonitis associated with cardiac ascites. Am J Gastroenterol. 1984;79:796.
5. Runyon BA. Low-protein concentration ascitic fluid is predisposed to spontaneous bacterial peritonitis. Gastroenterology. 1986;91:1343–1346.
6. Pinzello G, Simonetti RG, Craxi A, et al. Spontaneous bacterial peritonitis: A prospective investigation in predominantly nonalcoholic cirrhotic patients. Hepatology. 1983;3:545–549.
7. Almdal TP, Skinhoj P. Spontaneous bacterial peritonitis in cirrhosis: Incidence, diagnosis and prognosis. Scand J Gastroenterol. 1987;22:295–300.
8. Felisart J, Rimola A, Arroyo V, et al. Cefotaxime is more effective than is ampicillin-tobramycin in cirrhotics with severe infections. Hepatology. 1985;5:457–462.
9. Cabrera J, Arroyo V, Ballestra AM, et al. Aminoglycoside nephrotoxicity in cirrhosis: Value of urinary B2-microglobulin to discriminate functional renal failure from acute tubular damage. Gastroenterology. 1982;82:97–105.
10. Tito L, Rimola A, Gines P, et al. Recurrence of spontaneous bacterial peritonitis in cirrhosis: Frequency and predictive factors. Hepatology. 1988;8:27–31.
11. Runyon BA. Spontaneous bacterial peritonitis: An explosion of information. Hepatology. 1988;8:171–175. Editorial.
12. Runyon BA, McHutchison JG, Antillon MR, et al. Short-course versus long-course antibiotic treatment of spontaneous bacterial peritonitis: A randomized controlled study of 100 patients. Gastroenterology. 1991;100:1737–1742.
13. Boyer TD, Kahn AM, Reynolds TB. Diagnostic value of ascitic fluid lactate dehydrogenase, protein and WBC levels. Arch Intern Med. 1978;138:1103–1105.
14. Runyon BA, Hoefs JC. Culture-negative neutrocytic ascites: A variant of spontaneous bacterial peritonitis. Hepatology. 1984;4:1209–1211.
15. Runyon BA, Umland ET, Merlin T. Inoculation of blood culture bottles with ascitic fluid: Improved detection of spontaneous bacterial peritonitis. Arch Intern Med. 1987;147:73–75.
16. Runyon BA, Canawati HN, Akriviadis EA. Optimization of ascitic fluid culture technique. Gastroenterology. 1988;95:1351–1355.
17. Runyon BA, Canawati HN, Hoefs JC. Polymicrobial bacterascites: A unique entity in the spectrum of infected ascitic fluid. Arch Intern Med. 1986;146:2173–2175.
18. Rimola A, Soto R, Bory F, et al. Reticuloendothelial system phagocytic activity in cirrhosis and its relationship to bacterial infections and prognosis. Hepatology. 1984;4:53–58.
19. Wyke RJ. Problems of bacterial infection in patients with liver disease. Gut. 1987;28:623–641.
20. Barnes PF, Arevalo C, Chan L, et al. A prospective evaluation of bacteremic patients with chronic liver disease. Hepatology. 1988;8:1099–1103.
21. Fox RA, Dudley FS, Sherlock S. The serum concentrations of the third component of complement in liver disease. Gut. 1971;12:574–578.
22. Kourlisky O, LeRoy C, Peltier AP. Complement and liver cell function in 53 patients with liver disease. Am J Med. 1973;55:783–790.
23. Rajkovic IA, Williams R. Abnormalities of neutrophil phagocytosis, intracellular killing, and metabolic activity in alcoholic cirrhosis and hepatitis. Hepatology. 1986;6:252–262.
24. Hassner A, Kletter Y, Schlag D, et al. Impaired monocyte function in cirrhosis. Br Med J. 1981;282:1262–1263.
25. Mellencamp MA, Preheim LC. Effect of cirrhosis on bacteremia and capsular antigenemia during experimental pneumococcal pneumonia. Proceedings of the 26th Interscience Conference on Antimicrobial Agents and Chemotherapy; 1986:283. Abstract.
26. Schweinburg FB, Seligman AM, Fine J. Transmural migration of intestinal bacteria: A study based on the use of radioactive Escherichia coli. N Engl J Med. 1950;242:747–751.
27. Runyon BA, Squier SU. Translocation of gut bacteria of cirrhotic rats to mesenteric lymph nodes may partially explain the pathogenesis of spontaneous bacterial peritonitis. Hepatology. 1991;14:91A. Abstract.
28. Hamdani R, Chaparala R, Stauber RE, et al. PEG 600 absorption and urinary excretion identify cirrhotics likely to die during hospitalization. Hepatology. 1991;14:245A.
29. Hoefs JC, Runyon BA. Spontaneous bacterial peritonitis. Disease-a-Month. 1985;31:1–48.
30. Runyon BA, Hoefs JC. Ascitic fluid analysis in the differentiation of spontaneous bacterial peritonitis from gastrointestinal tract perforation into ascitic fluid. Hepatology. 1984;4:447–450.
31. Hoefs JC, Canawati HN, Sapico FL, et al. Spontaneous bacterial peritonitis. Hepatology. 1982;2:399–407.
32. Bar-Mier S, Lerner E, Conn HO. Analysis of ascitic fluid in cirrhosis. Dig Dis Sci. 1979;24:136–144.
33. Young L, Martin B, Meyer R, et al. Gram-negative rod bacteremia: Microbiologic, immunologic and therapeutic considerations. Ann Intern Med. 1977;86:456–471.
34. Runyon BA, Morrissey RL, Hoefs JC, et al. Opsonic activity of human ascitic fluid: A potentially important protective mechanism against spontaneous bacterial peritonitis. Hepatology. 1985;5:634–637.
35. Runyon BA. Patients with deficient ascitic fluid opsonic activity are predisposed to spontaneous bacterial peritonitis. Hepatology. 1988;8:632–635.
36. Correia JP, Conn HO. Spontaneous bacterial peritonitis in cirrhosis: Endemic or epidemic? Med Clin North Am. 1975;59:963–981.
37. Runyon BA. Monomicrobial nonneutrocytic bacterascites: A variant of spontaneous bacterial peritonitis. Hepatology. 1990;12:710–715.
38. Pelletier G, Lesur G, Ink O, et al. Asymptomatic bacterascites: Is it spontaneous bacterial peritonitis? Hepatology. 1991;14:112–115.

39. Gines P, Rimola A, Planas R, et al. Norfloxacin prevents spontaneous bacterial peritonitis in cirrhosis: Results of a double-blind placebo-controlled trial. Hepatology. 1990;12:716–724.

40. Wang SS, Tsai YT, Lee SD, et al. Spontaneous bacterial peritonitis in patients with hepatitis-B–related cirrhosis and hepatocellular carcinoma. Gastroenterology. 1991;101:1656–1662.

41. Weinstein MP, Iannini PB, Stratton CW, et al. Spontaneous bacterial peritonitis: A review of 28 cases with emphasis on improved survival and factors influencing prognosis. Am J Med. 1978;64:592–598.

42. Conn HO, Fessell JM. Spontaneous bacterial peritonitis in cirrhosis: Variations on a theme. Medicine. 1971; 50:161–197.

43. Garcia-Tsao G, Conn HO, Lerner E. The diagnosis of bacterial peritonitis: Comparison of pH, lactate concentration and leukocyte count. Hepatology. 1985;5:91–96.

44. Attali P, Turner K, Pelletier G, et al. pH of ascitic fluid: Diagnostic and prognostic value in cirrhotic and noncirrhotic patients. Gastroenterology. 1986;90:1255–1265.

45. Yang CY, Liaw YF, Chu CM, et al. White count, pH and lactate in ascites in the diagnosis of spontaneous bacterial peritonitis. Hepatology. 1985;5:85–90.

46. Kammerer J, Taleb M, Dupeyron C. Peritonites bacteriennes spontanées du cirrhotique: à propos de 26 episodes. Gastroenterol Clin Biol. 1979;3:709–718.

47. Grange JD, Amiot X, Grange V, et al. Amoxicillin–clavulanic acid therapy of spontaneous bacterial peritonitis: A prospective study of 27 cases in cirrhotic patients. Hepatology. 1990;11:360–364.

48. Ariza J, Xiol X, Esteve M. Aztreonam vs. cefotaxime in the treatment of gram-negative spontaneous peritonitis in cirrhotic patients. Hepatology. 1991;14:91–98.

49. Kline MM, McCallum RW, Guth PH. The clinical value of ascitic fluid culture and leukocyte count studies in alcoholic cirrhosis. Gastroenterology. 1976;70:408–412.

50. Cummings D, Hoefs JC, Runyon BA, et al. Determinants of the outcome of spontaneous bacterial peritonitis: Multivariate discriminant analysis of prognostic factors. Hepatology. 1984;4:1071. Abstract.

51. Xiol X, Castellote J, Baliellas C, et al. Spontaneous bacterial empyema in cirrhotic patients: Analysis of 11 cases. Hepatology. 1990;11:365–370.

52. Lieberman FL, Hidemura R, Peters RL, et al. Pathogenesis and treatment of hydrothorax complicating cirrhosis with ascites. Ann Intern Med. 1966;64:341–345.

53. Rimola A, Bory F, Teres J, et al. Oral nonabsorbable antibiotics prevent infection in cirrhosis with gastrointestinal hemorrhage. Hepatology. 1985;5:463–467.

54. Ho H, Zuckerman MJ, Wassen C. A prospective controlled study of the risk of bacteremia in emergency sclerotherapy of esophageal varices. Gastroenterology. 1991;101:1642–1648.

55. Schuman BM, Beckman JW, Tedesco FJ, et al. Complications of endoscopic injection sclerotherapy: A review. Am J Gastroenterol. 1987;82:823–830.

56. Tam F, Chow H, Prindiville T, et al. Bacterial peritonitis following esophageal injection sclerotherapy for variceal hemorrhage. Gastrointest Endosc. 1990;36:131–133.

57. Shorvon PJ, Eykyn SJ, Cotton PB. Gastrointestinal instrumentation, bacteremia and endocarditis. Gut. 1983;24:1078–1093.

58. Soriano G, Guarner C, Tomas A, et al. Norfloxacin prevents bacterial infections in cirrhotics with gastrointestinal hemorrhage: Final results. Hepatology. 1991; 14:85A. Abstract.

59. Rhodes RS, Depalma RG, Robinson AV. Intestinal barrier function in hemorrhagic shock. J Surg Res. 1973;14:305–312.

60. Pardy BJ, Spencer RC, Dudley HAF. Hepatic reticuloendothelial protection against bacteremia in experimental hemorrhagic shock. Surgery. 1971;81:193–197.

61. Mallory A, Schaefer JW. Complications of diagnostic paracentesis in patients with liver disease. JAMA. 1978;239:628–630.

62. Hoefs JC. Increase in ascites WBC and protein concentrations during diuresis in patients with chronic liver disease. Hepatology. 1981;1:249–254.

63. Runyon BA, Hoefs JC. Ascitic fluid analysis before, during and after spontaneous bacterial peritonitis. Hepatology. 1985;5:257–259.

64. Runyon BA, Van Epps DE. Diuresis of cirrhotic ascites increases its opsonic activity and may help prevent spontaneous bacterial peritonitis. Hepatology. 1986;6:396–399.

65. Castellote J, Xiol X, Verdaguer R, et al. Comparison of two ascitic fluid culture methods in cirrhotic patients with spontaneous bacterial peritonitis. Am J Gastroenterol. 1990;85:1605–1608.

66. Runyon BA, Antillon MR, Akriviadis EA, et al. Bedside inoculation of blood culture bottles with ascitic fluid is superior to delayed inoculation in the detection of spontaneous bacterial peritonitis. J Clin Microbiol. 1990;28:2811–2812.

67. Akriviadis EA, Runyon BA. Utility of an algorithm in differentiating spontaneous from secondary peritonitis. Gastroenterology. 1990;98:127–133.

68. Lindsay KL, Canawati HN. Spontaneous *Arizona hinshawii* peritonitis in cirrhosis with ascites. Gastroenterology. 1981;81:349–351.

69. Garcia V, Vidal F, Toda R, et al. Spontaneous bacterial peritonitis due to *Salmonella enteritidis* in cirrhotic ascites. J Clin Gastroenterol. 1990;12:663–666.

70. Woolf GM, Runyon BA. Spontaneous *Salmonella* infection of high-protein noncirrhotic ascites. J Clin Gastroenterol. 1990;12:430–432.

71. Brook I, Altman RS, Loebman WW, et al. Measurement of lactate in ascitic fluid: An aid in the diagnosis of peritonitis with particular relevance to spontaneous bacterial peritonitis of the cirrhotic. Dig Dis Sci. 1981;26:1089–1094.

72. Gitlin N, Stauffer JL, Silvestri RC. The pH of ascitic fluid in the diagnosis of spontaneous bacterial peritonitis in alcoholic cirrhosis. Hepatology. 1982;2:408–411.

73. Scemamma-Clergue JL, Doutrellot-Phillippon C, Metreau J-M, et al. Ascitic fluid pH in alcoholic cirrhosis: A reevaluation of its use in the diagnosis of spontaneous bacterial peritonitis. Gut. 1985;26:332–335.

74. Pinzello G, Virdone R, Lojacono F, et al. Is the acidity of ascitic fluid a reliable index in making the presumptive diagnosis of spontaneous bacterial peritonitis? Hepatology. 1986;6:244–247.

75. Stassen WN, McCullough AJ, Bacon BR, et al. Immediate diagnostic criteria for bacterial infection of ascitic fluid: Evaluation of ascitic fluid polymorphonuclear leukocyte count, pH and lactate concentration, alone and in combination. Gastroenterology. 1986;90:1247–1254.

76. Runyon BA, Antillon MR. Ascitic fluid pH and lactate: Insensitive and nonspecific tests in detecting ascitic fluid infection. Hepatology. 1991;13:929–935.

77. Albillos A, Cuervas-Mons V, Millan I, et al. Ascitic fluid polymorphonuclear cell count and serum to ascites albumin gradient in the diagnosis of spontaneous bacterial peritonitis. Gastroenterology. 1990;98:134–140.

78. Runyon BA. Bacterial peritonitis secondary to a perinephric abscess. Case report and differentiation from spontaneous bacterial peritonitis. Am J Med. 1986;80:997–998.

79. Runyon BA, Hoefs JC. Spontaneous versus secondary bacterial peritonitis. Differentiation by response of asci-

tic fluid neutrophil count to antimicrobial therapy. Arch Intern Med. 1986; 146:1563–1565.

80. Runyon BA. Ascitic fluid bilirubin concentration as a key to chyloperitoneum. J Clin Gastroenterol. 1987;9:543–545.

81. Gill MA, Kern JW. Altered gentamicin distribution in ascites patients. Am J Hosp Pharm. 1979;36:1704–1706.

82. Moore RD, Smith CR, Lietman PS. Increased risk of renal dysfunction due to interaction of liver disease and aminoglycosides. Am J Med. 1986;80:1093–1097.

83. Cherubin CE, Marr JS, Sierra MF, et al. *Listeria* and gram-negative bacillary meningitis. Am J Med. 1981;71:199–209.

84. McNamara PJ, Trueb V, Stoeckel K. Protein binding of ceftriaxone in extravascular fluids. J Pharm Sci. 1988;77:401–404.

85. Mercader J, Gomez J, Ruiz J, et al. Use of ceftriaxone in the treatment of bacterial infection in cirrhotic patients. Chemotherapy. 1989;35:23–26.

86. Van Gossum A, Quernon M, Van Gossum M, et al. Penetration of cefoperazone into ascites. Eur J Clin Pharmacol. 1989;37:577–580.

87. Fong T-L, Akriviadis EA, Runyon BA, et al. Polymorpho-

nuclear cell count response and duration of antibiotic therapy in spontaneous bacterial peritonitis. Hepatology. 1989;9:423–426.

88. Nord CE. Effect of new quinolones on human gastrointestinal microflora. Rev Infect Dis. 1988;10(suppl 1):S193–S196.

89. Karp JE, William GM, Hendrickson C, et al. Oral norfloxacin for prevention of gram-negative bacterial infections in patients with acute leukemia and granulocytopenia. Ann Intern Med. 1987;106:1–7.

90. Soriano G, Guarner C, Teixido M, et al. Selective intestinal decontamination prevents spontaneous bacterial peritonitis. Gastroenterology. 1991;100:477–481.

91. Such J, Guarner C, Soriano G, et al. Selective intestinal decontamination increases serum and ascitic fluid C3 levels in cirrhosis. Hepatology. 1990;12:1175–1178.

92. Rolando N, Gimson A, Sahathevan M, et al. Imipenem prophylaxis of infectious sequelae after sclerotherapy in cirrhotic patients with bleeding oesophageal varices. J Hepatol. 1991;13:S65.

93. Runyon BA, Sugano S, Kanel G, et al. A rodent model of cirrhosis, ascites and bacterial peritonitis. Gastroenterology. 1991;100:489–493.

5

Approaches to Gastrointestinal Infection Syndromes

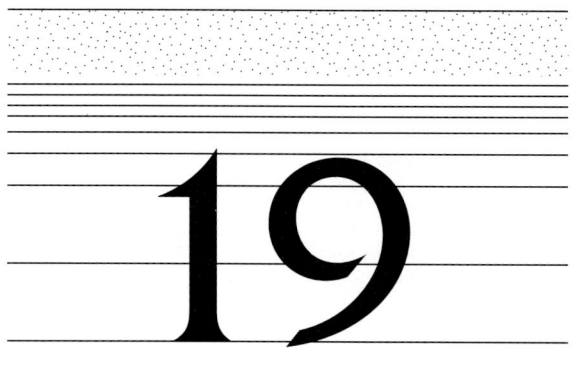

Laboratory Performance in the Diagnosis of Gastrointestinal Infections

PAUL E. STEELE, M.D.

CECILIA FENOGLIO-PREISER, M.D.

Optimal care for the patient with a suspected gastrointestinal infection depends upon an understanding of the role the laboratory can play in the diagnosis, including an appreciation of the performance quality of the laboratory in various settings. Clinicians may regard different types of laboratory results with the same degree of confidence, when in fact, substantial differences in precision, accuracy, and reproducibility may exist among them.

Laboratorians are responsible for overseeing a comprehensive quality assurance program that is designed to improve patient care by improving all aspects of specimen testing. The targets of quality assurance monitors certainly include laboratory analysis itself but also include a wide variety of pre- and postanalytic steps, ranging from test use, patient preparation, and specimen collection and transport to result reporting, medical record charting, and physician response.

This chapter emphasizes laboratory performance as it relates to analysis of specimens, but the pre- and postanalytic sources of error should not be underestimated as causes for suboptimal patient care. A variety of laboratory test methods are discussed with respect to the identification of causal agents in gastrointestinal infections: direct microscopy, culture, immunoassay, nucleic acid hybridization, and polymerase chain reaction (PCR). Examples are drawn from assay performance data on the identification of *Cryptosporidium* species, *Helicobacter pylori*, and rotavirus by laboratory methods.

DIRECT MICROSCOPY

Direct microscopy is a fundamental laboratory method that continues to provide challenges to laboratorians with respect to sensitivity and specificity. The difficulties associated with direct microscopy extend far beyond the usual concerns of reagent performance, instrument integrity, and methodologic accuracy. More than most laboratory methods, direct micros-

TABLE 19–1. COLLEGE OF AMERICAN PATHOLOGISTS SURVEYS RELATING TO GASTROINTESTINAL AND HEPATIC INFECTIONS

CLINICAL MICROBIOLOGY	SURGICAL PATHOLOGY
Parasitology	Lesions
Fecal suspension for wet mount	Colon
Slides for permanent stains	Liver
Bacteriology	Intestine
Bacterial identification	In situ hybridization
Gram stain	
Antimicrobial susceptibility testing	
Virology culture	**CLINICAL CHEMISTRY**
Virology: Antigen detection	ALT/SGPT
Virology: Antibody detection	AST/SGOT
Viral markers	Bilirubin
Hepatitis A, B, C markers	Total
Delta hepatitis antibody	Direct
CMV antibody	Lactate dehydrogenase
Virology: Western blot	LD isozymes

KEY: ALT/SGPT = alanine aminotransferase (formerly called serum glutamate pyruvate transaminase), AST/SGOT = aspartate aminotransferase (formerly called serum glutamic-oxaloacetic transaminase), LD = lactate dehydrogenase.

copy is critically dependent on operator experience and skill.

Individual laboratories may gauge their performance of laboratory tests, including direct microscopy, by participation in external proficiency testing programs, the largest of which are conducted by the College of American Pathologists (CAP). Table 19–1 lists CAP surveys that relate to the diagnosis of gastrointestinal and hepatic infections. Unidentified samples are submitted to participating laboratories as well as to referee laboratories whose expertise places them among the highest performing laboratories. CAP Microbiology Surveys offer laboratories the opportunity to select combinations of surveys most appropriate for the scope of microbiology testing performed. The laboratories receive individualized evaluations and an all-participant summary, which allows them to compare their results with those of other participating laboratories. In this way, an individual laboratory can determine whether it is performing at a comparable level.

Cryptosporidium

The identification of *Cryptosporidium* species is one of the laboratory skills surveyed by the CAP. These organisms may be visualized by modified acid-fast staining of intestinal biopsies,[1] but more commonly they are sought after by examination of stool. The organism is 3 to 6 μm in length and appears as a densely red-stained body with darker blue or brownish internal bodies seen, after acid-fast staining, with a modified Ziehl-Neelsen technique.[2] Some are lighter stained, perhaps representing a different life cycle stage.

The difficulty with the use of modified acid-fast staining for CAP Survey participating laboratories has been, in part, the incorrect identification of acid-fast fecal debris as *Cryptosporidium*. For instance, in a 1989 survey, a slide containing no parasites was submitted to participating laboratories with the request to identify using routine as well as *Cryptosporidium*-specific stains. One of 15 referee laboratories, 15% of laboratories that render definitive diagnoses or prepare permanent sections for referral, and 36% of laboratories that recognize the presence of parasites but may refer the slide to a reference laboratory for identification, mistakenly identified fecal debris as *Cryptosporidium*.* A similar problem had been seen in a 1987 CAP Survey, in which approximately one fifth of participants incorrectly reported the presence of *Cryptosporidium*.

The problem of false-positive identification of *Cryptosporidium* again appeared in a 1990 CAP Survey in which a slide containing *Isospora belli* oocysts was submitted. Since it is unlikely that *I. belli* would be mistaken for *Cryptosporidium*, the presence of acid-fast fecal artifacts could again be blamed for the false-positive results. In the following year, still another CAP Survey produced a substantial percentage of false-positives from participants asked to evaluate a slide that did not contain parasites; 6% (1/16) of referee laboratories, 16% (382/2349) of more sophisti-

---

*The results of the Surveys program are published and copyrighted publications of the College of American Pathologists and are referenced in this manuscript with the permission of the College.

cated laboratories, and 18% (89/484) of less sophisticated laboratories made the incorrect identification of *Cryptosporidium*.

Another source of false-positive findings is coccidia-like organisms associated with self-limited traveler's diarrhea, in which 8- to 9-μm organisms that stain red with modified acid-fast staining are encountered.[3]

In intestinal biopsies, the cryptosporidia appear as spherical bodies attached to the microvillus border of the small bowel[4, 5] or to the surface of epithelial cells in the colon. Especially in the specimens of epithelial cells, apical blebbing of the cells or mucin droplets may be mistaken for organisms.[5]

How well do laboratories identify an organism when it is, in fact, present? Again, the best source of information is the CAP Surveys. In Surveys from 1989 and 1990, correct recognition of the presence of *Cryptosporidium* oocysts was made by 100% of referee laboratories in both years, 86% and 95% of laboratories that render definitive identifications, 74% and 83% of laboratories that refer some slides for definitive identification, and 50% and 74% of laboratories that are expected to identify the presence of a parasite for each of the 2 years, respectively. The improvement in the percentage of correct responses among the participating laboratories from 1989 to 1990 may very well be the result of the CAP Survey process itself, through which laboratories endeavor to learn from their past errors.

The percentage of assays that are correctly performed by a laboratory in response to survey questionnaires obviously relates to the sensitivity of that assay as carried out by that particular laboratory, but it does not define the sensitivity of the test. Ideally, all laboratories would correctly note the presence of a parasite that is in fact present within the submitted specimen. The sensitivity of staining methods for the identification of *Cryptosporidium* is difficult to ascertain. Examination of results obtained on specimens from patients involved in outbreaks may lead to the best approximation of the sensitivity. In one outbreak involving 44 of 60 swimmers (73%) from five different groups using a pool in Los Angeles, *Cryptosporidium* was identified in 5 of 8 stool specimens (63%) examined with auramine O staining as a screen and confirmed by modified acid-fast staining.[6] In another outbreak, involving 20 of 59 children (34%) attending a daycare center in Philadelphia, 11 of 17 symptomatic children (65%) and 3 of 28 asymptomatic children (11%) had positive findings on stool samples using both phase-contrast and brightfield microscopy.[7] A much lower sensitivity was reported during a large outbreak involving two daycare centers when 703 stool examinations were performed using two different concentrating techniques. Of specimens prepared with Ritchie formalin-ethyl acetate sedimentation of 10% formalin-fixed samples, 129 were positive (18%), a finding similar to the 127 positive specimens (18%) prepared with Sheather sucrose flotation, giving an overall sensitivity of 23% (161 of 703).[8]

What improvements could be made in laboratory performance of *Cryptosporidium* identification? Education of laboratory workers is a key component of improvement, since this identification, and indeed all direct microscopy assays, is dependent on the skill and experience of the laboratorian. Questionnaires from the CAP in 1989 and 1990 revealed that approximately 40% of participating laboratories had fewer than 10 requests per year for *Cryptosporidium* identification and 33 to 36% had fewer than 50 such requests. Furthermore, the incidence of positive results was low, with most laboratories having no or fewer than 1% positive findings and only 3% of respondents reporting more than 5% positivity.

Given both this low rate of positive findings in specimens and the existence of acid-fast artifacts, a reasonable approach to improving the accuracy of *Cryptosporidium* identification is to incorporate the use of monoclonal antibodies in an indirect immunofluorescence assay. Garcia and coworkers adopted this approach and found that the immunofluorescence assay is more sensitive, in that fluorescent antibody-positive, acid-fast–negative cases were shown to be acid-fast–positive after additional slides had been prepared, and faster than conventional methods.[9] Only 17% of respondents to the 1990 CAP questionnaire reported using immunofluorescence to detect *Cryptosporidium*.

The importance of accurate *Cryptosporidium* identification will increase as the infection assumes more importance in human populations. The 1989 and 1990 CAP questionnaires revealed that 64% of positive results were encountered in AIDS patients, a growing population. Nonimmunocompromised children (16–20% of positive findings) form another important patient group with positive results. In a 1991 report from South Africa, 289 of 6870 specimens (4%) collected since 1985 were positive for *Cryptosporidium*, mostly from children younger than the age of 3, and cryptosporidiosis has replaced giardiasis as the most commonly encountered parasitic infection in the hospitalized population.[10]

Helicobacter pylori

Although microscopy of silver-stained gastric sections had revealed the presence of spiral bacteria many decades before,[11, 12] interest in these organisms as a cause of active chronic gastritis was stimulated in 1983 by a report that linked the two, noting that inflammatory cells appeared to be associated with the presence of the bacteria.[13] This microscopy observation led to attempts to cultivate the organism, which was shown to be microaerophilic.[14]

Originally called *Campylobacter pylori*, its name was changed to *Helicobacter pylori* in recognition of its differences from *Campylobacter* species. Laboratory testing for this organism, unlike testing for typical enteric bacteria, has emphasized microscopy, since the relatively unique appearance of the organism and the paucity of other gastric bacteria make microscopy one of the most sensitive techniques for its detection.[15–19]

The Warthin-Starry silver impregnation stain, which is difficult technically to perform, has been one of the major assays in direct microscopy of *H. pylori*. Although many laboratories have switched to a modified Giemsa stain as a reliable and easier staining method,[20] others believe that the Warthin-Starry is superior for quantification.[17] Large numbers of organisms can be seen on routine hemotoxylin and eosin (H & E) stains. Microscopy of smears from gastric biopsies can also be performed with the use of Gram staining or Papanicolaou staining.[21]

Laboratory performance in the identification of *H. pylori* has not been surveyed by organizations such as CAP, but the reported experience of a number of clinical microbiology laboratories is available to predict some issues of laboratory performance and quality assurance that arise with this identification. For example, culture may be unsuccessful if transport time to the laboratory or specimen processing is delayed longer than 2 hours.[16] Other preanalytic sources of error exist and may not be obvious; for example, the use of benzocaine rather than lidocaine as a topical anesthetic prior to endoscopy is said to be inhibitory to cultivation.[15] Since the organism is sensitive to high concentrations of oxygen and to desiccation, proper transport and handling are important.[16]

The problems associated with culture have resulted in the use of direct microscopy as well as culture to define true-positive results in method comparison studies. The sensitivity of microscopy is difficult to ascertain, but it appears to be fairly high, approximately 90%, for histologic staining[15, 19] and smear staining.[17–19, 22] This sensitivity may be optimal, given that the investigators reporting the data obviously would have made a concerted attempt to identify all positives. Small numbers of organisms can be overlooked, however, even in the context of one of these studies,[17] so it seems likely that the diligence and motivation of the microscopist would have an effect on sensitivity in routine clinical laboratory testing of this type.

A supplemental, rapid test to evaluate gastric biopsies for the presence of *H. pylori* is the urease test. Taking advantage of the high urease expression by these organisms, this test consists of incubating a crushed portion of the gastric biopsy in broth that contains phenol red as a pH indicator. The production of ammonium ions raises the pH and produces a yellowish brown-to-pink color change. Crushing of the biopsy is said by one group of investigators to be an important factor in avoiding false-negatives[23]; this group has achieved a higher level of sensitivity with this test (96%)[24] than have other groups (62–74%),[16, 18, 19] suggesting that laboratory technique, processing, transport, and other factors may be important.

Another auxiliary test that does not involve endoscopy is the breath test in which labeled urea is ingested and labeled carbon dioxide is measured in exhaled breath samples. The label can be either ^{13}C-urea, which is expensive and requires gas-isotope ratio mass spectrometry,[25, 26] or ^{14}C-urea, which is less expensive but results in radioisotope exposure of the patient.[27]

The high urease expression by *H. pylori* and its relative infrequency in the gastric mucosa produce high specificities for each of these urease tests (above 80% and as high as 100%). Whether this level of specificity characterizes routine clinical use of the tests remains in question.

Specificity of the microscopic identification of spiral bacteria in gastric biopsies or biopsy smears is considered high for *H. pylori*, but another spiral organism has also been observed in the gastric mucosa, if infrequently, with one study reporting that 6 of 1650 patients studied (0.4%) were positive.[28] An immunocytochemical stain has been described for *H. pylori* and could be used if the specificity of the microscopic identification were in question.[29]

Rotavirus

Electron microscopy (EM) provided the first evidence for the existence of rotavirus, which was seen in duodenal biopsies of children with acute nonbacterial gastroenteritis.[30] Further EM studies of feces from such patients revealed the presence of the distinctive viral particles; their association with patients younger than 6 years was also noted.[31] Although not available in many institutions, EM has become a laboratory standard for early assays of this agent since it offers speed, simplicity, and the possibility of morphologic confirmation.[32]

The integrity of the viral particles depends upon the staining method used. For example, the use of phosphotungstic acid (PTA) above pH 5 for 10 seconds or longer is associated with degradation of the specimen from characteristic double-shelled particles to single-shelled particles[33]; the use of PTA at pH values between 5.5 and 7.2 is common in published studies.[33] The use of uranyl acetate at an unadjusted pH of 4.3 or PTA at pH 4.5 has been recommended, with a preference for PTA for immune electron microscopy (IEM) when resolution of bound antibody is important.[33]

Other variables, including operator skill and perseverance, affect the sensitivity and reliability of the direct EM staining approach.[34] In one study, the percentage of positive EM results obtained at various microscopy reading time intervals increased from approximately 50% at 30 seconds to approximately 95% at 6 minutes.[35] The same authors found that rectal swabs were much inferior to stool specimens for direct EM studies; in some cases, microscopic searches of 30 minutes or longer were required to identify virus in specimens that were found positive by other assays.

Immune electron microscopy, which can include a solid-phase technique in which antibody-coated microscope grids are used, is described as a more sensitive technique than direct EM,[34] although as a practical method for clinical testing during outbreaks of rotavirus infection it may not be clearly superior to direct EM, which has the advantages of speed and simplicity.[35] Also, the specificity of the antibody used in IEM could limit the specificity of the test, whereas direct EM has the advantage that a variety of agents, including diverse serotypes of rotavirus as well as adenovirus and other viruses, could be visualized.[35]

An auxiliary test for rotavirus, polyacrylamide gel electrophoresis of viral genomic ribonucleic acid (RNA) obtained directly from stool samples, has been described.[36–41] In addition to providing useful epidemiologic data, these analyses have provided a glimpse at the sensitivity of the reference method EM, yielding a relative sensitivity of 95% in one study[41] and 83% in another.[39] Like EM, genome analysis by RNA electrophoresis is considered 100% specific since the band patterns produced are highly characteristic. Since false-positive results are not expected, the method is capable of detecting false-negative EM results. This method is unlikely to become popular in clinical laboratories, given the availability of the cheaper, faster, and easier enzyme-linked immunoassay (EIA). Assay results by EIA also suggest that EM is less sensitive than EIA, although the possibility of false-positives with EIA tempers this interpretation.

ENZYME IMMUNOASSAY

The EIAs are regarded as highly sensitive and specific laboratory assays. Ideally, when laboratory workers perform the assay exactly according to the manufacturer's directions, operator influence is minimal. In most cases, this appears to be true. For example, recent interlaboratory Surveys conducted by CAP have shown that the degree of agreement on the presence or absence of hepatitis B surface antigen or of antibody to human immunodeficiency virus (HIV) in survey samples examined by hundreds of participating laboratories often exceeds 99% and can be 100%.

Nevertheless, operator-dependent variation due to such factors as timing of incubation and washing steps can occur with EIAs. The speed of pipetting reagents can vary when varying numbers of samples are being tested, especially when a large number of specimens is involved. Operators vary with regard to manual dexterity and speed of pipetting, adequacy of reagent mixing, washing technique, and so forth. In addition, the assays themselves are subject to false-positives and false-negatives, depending upon the specificity and sensitivity of the antibody reagents used, the presence of interfering or cross-reacting substances within the sample, and the sensitivity of the detection scheme. The highly reproducible, sensitive, and specific assays mentioned earlier tend to be second-, third-, or fourth-generation assays that have been extensively refined. Using the three gastrointestinal infections already discussed, a review of the performance of EIAs in their identification follows.

Cryptosporidium Species

The use of immunoassays to detect *Cryptosporidium* antigen is still clearly in its developmental stages. In one report, sonicated oocysts were used to produce a rabbit polyclonal antiserum that was used in an enzyme-linked immunosorbent assay (ELISA).[42] Using two separate positive microscopic examinations as the reference method, the sensitivity of the ELISA was found to be 82.3% and the specificity 96.7%. The false-positive ELISAs were on patients with previously documented *Cryptosporidium* infections, so the ELISA may, in some instances, have greater sensitivity than a microscopic exam; the clinical relevance of such antigen persistence has not been explored. The cause of the false-negative ELISAs is unknown but could involve antigenic differences or technical factors such as specimen freeze-thaw artifact.[42]

The use of a monoclonal antibody to capture oocysts in investigations of bovine infection by *Cryptosporidium parvum* revealed a sensitivity of 3×10^5 oocysts per ml of feces, a level near the lower limit of organism density found in calves with clinical disease.[43] This ELISA was approximately 3 times more sensitive than is acid-fast staining, but half as sensitive as indirect immunofluorescence.[43]

Improvements in the sensitivity and specificity of ELISA testing for *Cryptosporidium* antigen can be expected, and it is likely that such an assay may find its way into clinical laboratories given the labor intensiveness and difficulty associated with microscopic identification.

Helicobacter pylori

The use of antibody reagents in the laboratory diagnosis of *H. pylori* has been confined to the immunocytochemical staining previously mentioned[29] and to serologic testing. Serologic testing is appealing because of its noninvasive nature.

The investigation of children with chronic abdominal pain has produced promising results in two reports. In a study of 60 children, 8 patients (13%) had evidence of *H. pylori* infection by microscopy, culture, or urease testing of an antral biopsy. The sensitivity of immunoglobulin G (IgG) and immunoglobulin A (IgA) antibodies in this group of 8 patients was 7 patients (87%) and 6 patients (75%), respectively, with specificities of 96% and 100%, respectively.[44] In a study of 100 children, 20 had positive findings by biopsy culture or modified Giemsa stain; all had elevated *H. pylori*–specific IgG levels, as did 2 additional patients with histopathologic changes characteristic of *H. pylori* disease.[45] In contrast to the first study, a lack of correlation between IgA levels and disease existed.

The usefulness of serodiagnosis in adults is less clear, since an age-related increase in the prevalence of antibodies occurs, reaching 50%

in persons older than 60 years.[46] Furthermore, the antibody appears to persist in patients who have been treated,[47] eliminating its usefulness in monitoring therapy. In one study, however, further investigation of false-positive IgG and IgA serologic findings by review of biopsy histologic examination revealed instances in which small numbers of *H. pylori* organisms originally overlooked in the initial biopsy were then detected.[17]

Given the prevalence of gastritis and ulcer disease in the population, it seems likely that EIAs will assume a greater role in the diagnosis and monitoring of patients with *H. pylori* infections. Technologic improvements may include the preparation of pure, specific antigens, rather than disrupted whole-cell preparations, and the development of an antigen assay.

Rotavirus

Of the three gastrointestinal infections used as examples in this chapter, rotavirus infections have received by far the greatest attention with respect to EIA development and refinement. The difficulty with growing this virus in tissue culture, its prevalence in neonatal and infant diarrheal patients, and the limited availability of EM stimulated the development of antigen detection by EIA as a useful approach for many clinical laboratories.

The development of EIA for rotavirus antigen in stool has evolved during several years, with many kits available commercially; in addition, latex agglutination tests are available for rapid diagnosis.[34, 35, 48–62]

A number of problems have surfaced with regard to the use of these tests in rotavirus detection. In an early report prior to the development of commercial kits, a high rate of false positivity was encountered, associated with a high rate of reactivity of samples with pre-immune sera. By using pre-immune sera as a control at a lower dilution than the post-immune sera, this problem was surmounted.[35] False-positivity has continued to be a problem, however, in some of the commercial kits. The basis for this problem is unclear, but certainly could include operator-dependent steps such as washing between or after antibody incubation steps. One example is a single commercially available assay with a reported specificity of only 50% in one study,[56] 71% in another,[55] and 90 to 100% in others.[34, 51, 57, 58, 62]

Several approaches are available to decrease false-positives, such as the use of negative controls for each patient specimen, the use of pre-immune serum as a negative control,[35] repeating all positive results, and confirmation assays. One widely used type of confirmation procedure involves blocking at least 50% of the positivity by preincubating the specimen with a high concentration of rotavirus antibodies.[34] Another confirmation step involves the use of indirect immunofluorescence to detect foci in African green monkey kidney cells infected with the specimen.[57]

It would be of great interest to see data relating to interlaboratory comparisons of EIAs for rotavirus-positive and rotavirus-negative specimens. The CAP is planning to introduce such surveys, but until they are available there will be little information on this topic. One revealing report from the University of Pennsylvania detailed a comparison of results obtained in their laboratory with those of a local reference laboratory.[63] Both laboratories used the same commercially available EIA to test 66 stool samples. The reference laboratory reported 46 positives (70%), of which only 30 actually were positive (45% of total) in the University of Pennsylvania laboratory. Twenty samples (30%) were negative in both laboratories. Investigation of the 16 samples (24%) that were positive in only one laboratory revealed negative findings by genomic RNA gel electrophoresis in all cases, suggesting strongly that these 16 were false-positive results. It is highly likely that laboratory performance in the reference laboratory, rather than reagent defects or specimen processing errors, was to blame for this disturbing discrepancy.

NUCLEIC ACID–BASED TESTS

Problems with antibody-based assays have led many to theorize that nucleic acid–based tests may offer greater sensitivity, specificity, speed, and convenience. Direct hybridization assays to detect pathogens in patients' specimens are very rarely employed in clinical laboratories, despite the fact that the technology to perform such assays has existed for many years. This fact betrays the difficulty and disappointing results that such assays have usually produced in developmental settings. Currently, enthusiasm exists for using such direct hybridization assays to detect pathogens once they have been amplified by culture or to detect pathogen nucleic acid once it has been amplified by polymerase chain reaction (PCR). The PCR technique is also only rarely employed in routine clinical laboratory assays but is considered very promising for di-

rect sample analyses and will undoubtably receive increasing attention as a clinical tool.

Little information exists about the performance of clinical laboratories in using this technology to diagnose the three gastrointestinal infections discussed in this chapter. For two of the organisms, *H. pylori* and rotavirus, nucleic acid–based tests have been developed and tested to a limited extent.

Helicobacter pylori

Early efforts to use deoxyribonucleic acid (DNA) probes for *H. pylori* included the use of genomic DNA from the organism as a probe in dot blot[64] or in situ hybridization[65] assays. Subsequent probe development has included 16S ribosomal RNA (rRNA)[66] and a gene segment identified in an expression library.[67] Further work has included the use of PCR assays that are directed to a variety of *H. pylori* gene targets.[68–72] These assays are described as highly sensitive and specific, but no data are available on laboratory performance.

Rotavirus

Dot blot hybridization[73] and complementary DNA (cDNA) PCR assays[74–76] have been described for rotavirus RNA detection. As with *H. pylori,* the assays appear promising with regard to sensitivity and specificity, but these reports are too recent to evaluate routine laboratory performance. Interestingly, a rotavirus PCR assay is sensitive enough to detect environmental sources of rotavirus and was used to demonstrate differences between daycare centers with and without rotavirus outbreaks.[75]

CONCLUSIONS

The reported performance of laboratory tests can be misleading, since issues of reproducibility and operator-dependent variability are rarely addressed. The range in laboratories from a single developmental laboratory staffed by highly motivated individuals who focus their attention on a single assay to many routine clinical laboratories in which workload demands may detract from the quality of individual assays may erode the accuracy of the reported sensitivity and specificity of an assay. Interlaboratory surveys such as those conducted by CAP, state and local health agencies, and others reveal that laboratory performance can fall short of theoretical expectations and that performance can improve once laboratorians become aware of defects in their testing procedures.

The quality of direct microscopy assays is highly operator-dependent, with motivation, experience, and skill having as much importance in the accuracy of the findings as the quality of the staining method. Even EIAs, which have the reputation of being highly sensitive and specific, may produce markedly different results depending upon operator-dependent steps in the procedure, particularly in first-generation assays. Optimism about sensitivity and specificity of nucleic acid–based tests such as PCR is justified, but it will be of great interest to see results of proficiency testing when they are placed into the routine clinical laboratory arena.

REFERENCES

1. Garcia LS, Bruckner DA, Brewer TC, Shimizu RY. Techniques for the recovery and identification of *Cryptosporidium* oocysts from stool specimens. J Clin Microbiol. 1983;18:185–190.
2. Henriksen SA, Pohlenz JFL. Staining of cryptosporidia by a modified Ziehl-Neelsen technique. Acta Vet Scand. 1981;22:594–596.
3. Connor BA, Shlim DR, Scholes JV, et al. Pathologic changes in the small bowel in nine patients with diarrhea associated with a coccidia-like body. Ann Intern Med. 1993;119:377–382.
4. Fenoglio-Preiser CM, Lantz PE, Listrom MB, et al. Gastrointestinal Pathology. An Atlas and Text. New York: Raven Press; 1989:313.
5. Soave R, Danner RL, Honig CL, et al. Cryptosporidiosis in homosexual men. Ann Intern Med. 1984;100:504–511.
6. Sorvillo FJ, Fujioka K, Nahlen B, et al. Swimming-associated cryptosporidiosis. Am J Public Health. 1992;82:742–744.
7. Alpert G, Bell LM, Kirkpatrick LD, et al. Cryptosporidiosis in a day-care center. N Engl J Med. 1984;311:860–861.
8. McNabb SJN, Hensel DM, Welch DF, et al. Comparison of sedimentation and flotation techniques for identification of *Cryptosporidium* sp. oocysts in a large outbreak of human diarrhea. J Clin Microbiol. 1985;22:587–589.
9. Garcia LS, Brewer TC, Bruckner DA. Fluorescence detection of *Cryptosporidium* oocysts in human fecal specimens by using monoclonal antibodies. J Clin Microbiol. 1987;25:119–121.
10. Fripp PJ, Bothma MT, Crewe-Brown HH. Four years of cryptosporidiosis at GaRankuwa Hospital. J Infect. 1991;23:93–100.
11. Doenges JL. Spirochetes in gastric glands of *Macacus rhesus* and humans without definite history of related disease. Proc Soc Exp Biol Med. 1938;38:536–538.
12. Freedberg AS, Barron LE. The presence of spirochetes in human gastric mucosa. Am J Dig Dis. 1940;7:443–445.
13. Warren JR, Marshall B. Unidentified curved bacilli on gastric epithelium in active chronic gastritis. Lancet. 1983;1:1273–1275.
14. Kasper G, Dickgiesser N. Isolation of *Campylobacter*-like bacteria from gastric epithelium. Infection. 1984;12:179–180.
15. Menge H, Warrelmann M, Loy V, et al. Comparison between cultural and histological techniques in diagnosis of *Campylobacter pylori* colonization. In: Menge H, Gregor M, Tytgat GNJ, Marshall BJ, eds. *Campylobacter pylori*. Berlin: Springer-Verlag; 1987:145–150.
16. Deltenre M, Glupczynski Y, De Prez C, et al. The reliability of urease tests, histology and culture in the diagnosis of *Campylobacter pylori* infection. Scand J Gastroenterol Suppl. 1989;160:19–24.
17. Strauss RM, Wang TC, Kelsey PB, et al. Association of *Helicobacter pylori* infection with dyspeptic symptoms in patients undergoing gastroduodenoscopy. Am J Med. 1990;89:464–469.
18. Van Horn KG, Dworkin BM. Direct Gram stain and urease test to detect *Helicobacter pylori*. Diagn Microbiol Infect Dis. 1990;13:449–452.
19. Nichols L, Sughayer M, DeGirolami PC, et al. Evaluation of diagnostic methods for *Helicobacter pylori* gastritis. Am J Clin Pathol. 1991;95:769–773.
20. Gray SF, Wyatt JI, Rathbone BJ. Simplified techniques for identifying *Campylobacter pyloridis*. J Clin Pathol. 1986;39:1279.
21. Pinto MM, Meriano FV, Afridi S, Taubin HL. Cytodiagnosis of *Campylobacter pylori* in Papanicolaou-stained imprints of gastric biopsy specimens. Acta Cytol. 1991;35:204–206.
22. Morris A, McIntyre D, Rose T, Nicholson G. Rapid diagnosis of *Campylobacter pyloridis* infection. Lancet. 1986;1:149.
23. McNulty CAM, Wise R. Rapid diagnosis of *Campylobacter pyloridis* gastritis. Lancet. 1986;1:387.
24. McNulty CA, Dent JC, Uff JS, et al. Detection of *Campylobacter pylori* by the biopsy urease test: An assessment of 1445 patients. Gut. 1989;30:1058–1062.
25. Graham DY, Klein PD, Evans DJ Jr, et al. *Campylobacter pylori* detected noninvasively by the ^{13}C-urea breath test. Lancet. 1987;1:1174–1177.
26. Dill S, Payne-James JJ, Misiewicz JJ, et al. Evaluation of ^{13}C-urea breath test in the detection of *Helicobacter pylori* and in monitoring the effect of tripotassium dicitratobismuthate in non-ulcer dyspepsia. Gut. 1990;31:1237–1241.
27. Henze E, Malfertheiner P, Clausen M, et al. Validation of a simplified carbon-14-urea breath test for routine use for detecting *Helicobacter pylori* noninvasively. J Nucl Med. 1990;31:1940–1944.
28. McNulty CAM, Dent JC, Curry A, et al. New spiral bacterium in gastric mucosa. J Clin Pathol. 1989;42:585–591.
29. Barbosa AJ, Queiroz DM, Mendes EN, et al. Immunocytochemical identification of *Campylobacter pylori* in gastritis and correlation with culture. Arch Pathol Lab Med. 1988;112:523–525.
30. Bishop RF, Davidson GP, Holmes IH, Ruck BJ. Virus particles in epithelial cells of duodenal mucosa from children with acute nonbacterial gastroenteritis. Lancet. 1973;2:1281–1283.
31. Flewett TH, Davies H, Bryden AS, Robertson MJ. Diagnostic electron microscopy of the faeces: II, Acute gastroenteritis associated with reovirus-like particles. J Clin Pathol. 1974;27:608–614.
32. Gomez-Barreto J, Palmer EL, Nahmias AJ, Hatch MH. Acute enteritis associated with reovirus-like agents. J Am Med Assoc. 1976;235:1857–1860.
33. Nakata S, Petrie BL, Calomeni EP, Estes MK. Electron microscopy procedure influences detection of rotaviruses. J Clin Microbiol. 1987;25:1902–1906.
34. Rubenstein AS, Miller MF. Comparison of an enzyme

immunoassay with electron microscopic procedures for detecting rotavirus. J Clin Microbiol. 1982;15:938–944.

35. Brandt CD, Kim HW, Rodriguez WJ, et al. Comparison of direct electron microscopy, immune electron microscopy, and rotavirus enzyme-linked immunosorbent assay for detection of gastroenteritis viruses in children. J Clin Microbiol. 1981;13:976–981.

36. Rodger SM, Bishop RF, Birch C, et al. Molecular epidemiology of human rotaviruses in Melbourne, Australia, from 1973 to 1979, as determined by electrophoresis of genome ribonucleic acid. J Clin Microbiol. 1981;13:272–278.

37. Follett EAC, Desselberger U. Cocirculation of different rotavirus strains in a local outbreak of infantile gastroenteritis: Monitoring by rapid and sensitive nucleic acid analysis. J Med Virol. 1983;11:39–52.

38. Dimitrov DH, Graham DY, Lopoez J, et al. RNA electropherotypes of human rotaviruses from North and South America. Bull World Health Organ. 1984;62:321–329.

39. Dolan KT, Twist EM, Horton-Slight P, et al. Epidemiology of rotavirus electropherotypes determined by a simplified diagnostic technique with RNA analysis. J Clin Microbiol. 1985;21:753–758.

40. Uhnoo I, Svensson L. Clinical and epidemiological features of acute infantile gastroenteritis associated with human rotavirus subgroups 1 and 2. J Clin Microbiol. 1986;23:551–555.

41. Pyndiah N, Beguin R, Richard J, et al. Accuracy of rotavirus diagnosis: Modified genome electrophoresis versus electron microscopy. J Virol Methods. 1988;20:39–44.

42. Ungar BLP. Enzyme-linked immunoassay for detection of Cryptosporidium antigens in fecal specimens. J Clin Microbiol. 1990;28:2491–2495.

43. Anusz KZ, Mason PH, Riggs MW, Perryman LE. Detection of Cryptosporidium parvum oocysts in bovine feces by monoclonal antibody capture enzyme-linked immunosorbent assay. J Clin Microbiol. 1990;28:2770–2774.

44. Glassman MS, Dallal S, Berezin SH, et al. Helicobacter pylori–related gastroduodenal disease in children: Diagnostic utility of enzyme-linked immunosorbent assay. Dig Dis Sci. 1990;35:993–997.

45. Thomas JE, Whatmore AM, Barer MR, et al. Serodiagnosis of Helicobacter pylori infection in childhood. J Clin Microbiol. 1990;28:2641–2646.

46. Perez-Perez GI, Dworkin BM, Chodos JE, Blaser MJ. Campylobacter pylori antibodies in humans. Ann Intern Med. 1988;109:11–17.

47. Hirschl AM, Hirschl MM, Berger J, Rotter ML. Evaluation of a commercial latex test for serological diagnosis of Helicobacter pylori infection in treated and untreated patients. Eur J Clin Microbiol Infect Dis. 1991;10:971–974.

48. Haikala OJ, Kokkonen JO, Leinonen MK, et al. Rapid detection of rotavirus in stool by latex agglutination: Comparison with radioimmunoassay and electron microscopy and clinical evaluation of the test. J Med Virol. 1983;11:91–97.

49. Yolken RH, Miotti P, Viscidi R. Immunoassays for the diagnosis and study of viral gastroenteritis. Pediatr Infect Dis J. 1986;5(Suppl):S46–S52.

50. Gerna G, Sarasini A, Passarani N, et al. Comparative evaluation of a commercial enzyme-linked immunoassay and solid-phase immune electron microscopy for rotavirus detection in stool specimens. J Clin Microbiol. 1987;25:1137–1139.

51. Brooks R, Brown L, Franklin R. Comparison of a protein-stabilized Rotazyme II test, with standard Rotazyme II, and electron microscopy for detection of rotavirus. Diagn Microbiol Infect Dis. 1988;11:205–208.

52. Chernesky M, Castriciano S, Mahony J, et al. Ability of TESTPAK ROTAVIRUS enzyme immunoassay to diagnose rotavirus gastroenteritis. J Clin Microbiol. 1988;26:2459–2461.

53. Marchlewicz B, Spiewak M, Lampinen J. Evaluation of Abbott TESTPAK ROTAVIRUS with clinical specimens. J Clin Microbiol. 1988;26:2456–2458.

54. Prey MU, Lorelle CA, Taff TA, et al. Evaluation of three commercially available rotavirus detection methods for neonatal specimens. Am J Clin Pathol. 1988;89:675–678.

55. Thomas EE, Puterman ML, Kawano E, Curran M. Evaluation of seven immunoassays for detection of rotavirus in pediatric stool samples. J Clin Microbiol. 1988;26:1189–1193.

56. Dennehy PH, Gauntlett DR, Tente WE. Comparison of nine commercial immunoassays for the detection of rotavirus in fecal specimens. J Clin Microbiol. 1988;26:1630–1634.

57. Lipson SM, Zelinsky-Papez KA. Comparison of four latex agglutination (LA) and three enzyme-linked immunosorbent assays (ELISA) for the detection of rotavirus in fecal specimens. Am J Clin Pathol. 1989;92:637–643.

58. Mathewson JJ, Winsor DK Jr, DuPont HL, Secor SL. Evaluation of assay systems for the detection of rotavirus in stool specimens. Diagn Microbiol Infect Dis. 1989;12:139–141.

59. Brooks RG, Brown L, Franklin RB. Comparison of a new rapid test (TestPack Rotavirus) with standard enzyme immunoassay and electron microscopy for the detection of rotavirus in symptomatic hospitalized children. J Clin Microbiol. 1989;27:775–777.

60. Lipson SM, Leonari GP, Salo RJ, et al. Occurrence of nonspecific reactions among stool specimens tested by the Abbott TestPack rotavirus enzyme immunoassay. J Clin Microbiol. 1990;28:1132–1134.

61. Dennehy PH, Gauntlett DR, Spangenberger SE. Choice of reference assay for the detection of rotavirus in fecal specimens: Electron microscopy versus enzyme immunoassay. J Clin Microbiol. 1990;28:1280–1283.

62. Christy C, Vosefski D, Madore HP. Comparison of three enzyme immunoassays to tissue culture for the diagnosis of rotavirus gastroenteritis in infants and young children. J Clin Microbiol. 1990;28:1428–1430.

63. Forrer CB, Rodden JM, Clark HF, Friedman HM. Discrepant rotavirus results in two laboratories using the same enzyme immunoassay. Am J Clin Pathol. 1989;91:85–87.

64. Wetherall BL, McDonald PJ, Johnson AM. Detection of Campylobacter pylori DNA by hybridization with non-radioactive probes in comparison with a ^{32}P-labelled probe. J Med Microbiol. 1988;26:257–263.

65. Van den berg FM, Zijlmans H, Langenberg W, et al. Detection of Campylobacter pylori in stomach tissue by DNA in situ hybridization. J Clin Pathol. 1989;42:995–1000.

66. Morotomi M, Hoshina S, Green P, et al. Oligonucleotide probe for detection and identification of Campylobacter pylori. J Clin Microbiol. 1989;27:2652–2655.

67. Clayton CL, Wren BW, Mullany P, et al. Molecular cloning and expression of Campylobacter pylori species-specific antigens in Escherichia coli K12. Infect Immun. 1989;57:623–629.

68. Valentine JL, Arthur RR, Mobley HL, Dick JD. Detection of Helicobacter pylori by using the polymerase chain reaction. J Clin Microbiol. 1991;29:689–695.

69. Ho S-A, Hoyle JA, Lewis FA, et al. Direct polymerase chain reaction test for detection of Helicobacter pylori in humans and animals. J Clin Microbiol. 1991;29:2543–2549.

70. Foxall PA, Hu L-T, Mobley HLT. Use of polymerase chain reaction–amplified Helicobacter pylori urease structural genes for differentiation of isolates. J Clin Microbiol. 1992;30:739–741.

71. Hammar M, Tyszkiewicz T, Wadstrom T, O'Toole PW. Rapid detection of *Helicobacter pylori* in gastric biopsy material by polymerase chain reaction. J Clin Microbiol. 1992;30:54–58.

72. Clayton CL, Kleanthous H, Coates PJ, et al. Sensitive detection of *Helicobacter pylori* by using polymerase chain reaction. J Clin Microbiol. 1992;30:192–200.

73. Eiden J, Sato S, Yolken R. Specificity of dot hybridization assay in the presence of rRNA for detection of rotaviruses in clinical specimens. J Clin Microbiol. 1987;25:1809–1811.

74. Gouvea V, Glass RI, Woods P, et al. Polymerase chain reaction amplification and typing of rotavirus nucleic acid from stool specimens. J Clin Microbiol. 1990;28:276–282.

75. Wilde J, Van R, Pickering L, et al. Detection of rotaviruses in the day care environment by reverse transcriptase polymerase chain reaction. J Infect Dis. 1992;166:507–511.

76. Gentsch JR, Glass RI, Woods P, et al. Identification of group A rotavirus gene 4 types by polymerase chain reaction. J Clin Microbiol. 1992;30:1365–1373.

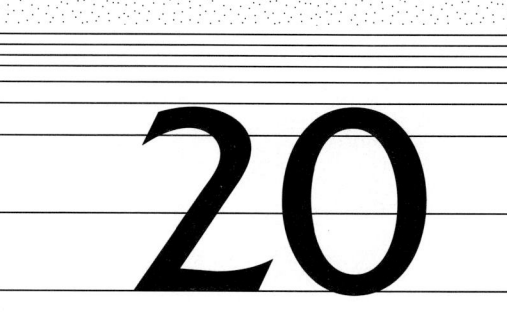

Evaluation of Diarrhea, Including Molecular Diagnostic Methods and Interpretation of Diagnostic Tests

GRACE M. THORNE, Ph.D.
JANE S. GREATOREX, F.I.M.L.S.

Worldwide, diarrheal diseases constitute the greatest single cause of morbidity and mortality. The highest mortality rate from diarrheal disease is seen in infants and children, especially in developing countries, accounting for an estimated 4 million to 4.5 million deaths per year.[1] The attack rates of acute gastrointestinal illnesses range from 2 to 12 or more illnesses per person per year in developed and developing countries.[2] In the last decade, in appropriately equipped laboratories, a causal diagnosis could be established in 68% of pediatric patients seeking treatment in developing countries versus 70 to 75% in developed countries.[3]

The 1980s and early 1990s saw many new organisms added to the list of identifiable bacterial, viral, and parasitic agents causing diarrheal disease. The list now includes *Salmonella, Shigella, Campylobacter, Escherichia coli* (enterotoxigenic (ETEC), enteroinvasive (EIEC), entero-

pathogenic (EPEC), enterohemorrhagic (EHEC), and enteroadherent (EAEC)), *Yersinia, Vibrio cholerae* and other vibrios, *Aeromonas, Plesiomonas, Clostridium difficile, Staphylococcus aureus,* and *Bacillus cereus;* it also includes the parasites *Entamoeba histolytica, Giardia lamblia,* and *Isospora belli;* the newly recognized enteropathogenic sporozoan *Cryptosporidium;* and the microsporidian parasite *Enterocytozoon bieneusi.* The enteric viruses now include rotavirus, coronavirus, calicivirus, astrovirus, certain adenoviruses, and the Norwalk agent. Often, specimens are found to contain more than one of the aforementioned pathogenic agents.

Some rapid diagnostic methods have been developed, but most of the identification methods in the laboratory are still time-consuming and require a battery of media. Thus, the present conventional approach toward identification of enteric pathogens may take several days before

TABLE 20–1. FECAL LEUKOCYTES IN INTESTINAL INFECTIONS

PRESENT	VARIABLE	ABSENT
Shigella	*Salmonella*	*Vibrio cholerae*
Campylobacter	*Yersinia*	Enterotoxigenic *E. coli* (ETEC)
Enteroinvasive *Escherichia*	*Vibrio*	Enteropathogenic *E. coli* (EPEC)
coli (EIEC)	*parahaemolyticus*	Adenovirus 40/41
	Clostridium difficile	Rotavirus
	Enterohemorrhagic	Coronavirus
	E. coli (EHEC)	Norwalk virus
		Astrovirus
		Giardia lamblia
		Entamoeba histolytica
		Staphylococcus aureus
		Clostridium perfringens
		Bacillus cereus

a diagnosis can be made. In addition to summaries of routine approaches used to diagnose infectious diarrheas, this chapter includes information on new, reliable, and rapid test techniques. New technologies, such as deoxyribonucleic acid (DNA) probes and polymerase chain reaction (PCR) assays, are also described. These new procedures have revolutionized the approach to identification of enteric pathogens in feces, and will have a tremendous impact on the diagnosis of enteric infectious disease in the future.

COLLECTION AND TRANSPORT OF SPECIMENS

Fecal specimens should be collected as early as possible in the course of the disease, when enteric pathogens are present in the stool in high numbers, and preferably before antibiotic therapy is started. Stool specimens are preferred over rectal swabs for the isolation of most pathogens. Some pathogens, such as *Shigella* species, however, which invade the mucosa of the colon, are best isolated from a carefully collected rectal swab. Adkins and Santiago[4] showed that sensitivity of culture for enteric pathogens improved by 11% when both stools and rectal swabs were cultured. Testing of multiple specimens is also advantageous.

Stool specimens should be collected in a clean, nonabsorbent container and processed in the laboratory as soon as possible. If there is a delay of more than 2 hours, the specimens should be refrigerated (4°C) or placed into a transport medium. If stools or fecal suspensions are to be held for longer times, that is, for weeks, they should be frozen, preferably at −70°C.

Cary-Blair transport medium is very useful for long-term survival and transport of specimens

for the isolation of *Salmonella, Shigella, E. coli, V. cholerae, Vibrio parahaemolyticus,* and *Yersinia.* Thioglycolate broth sustains *Campylobacter* for a longer time than does Cary-Blair medium.

DIRECT EXAMINATION

Microscopic Examination of Feces

Microscopic examination of fecal smears can be very useful (Table 20–1). The detection of abundant polymorphonuclear leukocytes suggests an invasive inflammatory process involving the colon, such as *Shigella* or *Campylobacter* infection. Other disorders associated with colonic mucosal inflammation and destruction, such as ulcerative colitis and *C. difficile*–related antibiotic-associated colitis, are often associated with a fecal exudate containing leukocytes.

Fecal examination is performed by placing a small fleck of stool, and blood or mucus if present, on a clean glass slide and mixing it thoroughly with two drops of Löffler's methylene blue stain. A coverslip is placed over the specimen, which is then ready for microscopic viewing.

There is also evidence that examination of feces by darkfield or phase-contrast microscopy can reveal a characteristic described as the darting motility of *Campylobacter* or *Vibrio* in cases of gastroenteritis.[5] Gram stain of a fecal smear may provide clues to the possible agent, as, for example, in staphylococcal enteritis.

Microscopic Search for Parasites

Examination of wet mounts is the simplest and most widely used method to search for parasites. A small fleck of feces is emulsified in saline on one half of a slide, and the other half is used for a similar preparation stained with a drop of iodine solution. The mounts are screened with low-power microscopic magnification ($\times$ 10) to detect eggs, larvae, cysts, and trophozoites. Higher ($\times$ 40) magnification is used for speciation.

If trophozoites of amebae are suspected or observed to be present, additional staining of the preparation with buffered methylene blue (BMB) solution, merthiolate iodine formaldehyde (MIF), or trichrome stain may be performed. The trichrome stain is a permanent stain, and the reagents have a long shelf life. Expertise is required to identify the protozoal pathogens among the commensals and cellular artifacts. Macrophages are often mistaken for *E. histolytica* when MIF staining is used.

Giardia

Giardia lamblia is an important cause of diarrhea in children and adults. In the United States, this organism is the most common protozoal pathogen. Outbreaks occur in daycare settings by person-to-person contact and also by consumption of contaminated water. The diagnosis of giardiasis is usually made by microscopic examination of stool for cysts or trophozoites. Since infected individuals excrete the cysts intermittently, specimens collected over 3 days are examined to detect the parasite. This method has been reported to be 50 to 70% sensitive when only 1 specimen is examined.[6] Usually individual stool specimens are examined, but Wahlquist and colleagues have shown that examination of pooled stool specimens is efficient, practical, and cost-effective.[7] Pooling of specimens should be performed at the laboratory, since individual samples need to be available for further diagnostic testing in cases in which *G. lamblia* is strongly suggested clinically but the pool is negative. A monoclonal antibody to *Giardia* cyst wall is available commercially in an indirect immunofluorescence assay.[8] This product does not detect *Giardia* trophozoites, however, and therefore cannot identify individuals excreting only the trophozoite forms at the time the specimen is obtained.

A new enzyme immunoassay (EIA) has been evaluated by Rosoff and colleagues and compared with conventional ova and parasite (O & P) microscopic examination.[9] This assay is based on the detection of Giardia-specific antigen, associated with the cyst wall and to a lesser extent with trophozoites, in aqueous extracts of stool specimens, with a monospecific polyclonal serum. In this study, the EIA had a sensitivity of 94% and specificity of 97%. The sensitivity and specificity of the EIA may be better than those of an O & P examination, since several assay-positive but microscopic-negative specimens were from individuals who had contact with *Giardia* patients and were probably true cases of disease.

Addiss and colleagues evaluated the performance of this EIA as part of a large epidemiologic study of endemic giardiasis in diapered children attending daycare centers.[10] Compared with microscopic O & P examination, the EIA was highly sensitive and 100% specific for *G. lamblia*. The sensitivity of both microscopy and EIA improved as the number of specimens per child increased. These results suggest that the shedding in stool of *Giardia* antigen, like that of cysts, may be intermittent. This test is not a replacement for routine microscopic O & P examinations, since other potential pathogens would be missed. It does, however, fill a role in confirming the clinical diagnosis of giardiasis and in testing family members of *Giardia*-positive patients. It should also be useful as an epidemiologic tool, particularly during outbreaks in daycare settings.

Two assays by DNA probe have been reported, one with a sensitivity of 5×10^3 trophozoites ($\sim$1 mg DNA),[11] the other with a sensitivity of 1 cyst.[12] Mahbubani and colleagues developed a PCR-based assay with a gene probe detection system able to detect a single *Giardia* cyst (Table 20–2).[13] Although the level of sensitivity of this test makes it suitable for clinical application, only environmental testing was performed.

Entamoeba histolytica

Entamoeba histolytica causes amebiasis and is the only ameba pathogenic for humans. Isoenzyme analysis has shown that strains isolated from patients with clinical disease differ from commensal isolates. The strain-specific differences have also been demonstrated by biologic assays, monoclonal antibodies, DNA probes,[14] and most recently by gene amplification.

Tannich and Burchard reported using a PCR-amplification and subsequent restriction fragment analysis to detect genomic DNA differences between pathogenic and nonpathogenic *E. histolytica* (see Table 20–2).[15] The assay allowed for rapid detection and classification of these organisms; fewer than 10 amebae were identified within a few hours. Samples underwent short-term culture prior to the PCR testing, and the authors are working on procedures to amplify the target DNA directly out of stool specimens. The authors studied 48 fresh clinical

TABLE 20–2. POLYMERASE CHAIN REACTION–BASED ASSAYS FOR ENTERIC PATHOGENS

PATHOGEN	TARGET	REFERENCE
Clostridium difficile	Toxin A	Wren (1990)[213]
	Repeat sequence	
	Toxin A	Kato (1991)[215]
	Repeat and nonrepeat sequences	
ETEC	LT (A subunit)	Olive (1989)[68]
	LT (B subunit)	Victor (1991)[69]
EHEC	SLT-I, SLT-II	Karch (1989)[93]
	SLT-II, SLT-IIv	Johnson (1990)[94]
	SLT-I	Jackson (1991)[97]
EIEC and *Shigella*	Invasion-associated locus	Frankel (1990)[72]
Yersinia enterocolitica	Attachment invasion locus	Wren (1990)[136]
	pYvir plasmid	Fenwick (1991)[137]
Entamoeba histolytica	482-bp chromosomal sequence	Tannich (1991)[15]
Giardia duodenalis	Giardia gene	Mahbubani (1992)[13]
Adenovirus		
Type 40	E1a	Allard (1990)[232]
Types 40 and 41	E1b	
Rotavirus*		
Group A	Gene 9	Gouvea (199)[242]
	Gene 6	Wilde (1990)[244]
Group B	Gene 8	Gouvea (1991)[243]
	Gene 11	Eiden (1991)[245]
Group C	Gene 6	Gouvea (1991)[243]

*Detection of rotavirus group A, B, and C RNA was achieved using reverse transcription, followed by polymerase chain reaction amplification.
KEY: EHEC = enterohemorrhagic *Escherichia coli;* EIEC = enteroinvasive *E. coli,* ETEC = enterotoxigenic *E. coli;* LT = heat-labile enterotoxin; SLT = Shiga-like cytotoxins.
SOURCE: Thorne GM. Diagnostic tests in gastrointestinal infection. Curr Op Gastroenterol. 1992;8:134–145.

isolates and found nearly complete correlation (47/48) with clinical status of the infected individual and other markers of pathogenicity (i.e., strains' isoenzyme mobility, patients' anti-amebic antibodies). These studies provide further support for the theory that *E. histolytica* contains distinct subspecies of pathogenic and nonpathogenic strains.

Enterocytozoon bieneusi

The microsporidian parasite *E. bieneusi* has been reported in acquired immunodeficiency syndrome patients with persistent diarrhea when no other enteric pathogen was identified.[16–18] Diagnosis has in the past depended on light or electron microscopic examination of biopsy tissue. In 1990, van Gool and colleagues reported the isolation of *E. bieneusi* spores from feces.[19] These authors used a standard stool concentration process, followed by staining with 10% Giemsa stain for 35 minutes. Under 1250 × magnification, the small spores (1–2 μm) were broadly oval, with the cytoplasm staining light grey-blue and the nucleus staining an intense purple. In another study, Weber and colleagues demonstrated the use of a new chromotropic staining technique.[20] Their method involved an approximately 2-hour staining proc-

ess, followed by examination of the stained smear under 1000 × magnification for 10 minutes. *Enterocytozoon bieneusi* spores appeared ovoid and refractile, and the spore wall stained bright pinkish red. They advised the use of unconcentrated specimens after testing a range of concentration techniques and showing that none improved the detection of microsporidial spores. Use of such a simple diagnostic procedure should facilitate studies of the prevalence and significance of *E. bieneusi* in both acquired immunodeficiency syndrome and immunocompetent patients, until a fluorescent antibody or enzyme-linked immunosorbent assay (ELISA) detection system is available.

Cryptosporidium

Cryptosporidium, a well-known cause of diarrhea in animals, has only recently been recognized as a cause of disease in humans. Since the first case was reported in 1976, numerous reports have documented the disease in immunocompromised patients, including those with AIDS, and more recently in immunocompetent individuals.[21–25] Outbreaks have been documented that were either waterborne or spread in hospitals and daycare centers.[26]

The organism is a small, 2- to 6-μm coccidian

that usually undergoes its life cycle within the microvillus border of the intestine. Initially, identification of the organism was made by microscopic examination of intestinal biopsy specimens. More recently, it has been determined that infective oocysts shed in the feces may also be detected using various acid-fast (AF) stains.[27] Modified Kinyoun's AF stains have worked well. Upon examination under high power and oil immersion, the cryptosporidial oocysts stain bright red against a blue or green background. The modified AF stains are more specific than an iodine wet mount because as little as 15 minutes of exposure to iodine stains both the oocysts and the yeasts, which may cause confusion in differentiating between the two. Concentration procedures are not usually necessary to find oocysts in specimens from immunosuppressed patients, but either Sheather sucrose flotation or modified formalin–ethyl acetate (FEA) stool concentration method may be used for detection of small numbers of organisms.[28] As in most parasitic infections, the presence of the parasites in fecal specimens can be intermittent; therefore, a stool examination that produces negative findings should be repeated in 3 or 4 days, the life cycle of the organism.[29]

Garcia and colleagues have reported an excellent screening method using a monoclonal antibody raised against oocyst walls.[30] When a fluorescein isothiocyanate–labeled mouse antibody (Meridian Diagnostics, Cincinnati OH) was used for antigen detection, the sensitivity and specificity were found to be 100%. The study included 99 positive and 198 negative human fecal specimens tested in blind trials. The fluorescent antibody technique detected an additional 7 specimens previously considered negative by AF techniques. The authors suggested that this technique was at least 10 times more sensitive than the AF method, and the slides could be viewed quickly to look for the distinctive fluorescence. Weber and colleagues studied the efficiency of the FEA techniques for concentrating oocysts using detection by AF or immunofluorescence (IF) staining.[31] Although the IF stain was more sensitive than the AF staining method, the study revealed oocyte losses of 50 to 90% during the FEA concentration procedure. These results suggest that commonly used techniques may fail to detect this pathogen. *Cryptosporidium* antigen detection systems may eventually provide improved diagnostic sensitivity. Nevertheless, two first-generation tests were able to detect 2 to 4 $\times$ 10^3 purified oocysts[32] or 10^5 oocysts per gram of feces.[33] Both these assays

were outperformed by IF staining of fecal smears. The limitation of current methods needs to be recognized, and new, more sensitive methods should be sought.

Isospora belli

Isospora belli is the only sporozoan that is an obligate tissue parasite in the intestinal tract. It is infrequently diagnosed in the United States, where it is isolated most commonly from patients with AIDS. Even so, fewer than 2% of AIDS patients in the United States have the organism.[34] In other parts of the world, it is more prevalent; in Haiti and Africa, for example, 15% of AIDS patients have isosporiasis.[35]

In immunocompetent hosts, isosporiasis is characterized by acute onset of watery diarrhea, usually occurring 7 days after ingestion, and by fever, malaise, abdominal pain, and weight loss.[36] Infections are self-limiting and resolve in several weeks. In immunodeficient patients, the disease is characterized by chronic, profuse, watery diarrhea associated with malabsorption and the continuous passage of oocysts. The symptoms may persist for weeks or months, and there is a report of 1 case that persisted for 15 years.[37] Isosporiasis with diarrhea persisting for more than 1 month is an indicator for the diagnosis of AIDS.[38]

Exactly how *I. belli* is transmitted is poorly understood. There is no evidence that *I. belli* is capable of infecting nonhuman hosts,[39] nor is there evidence that *Isospora* species of other animals, mainly birds and carnivorous mammals, are capable of infecting human beings.

Diagnosis of isosporiasis is made by the detection of mature or immature oocysts in fecal specimens. The mature oocyst, which is rarely observed, is ellipsoidal, 20 to 30 μm in length, and 10 to 19 μm in width and contains two spherical sporocysts with 4 sporozoites in each. More common are the immature oocysts, which are 20 to 30 μm in length and 10 to 19 μm in width, and contain only a single, round sporoblast. Charcot-Leyden crystals and mucus may also be present in the specimen. In saline preparations, *I. belli* may be missed by the inexperienced microscopist. The specimen is usually prepared by the sugar flotation procedure[40] or the FEA. Iodine-stained wet mounts may be prepared directly from the specimen or after concentration. The stains less commonly used to detect the oocysts include modified AF[41] (oocyst stains pink, with bright red sporocysts), Kinyoun's[41] (same staining as the modified AF stain), rhodamine–auramine[41, 42] (oocyst and sporocyst fluoresce bright yellow), and Giemsa (oocyst and sporocyst stain pale blue). Unlike cryptosporidiosis, *I. belli* has no specific methods of detection.

Cyclospora Species—A New Coccidian Enteric Pathogen

Since 1986,[42a] numerous reports have described spherical organisms that appear as granule-containing cysts 10 μm in diameter in stools of both immunocompetent and immunocompromised patients with diarrhea. The cyst forms have been described in these reports as possibly a large *Cryptosporidium*, a flagellate, an unsporulated coccidian, a blue-green alga (*Cyanobacterium*-like body), a *Cryptosporidium muris*–like cyst, or a coccidian-like body. Recently Ortega and coworkers[42b] have identified the organisms as belonging to the genus *Cyclospora*, based on observations made during sporulation and excystation. Complete excystation resulted in release of two sporozoites from each oocyst, in contrast to cryptosporidia, which have four sporozoites within each oocyst. These authors identified these organisms in the feces of Peruvian infants and children; consequently, it appears that persons of all ages can become infected. This study also provides evidence that the organisms recently described as *Cyanobacterium*-like bodies[43] in outbreaks in Chicago and Nepal[44] and in travelers returning from Central and South America, Caribbean countries, and Southeast Asia[45–45d] are in fact a new coccidian pathogen.

In freshly passed stool, the organisms are readily identified by their intense blue autofluorescence under ultraviolet light.[43] This method may be more sensitive and reliable than the modified acid-fast or phenosafranin stain, since both are highly variable in their ability to stain the cyst. Since the organism has been seen in patients with AIDS who have experienced intractable diarrhea, this infection should be distinguished from cryptosporidiosis by precise cyst measurement or by immunofluorescence with a *C. parvum*–specific monoclonal antibody (Merifluor, Meridian Diagnostics, Cincinnati, OH). This is particularly important because successful treatment of *Cyclospora* with co-trimoxazole has been reported.[45e]

Although knowledge of the complete life cycle and epidemiology of this new pathogen awaits additional studies, this organism should be considered in cases of unexplained diarrhea, particularly in AIDS patients, and in affected individuals returning from travel in tropical countries.

ROUTINE STOOL CULTURE

Laboratory studies of stool specimens are among the most laborious and expensive tests performed in clinical bacteriology laboratories. Consequently, from a cost-benefit standpoint, a routine stool culture on all patients with mild, self-limiting illness cannot be justified. Children younger than 1 year may not need to have a stool culture unless there are other important clinical findings, such as fecal leukocytes, presence of blood in stool, or high fever. These patients can be managed with fluids, electrolyte treatment, and diet modifications.

If white blood cells are seen in the patient's diarrheal stools, the invasive colonic pathogens should be sought. If *Vibrio, Yersinia, Campylobacter,* or viruses are suspected as causative agents from the patient's history, the laboratory should be notified so that the appropriate culture or testing is performed.

Inoculation of Primary Isolation Media

Specimens should be plated immediately on arrival in the laboratory; if this is not possible, they should be stored at 4°C. There are several suitable media of varying selectivity that can be used for primary plating that will allow certain enteric pathogenic bacteria to grow while inhibiting the growth of gram-positive bacteria and some gram-negative bacteria. These media have been designed to permit initial differentiation of bacterial species by colony color and morphology (Table 20–3). Media of low selectivity should be inoculated with a light loopful of stool, whereas the media of high selectivity should be inoculated more heavily, that is, with several loopfuls of stool.

Quality-control testing of each new batch or new lot number of media should be undertaken in the bacteriology laboratory. Testing should include inoculation with reference strains, to test for growth and colony characteristics of pathogens as well as suppression of breakthrough of representative cultures of the normal fecal flora. In particular, daily quality-control testing should be performed on *Campylobacter* isolation media and gas mixtures, using control strains of *C. jejuni* for those cultures with growth and *E. coli* for those without growth.

Enrichment Procedures

Broth enrichments are useful for the culture of stool specimens because they provide for the

TABLE 20–3. GROWTH AND COLONY MORPHOLOGY OF ENTERIC ORGANISMS ON SELECTIVE AND DIFFERENTIAL MEDIA

ORGANISM	EOSIN–METHYLENE BLUE (EMB) AGAR	MacCONKEY'S AGAR (MAD)	SALMONELLA-SHIGELLA (SS) AGAR	XYLOSE LYSINE DESOXYCHO-LATE AGAR	HEKTOEN'S ENTERIC AGAR	CEFSULODIN–IRGASAN–NOVOBIOCIN (CIN) AGAR	BISMUTH SULFITE AGAR	BRILLIANT GREEN AGAR	THIOSULFATE–CITRATE–BILE SALTS–SUCROSE (TCBS) AGAR
	MILDLY SELECTIVE		MODERATELY SELECTIVE				HIGHLY SELECTIVE		
Escherichia coli	Blue-purple metallic sheen	Red* 2–3 mm	Red	Yellow	Salmon-orange	±	–	–	–
Salmonella sp.	Colorless 2–3 mm	Colorless 2–3 mm	Colorless	Red	Blue-green		Black center, translucent edge, metallic sheen	Pink-white 1–3 mm	–
Salmonella typhi	Colorless 2–3 mm	Colorless 2–3 mm	Colorless	Red	Blue-green		Black	–	
Shigella	Colorless	Colorless	Colorless	Red	Blue-green		–	–	–
Yersinia enterocolitica	Colorless 0.5 mm (48 h)	Colorless or light pink 1–2 mm (48 h)	Colorless 0.5 mm (48 h) 22–30°C	–	–	Pink	–	–	–
Vibrio cholerae	Colorless	–	–	–	–		–	–	Yellow to yellow-green, large
Vibrio parahaemolyticus	Colorless	–	–	–	–		–	–	Blue-green 3–5 mm
Aeromonas hydrophila	±	+	±	+	±		±	Pink	
Plesiomonas shigelloides	+	Colorless to light pink	+	+	±		–	–	Variable growth

*Sorbitol MacConkey agar, used for detection of *E. coli* O157 which are pale (sorbitol negative, i.e., nonfermenting) while other *E. coli* are pink.

493

growth of enteric pathogens while retarding the growth of normal flora. These media are particularly useful when pathogens are present in low numbers, that is, in the later stages of illness, in asymptomatic or convalescing patients screened for epidemiologic studies, and in carriers. Gram-negative tetrathionate and selenite broths have been used for many years for *Salmonella*. As yet, there is no suitable enrichment medium for *Shigella*. For *Y. enterocolitica*, fecal material can be placed in phosphate-buffered saline and refrigerated for 2 to 3 weeks before plating on MacConkey or *Salmonella-Shigella* (SS) agar. Cold enrichment for *Yersinia* is not necessary for culture in acute disease, but is useful in cultures of specimens from convalescent or asymptomatic persons. For *Vibrio*, a brief enrichment for 6 to 8 hours of fecal suspension or rectal swab in alkaline peptone water prior to plating can enhance isolation.

ISOLATION AND IDENTIFICATION OF ENTERIC BACTERIAL PATHOGENS

Several media should be included for routine use in the culture of Enterobacteriaceae from stool specimens. The set of media should include a nonselective medium, for example, blood agar; a mildly selective differential medium, for example, MacConkey agar; a moderately selective differential medium, for example, xylose–lysine–deoxycholate [XLD] or Hektoen's enteric [HE], Table 20–3; and a broth enrichment. Such an approach will allow for effective detection of organisms commonly associated with enteric infections. Use of additional media for isolation of *Yersinia*, *Aeromonas* species, *Vibrio*, and *C. difficile* is usually done at the physician's request.

Members of the family Enterobacteriaceae are identified by both biochemical and serologic tests, but the extent to which such testing is carried out varies with the capabilities of the laboratory.

Salmonella

Salmonella organisms are the causal agents of a wide variety of infections, ranging from simple gastroenteritis to very severe illnesses such as enteric fever with bacteremia. In addition, the organisms can cause local infections in virtually any organ as a result of the bacteremia. *Salmonella* typically invades through the intestinal mu-

cosa and multiplies within the submucosa. Depending on the virulence of the strain and the host response, the organism can invade and multiply in the bloodstream or lymphatic tissues or both.

Typically, *Salmonella* are urease-negative, and on Kliger's iron agar (KIA) they produce the characteristic alkaline (K) slant, acid (A) butt, and gas (G), known as the K/A,G reaction. These organisms are usually motile but negative for indole. Because *Citrobacter* strains also produce these reactions, they can be mistaken for *Salmonella*. Unlike *Salmonella*, *Citrobacter* ferments glycerol in 24 hours and can be excluded by this test. *Edwardsiella* also mimics *Salmonella* in some reactions but is rarely isolated from human feces. When presumptive tests indicate typical *Salmonella*, the isolate should be tested with *Salmonella* group A through E antisera.

Use of a new fluorescent reagent (MUCAP test, Biolife Italian, Milan, Italy) in conjunction with the oxidase test results in rapid presumptive identification of *Salmonella* species.[46] The MUCAP test reagent detects the C9 esterase enzyme present in *Salmonella* species and in other bacteria. The 4-methylumbelliferone (MUG) liberated by this esterase is strongly fluorescent. Ruiz and colleagues tested 4284 H_2S-positive colonies isolated on SS agar and 4350 isolated on Hektoen's agar.[47] The MUCAP test was 100% sensitive and 99.8% specific.

In this study, only 6 isolates identified as *Proteus vulgaris* produced positive findings on the MUCAP test. These findings confirm the results of Aguirre and colleagues.[48] The test is performed by directly flooding H_2S-positive colonies with 5 μl of the sterile MUCAP reagent and observing the colony after 3 to 5 minutes under a Wood's lamp (366 nm). The reagent has no effect on the viability of the colonies, but testing has not been performed using XLD, bismuth sulfite, or brilliant green agar selective media.

A noncommercial esterase spot test (methylumbelliferyl caprylate dissolved in ethanol at 1 mg/mL final concentration) was also evaluated using Rombach's agar, a new medium for detection of foodborne salmonellae.[49] All 190 *Salmonella* isolates tested were positive for the esterase after 24 hours of growth on Rombach's medium. The test was negative for all β-galactosidase–negative members of the Enterobacteriaceae but positive for *Pseudomonas* and *Acinetobacter* species. The authors also found Rombach's agar useful for coproculture in the clinical microbiology laboratory for detection of non-*typhi* *Salmonella* species.

A rapid new DNA hybridization procedure has been described for the detection of salmonellae in clinical fecal specimens.[50] The 1600–base-pair probe used in the assay was cloned from *Salmonella enteritidis* DNA and is unique. The probe had high sensitivity, hybridizing to all 70 *Salmonella* serotypes tested. The hybridizations were performed according to a novel specimen-processing protocol called wicking. The test did, however, use a radiolabeled probe, which limits its use in clinical laboratories.

Shigella

Shigella species cause bacillary dysentery, which is characterized by blood and mucus in stools. The organisms invade the intestinal mucosal epithelial cells and multiply within, causing host cell destruction. They rarely invade beyond the mucosa. *Shigella* remains one of the most common agents of bacterial diarrhea in the United States. An average of significantly more than 12,000 isolates are reported to the federal Centers for Disease Control (CDC) in Atlanta each year.[51] The genus consists of 39 serotypes or subtypes, which are divided antigenically on the basis of O antigenic groups into four species, or groups: *Shigella dysenteriae* (group A), *Shigella flexneri* (group B), *Shigella boydii* (group C), and *Shigella sonnei* (group D). Although slide agglutination tests used to serotype *Shigella* are easy and rapid, the success does depend on the quality of the antisera. A study from the CDC found that only 31 of the 73 grouping and typing sera tested (42%) from United States manufacturers were satisfactory.[52]

The organism can be detected on several of the enteric media (see Table 20–3) as lactose-negative colonies. On KIA, *Shigella* is nonmotile and urease-negative and produces no H_2S. With few exceptions, gas is not produced during sugar fermentations. Enteroinvasive *E. coli* resembles *Shigella* in that it may not be able to ferment lactose and it expresses identical surface antigenic structures. Invasive strains of *Shigella* and EIEC have been shown to carry a 120- to 140-MDa plasmid, the invasiveness (inv) plasmid, which encodes genes necessary for virulence.[53, 54] These findings have led to a number of independently developed probes and to a PCR system for the detection of these pathogens.

Escherichia coli

Four groups of *Escherichia coli* are well recognized as causes of infectious diarrhea: classic enteropathogenic serotypes (EPEC); those that produce the heat-labile enterotoxin (LT) or heat-stable enterotoxin (ST), (ETEC); enteroinvasive organisms that mimic *Shigella* (EIEC); and strains that produce Shiga-like cytotoxins (SLT) and cause enterohemorrhagic colitis (EHEC). Other groups of *E. coli*, defined by their adherence patterns as diffuse adhering *E. coli* (DAEC) and enteroaggregative *E. coli* (EAggEC) in assays of tissue culture, have been described, but their pathogenic capability is still controversial. These 4 accepted groups are distinguished on the basis of their pathogenic, clinical, and epidemiologic features and their association with certain O:H serotypes (Table 20–4). With the exception of the EHEC 0157:H7 strains, there are no reliable and specific biochemical tests that allow the differentiation of strains of any one of these groups from other commensal *E. coli*. Identification of these diverse groups of pathogens has been greatly facilitated by DNA probes (Table 20–5) and PCR-based tests (see Table 20–2).

Detection of Enteropathogenic *Escherichia coli*

Historically, EPEC was the first group of this genus to be identified as causal agents of diar-

TABLE 20–4. COMMON SEROTYPES OF DIARRHEAGENIC *ESCHERICHIA COLI**

ASSOCIATED WITH ENTEROPATHOGENIC *E. COLI*		
026:H11	0111:NM	0127:H9
026:NM	0111:H2	0127:H21
055:NM	0111:H12	0127:NM
055:H6	0111:H21	0127:H6
055:H7	0114:H2	0128ab:H2
086:NM	0119:H6	0142:H6
086:H34	0125ac:H21	0158:H23
086:H2	0126:H27	
ASSOCIATED WITH ENTEROTOXIGENIC *E. COLI*		
06:H16	025:H42	078:H11
06:H-	025:H-	078:H12
08:H9	026:H-	078:H-
015:H11	063:H12	0115:H40
015:H-	063:H-	0115:H51
		0149:H10
ASSOCIATED WITH ENTEROINVASIVE *E. COLI*		
028ac:H-	0112ac:H-	0143:H-
029:H-	0124:H-	0144:H-
032:H-	0136:H-	0152:H-
042:H-		0164:H-
ASSOCIATED WITH ENTEROHEMORRHAGIC *E. COLI* 0157:H7 (TYPE STRAIN)		
04:NM	0113	0126:H11
045:H2		0145:NM
0111:H8	0125:NM	
05:NM	0113:K75:H2	
091:H21	0121:H19	
0103:H2	0125:NM	

*More complete listing of serotypes can be found in Farmer JJ, III, Kelly MT. Enterobacteriaceae. *In*: Balows A, Hausler WJ Jr, Herrmann KL, *et al.*, eds. Manual of Clinical Microbiology, 5th ed. American Society for Microbiology, Washington DC, 1991:368.

TABLE 20–5. PROBES FOR DIARRHEAGENIC *ESCHERICHIA COLI*

PATHOGEN	PROBES	VIRULENCE PROPERTY DETECTED	REFERENCE
EPEC	EAF fragment	EPEC adherence factor (localized adherence to HEp-2 cells)	Scaletsky (1985)[55]
ETEC	LT_h -ST_{A1} -ST_{A1} -ST_{B1}	LT, ST enterotoxins	Scotland (1989)[66]
	ST_{A1}	ST enterotoxin	References 103–107
	ST_{A2}	ST enterotoxin	References 108–112
	LT	LT enterotoxin	
EIEC	*ipa* H	invasive ability	Venkatesan (1989)[113]
Shigella	*ipa* B, C, D	invasive ability	Venkatesan (1988)[114]
	17kb EcoR1 fragment	invasive plasmid	Venkatesan (1988)[114]
	2.5kb HindIII fragment	invasive plasmid	
EHEC	SLT-I	Shiga-like toxin I	Taylor (1988)[115]
	SLT-II	Shiga-like toxin II	Newland (1988)[116]
	CVD419	fimbrial adhesin plasmid	Brown (1989)[117]
EAggEC	1kb	aggregative HEp-2 cell adherence pattern	Levine (1987)[118] Baudry (1990)[101]

KEY: EAggEC = enteroaggregative *E. coli*, EHEC = enterohemorrhagic *E. coli*, EIEC = enteroinvasive *E. coli*, EPEC = enteropathogenic *E. coli*, ETEC = enterotoxigenic *E. coli*, LT = heat labile toxin, ST = heat stable toxin.
NOTE: LT probes also detect *V. cholerae* toxin.

rhea, and until recently, the organisms were defined by belonging to certain O:H serotypes, by not producing LT or ST, and by not having invasive ability. EPEC have declined in industrialized countries, and routine serotyping has been discontinued in most laboratories. In developing countries, however, EPEC are important pathogens. Polyvalent sera are available for serologic screening of strains. Strains that agglutinate in the sera must be confirmed by titration and H-antigen determination, usually at a reference laboratory.

More recently the adherence ability of EPEC in tissue culture assays, in a manner described as localized adherence, has been recognized as an important characteristic of this group.[55] The adherence to HEp-2 cells in a localized pattern is known to be associated with a high molecular weight plasmid. A 21 base pair oligonucleotide probe has been developed from a cloned fragment of plasmid and termed EPEC adherence factor (EAF). The oligonucleotide probe detected EPEC with localized adherence with greater sensitivity and specificity than did the previous EAF fragment probe.[56] This probe appeared to show great promise for detecting EPEC in future studies.

Detection of Enterotoxigenic *Escherichia coli*

Enterotoxigenic *E. coli* is a common cause of diarrhea in children in developing countries, and is responsible for traveler's diarrhea and occasional outbreaks due to heavily contaminated food and drink.[57] Patients with voluminous watery, cholera-like diarrhea should have 10 colonies picked from primary isolation plates to nutrient slants for storage until they can be tested for enterotoxin production. Two types of enterotoxin are produced: LT, which is destroyed by heating at 60°C for 15 minutes, and ST, which resists heating at 100°C for 15 minutes. ETEC may produce one or both of these enterotoxins. The *E. coli* LT is a complex, high molecular weight protein that is closely related structurally and functionally to cholera toxin. The immunologic cross-reactivity of the two toxins and their specific binding to GM_1 ganglioside have been utilized in the design of serologic detection systems. There are numerous assays for the enterotoxins produced by these strains (Table 20–6). Among the most sensitive and simple tests for LT are the Chinese hamster ovary (CHO) cell or mouse Y1 adrenal cell assays.[58,59] Three simple and rapid immunologic methods are the modified GM_1–horseradish peroxidase (HRP) ELISA,[60] the modified Biken (Elek) test,[61] and the modified staphylococcal coagglutination test.[62]

A commercial test is available for detecting LT. Scotland and colleagues evaluated a reverse passive latex agglutination (RPLA) test (VET-RPLA, Oxoid USA, Columbia, MD) designed to detect the LT.[63] In this study of 100 well-characterized ETEC isolates, there was 100% correlation between the new test and the Y1 mouse adrenal cell cytotoxicity assay. This test has also been found to assist in the detection of cholera toxin.

Fewer tests are available for ST, and the suckling mouse assay remains the gold standard for this toxin assay.[64] A new GM_1 ELISA was 100%

TABLE 20–6. ASSAYS FOR DETECTION OF LT AND ST ENTEROTOXINS

ASSAY	REFERENCE
HEAT-LABILE ENTEROTOXIN (LT)	
Cell culture assays	
Chinese hamster ovary (CHO)	Guerrant (1974)[58]
Y1 mouse adrenal cell	Sack (1975)[59]
Enzyme immunoassay (EIA) methods	
GM₁ ELISA	Svennerholm (1983)[60]
Biken (Elek) test	Honda (1981)[61]
Modified staphylococcal coagglutination	Ronnberg (1983)[62]
Latex agglutination test (LAT)	
VET-RPLA	Scotland (1989)[63]
HEAT-STABLE ENTEROTOXIN (ST)	
Suckling mouse	Dean (1972)[64]
GM₁ ELISA	Sanchez (1988)[65]
COLI-ST-EIA	Scotland (1989)[66]

NOTE: Not an exhaustive list.
KEY: ELISA = enzyme-linked immunosorbent assay.

sensitive and specific in the detection of ST-producing *E. coli*.[65] Scotland and colleagues have evaluated a commercial ELISA product for the detection of ST (COLI ST EIA, Denka Seiken, Tokyo, Japan).[66] The test used a peroxidase-conjugated monoclonal antibody to ST_A together with ST_A prepared by peptide synthesis. The test was positive for 100 strains of *E. coli* that carried ST_AI or ST_AII genes when compared with the infant mouse assay. The authors also tested the strains with an alkaline phosphatase conjugated mix of oligonucleotide probes for both ST_{A1} and ST_{A2} (DuPont, NEN Research Products, Boston MA). There was agreement among all three tests for the 100 toxin-producing isolates. Two additional strains were found to be positive only by the probes, however, and they produced LT and carried ST_{A1} gene sequences. It is not uncommon for a probe toxin assay to detect strains with toxin gene sequences that do not produce biologically active toxins.

The construction and use of an enzyme-labeled trivalent LT and ST probe for the detection of ETEC by hybridization has been described by Abe and colleagues.[67] They first constructed a so-called cassette-probe plasmid that contained copies of the enterotoxins most frequently found in human ETEC arranged in a tandem array (LT_h-ST_{A1}-ST_{A1}-ST_{B1}). Two copies of the ST_{A1} gene were incorporated to enhance the hybridization signal for this gene. This easily prepared probe specifically identified bacterial colonies of ETEC that produced the enterotoxins singly or in combination. The binding of the probe to the target has been assayed without

the use of radioisotopes. The enzyme-labeled probe detected 10^2 colony-forming units contained in 5 mg of feces, whereas the radiolabeled trivalent probe could detect only 10 colony-forming units. The trivalent probe also had 78% base sequence homology with the subunit A gene of *V. cholerae* enterotoxin and was able to detect strains of serotype Inaba or Ogawa. The cassette-probe plasmid offers several advantages, from ease of rapid probe preparation to simultaneous detection of multiple toxin genes. The results of this study suggested that such a trivalent probe could speed recognition of ETEC in stool specimens of diarrheal patients.

A PCR-based assay for detection of LT producing *E. coli* was first described by Olive, who reported amplification of the B subunit of the LT gene (Table 20–2).[68] Victor and colleagues successfully amplified a conserved region of the A subunit of the LT gene directly from a bacterial suspension without DNA extraction.[69] The amplified product (110-bp fragment) was detected by agarose gel electrophoresis. The sensitivity of the assay using visual detection of the DNA fragment with ethidium bromide staining was 100 LT⁺ colony-forming units per assay. Use of a radioisotope heightened the sensitivity to 1 LT⁺ colony-forming units per assay. An alkaline phosphatase–labeled probe detection system has also been examined and has been found to be more sensitive than the visual, but less sensitive than the radioisotopic, detection method.

Detection of Enteroinvasive *Escherichia coli*

There is a widespread sharing of antigens between EIEC and *Shigella*. These *E. coli* are frequently delayed or nonlactose fermenters, anaerogenic, nonmotile, and lysine decarboxylase–negative; thus, they are readily confused with *Shigella*. In addition, isolates with the above biochemical profile may sometimes cross-react with *Shigella* antisera. Patients with dysenteric diarrhea should be screened for EIEC serotypes (see Table 20–4) by preserving 5 to 10 colonies with the previously described biochemical characteristics for testing at a research center by the Sereny test,[70] an ELISA assay,[71] or DNA probe assays[113, 114] (see Table 20–5). None of these tests are available commercially.

Polymerase chain reaction–based tests have also been performed directly on crude DNA isolated from feces, with successful detection of *Shigella* and EIEC. Frankel and colleagues identified DNA sequences within an invasion-associated locus *(ial)* of the invasion plasmid that were specific for these pathogens (see Table 20–2).[72] Two unique sequences flanking the sequence corresponding to the *ial* region were used as primers. The 320–base pair amplification product could be detected by gel electrophoresis or DNA hybridization using the *ial* gene probe. The assay was found to be 10^2 times more sensitive than the macrocolony hybridization assay (fecal blot) using the same *ial* probe, and 10^5 times more sensitive than conventional biochemical tests. The assay could be completed in 7 hours and could detect as few as 10 colony-forming units.

Detection of Enterohemorrhagic *Escherichia coli*

Escherichia coli was first associated with hemorrhagic colitis after an investigation of two outbreaks in 1982.[73, 74] These *E. coli* organisms, which are now known as EHEC, produce cytotoxins active against Vero cells (Verotoxins, also known as Shiga-like toxins [SLTs]) and HeLa cells in much the same manner as Shiga toxin is produced by *S. dysenteriae* type 1. More than 30 serotypes of *E. coli* are known to produce SLTs, although *E. coli* serotype 0157:H7 is the most prevalent in North America and Europe (see Table 20–4). The incidence rate of *E. coli* 0157:H7 in the Puget Sound area of Washington State is 8 per 100,000 person-years compared with 150 for *Campylobacter* and 21 for *Salmonella*.[75] The organism is highly infectious and should be handled with care, since laboratory and hospital infections have occurred. The EHEC have also been shown to have an association with the development of hemolytic-uremic syndrome (HUS) and possibly thrombocytopenic purpura (TTP).[76] Because of the seriousness of complication of EHEC infections, it is important that early identification be made in the clinical laboratory. At present, *E. coli* 0157:H7 should be sought in stool cultures of patients with acute bloody diarrhea. The organism appears to be rapidly shed during the disease, and early culture is more successful. Tarr and colleagues showed the importance of early detection of *E. coli* 0157:H7 in establishing this organism as the causal agent.[77]

Certain biochemical characteristics of *E. coli* 0157:H7 allow these strains to be more rapidly identified in clinical laboratories. The majority fail to ferment D-sorbitol within 18 hours, and this trait allowed for development of a rapid screening medium using MacConkey agar with sorbitol substituted for lactose in the formulation. The sorbitol-negative colonies, which appeared colorless, could then be identified as *E. coli* and tested for agglutination with specific antisera. Sorbitol MacConkey agar is available

commercially. The commercially available 0157 and H7 antisera (Difco Laboratories, Detroit MI) work well if the manufacturer's instructions are followed; the organisms need to be subcultured for testing. Two new latex products (Oxoid USA, Columbia MD and Pro-Lab Diagnostic, Round Rock TX) can be used to screen non–sorbitol-fermenting *E. coli*–like colonies directly from the sorbitol MacConkey plate. Both these kits include control latex reagents, which greatly reduce the frequency of false-positive reactions.[78] The MUG test can be performed to assist in the recognition of this group of pathogens. Ninety-six percent of *E. coli* isolates produce the enzyme β-D-glucuronidase, which cleaves the substrate MUG, producing the fluorescent end product. *Escherichia coli* 0157:H7 organisms have been known to be uniformly MUG-negative. Thompson and colleagues developed a rapid (20 min) MUG test and screened 879 clinical *E. coli* isolates.[79] Included in this sample were various *E. coli* serotype 0157 strains, of which 155 were toxin-positive and 22 were toxin-negative. This study demonstrated that all 0157 serotypes that were toxin-positive were MUG-negative, and all toxin-negative 0157 isolates were MUG-positive. Thus, the MUG test could be used to predict toxin production by 0157 isolates. The authors also noted that inocula used for MUG testing should be taken from blood agar media, rather than directly from MacConkey and triple sugar iron agar, since both these media can interfere in the enzyme reaction. Use of the latex agglutination test (LAT)[80] or a fluorescent antibody test[81] along with a rapid MUG test should allow for fast and accurate detection of *E. coli* serotype 0157:H7 involved in disease.

Other assays have been aimed at detection of the toxins produced by EHEC. Shiga-like toxins are classified in two antigenically distinct groups: SLT-I and SLT-II. The SLT-I type appears to be an antigenically homogeneous group more closely related to Shiga toxin. The SLT II group (i.e., SLT-II, SLT-IIv, SLT-IIva) appears to be more diverse antigenically. *Escherichia coli* producing SLT-IIv are the causative agents of edema disease in pigs,[82] which resembles, but is not identical to, HUS in humans. Edema disease has been reproduced in pigs with purified SLT-IIv.[83] The SLT-IIva has been associated with diarrhea in a human infant.[84] At present, it seems that strains producing one or both SLT-I and SLT-II are pathogenic. Nevertheless, the role that these potent toxins play in shigellosis, other diarrheal diseases, and possibly HUS and TTP, is still unclear.

Both SLTs can be rapidly detected using Vero cell or HeLa cell cytotoxicity assays. Test material can be stool filtrates or broth supernatants from colony sweeps. Ideally, the stool should undergo testing of several hundred colonies in order to search adequately for this pathogen. For such screenings, monoclonal immunoblot techniques[85] or DNA toxin probes are most efficient,[86-90] but they are not commercially available and are relatively time-consuming. The ELISA developed by Basta and colleagues for the rapid detection of SLT-I employs the deacylated globotriosyl ceramide Gb_3 as the capture molecule for the toxin.[91] In comparison with the cytotoxicity assay, a 98% correlation was found. A new sandwich ELISA was developed by Acheson and colleagues using preparations of P_1 glycoprotein as the toxin capture molecule.[92] The glycoprotein was prepared from hydatid cyst fluid isolated from sheep infected with *Echinococcus granulosus*. The hydatid cyst protein-based ELISAs detected as little as 80 pg of Shiga toxin, or 132 pg of SLT-II. Neither of these methods has been adapted for detection of free fecal toxins.

Polymerase chain reaction techniques have been developed to speed identification of strains capable of producing serologically distinct SLTs (see Table 20–2). Karch and Meyer developed a single primer pair of so-called degenerate sequence primers, which functioned in the cytotoxin-producing *E. coli* irrespective of the type of toxin produced.[93] The test required the use of detection probes for SLT-I and SLT-II. Using two sets of synthetic oligonucleotide primers, Johnson and colleagues were able to distinguish between the closely related genes for SLT-II and the toxin associated with porcine edema disease, SLT-IIv.[94] EHEC that produce SLT-II variants have been reported in human disease,[84, 95] although analysis of these isolates by PCR and restriction length polymorphism analysis indicated that a human SLT-IIv–producing strain has yet to be described.[96]

Jackson reported a technique for SLT-I detection that centered on PCR testing with simultaneous incorporation of digoxigenin-11-dUTP (uridine 5′-triphosphate) into the amplification products.[97] A spot blot detection system was used to detect the PCR product. The technique did not require gel electrophoresis or radioactive DNA probes. This type of assay appears well suited for clinical detection of EHEC that produce SLT-I.

Detection of Adherent *Escherichia coli*

Studies of certain diarrheagenic *E. coli* in an HEp-2 cell assay revealed three distinct patterns of adherence: diffuse, localized, and aggregative.

The localized phenotype was found to be a characteristic of the EPEC. Isolates exhibiting the diffuse and aggregative attachment are two new categories of adherent *E. coli*. Epidemiologic studies of enteroaggregative *E. coli* (EAggEC) have found an association with diarrheal disease. Evidence implicating the DAEC is, however, less clear.[98-100]

The EAggEC derive their name from a stacked-brick–like lattice adherence pattern observed in HEp-2 cell culture. This group shares some characteristics in common with other categories of diarrheagenic *E. coli*. Certain O:H serotypes are common, and a ~60 MDa plasmid is required for expression of the adherence phenotype.

Baudry and colleagues isolated and cloned a 1-Kb fragment from the plasmid of an EAggEC strain (see Table 20–5).[101, 103-118] This fragment functioned as well as a probe. In a survey of 439 strains, the fragment proved to be 89% sensitive and 99% specific for EAggEC identification. This probe, or a DNA sequence from a newly described ST enterotoxin,[102] should greatly facilitate epidemiologic studies to assess the role of EAggEC in diarrheal disease.

Yersinia enterocolitica

Yersinia enterocolitica is well recognized as a human pathogen implicated in acute gastroenteritis, and a severe form is also seen that mimics appendicitis. While diarrhea is the most commonly recognized clinical presentation, this pathogen can also cause invasive disease and has been associated with a variety of autoimmune manifestations such as arthritis and erythema nodosum.

Infections due to this organism occur primarily in infants and young children living in temperate climates. Sporadic cases as well as food- and waterborne outbreaks have occurred.[119] Because the organism has low prevalence in certain geographic areas, each laboratory needs to determine whether every stool sample should be screened for the organism or whether such cultures will be performed only on request.[120]

Metchock and colleagues reported an isolation rate of 1% at an urban hospital serving a large pediatric population in the southeast United States.[121] Similarly, in an outpatient study conducted in Baltimore MD, *Y. enterocolitica* was isolated from 2% of children younger than 2 years who had diarrhea.[122] These studies suggest that institutions with large pediatric populations, especially those with children younger than 2 years, should reassess the need for routine screening for this organism.

Although there are more than 50 serogroups in the species, only five, designated 0:1,2a, 3; 0:3; 0:5,27; 0:8; and 0:9, are generally regarded as pathogenic for humans. Characteristics shared by these groups and believed to be associated with virulence include carriage of a virulence plasmid, which confers calcium dependence and the ability to bind Congo red dye[123]; a negative pyrazinamidase reaction[124]; production of *Yersinia* ST[125]; and invasive ability, assayed by invasion of HEp-2 cells,[126] or the presence of chromosomal loci involved in invasion, termed *ail* and *inv*.[127–129]

Yersinia enterocolitica can be isolated from MacConkey's medium, although the colonies are much smaller than those of other enteric organisms. Growth of *Yersinia* on SS or Hektoen's agar can be variable. A *Yersinia* selective agar is available, cefsulodin–Irgasan–novobiocin (CIN) medium. This medium should be incubated at room temperature (22–25°C) and inspected at 24 and 48 hours for characteristic colonies (see Table 20–3). Cold enrichment is also effective, but it is time-consuming and, consequently, may not allow for detection of the organism within a clinically relevant time frame.[130] Once the organism is identified, a number of simple tests can be used to identify virulent strains. On Congo red–magnesium oxalate (CRMOX) agar, *Y. enterocolitica* produces red colonies, indicating the presence of the *Yersinia* virulence plasmid, or large colorless colonies, indicating loss of the plasmid. The red colonies can be tested with the pyrazinamidase test, and salicin–esculin fermentation, both of which produce negative findings for virulent isolates.

Since isolation of *Yersinia* from feces is not always successful, the laboratory diagnosis is often dependent on detection of specific antibodies in serum. Currently, the serologic diagnosis is made primarily by ELISA[131] or tube agglutination.[132] *Yersinia* infections are usually associated with a strong antibody response. Separate quantification of serotype-specific *Yersinia* antibodies of different immunoglobulin classes is considered important.[131, 133, 134] The multiple *Yersinia* serotypes and their wide antigenic diversity have made the routine separate testing against various common serotypes laborious and expensive.

An ELISA using a combined antigen (virulence plasmid encoded released *Yersinia* proteins and *Y. enterocolitica* 0:3 LPS) was designed.[135] Used on the sera of 43 patients infected with different *Yersinia* serotypes, this test was more sensitive (93%) than a routine battery of 6 serotype-specific ELISAs (88% sensitivity). This test shows promise as a screening ELISA.

Two PCR-based assays have been described. Using primers based on a nucleotide sequence for the *virF* gene located on the virulence plasmid pYV, Wren and Tabaqchali were able to obtain a 590 base pair product when 51 of 59 pathogenic *Y. enterocolitica* strains were tested.[136] The eight PCR-negative strains were found to have lost the pYV plasmid, as evidenced by lack of uptake of Congo red. In addition, five pathogenic strains of *Yersinia pseudotuberculosis* that contained the plasmid were also PCR-positive. This technique did not require hybridization or use of a radioisotope and could be performed in 3 hours. A potential drawback to this method is plasmid loss on subculture prior to PCR testing. Fenwich and Murray have developed a PCR-based test that avoids such false-negatives by targeting a sequence within the *ail* gene specific for pathogenic *Yersinia*.[137, 138] A 359 base pair amplification product was found when *Y. enterocolitica* biotypes 2, 3, and 4 were tested. Nonpathogenic *Y. enterocolitica* as well as other *Yersinia* species and six common enteric bacterial species were all negative in this test. Neither of these two PCR-based tests has been applied directly to fecal specimens.

Aeromonas

Aeromonas species occur widely in soil and natural waters; they have long been recognized as the cause of disease in fish and amphibians. These organisms have been found in chlorinated as well as untreated drinking water and in a variety of foods such as ground beef and pork, fish, shellfish, poultry, and raw milk.[139, 140]

Human infections can range from cellulitis in patients with traumatic wounds infected in aquatic areas to bacteremia in immunocompromised patients. Although the wound and blood infections caused by these organisms are well described, *Aeromonas* species were only recently recognized as a potentially important cause of gastrointestinal disease, particularly in certain geographic areas.[141–146]

A range of symptoms has been described, from mild, self-limiting diarrhea to acute dysentery or chronic watery diarrhea persisting for weeks or months. The breadth of this range of symptoms suggests a complex cause in which strains can possess a variety of virulence factors, as has been documented for the various classes of diarrheagenic *E. coli*.

The role of these organisms in gastrointestinal disease is still controversial, in part owing to the confusion that has existed concerning the species within the genus *Aeromonas*. Difficulties also exist in correlating the potential virulence properties of clinical isolates, including enterotoxin, cytotoxin, hemolysin, hemagglutinin, and invasive ability, with the production of specific symptoms of disease. At present, no consistent pattern of biochemical reactions or virulence properties can reliably predict the pathogenicity of a particular strain.

The taxonomy of this group of organisms has undergone a revision. On the basis of biochemical reactions, human diarrheal isolates of *Aeromonas* are now divided into 4 phenospecies, *A. hydrophila*, *A. caviae*, *A. sobria* (consisting of two genospecies: *A. veronii* and *A. jandaei,* differentiated by sucrose fermentation[147]), and *A. veronii* (Table 20–7). The range of tests required to differentiate these phenospecies is extensive, however, and most rapid identification systems used in clinical laboratories identify only to the genus level.[148, 149]

Using DNA hybridization, the *Aeromonas* species have been divided into 13 DNA hybridization groups (see Table 20–7).[150, 151] Of these, groups 1, 4, and 8 are those predominantly associated with diarrhea in humans.[152] Using multilocus enzyme electrophoresis, Altwegg and colleagues showed that electromorphic variation at 4 enzymatic loci could be used to assign 98% of the *Aeromonas* strains to the correct DNA hybridization group.[153]

In the routine clinical laboratory, *Aeromonas* species may be grown on the usual enteric agar. It may be difficult, however, to distinguish *Aeromonas* from other nonaeromonad fecal flora. As a result, it has been suggested that ampicillin at a concentration of 30 mg/L be added to blood agar.[154] This would have the effect of suppressing the other flora, and hemolysis of certain strains of *Aeromonas* could be observed. A small proportion of *A. caviae* would be inhibited by this concentration of ampicillin, and although the pathogenicity of *A. caviae* is still in question, Namdari and Buttone have reported *A. caviae* in cases of pediatric gastrointestinal infections.[155] The addition of bile salts to media at a level required to inhibit the growth of *E. coli* would also inhibit the growth of *Aeromonas* species[154] and is, therefore, not recommended. *Aeromonas* species are distinguished from the Enterobacteriaceae, which they most closely resemble, by the oxidase test; Enterobacteriaceae are oxidase-negative. *Aeromonas* species are differentiated from oxidase-positive vibrios by their resistance to the vibriostatic agent 2,4-diamino-6,7-diisopropylpteridine phosphate (referred to as 0/129). The growth of all vibrios is inhibited at a 150 μg/ml concentration of 0/129. The commercial biochemical and enzymatic identification systems routinely used for characterization of Enterobacteriaceae identify *Aeromonas* and *Plesiomonas* to at least the genus level with the addition of the oxidase test to the panel of tests used.

With the continuing clarification of the subdivisions of the genus *Aeromonas* it may be possible in the future to look at potential virulence factors produced by these organisms, and to determine the clinical significance of each species. Examination of clinical isolates at the DNA level should resolve some of the conflicting reports produced by investigators using different biochemical approaches to identifying the *Aeromonas* species. Until more rapid techniques are developed for the identification of the various *Aeromonas* species and until the pathogenicity of each is determined, laboratories should continue to identify and report *Aeromonas* as a probable cause of human diarrheal disease.

Plesiomonas

The genus *Plesiomonas* consists of one species only, *P. shigelloides*. Like *Aeromonas* species, it is

TABLE 20–7. *AEROMONAS* SPECIES ASSOCIATED WITH HUMAN DIARRHEAL DISEASE

GENOSPECIES	PHENOSPECIES	DNA GROUPS	DISCRIMINATING BIOCHEMICAL TESTS
A. hydrophila	*A. hydrophila*	1	
	A. hydrophila	2	
A. salmonicida	*A. hydrophila*	3	Sorbitol+
A. caviae	*A. caviae*	4	
A. media	*A. caviae*	5	
A. veronii	*A. sobria*	8/10	
A. jandaei	*A. sobria*	9	Sucrose−
A. veronii	*A. veronii*	10/8	Ornithine decarboxylase+ Arginine dihydrolase−
Unnamed	*A. veronii*	11	Ornithine decarboxylase+

found in fresh water, mud, and coastal waters. The aquatic distribution of this organism, however, is limited by its minimum growth temperature of 8°C and the fact that it is not halophilic. The organism has been associated with several outbreaks of human gastroenteritis[156] and with sporadic cases of gastritis[157–159] occurring mainly in tropical regions.[160] *Plesiomonas shigelloides* organisms grow on most of the enteric isolation media, apart from thiosulphate–citrate–bile salts–sucrose TCBS or bismuth sulphite agar. On eosin–methylene blue (EMB) or MacConkey's agar it appears as a non–lactose-fermenting or late lactose-fermenting colony. Like *Aeromonas* species, *Plesiomonas* is oxidase-positive, catalase-positive, and H_2S-negative. Unlike *Aeromonas* species, *Plesiomonas* is DNase-positive and sensitive to 0/129 at a concentration of 150 μg/ml. *Plesiomonas* is differentiated from *Vibrio* species by its failure to grow on TCBS agar and in 6% NaCl. Infections due to *P. shigelloides* should be considered in patients returning from tropical regions with a history of diarrhea. In particular, it should be considered in patients who may have been exposed to untreated water in those locations.

Vibrio

Classic cholera is caused by enterotoxin-producing *Vibrio cholerae* 01, a waterborne pathogen. After an incubation time of 1 to 4 days after ingestion of infected substance, the enterotoxigenic organisms produce the severe, large-volume, watery diarrhea, termed rice water stool. This disease, responsible for seven pandemics since the 1850s, is increasing in incidence again in South America and causes tens of thousands of deaths annually in the Indian subcontinent. The mechanisms by which cholera toxin produces the characteristic symptoms of cholera have been studied extensively.[161] In addition to cholera toxin, *V. cholerae* has been demonstrated to produce a second LT moiety, 10 to 30 kDa in mass.[162] Using rabbit ileum, the toxin was found to alter intestinal permeability rapidly by acting on intestinal epithelial cell tight junctions (zonula occludens) and has, therefore, been named ZOT. *Vibrio cholerae* serogroup 1 may be divided into 2 or 3 subtypes and into 2 biogroups, classical and el Tor. The el Tor variant is currently predominant, and with this biogroup a milder form of illness, characterized by diarrhea lasting 1 to 5 days and followed by spontaneous recovery, is more common than is severe cholera. The two biogroups are distinguishable by biochemical tests and specific bacteriophage lysis.

Any noncholera vibrio (NCV), also referred to as a nonagglutinable vibrio (NAG), is biochemically identical to *V. cholerae*, but NCVs are not agglutinable in *Vibrio* O group 1 antiserum. The NCV strains may produce a similar enterotoxin and cause a similar illness. *Vibrio mimicus* is almost identical to *V. cholerae* biochemically, but DNA hybridization studies show homology of only 24 to 54%. It appears to be a less common cause of infection than other *Vibrio* species but has been associated with cases of diarrhea.[163] *Vibrio parahaemolyticus*, although rare in North America, is a common cause of foodborne outbreaks of gastroenteritis in Japan and other areas of the world.[164] Typically, it is associated with contaminated raw seafood. Outbreaks have occurred on cruise ships when cooked foods have been contaminated by infected raw foodstuffs. The diarrhea is watery and sometimes bloody.

Vibrio vulnificus is one of the group of ornithine decarboxylase–negative, lysine decarboxylase–positive *Vibrio* species. It is thought to be a rare cause of diarrhea in humans. Sporadic cases of diarrhea due to *Vibrio fluvialis* infection have been reported, and it may be capable of causing outbreaks.[165] Diarrhea is watery and may be accompanied by vomiting, abdominal pain, and, sometimes, severe dehydration. *Vibrio furnissii* has, likewise, been isolated from patients with diarrhea, but the pathogenic significance of this organism has yet to be elucidated.[166]

The remaining *Vibrio* species associated with diarrhea in man is *V. hollisae*. This organism has been demonstrated to be a rare cause of diarrhea in humans, although increased awareness may reveal the organism to be more common than originally recognized.[167]

When the presence of *Vibrio* species is suspected, stool specimens should, ideally, be collected within the first 24 hours of illness. Rectal swabs or fecal material may be placed in semisolid Cary-Blair transport medium if there is to be a delay in processing a specimen. In the field, tellurite–taurocholate–peptone broth has been used successfully as an enrichment transport medium. The fecal specimen should be plated on TCBS medium, which is both selective and differential. If small numbers of organisms are anticipated, the specimens should first be incubated in enrichment broth. An alkaline peptone water (1.5% peptone and 0.5% NaCl adjusted to pH 9.0 before autoclaving) is incubated at 35°C for 12 hours and subcultured to TCBS agar.

On TCBS, *V. cholerae* forms large (2 mm in diameter), flat, yellow colonies (Table 20–8). There are many commercial sources of TCBS

TABLE 20–8. TESTS DISTINGUISHING AMONG *VIBRIO* SPECIES ISOLATED FROM PATIENTS WITH DIARRHEA

TEST	V. CHOLERAE	V. MIMICUS	V. HOLLISAE	V. FLUVIALIS	V. FURNISSII	V. PARA-HAEMOLYTICUS	V. VULNIFICUS
Growth in nutrient broth without NACl	+	+	–	–	–	–	–
Sucrose	+	–	–	+	+	–	–
Arginine dihydrolase	–	–	–	+	+	–	–
Lysine decarboxylase	+	+	–	–	–	+	+
D-glucose gas-production			–	+			
Salicin						–	+
Cellobiose						–	+
Swarming (marine agar, 25°C)						+	–
Motility						+	–

medium, of variable quality, making laboratory quality control mandatory. Typical *V. cholerae* colonies should be subcultured to nutrient agar before performing a slide agglutination test with O group 1 serum. An inoculum can also be transferred to KIA, and after overnight incubation, a K/A reaction without gas or H_2S production is indicative of *V. cholerae*. If the strain does not agglutinate in the group 01 serum, an oxidase test and a string test should be performed. In a string test, 18- to 24-hour growth is suspended in a drop of 0.5% aqueous solution of sodium deoxycholate. The suspension should become less turbid and very mucoid immediately, and form strings when a loop is drawn slowly away from the solution. String test–positive and oxidase-positive isolates can be identified as *V. cholerae* non-01. Table 20–8 shows the tests described above and additional biochemical reactions that differentiate the *Vibrio* species described. The use of vibriostatic compound 0/129 as a primary screening agent for vibrios may warrant further investigation after a report from Bangladesh of *Vibrio cholerae* 01 isolates resistant to 0/129.[168]

An RPLA assay (VET-RPLA Oxoid USA, Columbia MD) mentioned above, is available commercially and offers the potential for a simple, rapid diagnostic assay for cholera toxin and *E. coli* LT enterotoxin, with which cholera toxin is virtually identical. This was found to be comparable in sensitivity and specificity to an ELISA for cholera toxin.[169] DNA probe assays for cholera toxin have been developed as research tools, but as yet such tests are labor-intensive, lengthy, and not available commercially.

Campylobacter

Campylobacter species are widely distributed in nature in both animals and humans and in water contaminated with feces. *Campylobacter* enteritis has received much attention since Butzler and colleagues isolated *C. jejuni*, previously called *C. fetus* subspecies *jejuni*, at a higher rate from feces of children with diarrhea than from controls.[170] Since then, this pathogen has been shown by a number of investigators to be as common a cause of diarrhea as *Salmonella* and *Shigella* combined.[171–173]

Among the so-called true *Campylobacter* species causing enteric disease are the thermophilic *Campylobacter*: *C. jejuni*, *C. coli*, *C. lari*, and the less common *C. upsaliensis*. The first two may be differentiated from *C. jejuni* on the basis of nalidixic acid sensitivity and hippurate hydrolysis (Table 20–9). *Campylobacter upsaliensis* was first isolated from dogs but has been found to have a wider habitat, and using a filtration isolation system, it has been shown to be a frequent pathogen in humans.[174]

Campylobacter fetus subspecies *fetus*, *C. hyointestinalis*, *C. butzleri*, and some organisms previously classified as *Campylobacter*, namely *Helicobacter cinaedi*, *Helicobacter fennelliae*, and *Arcobacter cryaerophilus*, have also been associated with human disease. *Helicobacter cinaedi* and *H. fennelliae* have been isolated from the rectal cultures of homosexual males with proctitis or proctocolitis and from the blood of patients with AIDS.[175] *Campylobacter butzleri* and *A. cryaerophilus* (previously *Campylobacter cryaerophila*[175a]) grow at low temperatures. *Campylobacter butzleri* has been associated with diarrhea in humans.[176] The pathogenicity of the heterogeneous *A. cryaerophilus* has yet to be fully determined.

In general, there are several selective media consisting of blood or charcoal agars supplemented with antibiotics. Media for the isolation of *Campylobacter* species containing cephalothin do not support the growth of *C. fetus* subspecies

TABLE 20–9. SUMMARY OF DIFFERENTIAL TEST REACTIONS AND CHARACTERISTICS OF NINE CAMPYLOBACTER SPECIES ISOLATED FROM HUMAN FECES

TEST	C. JEJUNI SUBSP JEJUNI	C. COLI SUBSP DOYLEI	C. LARI	C. UPSALIENSIS	C. FETUS SUBSP FETUS	C. HYOINTESTINALIS	AR.* BUTZLERI	AR.* CRYAEROPHILUS	C. CINAEDI	C. FENNELLIAE
Growth										
25°C	−	−	−	−	+	+	+	+		−
37°C	+	+	+	+	+	+	+	+	+	+
42°C	+	+	+	+	d	+	−	d	−	−
1% glycine	+	+	+	−	+	+	+	+		
3.5% NaCl	−	−	−	+	+	+	−	d	−	−
Motility	+	+	+	+	+	−	d	d	+	+
Oxidase	+	+	+	+	+	+	+	+	+	−
Catalase	+	+	+	e	+	+	d	d	+	+
Nitrate reduction	+	+	+	+	+	+	−	−	+	+
H₂S (TSI medium)	−	−	−	+	−	+	−	−	+	+
H₂S (cystein medium with lead acetate strip)	+	+	+	−	d	+	d	d	−	−
Hippurate hydrolysis	+	−	−	−	−	−	−	−	−	−
Odor (hypochlorite)	−	−	−	−	−	−	−	−	+	+
Susceptibility										
Cephalothin	R	R	R	S	S	S	R	d	±	S
Nalidixic acid	S	S	R	S	R	R	S	d	S	S

*Organisms previously known as aero-tolerant *Campylobacter* are now included in the genus *Arcobacter*.

KEY: + = Positive reaction for 90% or more of strains; − = negative reaction for 90% or more of strains; d = positive reaction for 11 to 89% of strains; R = resistant; S = susceptible; e = most strains negative, a few strains positive; I = intermediate (30 μg disks).

fetus.[177] The obvious advantage of the selective media is their ease of handling compared with the difficulty in organizing a filtration procedure. The disadvantages, however, include decay of inhibitors and growth of many fecal organisms other than *Campylobacter* species. Use of two differing selective media for direct inoculation can increase the isolation rates of these organisms.[178]

Campylobacter jejuni remains viable in stool specimens at 25°C for a few hours but can survive for at least 2 weeks at 4°C in feces, water, milk, and urine.[179] Thus, fecal specimens should be refrigerated if they cannot be processed within a few hours. In a study of 1249 fecal specimens cultured by direct inoculation on both selective Columbia medium and liquid enrichment medium, Hodge and Terro showed that the use of liquid medium provided a 30% higher isolation rate for *C. jejuni.*[180] A filtration technique that also proved effective involved placing drops of heavy fecal suspension on a Millipore filter (0.65 μm, pore size) on the surface of a chocolate agar plate. This plate was incubated for 1 hour at 37°C, the filter was removed, and the plate was incubated as usual in appropriate atmosphere at 42°C or 37°C.[181] As mentioned above, filtration in the isolation of *C. upsaliensis* greatly increases the yield of positive cultures.[174]

In general, after plates are streaked for isolation, they should be incubated at 42°C. *Campylobacter jejuni* is microaerophilic and grows best in an atmosphere containing no greater than 6% oxygen, 10% hydrogen, and 85% nitrogen. There are commercial systems available for growth of these organisms: CampyPak I, which requires the addition of the catalyst to the jar, or CampyPak II, which has a self-contained catalyst (BBL Microbiology Systems, Cockeysville MD). Although it is possible to achieve the correct atmosphere using a GasPak (Becton Dickinson, Cockeysville MD) hydrogen and CO_2-generator envelope in a GasPak jar with the catalyst removed, this method should be avoided, since the hydrogen generated under these conditions may be potentially explosive. The jars or gas-filled bags should not be overfilled. Plates should be examined at 24 and 48 hours for typical colonies, and if absent, they should be reincubated for another day. Subcultures should be made immediately because the organism may lose viability after prolonged (72 hours) incubation at 42°C.

Campylobacter colonies can be flat, greyish, and glistening, with an irregular or entirely convex edge. In the Gram stain protocol, 0.06% carbolfuchsin should be substituted as the counterstain. Prolonged staining time also improves the quality of the staining reaction.

For all practical purposes, the genus *Campylobacter* is identified by the following criteria: small gram-negative curved rods with occasional seagull-like forms, characteristic darting movements by darkfield or phase-contrast microscopy, inability to ferment or oxidize glucose, and positive findings on oxidase test. Biochemical confirmation and identification of various species is shown in Table 20–9. Identification and differentiation of clinical isolates is based on a limited number of morphologic and biochemical reactions, and misidentification may result when atypical reactions occur.

A commercial rapid LAT (Campyslide, BBL Microbiology Systems, Cockeysville MD) is also available for confirmatory genus-level identification of the three major *Campylobacter* human enteric pathogens as well as of *C. fetus* subspecies *fetus.* The test cross-reacts with some isolates of *Pseudomonas aeruginosa*, which could cause confusion, since *Pseudomonas* is also oxidase-positive.[182]

Campylobacter hyointestinalis grows at 42°C, but some strains grow more abundantly at 37°C. Colonies are yellow, smooth, and nonswarming. The previously designated *Campylobacter* species *C. cinaedi* and *C. fennelliae* are fastidious, often requiring 4 to 7 days for growth, and prefer a more hydrogen-rich atmosphere than do *C. jejuni* and *C. coli*. The previously designated *C. cryaerophila* has the ability to grow at low temperatures and in the presence of air after isolation. Cultivation of this organism is complicated, however, requiring two stages: an initial isolation in leptospira medium (with 5-fluorouracil and 1% rabbit serum) incubated aerobically at 30°C for 4 to 5 weeks, followed by subculture to blood agar supplemented with 7% lysed horse blood and carbenicillin (125 μg/ml), microaerophilic incubation at 30°C for 48 to 72 hours. A strain has also been isolated by using blood agar containing 6% lysed horse blood, vancomycin (10 mg/ml), polymyxin B (1250 IU/ml), and trimethoprim (10 mg/ml). Colonies appeared after 3 days of incubation at 37°C but not at 42°C.[183]

Assays using DNA probes are available for detection of some of these pathogens.[184–186] The specificity of these assays is excellent, making them ideal tools for culture confirmation. Improvements still need to be made in order to increase the sensitivity of these tests so that they can be used for the direct detection of *Campylobacter* species in stool specimens. Species-specific DNA probes remain a research tool, however, and serology is the usual means of epidemiologic investigation.

Clostridium

Recognized since the 1890s, pseudomembranous colitis may occur in association with gastrointestinal surgery, staphylococcal infection, bowel obstruction, vascular insufficiency, and uremia; it is also seen in high-risk newborn infants. The vast majority of cases described since the 1960s, however, have occurred in association with antibiotic usage. The precise mechanism involved in this disease, found in association with a number of clinical settings, has recently become apparent with the recognition of the toxins produced by *C. difficile*. This organism is only rarely present (0–4%) in the colonic flora of adults. When present, therapy with certain antibiotics apparently sets the stage for overgrowth by this organism, production of toxins, and development of pseudomembranous colitis.

Clostridium difficile produces at least two distinct toxins, A and B,[187, 188] and a little-described motility factor.[189] Toxin A has been described as an enterotoxin because it causes a fluid response in rabbit ileal loops. Toxin B has minimal enterotoxin activity but is the primary cytotoxin. The cytotoxic activity of toxin B is approximately 1000 times greater than that of toxin A. Several methods that are currently available for the diagnosis of *C. difficile*–mediated disease include isolation of the organism and detection of toxin A or B. The cytotoxicity assay first developed by Chang and colleagues,[190, 191] has become the primary method of testing for *C. difficile* toxin in diagnostic and research laboratories. The cytotoxicity assay has high specificity and sensitivity, detecting more than 1 pg of toxin B and consequently has been considered the gold-standard method.[192] The test involves detection of a cytopathic effect on any of a variety of tissue culture cell lines (HeLa 229, McCoy, Vero, Y1 adrenal cells). Specific neutralization assays using *Clostridium sordellii* or specific *C. difficile* antitoxins are performed on each patient's specimen. The test can require 48 hours for detection of some slow-growing specimens, although often a positive identification can be made in 6 to 8 hours. Aronsson and colleagues have found the testing of consecutive stool specimens to be advantageous when *C. difficile* is suspected as the cause of antibiotic-associated diarrhea or colitis.[193] According to these authors, a second stool sample on a subsequent day can improve detection of infected patients by 7%, or by 10% if 3 samples are tested.

A complete microtiter plate cell culture system is available commercially (Bartels Immunodiagnostic Supplies, Bellevue WA) for the detection of *C. difficile* toxin B. The system is supplied complete with a microtiter plate containing human foreskin fibroblast cells, diluent, positive and negative controls, and specific antitoxin. The system requires a 35 to 37°C incubator and a brightfield or inverted microscope. Wu and Gersch have found it to be an acceptable alternative to the conventional cell culture assay.[194]

Isolation of *C. difficile* from stool specimens has become feasible since the development of a selective medium consisting of an egg yolk–fructose base with cycloserine and cefoxitin.[195] Compared with toxin detection by tissue assay, isolation of the organism has yielded a higher frequency of positivity for *C. difficile* from stools of patients with antibiotic-associated diarrhea.[196] The procedure for complete identification of the organism and confirmation of toxin production is time-consuming, however, and thus beyond the testing capacities of most clinical laboratories.

Chang and Gorbach have developed a rapid method for identifying *C. difficile* by toxin detection.[197] Stool samples were inoculated directly into agar or broth culture containing cycloserine and cefoxitin. By the inoculation of an agar piece adjacent to a suspicious colony or of a cell-free broth supernatant into tissue culture wells with and without *C. sordellii* antitoxin, identification of *C. difficile* could often be accomplished within 24 hours.

Obviously, there remains a need for a rapid, simple, and efficient test for *C. difficile* that could replace culture of stool specimens and tissue culture cytotoxicity assay. In the past, other types of assays, such as counterimmunoelectrophoresis (CIEP), LAT, and more recently ELISA, have been tried. The CIEP assays suffered from a lack of sensitivity and specificity.[198–201] A LAT was introduced in the mid-1980s as being capable of detecting toxin A as characterized by Banno and colleagues.[187, 188] Shortly after, Lyerly and colleagues showed that the test detected a nontoxic bacterial antigen produced by *C. difficile* (both toxigenic and nontoxigenic) as well as other species of *Clostridium*.[202] Evaluations of the commercially available LAT have found a wide range of sensitivities and specifics.[203–208] Although sensitivity of the LAT is less than that of the cytotoxicity assay, the test is frequently recommended for use as a screening test, with all positive results confirmed by another method.[208, 209] The ELISA methods have been used for detection of both the enterotoxin A and cytotoxin B. Laughon and colleagues developed an ELISA for toxin A that detected 91% of the cytotoxin-positive specimens included in their study.[210]

The ELISA methods for detection of toxins A and toxins A/B have become available commercially. DiPersio and colleagues developed a rapid (2.5 h) direct ELISA for toxin A.[211] In their study of 313 fresh specimens from patients suspected of *C. difficile*–associated disease, the ELISA had a sensitivity of 85% and specificity of 98%, whereas the cytotoxin assay and the LAT had sensitivities of 94% and 59% and specificities of 98% and 96%, respectively. In a second multicenter evaluation of this same test, De-Girolami and colleagues achieved comparable results, finding that the EIA had a sensitivity and specificity of 86% and 99%, respectively, whereas tissue cytotoxicity testing had sensitivity and specificity of 94% and 99.8%, respectively.[212]

Toxin A has been linked with disease in animal models and may prove to be the most important marker for *C. difficile*–associated disease. The first of the new EIA tests do not, however, appear to have the necessary sensitivities to replace completely the cytotoxicity assay, although they may prove valuable as rapid screening tests, particularly in laboratories with a high volume of tests. Future studies of other new assays for detection of the toxins produced by *C. difficile* should be carefully compared with findings of cytotoxicity tests, culture, and individual patient case review.

Two groups have developed PCR-based assays. Wren and colleagues used PCR to amplify a fragment of the repeating sequence of the *C. difficile* toxin A (enterotoxin) gene.[213] Their assay was able to distinguish toxigenic from nontoxigenic strains of *C. difficile,* but amplification was also reported with the DNA of *C. sordellii.* The *C. sordellii* organism produces hemorrhagic toxin, which is related immunologically to the toxin A of *C. difficile.*[214]

Kato and colleagues have described a PCR-based assay that differentiates between toxigenic and nontoxigenic strains of *C. difficile* with apparent specificity.[215] The authors used two sets of oligonucleotide primer pairs. Primers from the nonrepeating sequences of the toxin A gene amplified 546– and 252–base pair DNA fragments, whereas a primer pair from the repeating sequences of the toxin A gene amplified a 1266–base pair DNA fragment. Using the PCR assay, the authors found production of fragments from repeating and nonrepeating sequences of all 35 *C. difficile* toxin A producers

and none of 26 cytotoxin-negative strains. Of 20 other clostridial species tested, none was PCR positive; neither cytotoxic nor noncytotoxic strains of *C. sordellii* were amplified in this system. The authors stated that preliminary results indicate that the toxin A gene of *C. difficile* can be directly amplified from stool samples after only minimal processing.

Staphylococcal Enterocolitis

Normally, *Staphylococcus aureus* is a very minor component of the fecal flora of humans. The organism can proliferate, however, and become the predominant aerobic organism when normal bowel flora are suppressed by antimicrobial agents. When the organism predominates in the fecal flora, diarrhea almost always occurs.

The antibiotics most commonly associated with staphylococcal enterocolitis have been chloramphenicol, tetracycline, and neomycin. Other agents less frequently involved include penicillin, streptomycin, and the sulfonamides. Only a minority of patients receiving antimicrobial drugs ever develop the syndrome, and the underlying pathogenesis is still unclear. The lesions are generally localized to the mucosa. In severe cases, mucosal ulceration can progress to mucosal necrosis and the formation of pseudo-membranes.

Confirmation is made by the isolation of *S. aureus* in large numbers from the stool. After overnight incubation at 37°C on blood agar, *S. aureus* forms smooth, circular, opaque, buff-to-orange or occasionally white colonies 1 to 2 mm in diameter. The colonies may or may not be hemolytic. Early detection can be made by microscopic examination of gram-stained smear of feces. An abundance of gram-positive cocci in clusters suggests staphylococcal enterocolitis.

It should also be noted that patients who develop diarrhea while receiving antibiotics may yield stool cultures with pure or predominant growth of other organisms, such as *Streptococcus faecalis, Pseudomonas aeruginosa, Proteus mirabilis,* or *Candida albicans.* Under these conditions, the microorganisms have been presumed to be the causal agent. Thus, overgrowth of a single resistant organism after suppression of the normal intestinal flora is thought to be important.

FOODBORNE BACTERIAL DIARRHEAL DISEASES

Foodborne illness is an important public health concern worldwide and has immense costs in terms of both human illness and economics. Estimates for the cost of all foodborne illness in the United States, including diarrheal disease, range from US $7.7 to $23 billion annually. Bacterial illness accounts for about 80% of this cost, and salmonellosis alone, for about 47% of this total.[216]

Common foodborne pathogens include *Salmonella*, *Campylobacter*, *S. aureus*, *Clostridium perfringens*, *V. parahaemolyticus*, *B. cereus*, *Shigella*, and possibly *Aeromonas*. Several of these pathogens have already been discussed along with their isolation and identification. *Staphylococcus aureus*, *C. perfringens*, and *B. cereus* cause disease when contaminated foods containing toxins elaborated by the microorganisms are ingested. The diarrheal diseases and vomiting are due to the toxins present. Hence, these diseases are often described as food poisoning.

Staphylococcus aureus

The enterotoxins of *S. aureus* form a group of six serologically distinct extracellular proteins designated A, B, C, C^2, D, and E. These are the direct causes of staphylococcal food poisoning. Only approximately 100 to 200 ng of the enterotoxins is required to produce disease. Ingestion of the preformed enterotoxin in contaminated food leads to the rapid development within 6 hours of symptomatic nausea, vomiting, abdominal pain and diarrhea, but not fever. The illness is usually mild, lasting as long as 24 hours, and unless the intoxication involves a group of persons, it is often unrecognized and rarely fatal.

Foods often implicated in staphylococcal foodborne disease are prepared foods like custards, cream desserts, ice cream, or cooked meats that are eaten cold, such as chicken and ham. A food handler with *S. aureus* in a skin lesion or colonizing the nares is the usual source of contamination. If contaminated food is stored at ambient temperature for too long, the organisms multiply and produce toxin. Additional cooking may kill the staphylococci after they have multiplied, but the enterotoxin, which is highly heat-stable, will remain biologically active in the food.

Diagnosis of this disease is made after the detection of a staphylococcal enterotoxin in the suspected food or by the production of enterotoxin by strains of *S. aureus* cultured from these foods. Such investigations are usually undertaken by health department laboratories. Phage typing is also an important epidemiologic tool that can be used to link strains from food with those isolated from the feces and vomitus of patients and the skin of food handlers. In the instance of an isolated case, growth of *S. aureus* in almost pure culture from feces or vomitus can be sufficient evidence of staphylococcal disease.

Blood agar can be used to culture the organism. The strains are identified as *S. aureus* by testing for coagulase production and detection of the enterotoxin in broth cultures. Toxin detection has been facilitated by the development of ELISA and RPLA tests.[217]

Clostridium perfringens

Clostridium perfringens has remained a leading cause of foodborne disease in the United States, ranking third most common behind *Salmonella* species and *S. aureus*.[218] The disease is associated with ingestion of strains of *C. perfringens* type A that are capable of producing heat-resistant spores. Almost all outbreaks in the United States and cases of *C. perfringens* foodborne disease appear to be due to type A strains. These strains are widespread in nature and often isolated from raw meats, animal feces, and the feces of healthy humans. The disease is most often associated with food dishes containing meat, poultry, and gravy that are stored and served in large quantities. Onset of symptoms of the disease, diarrhea and abdominal cramps, usually occurs 10 to 24 hours after ingestion of the tainted food and can last for 12 to 24 hours. Approximately 10^8 vegetative cells are required for disease, and the organisms undergo sporulation in the stomach and produce the enterotoxin. The illness is usually mild, and patients recover in 2 to 3 days. Despite its prevalence, *C. perfringens* is infrequently isolated from gastrointestinal infections because most laboratories do not include anaerobic culture in their standard enteric workup. A diagnosis, therefore, relies upon close collaboration between public health epidemiologists and the microbiology laboratory. This may lead initially to misleading findings, as was the case in a report of gastroenteritis due to *Klebsiella pneumoniae*, a very rare cause of diarrheal disease, masked by *C. perfringens*.[219]

Confirmation of *C. perfringens* as the cause of the disease requires the quantitative assay of incriminated food (1×10^5 CFU/g). In addition, quantitative stool cultures (10^6 spores/g) from ill and healthy individuals with serologic confirmation are required to distinguish between normal bowel flora and the infecting organism.

Gross and colleagues claimed that these criteria alone may be inadequate to confirm a diagnosis of *C. perfringens,* particularly if there is a lack of satisfactory food samples.[220] They found that enumeration of *C. perfringens* from a suitable number of fecal specimens (at least 5) from patients and subsequent serotyping of the isolates was helpful in implicating *C. perfringens* as the cause of foodborne illness. Such investigations are a function of health department laboratories. The counts are performed using egg yolk–free tryptose sulfite–cycloserine agar.[221]

The availability of an RPLA test kit for *C. perfringens* enterotoxin (Oxoid USA, Columbia, MD) may hold promise for the quick identification of toxin.[222] Other investigators have developed cytotoxicity assays and synthetic DNA probes for detection of the enterotoxin,[223, 224] but they are not available commercially and are beyond the range of most diagnostic laboratories.

Clostridium perfringens type F strains can cause a rare type of clostridial food poisoning termed enteritis necroticans. This illness is characterized by acute onset of severe abdominal pain, vomiting, diarrhea, prostration, and shock, and it can be rapidly fatal.

Bacillus cereus

In recent years *B. cereus* received recognition as an etiologic agent of food poisoning. Two syndromes have been described. A diarrheal type of syndrome, characterized predominantly by diarrhea and abdominal cramps, was noted to occur 8 to 16 hours after eating incriminated food. A wide variety of foods have been involved, ranging from meats and vegetable dishes to milk, sauces, pasta, and desserts.[225, 226] A second distinct type of food poisoning, termed the emetic type of syndrome, has also been accepted as due to *B. cereus.* This syndrome is characterized by vomiting after a short incubation period of less than 1 to 5 hours, and all but a few instances have been associated with rice dishes.

Two distinct enterotoxins have been proposed in relation to the two types of food poisoning.[227] The toxin thought to be responsible for the diarrheal type of *B. cereus* food poisoning has been partially purified and characterized. It appears to be a toxin complex and is the basis for assays designed to detect the toxin in food and feces (Central Public Health Laboratory, London, England; US FDA, Washington DC).

The emetic factor or factors are equally elusive and may be associated with sporulation or rice breakdown products. Much more study is needed to unravel the role of certain toxic metabolites with the related clinical syndrome.

Diagnosis of this disease can be confirmed by isolation of 10^5 colony-forming units or more of *B. cereus* per gram of incriminated food, feces, or vomitus of patients. Presence of low numbers of organisms is of no significance since *B. cereus* is distributed widely in nature and can be readily isolated from foods such as milk, cereals, spices, meat, and poultry and can sometimes be found in stools of well persons. Obtaining counts of *B. cereus* from foods, feces, or vomitus involves the preparation of a 10% weight in volume homogenate in one-quarter strength Ringer's solution or 0.1% peptone water. Aliquots (0.1 ml) of each dilution (serial tenfold dilutions, 10^{-2} to 10^{-4}) should be spread on mannitol–egg yolk–phenol red–polymyxin agar (MYPA). The number of colony-forming units per gram of sample is determined after the aerobic incubation of the plates for 18 to 24 hours at 35° to 37°C. The colonies of *B. cereus* are flat, grey-white, and dry and are surrounded by a zone of white precipitate that is due to lecithinase production. The background medium around the colony remains violet-red because *B. cereus* does not ferment mannitol. A blood agar plate (BAP) can also be used. Colonies of *B. cereus* on BAP are flat, 2 to 6 mm, irregularly edged, matte, and opaque grey-green. Zones of hemolysis will be present, particularly on sheep BAP. Confirmatory tests for *B. cereus* include positivity on glucose and negativity on mannitol, xylose, and arabinose ammonium salt sugar slants. Identification of *Bacillus* isolates to species level has been greatly facilitated by the use of the API 50CH test strip (API Laboratory Products, marketed by Analytab Products, Plainview NY). This strip is designed for use in conjunction with the API 20E.

A strain differentiation system for *B. cereus,* based on the recognition of greater than 40 flagella H antigens, was developed at the Food Hygiene Laboratory, Central Public Health Laboratory, Colindale, London, England.[228, 229]

In addition, *Bacillus subtilis, Bacillus licheniformis,* and occasionally other *Bacillus* species have been increasingly incriminated in foodborne illness.

ENTERIC VIRUSES

Adenovirus types 40 and 41

Adenovirus types 40 and 41 (AD 40/41) have been recognized as the second most frequently identified agents in the stools of infants and young children with viral gastroenteritis in temperate climates. The viruses are shed in high numbers in stool during the acute infection, but unlike conventional adenoviruses, they grow inefficiently in cell cultures. The diagnosis of these agents has been simplified by the development of a commercial EIA (Cambridge Biotech Corp., Worcester MA) that utilizes a monoclonal antibody able to identify AD 40/41. The test was evaluated for the detection of enteric adenoviruses in Manitoba, Canada.[230] The stool specimens from 21 pediatric gastroenteritis patients, which contained adenovirus particles visible by EM as well as AD 40/41 reference strains, were tested by the new AD 40/41–specific adenovirus group-reactive immunoassays. Of the 21 specimens, 15 (71%) were negative in the specific immunoassay. These specimens were shown by restriction analysis of the DNA to contain a genomic variant of AD 41. Apparently, genetic variation within one type of adenovirus, which results in an altered antigenic epitope, can interfere with the reactive ability of specific monoclonal antibodies. The AD 40/41 specific monoclonal antibody used for this assay was shown to react with a hexon epitope.[231] The AD 41 variant had restriction site changes within the hexon gene. It would appear likely that enteric adenoviruses undergo strain succession, like other adenoviruses, that could affect the long-term usefulness of species-specific monoclonal-based tests. Consequently, the ideal targets for reagent antibodies need to be more highly conserved epitopes. In an addendum, the authors reported that the company had developed other antibodies that were able to detect 15 of 16 isolates of AD 41.

Allard and colleagues have developed three different PCR systems for the detection of human adenoviruses.[232] One system utilized general hexon region primers and successfully amplified 18 different adenovirus types from all six subgenera. The two PCR systems specific for enteric AD 40/41 targeted the early E1 area and detected AD 40/41 or AD 40 specifically. The AD 40/41 PCR assay was also able to detect enteric adenovirus in a small number of stool samples.

Rotavirus

Rotavirus gastroenteritis is a worldwide disease affecting humans as well as a variety of mammalian and avian species. The rotavirus genus is divided into six different groups, serogroups A to F; three of these groups infect humans. The group A rotaviruses were first recognized in 1979 and are the most studied and best understood. An inability to grow the virus efficiently in simple tissue culture systems has led to the development of a variety of diagnostic methods. Rotavirus was first detected by direct EM of fecal samples.[233] The sensitivity of this diagnostic method was improved by the use of immune electron microscopy (IEM), based on the interaction between virus and antibody.

Other direct detection systems have involved various immunologic assays to detect virus-associated antigen.[234–237] Currently, a battery of rapid tests is available, including LAT and EIA kits, utilizing either polyclonal or monoclonal antibodies in their detection systems. Nine of these products from seven manufacturers were compared for rapid detection of rotavirus in 100 fecal specimens.[238] Four of the five EIA products were found to have good sensitivities and specificities of 95 to 100%. The four LAT kits, although more rapid, were often less sensitive and less specific than the EIA kits.

Two of the EIA kits were compared with direct EM, the current reference laboratory standard.[239] The findings of this study indicated that direct EM, although very specific, had a sensitivity of only 80% compared with the highly sensitive and specific monoclonal antibody–based ELISA. The authors recommended that an ELISA with high sensitivity and specificity, such as Rotaclone (Cambridge Biotech Corp., Worcester MA), was a more appropriate reference standard for rotavirus testing.

Group B rotavirus, also called adult diarrhea rotavirus, has caused major outbreaks of diarrhea in adults in the People's Republic of China.[240, 241] Outbreaks appear to have been confined to China, since seroepidemiologic evidence indicates that the virus is rarely found outside of that country. Group C rotavirus has been isolated from humans as well as piglets with diarrheal disease. Both group B and C rotavirus are noncultivatable, and since they are antigenically and genetically distinct from group A rotaviruses, they cannot be detected with any of the commercial immunoassays available. Immunoassays and IEM have been developed for group B rotaviruses, but these are research tools and not available commercially. Future studies may make possible the development of similar products to aid in the rapid identification of the growing list of enteric viruses.

Polymerase chain reaction–based assays have been reported by two groups to achieve sensitive detection of rotavirus of groups A, B, and C. Gouvea and colleagues developed a method for typing rotaviruses from clinical specimens using a gene 9 segment, coding for the major outer capsid glycoprotein (VP7) as the target sequence.[242] Rotavirus double-stranded RNA (dsRNA) was extracted from feces and used as a template for reverse transcriptase (RT). This group also described type-specific primers to identify human rotavirus serotypes in the specimen.

Gouvea and colleagues adapted their group A-specific RT-PCR assay to detect groups B and C rotavirus.[243] The assays's primer pairs were used separately in individual PCR assays and also functioned when pooled in a combined PCR assay for the simultaneous detection of all three rotavirus groups.

Wilde and colleagues reported the development of a different PCR-based system aimed at the detection of a rotavirus gene 6 target.[244] These investigators developed an extraction process that used chromatographic cellulose fiber powder to purify the viral RNA from the specimen. The sensitivity of the PCR system allowed detection of less than 1 pg of genomic rotavirus RNA in the sample. In addition, this group has developed a PCR detection system for group B rotavirus that has comparable sensitivity to the group A test.[245]

SUMMARY

The diagnosis of gastrointestinal infections is undergoing a period of rapid expansion. New technologies employing monoclonal antibodies, DNA probes, and PCR allow for the rapid detection of antigens and specific nucleic acid sequences of enteric pathogens, often directly from feces. Although the antibody-based tests have been rapidly incorporated into the clinical laboratory, DNA probe techniques have not made so great an impact. The sensitivity of probe methods is greatly increased when linked to PCR amplification of specific, often virulence-related, targets. The combination of these two methods holds great promise for rapid, sensitive, and specific detection of the many diarrheal disease agents. At least 19 new PCR-based assays (see Table 20–2) have been reported for a variety of bacterial, viral, and protozoan enteric pathogens. The targets of the various tests are toxin genes of *C. difficile*, ETEC, and EHEC; virulence genes of *Shigella*, EIEC, *Yersinia*, and *E. histolytica;* the gene for urease enzyme of *H. pylori;* and genes for the major outer capsid glycoproteins of rotaviruses. Two of the major problems associated with early PCR methods, that is, radio-isotopes and crossover contamination, have been overcome by the development

of nonisotopic enzyme-labeled detection systems and by the pretreatment of amplification mixes with the enzyme uracil *N*-glycosylase, which nicks DNA products with uridine-substituted bases if they contaminate the reaction mixture. Even with these improvements, additional criteria related to cost, time, specificity, sensitivity, and interpretation of results must be met before PCR will be incorporated into the clinical laboratory. It is also essential that improvements be made in ease of isolation of nucleic acids from clinical samples. We look to the future for new applications and further refinements of these techniques.

ACKNOWLEDGMENT

The authors wish to thank Sally Bynoe for her excellent secretarial assistance. We also acknowledge that sections of this paper are reprinted from Thorne GM, Diagnosis of infectious diarrheal diseases. In: Infectious Disease Clinics of North America. 1988; 2. With permission from the publisher.

REFERENCES

1. Snyder JD, Marson MH. The magnitude of the global problem of acute diarrheal disease: A review of active surveillance data. Bull World Health Organ. 1982; 60:603–613.
2. Guerrant RL, Hughes JM, Lima NL, *et al.* Diarrhea in developed and developing countries: Magnitude, special settings, and etiologies. Rev Infect Dis. 1990; 12:S41–S50.
3. Huilan S, Zhen LG, Mathan MM, *et al.* Etiology of acute diarrhea among children in developing countries: A multicentre study in five countries. Bull World Health Organ. 1991;69:549–555.
4. Adkins HJ, Santiago LT. Increased recovery of enteric pathogens by use of both stool and rectal swab specimens. J Clin Microbiol. 1987;25:158–159.
5. Karmali MA, Fleming PC. *Campylobacter* enteritis in children. J Pediatr. 1979;94:527–533.
6. Burke JA. Giardiasis in childhood. Am J Dis Child. 1975;129:1304–1310.
7. Wahlquist SP, Williams RM, Bishop H, *et al.* Use of pooled formalin-preserved fecal specimens to detect *Giardia lamblia.* J Clin Microbiol. 1991;29:1725–1726.
8. Kneip J, Topping J. Comparison of the Merifluor *Giardia* indirect immunofluorescent procedure and standard ova and parasite detection methods for *Giardia* cysts in feces. American Society for Microbiology. Annual Meeting Abstract 1988:116.
9. Rosoff JD, Sanders CA, Sonnad SS, *et al.* Stool diagnosis of giardiasis using a commercially available enzyme immunoassay to detect *Giardia*-specific antigen 65 (GSA65). J Clin Microbiol. 1989;27:1997–2002.
10. Addiss DG, Matthews HM, Stewart JM, *et al.* Evaluation of a commercially available enzyme-linked immunosorbent assay for *Giardia lamblia* antigen in stool. J Clin Microbiol. 1991;29:1137–1142.

11. Butcher PD, Farthing MJG. DNA probes for the faecal diagnosis of *Giardia lamblia* infections in man. Biochem Soc Trans. 1989;17:363–364.

12. Abbaszadegan M, Gerba CP, Rose JB. Detection of *Giardia* cysts with a cDNA probe and applications to water samples. Appl Environ Microbiol. 1991;57:927–931.

13. Mahbubani MH, Bej AK, Perlin MH, et al. Differentiation of *Giardia duodenalis* from other *Giardia* spp. by using polymerase chain reaction and gene probes. J Clin Microbiol. 1992;30:74–78.

14. Garfinkel LI, Giladi M, Huber M, et al. DNA probes specific for *Entamoeba histolytica* possessing pathogenic and nonpathogenic zymodemes. Infect Immun. 1989;57:926–931.

15. Tannich E, Burchard GD. Differentiation of pathogenic from nonpathogenic *Entamoeba histolytica* by restriction fragment analysis of a single gene amplified in vitro. J Clin Microbiol. 1991;29:250–255.

16. Rijpstra AC, Canning EU, van Ketel RJ, et al. Use of light microscopy to diagnose small-intestinal microsporidiosis in patients with AIDS. J Infect Dis. 1988;157:827–831.

17. Cali A, Owen RL. Intracellular development of *Enterocytozoon*, a unique microsporidian found in the intestine of AIDS patients. J Protozool. 1990;37:145–155.

18. Orenstein JM, Chiang J, Steinberg W, et al. Intestinal microsporidiosis as a cause of diarrhea in human immunodeficiency virus–infected patients: A report of 20 cases. Human Pathol. 1990;21:475–481.

19. van Gool V, Hollister WS, Schattenkerk JE, et al. Diagnosis of *Enterocytozoon bieneusi* microsporidiosis in AIDS patients by recovery of spores from faeces. Lancet. 1990;336:697–698.

20. Weber R, Bryan RT, Owen RL, et al. Improved light-microscopical detection of microsporidia spores in stool and duodenal aspirates. N Engl J Med. 1992;326:161–166.

21. Centers for Disease Control. Cryptosporidiosis among children attending daycare centers—Georgia, Pennsylvania, Michigan, California, New Mexico. MMWR Morb Mortal Wkly Rep. 1984;33:599.

22. Holley HP Jr, Dover C. *Cryptosporidium:* A common cause of parasitic diarrhea in otherwise healthy individuals. J Infect Dis. 1986;153:365–368.

23. Navin TR, Juranek DD. Cryptosporidiosis: Clinical, epidemiologic and parasitologic review. Rev Infect Dis. 1984;6:313–327.

24. Nime FA, Burek JD, Page DL, et al. Acute enterocolitis in a human being infected with the protozoan *Cryptosporidium.* Gastroenterology. 1976;70:592.

25. Soave R, Ma P: Cryptosporidiosis: Traveler's diarrhea in two families. Arch Intern Med. 1985;145:70–72.

26. Crawford FG, Vermund SH. Human cryptosporidiosis. Crit Rev Microbiol. 1988;16:113–159.

27. Garcia LS, Bruckner DA, Brewer TC, et al. Techniques for the recovery and identification of *Cryptosporidium* oocysts from stool specimens. J Clin Microbiol. 1983;18:185–190.

28. McNabb SJN, Hensel DM, Welch DF, et al. Comparison of sedimentation and flotation techniques for identification of *Cryptosporidium* sp. oocysts in a large outbreak of human diarrhea. J Clin Microbiol. 1985;22:587–589.

29. Reese NC, Current WL, Ernst JV, et al. Cryptosporidiosis of man and calf: A case report and results of experimental infections in mice and rats. Am J Trop Med Hyg. 1982;31:226–229.

30. Garcia LS, Brewer TC, Bruckner DA. Fluorescence detection of *Cryptosporidium* oocysts in human fecal specimens by using monoclonal antibodies. J Clin Microbiol. 1987;25:119–121.

31. Weber R, Bryan RT, Bishop HS, et al. Threshold of detection of *Cryptosporidium* oocysts in human stool specimens: Evidence for low sensitivity of current diagnostic methods. J Clin Microbiol. 1991;29:1323–1327.

32. Unger BLP. Enzyme-linked immunoassay for detection of *Cryptosporidium* antigens in fecal specimens. J Clin Microbiol. 1990;28:2491–2495.

33. Anusz KZ, Mason PH, Riggs MW, et al. Detection of *Cryptosporidium parvum* oocysts in bovine feces by monoclonal antibody capture enzyme-linked immunosorbent assay. J Clin Microbiol. 1990;28:2770–2774.

34. Soave R, Johnson WD Jr. *Cryptosporidium* and *Isospora belli* infections. J Infect Dis. 1988;157:225–229.

35. DeHovitz JA, Pape JW, Boncy M, et al. Clinical manifestations and therapy of *Isospora belli* infection in patients with the acquired immunodeficiency syndrome. N Engl J Med. 1986;315:87–90.

36. DeHovitz JA. Management of *Isospora belli* infections in AIDS patients. Infect Med. 1988;437–440.

37. Brandborg LL, Goldberg SB, Breidenbach WC. Human coccidiosis—a possible cause of malabsorption: The life cycle in small bowel mucosal biopsies as a diagnostic feature. N Engl J Med. 1970;283:1306–1313.

38. Centers for Disease Control. Revision of the case definition of acquired immunodeficiency syndrome for national reporting—United States. MMWR Morb Mortal Wkly Rep. 1985;34:373–375.

39. Kirkpatrick CE. Animal reservoirs of *Cryptosporidium* spp. and *Isospora belli.* J Infect Dis. 1988;158:909.

40. Garcia LS, Bruckner DA. In: Diagnostic Medical Parasitology. New York: Elsevier; 1988:389–390.

41. Forthal DN, Guest SS. *Isospora belli* enteritis in 3 homosexual men. Am J Trop Med Hyg. 1984;33:1060–1064.

42. Garcia LS. Laboratory methods for diagnosis of parasitic infections. In: Baron JE, Finegold S, eds. Bailey and Scott's Diagnostic Microbiology. 8th ed. 1990:776–861.

42a. Soave R, Dubey JP, Ramos LJ, et al. A new intestinal pathogen? Abstract. Clin Res. 1986;34:533A.

42b. Ortega YR, Sterling CR, Gilman RH, et al. *Cyclospora* species—A new protozoan pathogen of humans. N Engl J Med. 1993;328:1308–1312.

43. Long EG, White EH, Carmichael WW, et al. Morphologic and staining characteristics of a *Cyanobacterium-* like organism associated with diarrhea. J Infect Dis. 1991;164:199–202.

44. Kocka F, Peters C, Dacumos E, et al. Outbreaks of diarrheal illness associated with cyanobacteria (blue-green algae)–like bodies. Chicago and Nepal, 1989 and 1990. MMWR Morb Mortal Wkly Rep. 1991;40:325–327.

45. Long EG, Ebrahimzadeh A, White EH, et al. Alga associated with diarrhea in patients with acquired immunodeficiency syndrome and in travelers. J Clin Microbiol. 1990;28:1101–1104.

45a. Shlim DR, Cohen MT, Eaton M, et al. An algae-like intestinal organism associated with an outbreak of prolonged diarrhea among foreigners in Nepal. Am J Trop Med Hyg. 1991;45:383–389.

45b. Pollok RC, Bendall RP, Moody A, et al. Traveller's diarrhoea associated with cyanobacterium-like bodies [letter]. Lancet 1992;340:5516–5517.

45c. Gascon J, Corachan M, Valls ME, et al. Cyanobacteria-like bodies (CLB) in travellers with diarrhea. Scand J Infect Dis. 1993;25:253–257.

45d. Smith PM. Traveller's diarrhoea associated with a cyanobacterium-like body [letter]. Med J Australia 1993;158:724.

45e. Madico G, Gilman RH, Miranda E, et al. Treatment of cyclospora infections with co-trimoxazole [letter]. Lancet. 1993;342:122–123.

46. Ruiz J, Varela MC, Sempere, MA, et al. Presumptive

identification of *Salmonella enterica* using two rapid tests. Eur J Clin Microbiol Infect Dis. 1991;10:649–651.

47. Ruiz J, Sempere MA, Varela MC, *et al.* Modification of the methodology of stool culture for *Salmonella* detection. J Clin Microbiol. 1992;30:525–526.

48. Aguirre PM, Cacho JB, Folgueira L, *et al.* Rapid fluorescence method for screening *Salmonella* spp. from enteric differential agars. J Clin Microbiol. 1990;28:148–149.

49. Freydiere AM, Gille Y. Detection of salmonella by using Rombach agar and by a C8 esterase spot test. J Clin Microbiol. 1991;29:2357–2359.

50. Scholl DR, Kaufman C, Jollick JD, *et al.* Clinical application of novel sample processing technology identification of salmonellae by using DNA probes. J Clin Microbiol. 1990;28:237–241.

51. Centers for Disease Control. Shigellosis in the United States, 1984. MMWR Morb Mortal Wkly Rep. 1985;34:600.

52. Evins GM, Gheesling LL, Tauxe RV. Quality of commercially produced *Shigella* serogrouping and serotyping antisera. J Clin Microbiol. 1988;26:438–442.

53. Hale TL, Sansonetti PJ, Schad PA, *et al.* Characterization of virulence plasmid-associated outer membrane proteins in *Shigella flexneri, Shigella sonnei,* and *Escherichia coli.* Infect Immun. 1983;40:340.

54. Harris JR, Wachsmuth IK, Davis BR, *et al.* High-molecular-weight plasmid correlates with *Escherichia coli* enteroinvasiveness. Infect Immun. 1982;37:1295.

55. Scaletsky ICA, Silva, Toledo MRF, *et al.* Correlation between adherence of HeLa cells and serogroups, serotypes and bioserotypes of *Escherichia coli.* Infect Immun. 1985;49:528–532.

56. Jerse AE, Martin WC, Galen JE, *et al.* Oligonucleotide probe for detection of the enteropathogenic *Escherichia coli* (EPEC) adherence factor of localized adherence EPEC. J Clin Microbiol. 1990;28:2842–2844.

57. DuPont HL, Pickering LK. Relative importance of enteropathogens in acute endemic diarrhea and foodborne diarrheal illness. In: Infections of the Gastrointestinal Tract. New York: Plenum Publishing; 1980: 195–213.

58. Guerrant RL, Brunton LL, Schnaitman TC, *et al.* Cyclic adenosine monophosphate and alteration of the Chinese hamster ovary cell morphology: A rapid sensitive in vitro assay for enterotoxins of *Vibrio cholerae* and *Escherichia coli.* Infect Immun. 1974;10:320–327.

59. Sack DA, Sack RB. Test for enterotoxigenic *Escherichia coli* usuing Y-1 adrenal cells in miniculture. Infect Immun. 1975;11:334–336.

60. Svennerholm AM, Wiklund G. Rapid GM₁-enzyme-linked immunosorbent assay with visual reading for identification of *Escherichia coli* heat-labile enterotoxin. J Clin Microbiol. 1983;17:596–600.

61. Honda T, Taga S, Takeda Y, *et al.* Modified Elek test for detection of heat-labile enterotoxin of enterotoxigenic *Escherichia coli.* J Clin Microbiol. 1981;13:1.

62. Ronnberg B, Wadstrom T. Rapid detection by a coagglutination test of heat-labile enterotoxin in cell lysates from blood agar–grown *Escherichia coli.* J Clin Microbiol. 1983;17:1021–1025.

63. Scotland SM, Flomen RH, Rowe B. Evaluation of a reversed passive latex agglutination test for detection of *Escherichia coli* heat-labile toxin in culture supernatants. J Clin Microbiol. 1989;27:339–340.

64. Dean AG, Ching Y, Williams RG, *et al.* Test for *Escherichia coli* enterotoxin using infant mice application in a study of diarrhea in children in Honolulu. J Infect Dis. 1972;125:407–411.

65. Sanchez J, Svennerholm AM, Holmgren J. Genetic fusion of nontoxic heat-stable enterotoxin-related decapeptide to cholera toxin B-subunit. FEBS Lett. 1988;241:110–114.

66. Scotland SM, Willshaw GA, Said B, *et al.* Identification of *Escherichia coli* that produces heat-stable enterotoxin ST_A by a commercially available enzyme-linked immunoassay and comparison of the assay with infant mouse and DNA probe tests. J Clin Microbiol. 1989;27:1697–1699.

67. Abe A, Komase K, Bangtrakulnoth A, *et al.* Trivalent heat-labile and heat-stable enterotoxin probe conjugated with horseradish peroxidase for detection of enterotoxigenic *Escherichia coli* by hybridization. J Clin Microbiol. 1990;28:2616–2620.

68. Olive DM. Detection of enterotoxigenic *Escherichia coli* after polymerase chain reaction amplification with a thermostable DNA polymerase. J Clin Microbiol. 1989;27:261–265.

69. Victor T, duToit R, van Zyl J, *et al.* Improved method for the routine identification toxigenic *Escherichia coli* by DNA amplification of a conserved region of the heat-labile toxin A subunit. J Clin Microbiol. 1991;29:158–161.

70. Sereny B. Experimental *Shigella* keratoconjunctivitis. Acta Microbiol Acad Sci Hung. 1955;2:293.

71. Pal T, Pacsa AS, Emody L, *et al.* Modified enzyme-linked immunosorbent assay for detecting enteroinvasive *Escherichia coli* and virulent *Shigella* strains. J Clin Microbiol. 1985;21:415–418.

72. Frankel G, Riley L, Giron JA, *et al.* Detection of *Shigella* in feces using DNA amplification. J Infect Dis. 1990;161:1252–1256.

73. Riley LW, Remis RS, Helgerson SD, *et al.* Hemorrhagic colitis associated with a rare *Escherichia coli* serogroup. N Engl J Med. 1983;308:681–685.

74. Wells JG, Davis BR, Wachsmuth TK, *et al.* Laboratory investigation of hemorrhagic colitis outbreaks associated with a rare *Escherichia coli* serotype. J Clin Microbiol. 1983;18:512–520.

75. Ostroff SM, Kobayashi JM, Lewis HH. *Escherichia coli* 0157:H7 infections in Washington State: The first year of statewide disease surveillance. JAMA. 1988;262:355–359.

76. Karmali MA. Infection by Verocytotoxin-producing *Escherichia coli.* Rev Clin Microbiol. 1989;2:15–38.

77. Tarr PI, Neill MA, Clausen CR, *et al. Escherichia coli* 0157:H7 and the hemolytic-uremic syndrome: Importance of early cultures in establishing etiology. J Infect Dis. 1990;162:553–556.

78. Borczyk AA, Harnett N, Lombos M, *et al.* False-positive identification of *Escherichia coli* 0157 by commercial latex agglutination tests. Lancet. 1990;336:946–947.

79. Thompson JS, Hodge DS, Borczyk AA. Rapid biochemical test to identify Verocytotoxin-positive strains of *Escherichia coli* serotype 0157. J Clin Microbiol. 1990;28:2165–2168.

80. March SB, Ratnam S. Latex agglutination test for detection of *Escherichia coli* serotype 0157. J Clin Microbiol. 1989;27:1675–1677.

81. Tison D. Culture confirmation of *Escherichia coli* serotype 0157:H7 by direct immunofluorescence. J Clin Microbiol. 1990;28:612–613.

82. Marques LRM, Peiris JSM, Cryz JS, *et al. Escherichia coli* strains isolated from pigs with edema disease produce a variant of Shiga-like toxin II. FEMS Microbiol Lett. 1987;44:33–38.

83. MacLeod DL, Gyles CL, Wilcock BP. Reproduction of edema disease of swine with purified Shiga-like toxin II variant. Vet Pathol. 1991;28:66–73.

84. Gannon VPJ, Teerling C, Masrei SA, *et al.* Molecular cloning and nucleotide sequence of another variant of the *Escherichia coli* Shiga-like toxin II family. J Gen Microbiol. 1990;136:1125–1135.

85. Strockbine NA, Marques LRM, Holmes RK, et al. Characterization of monoclonal antibodies against Shiga-like toxin from Escherichia coli. Infect Immun. 1985;50:695–700.

86. Huang A, DeGrandis S, Friesen J, et al. Cloning and expression of the genes specifying Shiga-like toxin production in Escherichia coli H19. J Bacteriol. 1986;166:375–379.

87. Jackson MP, Newland JW, Holmes RK, et al. Nucleotide sequence analysis of the structural genes for Shiga-like toxin 1 encoded by bacteriophage 933J from Escherichia coli. Microbial Pathogen. 1987;2:147–153.

88. Scotland SM, Smith HR, Willshaw GA, et al. Vero cytotoxin production in strain of Escherichia coli is determined by genes carried on bacteriophage. Lancet. 1983;2:216.

89. Smith HR, Rowe B, Gross RJ, et al. Haemorrhagic colitis and Vero-cytotoxin–producing Escherichia coli in England and Wales. Lancet. 1987;1:1062–1065.

90. Willshaw GA, Smith HR, Scotland SM, et al. Heterogeneity of Escherichia coli phage encoding Vero cytotoxins: Comparison of cloned sequences determining VT1 and VT2 and development of specific gene probes. J Gen Microbiol. 1987;133:1309–1317.

91. Basta M, Karmali M, Lingwood C. Sensitive receptor-specified enzyme-linked immunosorbent assay for Escherichia coli verocytotoxin. J Clin Microbiol. 1989;27:1617–1622.

92. Acheson DWK, Keusch GT, Lightowler M, et al. Enzyme-linked immunosorbent assay for Shiga toxin and Shiga-like toxin II using P1 glycoprotein from hydatid cysts. J Infect Dis. 1990;161:134–137.

93. Karch H, Meyer T. Single primer pair of amplifying segments of distinct Shiga-like toxin genes by polymerase chain reaction. J Clin Microbiol. 1989;27:2751–2757.

94. Johnson WM, Pollard DR, Lior H, et al. Differentiation of genes coding for Escherichia coli Verotoxin 2 and Verotoxin associated with porcine edema disease (VTe) by the polymerase chain reaction. J Clin Microbiol. 1990;28:2351–2353.

95. Ho H, Terai A, Kurazono H, et al. Cloning and nucleotide sequencing of verotoxin 2 variant genes from Escherichia coli 091:H21 isolated from a patient with hemolytic-uremic syndrome. Microb Pathog. 1990;8:47–60.

96. Tyler SD, Johnson WM, Lior H, et al. Identification of Verotoxin type 2 variant B subunit genes in Escherichia coli by the polymerase chain reaction and restriction fragment length polymorphism analysis. J Clin Microbiol. 1991;29:1339–1343.

97. Jackson MP. Detection of Shiga toxin–producing Shigella dysenteriae type 1 and Escherichia coli by using polymerase chain reaction with incorporation of digoxigenin-11-dUTP. J Clin Microbiol. 1991;29:1910–1914.

98. Levine MM, Prado V, Robins-Browne R, et al. Use of DNA probes and HEp-2 cell adherence assay to detect diarrheagenic Escherichia coli. J Infect Dis. 1988;158:224–228.

99. Gomes TAT, Blake PA, Trabulsi LR. Prevalence of Escherichia coli strains with localized, diffuse, and aggregative adherence to HeLa cells in infants with diarrhea and matched controls. J Clin Microbiol. 1989;27:266–269.

100. Tacket CO, Moseley SL, Kay B, et al. Challenge studies in volunteers using Escherichia coli strains with diffuse adherence to HEp-2 cells. J Infect Dis. 1990;162:550–552.

101. Baudry B, Savarino SJ, Vial P, et al. A sensitive specific DNA probe to identify enteroaggregative Escherichia coli, a recently discovered diarrheal pathogen. J Infect Dis. 1990;161:1249–1251.

102. Savarino SJ, Fasano A, Robertson DC, et al. Enteroaggregative Escherichia coli elaborate a heat-stable enterotoxin demonstrable in an in vitro rabbit intestinal model. J Clin Invest. 1991;87:1450–1455.

103. Kirii YH, Danbara K, Arita KH, et al. Detection of enterotoxigenic Escherichia coli by colony hybridization with biotinylated enterotoxin probes. J Clin Microbiol. 1987;25:1962–1965.

104. Seriwatana J, Echeverria DN, Taylor T, et al. Identification of enterotoxigenic Escherichia coli with synthetic alkaline phosphatase conjugated oligonucleotide DNA probes. J Clin Microbiol. 1987;25:1438–1441.

105. Olive DM, Khalik DA, Sethi SK. Identification of enterotoxigenic Escherichia coli isolates using alkaline phosphatase labelled synthetic oligodeoxyribonucleotide probes. Eur J Clin Microbiol Infect Dis. 1988;7:161–171.

106. Sommerfelt H, Grewal HMS, Bhan MK. Simplified and accurate non-radioactive polynucleotide gene probe assay for identification of enterotoxigenic E coli. J Clin Microbiol. 1990;28:49–54.

107. Sommerfelt H, Svennerholm AM, Kalland KH, et al. Comparative study of colony hybridization using synthetic oligonucleotide enterotoxigenic Escherichia coli. J Clin Microbiol. 1988;26:530–534.

108. Moseley SL, Echeverria P, Seriwatan J, et al. Identification of enterotoxigenic Escherichia coli by colony hybridization using three enterotoxin gene probes. J Infect Dis. 1982;145:863–869.

109. Murray BE, Mathewson JJ, Du Pont HL, et al. Utility of oligodeoxyribonucleotide probes for detecting enterotoxigenic Escherichia coli. J Infect Dis. 1987;155:809–811.

110. Medon PP, Lancer JA, Monckton PR, et al. Identification of enterotoxigenic Escherichia coli isolates with enzyme-labelled synthetic oligonucleotide probes. J Clin Microbiol. 1988;26:2173–2176.

111. Nishibuchi M, Arita M, Honda T, et al. Evaluation of non-isotopically labelled oligonucleotide probe to detect the heat stable enterotoxin gene of E. coli by the DNA colony hybridization test. J Clin Microbiol. 1988;26:784–786.

112. Echeverria P, Taylor DN, Seriwatan J, et al. Examination of colonies and stool blots for detection of enteropathogens by DNA hybridization with eight DNA probes. J Clin Microbiol. 1989;27:331–334.

113. Venkatesan MM, Buysse JM, Kopecko DJ. Use of Shigella flexneri ipa C and ipa H gene sequences for the general identification of Shigella spp. and enteroinvasive Escherichia coli. J Clin Microbiol. 1989;27:2687–2691.

114. Venkatesan MM, Buysse JM, Vandendries EV, et al. Development and testing of invasion-associated DNA probes for the detection of Shigella spp. and enteroinvasive Escherichia coli. J Clin Microbiol. 1988;26:261–266.

115. Taylor DN, Echeverria P, Sethabula O, et al. Clinical and microbiologic features of Shigella and enteroinvasive Escherichia coli infections detected by DNA hybridization. J Clin Microbiol. 1988;26:1362–1366.

116. Newland JW, Neill RJ. DNA probes for Shiga-like toxins I and II and for toxin-converting bacteriophages. J Clin Microbiol. 1988;26:1292–1297.

117. Brown JE, Echeverria P, Taylor DN, et al. Determination of DNA hybridization of Shiga-like toxin–producing Escherichia in children with diarrhoea in Thailand. J Clin Microbiol. 1989;27:291–294.

118. Levine MM, Xu JG, Kaper JB, et al. A DNA probe to identify enterohemorrhagic Escherichia coli of 0157:H7 and other serotypes that cause hemorrhagic colitis and hemolytic-uremic syndrome. J Infect Dis. 1987;156:175–182.

119. Bissett ML, Powers C, Abbott SL, et al. Epidemiologic investigations of Yersinia enterocolitica and related species: Sources, frequency, and serogroup distribution. J Clin Microbiol. 1990;28:910–912.

120. Kachoris M, Ruoff KL, Welch K, et al. Routine culture of stool specimens for Yersinia enterocolitica is not a cost-effective procedure. J Clin Microbiol. 1988;26:582–583.

121. Metchock B, Lonsway DR, Carter GP, et al. Yersinia enterocolitica: A frequent seasonal stool isolate from children at an urban hospital in the southeast United States. J Clin Microbiol. 1991;29:2868–2869.

122. Kotloff KL, Wasserman SS, Steciak JY, et al. Acute diarrhea in Baltimore children attending an outpatient clinic. Pediatr Infect Dis J. 1988;7:753–759.

123. Prpic JK, Robins-Browne RM, Davey RB. Differentiation between virulent and avirulent Yersinia enterocolitica isolates by using Congo red agar. J Clin Microbiol. 1983;18:486–490.

124. Kandolo K, Wauter G. Pyrazinamidase activity in Yersinia enterocolitica and related organisms. J Clin Microbiol. 1985;21:980–982.

125. Delor I, Kaeckenbeeck A, Wauter G, et al. Nucleotide sequence of yst, the Yersinia enterocolitica gene encoding the heat-stable enterotoxin, and prevalence of the gene among pathogenic and nonpathogenic Yersiniae. Infect Immun. 1990;58:2983–2988.

126. Prpic JK, Robins-Browne RM, Davey RB. In vitro assessment of virulence in Yersinia enterocolitica and related species. J Clin Microbiol. 1985;22:105–110.

127. Miller VL, Falkow S. Evidence for two genetic loci in Yersinia enterocolitica that can promote invasion of epithelial cells. Infect Immun. 1988;56:1242–1248.

128. Miller VL, Farmer JJ III, Hill WE, et al. The ail locus is found uniquely in Yersinia enterocolitica serotypes commonly associated with disease. Infect Immun. 1989;57:121–131.

129. Robins-Browne RM, Miliotis MD, Cianciosi S, et al. Evaluation of DNA colony hybridization and other techniques for detection of virulence in Yersinia species. J Clin Microbiol. 1989;27:644–650.

130. Pai CH, Sarger S, Lafleur L, et al. Efficacy of cold enrichment techniques for recovery of Yersinia enterocolitica from human stools. J Clin Microbiol. 1979;9:712–715.

131. Granfors K, Viljanen M, Tiilikainen A, et al. Persistence of IgM, IgG, and IgA antibodies to Yersinia in yersinia arthritis. J Infect Dis. 1980;141:424–429.

132. Bottone EJ, Sheehan DJ. Yersinia enterocolitica: Guidelines for serologic diagnosis of human infections. J Infect Dis. 1983;5:898–906.

133. Tertti R, Granfors K, Lehtonen OP, et al. An outbreak of Yersinia pseudotuberculosis infections. J Infect Dis. 1984;149:245–250.

134. Hessemann J, Eggers CH, Schroder J, et al. Serological diagnosis of yersiniosis by the immunoblot technique using plasmid-encoded antigens of Yersinia enterocolitica. In: Simon C, Wilkinson P, eds. Diagnosis of infectious diseases: New aspects. Stuttgart, FRG: Schattauer; 1986:79–88.

135. Maki-Ikola O, Heesemann J, Lahesmaa R, et al. Combined use of released proteins and lipopolysaccharide in enzyme-linked immunosorbent assay for serologic screening of Yersinia infections. J Infect Dis. 1991;163:409–412.

136. Wren BW, Tabaqchali S. Detection of pathogenic Yersinia enterocolitica by the polymerase chain reaction. Lancet. 1990;337:693.

137. Fenwick SG, Murray A. Detection of pathogenic Yersinia enterocolitica by polymerase chain reaction. Lancet. 1991;337:496–497. Letter.

138. Muller VL, Bliska JB, Falkow S. Nucleotide sequence of

the Yersinia enterocolitica by polymerase chain reaction. Lancet. 1991;337:496–497.

139. Buchanan RL, Palumbo SA. Aeromonas hydrophila and Aeromonas sobria as potential food poisoning species: A review. J Food Safety. 1985;7:15–29.

140. Burke V, Robinson J, Gracey M, et al. Isolation of Aeromonas hydrophila from a metropolitan water supply: Seasonal correlation with clinical isolates. Appl Environ Microbiol. 1984;48:361–366.

141. Baman SI. Aeromonas hydrophila as the etiologic agent in severe gastroenteritis: Report of a case. Am J Med Technol. 1980;46:179–181.

142. Champsaur H, Andremont A, Mathieu D, et al. Cholera-like illness due to Aeromonas sobria. J Infect Dis. 1982;145:248–254.

143. Freij BJ. Aeromonas: Biology of the organism and diseases of children. Pediatr Infect Dis. 1984;3:164–175.

144. Gracey M, Burke V, Robinson J. Aeromonas-associated gastroenteritis. Lancet. 1982;2:1304–1306.

145. Gracey M, Burke V, Robinson J. Aeromonas spp. in traveller's diarrhea. Br Med J. 1984;289:658.

146. Palfreeman SJ, Waters LK, Norris M. Aeromonas hydrophila gastroenteritis. Aust N Z J Med. 1983;13:524–525.

147. Carnahan A, Fanning GR, Joseph SW. Aeromonas jandaei (formerly genospecies DNA Group 9 A. sobria), a new sucrose-negative species isolated from clinical specimens. J Clin Microbiol. 1991;29:560–564.

148. Altwegg M, Steigerwalt AG, Altwegg-Bissig R, et al. Biochemical identification of Aeromonas geno-species isolated from humans. J Clin Microbiol. 1990;28:258–264.

149. Popoff M. Genus III: Aeromonas Kluyver and Van Niel 1936. In: Krieg NR, Holt JG, eds. Bergey's Manual of Systemic Bacteriology. Baltimore: Williams & Wilkins 1984;1:545–548.

150. Hickman-Brenner FW, MacDonald KL, Steigerwalt AG, et al. Aeromonas veronii, a new ornithine decarboxylase-positive species that may cause diarrhea. J Clin Microbiol. 1987;25:900–906.

151. Kuijper EJ, Steigerwalt AG, Schoenmakers BS, et al. Phenotypic characterization and DNA relatedness in human fecal isolates of Aeromonas spp. J Clin Microbiol. 1989;27:132–138.

152. Janda JM. Recent advances in the study of the taxonomy, pathogenicity and infectious disease syndromes associated with the genus Aeromonas. Clin Microbiol Rev. 1991;4:397–410.

153. Altwegg M, Steigerwalt AG, Janda JM, et al. Identification of Aeromonas species by isoenzyme analysis. American Society for Microbiology. Annual Meeting Abstract. 1989;253:435.

154. Want SV, Millership SE. Effects of incorporating ampicillin, bile salts and carbohydrates in media on the recognition and selection of Aeromonas spp. from faeces. J Med Microbiol. 1990;32:49–54.

155. Namdari H, Buttone EJ. Cytotoxin and enterotoxin production as factors delineating enteropathogenicity of Aeromonas caviae. J Clin Microbiol. 1990;28:1796–1798.

156. Arai T, Ikejima N, Itoh T, et al. A survey of Plesiomonas shigelloides from aquatic environments, domestic animals, pets and humans. J Hyg. 1980;84:203–211.

157. Holmberg SD, Wachsmuth IK, Hickman-Brenner FW, et al. Plesiomonas enteric infections in the United States. Ann Intern Med. 1986;105:690–694.

158. Sack DA, Chowdhury KA, Hug A, et al. Epidemiology of Aeromonas and Plesiomonas diarrhea. J Diarrhoeal Dis Res. 1988;6:107–112.

159. Brendan RA, Miller MA, Janda JM. Clinical disease spectrum and pathogenic factors associated with Plesiomonas shigelloides infection in humans. Rev Infect Dis. 1988;10:303–316.

160. Alabi SA, Odugbemi T. Occurrence of *Aeromonas* species and *Plesiomonas shigelloides* in patients with and without diarrhea in Lagos, Nigeria. J Med Microbiol. 1990;32:45–48.

161. O'Loughlin EV, Scott RB, Gall DG. Pathophysiology of infectious diarrhea: Changes in intestinal structure and function. J Pediatr Gastroenterol Nutr. 1991;12:5–20.

162. Fasano A, Baudry B, Pumplin DW et al. *Vibrio cholerae* produces a second enterotoxin, which affects intestinal tight junctions. Proc Natl Acad Sci U S A. 1991; 88:5242–5246.

163. Shandera WX, Johnston JM, Davis BR, et al. Disease from infection with *Vibrio mimicus*, a newly recognized *Vibrio* species. Ann Intern Med. 1983;99:169–171.

164. Joseph SW, Kaper JB, Colwell RR. *Vibrio parahaemolyticus* and related halophilic vibrios. Crit Rev Microbiol. 1982;10:77–124.

165. Tacket CO, Hickman F, Pierce GV, et al. Diarrhea associated with *Vibrio fluvialis* in the United States. J Clin Microbiol. 1982;16:991–992.

166. Brenner DJ, Hickman FW, Lee JV, et al. *Vibrio furnissii* (formerly aerogenic biogroup of *Vibrio fluvialis*), a new species isolated from human feces and the environment. J Clin Microbiol. 1983;18:816–824.

167. Hickman FW, Farmer III JJ, Hollis DG, et al. Identification of *Vibrio hollisae* sp. nov. from patients with diarrhea. J Clin Microbiol. 1982;15:395–401.

168. Huq A, Alam M, Parveen S, et al. Occurrence of resistance to vibriostatic compound 0/129 in *Vibrio cholerae* 01 isolated from clinical and environmental samples in Bangladesh. J Clin Microbiol. 1992;30:219–221.

169. Almeida RJ, Hickman-Brenner FW, Sowers EG, et al. Comparison of a latex agglutination assay and an enzyme-linked immunosorbent assay for detecting cholera toxin. J Clin Microbiol. 1990;28:128–130.

170. Butzler JP, Dekeysen P, Detrain M, et al. Related *Vibrio* in stools. J Pediatr. 1973;82:493–495.

171. Blaser MJ, Berkowitz ID, La Force FM, et al. *Campylobacter* enteritis: Clinical and epidemiological features. Ann Intern Med. 1979;91:179–185.

172. Pai CH, Sorger S, Lackman L, et al. *Campylobacter* gastroenteritis in children. J Pediatr. 1979;94:589–591.

173. Smith JP, Durfee K, Marymount JH. Incidence of *Campylobacter* enteritis in the midwestern United States. Am J Med Technol. 1980;46:81–84.

174. Goossens H, Vlaes L, Butzler JP, et al. *Campylobacter upsaliensis* enteritis associated with canine infections. Lancet. 1991;337:1486–1487.

175. Totten PA, Gennell CL, Tenover FC, et al. *Campylobacter cinaedi* (sp. nov.) and *Campylobacter fennelliae* (sp. nov.): Two new *Campylobacter* species associated with enteric disease in homosexual men. J Infect Dis. 1985;151:131–139.

175a. Vandamme P, Falsen E, Rossau R, et al. Revision of *Campylobacter*, *Helicobacter* and *Wolinella* Taxonomy: Emendation of generic descriptions and proposal of *Arcobacter* gen. nov. Int J Sys Bact. 1991;41:88–103.

176. Kiehlbauch JA, Brenner DJ, Nicholson MA, et al. *Campylobacter butzleri* sp. nov. isolated from humans and animals with diarrheal illness. J Clin Microbiol. 1991;29:376–385.

177. Harvey SM, Greenwood JR. Probable *Campylobacter fetus* subsp. *fetus* gastroenteritis. J Clin Microbiol. 1983;18:1278–1279.

178. Ng LK, Taylor DE, Stiles ME. Characterization of freshly isolated *Campylobacter coli* strains and suitability of selective media for their growth. J Clin Microbiol. 1988;26:518–523.

179. Doyle MP: *Campylobacter* in Foods. In: Butzler J-P, ed. Campylobacter Infection in Man and Animals. Boca Raton, FL: CRC Press Inc, 1984:163–179.

180. Hodge DS, Terro R: Comparative efficacy of liquid enrichment medium for isolation of *Campylobacter jejuni*. J Clin Microbiol. 1984;19:434.

181. Steele TW, McDermott SN. Technical note: The use of membrane filters applied directly to the surface of agar plates for the isolation of *Campylobacter jejuni* from feces. Pathology. 1984;16:263–265.

182. Hodinka RL, Gilligan PH. Evaluation of the Campyslide agglutination test for confirmatory identification of selected *Campylobacter* species. J Clin Microbiol. 1988;26:47–49.

183. Penner VL. *Campylobacter, Helicobacter* and related spiral bacteria. In: Manual of Clinical Microbiology. 5th ed. Washington DC: American Society for Microbiology 1991:402–409.

184. Olive DM, Johny M, Sethi SK. Use of an alkaline phosphatase–labeled synthetic oligonucleotide probe for the detection of *Campylobacter jejuni* and *Campylobacter coli*. J Clin Microbiol. 1990;28:1565–1569.

185. Tenover FC, Carlson L, Barbagallo S, et al. DNA probe culture confirmation assay for identification of thermophilic *Campylobacter* species. J Clin Microbiol. 1990;28:1284–1287.

186. Thorne GM, Macone A, Goldmann DA. Enzymatically labelled nucleic acid (NA) probe assays for detection of *Campylobacter* species in human fecal specimens and in culture. Mol Cell Probes. 1990;4:133–142.

187. Banno Y, Kobayashi T, Kono H, et al. Biochemical characterization and biologic actions of two toxins (D-1 and D-2) from *Clostridium difficile*. Rev Infect Dis. 1984;6:S11–S20.

188. Banno Y, Kobayashi T, Watanabe K, et al. Two toxins (D-1 and D-2) of *Clostridium difficile* causing antibiotic-associated colitis: Purification and some characterization. Biochem Int. 1981;2:629–635.

189. Justus PG, Martin JL, Goldberg DA, et al. Myoelectric effects of *Clostridium difficile*: Motility-altering factors distinct from its cytotoxin and enterotoxin in rabbits. Gastroenterology. 1982;83:836–843.

190. Chang T-W, Lauermann M, Bartlett JG. Cytotoxicity assay in antibiotic-associated colitis. J Infect Dis. 1979;140:765–770.

191. Chang T-W, Lin PS, Gorbach SL, et al. Ultrastructural changes of cultured human amnion cells by *Clostridium difficile* toxin. Infect Immun. 1979;23:795–798.

192. Lyerly DM, Krivan HC, Wilkins TD. *Clostridium difficile*: Its disease and toxins. Clin Microbiol Rev. 1988;1:1–18.

193. Aronsson B, Mollby R, Nord CE. Diagnosis and epidemiology of *Clostridium difficile* enterocolitis in Sweden. J Clin Microbiol. 1984;14(suppl D):85–95.

194. Wu TC, Gersch SM. Evaluation of a commercial kit for the routine detection of *Clostridium difficile* cytotoxin by tissue culture. J Clin Microbiol. 1986;23:792–793.

195. George WL, Sutter VL, Citron D, et al. Selective and differential medium for isolation of *Clostridium difficile*. J Clin Microbiol. 1979;9:214–219.

196. Bartlett JG, Taylor NS, Chang TW. *Clostridium difficile*: A new toxigenic clostridium. In: Proceedings of International Conference: Les Anaérobies. Paris: Masson; 1981:383–391.

197. Chang TW, Gorbach SL. Rapid identification of *Clostridium difficile* by toxin detection. J Clin Microbiol. 1982;15:465–467.

198. Peterson LR, Holter JJ, Shanholtzer CJ, et al. Detection of *Clostridium difficile* toxins A (enterotoxin) and B (cytotoxin) in clinical specimens. Am J Clin Pathol. 1986;86:208–211.

199. Poxton IR, Byrne MD. Detection of *Clostridium difficile* toxin by counterimmunoelectrophoresis: A note of caution. J Clin Microbiol. 1981;14:349.

200. Sands M, Yungbluth M, Sommers HM. The non-value

of counterimmunoelectrophoresis for the direct rapid detection of *Clostridium difficile* toxin in stool filtrates. Am J Clin Pathol. 1983;79:375–377.

201. West SEH, Wilkins TD. Problems associated with counterimmunoelectrophoresis assays for detection of *Clostridium difficile* toxin. J Clin Microbiol. 1982;15:347–349.

202. Lyerly DM, Ball DW, Toth J, *et al.* Characterization of cross-reactive proteins detected by Culturette Brand Rapid Latex Test for *Clostridium difficile.* J Clin Microbiol. 1988;26:397–400.

203. Kelly MT, Champagne SG, Sherlock CH, *et al.* Commercial latex agglutination test for detection of *Clostridium difficile*–associated diarrhea. J Clin Microbiol. 1987;25:1244–1247.

204. Kamiya S, Nakamura S, Yamakawa K, *et al.* Evaluation of a commercially available latex immunoagglutination test kit for detection of *Clostridium difficile* D-1 toxin. Microbiol Immunol. 1986;30:177–181.

205. McFarland LV, Mulligan ME, Kwok RYY, *et al.* Nosocomial acquisition of *Clostridium difficile* infection. N Engl J Med. 1989;320:204–210.

206. Miles Bl, Siders JA, Allen SD. Evaluation of a commercial latex test for *Clostridium difficile* for reactivity with *C difficile* and cross-reactions with other bacteria. J Clin Microbiol. 1988;26:2452–2455.

207. Peterson LR, Olson MM, Shanholtzer CJ, *et al.* Results of a prospective, 18-month clinical evaluation of culture, diagnosis of *Clostridium difficile*–associated diarrhea. Diagn Microbiol Infect Dis. 1988;10:85–91.

208. Ryan RW, Kwasnik I, Clout D, *et al.* Utility of a rapid latex test for the detection of *Clostridium difficile* in fecal specimens. Ann Clin Lab Sci. 1987;17:232–235.

209. Sherman ME, DeGirolami PC, Thorne GM, *et al.* Evaluation of a latex agglutination test for diagnosis of *Clostridium difficile*–associated colitis. Am J Clin Pathol. 1988;89:228–233.

210. Laughon BE, Viscidi RP, Gdovin SL, *et al.* Enzyme immunoassay for the detection of *Clostridium difficile* toxins A and B in fecal specimens. J Infect Dis. 1984;149:781–788.

211. DiPersio JR, Varga FJ, Conwell DL, *et al.* Development of a rapid enzyme immunoassay for *Clostridium difficile* toxin A and its use in the diagnosis of *C. difficile*–associated disease. J Clin Microbiol. 1991;29:2724–2730.

212. DeGirolami PC, Hanff PA, Eichelberger K, *et al.* Multicenter evaluation of a new enzyme immunoassay for detection of *Clostridium difficile* enterotoxin A. J Clin Microbiol. 1992;30:1085–1088.

213. Wren B, Clayton C, Tabaqchali S. Rapid identification of toxigenic *Clostridium difficile* by polymerase chain reaction. Lancet. 1990;335:423.

214. Martinez RD, Wilkins TD. Purification and characterization of *Clostridium sordellii* hemorrhagic toxin and cross-reactivity with *Clostridium difficile* toxin A (enterotoxin). Infect Immun. 1988;56:1215–1221.

215. Kato N, Ou CY, Kato H, *et al.* Identification of toxigenic *Clostridium difficile* by the polymerase chain reaction. J Clin Microbiol. 1991;29:33–37.

216. Todd ECD. Preliminary estimates of costs of foodborne disease in the United States. J Food Protect. 1989; 52:595–601.

217. Rose S, Bakes P, Stringer M. Detection of staphylococcal enterotoxins in dairy products by the reversed passive latex agglutination (SET-RPLA) kit. Int J Food Microbiol. 1989;8:65–72.

218. Centers for Disease Control. Foodborne disease outbreaks annual summary 1981. Atlanta GA:CDC;1983.

219. Rennie RP, Anderson CM, Wensley BG, *et al. Klebsiella pneumoniae* gastroenteritis masked by *Clostridium perfringens.* J Clin Microbiol. 1990;28:216–219.

220. Gross TP, Kamara LB, Hatheway CL, *et al. Clostridium perfringens* food poisoning: Use of serotyping in an outbreak setting. J Clin Microbiol. 1989;27:660–663.

221. Harmon SM, Kautter DA, Hatheway CL. Enumeration and characterization of *Clostridium perfringens* in the feces of food poisoning patients and normal controls. J Food Protect. 1986;49:23–28.

222. Harmon SM, Kautter DA. Evaluation of a reversed passive latex agglutination test kit for *Clostridium perfringens* enterotoxins. J Food Protect. 1986;49:523–525.

223. Mahony DE, Gilliatt E, Dawson SV, *et al.* Vero cell assay for rapid detection of *Clostridium perfringens* enterotoxin. Appl Environ Microbiol. 1989;55:2141–2143.

224. Van Damme-Jongsten M, Rodhouse J, Gilbert RJ, *et al.* Synthetic DNA probes for detection of enterotoxigenic *Clostridium perfringens* strains isolated from outbreaks of food poisoning. J Clin Microbiol. 1990;28:131–133.

225. Giannella RA, Brasile L. A hospital-borne outbreak of diarrhea caused by *Bacillus cereus:* Clinical, epidemiologic and microbiologic studies. J Infect Dis. 1979;139:366–370.

226. Gilbert RJ. *Bacillus cereus* gastroenteritis. In: Riemann H, Bryan FL, eds. Food-borne Infections and Intoxications. 2nd ed. New York: Academic Press; 1979;495–518.

227. Turnbull PCB. *Bacillus cereus* toxins. In: Dorner F, Drews J, eds. International Encyclopedia of Pharmacology and Therapeutics: Section 119, pharmacology of bacterial toxins. New York: Pergamon Press; 1986.

228. Kramer JM, Gilbert RJ. *Bacillus cereus* and other *Bacillus* species. In: Doyle MP, ed. Foodborne Bacterial Pathogens. New York: Marcel Dekker; 1989;21–70.

229. Kramer JM, Turnball PCB, Munshi G, *et al.* Identification and characterization of *Bacillus cereus* and other *Bacillus* species associated with food poisoning. In: Corry JEL, Roberts D, Skinner FA, eds. Isolation and identification methods for food poisoning organisms. Society for Applied Bacteriology Technical Series. London: Academic Press. 1982;17:261–286.

230. Scott-Taylor T, Ahluwalia G, Klisko B, *et al.* Prevalent enteric adenovirus variant not detected by monoclonal antibody enzyme immunoassay. J Clin Microbiol. 1990;28:2797–2801.

231. Hermann JE, Perron-Henry DM, Stobbs-Walro D, *et al.* Preparation and characterization of monoclonal antibodies to enteric adenovirus types 40 and 41. Arch Virol. 1987;94:259–265.

232. Allard A, Girones R, Juto P, *et al.* Polymerase chain reaction for detection of adenoviruses in stool samples. J Clin Microbiol. 1990;28:2659–2667.

233. Bishop RF, Davidson GP, Holmes IH, *et al.* Detection of a new virus by electron microscopy of fecal extracts from children with acute gastroenteritis. Lancet. 1974;1:149–151.

234. Kalica AR, Purcell RH, Screno MM, *et al.* A microtiter solid-phase radioimmunoassay for detection of the human reovirus-like agent in stools. J Immunol. 1977;118:1275–1279.

235. Matsuno S, Nagayoshi S. Quantitative estimation of infantile gastroenteritis virus antigens in stools by immune adherence hemagglutination test. J Clin Microbiol. 1978;7:310–311.

236. Middleton PJ, Petric M, Hewitt CM, *et al.* Counterimmunoelectrophoresis for the detection of infantile gastroenteritis virus (orbi-group) antigen and antibody. J Clin Pathol. 1976;29:191–197.

237. Yolken RH, Kim HW, Clem T, *et al.* Enzyme-linked immunosorbent assay (ELISA) for detection of human reovirus-like agent of infantile gastroenteritis. Lancet. 1977;2:263–267.

238. Dennehy P, Gauntlett DR, Tente WE. Comparison of

nine commercial immunoassays for the detection of rotaviruses in fecal specimens. J Clin Microbiol. 1988;26:1630–1634.

239. Dennehy PH, Gauntlett DR, Spagenberger SE. Choice of reference assay for the detection of rotavirus in fecal specimens: Electron microscopy versus enzyme immunoassay. J Clin Microbiol. 1990;28:1280–1283.

240. Huang T, Chen G, Wang C, *et al.* Waterborne outbreak of rotavirus diarrhea in adults in China caused by a novel rotavirus. Lancet. 1984;1:1139–1142.

241. Saif LJ. Nongroup A rotaviruses. In: Saif LJ, Theil KW, eds. Viral Diarrheas of Man and Animals. Boca Raton FL: CRC Press; 1989:73–95.

242. Gouvea V, Glass RI, Woods P, *et al.* Polymerase chain reaction amplification and typing of rotavirus nucleic acid from stool specimens. J Clin Microbiol. 1990;28:276–282.

243. Gouvea V, Allen JR, Glass RI, *et al.* Detection of group B and C rotaviruses by polymerase chain reaction. J Clin Microbiol. 1991;29:519–523.

244. Wilde J, Eiden J, Yolken R. Removal of inhibitory substances from human fecal specimens for detection of group A rotaviruses by reverse transcriptase and polymerase chain reactions. J Clin Microbiol. 1990;28:1300–1307.

245. Eiden JJ, Wilde J, Firoozmand F, *et al.* Detection of animal and human group B rotaviruses in fecal specimens by polymerase chain reaction. J Clin Microbiol. 1991;29:539–543.

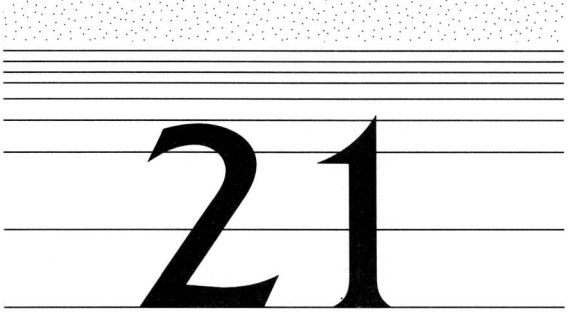

The Treatment of Acute Diarrhea

MYRON M. LEVINE, M.D.,
D.T.P.H.
STEVEN SAVARINO, M.D.

Acute diarrheal disease is a common clinical illness, particularly in less developed areas of the world where potable water and sanitation are not readily available and where personal hygiene practices are often primitive. In such areas, bacterial and protozoal enteropathogens account for a large proportion of diarrheal illness. In industrialized countries, viral pathogens are of relatively greater importance, although in situations such as custodial institutions and daycare centers for young children, where personal hygiene is compromised, bacterial and protozoal infections such as shigellosis, giardiasis, and cryptosporidiosis are readily transmitted.

Diarrheal infections present clinically in a number of distinct syndromes, depending on the causative agent. In general, most episodes of diarrheal disease are mild and self-limited and require no specific therapy. By contrast, some diarrheal infections result in severe clinical illness and require aggressive rehydration and specific antibiotic therapy. In this chapter, we consider the clinical presentations of diarrheal illness in the immunocompetent host, the importance of rehydration therapy, the indications for specific antibiotic therapy, clinically important complications of certain diarrheal infections, and the role of nonspecific therapy that aims to diminish intestinal secretion and discomfort due to abdominal cramping.

Twenty-five years ago, most of the microorganisms that we now recognize as important causal agents of acute diarrhea were not yet identified, and there was no appreciation of the virulence properties (e.g., fimbrial attachment factors and enterotoxins) that mediate diarrheal illness and that many such pathogens possess to overcome host defenses. Today, however, if comprehensive techniques are employed, including some available only as research tools, it is possible to identify a putative pathogen in the majority of episodes of acute diarrhea. Despite the large number of agents that can cause diarrheal illness, a relatively small number of them account for most disease of clinical and public health importance. Most of the important causal agents of diarrheal illness in immunocompetent hosts are shown in Table 21–1, with a comment on whether specific antimicrobial agents are indicated in the treatment of such infections. Clinical illness caused by the various enteric pathogens typically falls into one or more of the six clinical syndromes described in Table 21–2, depending on the pathogen.

TABLE 21–1. RELATIVE INDICATIONS FOR ANTIMICROBIALS IN DIARRHEAL DISEASE DUE TO SPECIFIC CAUSAL AGENTS IN IMMUNOCOMPETENT HOSTS

CLEARLY INDICATED	SOMETIMES INDICATED	NOT INDICATED
Shigellosis	Nontyphoidal salmonellosis	Rotavirus
Cholera	(in infants younger than 12 wk)	Other viral agents
Enterotoxigenic *Escherichia coli*	Enteropathogenic *E. coli*	Nontyphoidal salmonellosis
(traveler's diarrhea)*	(nursery outbreaks or persistent	(except in infants younger
Amebiasis	infection)	than 12 wk)
Giardiasis	Enteroinvasive *E. coli*	Cryptosporidiosis
Clostridium difficile colitis	*Campylobacter* (early treatment of	
	dysentery)	
	Clostridium difficile diarrhea	
	Non-*Vibrio cholerae* vibrios	
	Enteroaggregative *E. coli*	
	(persistent diarrhea)	

*Enterotoxigenic *E. coli* is the most common cause of acute traveler's diarrhea, and certain antibiotics are highly effective.

FLUID THERAPY

Diarrhea and vomiting constitute abnormal losses of body water and electrolytes. The most common complication of acute diarrheal illness is dehydration, which if severe, can lead to hypovolemia, acidosis, shock, and death. Diarrheal illness from many causes can lead to dehydration in infants. The greater surface area per kilogram of body weight of infants leads to relatively greater water losses through transpiration, and as a result, the daily fluid and electrolyte requirements per kilogram of body weight are greater in infants than in older children or adults. Abnormal losses due to diarrhea and vomiting are of relatively greater consequence in infants, but elderly adults and individuals of any age who are debilitated by underlying disease states (e.g., diabetes, heart disease) are also vulnerable to dehydration or to abnormalities in electrolytes. By contrast, it takes severe purging, such as that due to cholera, before severe dehydration is seen in an otherwise healthy adult.

Rehydration that aims to correct fluid and electrolyte deficits and to replace continuing losses serves as the cornerstone of therapy for all diarrheal diseases. Early rehydration initiated at the onset of diarrhea can usually prevent dehydration except in severe cholera. If the patient is already overtly dehydrated at the time of clinical presentation, rehydration must be instituted promptly to replace the deficits in body water and electrolytes.

Intravenous Fluid Therapy

Prompt intravenous fluid therapy is necessary in patients with severe dehydration and hypovolemic shock. Intravenous fluids may also be useful in patients with diminished mental status, symptomatic electrolyte disturbances, paralytic ileus, excessive purge rates, or intractable vom-

TABLE 21–2. CLINICAL PRESENTATIONS AND LIKELY AGENTS OF ACUTE DIARRHEAL DISEASE

CLINICAL TYPE	~ % OF PATIENTS	LIKELY AGENT	
		INDUSTRIALIZED COUNTRIES	DEVELOPING COUNTRIES
Simple diarrhea	90	Rotavirus, other viruses, *Salmonella*, *C. jejuni*	Rotavirus, ETEC, *Campylobacter jejuni*
Dysentery	5–10	*Shigella*, *C. jejuni*, EIEC, *Yersinia*	*Shigella*, *C. jejuni*, *Entamoeba histolytica*, EIEC
Persistent diarrhea (longer than 14 days)	3–4	*Giardia*, *Salmonella*, *Yersinia*	EPEC, *Giardia*, EAggEC
Severe purging of rice water stools	1*	Rotavirus, *Salmonella*	*Vibrio cholerae*, ETEC
Hemorrhagic colitis	<1	EHEC	EHEC, *Shigella dysenteriae* 1
Repeated vomiting without diarrhea	1–2		
Acute	1	Norwalk agent, other viruses	*Giardia*, *Strongyloides*
Persistent	<0.5	*Giardia*	

*More common in cholera-endemic areas.
KEY: EAggEC = enteroaggregative *Escherichia coli*, EHEC = enterohemorrhagic *E. coli*, EIEC = enteroinvasive *E. coli*, EPEC = enteropathogenic *E. coli*, ETEC = enterotoxigenic *E. coli*.

TABLE 21–3. CARBOHYDRATE AND ELECTROLYTE CONCENTRATIONS OF ORAL REHYDRATION AND MAINTENANCE SOLUTIONS

	Na$^+$ (mmol/L)	K$^+$ (mmol/L)	Cl$^-$ (mmol/L)	BICARBONATE (mmol/L)	CITRATE (mmol/L)	CARBOHYDRATE (g/L)
REHYDRATION						
WHO Solution	90	20	80	—	30	20
Pedialyte RS (Ross)	75	20	65	—	30	25
MAINTENANCE						
Resol (Wyeth)	50	20	50	—	34	20
Lytren (Mead-Johnson)	50	25	45	—	30	20
Pedialyte (Ross)	45	20	35	—	30	25
Infalyte (Penwalt)	50	20	40	30	—	20
OTHER FREQUENTLY USED SOLUTIONS						
Gatorade	23.5	<1	17	—	—	40
Coca-Cola	1.6	<1	—	13.4	—	100
Apple juice	<1	25	—	—	—	120
Orange juice	<1	50	—	50	—	120

iting. Overall, however, these instances represent a relatively small proportion of all patients with diarrheal disease, even in pediatric practice. Severely dehydrated patients are rapidly infused with an appropriate solution such as Ringer's lactate to expand vigorously the intravascular volume; this is followed by additional rehydration fluids, preferably by the oral route, to replace the remaining deficit and to provide for continuing losses and maintenance requirements.

Oral Rehydration

Glucose–Electrolytes Solution

Since the late 1970s it has been repeatedly shown that the vast majority of patients with diarrheal dehydration in either developing or industrialized areas can be effectively treated with oral rehydration; this therapy is simple to administer, inexpensive, and highly efficacious.[1–5] The introduction of glucose-based oral rehydration therapy (ORT) followed the observation that the active transport of glucose is coupled with sodium transport in the small intestine,[6] a process that is preserved during diarrheal illness.

For both the treatment and prevention of diarrheal dehydration, in less developed countries, irrespective of its cause or the age of the patient, the World Health Organization (WHO) recommends the use of a single oral solution (WHO-ORS) with a sodium concentration of 90 mEq/L.[7] The WHO-ORS is used both early in diarrheal illness to prevent dehydration and late to rehydrate dehydrated patients who are not in overt shock. When used to prevent dehydration

in patients who are not clinically dehydrated, appropriate amounts of low solute fluids must be administered along with WHO-ORS. Given in this way, there is no tendency for serum sodium concentrations to become elevated.[1–3, 8–11]

In treating patients with overt clinical dehydration, WHO-ORS ORT is as efficacious as intravenous fluid therapy in treating hyponatremic and isotonic dehydration, and in hypernatremic dehydration it is associated with a lower incidence of seizures than is intravenous fluid therapy.[4, 5] Some pediatricians in industrialized countries have been reluctant to use WHO-ORS with its sodium concentration of 90 mEq/L, believing it to be too high.[12] As an alternative therapy in such environments, two different oral rehydration solutions have been made available. One solution, with a sodium concentration 60 to 75 mEq/L, is used for replacement of deficits in overtly dehydrated patients. A solution of lower sodium concentration (45–50 mEq/L) is employed to prevent dehydration by replacing continuing losses in the patient who is not clinically dehydrated. Some oral rehydration solutions available in the United States are shown in Table 21–3, where they are compared with WHO-ORS.

Super Solutions

Although glucose-based ORS effectively replaces diarrheal losses, it does not abate stool output. Other solutes such as the neutral amino acids glycine and alanine[13] and dipeptides such as glycylglycine[14] are also actively and independently cotransported with sodium and are effective clinically in oral rehydration.[15–20] These observations have led to the concept of a so-called super solution that would contain multiple actively transported substrates and would be so potent in stimulating absorption that it actually diminishes diarrheal losses while rehydrating the patient.[1, 21] Regrettably, no multiple substrate solution has consistently achieved such results in clinical studies.[15-20, 22]

A natural oral rehydration solution, rice powder–electrolyte solution, sometimes behaves like a super solution, particularly in diarrheal infections due to enterotoxigenic bacteria such as *Vibrio cholerae* O1 and enterotoxigenic *E. coli* (ETEC).[21, 23-28] Rice powder–electrolyte solutions deliver higher densities of glucose to the small intestine in the form of complex starches and also provide amino acids and small peptides; a solution containing 50 g/L of rice powder is optimal. In some direct comparisons with WHO-ORS in treating dehydration due to cholera and ETEC diarrhea, rice powder–electrolyte solution proved quantitatively superior: Oral intake requirements, stool output, and duration of diarrhea were all significantly reduced in the rice powder–electrolyte group.[21, 23-25, 28] By contrast, rice powder–electrolyte solution has not proved superior in the treatment of noncholera diarrhea.[26, 28, 29]

Early Realimentation

The administration of food during the treatment of diarrheal illness has been a point of contention for many years.[30-32] In the past, it was common practice to withhold food from infants and young children and rest the gut during treatment of diarrheal illness, while water and electrolyte needs were provided by parenteral fluids. Others argued that the administration of food during active diarrheal illness could result in food allergies. Even with the advent of oral rehydration, the point at which feeding should be initiated and the type of food that should be given have been the source of much contention. Advocates of early feeding contend that from a nutritional standpoint, the benefits of early refeeding after the initial period of rehydration generally outweigh the risks. This is especially true in situations in which the nutritional consequences of diarrheal diseases are high, as for example, in young children in less developed areas who may experience as many as 6 to 8 episodes of diarrhea each year. The pendulum has swung to the point where feeding during the treatment of diarrheal illness is considered correct and the administration of appropriate foods is deemed an integral component of the treatment of diarrhea.

SPECIFIC ANTIMICROBIAL THERAPY

In general, antimicrobial agents are prescribed too liberally in the treatment of diarrheal diseases. In fact, most illness is mild and self-limited and can be treated with fluid therapy alone. The widespread use of antibiotics in some areas has contributed selective pressures leading to antibiotic resistance among enteropathogens, complicating the treatment of patients whose condition warrants the use of antibiotics. For a number of bacterial pathogens that cause diarrhea, controlled studies have not been carried out to establish the efficacy of specific antibiotics, whereas in other instances, studies have been performed but show no benefit.[33] Obviously, viral diarrheas do not respond to antibiotic treatment, but antibiotic treatment is of proven efficacy for certain bacterial and protozoan enteropathogens and may be warranted in treating others when the illness is complicated or severe.

Shigellosis

Shigella is the most common cause of dysentery. One serotype, *Shigella dysenteriae* 1 (also called Shiga's bacillus), causes a particularly fulminant illness and in less developed countries is associated with a high case fatality rate. In controlled clinical trials, several antibiotics have been shown to diminish significantly the duration and severity of the illness and to curtail excretion of *Shigella*. Information from such trials is critical since in vitro susceptibility does not necessarily correlate with in vivo efficacy. Some antibiotics, including oral cephalexin,[34] cefaclor,[35] and amoxicillin[36] and parenteral kanamycin,[37] are of little value clinically, despite favorable in vitro activity. Moreover, as effective antibiotics have achieved broad usage, resistant strains of organisms have increasingly appeared. Successively, from the 1940s through the mid-1970s, sulfa drugs, tetracycline, and ampicillin were each used as the drug of choice for treating shigellosis until resistant strains became highly prevalent.[33] Until recently, trimethoprim-sulfamethoxazole (TMP/SMZ) was the drug of choice in many areas,[38-41] but its utility has been eroded worldwide by increasing levels of resistance.[42-47] Often TMP/SMZ resistance genes are found on plasmids that code multiple other antibiotic resistances. A summary of effective treatment regimens for shigellosis, depending on the resistance pattern of the *Shigella* strains, is given in Table 21–4.

Consequent to the increasing resistance to

TABLE 21–4. RECOMMENDED ANTIBIOTIC DOSAGE REGIMENS FOR THE TREATMENT OF SHIGELLOSIS

| ANTIBIOTIC | DOSE AND DURATION | |
	INFANTS AND CHILDREN	ADULTS AND ADOLESCENTS
ORAL		
TMP-SMZ	10–50 mg/kg/d in 4 divided doses for 5 d	160–800 mg q 6 h for 5 d
Ampicillin	100 mg/kg/d in 4 divided doses for 5 d	500 mg q 6 h for 5 d
Norfloxacin		400 mg q 12 h for 5 d Stoss therapy 100 mg/kg in 1 dose
Tetracycline		500 mg q 6 h for 5 d Stoss therapy 2.5 g in 1 dose
Ciprofloxacin		500 mg q 12 h for 5 d
Nalidixic acid	55 mg/kg/d in 4 divided doses for 5–7 d	1 g q 6 h for 5–7 d
PARENTERAL		
Ceftriaxone	50 mg/kg single daily dose for 5 d	

KEY: TMP-SMZ = trimethoprim-sulfamethoxazole.
SOURCE: Adapted from DiJohn D, Lovino MM. Treatment of diarrhea. Infect Dis Clin North Am. 1985; 2:723.

TMP/SMZ, the newer quinolone derivatives are now often employed to initiate treatment in severely ill adults when a *Shigella* infection is suspected or when a strain is isolated that is resistant to other antibiotics. Because use of the new fluoroquinolones is contraindicated in pediatrics, the venerable quinolone nalidixic acid must be used to treat such infections in children. In Bangladesh, where nalidixic acid is a drug of choice, isolates of *S. dysenteriae* 1 resistant to this antibiotic have been reported.[48] Antibiotics must be used judiciously in treating moderate to severe shigellosis, must be used with antibiotic susceptibility testing, and must be guided by information from epidemiological surveillance that tracks the prevalence of resistance to clinically important antibiotics.

For treatment of infection in adults due to strains known to be sensitive, as in an outbreak, a 5-day course of oral tetracycline, given in 500-mg doses every 6 hours, shortens and mitigates the course of shigellosis and diminishes the duration of pathogen excretion.[49] A single large (2.0 mg) dose of tetracycline, so-called stoss therapy or bolus therapy, has comparable efficacy.[49–51] In one study, curiously, clinical and

bacteriologic cures were obtained with stoss therapy even against strains demonstrating in vitro resistance to tetracycline.[50] Tetracycline is contraindicated in pregnancy and in children younger than 7 years because of its associated tooth discoloration; the safety of stoss therapy has not been evaluated in these groups.

In all age groups, infection due to ampicillin-sensitive strains is amenable to a 5-day regimen of either oral or parenteral ampicillin.[37, 52, 53] Although the clinical response to stoss therapy with ampicillin compares favorably with a 5-day regimen, in a study in Bangladesh it was associated with significantly higher rates of bacteriologic failure.[54] Amoxicillin is ineffective in the treatment of shigellosis for reasons that are not well understood.[36]

A 5-day course of TMP/SMZ effectively treats shigellosis due to sensitive strains.[38–41] This continues to be the regimen of choice in many areas where resistant strains remain uncommon or where the relatively high cost of the new quinolone antibiotics precludes their routine use.

A study in the United States comparing the efficacy of nalidixic acid versus ampicillin in treating severe childhood shigellosis demonstrated a significantly slower clinical response to nalidixic acid.[55] By contrast, a study conducted in Bangladeshi children demonstrated similar clinical and bacteriologic cure rates when strains were sensitive in vitro to both drugs and when patients were treated within 72 hours of the onset of symptoms.[42] On the Indian subcontinent, where TMP/SMZ-resistant *Shigella* strains are common and drug costs are of paramount importance in guiding therapy, nalidixic acid has become a drug of choice.[42]

Three fluoroquinolones, norfloxacin, ciprofloxacin, and ofloxacin, show excellent in vitro activity against *Shigella*.[56, 57] The clinical efficacy of norfloxacin and ciprofloxacin matches their high in vitro activity.[57–60] In Thai adults with shigellosis, a norfloxacin regimen of 400 mg 2 times a day for 3 days provided good clinical and bacteriologic outcomes.[58] In the course of seven separate trials in Latin America, two regimens of 400 mg of norfloxacin, given either 2 or 3 times a day for 5 days, were compared with TMP/SMZ (160 mg TMP and 800 mg SMZ), given 2 times a day for 5 days, in the treatment of acute bacterial diarrhea in patients older than 11 years.[61] Both norfloxacin regimens showed 100% eradication of *Shigella* 2 to 4 days after treatment. In these studies, the clinical efficacy was high against all bacterial pathogens.

Ciprofloxacin, given in 500-mg doses every 12 hours, was superior to ampicillin in treating patients with severe shigellosis in Bangladesh.[59] In Peruvian adults, a single 800-mg dose of norfloxacin was as effective as 5 days of TMP/SMZ in treating shigellosis.[60] In areas where resistance has substantially eroded the utility of other available antibiotics and where these new antimicrobials can be afforded, the fluoroquinolones have become the drugs of choice, but the relatively high cost of these agents limits their usefulness and their availability in less developed countries.

Several of the quinolones have been associated with arthropathies in young animals,[62] and rare case reports of ciprofloxacin-associated arthropathy in children have appeared.[63] For this reason, the quinolones, except nalidixic acid, have not been approved for use in children and pregnant or nursing women. Nalidixic acid also causes such arthropathies in juvenile animal models, however, and there are strong advocates for the initiation of careful clinical studies to assess the role of these antimicrobials in the treatment of severe shigellosis in pediatrics.[64] Limited use of the new fluoroquinolones in other pediatric infections such as *Pseudomonas* pulmonary infections in children with cystic fibrosis has shown that they are tolerated well.[64]

Salmonella Gastroenteritis

The effect of antibiotic treatment on uncomplicated non-*typhi Salmonella* gastroenteritis has been studied in several randomized placebo-controlled trials. Chloramphenicol,[65] neomycin,[66] TMP/SMZ, ampicillin, and amoxicillin[68, 69] have not shown benefit by significantly diminishing the duration or the severity of diarrheal illness or the length of pathogen excretion in comparison with a placebo. One study found that children treated with oral amoxicillin or ampicillin had a significantly higher incidence of bacteriologic relapse, not infrequently associated with recurrence of diarrhea.[69] On the basis of these studies, these antibiotics are not recommended for treatment of uncomplicated *Salmonella* gastroenteritis.

With the advent of the new fluoroquinolones, the question has once again been raised whether these antimicrobials may play a beneficial role in altering the course of non-typhoidal *Salmonella* gastroenteritis in the immunocompetent adult. In a randomized, placebo-controlled trial using ciprofloxacin to treat acute bacterial diarrhea in adults, *Salmonella* was the most commonly isolated pathogen.[70] In this subset, the duration of diarrhea was significantly shorter in the ciprofloxacin group. Although none were

excreting the pathogen by 48 hours into treatment, 4 of 16 patients subsequently had bacteriologic relapse. A placebo-controlled clinical study that investigated the effectiveness of ciprofloxacin, given in 750-mg doses 2 times a day for 14 days, to eradicate the excretion of nontyphoidal *Salmonella* in individuals infected after a common-source outbreak, showed initial success followed by a high rate of bacteriologic relapse.[71] Since the peak age incidence of salmonellosis occurs in childhood and most illness is self-limited, the future role of fluoroquinolones in treating this entity may be limited.

Infants younger than 12 weeks and patients with hemoglobinopathies who develop *Salmonella* gastroenteritis are at increased risk of developing bacteremia and metastatic infectious complications such as meningitis, septic arthritis, and osteomyelitis.[72, 73] These high-risk groups should be vigorously treated with antibiotics. Therapy may be initiated with ampicillin or amoxicillin, given in a dosage of 100 mg/kg of body weight per day, or chloramphenicol, given in a dosage of 80 mg/kg of body weight per day, although in vitro susceptibility patterns should guide the choice. Some extend this recommendation to include patients with malignancies and other immunosuppressive conditions.[74]

Campylobacter jejuni Enteritis

Since the late 1970s, *Campylobacter* enteritis has become recognized as a common diarrheal disease in both developed and underdeveloped areas, with a spectrum of illness ranging from watery diarrhea to frank dysentery. Several placebo-controlled trials with erythromycin in children and adults have demonstrated significant curtailment of pathogen excretion in treated groups.[75–79] In only one study, however, in which infants with dysentery were treated early in their illness with erythromycin, in a dosage of 50 mg/kg of body weight per day for 5 days, was a significant mitigation of diarrheal illness demonstrated.[79] A 1987 study from Bangkok noted a high proportion of erythromycin-resistant *Campylobacter* isolates.[80]

The new fluoroquinolones show excellent in vitro activity against *Campylobacter* isolates, and initial results suggest that ciprofloxacin may be efficacious in treating adults with *Campylobacter* diarrheal infections.[70, 31]

Enterotoxigenic Escherichia coli Infections

Enterotoxigenic *E. coli*, which produces a toxin-mediated secretory diarrhea, is a frequent cause of diarrhea in travelers to developing areas and is also endemic among children in those areas. In a placebo-controlled trial, the effect of tetracycline on the clinical course of ETEC diarrhea in Bangladeshi adults differed according to the toxin phenotype of the infecting strain. Among patients infected with strains elaborating both heat-labile toxin (LT) and heat-stable toxin (ST), the duration of diarrhea was slightly shortened, but there was no clinical effect in patients infected with strains producing only ST; abbreviated excretion occurred in both groups.[82] The use of TMP/SMZ proved efficacious for ETEC diarrhea in three well-designed studies in which the infecting strains were sensitive. In an experimental challenge study in adult volunteers in the United States[83] and in a field trial of traveler's diarrhea in Mexico,[84] TMP/SMZ significantly shortened the duration and severity of diarrhea and curtailed ETEC excretion compared with a placebo. In young Mexican children, this agent significantly shortened ETEC-induced diarrhea.[85]

As resistance to tetracycline, ampicillin, and TMP/SMZ has increased in many areas,[86, 87] the fluoroquinolones, which are active in vitro against ETEC,[56] have become drugs of choice for treatment of adults with ETEC traveler's diarrhea. Ciprofloxacin was found to be as efficacious as TMP/SMZ in interrupting diarrhea due to ETEC in a study of traveler's diarrhea in Mexico.[61] Many authorities recommend that in areas where ETEC is prevalent, adult traveler's diarrhea should be treated promptly with ciprofloxacin, given in a dosage of 500 mg 2 times a day for 5 days. Although data from definitive studies are not available, pediatric travelers should also be treated early in their course of diarrheal illness with TMP/SMZ, given in a dosage of 4 mg/kg of body weight for TMP and 20 mg/kg of body weight for SMZ 2 times a day. Antibiotics are not routinely recommended for suspect ETEC diarrhea in indigenous persons living in areas where ETEC is endemic. A vast clinical experience from oral rehydration studies where etiologic agents were identified supports this contention. In individuals from endemic areas, degrees of background immunity tend to make the ETEC infections self-limited and treatable with oral rehydration alone.

Enteropathogenic *Escherichia coli* Infections

Enteropathogenic *E. coli* (EPEC) infections are an important cause of diarrhea in infants younger than 6 months in many developing areas of the world, and occasional nursery and community outbreaks still occur in industrialized countries. In the 1960s, oral neomycin was sometimes used to treat EPEC diarrhea,[88] but its use is now discouraged because neomycin commonly causes intestinal malabsorption and diarrhea as side effects in a proportion of recipients. In an Ethiopian trial, infants receiving either mecillinam or TMP/SMZ for 5 days had significant clinical improvement and diminished excretion compared with an untreated control group.[89] Two studies in EPEC-infected infants and children that employed ampicillin differed in their outcome, one showing a favorable clinical and bacteriologic response[52] and the other no differences[68] when compared with a placebo. A reasonable approach is to employ an antibiotic such as TMP/SMZ when EPEC is implicated as the cause of severe or persistent diarrhea in a young infant or in a nursery outbreak situation.

Enteroinvasive *Escherichia coli* Infections

Enteroinvasive *E. coli* (EIEC) closely resembles *Shigella* in the virulence properties that it possesses and in its pathogenesis. Both harbor large invasiveness plasmids that are required for the invasion of epithelial cells. Clinically, the vast majority of patients with EIEC infection manifest watery, nonbloody diarrhea as their main complaint accompanied by low-grade fever. An analysis of the clinical pictures observed in several outbreaks of EIEC shows that only 2 to 7% of patients manifest bloody diarrhea.[90, 91] Enteroinvasive *E. coli* infections are thought to be responsive to the same agents as are used in shigellosis, but there have been no controlled trials to support this belief and there are few published antibiotic susceptibility data available.

Enterohemorrhagic *Escherichia coli* Infections

Enterohemorrhagic *E. coli* (EHEC) possess three notable virulence properties, the elaboration of potent Shiga-like toxins (also referred to as Verotoxins), the expression of plasmid-associated fimbriae, and an ability to attach intimately to, and to efface, microvilli of enterocytes. Infections from EHEC cause a spectrum of clinical illness that includes simple diarrhea, hemorrhagic colitis, and the hemolytic-uremic syndrome (HUS). No controlled trials of antibiotic therapy of EHEC infection have been conducted. Results of retrospective analyses are conflicting. Some studies suggest that the administration of antibiotics enhances the propensity for HUS to occur as a complication of EHEC diarrhea.[92, 93] It has been noted that exposure of EHEC to sublethal doses of certain antimicrobial agents in vitro results in the release of Shiga-like toxins from the periplasmic space of the bacteria.[94] Data from other retrospective analyses support a conflicting conclusion. For example, a report from Washington State, where EHEC infections are common, suggests that antibiotic therapy does not influence the course of illness or the risk of post-infectious sequelae.[95]

Yersinia enterocolitica Enteritis

Yersinia enterocolitica is a common cause of enteritis and dysentery in young children, particularly in certain cooler climates such as northern Europe. Infected adolescents frequently present with mesenteric lymphadenitis, whereas extraintestinal infections, including septicemia, have been reported, albeit infrequently, in patients with certain underlying conditions, most notably iron overload states. Generally, isolates are susceptible in vitro to aminoglycosides, tetracycline, chloramphenicol, TMP/SMZ, third-generation cephalosporins, and quinolones,[96] but data are lacking to support their use in uncomplicated diarrhea. In the only placebo-controlled trial, in which children with enteritis were treated on average 12 days after onset of their illness, TMP/SMZ offered no beneficial clinical or bacteriologic effect.[97] Based on available information, it is recommended that antibiotic therapy be limited to patients with severe or chronic Y. enterocolitica enteritis and those with focal extra-intestinal or systemic infections, with the choice of antibiotics guided by in vitro susceptibility testing.

Cholera

Vibrio cholerae O1 causes a secretory diarrhea characterized by voluminous purging. As an adjunct to fluid therapy, antibiotics are of proven benefit. Tetracycline, the drug of choice, markedly diminishes the volume and duration of the diarrhea itself and of the fluid replacement requirements, and it curtails the excretion of vibrios.[98-100] Adults may be given 500 mg 4 times a day or 2 g once daily for 2 days with equivalent

results. Because the duration of therapy is short, its use in children is considered safe, and it is given in a dosage of 125 mg 4 times a day for 2 to 4 days. In the face of outbreaks due to tetracycline-resistant V. cholerae O1, alternative regimens of proven efficacy include erythromycin,[101] TMP/SMZ,[101, 102] furazolidone,[100] and chloramphenicol.[93] Erythromycin or furazolidone may be used as a treatment in childhood and pregnancy. Tetracycline-resistant strains are prevalent in eastern Africa and occasional outbreaks have also been reported from Bangladesh.

Clostridium difficile Diarrhea and Colitis

Clostridium difficile is the most frequent causative agent of antibiotic-associated pseudomembranous colitis, but it is also implicated in antibiotic-associated diarrhea without colitis.[103] In patients with C. difficile–induced colitis and in those with diarrhea not responding simply to discontinuation of the offending antibiotic, specific therapy is warranted. Multiple studies, including one placebo-controlled trial, have documented the efficacy and safety of oral vancomycin,[104-108] which is considered the drug of choice. A dosage of 125 mg 4 times a day for 10 to 14 days is generally adequate, although some patients may require up to 2 g daily. Because of its high cost and the frequency of clinical relapse (6 to 39%), other agents have been sought. Both oral metronidazole (in a dosage of 250 mg 4 times a day)[109-111] and bacitracin, (given in a dosage of 20,000 U 4 times a day),[112, 113] appear clinically comparable to vancomycin and provide inexpensive alternatives, although relapse rates are similar to those with vancomycin in all. Metronidazole is contraindicated in pregnant and nursing women because of its theoretical potential for human teratogenesis. Moreover, because of its disulfiram-like effect, concomitant use of alcohol is proscribed. A preliminary report suggests that oral teicoplanin may benefit patients with pseudomembranous colitis.[114] Documented relapses and cases unresponsive to alternative antimicrobials should be treated with a course of vancomycin. Patients with multiple relapses or those with associated adynamic ileus are especially difficult to treat. In patients who have many relapses, uncontrolled studies have shown favorable response to an extended course of cholestyramine together with oral vancomycin and the use of bacteriotherapy, although optimal therapy has not been established. In patients unable to tolerate oral therapy, limited anecdotal experience using parenteral metronidazole and vancomycin suggests both success and failure with each agent.[115] Demonstrable achievement of therapeutic intracolonic metronidazole levels after parenteral dosing[111] favors its usage, although more controlled studies with these agents and a search for other potential therapies need to be pursued.

Amebiasis

Entamoeba histolytica causes a spectrum of intestinal infection ranging from asymptomatic cyst excretion to amebic colitis, which is sometimes complicated by metastatic spread that usually involves the liver. Amebiasis is a recognized health problem in many parts of the developing world, where it is endemic. While amebiasis is infrequent in industrialized countries, travelers and homosexual males compose sub-populations at increased risk. Current use of amebicidal agents is based mostly on uncontrolled experience, and although apparently effective, some drugs carry the risk of serious adverse reactions. Table 21–5 lists recommended therapy for amebic infections, and the reader is referred to recent reviews for a more detailed discussion.[116, 117] Although disputed, most authorities recommend treatment for asymptomatic infection with an antiamebic agent having intraintestinal activity in an effort to halt transmission and prevent invasive disease. Such agents include diloxanide furoate which is available in the United States only through the federal Centers for Disease Control and Prevention (CDC) in Atlanta and which some consider the drug of choice. Other agents include iodoquinol, and paromomycin. The nitroimidazoles metronidazole and tinidazole show amebicidal activity both in the intestinal lumen and in tissues, and they are drugs of choice for intestinal and extraintestinal disease. Both are contraindicated during pregnancy and lactation. Although these agents usually ablate intestinal carriage, an agent that is active in the intestinal lumen may be added if cyst excretion persists after therapy. Some studies show tinidazole to be safer and more efficacious than metronidazole for treatment of invasive disease,[118, 119] but tinidazole is not available in the United States. Dehydroemetine and emetine, with only tissue amebicidal activity, are less attractive alternatives in that a painful intramuscular injection is the only route of administration; they are frequently accompanied by marked gastrointes-tinal adverse effects and, less frequently, by cardiac toxicity; furthermore, the concomitant treatment with a luminal amebicide is required.

Giardiasis

Giardia lamblia can cause acute or chronic diarrhea that may be accompanied by malabsorption. Giardiasis is endemic in both industrialized and developing areas. The nitroimidazoles (tinidazole and metronidazole), quinacrine, and furazolidone are the most active and frequently used anti-giardial agents.[120, 121] Quinacrine is perhaps the most efficacious, with cure rates above 90%, but it can cause adverse reactions that include gastrointestinal side effects, dermatologic reactions, and, rarely, reversible toxic psychosis. The nitroimidazoles are comparable in efficacy to quinacrine and have fewer side effects,[122] but they are not approved by the federal Food and Drug Administration (FDA) for use in the United States. Tinidazole is attractive because of the effectiveness of single-dose therapy.[123] Furazolidone is the least efficacious, with cure rates of about 80%, although the available suspension is frequently prescribed for children because of convenience and tolerability. Both quinacrine and furazolidone may induce hemolysis in glucose-6-phosphate dehydrogenase (G6PD)–deficient persons, and metronidazole and furazolidone have disulfiram-like effects. Paromomycin has been used when treatment is required during pregnancy, although no studies have been done to establish efficacy. A summary of recommended dosage regimens appears in Table 21–5.

Cryptosporidiosis

Cryptosporidium parvum is increasingly recognized as a relatively common cause of diarrhea in humans. In immunocompetent individuals, illness is usually self-limited, whereas immunodeficient hosts may experience prolonged, severe, watery diarrhea that can be fatal. Little success has been achieved with antimicrobial therapy. Limited benefits were anecdotally reported with spiramycin in patients with acquired immunodeficiency syndrome (AIDS),[124] those on immunosuppressive therapy,[125] and the elderly.[126] Controlled trials of spiramycin therapy in immunocompetent children with *Cryptosporidium* diarrhea have shown no benefit.[127, 128]

TABLE 21–5. ANTIMICROBIAL TREATMENT REGIMENS FOR PARASITIC DIARRHEAS

INDICATION	PEDIATRIC DOSE	ADULT DOSE
GIARDIASIS		
Tinidazole		150 mg bid × 7 d
Metronidazole	15 mg/kg/d in 3 doses × 5 d	250 mg tid × 5 d
Furazolidone	5 mg/kg/d in 4 doses × 10 d	100 mg qid × 7 d
Quinacrine	6 mg/kg/d in 3 doses × 5 d	100 mg tid × 5 d
AMEBIASIS ASYMPTOMATIC INFECTION		
Diloxanide furoate	20 mg/kg/d in 3 doses × 10 d	500 mg tid × 10 d
Iodoquinol	30–40 mg/kg/d in 3 doses × 20 d (max 2 g/d)	650 mg tid × 20 d
Metronidazole	35–50 mg/kg/d in 3 doses × 10 d	750 mg tid × 5–10 d
MILD TO MODERATE INTESTINAL DISEASE		
Metronidazole	250 mg tid × 5 d	15 mg/kg/d in 3 doses × 5 d
Tetracycline	10 mg/kg/d in 4 doses × 10 d (max 2 g/d)	500 mg qid × 10 d
followed by iodoquinol	30–40 mg/kg/d in 3 doses × 20 d max 2 g/d)	650 mg tid × 20 d
Paromomycin sulfate	25–30 mg/kg/d in 3 doses for 5–10 d	25–30 mg/kg/d in 3 doses for 5–10 d
followed by iodoquinol	30–40 mg/kg/d in 3 doses × 20 d (max 2 g/d)	650 mg tid × 20 d
SEVERE INTESTINAL DISEASE		
Metronidazole	15 mg/kg/d in 3 doses × 5 d	500 mg tid × 5–20 d
Tetracycline	10 mg/kg/d in 4 doses × 10 d (max 2 g/d)	500 mg qid × 10 d
followed by iodoquinol	30–40 mg/kg/d in 3 doses × 20 d (max 2 g/d)	650 mg tid × 20 d
Emetine hydrocholoride	0.5 mg/kg/d in 2 doses (max 60 mg/d) for up to 5 d	1 mg/kg/d (max 60 mg/d) up to 5 d
followed by iodoquinol	30–40 mg/kg/d in 3 doses × 20 d (max 2 g/d)	650 mg tid × 20 d
Dehydroemetine HCl	1.0–1.5 mg/kg/d (max 90 mg/d) for up to 5 d	1.0–1.5 mg/kg/d (max 90 mg/d) for up to 5 d
followed by iodoquinol	30–40 mg/kg/d in 3 doses × 20 d (max 2 g/d)	650 mg tid × 20 d
HEPATIC ABSCESS		
Metronidazole	35–50 mg/kg/d in 3 doses × 10 d	750 mg tid × 5–10 d
Dehydroemetine HCl and	1.0–1.5 mg/kg/d (max 90 mg/d) for up to 5 d	1.0–1.5 mg/kg/d (max 90 mg/d) for up to 5 d
chloroquine phosphate	10 mg (base)/kg/d for 21 d (max 600 mg/d)	9 g (600 mg base) q d × 2 wk, then 500 mg q d × 2–3 wk

Strongyloides stercoralis Infection

Strongyloides stercoralis infection is occasionally diagnosed in patients with persistent vomiting or diarrhea. Such patients should be treated with thiabendazole, given in a dosage of 50 mg/kg of body weight per day in 2 doses for 2 days.[129]

NONSPECIFIC ADJUNCTIVE THERAPIES FOR DIARRHEAL ILLNESS

Throughout the world, in industrialized as well as less developed countries, a wide array of nonspecific antidiarrheal agents are given to patients in the hope of attaining symptomatic relief from diarrheal illness by diminishing diarrheal losses and alleviating abdominal cramps. Regrettably, few of these agents are effective yet innocuous. In less developed countries, the use of such medications often means unnecessary expenditure for families with little income and detracts attention from the all-important use of oral rehydration solutions.

Adsorbents

Kaolin-pectin preparations increase the consistency of the diarrheal stool, but the effect is only cosmetic, since the water and electrolyte content of the stools is unchanged.[130] While not effective, kaolin-pectin preparations are innocuous and thus may be prescribed by the clinician for their placebo effect.

Attapulgite (Diasorb, Schering) a naturally occurring hydrous magnesium aluminum silicate in a three-layer, crystalline structure, adsorbs up to eight times its weight in water and is 33 times more adsorbent than kaolin. The FDA recognizes attapulgite as a safe and effective adsorbent type of antidiarrheal compound.[131] Another adsorbent that is recognized by the FDA as a safe and effective over-the-counter antidiarrheal compound is polycarbophil, a hydrophilic polyacrylic resin that adsorbs 60 times its weight in water.[131-133]

Cholestyramine, a nonadsorbable exchange resin, has been studied in several settings.[134-139] It significantly shortened the duration of acute diarrhea in infants, most of whom had rotavirus gastroenteritis.[134] A few small uncontrolled studies suggest that cholestyramine may have a beneficial effect in treating persistent diarrhea in infants in less developed countries[138, 139] and antibiotic-associated diarrhea and colitis, particularly in patients who relapse after oral vancomycin therapy.[137, 140] Potential adverse effects include the development of hyperchloremic acidosis in very young patients and in those with renal insufficiency. Cholestyramine may interfere with the adsorption of other drugs.

Antisecretory Drugs

Chlorpromazine diminishes the secretory effect of cholera toxin and *E. coli* LT in animal models.[141] Clinical trials in cholera patients showed that chlorpromazine can significantly diminish the voluminous diarrhea of cholera.[142] At the dosage required to achieve a therapeutic effect, however, the patients suffer from somnolence, which interferes with their ability to ingest oral rehydration solutions. For this reason, chlorpromazine has not been added to the armamentarium of drugs used to treat cholera.

In two small inpatient studies in developing countries, in which moderate dosages of aspirin (25 mg/kg/d) were used to treat acute diarrhea in infants and children, intestinal fluid losses were diminished.[143, 144] Aspirin, given in a dosage of 25 mg/kg of body weight per day, decreased the mean daily diarrheal stool volume by approximately 100 ml compared with that of the placebo group; the magnitude of this difference was statistically significant but so small as to be of no clinical therapeutic relevance. In another

study, in which EPEC was the most commonly identified pathogen, no beneficial effect was demonstrated.[145]

Despite promising animal data,[146] the few studies using indomethacin as an antidiarrheal agent have either been poorly controlled[147] or have failed to demonstrate efficacy.[148] Nicotinic acid, given in a dosage of 500 mg every 6 hours for 1 day, significantly lowered purging rates in patients with cholera.[149] Flushing was a side effect. Until more safety and efficacy data are available, the use of aspirin, indomethacin, or nicotinic acid in the symptomatic treatment of diarrhea cannot be advocated.

Berberine, a plant alkaloid that has been used in China and India for millennia for the treatment of diarrhea, has been recommended for several decades as an adjunct to the therapy of cholera in the Indian subcontinent.[150] A controlled clinical trial demonstrated that berberine, given as a single 400-mg dose, significantly reduced the stool volume of ETEC diarrhea but was of little value, either alone or coadministered with tetracycline, in the treatment of cholera.[151]

Aciduric Bacteria

Normal intestinal flora can markedly inhibit certain pathogenic bacteria. This observation has renewed interest in the use of nonpathogenic flora to treat enteric infections. *Lactobacillus acidophilus* is inhibitory for many bacterial enteropathogens in vitro and in animal models and is commonly prescribed in the treatment of acute diarrhea. There is no evidence from controlled studies, however, that *Lactobacillus* preparations can prevent or alleviate infectious diarrheas.[152-154]

Other examples of bacteriotherapy include the use in uncontrolled studies of a particular strain of *Enterococcus faecium*, designated SF68, in children and adults with acute diarrhea[155, 156] and the rectal instillation of a mixture of 10 different bacteria, including three *Bacteroides* species in several patients with chronic relapsing *difficile*-associated diarrhea.[157] The mixture of 10 bacteria led to the recolonization by *Bacteroides*, which had been absent in all patients before treatment, and to the loss of *C. difficile*, and it was accompanied by cessation of the diarrhea.

Antimotility Agents

Opioids, including paregoric and codeine, have long been employed to relieve diarrhea and to reduce cramping. One of their most prominent effects is to decrease intestinal motility. Newer licensed antimotility agents include diphenoxylate and loperamide; these may also have antisecretory effects. The advisability of using antimotility agents is the subject of considerable debate among physicians experienced in the treatment of diarrheal disease. Some evidence from animal models and clinical studies suggests that antimotility agents may be contraindicated in patients with invasive bacterial infections such as shigellosis. For example, guinea pigs are normally quite resistant to *Shigella*, but if the guinea pigs are pretreated with paregoric, fatal enteritis follows oral inoculation with *Shigella*.[158] Moreover, volunteers experimentally challenged with pathogenic *Shigella* and then treated with diphenoxylate upon developing clinical illness exhibited increased fever and prolonged excretion of *Shigella* compared with infected volunteers who did not receive that antimotility agent. A recent report suggests that if loperamide is administered as a single dose in conjunction with a single dose of an effective antimicrobial such as TMP/SMZ in the treatment of acute traveler's diarrhea, it is superior to 3 days' therapy with the antimicrobial alone and to 3 days' therapy with loperamide alone in diminishing the duration of diarrhea.[159] Some of the patients who received combination therapy had *Shigella* infections, and their clinical response was not impaired. Notably, of 5 patients with *Shigella* infection who received loperamide alone in this randomized, blinded trial, 3 (60%) were deemed treatment failures and were administered effective antimicrobials.

The following recommendations appear to be both conservative and reasonable with respect to the use of antimotility agents in patients with diarrheal disease:

1. These drugs should not be used in the treatment of diarrheal disease in children or adults living in less developed countries, since in such areas invasive bacterial diarrheas are common, the monetary cost of therapy must be as economical as possible, and any diversion from an emphasis on oral rehydration is considered ill advised.

2. Loperamide, apparently the safest of the antimotility agents, may be used as an adjunct to therapy in adults or older children with diarrhea in industrialized countries if appropriate precautions are taken (e.g., exclusion of patients with frank dysentery and a stool examination to detect fecal leukocytes) to show that the diarrhea is not likely to be due to an invasive bacterial enteropathogen such as *Shigella*.

3. While some advocate the use of loperamide in adult travelers with mild to moderate watery diarrhea,[159, 160] we still prefer a conservative approach that refrains from the use of antimotility agents. If the practitioner elects to use loperamide in this situation, we advise that only 1 or 2 doses be administered, always in conjunction with effective antibiotics. If there is clinical evidence of dysentery, loperamide should be withheld.

Other Agents

Bismuth subsalicylate (BSS) has been widely studied as an antidiarrheal agent. It may function both as an adsorptive and as an antisecretory agent. Its effects are probably mediated by the aspirin component, although studies with ETEC-induced diarrhea suggest that the bismuth compound may act to inhibit intraluminal attachment and growth. Field studies in adults with traveler's diarrhea have shown that the liquid suspension of BSS provides moderate relief of symptoms[161, 162] and diminishes the number of stools by one half. Because of the inconvenient dosing regimen with the liquid formulation, BSS in tablet form has been studied. The BSS tablets reduce the occurrence of traveler's diarrhea when used in a prophylactic fashion for up to 3 weeks but have not been efficacious in relieving diarrhea once established.[163, 164] The salicylate component of BSS is readily absorbed, and serum levels in the range of 70 to 80 μg/ml have been recorded after multiple doses in adults. Therefore, patients taking aspirin, those with aspirin hypersensitivity or bleeding diathesis, and young children should avoid its use.

A CLINICAL APPROACH TO THE TREATMENT OF DIARRHEAL DISEASE

The therapeutic approach to be followed in an individual patient depends upon the clinical syndrome manifested by the patient, the causal agents deemed most likely to be responsible or actually demonstrated by laboratory tests, evidence of the existence of an effective specific therapy against the suspected agents, and the likelihood of complications. The likelihood that a particular agent is responsible for an individual case of diarrheal illness greatly depends on the age of the patient, the time of the year, and the epidemiologic history, covering factors such as industrialized versus less developed setting, community versus nosocomial infection, and whether the patient is a traveler.

When the clinician is confronted by a patient suffering from diarrheal disease, a series of therapeutic decisions arise that include an assessment of the patient's state of hydration and a determination of the appropriate fluid therapy to institute, if necessary. The indication for antimicrobial therapy depends on ascertaining the probable identity of the causative agent and on whether that pathogen is likely to respond to such therapy. It is helpful to categorize the patient's disease into one of the six clinical types shown in Table 21–2. The most frequent pathogens causing each of these types of diarrhea vary somewhat depending on the geographic setting.

Simple Diarrhea

The vast majority of patients present with simple diarrhea, characterized by watery stools without blood, low-grade fever, abdominal cramps, malaise, and occasionally vomiting. Viral pathogens are the most frequent causal agents of diarrhea in industrialized areas and clearly do not warrant antibiotics. The most important viruses include rotavirus, enteric adenovirus, and astroviruses in infants and toddlers, and Norwalk agent and related 27-nm gastroenteritis viruses in older children and adults. In developing countries, bacterial pathogens, including ETEC and EPEC, are more frequent offenders. Hence, adult travelers to such areas with moderate to severe watery diarrhea are likely to respond to early institution of ciprofloxacin, which is active against ETEC.

Dysentery

Dysentery refers to the occurrence of gross blood and mucus in diarrheal stools, often following a clinical onset that includes high fever, malaise, and some hours of watery diarrhea. In any setting, when a patient presents with dysentery, one must consider that an invasive bacterial pathogen such as *Shigella, C. jejuni*, EIEC, or *Y. enterocolitica* is responsible. In most geographic areas, *Shigella* is the most common causal agent of bacillary dysentery, and empiric therapy with ciprofloxacin or norfloxacin in adults and cotrimoxazole or nalidixic acid in children is generally indicated. In adults, the use of fluoroquinolones may also alleviate dysentery due to *C. jejuni*, since these antimicro-

bials are active against this pathogen. By contrast, in children, an age group for which use of the new generation of fluoroquinolones is contraindicated, early treatment of *C. jejuni* dysentery requires the administration of erythromycin.[79] In developing areas where *E. histolytica* is endemic, stool examination for ameba must determine whether antiprotozoal therapy is warranted.

Rice Water Stools

In situations in which cholera is endemic or epidemic, tetracycline therapy is warranted for patients who present with voluminous rice water purging. Appropriate antibiotics diminish by approximately 50% the total diarrheal stool volume, thereby diminishing the volume of intravenous and oral fluids that are required to rehydrate the patient. Fecal excretion is also rapidly curtailed by appropriate antibiotics. If tetracycline-resistant *V. cholerae* O1 strains are known to be prevalent, TMP/SMZ, erythromycin, and furazolidone are popular alternative antimicrobials that can be used.

Persistent Diarrhea

An episode of acute diarrheal illness that continues for more than 14 days is considered persistent diarrhea. Patients with persistent diarrhea may suffer profound nutritional losses. In less developed countries, approximately 5% of patients with diarrheal illness who present to health care facilities are suffering from the syndrome of persistent diarrhea. In infants in such areas, this carries a poor prognosis and is associated with high case fatality. Causal agents associated with persistent diarrhea include enteroaggregative *E. coli*, EPEC, and *Giardia*. A detailed microbiological workup for an infectious agent should always be undertaken in patients with persistent diarrhea.

Hemorrhagic Colitis

The syndrome of hemorrhagic colitis caused by EHEC is characterized by the passage of bloody liquid stools and can be distinguished from bacillary dysentery by the facts that the stools in hemorrhagic colitis tend to be more voluminous than the scanty stools of dysentery; few fecal leukocytes are seen in hemorrhagic colitis stools, whereas sheets of fecal leukocytes are seen in the mucus from dysenteric stools; and high fever is an unusual occurrence in hemorrhagic colitis, whereas a history of high fever is common in patients with bacillary dysentery.

There are no rigorous data to support a beneficial role for antimicrobials in the treatment of hemorrhagic colitis. Moreover, the use of antimicrobials is controversial in that some retrospective surveys suggest that such therapy may increase the likelihood of HUS as a complication.[92, 93]

Vomiting Syndrome

An acute, short-lived episode of vomiting, with no diarrhea or little diarrhea, is most often due to infection with Norwalk or Norwalk-like viruses or to ingestion of preformed enterotoxins such as staphyloccoal enterotoxin. Antimicrobials are not indicated in these instances. Occasionally, the syndrome of vomiting accompanied by little or no diarrhea is persistent. In this instance, one should investigate the possibility of duodenal or proximal jejunal infection due to *Giardia* or *S. stercoralis;* if these pathogens are identified, specific antimicrobial therapy should be instituted.

REFERENCES

1. Levine MM, Pizarro D. Advances in therapy of diarrheal dehydration: Oral rehydration. Adv Pediatr. 1984;31:207–234.
2. Santosham M, Daum RS, Dillman L, et al. Oral rehydration therapy of infantile diarrhea: A controlled study of well-nourished children hospitalized in the United States and Panama. N Engl J Med. 1982; 306:1070–1076.
3. Nalin DR, Levine MM, Mata L, et al. Oral rehydration and maintenance of children with rotavirus and bacterial diarrhoeas. Bull World Health Organ. 1979; 57:453–459.
4. Pizarro D, Posada G, Villavicencio N, et al. Oral rehydration in hypernatremic and hyponatremic diarrheal dehydration: Treatment with oral glucose/electrolyte solution. Am J Dis Child. 1983;137:730–734.
5. Pizarro D, Posada G, Levine MM. Hypernatremic diarrheal dehydration treated with "slow" (12 hour) oral rehydration therapy: A preliminary report. J Pediatr. 1984;104:316–319.
6. Schedl HP, Clifton JA. Solute and water absorption by human small intestine. Nature. 1963;199:1264.
7. World Health Organization. The Treatment and Prevention of Acute Diarrhoea: Practical Guidelines. 2nd ed. Geneva: World Health Organization; 1989:39.
8. Ahmed SM, Islam MR, Butler T. Effective treatment of diarrhoeal dehydration with an oral rehydration solution containing citrate. Scand J Infect Dis. 1986;18:65–70.
9. Sack DA, Islam S, Brown KH, et al. Oral therapy in children with cholera: A comparison of sucrose and glucose electrolyte solutions. J Pediatr. 1980;96:20–25.
10. Nalin DR, Harland E, Ramlal A, et al. Comparison of low and high sodium and potassium content in oral rehydration solutions. J Pediatr. 1980;97:848–853.
11. Cutting WAM, Belton NR, Gray JA, et al. Safety and efficacy of three oral rehydration solutions for children with diarrhoea (Edinburgh 1984–1985). Acta Paediatr Scand. 1989;78:253–258.
12. Nichols B, Soriano HA. A critique of oral therapy of dehydration due to diarrhoeal syndromes. Am J Clin Nutr 1977;30:1457–1472.
13. Schultz SG. Sodium-coupled solute transport by small intestine: A status report. Am J Physiol. 1977;233:249–254.
14. Matthews DM. Intestinal absorption of peptides. Physiol Rev. 1975;55:537–608.
15. Nalin DR, Cash RA, Rahman M, et al. Effect of glycine and glucose on sodium and water absorption in patients with cholera. Gut. 1970;11:768–772.
16. Patra FC, Sack DA, Islam A, et al. Oral rehydration formula containing alanine and glucose for treatment of diarrhoea: A controlled trial. Br Med J. 1989; 298:1353–1356.
17. Santosham M, Burns BA, Reid R, et al. Glycine based oral rehydration solution: Reassessment of safety and efficacy. J Pediatr. 1986;109:795–801.
18. Pizarro D, Levine MM, Posada G, et al. Comparison of glucose/electrolyte and glucose/glycine/electrolyte oral rehydration solutions in hospitalized children with diarrhea in Costa Rica. J Pediatr Gastroenterol Nutr. 1988;7:411–416.
19. Vesikari T, Isolauri E. Glycine-supplemented oral rehydration solutions for diarrhoea. Arch Dis Child. 1986; 61:372–376.
20. Bhan MK, Sazawal S, Bhatnagar S, et al. Glycine, glycylglycine and malodextrin-based oral rehydration solution. Acta Paediatr Scand. 1990;79:518–526.
21. Patra FC, Mahalanabis D, Jalan KN, et al. Is oral rice electrolyte solution superior to glucose electrolyte solution in infantile diarrhoea? Arch Dis Child. 1982; 57:910–912.
22. Mahalanabis D, Patra FC. In search of a super oral rehydration solution: Can optimum use of organic solute-mediated sodium absorption lead to the development of an absorption-promoting drug? J Diarrhoeal Dis Res. 1983;1:76–81.
23. Molla AM, Ahmed SM, Greenough WB. Rice-based oral rehydration solution decreases the stool volume in acute diarrhoea, Bull World Health Organ. 1985; 63:751–756.
24. Molla AM, Molla A, Rohde J, et al. Turning off the diarrhea: The role of food and ORS. J Pediatr Gastroenterol Nutr. 1989;8:81–84.
25. Molla AM, Sarker SA, Hossain M, et al. Rice-powder electrolyte solution as oral therapy in diarrhoea due to *Vibrio cholerae* and *Escherichia coli*. Lancet. 1982;i:1317–1319.
26. El-Mougi M, Hegazi E, Gala O, et al. Controlled clinical trial on the efficacy of rice powder–based oral rehydration solution on the outcome of acute diarrhea in infants. J Pediatr Gastroenterol Nutr. 1988;7:572–576.
27. Pizarro D, Posada G, Sandi L, et al. Rice-based oral electrolyte solutions for the management of infantile diarrhea. N Engl J Med. 1991;324:517–521.
28. Khin-Maung U, Greenough WB III. Cereal-based oral rehydration therapy. I. Clinical studies. J Pediatr. 1991;118:S72–S79.
29. Mohan M, Sethi JS, Daral TS, et al. Controlled trial of rice powder and glucose rehydration solutions as oral therapy for acute dehydrating diarrhea in infants. J Pediatr Gastroenterol Nutr. 1986;5:423–427.

30. Chung AW, Viscorova B. The effect of oral feeding versus early starvation on the course of infantile diarrhoea. J Pediatr. 1948;33:14–22.

31. Torres-Pinedo R, Lavastida M, Rivera CI. A comparison of the effects of milk feeding and intravenous therapy upon the composition and volume of the stool and urine. J Clin Invest. 1966;45:469–480.

32. Brown KH, MacLean WC Jr. Nutritional management of acute diarrhea: An appraisal of the alternatives. Pediatrics. 1984;73:119–125.

33. Levine MM. Antimicrobial therapy for infectious diarrhea. Rev Infect Dis. 1986;8(suppl):S207–S216.

34. Nelson JD, Haltalin KC. Comparative efficacy of cephalexin and ampicillin for shigellosis and other types of acute diarrhea in infants and children. Antimicrob Agents Chemother. 1975;7:415–420.

35. Ostrower VG. Comparison of cefaclor and ampicillin in the treatment of shigellosis. Postgrad Med J. 1979; 55(suppl):82–84.

36. Nelson JD, Haltalin KC. Amoxicillin less effective than ampicillin against Shigella in vitro and in vivo: Relationship of efficacy to activity in serum. J Infect Dis. 1974;129(suppl):S222–227.

37. Tong MJ, Martin DG, Cunnugham JJ, et al. Clinical and bacteriological evaluation of antibiotic treatment in shigellosis. JAMA. 1970;214:1841–1844.

38. Chang MJ, Dunkie LM, Reken DV, et al. Trimethoprim/sulfamethoxazole compared to ampicillin in the treatment of shigellosis. Pediatrics. 1977;59:726–729.

39. Lexomboon U, Mansuwan P, Duangmani C, et al. Clinical evaluation of co-trimoxazole and furazolidone in the treatment of shigellosis in children. Br Med J. 1972;3:23–26.

40. Nelson JD, Kusmiesz H, Jackson LH. Comparison of trimethoprim-sulfamethoxazole and ampicillin therapy for shigellosis in ambulatory patients. J Pediatr. 1976; 89:491–493.

41. Nelson JD, Kusmiesz H, Jackson LH, et al. Trimethoprim-sulfamethoxazole therapy for shigellosis. JAMA. 1976;235:1239–1243.

42. Salam MA, Bennish ML. Therapy for shigellosis: I, Randomized, double-blind trial of nalidixic acid in childhood shigellosis. J Pediatr. 1988;113:901–907.

43. Griffin PM, Tauxe RV, Redd SC, et al. Emergence of highly trimethoprim-sulfamethoxazole–resistant Shigella in a native American population: An epidemiologic study. Am J Epidemiol. 1989;129:1042–1051.

44. Centers for Disease Control. Nationwide dissemination of multiple resistant Shigella sonnei following a common source outbreak. MMWR Morb Mortal Wkly Rep. 1987;36:633–634.

45. Taylor DE, Keystone JS, Devlin HR. Resistance to trimethoprim and other antibiotics in Ontario Shigellae. Lancet. 1980;i:425–426.

46. Tiemens KM, Shipley PL, Correia RA, et al. Sulfamethoxazole-trimethoprim–resistant Shigella flexneri in northeastern Brazil. Antimicrob Agents Chemother. 1984;25:653–654.

47. Frost JA, Willshaw GA, Barclay EA, et al. Plasmid characterization of drug-resistant Shigella dysenteriae 1 from an epidemic in central Africa. J Hyg Camb. 1985; 94:163–172.

48. Munshi MH, Sack DA, Haider K, et al. Plasmid-mediated resistance to nalidixic acid in Shigella dysenteriae type 1. Lancet. 1987;2:419–421.

49. Lionel NDW, Abeyasekera FJB, Samarasinghe HG, et al. A comparison of a single dose and a five day course of tetracycline therapy in bacillary dysentery. J Trop Med Hyg. 1969;72:170–172.

50. Pickering LK, DuPont HL, Olarte J. Single-dose tetracycline therapy for shigellosis in adults. JAMA. 1978; 239:853–854.

51. Stoker DJ. Treatment of bacillary dysentery with special reference to stosstherapy. Br Med J. 1962;1:1179–1181.

52. Haltalin KC, Kusmiesz HT, Hinton LV, et al. Treatment of acute diarrhea in outpatients: Double-blind study comparing ampicillin and placebo. Am J Dis Child. 1972;124:554–561.

53. Haltalin KC, Nelson JD, Ring R III, et al. Double-blind treatment study of shigellosis comparing ampicillin, sulfadiazine, and placebo. J Pediatr. 1967;70:970–981.

54. Gilman RH, Spira W, Rabbani H, et al. Single-dose ampicillin therapy for severe shigellosis in Bangladesh. J Infect Dis. 1981;143:164–169.

55. Haltalin KC, Nelson JD, Kusmiesz HT. Comparative efficacy of nalidixic acid and ampicillin for severe shigellosis. Arch Dis Child. 1973;8:305–312.

56. Goossens H, Mol PD, Coignau J, et al. Comparative in vitro activities of aztreonam, ciprofloxacin, norfloxacin, ofloxacin, HR 810 (a new cephalosporin), RU28965 (a new macrolide), and other agents against enteropathogens. Antimicrob Agents Chemother. 1985;27:388–392.

57. Bergan T, Lolekha S, Cheong MK, et al. Effect of recent antibacterial agents against bacteria causing diarrhoea. Scand J Infect Dis. 1988;56(suppl):7–10.

58. Lolekha S, Patanacharoen S, Thanangkul B, et al. Norfloxacin versus co-trimoxazole in the treatment of acute bacterial diarrhoea: A placebo controlled study. Scand J Infect Dis. 1988;56(suppl):35–45.

59. Bennish ML, Salam MA, Haider R, et al. Therapy for shigellosis. II, Randomized, double-blind comparison of ciprofloxacin and ampicillin. J Infect Dis. 1990; 162:711–716.

60. Gotuzzo E, Oberhelman RA, Maguina C, et al. Comparison of single-dose treatment with norfloxacin and standard 5-day treatment with trimethoprim-sulfamethoxazole for acute shigellosis in adults. Antimicrob Agents Chemother. 1989;33:1101–1104.

61. Ericsson CD, Johnson PC, DuPont HL, et al. Ciprofloxacin or trimethoprim-sulfamethoxazole as initial therapy for travellers' diarrhea. Ann Intern Med. 1987; 106:216–220.

62. Schluter G. Ciprofloxacin: Review of potential toxicologic effects. Am J Med. 1987;82(suppl 4A)91–93.

63. Alfaham M, Holt ME, Goodchild MC. Arthropathy in a patient with cystic fibrosis taking ciprofloxacin. Br Med J. 1987;295:699.

64. Fontaine O. Antibiotics in the management of shigellosis in children: What role for the quinolones? Rev Infect Dis. 1989;11:(suppl 5):S1145–S1150.

65. MacDonald WB, Friday F, McEacharn M. The effect of chloramphenicol on Salmonella enteritis of infancy. Arch Dis Child. 1954;29:238–241.

66. Association for the Study of Infectious Disease. Effect of neomycin in non-invasive Salmonella infections of the gastrointestinal tract. Lancet. 1970;2:1159–1161.

67. Kazemi M, Gumpert TG, Marks MI. A controlled trial comparing sulfamethoxazole-trimethoprim, ampicillin, and no therapy in the treatment of Salmonella gastroenteritis in children. J Pediatr. 1973;83:646–650.

68. de Olarte DG, Trujillo H, Agudelo N, et al. Treatment of diarrhea in malnourished infants and children: A double-blind study comparing ampicillin and placebo. Am J Dis Child. 1974;127:379–388.

69. Nelson JD, Kusmiesz H, Jackson LH, et al. Treatment of Salmonella gastroenteritis with ampicillin, amoxicillin, or placebo. Pediatrics. 1980;65:1125–1130.

70. Pichler HET, Divide G, Stickler K, et al. Clinical efficacy of ciprofloxacin compared with placebo in bacterial diarrhea. Am J Med. 1987;82(suppl 4A):329–332.

71. Neill MA, Opal SM, Heelan J, et al. Failure to eradicate convalescent fecal excretion after acute salmonellosis:

Experience during an outbreak in health care workers. Ann Int Med. 1991;114:195–199.

72. Torrey S, Fleisher G, Jaffe D. Incidence of *Salmonella* bacteremia in infants with *Salmonella* gastroenteritis. J Pediatr. 1986;108:718–721.

73. Vichinsky EP, Lubin BH. Sickle cell anemia and related hemoglobinopathies. Pediatr Clin North Am. 1980; 27:429–447.

74. Report of the Committee on Infectious Diseases. 21st ed. Elk Grove Village IL: American Academy of Pediatrics; 1989:372.

75. Pitkanen T, Petterson T, Ponka A. Effect of erythromycin on the fecal excretion of *Campylobacter fetus* subspecies *jejuni*. J Infect Dis. 1982;145:128.

76. Anders BJ, Lauer BA, Paisley JW, et al. Double-blind placebo controlled trial of erythromycin for treatment of *Campylobacter* enteritis. Lancet. 1982;1:131–132.

77. Pai CH, Gillis F, Tuomanen E, et al. Erythromycin in treatment of *Campylobacter* enteritis in children. Am J Dis Child. 1983;137:286–288.

78. Williams D, Schorling J, Barrett, et al. Early treatment of *Campylobacter jejuni* enteritis. Antimicrob Agents Chemother. 1989;33:248–250.

79. Salazar-Lindo E, Sack RB, Chea-Woo E, et al. Early treatment with erythromycin of *Campylobacter jejuni*–associated dysentery in children. J Pediatr. 1986;109:355–360.

80. Taylor DN, Blaser MJ, Echeverria P, et al. Erythromycin-resistant *Campylobacter* infections in Thailand. Antimicrob Agents Chemother. 1987;31:438–442.

81. Goodman LJ, Trenholme GM, Kaplan RL, et al. Empiric antimicrobial therapy of domestically acquired acute diarrhea in urban adults. Arch Intern Med. 1990;150:541–546.

82. Merson MH, Sack RB, Islam S, et al. Disease due to enterotoxigenic *Escherichia coli* in Bangladeshi adults: Clinical aspects and a controlled trial of tetracycline. J Infect Dis. 1980;141:702–710.

83. Black RE, Levine MM, Clements ML, et al. Treatment of experimentally induced enterotoxigenic *Escherichia coli* diarrhea with trimethoprim, trimethoprim-sulfamethoxazole, or placebo. Rev Infect Dis. 1982;4:540–545.

84. DuPont HL, Reves RR, Galindo E, et al. Treatment of traveller's diarrhea with trimethoprim/sulfamethoxazole and with trimethoprim alone. N Engl J Med. 1982;307:841–844.

85. Oberhelman RA, de la Cabada J, Garibay EV, et al. Efficacy of trimethoprim-sulfamethoxazole in treatment of acute diarrhea in a Mexican pediatric population. J Pediatr. 1987;110:960–965.

86. Echeverria P, Verhaert L, Ulyangco CV, et al. Antimicrobial resistance and enterotoxin production among isolates of *Escherichia coli* in the Far East. Lancet. 1978;2:589–592.

87. Sack RB, Santosham M, Froehlich JL, et al. Doxycycline prophylaxis of traveler's diarrhea in Honduras, an area where resistance to doxycycline is common among enterotoxigenic *Escherichia coli*. Am J Trop Med Hyg. 1984;33:460–466.

88. Nelson JD. Duration of neomycin therapy for enteropathogenic *Escherichia coli* diarrheal disease: A comparative study of 113 cases. Pediatrics. 1971;48:248–258.

89. Thoren A, Wolde-Mariam T, Stintzing G, et al. Antibiotics in the treatment of gastroenteritis caused by enteropathogenic *Escherichia coli*. J Infect Dis. 1980; 141:27–31.

90. Marier R, Wells JG, Swanson RC. An outbreak of enteropathogenic *Escherichia coli* foodborne disease traced to imported French cheese. Lancet. 1973;2:1376–1378.

91. Snyder JD, Wells JG, Yashuk Y, et al. Outbreak of invasive *Escherichia coli* gastroenteritis on a cuise ship. Am J Trop Med Hyg. 1984;33:281–284.

92. Ostroff SM, Kobayashi JM, Lewis JH. Infections with *Escherichia coli* 0157:H7 in Washington State: The first year of statewide disease surveillance. JAMA. 1989; 262:355–359.

93. Pavia AT, Nichols CR, Green DP, et al. Hemolytic-uremic syndrome during an outbreak of *Escherichia coli* 0157:H7 infections in institutions for mentally-retarded persons. J Pediatr. 1990;116:544–551.

94. Karch H, Strockbine NA, O'Brien AD, et al. Growth of *Escherichia coli* in the presence of trimethoprim-sulfamethoxazole facilitates detection of Shiga-like toxin producing strains by colony blot assay. FEMS Microbiol Lett. 1986;35:141–145.

95. Ostroff SM, Kobayashi JM, Lewis JH. Infections with *Escherichia coli* 157:H7 in Washington State: The first year of statewide disease surveillance. JAMA. 1989; 262:355–359.

96. Hoogkamp-Korstanje JA. Antibiotics in *Yersinia enterocolitica* infections. J Antimicrob Chemother. 1987; 20:123–131.

97. Pai CH, Gillis F, Tuomanen E, et al. Placebo-controlled double-blind evaluation of trimethoprim-sulfamethoxazole treatment of *Yersinia enterocolitica* gastroenteritis. J Pediatr. 1984;104:308–311.

98. Lindenbaum J, Greenough WB, Islam MR. Antibiotic therapy of cholera in children. Bull World Health Organ. 1967;37:529–538.

99. Wallace CK, Anderson PN, Brown TC, et al. Optimal antibiotic therapy in cholera. Bull World Health Organ. 1968;39:239–245.

100. Pierce NF, Banwell JG, Mitra RC, et al. Controlled comparison of tetracycline and furazolidone in cholera. Br Med J. 1968;3:277–280.

101. Burans JP, Podgore J, Mansour MM, et al. Comparative trial of erythromycin and sulphatrimethoprim in the treatment of tetracycline-resistant *Vibrio cholerae* 01. Trans R Soc Trop Med Hyg. 1989;83:836–838.

102. Pastore G, Rizzo G, Fera G, et al. Trimethoprim-sulfamethoxazole in the treatment of cholera. Chemotherapy. 1977;23:121–128.

103. Fekety R, Silva J, Armstrong J, et al. Treatment of antibiotic-associated enterocolitis with vancomycin. Rev Infect Dis. 1981;3(Suppl):S273–S281.

104. Tedesco F, Markham R, Gurwith M, et al. Oral vancomycin for antibiotic-associated pseudomembranous colitis. Lancet. 1978;2:226–228.

105. Keighley MRB, Burdon DW, Arabi Y, et al. Randomised controlled trial of vancomycin for pseudomembranous colitis and postoperative diarrhoea. Br Med J. 1978; 2:1667–1669.

106. Silva J Jr, Batts DH, Fekety R, et al. Treatment of *Clostridium difficile* colitis and diarrhea with vancomycin. Am J Med. 1981;71:815–822.

107. Bartlett JG. Treatment of antibiotic-associated pseudomembranous colitis. Rev Infect Dis. 1984;6(suppl 1): S235–S241.

108. Fekety R, Silva J, Kuffman C, et al. Treatment of antibiotic-associated *Clostridium difficile* colitis with oral vancomycin: Comparison of two dosage regimens. Am J Med. 1989;86:15–19.

109. Cherry RD, Portnoy D, Jabbari M, et al. Metronidazole: An alternative therapy for antibiotic-associated colitis. Gastroenterology. 1982;82:849–851.

110. Teasley DG, Gerding DN, Olson MM, et al. Prospective randomised trial of metronidazole versus vancomycin for *Clostridium difficile*–associated diarrhoea and colitis. Lancet. 1983;2:1043–1046.

111. Bolton RP, Culshaw MA. Faecal metronidazole concentrations during oral and intravenous therapy for anti-

biotic-associated colitis due to *Clostridium difficile*. Gut. 1986;27:1169–1172.

112. Young GP, Ward OB, Bayley N, et al. Antibiotic-associated colitis due to *Clostridium difficile:* Double-blind comparison of vancomycin with bacitracin. Gastroenterology. 1985;89:1038–1045.

113. Dudley MN, McLaughlin JC, Carrington G, et al. Oral bacitracin vs vancomycin therapy for *Clostridium difficile*-induced diarrhea: A randomized double-blind trial. Arch Intern Med. 1986;146:1101–1104.

114. De Lalla F, Privitera G, Rinaldi E, et al. Treatment of *Clostridium difficile*-associated disease with teicoplanin. Antimicrob Agents Chemother. 1989;33:1125–1127.

115. Oliva SL, Guglielmo BJ, Jacobs R, et al. Failure of intravenous vancomycin and intravenous metronidazole to prevent or treat antibiotic-associated pseudomembranous colitis. J Infect Dis. 1989;159:1154–1155.

116. Ravdin J. Intestinal disease caused by *Entamoeba histolytica*. In: Ravdin J. Amebiasis: Human Infection by *Entamoeba histolytica*. New York: John Wiley & Sons; 1988:495–510.

117. Tanowitz HB, Weiss LM, Wittner M. Diagnosis and treatment of protozoan diarrheas. Am J Gastroenterol. 1988;83:339–350.

118. Misra NP. A comparative study of tinidazole and metronidazole as a single daily dose for three days in symptomatic intestinal amoebiasis. Drugs. 1978; 15(suppl 1):19–22.

119. Islam N, Hasan K. Tinidazole and metronidazole in hepatic amoebiasis. Drugs. 1978;15(suppl 1):26–29.

120. Levi GC, Armando de Avila C, Neto VA. Efficacy of various drugs for treatment of giardiasis. Am J Trop Med Hyg. 1977;26:564–565.

121. Davidson RA. Issues in clinical parasitology: The treatment of giardiasis. Am J Gastroenterol. 1984;79:256–261.

122. Kavousi S. Giardiasis in infancy and childhood: A prospective study of 160 cases with comparison of quinacrine (Atabrine) and metronidazole (Flagyl). Am J Trop Med Hyg. 1979;28:19–23.

123. Gazder AJ, Banerjee M. Single dose therapy of giardiasis with tinidazole and metronidazole. Drugs. 1978; 15(suppl 1):30–32.

124. Portnoy D, Whiteside ME, Buckley E, et al. Treatment of intestinal cryptosporidiosis with spiramycin. Ann Intern Med. 1984;101:202–204.

125. Collier AC, Miller RA, Meyers JD. *Cryptosporidium* after marrow transplantation: Person-to-person transmission and treatment with spiramycin. Ann Intern Med. 1984; 101:205–206.

126. Bannister P, Mountford RA. *Cryptosporidium* in the elderly: A cause of life-threatening diarrhea. Am J Med. 1989;86:507–508.

127. Wittenberg DF, Miller NM, van den Ende J. Spiramycin is not effective in treating *Cryptosporidium* diarrhea in infants: Results of a double-blind randomized trial. J Infect Dis. 1989;159:131–132.

128. Saez-Llorens X, Odio CM, Umana MA, et al. Spiramycin vs. placebo for treatment of acute diarrhea caused by *Cryptosporidium*. Pediatr Infect Dis J. 1989;8:136–140.

129. Grove DI. Treatment of strongyloidiasis with thiabendazole: An analysis of toxicity and effectiveness. Trans R Soc Trop Med Hyg. 1982;76:114–118.

130. Portnoy BL, DuPont HL, Pruitt D, et al. Antidiarrheal agents in the treatment of acute diarrhea in children. JAMA. 1976;236:844–846.

131. Dukes GE. Over-the-counter antidiarrheal medications used for the self-treatment of acute nonspecific diarrhea. Am J Med. 1990;88(suppl 6A):24S–26S.

132. Rutledge ML, Wilner MM, King JT. Calcium polycarbophil in acute childhood diarrhea. Clin Pediatr. 1963;2:61–63.

133. LaCorte WSJ, Chapman J, Gotzowsky S, et al. A rapid new double-blind method for evaluating antidiarrheal agents. Clin Pharmaol Ther. 1980;27:263–264.

134. Isolauri E, Vesikari T. Oral rehydration, rapid feeding, and cholestyramine for treatment of acute diarrhea. J Pediatr Gastroenterol Nutr. 1985;4:366–374.

135. McCloy RM, Hoffman AF. Tropical diarrhea in Vietnam: A controlled study of cholestyramine therapy. N Engl J Med. 1971;284:139–140.

136. Berant M, Wagner Y, Cohen N. Cholestyramine in the management of infantile diarrhea. J Pediatr. 1976; 88:153–154.

137. Kreutzer EW, Milligan FD. Treatment of antibiotic-associated pseudomembranous colitis with cholestyramine resin. Johns Hopkins Med J. 1978;143:67–72.

138. Bowie MD, Mann MD, Hill ID. The bowel cocktail. Pediatrics. 1981;67:920.

139. Hill ID, Mann MD, Househam KC, Bowie MD. Use of oral gentamicin, metronidazole, and cholestyramine in the treatment of severe persistent diarrhea in infants. Pediatrics. 1986;77:477–481.

140. Pruksananonda P, Powell KR. Multiple relapses of *Clostridium difficile*-associated diarrhea responding to an extended course of cholestyramine. Pediatr Infect Dis J. 1989;8:175–178.

141. Lonnroth I, Holmgren J, Lange S. Chlorpromazine inhibits cholera toxin induced intestinal hypersecretion. Med Biol. 1977;55:126–129.

142. Rabbani GH, Greenough WB, Holmgren J, et al. Controlled trial of chlorpromazine as antisecretory agent in patients with cholera hydrated intravenously. Br Med J. 1982;284:1361–1364.

143. Burke V, Gracey M, Suharyono, Sunoto. Reduction by aspirin of intestinal fluid-loss in acute childhood gastroenteritis. Lancet. 1980;1:1329–1330.

144. Gracey M, Phadke MA, Burke V, et al. Aspirin in acute gastroenteritis: A clinical and microbiological study. J Pediatr Gastroenterol Nutr. 1984;3:692–695.

145. Mohan M, Daral TS, Singh JP, et al. Aspirin in childhood gastroenteritis. J Diarrhoeal Dis Res. 1985;3:215–218.

146. Wald A, Gotterer GS, Rajendra GR, et al. Effect of indomethacin on cholera-induced fluid movement, unidirectional sodium fluxes, and intestinal cAMP. Gastroenterology. 1977;72:106–110.

147. Neumann SZ. Childhood diarrhoea and its treatment with indomethacin in Libya. Trop Doct. 1980;10:24–28.

148. Rabbani GH, Butler T. Indomethacin and chloroquine fail to inhibit fluid loss in cholera. Gastroenterology. 1985;89:1035–1037.

149. Rabbani GH, Butler T, Bardhan PK, et al. Reduction of fluid-loss in cholera by nicotinic acid: A randomised controlled trial. Lancet. 1983;2:1439–1442.

150. Lahiri SC, Dutta NK. Berberine and chloramphenicol in the treatment of cholera and severe diarrhoea. J Ind Med Assoc. 1967;48:1–11.

151. Rabbani GH, Butler T, Knight J, et al. Randomized controlled trial of berberine sulfate therapy for diarrhea due to enterotoxigenic *Escherichia coli* and *Vibrio cholerae*. J Infect Dis. 1987;155:979–984.

152. Pozo-Olano JD, Warram JH Jr, Gomez RG, et al. Effect of lactobacilli preparation on traveler's diarrhea: A randomized double blind clinical trial. Gastroenterology. 1978;74:829–830.

153. Zoppi G, Balsamo V, Deganello A, et al. Oral bacteriotherapy in clinical practice: II. The use of different preparations in the treatment of acute diarrhoea. Eur J Pediatr. 1982;139:22–24.

154. Clements ML, Levine MM, Black RE, et al. Lactobacillus prophylaxis for diarrhea due to enterotoxigenic

Escherichia coli. Antimicrob Agents Chemother. 1981; 20:104–108.

155. Bellomo G, Mangiagle A, Nicastro L, et al. A controlled double-blind study of SF68 strain as a new biological preparation for the treatment of diarrhoea in pediatrics. Curr Therap Res. 1980;28:927–936.

156. Camarri E, Belvisi A, Guidoni G, et al. A double-blind comparison of two different treatments for acute enteritis in adults. Chemotherapy. 1981;27:466–470.

157. Tvede M, Rask-Madsen J. Bacteriotherapy for chronic relapsing *Clostridium difficile* diarrhoea in six patients. Lancet. 1989;1:1156–1160.

158. Formal SB, Abrams GD, Schneider H, et al. Experimental *Shigella* infections: VI, Role of the small intestine in an experimental infection in guinea pigs. J Bacteriol. 1963;85:119–125.

159. Ericsson CD, DuPont HL, Mathewson JJ, et al. Treatment of traveler's diarrhea with sulfamethoxazole and trimethoprim and loperamide. JAMA. 1990;263:257–261.

160. Van Loon FPL, Bennish M, Speelman P, et al. Double-blind trial of loperamide for treating acute watery diarrhoea in expatriates in Bangladesh. Gut. 1989;30:492–495.

161. DuPont HL, Sullivan P, Pickering LK, et al. Symptomatic treatment of diarrhea with bismuth subsalicylate among students attending a Mexican university. Gastroenterology. 1977;73:715–718.

162. Steffen R, Mathewson JJ, Ericsson CD, et al. Travelers' diarrhea in West Africa and Mexico: Fecal transport systems and liquid bismuth subsalicylate for self-therapy. J Infect Dis 1988;157:1008–1013.

163. Graham DY, Estes MK, Gentry LO. Double-blind comparison of bismuth subsalicylate and placebo in the prevention and treatment of enterotoxigenic *Escherichia coli*–induced diarrhea in volunteers. Gastroenterology. 1983;85:1017–1022.

164. DuPont HL, Ericsson CD, Johnson PC, et al. Prevention of travelers' diarrhea by the tablet formulation of bismuth subsalicylate. JAMA. 1987;257:1347–1350.

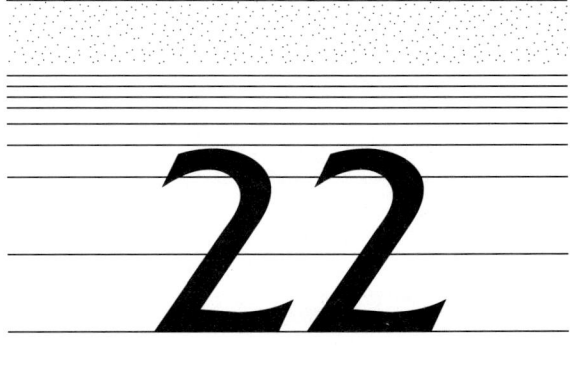

Diarrhea in Infants and Children

MELVIN B. HEYMAN, M.D., M.P.H.
ABIODUN O. JOHNSON, M.D., F.R.C.P.
JOHN D. SNYDER, M.D.

Diarrheal diseases are major causes of morbidity and mortality worldwide, with attack rates of 2 to 12 or more per person per year.[1, 2] Infants and young children in developing countries are particularly susceptible to infectious diarrhea because of poor standards of sanitation and hygiene as well as a high prevalence of malnutrition. It is estimated that children in these countries have approximately 1 billion episodes of acute diarrhea per year, resulting in 5 million deaths.[3] The magnitude and severity of diarrheal disease are less in developed countries, but costly hospital admissions are still frequent, with an estimated 13.8 per 1000 infants in the United States in 1984,[4] and diarrheal illness accounts for about 400 infant deaths in the United States each year.[5, 6] The current rates of diarrheal illness in developing countries are similar to those in the United States at the turn of the twentieth century.[7] The mortality in infants hospitalized with diarrhea in many other industrialized countries remains significant.[8]

The definition of diarrhea varies by culture and convention. Diarrhea is generally defined as an increased frequency and altered form of stool.[6] What is normal varies with each individual and is often diet-related. Infants with diarrhea often have more than 20 g stool/kg of body weight per day.

EPIDEMIOLOGY

Acute diarrheal illnesses are very common worldwide and are second only to acute upper respiratory tract illnesses as causes of childhood morbidity and mortality.[1] Attack rates in developing countries range from 2 to 12 episodes per child per year, with peak attack rates occurring in the first 2 years of life.[1, 2, 9, 10] Community-based studies in industrialized countries reveal about 1.5 episodes of diarrhea per person per year, with slightly higher attack rates in young schoolchildren and preschool siblings of schoolchildren.[1] In the United States, acute diarrheal illnesses account for 7% of all ambulatory clinic visits and 7 to 8% of all inpatient hospitalizations in children younger than 15 years.[11] The two sexes are equally affected.

Breast-feeding is associated with decreased morbidity from diarrheal disease, perhaps due to the reduced exposure to external pathogens and to the anti-infective agents in breast milk.[12-14] Increased prevalence of diarrheal disease is often observed when young children are placed in group settings, such as in daycare centers.[15, 16]

In industrialized countries, diarrheal illnesses are more frequent during the cold months, when viral causes are most common.[17, 18] The hot climate of many developing countries is associated with more bacterial enteric pathogens. The incidence of diarrheal illness caused by bacterial organisms is extremely variable and may be as high as 45% of episodes in some developing countries compared with approximately 15% in developed countries.[9, 19, 20] Although most bacterial infections occur during the summer, *Yersinia* infections appear to be more common in the winter.[21] *Vibrio cholerae* and enterotoxigenic *Escherichia coli* (ETEC) account for more illness in developing countries, whereas *Campylobacter jejuni* is the most common bacterial agent of acute diarrhea in the United States and the United Kingdom.[22-24] Most organisms that cause infectious diarrhea are spread by the fecal-oral route. Organisms with low infectivity, however, such as *Shigella* species, *Giardia lamblia*, and possibly *Campylobacter* species and *Cryptosporidium*, are spread by direct contact found, for example, in daycare centers.

The causal agent and severity of infectious diarrhea are often related to age, geographical location, social circumstances, lifestyle habits, associated medical conditions, and use of antibiotics. Thus, although enteropathogenic *E. coli* (EPEC) is an important pathogen in nurseries, rotavirus, a common cause of winter diarrhea in children younger than 2 years,[17, 25] is frequently found in the stools of healthy neonates in whom it usually causes only a silent or mild infection.[21] Nevertheless, rotavirus-associated hemorrhagic gastroenteritis and necrotizing enterocolitis have also been reported in the neonate.[26] Bacterial pathogens are relatively uncommon but can cause severe disease in this age group.[27, 28] Rotaviral diarrhea is most commonly seen in infants, while *G. lamblia*, *Shigella*, *Yersinia*, and *Campylobacter* are common enteropathogens in the 13 to 36-month toddler age group.[29, 30] *Yersinia* also causes acute watery diarrhea in children younger than 5 years. In school-aged children and adolescents, infection with *Yersinia* is more likely to present as pseudoappendicitis or mesenteric adenitis.[31] The increase in *Salmonella enteritidis* diarrhea during the 1980s in the United States has been linked to the consumption of undercooked eggs.[32] Close person-to-person contact, such as in institutions or daycare centers, facilitates the spread of infections with enteropathogens such as rotavirus, *Salmonella*,

Shigella, *G. lamblia*, *Campylobacter*, *Clostridium difficile*, and *Cryptosporidium*.[8, 15]

Other special situations in which diarrhea is increasingly recognized include nosocomial or hospital-acquired diarrhea and diarrhea in immunocompromised patients, including those with the acquired immunodeficiency syndrome (AIDS).[1]

ETIOLOGY

Acute diarrhea is often caused by enteric pathogens, including bacterial, viral, and parasitic agents (Table 22–1). The leading bacterial cause of acute infectious noninflammatory diarrhea in children worldwide is ETEC.[21] It is also the major cause of traveler's diarrhea in North Americans, with attack rates estimated to be 20 to 60% of travelers to endemic areas.[33, 34] In infants, EPEC is an important cause of diarrhea in the tropics,[35] while *Escherichia coli* are uncommon pathogens in the United States except enterohemorrhagic (EHEC) 0157:H7. This serotype is associated with nonbloody diarrhea, hemorrhagic colitis, and the hemolytic-uremic

TABLE 22–1. INFECTIOUS CAUSES OF ACUTE DIARRHEA

ORGANISM	% OF PATIENTS WITH DIARRHEA INFECTED WITH INDICATED ORGANISM	
	DEVELOPED AREAS	DEVELOPING AREAS
Viruses		
Enteric adenoviruses	2 (<2 y)	5–10 (<4 y)
Norwalk-like virus	10–27	1–2
Rotaviruses*	8–50	5–45
Bacteria		
Campylobacter spp.	1.0–1.7	2–14
Enteropathogenic *E. coli*	<5	4–8
Enterotoxigenic *E. coli*	1–7 (16)†	7–50
Salmonella	2–4	0–15
Shigella	1–25 (39)†	5–16
Aeromonas spp., *Bacillus fragilis*, *Clostridium difficile*, *Vibrio* spp., *Yersinia* spp.	1–3	1–6
Parasites		
Cryptosporidium parvum	2.8–4.1	4–11
Entamoeba histolytica	0.6	2–15
Giardia lamblia	3.7	1–44‡
Strongyloides stercoralis	0.2	5

*Higher rates reflect hospital-based studies of children younger than 2 years.

†Numbers in parentheses are from studies of summer diarrhea on Indian reservations of the southwestern United States.

‡In children younger than 4 years, the rates were 5–20%.

SOURCE: Guerrant RL, Hughes JM, Lima NL, et al. Diarrhea in developed and developing countries: Magnitude, special settings, and etiologies. Rev Infect Dis. 1990;12(suppl 1):541–550.

syndrome (HUS). It has been found to contaminate beef and poultry.[36–39]

Salmonella typhimurium and *S. enteritidis* are the most common of more than 1500 serotypes of nontyphoidal *Salmonella* that account for most of the diarrhea due to *Salmonella*. *Salmonella* organisms invade the mucosal cells of the distal small intestine and cause an inflammatory response in the lymphoid tissue, including Peyer's patches. Further invasion into the circulation may lead to bacteremia and metastatic infection in the central nervous system, bones, and joints, and at intravascular sites, as for example, in aortic aneurysms.[40, 41]

Of the *Shigella* serotypes, *Shigella sonnei* and *Shigella flexneri* are the most common. *Shigella sonnei* (group D), the most common cause of shigellosis in the United States, is frequently found in outbreaks in daycare centers or among institutionalized individuals.[42] The incidence of *Shigella* infections in the United States is declining, in contrast to infections with *Campylobacter* and *Salmonella* organisms.[43] Infection with *Shigella* is usually mucosal, although cytotoxins and enterotoxins may lead to extraintestinal involvement.[44] For example, a neurotoxin is thought to be responsible for seizures occasionally observed in patients with shigellosis, and the Shiga toxin produced by *Shigella dysenteriae* type 1 has been implicated in the development of HUS.[45]

Campylobacter organisms, in particular *C. jejuni*, cause illness ranging from mild diarrhea to fulminant colitis.[46] Although most episodes are sporadic, occasional outbreaks have been reported after ingestion of undercooked chicken and contaminated water.[47, 48] Most infections with *Campylobacter* are self-limited, although recurrent or chronic episodes and systemic complications such as meningitis, abscesses, pancreatitis, Reiter's syndrome, and Guillain–Barré syndrome have been reported.[46, 49]

Infection with *Y. enterocolitica* can cause an acute, self-limited diarrhea, although children may present with fever and severe, cramping, abdominal pain. *Yersinia enterocolitica* typically produces illness involving the distal ileum and colon, and it has been associated with aphthous ulcerations, mesenteric adenitis, appendicitis, erythema nodosum, arthritis, and signs and symptoms resembling Crohn's disease, including nodularity and mucosal thickening of the terminal ileum and colon.[50, 51] Outbreaks of *Y. enterocolitica* infection have been reported in association with contaminated milk and other foods.[52]

As in adults, *C. difficile* causes antibiotic-associated (pseudomembranous) colitis, which has been associated with all widely used antibiotics.[46] *Clostridium difficile* is commonly found in stool cultures of normal neonates, however, and *C. difficile* toxin can be obtained from feces of 10 to 50% of asymptomatic infants and young children.[53] By age 1 year, fewer than 5% have the organism or toxin in their stool.[54] *Clostridium difficile* also causes a mild diarrheal illness that may be self-limited or chronic.

Vibrio species are responsible for outbreaks of severe secretory diarrhea, primarily in developing countries. Occasional outbreaks are reported in the United States, often due to infected travelers or exposure to sewage or ingestion of contaminated uncooked oysters and crabs.[55–57] Infection may cause a mild and self-limited illness or a severe purging, resulting in rapid dehydration, vascular collapse, and death.

Aeromonas hydrophila has been reported to cause illness associated with fever, watery stools, occasionally with blood, and cramping abdominal pain.[58] It is usually self-limited, although it can cause a chronic diarrhea that is sometimes associated with colitis.[58, 59] *Plesiomonas shigelloides* infection is associated with similar but milder disease.[41, 60]

Viral enteritis is the most common cause of diarrhea in infants and children up to 2 years of age.[1] A variety of viral agents cause diarrhea by invading the small intestine. Rotavirus may account for up to 50% of cases in young children.[1] Other viral agents include Norwalk-like agents, enteric adenoviruses, and possibly calicivirus and astrovirus.[61, 62]

Parasitic causes of acute diarrhea include *G. lamblia, Entamoeba histolytica, Strongyloides stercoralis, Cryptosporidium,* and possibly *Blastocystis hominis*. In the United States, parasites are unusual causes of diarrhea except in high-risk groups, which include children in daycare centers or institutions, travelers, immigrants, migrant workers, and homosexuals. *Giardia lamblia* is the most common parasitic infection in the United States and has been reported in up to 54% of children in daycare centers where fecal-oral transmission is facilitated, compared with 2% of children not in daycare centers.[15] Many infections are acquired from contaminated drinking water and streams. Giardiasis is often asymptomatic or mild and self-limited, although persistent infection, seen in some normal subjects and particularly among immunodeficient patients, may lead to chronic diarrhea, abdominal cramping, flatulence, malabsorption, and failure to thrive. Recently it has also been reported to present with symptoms resembling those seen in patients with an inflammatory bowel disease.[63] *Cryptosporidium* was first recognized as a

TABLE 22–2. INFECTIOUS CAUSES OF DIARRHEA IN IMMUNE DEFICIENT INFANTS AND CHILDREN

BACTERIA
Campylobacter spp.
Clostridium difficile
Escherichia coli
Mycobacterium (M. avium-intracellulare, M. tuberculosis)
Salmonella spp.
Shigella spp.

VIRUSES
Cytomegalovirus
Herpes simplex virus
Rotavirus

PARASITES
Cryptosporidium parvum
Entamoeba histolytica
Giardia lamblia
Isospora belli
Microsporidia
Strongyloides stercoralis

FUNGUS
Candida albicans

significant cause of intractable watery diarrhea in patients with congenital immunodeficiency syndromes and was subsequently recognized as a cause of self-limiting diarrhea in normal subjects.[64] A common pathogen in daycare centers, *Cryptosporidium* accounts for more than 50% of diarrheal illnesses in some centers.[1, 15] It also is a serious complication in human immunodeficiency virus (HIV) infection, causing intractable diarrhea, and to date no treatment has proved to be effective. Other causes of diarrhea in immunodeficient patients are listed in Table 22-2.[65–67]

Diarrhea is also a common manifestation of nosocomial illnesses. Although *Salmonella* is the most commonly reported cause of epidemic nosocomial infection, viruses and *C. difficile* are more common causes of sporadic nosocomial diarrhea.[1] *Histoplasma* is an uncommon fungal cause of diarrhea, presenting as a granulomatous colitis or chronic diarrhea with protein-losing enteropathy.

PATHOPHYSIOLOGY

Several protective mechanisms help prevent infection by pathogenic organisms. These include gastric acid, mucosal surface barrier, intestinal motility, the indigenous florae that produce short-chain fatty acids and other factors that minimize pathogenic organisms, a normal state of nutrition, and the gut immune system, which involves secretory, humoral, and cell-mediated immune mechanisms.[68–71] Other mucosal protective factors important especially for infants are breast-feeding, weaning practices, and hygiene and sanitation practices that avoid excessive fecal contact.[3, 72] Infants are particularly susceptible to diarrheal infections owing to immaturity and abnormalities of some of these protective mechanisms, such as inadequate gastric acid secretion in early infancy,[73] antibiotic administration that alters intestinal flora,[74] and insufficient immunoglobulin levels to provide mucosal or systemic protection.[75]

Diarrheal disease due to infectious agents is caused by four general mechanisms that perturb normal physiologic mechanisms. Most organisms directly invade the intestinal mucosa. Some organisms produce enterotoxins or cytotoxins, and some pathogens injure the microvillous surface via mucosal adherence but do not invade the mucosa (Fig. 22–1).

Invasive organisms usually cause dysentery by infecting the distal small intestine and colon. Invasive organisms include *Shigella*, *S. enteritidis*, *C. jejuni*, enteroinvasive *E. coli* (EIEC), and *Y. enterocolitica*. Invasion of the surface epithelium causes edema, ulceration, bleeding, and leukocytic infiltration of the mucosa. Stools may consist only of leukocytes, erythrocytes, and mucus discharged into the lumen from the inflamed mucosa. Frequent stools result from the increased motility and reduced fluid absorption in the colon.

Bacterial enterotoxins are the most common cause of secretory diarrhea, although several

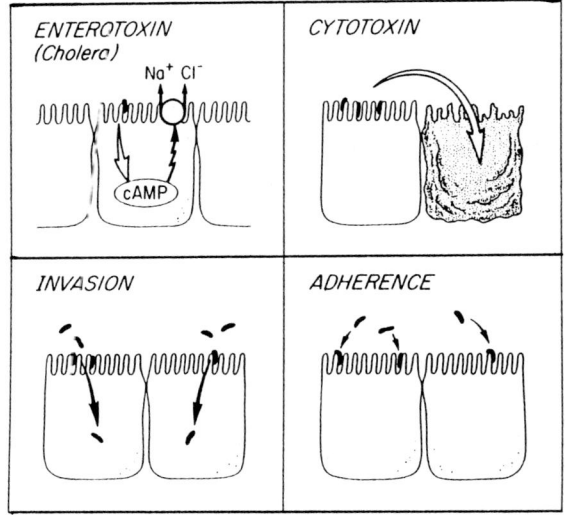

FIGURE 22–1.
Mechanisms of diarrhea due to infectious agents. SOURCE: Snyder JD. Bacterial infections. In: Walker WA, Durie PR, Hamilton JR, et al., eds. Pediatric Gastrointestinal Disease. 1st ed. Philadelphia: BC Decker; 1991:527.

TABLE 22–3. ETIOLOGY OF SECRETORY DIARRHEA IN INFANTS AND CHILDREN

ENTEROTOXINS
Cytotonic (*Vibrio cholera,* enterotoxigenic *Escherichia coli, Aeromonas hydrophila, Plesiomonas shigelloides, Bacillus cereus*)
Cytotoxic (*Shigella* spp., *Clostridium difficile,*
  enterohemorrhagic and enteropathogenic *Escherichia coli, Staphylococcus aureus, Campylobacter jejuni*)

VILLUS INJURIES ± CRYPT HYPERPLASIA
Infection
Celiac disease, food allergy
Inflammatory bowel disease (Crohn's disease)
Drugs: chemotherapy, neomycin
Radiation injury
Ischemic injury
Autoimmune disease, AIDS enteropathy
Collagen vascular disease

CONGENITAL ANOMALIES
Congenital microvillus atrophy
Congenital chloride diarrhea
Congenital bile acid malabsorption

LAXATIVES
Phenolphthalein
Docusate sodium
Senna
Danthron
Oxyphenisatin
Ricinoleic acid

FATTY ACIDS

BILE ACIDS

SECRETAGOGUES FROM TUMORS
Vasoactive intestinal polypeptide
Pancreatic polypeptide
Serotonin
Calcitonin
Gastrin
Somatostatin

other agents may stimulate intestinal fluid secretion (Table 22–3).[76] Cholera toxin is the prototype of this mechanism and binds to the mucosal cell surface, enters the cell, and activates the adenyl cyclase system. This leads to increased adenosine triphosphate (ATP) production, which then stimulates active fluid and electrolyte secretion, particularly chloride, from the crypt cells (in a cytotonic process). Cell injury does not occur. Enterotoxins also block absorption by villus cells. Thus, secretory diarrhea is due to increased intestinal secretion by the crypt cells and may be accompanied by inhibition of absorption of fluid by villus cells. Other enterotoxin-producing organisms include *A. hydrophila, P. shigelloides,* ETEC, and *C. difficile.*

Enhanced secretion resulting in secretory diarrhea may also be induced by cytotoxic processes that cause destruction of small intestinal mucosal cells and the villi. Cytotoxins, which are often released by infective agents such as *Shigella,* EHEC, EPEC, and *C. difficile,* may cause a

decrease in the number of absorptive cells of the intestine, whereas the secretory cells of the crypt are largely unaffected.[77] With few exceptions, in true secretory diarrhea, the diarrhea persists despite short-term fasting, because the diarrhea is due to increased secretion. Also, in pure forms of secretory diarrhea, the stool ionic contents account for the stool osmolality, since exogenous solute is not present and the stool contains no blood or pus.

Adherence occurs when organisms such as EPEC, *G. lamblia,* or *Cryptosporidium* attach to the surface of the enterocyte, disrupting normal absorptive processes and injuring the villus surface. Adherence of enteropathogenic *E. coli,* for example, causes dissolution of microvilli on the enterocytes, cupping of the outer membrane around the bacterium, and round cell inflammatory infiltrates in the lamina propria.[6, 78]

By contrast, osmotic diarrhea is caused by the presence in the intestinal lumen of unabsorbed osmotically active solutes, commonly a carbohydrate or a laxative salt such as magnesium sulfate (Table 22–4). Ingested nutrients in the small intestine produce osmotic forces that pull interstitial water into the lumen. As these nutrients are absorbed in the upper small intestine, luminal fluid becomes hypotonic, and water is absorbed along with the solute.[79] Destruction of villi by microorganisms or other

TABLE 22–4. ETIOLOGY OF OSMOTIC DIARRHEA IN INFANTS AND CHILDREN

VILLUS INJURY
Infection
Celiac disease
Food allergy
Inflammatory bowel disease (Crohn's disease)
Drugs: chemotherapy, neomycin
Radiation injury
Ischemic injury
Autoimmune disease
Collagen vascular disease
AIDS-associated intestinal infections

DISACCHARIDASE DEFICIENCY
Lactase deficiency (primary, secondary, congenital)
Sucrase–isomaltase deficiency

MONOSACCHARIDE MALABSORPTION
Fructose malabsorption
Sorbitol malabsorption
Congenital glucose–galactose malabsorption

MEDICATIONS, LAXATIVES
Lactulose
Magnesium sulfate (including antacids)
Products containing carbohydrates (e.g., sucrose, fructose, sorbitol, lactose)
Sodium sulfate
Sodium phosphate
Sodium citrate

processes that interfere with absorption can contribute to osmotic diarrhea. This action occurs in both secretory and cytotoxic mechanisms of diarrhea because of the inability of the intestine in both processes to function normally.[77] Osmotic diarrheas abate when ingestion of the offending agent is discontinued or infection is eliminated and mucosal epithelium regenerates. Because unabsorbed carbohydrate is metabolized by colonic bacteria to short-chain fatty acids with the release of carbon dioxide and hydrogen, osmotic diarrhea due to carbohydrate malabsorption is associated with flatulence and watery stools of low pH and high carbohydrate content. The stool pH is unaffected when osmotic diarrhea is caused by unabsorbed salts and ions such as magnesium and sulfate in Glauber's and Epsom salts, although it is high when milk of magnesia is the cause.[76]

Diarrhea can also result from abnormal intestinal motility that causes accelerated transit and reduced contact time between luminal contents and mucosal cells. This leads to delivery of a high solute and increased fluid load to the colon and to the ultimate passage of stools with increased volume and fluidity.[76] Increased motility may result from infections or from ingested substances such as fiber and medications, including laxatives and prokinetic agents such as metoclopramide, cisapride, erythromycin, and domperidone. It may also be caused by intrinsic neurohumoral abnormalities and may be observed intermittently in chronic nonspecific diarrhea in the young child, in irritable bowel syndrome in the older child and adolescent, and in neuromuscular disorders involving the gastrointestinal tract.

Chronic or protracted diarrhea is defined as diarrhea of 14 or more days' duration. Although the differential diagnosis in children is extensive (Table 22-5), the majority of patients with chronic diarrhea fit into specific categories, of which only a few are infectious in origin.[80, 81] The most common form of chronic diarrhea is idiopathic chronic nonspecific diarrhea, which manifests usually between 6 months and 4 years of age in otherwise well children without evidence of malabsorption, failure to thrive, or dehydration. It is frequently preceded by acute diarrhea that has been managed by administration of excessive clear fluids (high-carbohydrate) and reduced milk (low-fat) intake.[82] Disordered small intestinal motility has been reported in some children with chronic nonspecific diarrhea.[83] Diagnosis is by exclusion of other known causes of diarrhea. Failure to thrive becomes a problem in these children when they are placed on restricted diets that do not allow adequate nutritional intake to maintain normal growth and development.

Postviral gastroenteropathy syndrome is persistent diarrhea as a sequela of acute infectious gastroenteritis. Infectious diarrhea and many other causes of chronic diarrhea can be associated with patchy intestinal villus atrophy and consequent decrease in absorptive area, crypt cellular hypertrophy, and inflammatory infiltrates.[84, 85] Lactose intolerance, transient protein intolerance, dysmotility, and bacterial overgrowth can also contribute to the pathogenesis of chronic diarrhea in patients with persistent diarrhea after severe injury to the small intestine.

DIAGNOSIS

In infants and young children, diarrhea or vomiting may be a manifestation of a systemic illness, especially otitis media, pneumonia, or urinary tract infection. Other clinical features, such as fever, malaise, and irritability, are often evident. A detailed history and physical examination often suggest the systemic nature of the illness, which may be confirmed by appropriate diagnostic tests.

TABLE 22–5. CAUSES OF CHRONIC DIARRHEA IN YOUNG CHILDREN

Idiopathic chronic nonspecific diarrhea
Cystic fibrosis
Celiac disease
Disaccharidase deficiencies
Postviral gastroenteropathy
Infections (especially giardiasis)
Idiopathic inflammatory bowel disease: Crohn's disease, ulcerative colitis
Poisoning by drugs, surreptitious use of laxatives
Postoperative complication: short bowel syndrome
Blind loop syndrome
Shwachman–Diamond syndrome
Intestinal lymphangiectasia
Abetalipoproteinemia
Hormone secreting tumors: ganglioneuroma, ganglioneuroblastoma, nesidioblastosis (with vasoactive intestinal polypeptide secretion)
Milk or other food allergy
Immunodeficiency states: AIDS, severe combined immunodeficiency (SCID)
Congenital chloride malabsorption
Congenital glucose–galactose malabsorption
Enterokinase deficiency
Primary bile acid malabsorption
Dysautonomia syndromes

SOURCE: Adapted in part from: Ament ME. Malabsorption syndromes in infancy and childhood: J Pediatr. 1972;81:685–697, 867–884; and Fine KD, Krejs GJ, Fordtran JS. Diarrhea. In: Sleisenger MH, Fordtran JS, eds. Gastrointestinal Disease. 4th ed. Philadelphia: WB Saunders; 1989:313.

A careful history, noting duration, number of stools and their characteristics, risk factors, and amount and nature of fluid ingested, is essential for the diagnosis and treatment of the child with diarrhea (Fig. 22–2).[86]

Watery stools suggest a viral or toxin-induced diarrhea, whereas bloody mucoid stools suggest an inflammatory, often bacterial, cause. Non-bloody mucoid stools may occur in irritable bowel syndrome, whereas mushy, oily, and bulky stools are typical of malabsorption. Watery stools usually imply water, electrolyte, and osmotic agents, including carbohydrates. Stools that float suggest carbohydrate malabsorption,

since bacterial flora metabolize the carbohydrate into gases that remain in the stool. Fecal vegetable matter is not diagnostic of any condition, although many parents report its presence. Associated symptoms, such as emesis and abdominal pain and fever and factors such as changes in dietary patterns, growth, and medications, especially antibiotics and laxatives, must be noted. Information must also be obtained regarding any possible source of infection including daycare attendance, exposure to persons with symptoms or to animals, water sources, or recent travel to endemic areas.

Detailed dietary history is obtained, including

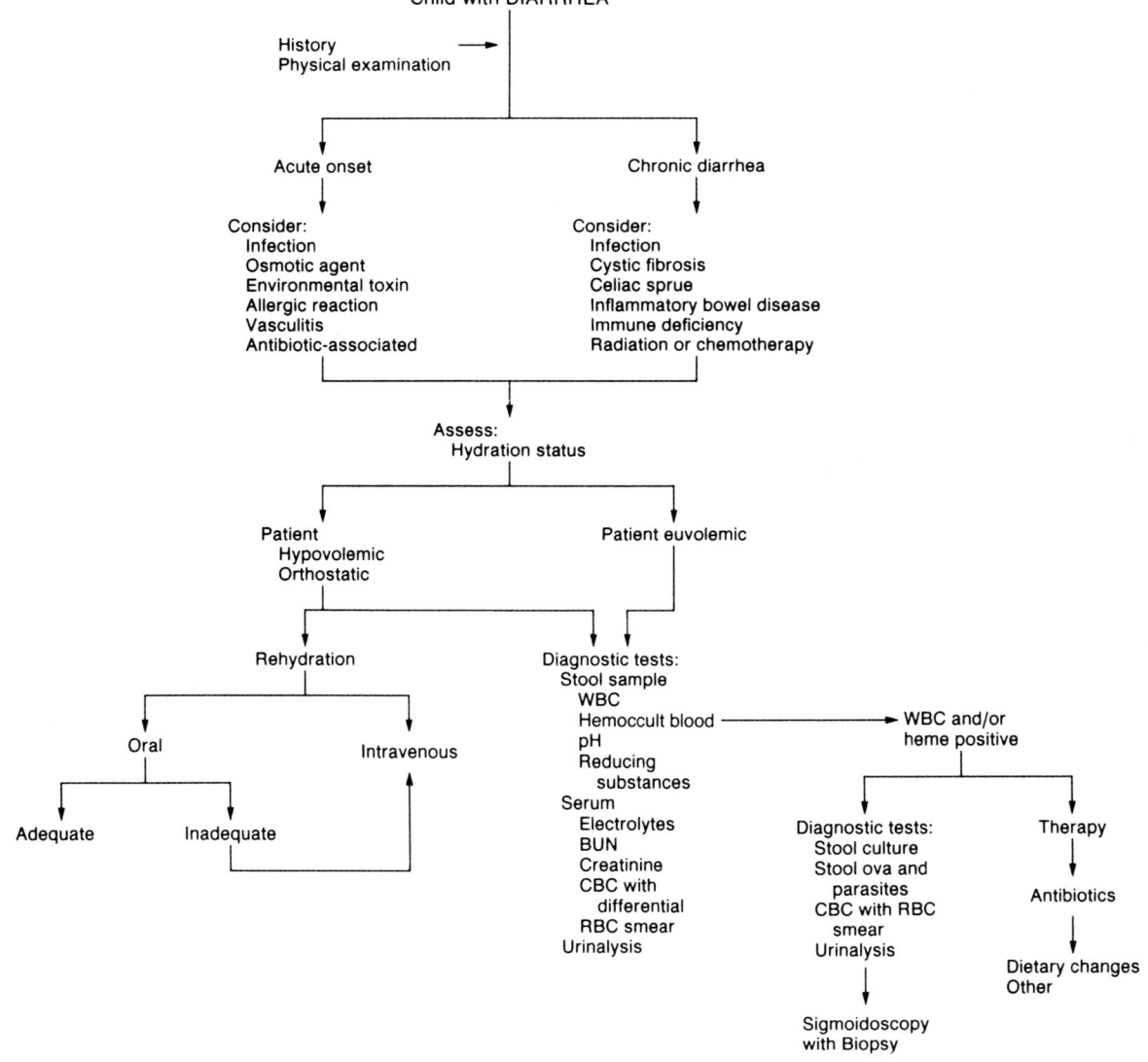

FIGURE 22–2.

Algorithm for the diagnosis and treatment of acute diarrhea in infants and children. SOURCE: Adapted from: Lavine JE, Heyman MB. Diarrhea in the child. In: Callaham ML, Barton CW, Schumaker HM, eds. Decision Making in Emergency Medicine. Philadelphia: BC Decker; 1990:343.

the use of well water and correlation of diarrhea with foods ingested. Preceding use of antimicrobial drugs predisposes to infection by *C. difficile*. Family history is important because of the familial occurrence of some disorders including inflammatory bowel disease, celiac sprue, cystic fibrosis, and irritable bowel syndrome, in which diarrhea may be a major symptom.

Disease of the small bowel and right colon usually manifests with large watery stools without gross blood and may be associated with borborygmi and cramping abdominal pain in the right lower abdominal quadrant or in the periumbilical area. Inflammatory disease involving the left colon and rectum usually manifests with small, frequent, mucoid, and bloody stools and with tenesmus.

A detailed physical examination is fundamental to assess a patient's general condition, including hydration and nutrition status. Vital signs, including blood pressure in all age groups, are necessary data in the initial evaluation of a patient with clinically significant diarrhea. Anthropometric measurements, particularly the weight, length or height, and weight-for-height assessments are important. The general physical should emphasize the abdominal and rectal examinations, but also include assessment of the skin and joints and the cardiopulmonary and other systems.

Depending on the severity of the illness, initial laboratory evaluation includes a complete blood count with differential and serum electrolytes, blood urea nitrogen and creatinine studies, which will give a further indication of the degree of dehydration as well as the presence and extent of any electrolyte imbalance (hypokalemia, acidosis) or renal disease. Anemia may result from hemolysis demonstrated on a red blood cell smear from a patient with HUS, gastrointestinal blood loss, or malabsorption. The findings on macroscopic and microscopic examinations of fresh stool specimens with Wright's or methylene blue stain establish presence or absence of blood or blood cells and leukocytes, indicating that the diarrhea is inflammatory having, most likely, a bacterial cause, or noninflammatory, having a viral or toxic cause (Table 22–6). Intestinal parasites such as *G. lamblia* or *Cryptosporidium* also cause noninflammatory diarrhea, and the less common *E. histolytica* may cause an inflammatory disease with mucoid bloody stools. Stool culture, for which a specimen can be obtained using a rectal swab, is only likely to have positive findings in inflammatory diarrhea with fecal leukocytes. Fecal leukocytes are also present in inflammatory bowel disease, in pseudomembra-

TABLE 22–6. CONDITIONS ASSOCIATED WITH FECAL LEUKOCYTES

ACUTE DIARRHEA	CHRONIC DIARRHEA
Shigella spp.	Inflammatory bowel disease
Escherichia coli (EIEC, EPEC)	Antibiotic-associated diarrhea
Entamoeba histolytica	*Entamoeba histolytica*
Salmonella spp.	Ischemic colitis
Gonococci	Mycobacteria
Campylobacter spp.	Radiation-induced colitis
Clostridium difficile	Schistosomiasis
Aeromonas hydrophila	
Balantidium coli	
Vibrio parahaemolyticus	
Yersinia spp.	
Rotavirus	
Cytomegalovirus	
Protein-induced colitis	
Hemolytic-uremic syndrome	
Henoch-Schönlein purpura	

KEY: EIEC = enteroinvasive *E. coli*, EPEC = enteropathogenic *E. coli*.

nous, ischemic, and radiation-induced colitis and in mycobacterial infection and schistosomiasis of the colon, all of which can cause chronic diarrhea. Other useful initial screening tests include stool test for pH and reducing sugars. A reduced pH associated with presence of reducing sugar in the stool is a hallmark of carbohydrate malabsorption. A breath hydrogen test confirms this finding.[87] Rotazyme, an enzyme-linked immunoassay, is a rapid clinic or office test to screen for rotavirus infection. An enzyme immunoassay (EIA) test for *G. lamblia* is now widely available to detect fecal antigen and is more sensitive than microscopic examination of stool samples.[88, 89] A gram-stained stool may show the characteristic gram-negative vibrio, in appearance a gull-winged organism, that is indicative of infection with *Campylobacter*. When the cause of disease is not detectable using other methods, flexible sigmoidoscopy is a minimally invasive method to screen for colitis and to obtain fresh stool specimens for cultures and other tests. Except in some children between 1 and 4 years of age, sedation is rarely necessary, and the procedure can be performed in less than 15 minutes, including obtaining mucosal biopsies for histology and culture. Since urinary tract infection may present with diarrhea, particularly in infancy, a urinalysis should also be done. The urinalysis is also useful to screen for renal involvement associated with HUS and Henoch-Schönlein purpura (HSP). A more detailed work-up may be necessary, particularly if diarrhea becomes prolonged or chronic (Table 22–7).

TABLE 22–7. DETAILED WORK-UP IN DIARRHEAL DISEASE

INITIAL EVALUATION

STOOL
Consistency
Frequency/24 h
Volume/24 h (estimated)
White blood cell count by Wright's stain
Cultures for enteric pathogens
Ova and parasites
Rotazyme
Clostridium difficile toxin (if clinically indicated)
pH
Reducing substances

BLOOD
Complete blood count with differential
Electrolytes, blood urea nitrogen, creatinine

URINE
Specific gravity
Urinalysis

SECONDARY EVALUATION
(for prolonged diarrhea, cause unknown)

STOOL
Volume/24 h (quantitated)
White blood cell count by Wright's stain
Quantitative fat/24 h
NaOH (for detection of phenolphthalein)
Osmolality
Na,K, Cl
Mg, SO_4, PO_4
α_1-Antitrypsin (protein-losing enteropathy)
Trypsin

PROCTOSCOPY
Mucosal appearance
Biopsy
Melanosis

BLOOD
Immunoglobulins, albumin
Triiodothyronine, thyroxine
Ameba serology
Folate, vitamin B_{12}
Cortisol
Ca, Mg, PO_4
Erythrocyte sedimentation rate
Eosinophil count

SPECIAL ASSAYS
Vasoactive intestinal polypeptide
Calcitonin
Gastrin
Other

GASTRIC ANALYSIS

IMAGING STUDIES
Upper gastrointestinal tract, small bowel, barium enema
Abdominal and pelvic sonogram, computed tomography
    scan
Abdominal angiogram

SMALL BOWEL STUDIES
Aspirate (ova and parasite, colony count, cultures)
Biopsy
Mucosal disaccharidase assays
D-xylose
Schilling's test with intrinsic factor
Bile acid absorption
Carbohydrate tolerance tests
Carbohydrate breath tests

EXOCRINE PANCREATIC FUNCTION
Sweat chloride

UPPER ENDOSCOPY WITH GASTRIC AND SMALL
    INTESTINAL BIOPSIES

COLONOSCOPY WITH BIOPSIES

URINE
Volume, Na, K
5-hydroxyindoleacetic acid
Metanephrines, vanilmandelic acid
NaOH (for phenolphthalein)
Heavy metals, drug screen

ROOM SEARCH FOR DRUGS

RECTAL MANOMETRY

INTESTINAL PERFUSION STUDIES

THERAPEUTIC TRIALS

SOURCE: Fine KD, Krejs GJ, Fordtran JS. Diarrhea. In: Sleisenger MH, Fordtran JS, eds. Gastrointestinal Disease. 5th ed. Philadelphia: WB Saunders; 1993.

TREATMENT

Most episodes of acute diarrhea in children are self-limited and require only oral therapy to correct dehydration and electrolyte imbalance and to provide appropriate nutrition early.[90] The oral rehydration therapy component of oral treatment, which uses glucose–electrolyte solutions, is effective in the great majority of patients. Clinical trials have documented the efficacy of oral rehydration therapy, with over 90% success in rehydrating patients with dehydration from all infectious causes of diarrhea.[6, 91]

It can be administered easily and safely in most environments, is inexpensive, and is associated with lower case-fatality ratios.[6, 91, 92] The physiologic basis for the use of these formulations is the coupled transport of glucose and sodium, resulting in enhanced absorption of salt and water across the intestinal membrane.[93] Coupled transport remains effective even in the presence of intestinal inflammation, as in bacterial enteritis.[94] Oral glucose and electrolyte solutions are useful for both deficit rehydration and maintenance fluid requirements. The American Academy of Pediatrics (AAP) Com-

TABLE 22–8. ORAL REHYDRATION THERAPY FOR ENTERITIS: SUMMARY OF AMERICAN ACADEMY OF PEDIATRICS (COMMITTEE ON NUTRITION) RECOMMENDATIONS

ORAL REHYDRATION

Glucose-electrolyte solutions are used for rehydration and maintenance therapy.
  Rehydration: 75–90 mEq/L of Na
  Maintenance: 40–60 mEq/L of Na

Rehydration solutions can be used to provide maintenance fluid and electrolytes when given with H_2O, breast milk, or low-carbohydrate juice.

Carbohydrate (CHO) to Na ratio should not exceed 2:1 in rehydration and maintenance solution.

Oral rehydrating solutions may be used to treat mild, moderate, and severe dehydration.

Successful therapy can be accomplished in a vomiting child.

Home mixing of dry ingredients and water is acceptable if a container of appropriate volume is distributed with the dry ingredients and water does not contain enteric infectious agents.

EARLY FEEDING THERAPY

Feeding should be reintroduced in the first 24 h of the episode.

Initial foods include:
  Infants: breast milk, diluted formula, or milk
  Older infants and children: rice cereal, bananas, potatoes, other nonlactose carbohydrate-rich foods.

Children should be followed closely to detect dehydration.

SOURCE: Adapted from: American Academy of Pediatrics (AAP) Committee on Nutrition. Use of oral fluid therapy and post-treatment feeding following enteritis in children in a developed country. Pediatrics. 1985;75:358–361.

mittee on Nutrition recommends that the sodium content should be 75 to 90 mEq/L for rehydration solutions and 40 to 60 mEq/L for maintenance solutions (Table 22–8).[95] A home-made rice cereal solution can be prepared by adding 1/2 to 1 cup precooked baby rice cereal plus 1/4 teaspoon salt to 2 cups of water.[96, 97] Several proprietary solutions are effective, but caution must be exercised and fluid and electrolyte abnormalities must be suspected when infants and young children are not tolerating oral solutions, especially when they are being hydrated with other (i.e., nonphysiologic clear liquid) solutions. (Table 22–9).[98]

Rehydration solutions can be used to provide maintenance fluid and electrolytes when given with water, breast milk or low-carbohydrate juice.[95] Close monitoring of fluid input and output is required during rehydration therapy.

Although oral rehydration therapy is effective in the majority of patients with diarrheal disease, intravenous rehydration is necessary for rapid expansion of intravascular volume if the patient has severe protracted vomiting or is in shock or has an ileus or altered state of consciousness. In hypernatremic dehydration, rehydration is effected more slowly to avoid cerebral edema and seizures.

Early reintroduction of feeding with age-appropriate foods is the second component of oral therapy. Early appropriate feeding facilitates healing of damaged intestinal mucosa, reduces nutritional deficits, and can shorten the duration of diarrhea.[99–102] Breast-fed infants can be fed safely through diarrhea, although they receive a higher concentration of lactose than do children receiving cow's milk or cow's milk formula.[103] Full strength animal milk or animal milk formula is usually tolerated well by children who have mild, self-limited diarrhea. Com-

TABLE 22–9. COMPOSITION OF ORAL REHYDRATION AND SOME CLEAR LIQUID SOLUTIONS

PRODUCT	CONCENTRATION (mmol/L)					
	CHO	Na	CHO/Na	K	BASE (CITRATE)	OSMOLALITY
Physiologic Solutions						
WHO/UNICEF ORS	111 (G)	90	1.2	20	30	310
Pedialyte (Ross)	140 (G)	45	3.1	20	30	249
Pediatric Electrolyte (NutraMax)	140 (G)	45	3.1	20	30	250
Naturalyte (Unlimited Beverages)	140 (G)	45	3.1	20	48	265
Rehydralyte (Ross)	140 (G)	75	1.9	20	30	304
Ricelyte (Mead Johnson)	70 (R)	50	1.4	25	34	200
Clear Liquids						
Gatorade	255 (S,G)	20	13	3	3	330
Chicken broth	0	250	—	8	0	500
Apple juice	690 (F,G,S)	3	230	32	0	730
Cola	700 (F,G)	2	350	0	13	750

KEY: CHO = carbohydrate, F = fructose, G = glucose, ORS = oral rehydration solution, R = glucose polymers from rice, S = sucrose, UNICEF = United Nations International Children's Emergency Fund, WHO = World Health Organization.
SOURCE: Snyder JD. Oral rehydration therapy for acute diarrhea. In: Hendricks KM, Walker WA, eds. Seminars in Pediatric Gastroenterology and Nutrition. Burlington, Ont.: BC Decker; 1990;1:7–9.

bining milk with staple foods like cereals is a successful regimen for children who are weaned.[104–108] As long as children are carefully monitored to identify the few who develop signs of intolerance, full strength milk or formula should be used.[109]

Most acute infectious diarrheal episodes with a recognized pathogen are mild and self-limited and do not require specific antimicrobial treatment. Enteritis caused by *Shigella, V. cholera,* and *C. difficile,* however, often require specific antimicrobial therapy because, particularly in the younger child, they tend to cause severe illness. Infections by *Campylobacter, Yersinia, Aeromonas,* and the several forms of *E. coli* may also require treatment, although reports are conflicting regarding the efficacy of antimicrobials in these infections (Table 22–10). The choice of antimicrobial drugs, when indicated, is based on in vitro sensitivity patterns and may be related to geographical prevalence of the infection.[110]

The use of antidiarrheal agents is not indicated in most diarrheal illnesses.[111] Both bismuth subsalicylate and loperamide have antiprostaglandin activity that counteracts the prostaglandin-mediated enhanced motility in enteritis. Bismuth subsalicylate also has antibacterial activity and in addition binds bile salts, which may contribute to the diarrheal process.[77, 94] The relatively large quantity of bismuth subsalicylate necessary for efficacy may, however, put the child at risk of toxic salicylism. Loperamide and narcotic-containing agents decrease gastrointestinal propulsion and should be avoided, especially in acute diarrhea.[111] Although they may relieve symptoms initially by decreasing peristalsis, intestinal secretion persists. Secretions may pool in distended loops of bowel, giving a false impression of decreasing diarrhea, and excretion of pathogens is prolonged. Paralytic ileus is a particularly significant concern as a complication of antimotility agents, including loperamide, in infants.[111–113] Use of adsorbents such as kaolin-pectin suspensions is also not recommended since they may cause increased sodium and potassium losses.

Because chronic diarrhea is commonly associated with prolonged injury to the intestinal villous processes, chronic malnutrition often results. The management of chronic malnutrition, therefore, includes nutritional replenishment of protein, calorie, and other nutrients by enteral or parenteral routes, as indicated, in addition to fluid and electrolyte replacement.[90, 114]

Diarrheal illness remains a major cause of morbidity in childhood worldwide. Preventive measures are essential to reduce its prevalence. Improved sanitation and careful hand washing, particularly in daycare settings, are essential to decrease the spread of intestinal pathogens. Although vaccines against rotavirus have been developed and are being tried clinically, the development of vaccines against other causative organisms has been extremely slow. Such vaccines may prove to be the most effective way to reduce the incidence of infectious diarrheal illnesses.[77]

REFERENCES

1. Guerrant RL, Hughes JM, Lima NL, et al. Diarrhea in developed and developing countries: Magnitude, special settings, and etiologies. Rev Infect Dis. 1990; 12(suppl 1):S41–S50.
2. Claeson M, Merson MH. Global progress in the control of diarrheal diseases. Pediatr Infect Dis J. 1990;9:345–355.
3. Snyder JD, Merson MH. The magnitude of the global problem of acute diarrhoeal disease: A review of active surveillance data. Bull World Health Organ. 1982; 60:605–613.
4. Kozak LJ, McCarthy E. Hospital use by children in the United States and Canada: Vital and health statistics. Comp Int Vital Health Stat Rep. 1984;5:1–59.
5. Ho MS, Glass RI, Pinsky PF, et al. Diarrheal deaths in American children: Are they preventable? JAMA. 1988;260:3281–3285.
6. Snyder JD. Bacterial infections. In: Walker WA, Durie PR, Hamilton JR, et al., eds. Pediatric Gastrointestinal Disease. 1st ed. Philadelphia: BC Decker; 1991:527–537.
7. Levine MM, Edelman R. Acute diarrheal infections in infants: I, Epidemiology, treatment and prospects for immunoprophylaxis. Hosp Pract. 1979;14:89–100.
8. Tripp JH, Wilmers MJ, Wharton BA. Gastroenteritis: A continuing problem of child health in Britain. Lancet. 1977;2:233–236.
9. Black RE, Brown KH, Becker S, et al. Longitudinal

TABLE 22–10. ANTIMICROBIAL TREATMENT FOR INFECTIOUS DIARRHEA

ORGANISM	DRUG
Aeromonas hydrophila	Amoxicillin, trimethoprim–sulfamethoxazole
Campylobacter spp.	Erythromycin
Clostridium difficile	Vancomycin, metronidazole
Clostridium perfringens	Penicillin, tetracycline
Escherichia coli	Trimethoprim-sulfamethoxazole
Entamoeba histolytica	Metronidazole, iodoquinol
Giardia lamblia	Metronidazole, furazolidone, quinacrine HCl
Salmonella	Tetracycline, chloramphenicol
Shigella	Amoxicillin, trimethoprim-sulfamethoxazole
Vibrio cholerae	Tetracycline, trimethoprim-sulfamethoxazole
Yersinia	Tetracycline, chloramphenicol

SOURCE: DeWitt TG: Acute diarrhea in children. Pediatr Rev. 1989; 11:6–13.

studies of infectious diseases and physical growth of children in rural Bangladesh: II, Incidence of diarrhea and association with known pathogens. Am J Epidemiol. 1982;115:315–324.

10. Bhatnagar S, Dosajh U. Diarrheal disease morbidity in children below 5 years in urban slums of Delhi. Indian J Med Res. 1986;84:53–58.

11. McCormick MC. Epidemiology of diarrhea in the United States. In: 13th Ross Roundtable Conference. Diagnosis and Management of Acute Diarrhea. 1982:1.

12. Larsen SA, Homer DR. Relation of breast versus bottle feeding to hospitalization for gastroenteritis in a middle class US population. J Pediatr. 1978;92:417–418.

13. Cunningham AS, Jelliffe DB, Jelliffe EF. Breast feeding and health in the 1980s: A global epidemiologic review. J Pediatr. 1991;118:659–666.

14. Feachem RG, Koblinsky MA. Interventions for the control of diarrhoeal diseases among young children: Promotion of breast-feeding. Bull World Health Organ. 1984;62:271–291.

15. Bartlett AV, Moore M, Gary GW, et al. Diarrheal illness among infants and toddlers in day care centers: I, Epidemiology and pathogens. J Pediatr. 1985;107:495–502.

16. Pickering LK, Bartlett AV, Wookward WE. Acute infectious diarrhea among children in day care: Epidemiology and control. Rev Infect Dis. 1986;8:539–547.

17. Blacklow NR, Cukor G. Viral gastroenteritis. N Engl J Med. 1981;304:397–406.

18. Rodriguez WJ, Kim HW, Brandt CD, et al. Fecal adenoviruses from a longitudinal study of families in metropolitan Washington, DC: Laboratory, clinical and epidemiological observations. J Pediatr. 1985;107:514–520.

19. Communicable Disease Surveillance Center. Campylobacter infections, 1977–80. Br Med J Clin Res Ed. 1981;282:1484.

20. Uhnoo I, Wadell G, Svensson L, et al. Aetiology and epidemiology of acute gastroenteritis in Swedish children. J Infect. 1986;13:73–89.

21. Guerrant RL, Lohr JA, Williams EK. Acute infectious diarrhea: I, Epidemiology, etiology and pathogenesis. Pediatr Infect Dis. 1986;5:353–359.

22. Blaser MJ, Wells JG, Feldman RA, et al. *Campylobacter* enteritis in the United States: A multicenter study. Ann Intern Med. 1983;98:360–365.

23. Kendall EJ, Tanner E. *Campylobacter* enteritis in general practice. J Hyg. 1982;88:155–163.

24. Edelman R, Levine MM. Acute diarrheal infections in infants: II, Bacterial and viral causes. Hosp Pract. 1980;15:97–104.

25. Kapikian AZ, Kim HW, Wyatt RG, et al. Human reovirus-like agent as the major pathogen associated with "winter" gastroenteritis in hospitalized infants and young children. N Engl J Med. 1976;294:965–972.

26. Dearlove J, Latham P, Dearlove B, et al. Clinical range of neonatal rotavirus gastroenteritis. Br Med J Clin Res Ed. 1983;286:1473–1475.

27. Nelson SJ, Granoff D. *Salmonella* gastroenteritis in the first 3 months of life. Clin Pediatr. 1982;21:708–712.

28. Anders BJ, Lauer BA, Paisley JW. *Campylobacter* gastroenteritis in neonates. Am J Dis Child. 1981;135:900–902.

29. San Joaquin VH, Welch DF. *Campylobacter* enteritis. Clin Pediatr. 1984;23:311–316.

30. Glass RI, Stoll B, Huq MI, et al. Epidemiological and clinical features of endemic *Campylobacter jejuni* infection in Bangladesh. J Infect Dis. 1983;148:292–296.

31. Kohl S, Jacobson JA, Nahmias A. *Yersinia enterocolitica* infections in children. J Pediatr. 1976;89:77–79.

32. Centers for Disease Control. Update: *Salmonella enteri-*

tidis infections and grade A shell eggs in the United States. MMWR 1990;39:909–912.

33. Merson MM, Morris GK, Sack DA, et al. Traveller's diarrhea in Mexico: A prospective study of physicians and family members attending a congress. N Engl J Med. 1976;294:1299–1305.

34. Guerrant RL, Rouse JD, Hughes JM, Rowe B. Turista among members of the Yale Glee Club in Latin America. Am J Trop Med Hyg. 1980;29:895–900.

35. Robins-Browne RM, Still CS, Miliotis MD, et al. Summer diarrhea in African infants and children. Arch Dis Child. 1980;55:923–928.

36. Remis RS, MacDonald KL, Riley LW, et al. Sporadic cases of hemorrhagic colitis associated with *Escherichia coli* 0157:H7. Ann Intern Med. 1984;101:624–626.

37. Karmali MA, Petric M, Lim C, et al. The association between idiopathic hemolytic-uremic syndrome and infection by verotoxin-producing *Escherichia coli*. J Infect Dis. 1985;151:775–782.

38. Griffin PM, Tauxe RV. The epidemiology of infections caused by *Escherichia coli* 0157:H7, other enterohemorrhagic *E coli*, and the associated hemolytic-uremic syndrome. Epidemiol Rev. 1991;13:68–90.

39. Siegler RL, Griffin PM, Barrett TJ, Strockbine NA. Recurrent hemolytic-uremic syndrome secondary to *Escherichia coli* 0157:H7 infection. Pediatrics. 1993;91:666–667.

40. Hyams JS, Durbin WA, Grand RJ. *Salmonella* bacteremia in the first year of life. J Pediatr. 1980;96:57–59.

41. Rennels MB, Levine MM. Classical bacterial diarrhea: Perspectives and update: *Salmonella, Shigella, Escherichia coli, Aeromonas* and *Plesiomonas*. Pediatr Infect Dis J. 1986;5:S91–S100.

42. Levine MM. Bacillary dysentery: Mechanisms and treatment. Med Clin North Am. 1982;66:623–638.

43. Blaser MJ, Pollard RA, Feldman RA. *Shigella* infections in the United States, 1974–1980. J Infect Dis. 1983; 147:771–775.

44. Middlebrook JL, Dorland RB. Bacterial toxins: Cellular mechanisms of action. Microb Rev. 1984;48:199–221.

45. Jadhav M, Verghese R, Bhat P, Webb JK. Clinical and microbiological features of shigellosis in 100 south Indian infants and children under 5 years. Indian J Pediatr. 1966;3:393–400.

46. Blaser MJ. Bacterial gastrointestinal infections. Gastroenterol Ann 1986;3:317–340.

47. Kist M, Keller KM, Niebling W, Kilching W. *Campylobacter coli* septicemia associated with septic abortion. Infection. 1984;12:88–90.

48. Taylor DN, McDermott KT, Little JR, et al. *Campylobacter* enteritis from untreated water in the Rocky Mountains. Ann Intern Med. 1983;99:38–40.

49. Blaser MJ, Reller LB. *Campylobacter* enteritis. N Engl J Med. 1981;305:1444–1452.

50. Black RE, Jackson RJ, Tsai T, et al. Epidemic *Yersinia enterocolitica* infections due to contaminated chocolate milk. N Engl J Med. 1978;298:76–79.

51. Ahvonen P. Human yersiniosis in Finland: II, Clinical features. Ann Clin Res. 1972;4:39–48.

52. Tacket CO, Narain JP, Sattin R, et al. A multistate outbreak of infections caused by *Yersinia enterocolitica* transmitted by pasteurized milk. JAMA. 1984;251:483–486.

53. Ellis ME, Mandal BK, Dunbar EM, Bundell KR. *Clostridium difficile* and its cytotoxin in infants admitted to hospital with infectious gastroenteritis. Br Med J Clin Res Ed. 1984;288:524–526.

54. Jarvis WR, Feldman RA. *Clostridium difficile* and gastroenteritis: How strong is the association in children? Pediatr Infect Dis. 1984;3:4–6.

55. Blake PA, Allegra DT, Snyder JD, et al. Cholera: A possible endemic focus in the United States. N Engl J Med. 1980;302:305–309.

56. Morris JG Jr, Black RE. Cholera and other vibrioses in the United States. N Engl J Med. 1985;312:343–350.

57. Finelli L, Swerdlow D, Mertz K, et al. Outbreak of cholera associated with crab brought from an area with epidemic disease. J Infect Dis. 1992;166:1433–1435.

58. Aggar WA, McCormick JD, Gurwith MJ. Clinical and microbiological features of *Aeromonas hydrophila*–associated diarrhea. J Clin Microbiol. 1985;21:909–913.

59. Gracey M, Burke V, Robinson J. *Aeromonas*-associated gastroenteritis. Lancet. 1982;2:1304–1306.

60. Holmberg SD, Farmer JJ. *Aeromonas hydrophila* and *Plesiomonas shigelloides* as causes of intestinal infections. Rev Infect Dis. 1984;6:633–639.

61. Mortensen ML, Ray CG, Payne CM, et al. Coronavirus-like particles in human gastrointestinal disease. Am J Dis Child. 1985;139:928–934.

62. Blacklow NR, Greenberg HB. Viral gastroenteritis. N Engl J Med. 1991;325:252–264.

63. Gunasekaran TS, Hassall E. Giardiasis mimicking inflammatory bowel disease. J Pediatr. 1992;120:424–426.

64. Current WL, Reese NC, Ernst JV, et al. Human cryptosporidia in immunocompetent and immunodeficient individuals: Studies of an outbreak and experimental transmission. N Engl J Med. 1983;308:1252–1257.

65. Gelb A, Miller S. AIDS and gastroenterology. Am J Gastroenterol. 1986;81:619–622.

66. Soave R, Johnson WD Jr. *Cryptosporidium* and *Isospora belli* infections. J Infect Dis. 1988;157:225–229.

67. Nelson JA, Wiley CA, Reynolds-Kohler C, et al. Human immunodeficiency virus detected in bowel epithelium from patients with gastrointestinal symptoms. Lancet. 1988;1:259–262.

68. Hill HR, Meier FA. Host defense factors in the gastrointestinal tract. Pediatr Infect Dis J. 1986;5:S144–S147.

69. Hentges DJ. The protective function of indigenous intestinal flora. Pediatr Infect Dis J. 1986;5:S17–S20.

70. Giannella RA, Broitman SA, Zamcheck N. Influence of gastric acidity on bacterial and parasitic enteric infections: A perspective. Ann Intern Med. 1973;78:271–276.

71. Walker WA. Antigen handling by the small intestine. Clin Gastroenterol. 1986;15:1–20.

72. Israel EJ, Walker WA. Development of intestinal mucosal barrier function to antigens and bacterial toxins. In: Mestecky J, McGhee JR, Bienenstock J, Ogra PL, eds. Recent Advances in Mucosal Immunology. New York: Plenum; 1987:673–683.

73. Grand RJ, Watkins JB, Forti FM. Development of human gastrointestinal tract: A review. Gastroenterology. 1976;70:790–810.

74. Hentges DJ. Role of the intestinal microflora in host defense against infection. In: Hentges DJ, ed. Human Intestinal Microflora in Health and Disease. New York: Academic Press; 1983:311.

75. Altemeier WA, Smith RT. Immunologic aspects of resistance in early life. Pediatr Clin North Am. 1965;12:663–686.

76. Fine KD, Krejs GJ, Fordtran JS. Diarrhea. In: Sleisenger MH, Fordtran JS, eds. Gastrointestinal Disease. 4th ed. Philadelphia: WB Saunders; 1989:290–316.

77. DeWitt TG. Acute diarrhea in children. Pediatr Rev. 1989;11:6–13.

78. Levine MM. *Escherichia coli* infections. N Engl J Med. 1987;313:445–447.

79. Fordtran JS, Rector RC, Carter NW. The mechanism of sodium absorption in the human small intestine. J Clin Invest. 1968;47:88–90.

80. Ament ME. Malabsorption syndromes in infancy and childhood. J Pediatr. 1972;81:685–697,867–884.

81. Ament ME, Barclay GN. Chronic diarrhea. Pediatr Ann. 1982;11:124–131.

82. Andres JM. Advances in understanding the pathogenesis of persistent diarrhea in young children. Adv Pediatr. 1988;35:483–498.

83. Fenton TR, Harries JT, Milla PJ. Disordered small intestinal motility: A rational basis for toddlers' diarrhea. Gut. 1963;24:897.

84. Rossi TM, Lebenthal E, Nord KS, Fazili RR. Extent and duration of small intestinal mucosal injury in intractable diarrhea of infancy. Pediatrics. 1980;66:730–735.

85. Brunser O. Effects of malnutrition on intestinal structure and function in children. Clin Gastroenterol. 1977;6:341–353.

86. Lavine JE, Heyman MB. Diarrhea in the child. In: Callaham ML, Barton CW, Schumaker HM, eds. Decision Making in Emergency Medicine. Philadelphia: BC Decker; 1990:342–343.

87. Barr RG, Perman JA, Schoeller DA, Watkins JB. Breath tests in pediatric gastrointestinal disorders: New diagnostic opportunities. Pediatrics. 1978;62:393–401.

88. Rosoff JD, Sanders CA, Sonnad SS, et al. Stool diagnosis of giardiasis using a commercially available enzyme immunoassay to detect *Giardia*-specific antigen 65 (GSA-65). J Clin Microbiology. 1989;27:1997–2002.

89. Addiss DG, Mathews HM, Stewart JM, et al. Evaluation of a commercially available enzyme-linked immunosorbent assay for *Giardia lamblia* antigen in stool. J Clin Microbiol. 1991;29:1137–1142.

90. Duggan C, Santosham M, Glass RI. The management of acute diarrhea in children: Oral rehydration, maintenance, and nutritional therapy. MMWR 1992;41:1–20.

91. Mahalanabis D, Choudhuri AB, Bagchi NG, et al. Oral fluid therapy of cholera among Bangladesh refugees. Johns Hopkins Med J. 1973;132:197–205.

92. Shepard DS. Procedures for assessing the cost effectiveness of a diarrheal disease control program based on oral rehydration therapy. In: Proceedings of International Conference on Oral Rehydration Therapy. Washington DC: Agency for International Development; 1983.

93. Hirschhorn N. The treatment of acute diarrhea in children: An historical and physiological perspective. Am J Clin Nutr. 1980;33:637–663.

94. Snyder JD. Oral therapy for acute diarrhea: An American perspective. Int Sem Paediatr Gastroent Nutr. 1992;1:9–12.

95. American Academy of Pediatrics (AAP) Committee on Nutrition. Use of oral fluid therapy and post-treatment feeding following enteritis in children in a developed country. Pediatrics. 1985;75:358–361.

96. Molla AM, Sarker SA, Hossain M, et al. Rice-powder electrolyte solution as oral-therapy in diarrhoea due to *Vibrio cholerae* and *Escherichia coli*. Lancet. 1982;1:1317–1319.

97. International Child Health Foundation Newsletter. Columbia, MD: International Child Health Foundation; 1992;10:3.

98. Snyder JD. Oral rehydration therapy for acute diarrhea. In: Hendricks KM, Walker WA, eds. Seminars in Pediatric Gastroenterology and Nutrition. Burlington, Ont.: BC Decker; 1990;1:7–9.

99. Knudsen KB, Bradley EM, Lecocq FR, et al. Effect of fasting and refeeding on the histology and disaccharidase activity of the human intestine. Gastroenterology. 1968;55:46–51.

100. Brown KJ, MacLean WC Jr. Nutritional management of acute diarrhea: An appraisal of the alternatives. Pediatrics. 1984;73:119–125.

101. Molla AM, Molla A, Rohde J, Greenough WB. Turning off the diarrhea: The role of food and ORS. J Pediatr Gastroenterol Nutr. 1989;8:81–84.
102. Santosham M, Fayad IM, Hashem M. A comparison of rice-based oral rehydration solution and "early feeding" for the treatment of acute diarrhea in infants. J Pediatr. 1990;16:868–875.
103. Khin-Maung-U, Nyunt-Nyunt-Wai, Myo-Khin, et al. Effect on clinical outcome of breast feeding during acute diarrhoea. Br Med J Clin Res Ed. 1985;290:587–589.
104. Gazala E, Weitzman S, Weizman Z, et al. Early versus late refeeding in acute infantile diarrhoea. Isr J Med Sci. 1988;24:175–179.
105. Rees L, Brooke CGD. Gradual reintroduction of full-strength milk after acute gastroenteritis in infants under 6 months old. Lancet. 1979;1:770–771.
106. Hjelt K, Paeeregard A, Petersen W, et al. Rapid versus gradual refeeding in acute gastroenteritis in childhood: Energy intake and weight gain. J Pediatr Gastroenterol Nutr. 1989;8:75–80.
107. Brown KH, Perez F, Gastanaduy AS. Clinical trial of modified whole milk, lactose-hydrolyzed whole milk, or cereal–milk mixtures for the dietary management of acute childhood diarrhea. J Pediatr Gastroenterol Nutr. 1991;12:340–350.
108. Alarcon P, Montcya R, Perez F, et al. Clinical trial of home available, mixed diets versus a lactose-free, soy-protein formula for the dietary management of acute childhood diarrhea. J Pediatr Gastroenterol Nutr. 1991;12:224–232.
109. Chew F, Penna FJ, Peret Filho LA, et al. Is dilution of cows' milk formula necessary for dietary management of acute diarrhoea in infants aged less than 6 months? Lancet. 1993;341:194–197.
110. Gorbach SL. Bacterial diarrhea and its treatment. Lancet. 1987;2:1378–82.
111. The rational use of drugs in the management of acute diarrhoea in children. Geneva: World Health Organization; 1990.
112. Murtaza A, Khan SR, Butt KS, et al. Paralytic ileus, a serious complication in acute diarrhoea disease among infants in developing countries. Acta Paediatr Scand. 1989;78:701–705.
113. Gussin RZ. Withdrawal of loperamide drops. Lancet. 1990;335:1603.
114. Lo CW, Walker WA. Chronic protracted diarrhea in infancy: A nutritional disease. Pediatrics. 1983;72:786–800.

23

Gastrointestinal Infections in the Elderly

ROBERT L. OWEN, M.D.
JUDY F. LEW, M.D.

In the United States, Japan, and other industrialized countries, the elderly are the most rapidly growing segment of the population. Elderly persons are at increased risk of intestinal infection because of frequent institutionalization in nursing homes and hospitals and increased exposure to infectious agents among those who are able to travel. In addition, waning immunity, behavior changes related to hygiene, and alterations in the natural physiologic barriers that can be protective against infectious agents increase the risk of acquiring infectious gastroenteritis in this age group. The elderly may be subject to more severe and prolonged response to intestinal infection because of immunodeficiency, and may have greater susceptibility to complications because of preexisting medical problems. The impoverished elderly often have inadequate facilities for storage and proper preparation of food, thereby increasing the possibilities of foodborne infection. As the elderly population grows, there is an increased need to evaluate the epidemiology and approaches to the diagnosis, treatment, and prevention of potentially severe gastroenteritis in this age group.

EPIDEMIOLOGY

Infectious gastroenteritis is a major cause of acute diarrhea in the elderly.[1] Studies have shown that approximately 35 to 55% of adults, including the elderly, with acute gastroenteritis had an enteric pathogen detected in their stools.[2, 3] Furthermore, these detection rates of infectious causes likely represent an underestimate, because many gastrointestinal viruses presently are difficult to detect. The elderly are especially at risk for hospitalization due to an acute episode of diarrhea, as suggested by a study where more than 50% of adults who required hospitalization for their acute illness were over 60 years of age.[3]

Hospitalizations involving gastroenteritis appear to be an important problem among the elderly. In a study based on hospital discharge records from a large national database, adults 70 years of age and older were more likely to have complications of gastroenteritis than younger adults, who similarly had gastroenteritis among their top three discharge diagnoses.[4] Over the 1-year study period, adults over 60

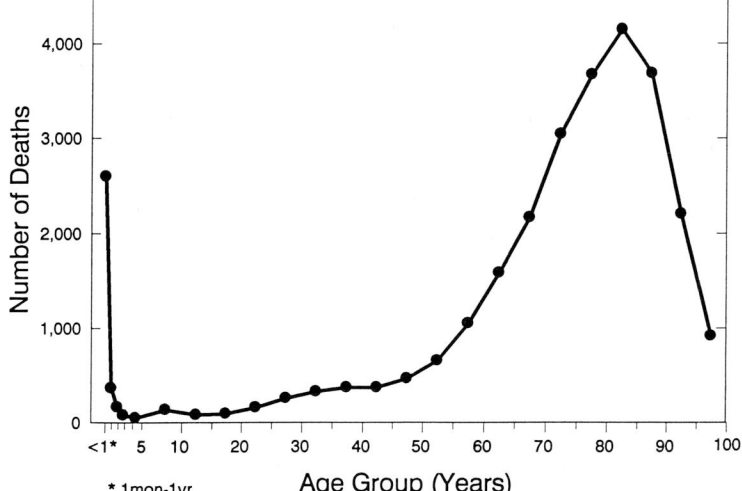

FIGURE 23–1.
Distribution of the ages of 28,538 persons dying from diarrhea, either as an immediate or underlying cause of death, in the United States from 1979 to 1987, showing peaks in numbers of deaths in the very young and the elderly. Over 51% of these deaths are in those over age 74 years. SOURCE: Death certificate information compiled by the National Center for Health Statistics, Hyattsville, MD.

years old comprised one fourth of all hospitalizations involving gastroenteritis, and this age group represented 85% of the diarrheal deaths. In addition, advanced age was found to be the most important risk factor for death subsequent to hospitalization that involved gastroenteritis.

Surprisingly, in industrialized countries, the elderly may be at highest risk of all age groups of death associated with diarrhea. The results of an analysis of national mortality data in the United States showed that the majority of the 28,538 deaths associated with diarrhea (diarrheal deaths) from 1979 to 1987 occurred in the elderly (older than 74 years of age).[5] For the 9-year study period, the majority of diarrheal deaths occurred in the old and the very young,

with the number of these deaths by age forming a J curve (Fig. 23–1). Fifty-one percent of all diarrheal deaths (14,603) were among the elderly (older than 74 years), 27% (7,827) were among adults 55 to 74 years of age, 11% (3,240) were among young children (1 month to 4 years), and the remaining 10% were among older children and adults 5 to 54 years of age. Age-specific mortality was also highest among the elderly (14.8 per 100,000 persons per year), second highest for adults 55 to 74 years of age (2.26/100,000), and next highest for children up to 4 years of age.

In the elderly, as in young children, deaths associated with diarrhea had clear winter seasonality (Fig. 23–2), even when diarrheal deaths

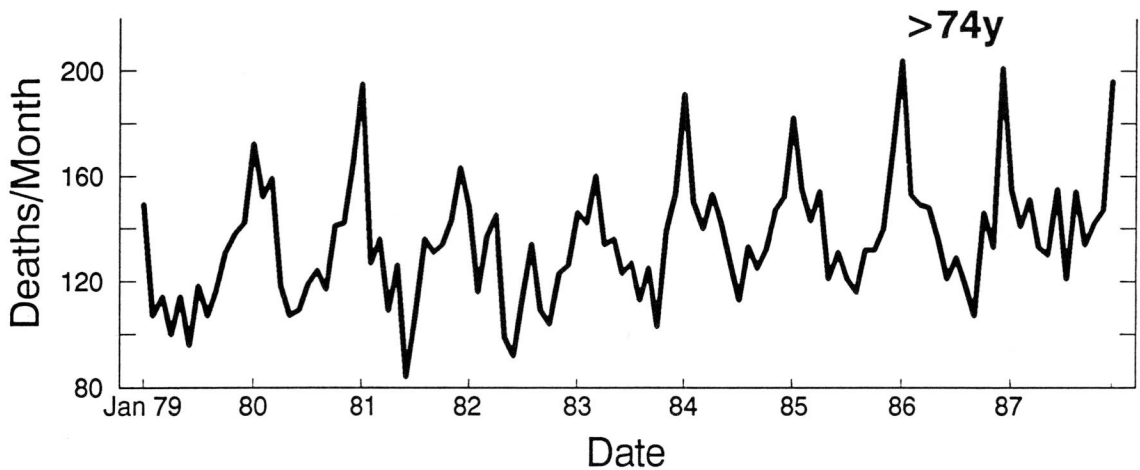

FIGURE 23–2.
Seasonality of diarrheal deaths in the elderly, over age 74 years, in the United States during the period 1979 to 1987. SOURCE: Death certificate information compiled by the National Center for Health Statistics, Hyattsville, MD.

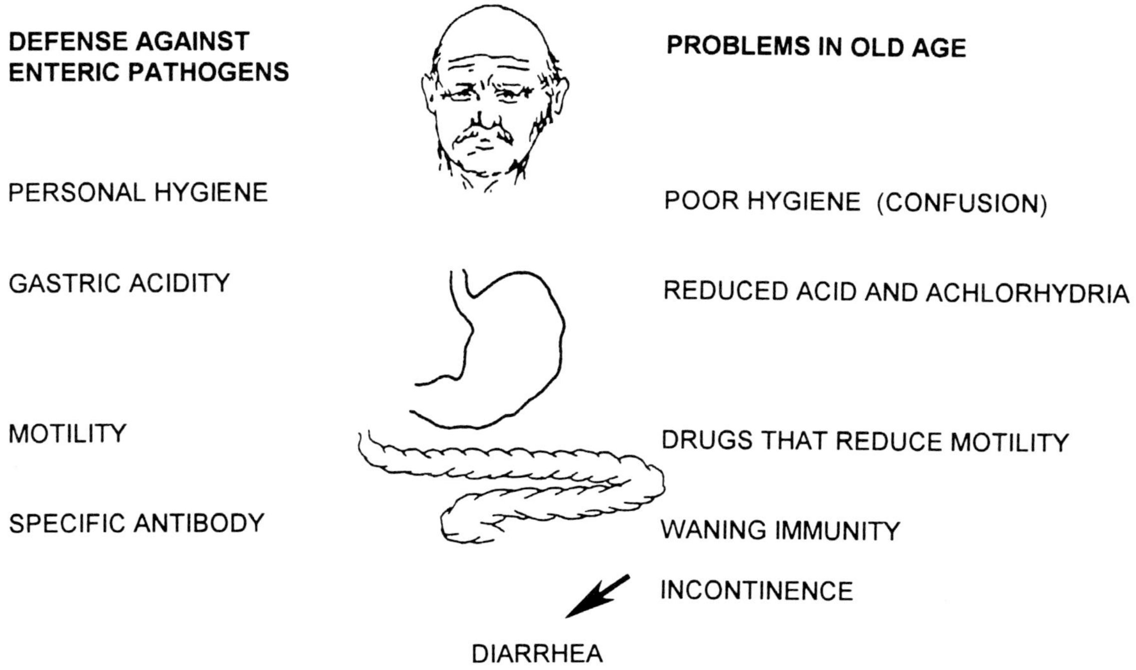

**DEFENSE AGAINST
ENTERIC PATHOGENS**

PROBLEMS IN OLD AGE

PERSONAL HYGIENE

POOR HYGIENE (CONFUSION)

GASTRIC ACIDITY

REDUCED ACID AND ACHLORHYDRIA

MOTILITY

DRUGS THAT REDUCE MOTILITY

SPECIFIC ANTIBODY

WANING IMMUNITY

INCONTINENCE

DIARRHEA

FIGURE 23–3.
Defenses against enteric pathogens and problems that can occur in the elderly, contributing to development of diarrheal diseases. SOURCE: Modified from Fox RA. Diarrhoea. In: Fox RA, ed. Immunology and Infection in the Elderly. Edinburgh: Churchill Livingstone; 1984:157–178.

that had a concurrent diagnosis of pneumonia were excluded, suggesting that infectious causes may be responsible for much of the diarrhea. Furthermore, diarrheal deaths in the elderly were disproportionately high for elderly white women, who form the bulk of the population in long-term care facilities, from which diarrheal outbreaks of presumed infectious origin are frequently reported.

Some of the physiologic and social factors that may predispose the elderly to acquiring infectious gastroenteritis and the associated complications are discussed below, as are special considerations concerning the clinical presentation and treatment of gastroenteritis in the elderly, and specific etiologic agents, including those that cause food poisoning and antibiotic-associated diarrhea. Faced with the potential of severe complications secondary to infectious gastroenteritis in the elderly, consideration should be given to more aggressive use of oral rehydration, reduction of nosocomial infections, and further evaluation of the epidemiology of enteric agents so that specific treatment and preventive strategies can be determined, if needed.

FACTORS PREDISPOSING TO INTESTINAL INFECTION

Physiologic Factors

Physiologic changes associated with aging may increase the rate of gastrointestinal infection. By definition, infections are acquired by ingestion of infectious agents and, with aging, many of the physiologic defenses that moderate growth of ingested bacteria and limit their proliferation within the gastrointestinal tract may be lost (Fig. 23–3).[6]

The major initial barrier to the entrance of pathogenic organisms into the gastrointestinal tract is the gastric acid barrier in the stomach. With a normal gastric pH of less than 4, most ingested bacteria will be killed. Consequently, at least 10^6 salmonellae must be ingested before there is a statistical likelihood that organisms will survive transit through the stomach in order to establish infection in the small intestine. With age and development of achlorhydia, ingestion of lower concentrations of microorganisms carries a risk of establishing intestinal infection, because of increased likelihood of transit of viable organisms through the stomach. Coliform counts in achlorhydric patients may be 1000 times greater than in normal subjects.[7] In addition to idiopathic achlorhydria, many elderly patients lack gastric acid because of prior gastric resections or because of medications taken to reduce gastric acid, including H_2 receptor antagonists (cimetidine, ranitidine) and proton pump blockers (omeprazole). There is a steady decline in acid production with age, which is more marked in females than in males, possibly on an autoimmune basis.

Viable infectious agents that pass through the stomach are prevented from reaching the mucosal surface by mucus that traps them in the lumen, where they are cleared by normal intestinal motility. Glycoproteins, which act as anchoring sites for microorganisms in the glycocalyx on enterocytes, are shed into the mucus, where they provide alternate microbial attachment sites. With age, the quality and quantity of mucus production may be adversely affected, facilitating microbial attachment and intestinal colonization. Motility is normally stimulated by fiber and bulk in the intestinal lumen and may consequently be reduced in patients on low-fiber diets, which are common in industrialized countries. Elderly patients concerned about intestinal gas production may also consciously choose a low-fiber diet, which contributes to reduced intestinal motility. Institutionalized patients on bed rest with little physical activity have prolonged intestinal transit times and frequent constipation, which may predispose to intestinal colonization and reduction in the normal intestinal clearance of microorganisms by peristalsis. Intestinal dysmotility may occur secondary to neurologic deterioration, prolonged diabetes, prior vagotomy, or prior surgical intestinal interruption with alteration in the normal intestinal pacemaker function. In addition, patients with chronic pain and frequent use of narcotic analgesics may suffer from reduced intestinal motility and impaired clearance of potential intestinal pathogens.

The intestinal immune system plays a major role in preventing and limiting intestinal symptoms following intestinal infection with pathogenic organisms. Infectious agents that reach the small intestine are taken up by M cells into lymphoid follicles in Peyer's patches or in isolated lymphoid follicles throughout the intestinal mucosa. Within lymphoid follicles, macrophages, dendritic cells, and other phagocytes break down microbes into antigenic components that are presented to lymphocytes, which then mount cellular and antibody immune responses. Sensitized lymphocytes replicate in lymphoid nodules and in mesenteric lymph nodes, pass through lymphatics to the general circulation, and distribute along the gastrointestinal tract in the lamina propria and in spaces between intestinal lining cells, where they are poised to produce secretory antibody, thereby limiting mucosal attachment, and are strategically positioned to destroy microorganisms that enter the epithelium. With age, the immunologic experience is great, but specific antibody production may be decreased, especially in patients with malnutrition or who are receiving immunosuppressive medications, including corticosteroids and chemotherapeutic agents. In elderly individuals, concentrations of IgA in serum and saliva are higher than in young subjects, and antibody in gut fluid is similar to that in younger age groups.[8] Secretory antibodies to common food antigens are of similar levels in the elderly as in younger controls. Primates were also found to have similar levels of total intestinal IgA in old and in young animals. However, when antigens to cholera were introduced for the first time, the specific IgA immune response in elderly (20 to 25 year old) primates was dramatically lower than in young (2 to 6 year old) monkeys.[9] This impaired ability to generate new specific antibody in response to encounters with new antigen may be related to inefficient T-helper cell function in the aged, or to precommitment of most available B cells.

Long-Term Care Facilities as Risk Factors for Intestinal Infection

Whenever groups of individuals are housed together, whether in day care centers, military barracks, or long-term care facilities for the aged, there is increased opportunity for exchange of infectious agents, with the possibility of epidemic spread of newly introduced pathogens. Retirement communities with separate living facilities but common eating accommodations, board and care facilities, nursing homes, and extended-care post-hospital facilities all offer opportunity for acquisition and spread of infectious agents. Crowding of residents and economic factors limiting the number of available caregivers increases the likelihood for nosocomial spread of enteric infections. Over-extended caregivers may have fewer opportunities for hand washing and must care for greater numbers of patients, which increases the likeli-

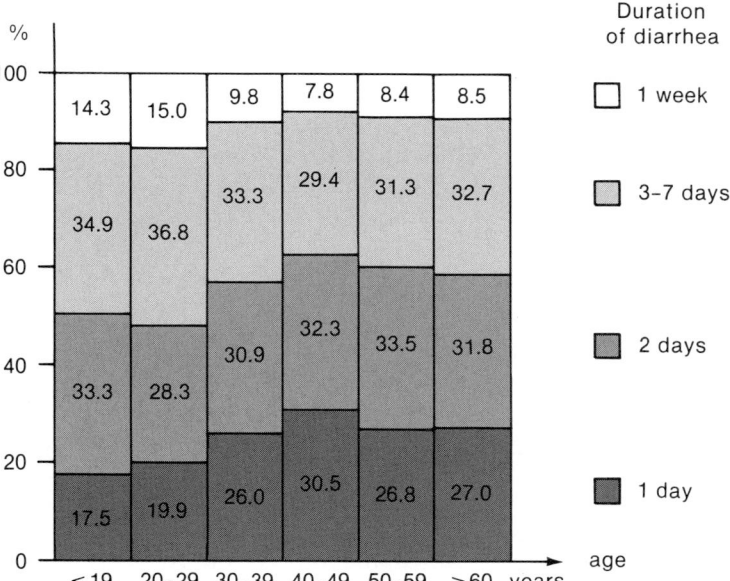

FIGURE 23–4.
Proportion of 3339 travellers to the tropics with travelers' diarrhea of various durations in six age groups. Travelers over age 60 years were less likely to have diarrhea lasting longer than 3 days than were travelers age 29 years and younger. SOURCE: Steffen R. Epidemiologic studies of travelers' diarrhea, severe gastrointestinal infections, and cholera. Rev Infect Dis. 1986; 8(suppl 2):S122–130.

hood of patient-to-patient spread of potential pathogens. Certain health characteristics that are commonly associated with the elderly also may increase the risk of significant enteric infection in this age group. For example, frequent use of antibiotics in elderly patients increases the likelihood that the normal enteric flora will be disturbed and replaced by enteropathogens of antibiotic-resistant strains. Incontinence in the elderly may increase the risk of fecal contamination of the environment in long-term geriatric facilities. Furthermore, because of dementia, depression, and economic deprivation, individual personal hygiene may deteriorate in elderly individuals, with reduced hand washing increasing the likelihood of hand-to-mouth transmission of infectious agents. Housing individuals in smaller living groups and restricting contact by caregivers to fewer patients may reduce the spread of infectious agents.

Travelers' Diarrhea in the Elderly

In contrast to the elderly infirm, who are exposed to risk of infection by housing in long-term care facilities, elderly individuals with relatively good health and adequate financial resources are at risk for different sorts of infections during travel. Popular tourist destinations in tropical and other unindustrialized areas have relatively limited sanitation facilities and water supply systems that are inadequate for ever-increasing populations. Travelers who hope to avoid infection risks by remaining on board cruise ships may also be at risk because of contamination of water supply facilities or food-borne outbreaks on board ship.

Surprisingly, the gastrointestinal infection rate may be lower in elderly travelers than in younger travelers. One study found that 33% of those less than 24 years of age experienced gastrointestinal infection, whereas only 18% of those over 55 years of age were so infected.[10] Several explanations have been proposed for this difference in infection rate. Possible reasons include greater immunologic experience among the elderly, less adventurous travel style, less likelihood of eating improperly prepared food on the street and in local restaurants with poor food preparation techniques, and smaller appetites that cause the consumption of fewer potential pathogens.[11] Patients older than 29 years of age are also inconvenienced for shorter periods of time than are younger travelers (Fig. 23–4). However, when travelers' diarrhea does strike, the consequences may be more severe in the elderly because of their greater susceptibility to dehydration due to poor general health and because of the increased likelihood of cardiovascular complications. A variety of infectious agents may be responsible for travelers' diarrhea, but in the elderly, as in the young, toxigenic *Escherichia coli* is the most commonly identified pathogen. Prophylactic use of antibiotics is ineffective during extended periods of travel, but a variety of antibiotics, if begun quickly after the initiation of symptoms, have proven effective in shortening the duration of episodes of travelers' diarrhea.[12] Patients with special susceptibility to dehydration should be given supplies of antibiotics such as ciprofloxacin or trimethoprim/sulfamethoxazole, to be taken as soon as travelers' diarrhea begins. Furthermore, bismuth subsalicylates have been shown to be of some use in treatment. Patients should be advised to avoid raw, unpeeled fruits and vegetables, food from street vendors, and ice. Beverages prepared from boiled water or bottled beverages should be consumed wherever possible in order to reduce risk of ingestion of pathogenic organisms.

SPECIAL CONSIDERATIONS IN THE ELDERLY

Clinical Presentation

In the elderly, as in younger patients, there is a progression of symptoms, beginning with upper gastrointestinal tract manifestations of infection (including nausea and vomiting), and progression to diarrhea as the infection moves more distally along the gastrointestinal tract. However, presentation of intestinal infections in the elderly may be less overt than in younger patients, with a different constellation of medical symptoms and a different range of complications.[13] Gastroenteritis in the elderly may not always be accompanied by diarrhea, especially in patients with chronic constipation, in whom there may instead be a "normalization" of bowel pattern with softer and more frequent stools, and without frank diarrhea. Although gastroenteritis may be accompanied by abdominal pain and leukocytosis, these manifestations may be relatively mild. In patients who do not develop diarrhea, or in whom diarrhea is either not noted or not reported, the first manifestation of acute gastroenteritis may be dehydration. Hypotension and confusion may be the only presenting symptoms.[11] Elderly patients who live alone may become dehydrated and disoriented and may be unable to give a relevant history when they are brought to medical attention. Similarly, institutionalized patients and others with short-term memory loss may not recall episodes of diarrhea, which may be overlooked unless noted by ancillary care providers.

The consequences of dehydration may be particularly severe in the elderly because of underlying health problems. Electrolyte depletion, especially loss of potassium, is of particular concern in patients who are taking diuretics and other cardiac medications. With vascular collapse and impaired perfusion of atherosclerotic blood vessels, patients may be susceptible to secondary myocardial infarction, cerebral infarction, and bowel ischemia. Infectious gastroenteritis with watery diarrhea thus can lead to ischemic colitis with mucoid or bloody diarrhea.

Fecal leukocytes may suggest an infectious cause; when fecal occult blood is present, an invasive enteropathogen such as Campylobacter, Salmonella, or Shigella should be considered. Stool cultures for bacterial pathogens and a stool rotavirus-specific enzyme-linked immunosorbent assay (ELISA) test for identification of intestinal rotavirus infection may be useful. Detection of specific infectious agents is of greatest concern in institutional settings, where there are serious epidemiologic considerations of the spread of diarrhea to other residents. In most cases, therapeutic intervention should focus on fluid replacement, regardless of the responsible etiologic agent.

Therapeutic Approach to Gastroenteritis in the Elderly

As in children, oral replacement of fluids is preferable to intravenous replacement, which can be complicated by line infections, overhydration, congestive failure, and development of fluid and electrolyte imbalance. Replacement solutions that contain glucose are more readily absorbed than those without glucose because of the beneficial effect of glucose on stimulating fluid transport by enterocytes. Patients should be advised to avoid drinking liquids containing caffeine, including coffee, tea, and cola drinks, which may stimulate peristalsis. During gastroenteritis, milk and milk products should also be avoided. Acute lactase deficiency may accompany gastroenteritis due to damage to mature enterocytes on villi, with temporary loss of lactase in the microvillous border. Patients should also avoid diet sodas, which lack glucose, and should generally avoid carbonated soft drinks, which may produce gastric distention and reflex colonic emptying, thereby exacerbating diarrhea.

If vomiting is not present, bismuth subsalicylate may be useful in absorbing enterotoxins, which may be contributing to infectious diarrhea. Antimotility agents such as diphenoxylate with atropine (Lomotil) or loperamide (Imodium) may prolong symptoms due to invasive bacteria, such as Shigella, and should be used with caution in elderly patients, particularly those with reduced hepatic and renal function. In elderly patients, drug levels may build up, producing lethargy. Loperamide, which is less permeable to the blood–brain barrier, may be less likely to produce central nervous system depression than diphenoxylate with atropine. There is also a theoretic risk that these antimotility agents may prolong infection by retarding clearance of infectious agents from the gastrointestinal tract by peristalsis.

SPECIFIC ETIOLOGIC AGENTS

Infectious agents that commonly cause gastroenteritis in the elderly may differ somewhat from those in the younger age groups; this is in part due to differences in immune status and exposure rates. For example, rotavirus is an important cause of diarrhea in infants and young children, but is only occasionally detected in the elderly. Brief descriptions of specific infectious agents as they pertain to gastroenteritis in the elderly follow, with an emphasis on those associated with epidemics in long-term care facilities. Furthermore, agents that cause foodborne or antibiotic-associated diarrhea, of which the elderly may be particularly at risk, are discussed.

Viral Gastroenteritis

Norwalk Virus

Norwalk and Norwalk-like viruses are the most common known viral etiologic agents of epidemic gastroenteritis in adults, including the elderly.[14] The incubation period for a Norwalk virus infection is 24 to 48 hours, with nausea, vomiting, nonbloody diarrhea, and abdominal cramps being common symptoms that typically last 12 to 60 hours. Vomiting can be a particularly prominent symptom in patients with Norwalk virus illness. In epidemics of self-limiting, nonbloody diarrhea, where vomiting occurs in approximately 50% or more of those who are ill, Norwalk and related viruses should be strongly considered as possible etiologic agents. Transmission can occur by person-to-person (fecal/oral) contact, food or water source contamination, and possibly by aerosol spread. Outbreaks of Norwalk virus diarrhea in nursing homes are a particular problem; in the elderly, persistence of constitutional symptoms for up to several weeks has been reported. Furthermore, outbreaks of Norwalk virus gastroenteritis in nursing homes have been associated with death in debilitated elderly patients with diffuse atherosclerosis.[15]

The results of past studies have shown that immunity to Norwalk virus infection appears to be transient.[16] In nursing homes, where both person-to-person transmission and common source transmission are major risk factors, attack rates can be quite high. In a geriatric convalescent facility in Los Angeles, 55% of patients and 25% of employees were affected during a midwinter outbreak of Norwalk virus gastroenteritis. However, although 55% of 188 geriatric convalescent facility patients became ill in a recent epidemic, there was no increase in death rate.[17] Detection by electron microscopy (EM) of the characteristic morphology of Norwalk virus, a 27-nm virus with an amorphous surface and a feathery edge, in the stool of a patient with gastroenteritis suggests a Norwalk or Norwalk-like virus infection. However, specific diagnosis of a Norwalk virus infection is usually only done at research centers where assays that require Norwalk virus stool antigen, Norwalk virus specific-antibody, or the recently expressed recombinant Norwalk virus capsid protein are available. ELISAs that make use of the recombinant capsid protein may make specific testing available for general medical use in the near future. In geriatric facilities and other institutions, enteric precautions, including restriction of visitors, emphasis on hand washing, and cohorting of ill patients and previously ill staff, may limit further spread of infection. Prevention of severe dehydration by oral hydration or, if necessary, intravenous fluid administration can avoid serious complications in the elderly.[17–19]

Caliciviruses

Other human caliciviruses besides the Norwalk virus, which has only recently been shown to be a member of the Caliciviridae family, have also been associated with diarrhea in the elderly.[20–22] These "classical" caliciviruses are distinguished by a different characteristic morphologic appearance and size than that of the Norwalk virus as seen by EM. The epidemiologic and immunologic relationships between Norwalk virus and classical caliciviruses have not yet been defined; for the purposes of this discussion, these classical caliciviruses will be called "caliciviruses." In outbreaks of gastroenteritis associated with calicivirus in long-term facilities for the elderly in England and in Canada, both residents and staff have been affected, with attack rates for the residents ranging from 27 to 100%.[20–23] In geriatric facilities, symptoms with calicivirus gastroenteritis have been relatively mild, and vomiting and diarrhea are described as the most common symptoms. Abdominal cramps, headaches, malaise, bodily aches, and fever were reported less frequently.[20, 22, 23] Duration of symptoms was usually from 12 to 48 hours[20-22]; however, two patients had symptoms lasting more than 3 days and required intravenous hydration.[23] These and other outbreaks of calicivirus infection have implicated person-to-person contact, food, or water as modes of transmission. Although illness in these outbreaks was not severe or long-standing, major commitment of health care resources was required, including time of physicians, nurses, and public health officers, along with laboratory expense in defining the nature of these outbreaks.

Identification of calicivirus as responsible for outbreaks of gastroenteritis in facilities for the elderly has been useful for avoiding unnecessary antibiotics, because no specific antiviral agents are presently available. Diagnosis is usually made by observation of the characteristic morphology (32- to 35-nm particles that appear to have 32 "cupped" depressions arranged in icosahedral symmetry as a surface feature) of these viruses in stool specimens by EM. Treatment is the same as for illness due to Norwalk virus, providing oral or intraveneous rehydration as needed. Institution of epidemiologic control measures, including careful personal hygiene, good food-handling techniques, limiting visitors, stopping new admissions, and confining symptomatic patients to one housing area, may be reasonable, although such measures have not been shown always to be effective in stopping epidemics within a given institution.

Astrovirus

A limited number of acute gastroenteritis outbreaks due to astrovirus among the elderly have been reported since 1981,[19, 21, 24] and the importance of these agents in causing disease in this age group is unknown. In the first reported outbreak, infections occurred over a 3-month period, with an overall attack rate of 51% in 187 convalescent hospital residents. However, symptoms were generally mild, usually consisting only of diarrhea, although nausea and vomiting did occur uncommonly. Illness in most residents lasted 3 days. There is some suggestion that prior viral gastroenteritis may predispose to astrovirus infection. In two other outbreaks in facilities for the elderly, astrovirus infection followed outbreaks with another intestinal virus—calicivirus[21] or rotavirus.[24] Routes of transmission that have been reported include water, food (shellfish-associated), and person-to-person contact. The identification of astrovirus as the cause of gastroenteritis is important in order

to determine the appropriate treatment and preventative measures. Diagnosis is usually made by observation of the characteristic 28-nm size and the five- to six- point, star-like form of these viruses in stool specimens by EM. Other methods of diagnosis, such as use of ELISAs specific for astrovirus, are usually available only at research centers. Treatment is mainly symptomatic, with oral or intravenous rehydration as needed.

Rotaviruses

Rotaviruses are double-stranded RNA viruses that can cause both endemic and epidemic gastroenteritis, most commonly during the winter months in temperate climates. Although group A rotavirus has been shown to be the most common single etiologic agent of severe diarrhea in infants and young children, little is known concerning the public health importance of this virus in causing disease in the elderly. Although typically 90% of children have acquired antibodies to rotavirus by the age of 5 years, infection with one of the four serotypes of group A rotavirus responsible for most of the human disease may not provide resistance to disease or infection from one of the others. Acquired immunity may be type-specific, although there may be a broadening of immunity (heterotypic immunity) with age and repeated infections. Hence, symptoms in young and middle-aged adults are usually milder than those in infants and are often asymptomatic, possibly because of previously acquired immunity. With the waning of acquired immunity, rotavirus infections may again become a problem among elderly persons, as suggested by several case reports of rotavirus gastroenteritis in nursing homes and other group care settings.

In contrast to the generally mild pattern of symptoms with group A rotavirus gastroenteritis in younger adults, severe gastroenteritis and death have been reported during epidemics in geriatric populations. In closed populations of the elderly, attack rates of up to 66% have been observed, with epidemics reported in geriatric wards, nursing homes, geriatric hospitals, and among elderly patients in a cardiology ward. Fecal/oral spread is presumed to involve both contaminated environmental surfaces and person-to-person transmission by staff members moving between patients in geriatric units.[25, 26] Patients over 60 years of age may have higher attack rates of illness with rotaviral infection than may younger adults, and older patients also appear to have more severe clinical manifestations. Deaths due to group A rotavirus infection in adults have only been observed in the elderly, possibly because of relative malnutrition and greater susceptibility to the consequences of dehydration.[27, 28] However, even when dehydration is severe in the elderly, if oral and intravenous rehydration is maintained, symptoms usually resolve within 2 to 6 days.

Diagnosis of group A rotavirus infections usually can be made by detecting the group antigen in stools by using commercially available enzyme immunoassays (EIAs). These EIAs have greatly facilitated the recognition of group A rotavirus as a cause of epidemic viral gastroenteritis in both nonpediatric and pediatric settings. Diagnosis of a rotavirus infection can also be made by detection of the rotavirus's characteristic 70-nm size and wheel-like (double-capsid) appearance by direct EM. However, the morphology of group A rotavirus cannot be distinguished by direct EM from groups B and C rotaviruses (groups that have only recently been associated with diarrheal disease in humans). Instead, these three groups of double-stranded RNA viruses can be distinguished by the characteristic electrophoretic patterns their 11-segmented genomes produce on polyacrylamide gels. Treatment, as for other viral gastrointestinal illnesses, primarily consists of prevention of severe dehydration by oral hydration or, if necessary, intravenous fluid administration to avoid serious complications.

Bacterial Gastroenteritis

Shigella

Outbreaks of shigellosis have been reported in geriatric facilities[29] but are uncommon. Among 116 adult patients hospitalized for sporadic shigellosis, 32 were older than 70 years of age (Table 23–1).[30] In this study, shigellosis occurred more frequently in the summer season, in contrast to the winter peaks of Norwalk virus and rotavirus. Diarrhea and fever were the most common symptoms in this population, followed in prevalence by abdominal pain and vomiting. Bloody diarrhea was present in only one third of the patients, and was somewhat more common in those with *Shigella flexneri* than in those with *S. sonnei*. Shigella infection produces symptoms in the small bowel by toxin production, which results in watery diarrhea. In the colon, tissue invasion produces bacillary dysentery that is characterized by frequent small movements of blood and mucus. The most virulent Shigella infections, with *S. dysenteriae* 1 (the Shiga bacillus), are infrequent in developed countries, but

TABLE 23–1. DEMOGRAPHIC DATA FOR PATIENTS HOSPITALIZED WITH SHIGELLOSIS FROM 1975 TO 1985, AT TEL AVIV MEDICAL CENTER

DISTRIBUTION	AGE (YRS), MEAN ± SD (RANGE)	NUMBER OF PATIENTS
All patients	48 ± 25.2 (15–91)	116
	<40	49
	40–70	35
	>70	32
Sex		
Men	48 ± 25.5	61
Women	49 ± 24.9	55
Ethnic origin		
European	57.6 ± 23.1	57
Middle Eastern	52.7 ± 21.6	50
Unknown		9

SOURCE: Halpern Z, Dan M, Giladi M, et al. Shigellosis in adults: Epidemiologic, clinical, and laboratory features. Medicine. 1989;68:210–217.

S. flexneri does produce a prolonged clinical course in patients over age 40 years, with persisting diarrhea and fever. The severity of symptoms with *S. flexneri* continues to increase with the age of the patient, unlike *S. sonnei* infections, which are relatively mild even in the elderly. Laboratory findings in adults include leukocytosis, hypokalemia, and other abnormalities of serum electrolytes. Elderly patients with shigellosis also develop elevation of blood urea nitrogen and liver enzyme abnormalities unrelated to the degree of fever. Cardiac arrhythmias, ischemic changes, and myocardial infarction have been observed in elderly patients with Shigella infection.[30] Fluid replacement is often adequate therapy in milder cases of shigellosis, but among elderly patients with relatively severe systemic infections, antibiotics are indicated, with choice of the specific antibiotic determined by local drug-resistance patterns.

Escherichia coli 0157:H7

In 1982, a new *E. coli* serotype, 0157:H7, was recognized as a major human intestinal pathogen to which elderly patients are particularly susceptible. This serotype and a variety of other *E. coli* strains, which produce verocytotoxins, also known as Shiga-like toxins (SLTs), are associated with a variety of syndromes, including nonbloody diarrhea, hemorrhagic colitis, the hemolytic uremic syndrome, and thrombotic thrombocytopenia purpura.[31] The very young and the very old seem to be at particular risk for *E. coli* 0157:H7 infections. Outbreaks of *E. coli* 0157:H7 diarrhea are usually foodborne and often associated with undercooked bovine meat. Such outbreaks commonly occur in nursing homes, with the highest attack rate among the oldest patients. Reported deaths from this agent have occurred primarily among the elderly, although deaths among young children have also occurred.

Due to its broad spectrum of clinical manifestations, *E. coli* 0157:H7 is often not recognized, especially because most clinical microbiology labs do not routinely culture stool specimens for this organism. Because of the severity of associated abdominal cramps and intestinal bleeding, the low number of fecal leukocytes, and the lack of fever, this infection is often mistaken for a noninfectious process, especially ischemic bowel disease in the elderly or inflammatory bowel disease in younger adults.[32] Sigmoidoscopy shows erythema and edema, with increasing frequency of abnormalities from the rectum to the cecum. There is often ileus on abdominal plain radiographs, and evidence of submucosal edema on barium enema.

These *E. coli* strains are sensitive to most antimicrobial agents; however, the duration of diarrhea is unchanged by treatment, and there is no clear evidence of a beneficial effect of their use. Some investigators have found that patients who die with this organism are more likely to have received antimicrobial therapy than those who survived. Previous gastrectomy and antimicrobial therapy prior to onset of illness have been associated with development of systemic infection. In a review of nine major outbreaks, all reported deaths occurred in the elderly, with a mortality rate of up to 35% in infected elderly nursing home residents.[32] Replacing fluid losses and correcting electrolyte imbalances are clearly of benefit in infections with this group of *E. coli* serotypes.

Salmonella

There are approximately 2000 recognized serotypes of Salmonella, many of which are potential pathogens for animals and humans. Because these intestinal microbes are common in a wide range of domesticated and wild animals, they frequently contaminate water and certain food items, especially eggs and chicken.[33] The majority of Salmonella infections cause gastroenteritis of varying severity, usually lasting 3 to 4 days. There is a wide clinical spectrum of Salmonella gastroenteritis symptoms in nursing home patients. Although some infections are asymptomatic or only mildly debilitating, Salmonella outbreaks can be a particular problem in nursing homes because the elderly are prone to have

underlying medical conditions that may complicate illness.[34] Use of antimicrobial agents both decreases resistance to initial infection and prolongs carriage of Salmonella strains.[35] Ciprofloxacin 500 mg twice daily for 7 days appears, however, to have been effective in eliminating Salmonella from both asymptomatic and symptomatic geriatric facility patients.[36]

Aeromonas hydrophila

Aeromonas hydrophila has been implicated in an outbreak of acute gastroenteritis in a long-term care facility for the aged.[37] Among 17 patients with an average age of 87 years, the majority of cases were mild, having two to four loose stools over a period of illness that persisted only 48 hours or less.[37] One patient, however, after 10 episodes of loose stools, developed tachycardia, tachypnea, and hypotension; death ensued, despite intravenous fluids for the last 8 hours of her 24-hour illness. In general, institutional outbreaks of *A. hydrophila* have occurred in the summer months, when aeromonads are increased in aquatic reservoirs, including pools and hospital sinks. Abrupt onset in groups of patients over a short period of time has been attributed to a foodborne or waterborne source of infection. In most cases of mild diarrhea, replacement of fluids and electrolytes is adequate therapy. In patients who are more seriously ill, antimicrobial agents may be necessary.

Campylobacter jejuni

Campylobacter jejuni has a peak incidence in preschool children but also has a second peak in young adults (see Chapter 6) and was the most commonly identified cause of diarrhea in a group of patients hospitalized on geriatric units and with community-acquired diarrhea (Table 23–2). Infections with *Campylobacter jejuni* often manifest as severe bloody diarrhea. In a community outbreak of *Campylobacter jejuni* in Norway associated with contaminated drinking water, patients of all ages reported symptoms. The highest attack rate (85.2%) was in the age group 5 to 14 years, followed by those older than 85 years (75%).[37a] Stool culture is required to identify *Campylobacter jejuni* infection, and symptoms have often subsided by the time culture results are available. Bacteremia with *Campylobacter jejuni* is, however, 20 times more common in those over 65 years of age (5.9 cases per 1000 intestinal Campylobacter infections) than in children ages 1 to 4 (0.3/1000).[37b] In septicemic patients, parenteral antibiotics are required (see Chapter 6).

TABLE 23–2. INCIDENCE OF ENTERIC PATHOGENS ISOLATED FROM 200 PATIENTS WITH INFECTIVE DIARRHEA*

FECAL PATHOGENS	NUMBER	(%)
Campylobacter jejuni	67	(33.5)
Salmonella spp.	57	(28.5)
Enterotoxigenic *C. perfringens*	25	(12.5)
Cryptosporidium	20	(10.0)
Shigella spp.	12	(6.0)
C. difficile	9	(4.5)
E. coli 0157:H7	7	(3.5)
Yersinia enterocolitica	2	(1.0)
Vibrio parahaemolyticus	1	(0.5)
Total	200	(100)

*Of the 25 patients with *C. perfringens*, only two were under age 60 years, and only seven had not received antibiotics preceding diarrhea.

SOURCE: Samuel SC, Hancock P, Leigh DA. An investigation into *Clostridium perfringens* enterotoxin-associated diarrhea. J Hosp Infect. 1991;18:219–230.

Parasitic Infection

Cryptosporidium

Intestinal infection with Cryptosporidium has been detected in many different groups of individuals, including infants in daycare centers, farmers exposed to domestic animals with diarrhea, immunodeficient patients, and the elderly. In immunocompetent patients, this infection usually produces illness of 5 to 14 days' duration and is usually characterized by watery diarrhea, abdominal cramps, nausea, mild fever, and weight loss; it is self-limiting. In the elderly, although disease symptoms with cryptosporidia infection may be similar to those of other age groups, more severe symptoms can also occur, with profuse diarrhea leading to dehydration, hypokalemia, and anemia.[38, 39] The severity of infection in elderly patients may resemble that seen in immunocompromised patients, even though no specific immunodeficiencies are noted.[39]

Giardia lamblia

An outbreak of giardiasis in a nursing home in Minnesota was associated with contact between nursing home residents and children attending a daycare center on the premises.[40] In this outbreak, 73% of 35 elderly participants in an "adopt-a-grandparent" program developed diarrhea. Although only a few of the ill patients reported other symptoms, such as vomiting and abdominal cramps, the morbidity was significant—the mean duration of diarrhea was 16 days with a mean weight loss of 1.4 kg. Transmission was thought to be caused by infected food handlers, as well as by person-to-person transmission from children visiting from the daycare center.

FOOD POISONING

The elderly are at particular risk for foodborne intestinal infections, both in nursing homes and in private residences. Between 1975 and 1987, 115 outbreaks of foodborne disease were reported in nursing homes in 26 states, with illness in 4944 individuals and death in 51.[41] These nursing home outbreaks represented 2% of all foodborne disease outbreaks reported to the Centers for Disease Control, but included 19% of all outbreak-associated deaths for this period. Salmonella accounted for 52% of these outbreaks and 81% of the deaths, with *Salmonella enteritidis* identified as the major serotype, usually associated with eggs or equipment contaminated by eggs. Staphylococcal foodborne disease accounted for 23% of outbreaks. *Clostridium perfringens* was identified in 5% of outbreaks. Other bacterial causes of foodborne disease outbreaks in nursing homes included *Bacillus cereus*, *Campylobacter jejuni*, *Shigella sonnei*, and *Escherichia coli* 0157:87, each of which was responsible for one outbreak. *Staphylococcus aureus* outbreaks were often associated with salad, *C. perfringens* outbreaks with different kinds of meats, and *E. coli* 0157:H7 with undercooked hamburger.

Factors in foodborne transmission in nursing homes included improper storage or holding temperatures for food, poor personal hygiene of food handlers, contaminated equipment, inadequate cooking, and food from unsafe sources. The case fatality rate in nursing homes was 10 times the case fatality rate for outbreaks in other settings.[40]

Elderly individuals living alone are also at risk of foodborne diseases, because of economic and social factors. Many retired elderly, especially in central cities, live in housing facilities without refrigeration or adequate cooking facilities. Economic limitations, reluctance to dispose of possibly inedible food, and lack of awareness of how long food should be kept without refrigeration, contribute to contamination with staphylococci or clostridia and their associated toxins. In the Netherlands, 214 self-supporting elderly between the ages of 65 and 80 years were investigated regarding food storage and preparation, and the prevalence of diarrhea and vomiting. In the 3 months prior to interview, 20% had diarrhea and 13% vomiting.[42] Among the 70% with hazardous food hygiene, 22% reported diarrhea. Among 35 persons without hazardous practices, the prevalence of diarrhea was only 6%, indicating a statistically significant association between food hygiene practices and diarrheal disease. Older people living alone reported more hazardous food storage and preparation practices than people living with someone else. Of those living alone, men were more likely than women to follow unsafe practices. The temperature of the refrigerators used by 20% of the elderly investigated in this survey was 8°C or higher, which is too warm for adequate food preservation.

ANTIBIOTIC-ASSOCIATED INFECTIONS IN THE ELDERLY

Clostridium difficile

C. difficile, a bacterium that in spore form persists on floors, clothes, hands, and throughout the environment, is a particular problem in chronic care facilities for the elderly. A high percentage of nursing home residents are given antibiotics that alter normal intestinal flora and permit overgrowth of antibiotic-resistant C. difficile strains, magnifying individual and environmental contamination with C. difficile. In one survey of stool specimens from patients treated with antibiotics in a long-term care facility, one third were infected with C. difficile. The incidence of postantibiotic infection was 70% on the chronic care ward, 26% in nursing home wards, and 0% on a rehabilitation ward.[43] Infected patients tended to be older, with dementia and stool incontinence. In this survey, nausea, vomiting, and abdominal pain were infrequent, and pseudomembranous colitis was not observed. Nonetheless, infected patients had a higher death rate at the end of 1 year than uninfected subjects. Although few had gastrointestinal symptoms, more than half of those infected with C. difficile had positive stool titers of C. difficile cytotoxin. Although C. difficile carriers may often be asymptomatic, many patients with C. difficile toxin in their stools will have diarrhea with severity varying from infrequent loose or watery stools, to severe diarrhea (up to 30 watery stools per day), usually without gross blood. Diarrhea can persist for weeks or months.

For those developing pseudomembranous colitis, C. difficile toxin is almost universally present. When C. difficile toxin assay is negative in this setting, endoscopy is indicated to look for other causes of bloody diarrhea. For patients with negative C. difficile toxin assay, it is important to discontinue implicated antibacterial agents.[44] When toxin is present, the usual treatment is to stop the prior antibiotic, if possible, and begin vancomycin 125 mg by mouth, four times a day for 7 to 14 days, or metronidazole 500 mg by mouth, twice a day for 7 to 14 days.

Clostridium perfringens

Elderly hospital patients are also at risk for diarrhea associated with the presence of enterotoxigenic Clostridium perfringens. In a survey in a geriatric hospital, 25 patients were identified with C. perfringens diarrhea, 18 of whom had received antibiotics prior to the onset of the diarrhea. C. perfringens was the third most commonly identified fecal pathogen in this population (Table 23–2). Cases often occurred in patients in close proximity to one another, and especially in patients 70 years of age or older. In patients in whom C. perfringens enterotoxin continued to be present, diarrhea also persisted. Diarrhea, enterotoxin, and clostridial counts all subsided after treatment with metronidazole.[45] Patient-to-patient cross infection with C. perfringens or C. difficile may occur. Hospital environments contaminated with clostridia may show persistence of the organism for 5 months or longer, particularly in the rooms of patients with severe diarrhea associated with these organisms. High rates of positivity are noted on toilets, sinks, bathroom floors, under patients' beds, and on patients' bedclothes.[46]

Candida albicans

Hospitalized patients receiving antibiotics may develop severe diarrhea associated with Candida overgrowth.[47] Candida diarrhea is usually watery, and without blood, mucus, or abdominal pain. It occurs predominantly in elderly, malnourished, and critically ill patients, as well as in those with chronic debilitating diseases. Colonoscopy is often unrevealing. Because Candida is so prevalent, it may be overlooked as a possible pathogen in elderly patients with diarrhea. When diarrhea is associated with Candida infection, it tends to be secretory, with stool volumes ranging up to 3 L per day, producing volume depletion, prerenal azotemia, and hyperchloremic metabolic acidosis that requires intravenous fluid replacement. The significance of Candida albicans in such patients can be clarified by response to oral nystatin, 500,000 U every 6 hours for 2 to 4 days. The role of Candida infection in the production of diarrhea is illustrated by the association of fecal Candida counts with numbers of stools per day, and the drop in both stool numbers and Candida counts following nystatin therapy.[48]

REFERENCES

1. Holt PR. Diarrhea and malabsorption in the elderly. Gastroenterol Clin North Am. 1990;19:345–359.
2. Pryor WM, Bye WA, Curran DH, Grohmann GS. Acute diarrhea in adults: A prospective study. Med J Aust. 1987;147:490–493.
3. Svanteson B, Thoren A, Castor B, et al. Acute diarrhea in adults: Aetiology, clinical appearance and therapeutic aspects. Scand J Infect Dis. 1988;20:303–314.
4. Gangarosa RE, Glass RI, Lew JF, Boring JR. Hospitalizations involving gastroenteritis in the United States, 1985: The special burden of the disease among the elderly. Am J Epidemiol. 1992;135:280–290.
5. Lew JF, Glass RI, Gangarosa RE, et al. Diarrheal deaths in the United States, 1979 through 1987. JAMA. 1991;265:3280–3284.
6. Fox RA. Diarrhoea. In: Fox RA, ed. Immunology and Infection in the Elderly. Edinburgh: Churchill Livingstone; 1984:157–178.
7. Giannella RA, Broitman SA, Zamcheck N. Influence of gastric acidity on bacterial and parasitic enteric infections. Ann Intern Med. 1973;78:271–276.
8. Arranz E, O'Mahony S, Barton JR, Ferguson A. Immunosenescence and mucosal immunity: Significant effects of old age on secretory IgA concentrations and intraepithelial lymphocyte counts. Gut. 1992;33:882–886.
9. Taylor LD, Daniels CK, Schmucker DL. Ageing compromises gastrointestinal mucosal immune response in the rhesus monkey. Immunology. 1992;75:614–618.
10. MacDonald KL, Cohen ML. Epidemiology of travelers' diarrhea: Current perspectives. Rev Infect Dis. 1986;8(suppl 2):S117–121.
11. Steffen R. Epidemiologic studies of travelers' diarrhea, severe gastrointestinal infections, and cholera. Rev Infect Dis. 1986;8(suppl 2):S122–130.
12. Patterson JE, Patterson TF, Bia FJ, Barry M. Assuring safe travel for today's elderly. Geriatrics. 1989;44:44–46, 49–53, 57.
13. Maasdam CF, Anuras S. Are you overlooking GI infections in your elderly patients? Geriatrics. 1981;36:127–134.
14. LeBaron CW, Furutan NP, Lew JF, et al. Viral agents of gastroenteritis: Public health importance and outbreak management. MMWR. 1990;39(RR5):1–24.
15. Kaplan JE, Gary GW, Baron RC, et al. Epidemiology of Norwalk gastroenteritis and the role of Norwalk virus in outbreaks of acute nonbacterial gastroenteritis. Ann Intern Med. 1982;96:756–761.
16. Parrino TA, Schreiber DS, Trier JS, et al. Clinical immunity in acute gastroenteritis caused by Norwalk agent. N Engl J Med. 1977;297:86–89.
17. Gellert GA, Waterman SH, Ewert D, et al. An outbreak of acute gastroenteritis caused by a small round structured virus in a geriatric convalescent facility. Infect Control Hosp Epidemiol. 1990;11:459–464.
18. Kaplan JE, Schonberger LB, Varano G, et al. An outbreak of acute nonbacterial gastroenteritis in a nursing home. Am J Epidemiol. 1982;116:940–948.
19. Oshiro LS, Haley CE, Roberto RR, et al. A 27-nm virus isolated during an outbreak of acute infectious nonbacterial gastroenteritis in a convalescent hospital: A possible new serotype. J Infect Dis. 1981;143:791–795.
20. Cubitt WD, Pead PJ, Saeed AA. A new serotype of calicivirus associated with an outbreak of gastroenteritis in a residential home for the elderly. J Clin Pathol. 1981;34:924–926.
21. Gray JJ, Wreghitt TG, Cubitt WD, Elliot PR. An outbreak of gastroenteritis in a home for the elderly associated with astrovirus type 1 and human calicivirus. J Med Virol. 1987;23:377–381.
22. Humphrey TJ, Cruickshank JG. An outbreak of calicivirus associated gastroenteitis in an elderly persons home. A possible zoonosis? J Hyg. (Lond.) 1984;92:293–299.
23. Calicivirus gastroenteritis in a long-term care facility for the elderly. Can Med Assoc J. 1991;144:1481–1482.
24. Lewis DC, Lightfoot NF, Cubitt WD, Wilson SA. Outbreaks of astrovirus type 1 and rotavirus gastroenteritis in a geriatric in-patient population. J Hosp Infect. 1989;14:9–14.
25. Holzel H, Cubitt DW, McSwiggan DA, et al. An outbreak of rotavirus infection among adults in a cardiology ward. J Infect. 1980;2:33–37.
26. Hrdy DB. Epidemiology of rotaviral infection in adults. Rev Infect. Dis. 1987;9:461–469.
27. Marrie TJ, Lee SHS, Faulkner RS, et al. Rotavirus infection in a geriatric population. Arch Intern Med. 1982;142:313–316.
28. Halvorsrud J, Orstavik I. An epidemic of rotavirus-associated gastroenteritis in a nursing home for the elderly. Scand J Infect Dis. 1980;12:161–164.
29. Horan MA, Gulati RS, Fox RA, et al. Outbreak of *Shigella sonnei* dysentery on a geriatric assessment ward. J Hosp Infect. 1984;5:210–212.
30. Halpern Z, Dan M, Giladi M, et al. Shigellosis in adults: Epidemiologic, clinical, and laboratory features. Medicine. 1989;68:210–217.
31. Ashkenazi S, Pickering LK. New *E. coli* serotype linked to GI disease. Contemp Gastroenterol. 1991;4:24–33.
32. Griffin PM, Ostroff SM, Tauxe RV, et al. Illnesses associated with *Escherichia coli* 0157:H7 infections: A broad clinical spectrum. Ann Intern Med. 1988;109:705–712.
33. Lightfoot NF, Ahmad F, Cowden J. Management of institutional outbreaks of salmonella gastroenteritis. J Antimicrob Chemother. 1990;26(suppl F):37–46.
34. Choi M, Yoshikawa TT, Bridge J, et al. *Salmonella* outbreak in a nursing home. J Am Geriatr Soc. 1990; 38:531–534.
35. Pavia AT, Shipman LD, Wells JG, et al. Epidemiologic evidence that prior antimicrobial exposure decreases resistance to infection by antimicrobial-sensitive *Salmonella*. J Infect Dis. 1990;161:255–260.
36. Ahmad F, Bray G, Prescott RWG, et al. Use of ciprofloxacin to control a salmonella outbreak in a long-stay psychiatric hospital. J Hosp Infect. 1991;17:171–178.
37. Bloom HG, Bottone EJ. *Aeromonas hydrophila* diarrhea in a long-term care setting. J Am Geriatr Soc. 1990;38:804–806.
37a. Melby K, Dahl OP, Crisp L, Penner JL. Clinical and serological manifestations in patients during a waterborne epidemic due to *Campylobacter jejuni*. J Infection. 1990;21:309–316.
37b. Skirrow MB, Jones DM, Sutcliffe E, Benjamin J. Campylobacter bacteraemia in England and Wales, 1981–91. Epidemiol Infect. 1993;110:567–573.
38. Bannister P, Mountford RA. *Cryptosporidium* in the elderly: A cause of life-threatening diarrhea. Am J Med. 1989;86:507–508.
39. Public Health Laboratory Service Study Group. Cryptosporidiosis in England and Wales: Prevalence and clinical and epidemiological features. Br Med J. 1990;300:774–777.

40. White KE, Hedberg CW, Edmonson LM, et al. An outbreak of giardiasis in a nursing home with evidence for multiple modes of transmission. J Infect Dis. 1989;160:298–304.

41. Levine WC, Smart JF, Archer DL, et al. Foodborne disease outbreaks in nursing homes, 1975–1987. JAMA. 1991;266:2105–2109.

42. Schouten EG, Pelt FL, Reitsma W, et al. Food hygiene and the prevalence of diarrhea and vomiting in independent elderly. Tijdschr Gerontol Geriat. 1988;19:7–10.

43. Thomas DR, Bennett RG, Laughon BE, et al. Postantibiotic colonization with *Clostridium difficile* in nursing home patients. J Am Geriatr Soc. 1990;38:415–420.

44. Bartlett JG. Antibiotic-associated diarrhea. Pract Gastroenterol. 1992;16:10–17.

45. Samuel SC, Hancock P, Leigh DA. An investigation into *Clostridium perfringens* enterotoxin-associated diarrhoea. J Hosp Infect. 1991;18:219–230.

46. Kim K-H, Fekety R, Batts DH, et al. Isolation of *Clostridium difficile* from the environment and contacts of patients with antibiotic-associated colitis. J Infect Dis. 1981;143:42–50.

47. Gupta TP, Ehrinpreis MN. *Candida*-associated diarrhea in hospitalized patients. Gastroenterology. 1990;98:780–785.

48. Danna PL, Urban C, Bellin E, Rahal JJ. Role of candida in pathogenesis of antibiotic-associated diarrhea in elderly inpatients. Lancet. 1991;337:511–514.

24

Traveler's Diarrhea and Foodborne Diseases

HERBERT L. DuPONT, M.D.

GEOGRAPHIC CONSIDERATIONS

An increased rate of occurrence of diarrhea is seen among travelers to all regions compared with the frequency of occurrence of diarrheal disease among persons who remain at home.[1] The world can be divided into three regions, depending upon the risk of diarrhea acquisition: high, low, and intermediate.[2] The high-risk areas include most countries of Latin America, Africa (except South Africa), and southern Asia. The low-risk areas include the United States, Canada, northwestern Europe, Japan, Australia, and New Zealand. The intermediate areas include the northern Mediterranean countries, eastern Europe, China, and the Soviet Union. Table 24–1 lists the approximate frequency of diarrhea occurrence among travelers in reference to countries of origin and destination. The rates are expressed in ranges derived from a number of published studies.[3–9] Within the high-risk areas of the world there is regional variation in risk. Some of the factors that are probably associated with a reduced risk include improved hygienic conditions, which are reflected in lower rates of endemic pediatric diarrhea (a barometer of environmental contamination); percentage of meals self-prepared[10, 11];

avoidance of high-risk foods[12]; and purpose and type of trip, whether for business, with a stay in a single hotel, or for adventure, with a more varied itinerary.[13]

Although natural immunity occurs as persons remain in a high-risk area,[6] the degree of immunity is only partial, and surprisingly high rates of illness persist over time in the local population.[6, 14] Despite our current understanding of the causes of acute diarrhea in developing tropical regions and our knowledge of how to decrease the threats of diarrhea by attention to water sanitation, sewage removal, and food hygiene, the rates of acute diarrhea among trav-

TABLE 24–1. EXPECTED RATE OF ACQUIRING DIARRHEA ACCORDING TO RISK AREAS OF ORIGIN AND DESTINATION

DIARRHEA RISK OF AREA OF ORIGIN	DIARRHEA RISK OF AREA VISITED		
	LOW (%)	INTERMEDIATE (%)	HIGH (%)
Low	2–5	10–15	40
Intermediate	Unknown	Unknown	10–20
High	2–10	Unknown	10

SOURCE: Adopted from References 3 through 9.

565

elers to these areas has not changed since the 1960s.[14-17]

ECONOMICS

Three hundred million travelers cross international boundaries each year, with 16 million entering tropical regions from industrialized countries.[18] With an average attack rate of 40%, approximately 6.4 million persons annually experience a diarrheal illness that translates into time lost from business or pleasure in addition to the cost of medication. Perhaps of greater economic consequence is the failed travel that does not develop because of the threat of enteric and other diseases. Many developing countries depend on the generation of revenue through their visitors. Of the more than 100 billion dollars spent in international travel each year, less than 20% goes to developing countries, where the need for such revenue is the greatest.[18] If the risk of acquiring infectious illnesses could be lessened through well-established principles of sanitation and hygiene, these relatively poor countries undoubtedly would see an increase in travel and revenue.

ETIOLOGY

Table 24–2 summarizes the approximate frequencies with which enteropathogens have been identified when all agents have been sought. The references providing the data used to make the estimates are included in this chapter.[16, 19-21] Seasonal and geographic factors influence the rates of occurrence of disease due to specific agents. Enterotoxigenic *Escherichia coli* (ETEC) is the single most important causal agent, accounting for approximately 40% of the disease, particularly during warm, rainy seasons in tropical regions, whereas during the dryer times of the year, it decreases in frequency at a time when *Campylobacter jejuni* becomes more common.[22] *Escherichia coli* that show the properties of attachment to intestinal epithelium and HEp-2 cells and others that resemble *Shigella* through their property of intestinal invasiveness account for approximately 10% of the disease.[23, 24] Noncholera vibrios are particularly common during warmer months along coastal areas of southeastern Asia.[20, 25] *Aeromonas* species and *Plesiomonas* species are common causes of the disease, showing regional variation.[26] The parasitic pathogens are not important causes of diarrhea in the usual traveler to tropical areas.[16, 27, 28] The intestinal protozoa are occasionally encountered in persons living under primitive hygienic conditions or during travel to Bangladesh[29] or St. Petersburg.[30] Viral gastroenteritis, especially that due to Norwalk virus, occurs in travelers.[8, 31] Rotavirus explains a measure of the disease, perhaps as high as 10% among travelers to Mexico.[8, 31-33] Approximately 80% of traveler's diarrhea is caused by a bacterial enteropathogen, explaining the effectiveness of antibacterial therapy in the illness.[34-36] During travel, alterations in intestinal flora occur in which *E. coli* of different serotypes cycle through the intestine[37] and antimicrobial-resistant flora may be acquired in these areas even in the absence of concomitant antimicrobial therapy.[38] It is not known whether these changes in flora result in diarrhea by themselves without intercurrent infection with a pathogenic microorganism.

TABLE 24–2. ETIOLOGY OF ACUTE DIARRHEA AMONG PERSONS TRAVELING FROM LOW-RISK AREAS TO DEVELOPING TROPICAL REGIONS

ENTEROPATHOGEN	RANGE OF OCCURRENCE (%)
Unidentified	20–50
Enterotoxigenic *Escherichia coli*	5–40
Shigella spp	3–25
Aeromonas spp and *Plesiomonas shigelloides*	10
Other diarrheagenic *E. coli*	10
Viral agents	10
Campylobacter jejuni	3–15
Noncholera vibrios	0–10
Salmonella enteritidis	0–5
Giardia and *Cryptosporidium*	2

NOTE: Approximate ranges based on limited studies.
SOURCE: Adopted from References 16, 18 through 26.

CLINICAL FEATURES AND PATHOGENESIS

The disease occurs at any time after arrival in the foreign country. The peak occurrence is between 3 days and 2 weeks after arrival. Fifteen percent of attacks occur after leaving the area of risk.[39] There is a wide variation in severity. In most cases, between 3 and 40 unformed stools are passed over a 3- to 5-day period, with abdominal cramps and pain being a nearly constant finding and fever, vomiting, or the passage of bloody stools occurring in from 10 to 20% of cases.[6, 9, 15] Since mechanisms of diarrhea production undoubtedly differ among the enteric pathogens, the vast majority of patients do not have a characteristic clinical picture.[40] Ten percent have diarrhea lasting longer than 1 week, and 2% report illness duration of more than 1 month.[9, 13, 18] The average duration of debility to the extent of confinement to a bedroom is 1 to 2 days.[15]

The source of the enteropathogen is usually food and occasionally water. Epidemiologic studies have consistently shown a relationship between place of food consumption or consumption of high-risk foods and occurrence of illness.[10–12, 41, 42] Food in these areas of high risk supports the growth of fecal coliforms and bacterial enteropathogens, including antimicrobial-resistant strains.[10, 11, 43] Water is probably the major source of viral gastroenteritis year-round and may contribute to the development of bacterial diarrhea during the rainy seasons.[44, 45] One of the curious published observations is that the illness risk relates to place where the majority of meals are eaten,[10, 11, 41] suggesting that the problem is related to the cumulative effect of multiple small exposures to enteropathogens rather than to a single large challenge. This is further supported by the finding of low numbers of bacterial enteropathogens in food when cultured quantitatively.[11]

PREVENTION

Ideally, the traveler to a high-risk area would attempt to minimize exposure by careful selection of food and beverages.[12] Unfortunately, less than 10% of travelers carefully select the safest food and beverage items when given the choice.[12] Improved methods of education in this area are needed. The generally safe foods include those served steaming hot (above 65°C)[46]; those with low pH such as citrus fruits; foods that are dry such as bread; those with high sugar content, such as syrup or jelly, and carbonated beverages.[2] Tap water and ice should be considered unsafe even if immersed in alcoholic drinks.[47] In the long run, it will be up to the developing countries to improve local hygienic conditions since they will be the beneficiaries when reduced rates of endemic enteric disease result in greater travel.

The second method of prevention is chemoprophylaxis. The various approaches have included regular use during the period of risk of antibacterial drugs active against the majority of the agents incriminated in the disease.[48–52] Bismuth subsalicylate (BSS)[53] and lactobacillus preparations[54] have been used as nonspecific measures to reduce the occurrence of disease. Of these nonspecific agents only BSS has been shown to be effective in reducing the disease,

with protection rates up to 65%. Undoubtedly, the most effective approach is the daily administration of an antibacterial drug active against most of the bacterial strains found in the area to be visited. Initially, sulfonamides and neomycin were used with success,[4, 15] but over the years resistance to these agents has become widespread. More recently, doxycycline,[50, 55] then trimethoprim–sulfamethoxazole (TMP/SMZ)[49] were used to prevent the illness during brief stays in areas of risk. Resistance acquisition to these drugs has limited their use in many parts of the world.[55] Undoubtedly, the most active and useful antibacterial drugs for adults for travel to all areas of high risk during all seasons are the new fluoroquinolones.[51, 52] When these drugs are used in areas where the local causal agents are susceptible, protection rates of 90% have been achieved. Considering a risk of acquiring diarrhea at 40% without prophylaxis and a protection rate with the use of an antibacterial drug of 90%, only 4 travelers in 100 put at risk would acquire diarrhea. The liabilities of using antimicrobial chemoprophylaxis are real. Minor side effects such as skin rash, vaginal yeast overgrowth, and insomnia with the quinolones occur in fewer than 10% of persons. Antimicrobial resistance of aerobic gut flora has occurred after TMP/SMX prophylaxis.[56] Although occurring in a very small percentage, potentially more serious reactions, such as anaphylaxis, Stevens-Johnson syndrome, and antimicrobial-associated colitis, will become important problems if all travelers to high-risk areas take these antibiotics. A reasonable estimate of these risks from taking an antibacterial agent to prevent diarrhea is .01% of exposed persons.[57] There is no available information about the best way to treat the unusual illness that might occur during chemoprophylaxis that should be due to an agent resistant to the preventive drug. Bismuth subsalicylate can be safely given to persons currently at risk for periods of up to 2 weeks, resulting in a 65% reduction in disease occurrence.[53] The prophylactic use of the drug is probably related to the antimicrobial effects of the drug and its intestinal reaction products.[58]

In deciding how to use or recommend antimicrobial chemoprophylaxis, the presence of underlying disease in the traveler, the nature of the planned trip and its duration all play a role in helping to determine the proper approach. If a 12- to 18-hour illness would have serious negative effects on the overall mission of the trip, BSS or antimicrobial chemoprophylaxis can be considered. For travelers likely to be more predisposed to enteric infection and its consequent chronic intestinal disease and immunodeficiency, this approach may be recommended. For most travelers, care with food and beverage selection and early therapy should illness occur is probably the optimal approach if they are willing to adhere strictly to recommended dietary precautions. The dose of BSS is 2 tablets qid with meals and at bedtime. When a more effective antibacterial is to be selected, TMP/SMX is satisfactory for travel to areas where TMP-resistant enteric bacterial pathogens are not common, such as the noncoastal areas of Mexico in the summertime. The minor adverse reactions to TMP/SMX therapy include skin rash, mouth sores, and vaginitis. For areas where susceptibility of the pathogens is unknown and an antibacterial is selected, a quinolone is probably preferred for adults. Each of the available fluoroquinolones appears to be appropriate for this use: norfloxacin at 400 mg, ciprofloxacin at 500 mg, or ofloxacin at 200 to 300 mg once a day for periods at risk of less than 2 to 3 weeks. Minor adverse effects of quinolone administration are insomnia, headache, and, rarely, skin rash. Although a consensus does not exist to indicate that chemoprophylaxis should be routinely employed,[18] the approach may be cost-effective during travel to high-risk areas.[57]

Several groups are currently working on the development and testing of immunoprophylactic measures to prevent traveler's diarrhea. Two general approaches are being pursued. The first is passive immunization, using bovine bacterial antibody given in multiple oral doses during the period of risk. Although field testing of this approach has not yet been carried out, successful studies of volunteers with experimental ETEC challenge[59] and infants exposed naturally to rotavirus infection have been reported.[60] This approach, although logistically difficult in terms of production problems (because regions would differ in preparation required) and requirements of compliance (the preparation would need to be taken multiple times daily as long as the individual was in the area of risk), may prove to be a practical means of preventing the major causes of diarrhea in areas where a limited number of predictable enteropathogens are responsible for a high percentage of the illness. A second, and equally exciting, approach has been active immunization with orally administered bacterial antigens. The first of the preparations developed and tested in a population of travelers was a mixture of heat-killed whole cells of *Vibrio cholerae* together with purified B subunit of cholera toxin, which has been evaluated in Finnish travelers to Morocco.[61] When given in 2 oral doses, the vaccine

had a 52% protection rate against ETEC diarrhea. It provided even better protection (71%) against disease associated with ETEC plus other pathogens. The vaccine stimulates intestinal immunity to many strains of ETEC owing to the similarity of the intestinal-binding portion of ETEC heat-labile enterotoxin to that of *V. cholerae* enterotoxin.

THERAPY

As with other forms of diarrhea, there are three forms of therapy to consider when diarrhea develops in a traveler. The first and most fundamental is fluid and electrolyte replacement. For intense and profuse watery diarrhea, a conventional oral rehydration solution is preferred and can generally be purchased locally in developing countries. For most traveler's diarrhea, flavored mineral water taken with saltine crackers should be sufficient to meet fluid and electrolyte needs. Travelers to cholera-endemic areas should be urged to pay particular attention to oral fluid therapy of intense diarrhea and to seek early medical attention should it be difficult to keep up with fluid losses. Symptomatic therapy shortens illness and helps the traveler return to nearly normal activities more quickly. Probably the most effective agent is loperamide,[62-64] which is given to adults in a dose of 4 mg initially, followed by 2 mg after passage of each subsequent unformed stool, but not to exceed 8 mg of the over-the-counter dosage or 16 mg of the prescription dosage per day. The agent should be taken for no more than 48 hours. Persons with fever or those passing bloody stools should not receive loperamide because of the rare potentiation of illness due to invasive enteropathogens.[65] Bismuth subsalicylate is a suitable alternative treatment,[66] although not quite so effective,[62, 64] and it is one that can be safely given to older children and adults. The adult dose is 30 ml (2 tablets of the solid formulation) taken orally every 30 minutes for 8 doses. This can be repeated 24 hours later if illness is continuing.

Antimicrobial therapy is the most important form of curative therapy of traveler's diarrhea in view of the bacterial cause of most cases of illness. As in antibacterial chemoprophylaxis, the destination of travel and the time of year may help to determine the best drug to administer. For the noncoastal areas of Mexico in summertime, TMP/SMX in a dose of 160 mg/800 mg 2 times a day for 3 days is the standard therapy.[34, 36, 67] As additional information becomes available concerning enteropathogen susceptibility in a variety of geographic locations, TMP/SMX may be satisfactory for therapy in other areas. Until such information is available, however, a fluoroquinolone is advised for most adults. All of the available agents appear to be equally effective.[35, 68, 69] The dosage schedule is norfloxacin 400 mg, ciprofloxacin 500 mg, or ofloxacin 200 to 300 mg 2 times a day for 3 days. If the patient is febrile or has dysentery, the antimicrobial should be given alone. For those without fever or dysentery, the antimicrobial can be given together with loperamide for both curative and more rapid responses.[36, 70] Although not so rapidly effective as TMP/SMX or the fluoroquinolones in treating enteric infection associated with susceptible strains, furazolidone, 100 mg 4 times a day for 5 days, can be used in the therapy of traveler's diarrhea.[71] Resistance to furazolidone has not occurred with significant frequency anywhere, and the drug is active against both bacterial enteropathogens and *Giardia,* for which it should be given for at least 7 days.

FOODBORNE DISEASE

When multiple cases of an illness occur following a common exposure, often a meal, a common-source outbreak is strongly suggested. Although a single case of botulism or chemical food poisoning in the proper setting is sufficient to incriminate a vehicle, in other situations multiple cases are required to implicate a meal or other common source as a vehicle of disease transmission. The development of symptoms after the ingestion of a contaminated material depends on one or more of four factors: number of organisms present; the virulence of the disease-producing microbe; host factors such as age, reduced gastric acidity or secretory immunoglobulin A (sIgA); or presence of a toxic substance. The causes of food- or waterborne illness can usually be divided into four groups: chemical, bacterial, viral, and parasitic. In approximately 60% of outbreaks of foodborne disease, a causal agent is not identified.[72]

Chemical Foodborne Illness

Chemical agents cause one fourth of the reported foodborne outbreaks, yet this amounts to only 2% of total cases.[72]

Heavy Metal Intoxication

In heavy metal intoxication, a food item has usually been stored in a tin, antimony, or copper container. Three minutes to 3 hours after ingesting the food, gastrointestinal symptoms, including diarrhea, develop. The person affected characteristically recalls a metallic taste to the item consumed.

Seafood Neurotoxins

There are three similar syndromes produced by neurotoxins that are ingested in a seafood vehicle. The toxins block voltage-gated sodium channels in myelinated and nonmyelinated nerves. The clinical illnesses produced by the three conditions cannot be distinguished. Variations in symptoms relate primarily to the amount of toxin ingested. Paralytic shellfish disease follows consumption of mollusks, usually oysters, or broth from cooked shellfish harvested in an area infested by dinoflagellates, known as red tide, and that contain saxitoxin, an alkaloid neurotoxin, or a related compound.[73] Ten minutes to 1 hour after eating the food, the person generally complains of paresthesias of the lips, mouth, and face. In more severe cases, ataxia, dysphagia, coma, muscular paralysis, and respiratory arrest can occur. As this is the most potent of the toxins, lethal cases are regularly reported.[74] It has been estimated that 1600 cases of paralytic shellfish poisoning occur worldwide each year, resulting in more than 300 deaths.[75] Rigid controls of fresh or canned shellfish are enforced since the toxin is heat-stable.

In ciguatera disease, a similar disease process, fish, oysters, or clams have been consumed minutes to 12 hours earlier. These fish or shellfish have previously ingested dinoflagellates containing the toxin that produces the gastrointestinal symptoms of dry mouth, pain in the teeth, and paresthesia. The condition, which is the most common form of fish poisoning, has occurred with increasing frequency among travelers to the Caribbean, and outbreaks may be quite large.[76] Deaths from this cause, although unusual, do occur. As in paralytic shellfish poisoning, the toxin is heat-stable, making ciguatera a problem for the canning industry. In typical cases of ciguatera fish poisoning, gastrointestinal symptoms occur first, within 3 to 6 hours, and include nausea, diarrhea, vomiting, and abdominal pain. They are followed within 12 to 72 hours of onset by neurologic symptoms such as a burning sensation on exposure of hands, feet, or mouth to cold as well as tingling, paresthesia, myalgia, arthralgia, itching, numbness of the jaw or toothache, and insomnia. Neurologic symptoms may last for months and may result in disability.[77]

Pufferfish intoxication occurs 10 minutes to 4 hours after the toxin-contaminated seafood is consumed. Again, the complaints are paresthesia and numbness. Pufferfish poisoning has been reported in recent years primarily in Japan. The fatalities that have been reported previously occurred predominantly among poorer persons who prepare the fish dish themselves, which is considered a delicacy. Meticulous professional preparation is required in order to avoid fish tissues that are high in toxin.

Treatment of any of the seafood neurotoxin diseases is supportive and symptomatic. With respiratory failure, assisted ventilation is required. Intravenous mannitol has been used successfully in ciguatera fish poisoning.[78]

Scombroid Poisoning

In scombroid poisoning, flushing, headache, dizziness, and nonspecific gastrointestinal symptoms occur 5 minutes to 1 hour after eating spoiled tuna or mackerel. The syndrome is produced by gram-negative enteric bacteria, characteristically *Proteus* species or *Klebsiella* species, which decarboxylate histidine-producing saurine, a histamine-like substance.[79, 80] Of the fish-associated poisonings in the United States, either ciguatera or scombroid fish can be implicated in over two thirds of the outbreaks.[72] Persons taking isoniazid are particularly susceptible. Affected patients invariably report a metallic, sharp, or peppery taste of the consumed fish.

Mushroom Toxin Poisoning

In this syndrome, gastrointestinal symptoms, perspiration, salivation or bradycardia develop 1 to 8 hours after consumption of the mushroom.[81] There is a characteristicly direct relationship between length of incubation period and severity of the intoxication. Patients with an incubation period of 6 hours or longer generally have a more serious course, which may be fatal. Interestingly, the syndrome characteristically occurs when mushrooms are picked by a person convinced of his ability to identify safe varieties. Rapid-acting toxins affect, usually within 1 hour, the autonomic nervous system, either the muscarinic group of autonomic nervous system receptors, to produce bradycardia, sweating, lacrimation, blurred vision, diarrhea, and abdominal pain, or the coprineic group of receptors, where symptoms occur only with concomitant alcohol consumption and produce dizziness, flushing, vomiting, and paresthesia. The mushrooms with a delayed onset of from 6 to 24 hours elaborate potent cytotoxins that produce muscle cramps, abdominal pain, and diarrhea that may be bloody. In severe cases, liver failure and convulsions, coma and death may occur. Depending upon the type of mushroom ingested in the longer incubation-period disease, therapy with pyridoxine or thioctic acid may be useful.[81]

Chinese Restaurant Syndrome

Five to 30 minutes after consuming food containing monosodium glutamate (MSG), the affected person characteristically complains of a burning sensation in the chest, neck, abdomen, and extremities and of sweating, bronchospasms, and tachycardia.[82] The syndrome, which affects all persons if they ingest sufficient quantities of MSG, is due to transient acetyl cholinergic responses. Between 15 and 25% of persons ingesting quantities normally present in many restaurants are susceptible. There is often a family history of the condition.

Bacterial Foodborne Disease

Bacterial foodborne disease is the most common of the food-associated disorders, accounting for two thirds of the foodborne outbreaks and 90% of total cases reported.[72] These outbreaks can be divided into two groups, depending upon whether fever occurs in a percentage of affected persons.

Subjects Experience Fever

When fever is reported in more than 20% of cases of an outbreak a mucosally invasive bacterial or viral pathogen should be suspected. Cultures of diarrheal stool and of the incriminated food, if still available, are usually required to determine the cause in the case of bacterial infection. The most frequent agent in this setting is a serotype of *Salmonella enteritidis* that characteristically has contaminated a meat item, often poultry. Other, less common, agents causing a similar clinical picture are *Shigella* species, *C. jejuni*, and *Vibrio parahaemolyticus*. In the case of *V. parahaemolyticus*, seafood is almost always the vehicle of transmission. A highly invasive organism, *Vibrio vulnificus* can be the cause of fatal septicemic disease in persons with liver disease who ingest raw seafood, typically shellfish.[83] Other illnesses may predispose to fulminant *V. vulnificus* infection, including hemochromatosis and the acquired immune deficiency syndrome (AIDS).

Subjects Experience Little or No Fever

In the case of noninvasive bacterial food-borne disease, the clinical manifestations generally depend upon whether an enterotoxin is produced in the food or whether the organism must first infect the small bowel before release of a secretory enterotoxin leads to fluid and electrolyte losses. The classic cause of an intoxication is *Staphylococcus aureus* food poisoning. The *S. aureus* strain introduced into the food by a colonized food handler elaborates the enterotoxin, which is heat-stable, and the enterotoxin subsequently leads to vomiting, often intense, 30 minutes to 4 hours after the food is consumed. *Clostridium perfringens* and ETEC must first infect the gut before releasing the enterotoxins that lead to intestinal secretion after stimulation of tissue cyclic nucleotides. *Bacillus cereus* produces both syndromes, resembling either *S. aureus* intoxication or *C. perfringens* infection, with their shorter or longer incubation period, respectively.

Viral Agents

Viruses cause 5% of the total number of reported cases of diarrhea identified with a food-borne illness in the United States.[72] In Norwalk gastroenteritis, 8 to 72 hours after ingesting the contaminated food, vomiting, fever and watery diarrhea occur. Vomiting is the most common feature. The presence of fever in a proportion of individuals plus a longer incubation period help to differentiate this disease from *S. aureus* food poisoning.

Parasitic Agents

Trichinella spiralis is the most important food-associated parasitic infection in the United States. Rarely, food is incriminated in the epidemiology of *Giardia lamblia* infection.

REFERENCES

1. Steffen R, Van der Linde F, Gyr K, et al. Epidemiology of diarrhea of travelers. JAMA. 1983;249:1176–1180.
2. DuPont HL, DuPont MW. Traveler's diarrhea. In: Travel with Health. New York: Appleton-Century-Crofts; 1981:148–156.
3. Dandoy S. The diarrhea of travelers: Incidence in foreign students in the United States. Calif Med. 1966;104:458–462.
4. Kean BH. Turista in Teheran: Travelers' diarrhea at the Eighth International Congress of Tropical Medicine and Malaria. Lancet. 1969;2:583–584.
5. Lowenstein MS, Balows A, Gangarosa EJ. Turista at an International Congress in Mexico. Lancet. 1973;1:529–531.
6. DuPont HL, Haynes GA, Pickering LK, et al. Diarrhea of travelers to Mexico: Relative susceptibility of United States and Latin American students attending a Mexican university. Am J Epidemiol. 1977;105:37–41.
7. Ryder RW, Wells JG, Gangarosa EJ. A study of traveler's diarrhea in foreign visitors to the United States. J Infect Dis. 1977;136:605–607.
8. Ryder RW, Oquist CA, Greenberg H. Traveler's diarrhea in Panamanian tourists in Mexico. J Infect Dis. 1981;144:442–448.
9. Steffen R. Epidemiologic studies of travelers' diarrhea, severe gastrointestinal infections and cholera. Rev Infect Dis. 1986;8(suppl 2):S122–S130.
10. Tjoa WS, DuPont HL, Sullivan P, et al. Location of food consumption and travelers' diarrhea. Am J Epidemiol. 1977;106:61–66.
11. Wood LV, Ferguson LE, Hogan P, et al. Incidence of bacterial enteropathogens in foods from Mexico. Appl Environ Microbiol. 1983;46:328–332.
12. Kozicki M, Steffen R, Schär M. "Boil it, cook it, peel it, or forget it": Does this rule prevent travellers' diarrhoea? Int J Epidemiol. 1985;14:169–172.
13. Steffen R. Epidemiology of travellers' diarrhoea. Scand J Gastroenterol. 1983;18(suppl 84):5–17.
14. Higgins AR. Observations on the health of United States personnel living in Cairo, Egypt. Am J Trop Med Hyg. 1955;4:970–979.
15. Kean BH. The diarrhea of travelers to Mexico: Summary of a five-year study. Ann Intern Med. 1963;59:605–614.
16. DuPont HL, Ericsson CD, DuPont MW. Emporiatric enteritis: Lessons learned from US students in Mexico. Trans Am Clin Climatol Assoc. 1986;97:32–42.
17. Haberberger RL Jr, Mikhail IA, Burans JP, et al. Travelers' diarrhea among United States military personnel during joint American–Egyptian Armed Forces exercises in Cairo, Egypt. Mil Med. 1991;156:27–30.
18. Gorbach SL, Edelman R, eds. Travelers' Diarrhea: National Institutes of Health Consensus Development Conference. Rev Infect Dis. 1986;8(suppl 2):S109–S233.
19. Black RE. Pathogens that cause travelers' diarrhea in Latin America and Africa. Rev Infect Dis. 1986;8(suppl 2):S131–S135.
20. Taylor DN, Echeverria P. Etiology and epidemiology of travelers' diarrhea in Asia. Rev Infect Dis. 1986;8(suppl 2):S136–S141.
21. Steffen R, Mathewson JJ, Ericsson CD, et al. Travelers' diarrhea in West Africa and in Mexico: Fecal transport systems and liquid bismuth subsalicylate for self-therapy. J Infect Dis. 1988;157:1008–1013.
22. Mattila L, Siitonen A, Kyrönseppä H, et al. Seasonal variation in etiology of travelers' diarrhea. J Infect Dis. 1992;165:385–388.
23. Mathewson JJ, Johnson PC, DuPont HL, et al. A newly recognized cause of travelers' diarrhea: Enteroadherent *Escherichia coli*. J Infect Dis. 1985;151:471–475.
24. Wanger AR, Murray BE, Echeverria P, et al. Enteroinvasive *Escherichia coli* in travelers with diarrhea. J Infect Dis. 1988;158:640–642.
25. Sriratanaba A, Reinprayoon S. *Vibrio parahaemolyticus:* A major cause of travelers' diarrhea in Bangkok. Am J Trop Med Hyg. 1982;31:128–130.
26. Echeverria P, Sack RB, Blacklow NR, et al. Prophylactic doxycycline for travelers' diarrhea in Thailand: Further supporting evidence of *Aeromonas hydrophila* as an enteric pathogen. Am J Epidemiol. 1984;120:912–921.
27. Frachtman RL, Ericsson CD, DuPont HL. Seroconversion to *Entamoeba histolytica* among short-term travelers to Mexico. Arch Intern Med. 1982;142:1299.
28. Mathewson JJ, Flores JF, DuPont HL, et al. Risk of ac-

quisition of *Entamoeba histolytica* infection during long-term travel to Mexico. Travel Med Int. 1990;8.2:65–68.

29. Speelman P, Struelens MJ, Sariyal SC, et al. Detection of *Campylobacter jejuni* and other potential pathogens in travellers' diarrhoea in Bangladesh. Scand J Gastroenterol. 1983;18(suppl 84):19–23.

30. Jokipii L, Pohjola S, Jokipii AMM. Cryptosporidiosis associated with traveling and giardiasis. Gastroenterol. 1985;89:838–842.

31. Johnson PC, Hoy J, Mathewson JJ, et al. Occurrence of Norwalk virus infections among adults in Mexico. J Infect Dis. 1990;162:389–393.

32. Bolivar R, Conklin RH, Vollet JJ, et al. Rotavirus in travelers' diarrhea: Study of an adult population in Mexico. J Infect Dis. 1978;137:324–327.

33. Vollet JJ, Ericsson CD, Gibson G, et al. Human rotavirus in an adult population with travelers' diarrhea and its relationship to the location of food consumption. J Med Virol. 1979;4:81–87.

34. DuPont HL, Reves RR, Galindo E, et al. Treatment of travelers' diarrhea with trimethoprim/sulfamethoxazole and with trimethoprim alone. N Engl J Med. 1982; 307:841–844.

35. Ericsson CD, Johnson PC, DuPont HL, et al. Ciprofloxacin and trimethoprim/sulfamethoxazole as initial therapy for acute travelers' diarrhea: A placebo-controlled randomized trial. Ann Intern Med. 1987;106:216–220.

36. Ericsson CD, DuPont HL, Mathewson JJ, et al. Treatment of travelers' diarrhea with sulfamethoxazole and trimethoprim and loperamide. JAMA. 1990;263:257–261.

37. Ørskov F, Black RB, Ørskov I, et al. Changing fecal *Escherichia coli* flora during travel. Eur J Clin Microbiol. 1984;3:306–309.

38. Murray BE, Mathewson JJ, DuPont HL, et al. Emergence of resistant fecal *Escherichia coli* in travelers not taking prophylactic antimicrobial agents. Antimicrob Agents Chemother. 1990;34:515–518.

39. Kendrick MA. Study of illness among Americans returning from international travel, July 11—August 24, 1971 (preliminary data). J Infect Dis. 1972;126:684–685.

40. Ericsson CD, Patterson TF, DuPont HL. Clinical presentation as a guide to therapy for travelers' diarrhea. Am J Med Sci. 1987;294:91–96.

41. Ericsson CD, Pickering LK, Sullivan P, et al. The role of location of food consumption in the prevention of travelers' diarrhea in Mexico. Gastroenterol. 1980;79:812–816.

42. Merson MH, Morris GK, Sack DA, et al. Travelers' diarrhea in Mexico: A prospective study of physicians and family members attending a congress. N Engl J Med. 1976;294:1299–1305.

43. Wood LV, Jansen DM, DuPont HL. Antimicrobial resistance of gram-negative bacteria isolated from foods in Mexico. J Infect Dis. 1983;148:766.

44. Deetz TR, Smith EM, Goyal SM, et al. Occurrence of rota- and enteroviruses in drinking and environmental water in a developing nation. Water Res. 1984;18:567–571.

45. Keswick BH, Gerba CP, DuPont HL, et al. Detection of enteric viruses in treated drinking water. Appl Environ Microbiol. 1984;47:1290–1294.

46. Bandres JC, Mathewson JJ, DuPont HL. Heat susceptibility of bacterial enteropathogens: Implications for the prevention of travelers' diarrhea. Arch Intern Med. 1988;148:2261–2263.

47. Dickens DL, DuPont HL, Johnson PC. Survival of bacterial enteropathogens in the ice of popular drinks. JAMA. 1985;253:3141–3143.

48. Carlson JR, Thornton SA, DuPont HL, et al. Comparative in vitro activities of ten antimicrobial agents against

bacterial enteropathogens. Antimicrob Agents Chemother. 1983;24:509–513.

49. DuPont HL, Galindo E, Evans DG, et al. Prevention of travelers' diarrhea with trimethoprim/sulfamethoxazole and trimethoprim alone. Gastroenterol. 1983;84:75–80.

50. Echeverria P, Sack RB, Blacklow NR, et al. Prophylactic doxycycline for traveler's diarrhea in Thailand: Further supportive evidence of *Aeromonas hydrophila* as an enteric pathogen. Am J Epidemiol. 1984;120:912–921.

51. Johnson PC, Ericsson CD, Morgan DR, et al. Lack of emergence of resistant fecal flora during successful prophylaxis of travelers' diarrhea with norfloxacin. Antimicrob Agents Chemother. 1986;30:671–674.

52. Rademaker CM, Hoepelman IM, Wolfhagen MJ, et al. Results of a double-blind placebo-controlled study using ciprofloxacin for prevention of travelers' diarrhea. Eur J Clin Microbiol Infect Dis. 1989;8:690–694.

53. DuPont HL, Ericsson CD, Johnson PC, et al. Prevention of travellers' diarrhea by the tablet formulation of bismuth subsalicylate. JAMA. 1987;257:1347–1350.

54. Oksanen PJ, Salminen S, Saxelin M, et al. Prevention of travellers' diarrhoea by *Lactobacillus* GG. Ann Med. 1990;22:53–56.

55. Sack RB, Santosham M, Froehlich JL, et al. Doxycycline prophylaxis of travelers' diarrhea in Honduras, an area where resistance to doxycycline is common among *Escherichia coli*. Am J Trop Med Hyg. 1984;33:460–466.

56. Murray BE, Rensimer ER, DuPont HL. Emergence of high-level trimethoprim resistance in fecal *Escherichia coli* during oral administration of trimethoprim or trimethoprim/sulfamethoxazole. N Engl J Med. 1982;306:130–135.

57. Reves RR, Johnson PC, Ericsson CD, et al. A cost-effectiveness comparison of the use of antimicrobial agents for treatment or prophylaxis of travelers' diarrhea. Arch Intern Med. 1988;148:2421–2427.

58. Graham DY, Estes MK, Gentry LO. Double-blind comparison of bismuth subsalicylate and placebo in the prevention and treatment of enterotoxigenic *Escherichia coli*-induced diarrhea in volunteers. Gastroenterol. 1983;85:1017–1022.

59. Tacket CO, Losonsky G, Link H, et al. Protection by milk immunoglobulin concentrate against oral challenge with enterotoxigenic *Escherichia coli*. N Engl J Med. 1988;318:1240–1243.

60. Ebina T, Sato A, Umezu K, et al. Prevention of rotavirus infection by oral administration of cow colostrum containing antihuman rotavirus antibody. Med Microbiol Immunol. 1985;174:177–185.

61. Peltola H, Siitonen A, Kyrönseppä H, et al. Prevention of travellers' diarrhoea by oral B-subunit/whole-cell cholera vaccine. Lancet. 1991;338:1285–1289.

62. Johnson PC, Ericsson CD, DuPont HL, et al. Comparison of loperamide with bismuth subsalicylate for the treatment of acute travelers' diarrhea. JAMA. 1986; 225:757–760.

63. Van Loon FB, Bennish ML, Speelman P, et al. Double-blind trial of loperamide for treating acute watery diarrhoea in ex-patriates in Bangladesh. Gut. 1989;30:492–495.

64. DuPont HL, Sanchez JF, Ericsson CD, et al. Comparative efficacy of loperamide hydrochloride and bismuth subsalicylate in the management of acute diarrhea. Am J Med. 1990;88(suppl 6A):S155–S195.

65. DuPont HL, Hornick RB. Adverse effect of Lomotil therapy in shigellosis. JAMA. 1973;226:1525–1528.

66. DuPont HL, Sullivan P, Pickering LK, et al. Symptomatic treatment of diarrhea with bismuth subsalicylate among students attending a Mexican university. Gastroenterol. 1977;73:715–718.

67. Bandres JC, Mathewson JJ, Ericsson CD, et al. Trimeth-

oprim/sulfamethoxazole remains active against enterotoxigenic *Escherichia coli* and *Shigella* spp in Guadalajara, Mexico. Am J Med Sci. 1992;303:289–291.

68. Wilstrom J, Jertborn M, Hedstrom SA, et al. Short-term self-treatment of travellers' diarrhoea with norfloxacin: A placebo controlled study. J Antimicrob Chemother. 1989;23:905–913.

69. DuPont HL, Ericsson CD, Mathewson JJ, et al. Five versus three days ofloxacin therapy of traveler's diarrhea: A placebo-controlled study. Antimicrob Agents Chemother. 1992;36:87–91.

70. Taylor DN, Sanchez JL, Candler W, et al. Treatment of travelers' diarrhea: Ciprofloxacin plus loperamide compared with ciprofloxacin alone: A placebo controlled, randomized trial. Ann Intern Med. 1991;114:731–734.

71. DuPont HL, Ericsson CD, Galindo E, et al. Furazolidone versus ampicillin in the treatment of traveler's diarrhea. Antimicrob Agents Chemother. 1984;26:160–163.

72. Bean NH, Griffin PM, Goulding JS, et al. Foodborne disease outbreaks: 5-Year summary, 1983–1987. MMWR Morb Mortal Wkly Rep. 1990;39:15–57.

73. Centers for Disease Control. Paralytic shellfish poisoning—Massachusetts and Alaska, 1990. MMWR Morb Mortal Wkly Rep. 1991;40:157–161.

74. Rodrigue DC, Etzel RA, Hall S, et al. Lethal paralytic shellfish poisoning in Guatemala. Am J Trop Med Hyg. 1990;42:267–271.

75. Mills AR, Passmore R. Pelagic paralysis. Lancet. 1988; 1:161–164.

76. Frenette C, MacLean JD, Gyorkos TW. A large common-source outbreak of ciguatera fish poisoning. J Infect Dis. 1988;158:1129–1131.

77. Morris JG, Lewin P, Hargrett NT, et al. Clinical features of ciguatera fish poisoning: A study of the disease in the US Virgin Islands. Arch Intern Med. 1982;142:1090–1092.

78. Palafox NA, Jaine LG, Pinano AZ, et al. Successful treatment of ciguatera fish poisoning with intravenous mannitol. JAMA. 1988;259:2740–2742.

79. Morrow JD, Margolies GR, Rowald J, et al. Evidence that histamine is the causative toxin of scombroid-fish poisoning. N Engl J Med. 1991;324:716–720.

80. Hughes JM, Potter ME. Scombroid-fish poisoning: From pathogenesis to prevention. N Engl J Med. 1991; 324:766–768.

81. Hanrahan JP, Gordon MA. Mushroom poisoning: Case report and a review of therapy. JAMA. 1984;251:1057–1061.

82. Settipane GA. The restaurant syndromes. Arch Intern Med. 1986;146:2129–2130.

83. Chin KP, Lowe MA, Tong MJ, et al. *Vibrio vulnificus* infection after raw oyster ingestion in a patient with liver disease and acquired immune deficiency syndrome–related complex. Gastroenterol. 1987;92:796–799.

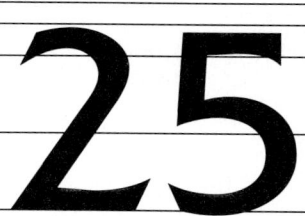

25

Approach to Gastrointestinal Infection in Immunosuppressed Patients

ROBERT C. BOLLINGER, M.D., M.P.H.

THOMAS C. QUINN, M.D., M.Sc.

The gastrointestinal (GI) tract is a multifunctional organ system. Many organisms are adapted to invade the human host through the GI tract, but to prevent the access of pathogens there are multiple defense mechanisms available, including gastric acid, proteolytic enzymes, the presence of normal bacterial flora, and bowel motility. In addition, the GI tract functions as one of the most important lymphatic organs, with the secretory and cellular immune systems providing an important barrier to infection. It is therefore no surprise that systemic defects in the immune system are manifest as a breakdown in the protective ability of the GI tract or that they are likely to lead to opportunistic infections.

SYSTEMIC IMMUNITY AND CONTROL OF INFECTION

The systemic immune response to infection relies on a cascade of coordinated components, including the cellular, humoral, and complement systems. T lymphocytes, as part of the cellular immune response, are of primary importance in the recognition and control of intracellular pathogens, such as viruses, most parasites, and some bacteria. The ability to recognize a host cell as infected depends upon the $CD4^+$ and $CD8^+$ T cell interaction with host cells that express foreign antigens on their surface in association with the appropriate major histocompatibility complex (MHC). One would predict, therefore, that defects in the $CD4^+$ or $CD8^+$ lymphocyte response would be manifested by an increased risk of intracellular opportunistic pathogens (Table 25–1). Monocytes and macrophages are also an important component of the cellular immune response to infections with mycobacteria, encapsulated bacteria, and many fungi. Neutropenia and other phagocytic defects increase susceptibility to these organism in particular. The humoral and complement components of the immune re-

TABLE 25–1. IMMUNOLOGIC DEFECTS AND ASSOCIATED OPPORTUNISTIC PATHOGENS

IMMUNOLOGIC DEFECT	CLINICAL SYNDROMES	OPPORTUNISTIC PATHOGENS
T cell abnormalities	AIDS Transplantation Steroids Lymphoma	Bacteria: *Mycobacterium, Nocardia, Listeria, Legionella, Salmonella* Viruses: herpes simplex virus, cytomegalovirus, varicella zoster virus, adenovirus Parasites: *Pneumocystis carinii, Toxoplasma,* microsporidia, *Strongyloides, Cryptosporidium* Fungi: *Candida, Mucor, Cryptococcus*
Neutropenia and phagocytic defects	Drug-induced Congenital	Bacteria: *Mycobacterium,* anaerobes, encapsulated gram-positive Fungi: *Aspergillus, Candida*
B cell abnormalities	Multiple myeloma Some leukemias Congenital	Bacteria: *Streptococcus pneumoniae, Haemophilus influenzae* Viruses: Enterovirus Parasites: *Giardia*
Complement defects	Congenital	Bacteria: *Streptococcus pneumoniae, H influenzae, Staphylococcus aureus, Neisseria, Salmonella*

sponse are particularly important for the control of many common enteric pathogens. Although these generalizations help to predict the pathogens that are most likely to be opportunistic for various immune defects, the picture is often clouded by the complexity and interdependence of the different components of the immune response.

HUMAN IMMUNODEFICIENCY VIRUS INFECTION

The GI tract is one of the primary portals of entry for human immunodeficiency virus (HIV) infection, especially in homosexual men, and it is the most symptomatic organ system in HIV-infected patients. The large lymphoid component of the GI tract may also be an important reservoir for HIV-infected cells. In addition, acute HIV seroconversion is often associated with a mononucleosis-like syndrome that may include nausea and transient diarrhea.[1]

The management of HIV-infected patients with enteric infections requires an appreciation of the multiple immune defects that are associated with HIV. In addition to the quantitative and qualitative CD4[+] T lymphocyte defects,[2–4] B cell abnormalities manifested by a generalized polyclonal activation,[5–7] hypergammaglobulinemia,[5] and reduced antibody response to new antigens[8, 9] have also been described in HIV infection. Evidence of a defect in phagocytosis and macrophage and monocyte function have also been described.[10, 11] In the GI tract, HIV infection is associated with a marked reduction of CD4[+] T cells and an increase in the CD8[+] T cells in the lamina propria of the GI mucosa.[12, 13] This is accompanied by a decrease in the number of immunoglobulin A (IgA) plasma cells

and secretory IgA2 in acquired immunodeficiency syndrome (AIDS).[14, 15] The wide range of enteric pathogens that affect HIV-infected patients is thus a reflection of the multiple immune defects, which also result in symptoms that may be seen throughout the GI tract.

Oral Lesions

Lesions of the oral mucosa are extremely common in HIV infection and include local pathologic conditions as well as oral manifestations of systemic infections.[16] Painful lesions include ulcerative lesions of herpes simplex virus (HSV) and the white plaquelike lesions of mucosal *Candida*. Herpes simplex virus is the more common cause of recurrent painful ulcerations with surrounding erythema and is diagnosed by culture of the lesions. Usually, HSV responds well to acyclovir therapy, and it is reasonable to begin empirical therapy for ulcerative lesions that are potassium hydroxide (KOH)–negative while viral cultures are pending.

Mucocutaneous *Candida* infection is extremely common in HIV-infected individuals and is often seen early in the disease process, frequently as the presenting complaint of HIV infection in high-risk populations.[17] The characteristic white plaquelike lesions of thrush or the erythematous lesions of mucocutaneous *Candida* are easily diagnosed with a simple swab and KOH smear. They are often associated with odynophagia or dysphagia, suggestive of esophagitis. Antifungal therapy with ketoconazole, clotrimazole, or nystatin provides predictable relief of symptoms in most patients.

Nonpainful lesions may include the characteristic syphilitic ulcer, the hyperpigmented nodular, and occasionally ulcerating, lesions of

TABLE 25–2. CAUSES OF ODYNOPHAGIA AND DYSPHAGIA IN HIV-INFECTED PATIENTS

ORGANISM	INITIAL THERAPY	SUPPRESSIVE THERAPY
Candida	Ketoconazole (200 mg po bid) or Fluconazole (100 mg po qd) or Amphotericin B (0.3–0.5 mg/kg/d IV)	Nystatin (500,000 units qid orally) or Clotrimazole (10 mg, qid orally) or Ketoconazole (200 mg qd or bid)
Herpes simplex virus	*Mild:* Acyclovir (200 mg po 5 ×/d) *Severe:* Acyclovir (15 mg/kg/d IV) or Vidarabine (15 mg/kg/d IV) or Experimental: Foscarnet (90 mg/kg/d IV)	Acyclovir (200 mg po tid)
CMV Cytomegalovirus	Ganciclovir (DHPG) (5 mg/kg/bid IV) or Foscarnet (90–120 mg/kg/8 hr IV)	Not established
Kaposi's sarcoma	Systemic chemotherapy Local sclerotherapy	
Lymphoma	Systemic chemotherapy Local irradiation	

Kaposi's sarcoma (KS), or the white, fibrinous lesions of hairy leukoplakia, typically located on the lateral aspects of the tongue. Hairy leukoplakia is a disorder that has only been seen in AIDS patients. It resembles leukoplakia but has fibrillar projections that extend outward from the surface of the lesion. Histopathologic findings resemble those of conventional leukoplakia without a mononuclear response; it is similar to a flat wart.[18] Hairy leukoplakia is often associated with oral thrush and although the etiology is unclear, a viral cause is suggested by the evidence of human papillomavirus (HPV), HSV, and Epstein-Barr virus (EBV) localized within this tissue.[19]

Dysphagia and Odynophagia

Candida esophagitis is responsible for more than 50% of dysphagia and odynophagia in HIV-infected patients.[20] Many patients with oral candidiasis have endoscopic evidence of esophageal invasion with minimal symptoms.[21] The diagnosis of *Candida* esophagitis is characterized by dilatation and abnormal esophageal motility. Endoscopic examination reveals a white exudate with the appearance of cottage cheese, often with deep ulcerations.[22] Biopsies of these lesions typically reveal hyphal invasion of the mucosa and submucosa. For most patients with symptomatic esophagitis who are able to tolerate oral medications and who do not have evidence of systemic candidiasis, ketoconazole, given in a dosage of 200 mg per day, or fluconazole, at a dosage of 100 mg per day, may be

prescribed. Occasionally, with severe invasive disease, when oral therapy is not tolerated initial therapy with intravenous amphotericin B at a dosage of 0.1 to 0.3 mg per kilogram body weight per day is indicated. *Candida* esophagitis is often a recurrent infection, and suppressive therapy with oral nystatin, clotrimazole, or ketoconazole is required.[23]

Other causes of odynophagia and dysphagia in HIV-infected patients include HSV, cytomegalovirus (CMV), KS, and lymphoma[20, 24, 25] (Table 25–2). Acute and chronic HSV esophagitis has been described in HIV-infected patients diagnosed histologically after endoscopic biopsy and by culture of the deep ulcerations observed. Successful therapy with acyclovir can be achieved in most patients with predictable symptom resolution. The esophageal ulcerations of CMV esophagitis may be discrete craters or extensive superficial lesions.[26, 27] Given the high frequency of esophageal colonization with CMV in HIV-infected patients, a more definitive diagnosis of CMV as the causative agent of esophagitis must be obtained using endoscopic biopsy specimens.[28] CMV in esophageal brushings or superficial cultures without a pathological diagnosis of CMV tissue involvement are insufficient. A proportion of patients with CMV esophagitis respond to ganciclovir (dehydroxyphenylglycol, DHPG) therapy, but treatment failures and relapses are well known.[28, 29]

Kaposi's sarcoma and lymphoma may rarely present with dysphagia and one or more nodular obstructive lesions. Gastrointestinal tract involvement with KS may occur in 50% of patients with cutaneous KS lesions. These include lesions of the oral mucosa, esophagus, stomach, small intestine, colon, and liver.[30] Kaposi's sarcoma lesions of the GI tract are typically vascular, submucosal tumors, but occult blood loss or bleeding complications of biopsy are rare. The endoscopic appearance of KS is characterized as a raised, red nodule, with an occasional central umbilication in larger lesions.[31] Kaposi's sarcoma of the GI tract is usually detected on routine endoscopy, and symptomatic disease is rare.

Diarrhea

In many developing countries, HIV infection frequently presents with a well-described clinical syndrome of weight loss and chronic diarrhea that is referred to as slim disease.[32-35] The high prevalence of enteric symptoms has lead to the development of a World Health Organization (WHO) provisional case definition for the diagnosis of AIDS in developing countries as the presence of two of the following three major symptoms: more than 10% weight loss, chronic diarrhea for more than 1 month, and prolonged fever for more than 1 month. These signs may occur in association with one or more of the following: chronic cough for more than 1 month, generalized pruritic dermatitis, recurrent zoster, oroesophageal candidiasis, chronic progressive HSV, generalized lymphadenopathy.[36]

Weight loss and chronic diarrhea are frequent complaints in HIV-infected patients in the industrialized world as well. Depending on the population studied, the overall frequency of chronic diarrhea reported in HIV-infected patients can range from 30 to 80%.[37-39] The importance of proper management of diarrhea has recently been underscored by the correlation of weight loss with survival in AIDS patients.[40] Recognizing the importance and frequency of diarrhea and weight loss in HIV-infected patients, the federal Centers for Disease Control and Prevention (CDC) in Atlanta included HIV-infected patients with a diarrhea–wasting syndrome to their surveillance criteria for AIDS in 1987.[41]

The management of chronic diarrhea in patients with HIV infection requires an appreciation of the common treatable causes of diarrhea (Table 25–3) as well as a rational approach to the workup (Fig. 25–1). Investigators of the etiologic agents of diarrhea in HIV-infected patients have been unable to identify a specific cause in 30 to 80% of cases, depending on the population studied and diagnostic methods used.[42-46]

Bacteria

Of the bacterial agents, *Mycobacterium avium-intracellulare* (MAI) is the most frequently identified cause of chronic diarrhea.[47-49] A frequent systemic opportunistic infection in AIDS, MAI is typically associated with chronic fever and weight loss.[50] Abdominal pain, diarrhea, malabsorption, and severe weight loss are seen with enteric MAI,[51, 52] with the small intestine typically more involved than the colon. Inoculation of rectal mucosa may also play a role in the pathogenesis of MAI infection, serving as the portal of entry and site for dissemination.[53] Mucosal changes visible by endoscopy include erythema, edema, and friability, and occasionally small erosions and fine white nodules. Although disseminated MAI infection can be identified by blood culture, the diagnosis of enteric MAI is established by demonstrating positive acid-fast bacteria (AFB) in stool or tissue specimens and culture of the organism for speciation.[54] Histologic examination of biopsy specimens typically reveals organisms within foamy, periodic acid-Schiff (PAS)–positive lamina propria macrophages, suggesting Whipple's disease.[55] Until recently, the therapeutic options for MAI yielded dismal results. Long-term combination therapy with isoniazid, ethambutol, rifabutin, and clofazimine have resulted in symptomatic improvement in 60 to 80% of patients in two small studies.[56, 57] Ethambutol, clofazimine, rifampin and ciprofloxacin have also shown encouraging results.[58] With either regimen, however, symptoms of diarrhea and weight loss are less likely to respond than are fever, malaise, and night sweats. Symptomatic and supportive care with antipyretics, antidiarrheal agents, and nutritional supplements are the standard therapies.

Of the enteric pathogens that can be routinely cultured from the stool, *Salmonella* species are the most important to consider since they are 20-fold more common in patients with AIDS than in the general population.[59, 60] Salmonellosis often presents early in HIV infection as enteric fever, with the acute onset of abdominal pain and watery diarrhea.[61-65] *Salmonella* bacteremia is 100-fold more common in AIDS patients and often presents without intestinal symptoms.[59] Chronic infection and relapse with typhoidal and nontyphoidal *Salmonella* is well described in HIV-infected patients throughout the world.[64, 66-68] *Salmonella* enteritis and bacteremia should be suspected in any HIV-infected patient who presents with the acute onset of abdominal pain and fever. Occasionally, patients develop an acute abdomen and bowel perforation prior to the onset of diarrhea. Thus, a high index of

TABLE 25–3. ETIOLOGY OF CHRONIC DIARRHEA IN HIV-INFECTED PATIENTS

ORGANISM		DIAGNOSIS	THERAPY

MAI		Bx	Experimental:
			  Clofazamine (300 mg/d po × 1 mo, then 300 mg/d)
			    and
			  Ethambutol (25 mg/kg/d × 2 mo, then 15 mg/kg/d)
			    and
			  Rifampin (600 mg/d) or rifabutin 300 mg/d +/−
			    ciprofloxacin (750 bid) +/− Amikacin (7.5 g/kg/
			    d IM or IV × 2 mo)

Bacteria	*Salmonella*	CX	Chloramphenicol
			  or
			TMP/SMX (5–10 mg/kg/d)
			  or
			Ampicillin/amoxicillin
			  or
			Ciprofloxacin (500–750 mg po bid)

	Shigella	Cx	Ampicillin or TMP/SMX or ciprofloxacin
	Campylobacter	Cx	Erythromycin or tetracycline or ciprofloxacin
Viruses	CMV	Bx & Cx	Ganciclovir (DHPG) or foscarnet
	HSV	Bx & Cx	Acyclovir or vidarabine or foscarnet
	Adenoviruses HIV?		Supportive

Parasites	*Cryptosporidium*	Stool acid-fast or
		  fluorescent monoclonal
			Supportive
			Experimental:
			  Spiramycin (1 gm tid) &/or
			  Octreotide (300–500 mcg every 8 h)

	microsporidia	SB Bx & chromotrope stain	+/− Metronidazole

	Isospora	Stool acid-fast Ziehl-
		  Neelsen
			TMP/SMX
			  or
			Pyrimethamine (50–75 mg po d) + folate (5 mg d)

	Giardia	Stool exam	Quinacrine HCl (100 mg tid × 5 d)
	Entameba histolytica		Metronidazole (750 mg tid × 10 d)
	Blastocystis hominis		Metronidazole (750 mg tid × 10 d)

KEY: Bx = biopsy, CMV = cytomegalovirus, Cx = culture, HSV = herpes simplex virus, IM = intramuscularly, IV = intravenously, MAI = *Mycobacterium avium-intracellulare,* SB = small bowel, TMP/SMX = trimethoprim-sulfamethoxazole.

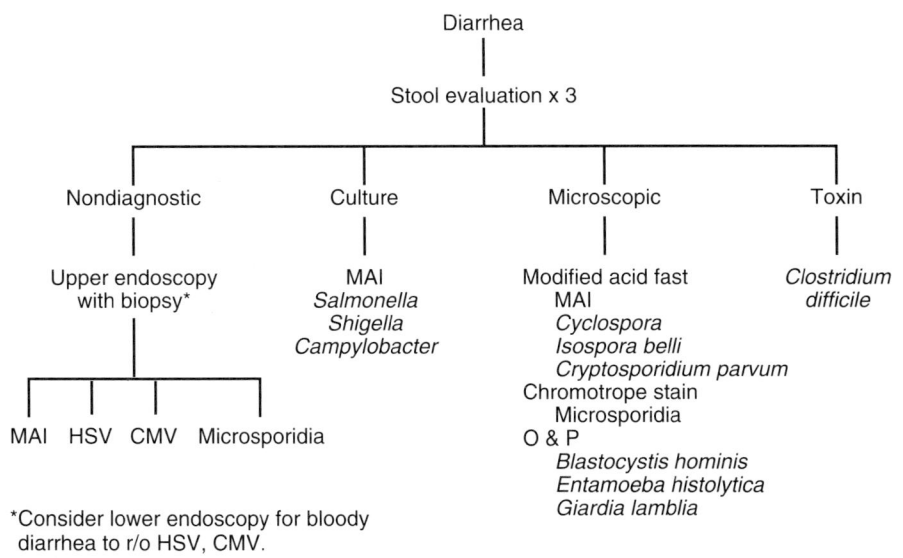

FIGURE 25–1.
Diagnostic evaluation of chronic diarrhea in HIV-infected patient. KEY: CMV = cytomegalovirus, HSV = herpes simplex virus, MAI = *Mycobacterium avium-intracellulare,* O + P = ova and parasite, r/o = rule out.

suspicion should be maintained to identify and manage this treatable and dangerous pathogen. Therapeutic options include chloramphenicol, ampicillin, ciprofloxacin, and trimethoprim-sulfamethoxazole (TMP/SMX). Owing to the high relapse rate in HIV-infected patients, long-term secondary prophylaxis with ciprofloxacin or ampicillin may be required.

Other bacterial causes of acute and chronic diarrhea associated with HIV can be diagnosed by stool culture and include *Shigella flexneri*, which causes intestinal illness ranging from mild diarrhea to severe dysentery.[69, 70] Bloody diarrhea, fever, abdominal cramps, and bacteremia may occur, and relapsing infections have been described. *Campylobacter jejuni* causes a persistent and severe diarrheal illness in patients with AIDS that contrasts with the mild, self-limited illness that typically occurs in immunocompetent persons.[49, 68, 71, 72] Recurrent bacteremia and multiple antibiotic-resistant organisms have been described, and although stool cultures are usually positive, chronic *C. jejuni* infection may require culture of biopsy specimens if multiple stool cultures produce negative findings.[72] *Shigella* may be treated with ampicillin, or TMP/SMX. Ciprofloxacin should be used only for resistant strains. *Campylobacter* is usually sensitive to erythromycin, doxycycline, or ciprofloxacin.

Viruses

Most HIV-infected patients in the United States are co-infected with CMV.[73, 74] Chorioretinitis continues to be the predominant pathologic condition caused by CMV, but esophagitis, enteritis, colitis, proctitis, intestinal perforation, toxic megacolon, and acalculous cholecystitis have also been described in HIV-infected patients.[49, 75, 76] The mucosal lesions associated with CMV infection of the GI tract are typically ulcerative on a background of hemorrhagic erythema. Histopathology shows the characteristic large intranuclear viral inclusions, chronic inflammation, and in some cases mucosal vasculitis.[77] In HIV-infected patients, positive CMV cultures from the GI tract are frequently found from individuals without GI symptoms or pathology. The diagnosis is best made histologically in specimens from ulcerative lesions with the characteristic inclusions and no evidence of other pathogens. Given the moderate success of treating symptomatic CMV GI infection with DHPG and, more recently, foscarnet,[78, 79] endoscopy and biopsy may be indicated in those individual in whom symptomatic CMV is suspected.

Other viruses have been implicated in the etiology of diarrhea in AIDS. Bloody diarrhea has been described in patients with HSV proctitis.[49, 68] Although acyclovir has been shown to benefit these patients, acyclovir-resistant strains of HSV have been described but have been shown to respond to foscarnet.[80] In other studies, adenovirus[80] and the direct effect of HIV[47, 82] have been suggested as potential viral pathogens in HIV-associated diarrhea. Although it has been suggested that the immunologic defects caused by HIV may be responsible, the finding of HIV virions infecting cells of the mucosa suggests a more direct effect of HIV.[83, 84] In addition, many symptomatic and asymptomatic HIV-infected patients have abnormal D-xylose absorption,[68, 85] abnormal findings on Schilling's test,[86] and altered mucosal histopathologic findings[85, 86] without evidence of other identified enteric infection, a condition that has been described as AIDS enteropathy.

Parasites

Parasitic pathogens are a large proportion of identifiable causes of diarrhea in AIDS patients worldwide. *Cryptosporidium* is one of the most important of this group and has been implicated as the cause of 10 to 20% of culture-negative diarrhea in United States AIDS patients[68, 85, 88–90] and up to 55% of diarrhea in the developing world.[91, 92] In addition, *Cryptosporidium* has been implicated as an important nosocomial infection in AIDS patients.[93] Although *Cryptosporidium* is a common cause of mild, self-limited diarrhea in the normal host,[94, 95] the parasite causes a severe, chronic diarrheal illness in AIDS patients. After an incubation period from 2 to 14 days, a clinical syndrome develops that is characterized by chronic, often voluminous, watery diarrhea, severe abdominal pain, weight loss, anorexia, malaise, low-grade fever, and often electrolyte imbalance.[96, 97] Various developmental forms of the *Cryptosporidium* protozoan have been found to inhabit the brush border surface of intestinal epithelial cells, particularly in the distal small intestine.[97] This results in histologic changes, including atrophy and distortion of the villi, increased crypt depth, and mononuclear cell infiltration of the lamina propria.[98] Diagnosis is based on identification of the protozoan in the stool smear with a modified acid-fast stain. Stool examination usually produces positive findings in infected patients, but an average of 3 specimens may be required before oocysts are identified, and concentration techniques may be required to optimize detection in some patients.[99, 100] Specific antimicrobial therapy for cryptosporidiosis is not available.

Spiramycin, an investigational drug with some promise, is under study, but its clinical efficacy in AIDS patients has not been clearly established.[101, 102]

Enterocytozoon bieneusi and *Septata intestinalis* are newly identified species of the phylum Microspora that has been associated with a chronic diarrheal syndrome in AIDS similar to that seen with *Cryptosporidium*. These important enteric pathogens are ubiquitous, small, obligate, intracellular, spore-forming protozoa that have been identified in up to 64% of AIDS patients with chronic unexplained diarrhea.[47, 85, 103–105] After ingestion of the microsporidia spore and its passage into the small intestine, a coiled polar tubule is stimulated to evert and penetrate the host villus epithelial cell. This leads to the injection of the initial infectious form, called the sporoplasm. Proliferation and maturation subsequently occur within the cytoplasm, leading to new spores capable of re-inoculation of the same host and passage into the environment. The typical clinical syndrome of chronic watery diarrhea, weight loss, and malaise is similar to that of cryptosporidiosis.[106] The diagnosis of microsporidiosis is difficult to arrive at due to the small size and poor staining qualities of the organisms. Although definitive diagnosis has required electron microscopic (EM) evaluation of small bowel biopsy specimens,[47, 85] light microscopic examination of duodenal biopsy specimens, using both Giemsa and hematoxylin and eosin (H & E) staining of tissue sections has shown promise.[105, 107] Occasionally, organisms may be detected in semi-thin plastic sections of biopsied tissue stained with basic fuchsin and eosin–methaline blue[106] or in Giemsa-stained, concentrated stool specimens.[108, 109] The gross features of microsporidiosis include the nonspecific appearance of diffuse erythema overlaid by a thin mucoid coating.[85] Microscopically, the characteristic, round-to-oval meront and sporont stages of microsporidia are seen in the supranuclear cytoplasm of villus, but not crypt, epithelial cells.[104, 106] This infection is associated with a degree of enterocyte degeneration, necrosis, and sloughing and partial villus atrophy that appears to parallel the intensity of the infection. As in the case of cryptosporidiosis, the therapeutic options for microsporidia infections are limited primarily to symptomatic and supportive care. Evidence suggests, however, that metronidazole may result in symptomatic improvement, but its therapeutic efficacy has not been clearly established and its use does not result in clearance of the organism.[105]

Isospora belli is an extremely rare pathogenic parasitic infection of the normal human host.[110]

Isosporiasis is, however, a relatively common problem in AIDS patients, particularly in the developing world.[111–113] As with cryptosporidiosis and microsporidiosis, the clinical manifestations of *Isospora* infection include watery diarrhea, cramping abdominal pain, weight loss, anorexia, and fever.[112] Patients may also present with steatorrhea and, in contrast to cryptosporidiosis, eosinophilia. *Isospora* is typically concentrated in the small intestine, but dissemination of this organism has been described in AIDS.[114] The diagnosis is established by identification of the large, oval oocysts in stool with a modified Kinyoun's acid-fast stain.[115] Occasionally, small-intestinal biopsy may be required, and the organism can be found within the enterocyte cytoplasm. Often an inflammatory cell infiltration of the lamina propria associated with mucosal atrophy can be seen on histopathologic examination. Unlike cryptosporidiosis or microsporidiosis, effective therapy for *Isospora* infection is available for AIDS patients. Isosporiasis responds to TMP–SMX therapy and secondary prophylaxis is recommended with TMP–SMX or pyrimethamine–sulfadoxine to prevent recurrence.[113, 116]

Giardia lamblia and *Entamoeba histolytica* are commonly detected in the stools of homosexual men, with infection rates of 20 to 35% in selected populations.[117, 118] Since AIDS patients do not have a significantly higher presence of these protozoa, their presence is not predictive of HIV infection. Giardiasis has been described in HIV-infected patients with diarrhea[68] but is not thought to be a significant problem. *Entamoeba histolytica* is commonly nonpathogenic in the majority of infected homosexual men,[119] but this protozoan has been associated with diarrhea in HIV-infected patients,[49, 68] and in rare instances it may cause fulminant invasive colitis.[120] Evidence suggests, however, that *E. histolytica* infection in most AIDS patients in developed countries may not be pathogenic.[121] There are few data regarding pathogenic *E. histolytica* in AIDS patients in developing countries.

Blastocystis hominis is a common commensal organism in the stool of asymptomatic individuals.[122] Prevalence rates in asymptomatic homosexual men (35%) and AIDS patients (15%) do not differ from the rates observed in symptomatic homosexual men and in AIDS patients.[123] Little epidemiologic or clinical evidence had suggested that *B. hominis* was pathogenic until a 1990 report described a syndrome of diarrhea, abdominal pain, tenesmus, fever, and eosinophilia in late-stage HIV-infected patients that was attributed to *B. hominis* and was responsive to metronidazole.[124] The identification of *G.*

lamblia, E. histolytica and *B. hominis* is made by standard examination of multiple stool samples for ova and parasites. Given the sensitivity of these organisms to antiprotozoal therapy, the presence of one of these organisms and the lack of other pathogens in an HIV-infected patient with symptomatic disease would justify a therapeutic trial of metronidazole.

As previously described, the most commonly identified enteric pathogens in HIV-associated chronic diarrhea include MAI, CMV, *Cryptosporidium,* and more recently various microsporidia. Few identifiable causes of HIV-associated chronic diarrhea can be treated successfully with specific antimicrobial therapy, and the mainstay of therapy continues to be symptomatic, with a combination of antidiarrheal agents, including opiates, loperamide, and diphenoxylate. Octreotide, a somatostatin analog, has been reported to provide symptomatic relief in a group of AIDS patients with diarrhea, but its efficacy has not been established in a randomized, placebo-controlled trial.[125] Nutritional supplements and occasionally short-term hyperalimentation have not been shown clearly to alter length of survival, but they can have a significant impact on the patient's quality of life and should be considered. The lack of specific therapeutic options for many AIDS patients with chronic diarrhea also suggests that the workup of chronic diarrhea should concentrate on diagnostic methods that would identify the treatable causes. The cost-effectiveness of an aggressive interventional approach to identifying the cause of diarrhea in these patients has been evaluated, and conclusions substantiate the view that most treatable causes of diarrhea can be identified with multiple stool examinations and cultures.[126, 127] Endoscopy with biopsy should be reserved for the patients for whom the cause of diarrhea has not been identified after multiple stool examinations and cultures.

The efficient management of chronic diarrhea in an HIV-infected patient should begin with at least three careful stool evaluations, including culture for *Salmonella, Shigella,* and *Campylobacter* and an ova and parasite examination (see Fig. 25–1). Owing to the frequent use of antibiotics in this population, a *Clostridium difficile* toxin assay should also be performed. If this proves nondiagnostic, upper gastrointestinal endoscopy should be considered, with small bowel biopsy for viral and AFB culture, histology, and possible EM for microsporidia. In patients with symptoms of colonic or rectal disease such as hematochezia or mucocutaneous lesions, lower intestinal endoscopy with biopsy and culture should be considered.

Anorectal Lesions

Proctitis, a well-described problem in homosexual men, is associated with HSV, syphilis, and sexual practices.[116] These problems tend to become more severe and less amenable to therapy in the HIV-infected patient. More than 95% of male homosexuals with AIDS have serologic evidence of HSV 2 infection,[128] which is reflected by the high frequency of chronic mucocutaneous HSV infection. Proctitis due to HSV is characterized by perianal or perineal ulcerations and painful herpetic vesicles. Occasionally, patients develop chronic, large, painful ulcers.[129] Bloody diarrhea, tenesmus, and fever can also be seen. Lumbosacral radiculopathy associated with urinary dysfunction, sacral paresthesias, and lower extremity pain comprise a syndrome that is well described in HSV-infected men.[130] Herpetic proctitis is diagnosed by a swab culture of the lesion or by cytologic evidence of intranuclear inclusions and multinucleated giant cells. Acyclovir, if initiated early in the course of the disease, is usually beneficial, and long-term suppression in HIV-infected patients may be required. Acyclovir-resistant HSV has become an increasing problem, but it has been shown to respond to foscarnet.[80]

Given the high frequency of syphilis in the population of homosexual men and HIV-infected individuals, the possibility of anal syphilis must be considered. Primary syphilis may be heralded by a chancre at the anal margin. It is often painful and may be confused with an anal fissure. Proctitis without anogenital lesions and inguinal adenopathy can also be seen. Any anal ulcer in an HIV-infected patient should be suspected as syphilitic. Darkfield examination of the chancre base and serology are then indicated.

Anal warts of condylomata acuminata are a common problem in homosexual men and in patients with HIV (see Chapter 11). Eradication in HIV-infected patients is similar to that for noninfected patients and includes local therapy with surgical excision, laser or cryotherapy, electrocoagulation, and topical podophyllum. Although indicated for immunocompetent patients, immunotherapy with condylomata vaccination[131] is contraindicated in HIV-infected patients, and interferon injection has no apparent benefit in these patients either.[132]

An association between nonspecific proctitis and HIV-infection has been described.[133] It is postulated that, in addition to the increased risk of HIV transmission in individuals with mucosal alteration due to proctitis, HIV may directly or indirectly alter the rectal mucosal inflammatory response.

Biliary Tract and Hepatic Disease

The frequency of cholestasis and gallbladder disease is increased in HIV-infected individuals above the normal population.[134, 135] Although rare in young immunocompetent patients, acalculous cholecystitis has been described in AIDS patients and is associated with histologic evidence of CMV, microsporidia, or cryptosporidia infection.[136, 137] In these patients, sonography has shown dilatation of intrahepatic and common bile ducts and thickened gallbladder walls.[138] Extrahepatic biliary obstruction, with a clinical syndrome resembling sclerosing cholangitis, has also been described.[139] An HIV-infected patient with serologic and clinical evidence of biliary obstruction should have a comprehensive diagnostic investigation with sonography, computed tomography (CT) scan, or endoscopic retrograde cholangiopancreatography (ERCP) to rule out the common treatable causes, including cholelithiasis. As in any other patient, in the HIV-infected patient a timely diagnosis and appropriate surgical intervention are indicated in the management of acute cholecystitis.

Hepatic dysfunction in the HIV-infected patient is also common, especially dysfunction due to the use of hepatotoxic medications such as sulfonamides or interferon-α.[139–141] Despite the high prevalence of hepatitis B, hepatitis C, and delta hepatitis in populations at risk for HIV,[142] symptomatic viral hepatitis is not so common as once believed. This may be owing to the role of immune-mediated cytolysis in viral hepatitis and the immune suppression of HIV. HIV-associated hepatic parenchymal disease is more typically caused by an infiltrative process such as MAI, *Mycobacterium tuberculosis*, histoplasmosis, *coccidiomycosis*, *Cryptococcus neoformans*, *Pneumocystis carinii*, KS, or lymphoma.[139, 143] Peliosis hepatis may also occur in some patients. Percutaneous liver biopsy is rarely indicated in HIV-infected patients with parenchymal liver disease. Usually, the hepatic pathologic findings reflect dissemination of a previously diagnosed opportunistic infection, or else the cause is suggested by positive findings on specific serology. In individuals without other evidence of a disseminating process such as MAI, CMV, lymphoma, or KS, however, a liver biopsy with viral, fungal, and mycobacterial cultures should be considered.

MALIGNANCY

The number of granulocytes per mm³ of blood is an important predictor of susceptibility to infection in patients with malignancies, particularly in those receiving marrow suppressive therapy. Other consequences of malignancy, such as leukemic cell tissue infiltration or leukostasis, may result in an increased risk of infection. In addition, certain malignancies are associated with qualitative immune defects that may increase the risk of infectious complications. These include hypogammaglobulinemia and B cell dysfunction associated with chronic lymphocytic leukemia (CLL) and myeloma, which result in defective opsonization and an increased risk of pyogenic infections.[144] Patients with T cell lymphomas such as Hodgkin's disease may have abnormal T cell function[145] and a higher risk for some fungal and mycobacterial infections. The phagocytic defects associated with some acute leukemias[146] may also increase the risk for pyogenic infections.[144]

Although specific infectious GI complications in the nonneutropenic cancer patient are rare, one syndrome described is the association between symptomatic *C. difficile* infection and hematological malignancies. Typically, *C. difficile* colitis is associated with antibiotic use, but in some patients with leukemia an unusual constellation of symptoms, including jaundice, abdominal pain, diarrhea, and large bowel ileus may occur.[147] The isolation of the organism from the stool does not by itself implicate *C. difficile* as the cause of colitis. Many healthy adults and newborns may be asymptomatic carriers.[148] Demonstration of *C. difficile* cytotoxin in the stools of symptomatic patients is diagnostic for this infection and would warrant specific therapy.[149] Therapeutic options for *C. difficile* include oral vancomycin[150] and metronidazole.[151]

Neutropenia

Patients with neutropenia are at a particular risk for infection and bacteremia. In one study of neutropenic patients with acute nonlymphocytic leukemia, 70% had a documented infection, 67% of which were caused by enteric gram-negative organisms.[152] This underscores the principle that neutropenic patients are at great risk from hospital-acquired gram-negative organisms that colonize the GI tract.

Because the risk of infection with organisms such as *Candida* and *Pseudomonas* has been associated with enteric colonization in neutropenic patients, surveillance cultures are performed in most institutions.[153, 154] This has led to the prophylactic administration of antibiotics such as ciprofloxacin or TMP/SMZ, with or without colistin, to patients with severe granulocytopenia since they have been shown to reduce the risk of acquired infection with enteric gram-negative organisms.[155–157]

Particular attention should be given to the oral mucosa and perirectal area as sources of infection in these patients. The presence of perirectal abscess in neutropenic patients is associated with a risk of septicemia that approaches 50%.[158] In addition, life-threatening necrotizing colitis can be a complication of neutropenia; it presents with fever, watery diarrhea, and abdominal pain.[159, 160] Bloody diarrhea can also occur in this syndrome. Bacteremia with enteric organisms including *Clostridium* species has been described in these patients,[161] but necrotizing colitis is not clearly associated with antibiotic use or previous colitis. Bowel rest and broad-spectrum antibiotics should be a component of the medical management of necrotizing colitis, and surgical resection of involved bowel may be necessary.[160]

BONE MARROW TRANSPLANTATION

Gastrointestinal symptoms are virtually expected after bone marrow transplantation (BMT) and are typically the result of drug toxicity, infections, or graft-versus-host disease (GVHD). Identifying infections due to other causes may be difficult, but timely diagnosis and appropriate treatment of these tenuous patients is extremely important. An understanding of the temporal association of certain infectious complications of BMT can be helpful in predicting which pathogens may be implicated (Table 25–4). In the immediate posttransplantation period, infectious complications are typically due to bacterial and fungal pathogens. Viral infections are more common later in the posttransplantation period, especially in patients on immunosuppressive therapy for GVHD. Although these classical generalizations may be helpful, complicated multidrug protocols may induce variable combinations of immunologic defects.

Immediate Complications

The preparative regimens of chemotherapy and whole-body radiation prior to BMT typically result in mucosal and hepatic damage within 3 weeks. The acute radiation syndrome of vomiting and diarrhea is radiation-dose–dependent.[162] Parotitis, vomiting, diarrhea, and particularly mucositis can occur and are usually self-limiting.[162, 163]

The mucosal insult of pretransplantation radiation and the prolonged posttransplantation neutropenia put the BMT patient at high risk for mucosal invasion and bacteremia by enteric gram-negative bacteria. Most transplant protocols include a prophylactic oral antibiotic regimen to reduce this risk, but the frequency of acute neutropenic colitis is still high, and patients with fever, abdominal pain, and neutropenia should be cultured and covered empirically with appropriate antibiotic therapy.

Owing to the frequent use of antibiotics in these patients, the possibility of *C. difficile* pseudomembranous colitis should also be investigated by assay of the stool for toxin production. Oral metronidazole or vancomycin is usually an effective therapy.

Prolonged neutropenia leads to a subsequent predisposition to *Candida* and *Aspergillus* infection in up to 40% of BMT recipients.[164] Muco-

TABLE 25–4. GASTROINTESTINAL COMPLICATIONS FOLLOWING BONE MARROW TRANSPLANTATION

TIMING	CAUSE
IMMEDIATE: LESS THAN 3 WK	
Enteric	
Vomiting & diarrhea	Pretransplant chemotherapy &
Neutropenic colitis	radiation
Clostridium difficile colitis	Antibiotics
Oroesophageal *Candida*	
Parotiditis	Neutropenia
Mucositis	
Hepatic	
Hepatitis	HVOD
EARLY: LESS THAN 2 MO	
Enteric	
Gastroenteritis	Adenovirus, acute GVHD
Diarrhea	Adenovirus, rotavirus, Cryptosporidium, *Giardia lamblia*, CMV, acute GVHD
Mucositis	HSV
Hepatic	
Hepatitis	Acute GVHD, HVOD, HSV, CMV, EBV, fungal, adenovirus
LATE: MORE THAN 2 MO	
Enteric	
Esophagitis	HSV, *Candida,* immunosuppression
Enteritis	CMV, giardiasis
	Adjuvant therapy, chronic GVHD
Hepatic	
Hepatitis	Chronic GVHD, viral

KEY: CMV = cytomegalovirus, EBV = Epstein-Barr virus, GVHD = graft-versus-host disease, HSV = herpes simplex virus, HVOD = hepatic veno-occlusive disease.

cutaneous *Candida* and esophagitis are the fungal GI complications of most concern. Most BMT prophylactic regimens also include oral antifungal agents such as clotrimazole, nystatin, and fluconazole.[165] In those patients with endoscopic evidence of invasive *Candida* esophagitis, amphotericin B, given in a dosage of 0.3 mg/kg of body weight per day, is indicated.

Hepatic veno-occlusive disease presenting as hepatomegaly, ascites, and jaundice is a well-recognized complication of BMT that occurs within 2 weeks of transplantation.[166, 167] This syndrome is more likely to occur in patients with active hepatitis at transplantation and is associated with a high mortality. Due to posttransplantation thrombocytopenia, diagnosis by liver biopsy is contraindicated. Supportive therapy, including fluid and electrolyte management, is the standard.

Early Complications

In addition to mucositis, often due to HSV,[168] gastroenteritis is a frequent problem in the early period after BMT and has been attributed to adenovirus infection in up to 15% of patients.[169] Adenovirus gastroenteritis typically presents with vomiting, diarrhea, and abdominal pain. The importance of this pathogen in these patients is accented by the high mortality associated with documented adenovirus infection. Diagnosis is made by culture, by demonstration of viral particles on histopathologic examination, or by serologic study. In addition to supportive care, patient isolation is important because adenovirus is highly contagious and of significant risk to other immunosuppressed patients.

Diarrhea occurs in up to 83% of children undergoing BMT, and recognized pathogens have been detected in 52% of diarrhea stools in one study.[170] Adenoviruses, rotaviruses, *Cryptosporidium* and *G. lamblia* were the organisms most frequently identified. Cytomegalovirus has been implicated as a frequent cause of GI disease in other studies.[171, 172] Rotavirus-associated diarrhea is of particular concern in the BMT recipient and is associated with increased mortality.[169] This infection is diagnosed readily by enzyme-linked immunosorbent assay (ELISA) or radioimmunoassay (RIA) of stool specimens,[173, 174] and therapy is supportive, with particular attention to electrolyte abnormalities, which can be associated with high mortality.[175] Cryptosporidiosis is relatively rare and causes a clinical syndrome in BMT recipients similar to, but milder than, that seen in AIDS patients. The clinical efficacy of spiramycin in BMT-associated cryptosporidiosis has not been clearly established, but there is one report of successful symptom management.[176]

The clinical syndrome of acute GVHD, including fever, pancytopenia, skin rash, abdominal pain, and diarrhea, typically presents 4 to 8 weeks after BMT.[177, 178] Massive diarrhea and hematochezia with metabolic and nutritional disturbances can also occur. Endoscopic examination in acute GVHD may initially detect mucosal erythema, but ulcerations and sloughing are seen with progressive disease.[179] The pathologic condition is typically concentrated in the small and large bowel, with sparing of the gastric mucosa.[180] Enteric GVHD is distinguished from infectious enteritis by negative findings on stool examination and histopathologic study of biopsy specimens, although secondary bacterial infection may contribute to the pathologic condition of GVHD.[181] Bowel rest with total parenteral nutrition (TPN) and treatment of any detectable pathogens are the initial therapy of acute enteric GVHD. In addition, somatostatin and its analogs have been used with some success in treating the diarrhea of GVHD.[182] An acute upper GI tract GVHD syndrome presenting as anorexia, dyspepsia, nausea, and vomiting has been recognized and confirmed histologically.[178]

Acute hepatic GVHD, presenting as cholestatic jaundice must be distinguished from viral hepatitis, veno-occlusive disease, HSV, CMV, EBV, or disseminated fungal infection.[181, 183] Hepatic GVHD is often heralded by the rash and diarrhea of systemic acute GVHD, although it may precede these symptoms and be difficult to diagnose. In the early stages, histologic study reveals small foci of lobular necrosis, with a lymphocytic infiltration that progresses to a more diffuse process and bile duct involvement.[180, 184] If liver enzymes are markedly elevated, viral hepatitis should be considered. Adenovirus hepatitis is a frequently recognized syndrome in BMT patients[185] that includes such symptoms as fever, anorexia, nausea, vomiting, and rising levels on liver function tests. Histopathologic examination reveals hepatocellular necrosis with intranuclear inclusions.

Late Complications

Esophagitis due to HSV and *Candida* can occur in the late posttransplantation period owing to immunosuppressive therapy and, as in HIV-infected patients, is diagnosed by upper intestinal endoscopy, biopsy, and culture. Cytomegalovirus enteritis, presenting with fever, diarrhea, and malabsorption and responsive to DHPG, has been described in BMT patients.[186] Giardiasis has been recognized as a complication of documented intestinal GVHD after BMT.[187]

Advanced hematologic malignancies are associated with high relapse rates after autologous BMT and adjuvant immunotherapy with cytokines and lymphokine-activated killer (LAK) cells are being used increasingly in these patients. Diarrhea, fever, rash, and nausea are common side effects of these therapies.[188]

Chronic GVHD occurring after 3 months, is usually preceded by acute GVHD[189] and has been associated with stomatitis, esophagitis, anorexia, chronic diarrhea, steatorrhea, weight loss, and nutrition-related problems.[190–192] Sicca syndrome, with dry mouth and eyes, is also a well-recognized component of chronic GVHD.[193] Histologic evidence of fibrosis of the lamina propria is characteristic of chronic GVHD.[194]

Chronic hepatic GVHD typically presents with cholestasis and fluctuating jaundice.[189, 194] Sonography or ERCP or both should be performed to rule out extrahepatic obstruction. Liver biopsy and viral serology should be considered to exclude viral hepatitis prior to initiation of long-term immunosuppressive therapy for GVHD. In chronic hepatic GVHD, a mixed cellular infiltrate of the portal triads and periportal regions may be seen, with portal fibrosis and occasionally cirrhosis.[194, 195] Bile duct infiltration and bile stasis have also been described.

SOLID ORGAN TRANSPLANTATION

The infectious complications of kidney, liver, and heart transplantations are the most important factors influencing the postoperative mortality and morbidity of the recipients. There are complications that affect all patients who undergo solid organ transplantations and others that are organ-specific.

Renal Transplantation

Renal transplantation patients are prone to stomatitis and esophagitis, usually due to HSV or *Candida albicans*.[196] Endoscopic biopsy of esophageal lesions is usually required to confirm the diagnosis of esophagitis from either organism. As in other immunosuppressed patients, acyclovir is the drug of choice for those with HSV. Amphotericin B should be used to treat most transplantation recipients with invasive *Candida* esophagitis. The clinical efficacy of

fluconazole or ketoconazole has not yet been established in these patients. It may be reasonable to treat the infection with amphotericin B until clinical improvement is apparent and to complete the course with one of these agents.

Cytomegalovirus esophagitis and enteritis have been described in renal transplant patients. Cecal ulcers can present with hematochezia.[197] Documented severe invasive GI tract disease due to CMV may respond to DHPG, which is a reasonable approach to therapy although its clinical efficacy in this setting has not been established.[198]

In addition to the usual pathogens associated with gastroenteritis in immunocompetent patients, renal transplant patients may also be at increased risk for salmonellosis[199] and for hemorrhagic enteritis due to *M. tuberculosis*.[200]

Strongyloides stercoralis is an endemic intestinal nematode that is asymptomatic in more than 50% of immunocompetent patients.[201] Symptomatic and more serious infections with strongyloides have been described in immunosuppressed patients, particularly renal allograft recipients.[202] The filariform larvae of strongyloides infect by penetrating the skin and then migrating through the circulation to the pulmonary veins and alveoli. They migrate up the endobronchial tree to the pharynx, are swallowed, and mature within the small intestine into adult forms. Adult females, attached to the wall of the small intestine, produce rhabditiform larvae,[203] which may mature into invasive filariform larvae prior to their excretion into the stool. This autoinfection process results in chronic infections. In immunosuppressed patients, hyperinfection can occur and is characterized by an increase in worm burden.[204] In addition to renal transplantation,[205] hyperinfection syndrome has been described in steroid use,[206, 207] lymphoma,[208] acute leukemia, and malnutrition. These patients typically present with abdominal pain, nausea, vomiting, diarrhea, and occasionally GI tract bleeding. These GI symptoms are often associated with fever, rash, and pulmonary manifestations.[202] Due to the nonspecific clinical presentation and the infrequency of infection, the diagnosis of strongyloidiasis in the immunosuppressed patient requires a high index of suspicion. Eosinophilia is a frequent finding in these patients and should initiate a more definitive diagnostic workup.[209, 210] The identification of strongyloides larvae in the stool is the definitive diagnostic evidence of infection, and the presence of the filariform larvae should raise the suspicion of autoinfection and hyperinfection.[211, 212] Thiabendazole, given in a dosage of 25 mg/kg of body weight 2 times a day, is the treatment of choice for stronglyloidiasis.[213] Therapy for intestinal disease is for 2 days and should be extended for a total of 5 to 14 days in disseminated disease.[214]

Liver Transplantation

The infectious complications of liver transplantation are especially severe. Up to 67% of liver transplant recipients develop a serious postoperative infection, with 89% of postoperative mortality associated with infection.[215] Intra-abdominal or liver abscess, peritonitis, cholangitis, pseudomembranous colitis, and invasive candidiasis are all frequent problems in these patients and are associated with a high mortality within the first 2 months of surgery.[215]

Of all solid organ transplantation patients, liver transplant recipients are the most susceptible to serious fungal infections with fungemia, and the abdomen and GI tract are the most common sites of infection. In some studies, 18 to 44% of liver transplant recipients developed a serious fungal infection, and up to 16% were fungemic.[215, 216] *Candida* is the most common source of infection, but *Aspergillus,* mucormycosis, and cryptococcal infections have been described. Most *Candida* infections occur within the first 2 months of surgery and are associated with high mortality.[215] Disseminated candidiasis is the most typical clinical presentation, with local pathologic conditions that include esophagitis, peritonitis, or intra-abdominal abscess.[215] These patients should be treated with a long course of amphotericin B. The roles of fluconazole and ketoconazole in these patients have not been established. Disseminated *Aspergillus* infections can occur in these patients, and in addition to pulmonary and central nervous system lesions, allograft infections have been described.[215] High-dose amphotericin B is the therapy of choice for aspergillosis.

Viral infections, particularly disseminated CMV infections, are common in liver transplant patients. Symptomatic disseminated CMV infection, associated with a mortality of 83%, was the most common serious infection in one study of liver transplantation.[215] Gastrointestinal tract involvement with CMV is rare relative to pulmonary complications but should be considered in postoperative patients with bloody diarrhea.[217]

Mucocutaneous HSV infections have been described in up to 34% of liver transplant recipients.[215] Rarely, disseminated HSV has caused allograft infection, esophagitis, and colitis in these patients, and it is associated with a high mortality despite acyclovir therapy. Most herpetic infections occur within the first 3 weeks of transplantation. After viral culture of the lesions, acyclovir is the therapy of choice in these patients, and it usually controls the mucocutaneous HSV complications.

Heart Transplantation

Up to 21% of heart and heart–lung transplant patients have significant postoperative GI pathologic changes, with 46% of these patients requiring posttransplantation abdominal surgical intervention.[218] Although most of the complications are noninfectious, problems such as visceral perforation and GI bleeding, diarrhea, cholecystitis, and abscess formation have been reported in 13% of transplant recipients.

Disseminated CMV infection is a well-described complication in transplant recipients of solid organs. Although most of these patients have symptomatic pulmonary disease, invasive, biopsy-confirmed CMV enteritis with diarrhea has been described and has been shown to respond symptomatically to DHPG.[217]

CONGENITAL IMMUNODEFICIENCY SYNDROMES

With the recognition and increasingly successful control of respiratory complications of primary disorders of the immune system, GI symptoms have become of greater importance. Congenital immune defects may present with GI manifestations of chronic, recurrent infections or with autoimmune disease (Table 25–5). For example, severe combined immunodeficiency (SCID) and agammaglobulinemia patients may present with chronic viral gastroenteritis. In addition, inflammatory bowel disease is associated with a number of primary immune disorders.

T Cell Disorders

DiGeorge's syndrome, resulting from abnormal development of the third and fourth pharyngeal pouches, is associated with cardiovascular deformities, abnormal facial development, and hypoparathyroidism.[219] In addition, thymic hypoplasia is reflected by a variable degree of cellular immune deficiency. These patients typically develop recurrent pneumonia and rhinitis. Gastrointestinal complications include recurrent oral and esophageal monilial infections, and chronic viral gastroenteritis is also de-

TABLE 25–5. GASTROINTESTINAL MANIFESTATIONS OF CONGENITAL IMMUNODEFICIENCY

		DEFECT	COMPLICATION
T cell disorders	DiGeorge's syndrome	Thymic hypoplasia	Recurrent oroesophageal *Candida* infection
	CMCC	Absent T-cell response to *Candida*	Oroesophageal *Candida* infection
B cell disorders	IgA deficiency	Low serum & secretory IgA	Giardiasis Milk allergy, IBD
	X-LA	Agammaglobulinemia	Chronic enteroviral diarrhea
	CVID	Hypogammaglobulinemia	Giardiasis, strongyloidiasis, cryptosporidiosis, IBD
Phagocytic defects	CGD		Perianal, hepatic and splenic abscesses
Combined deficiencies	SCID	Hypogammaglobulinemia Absence of T cells	Chronic viral diarrhea, oral/perirectal candidiasis

KEY: CGD = chronic granulomatous disease, CMCC = chronic mucocutaneous candidiasis, CVID = common variable immunodeficiency, IBD = inflammatory bowel disease, IgA = immunoglobulin A, SCID = severe combined immunodeficiency, X-LA = X-linked agammaglobulinemia.

scribed.[220] In many patients, the cause of diarrhea is unclear but may be related to hyperparathyroidism.[221]

Patients with an inability to develop a cellular immune response to *Candida* present with chronic mucocutaneous candidiasis (CMCC). Chronic mucocutaneous candidiasis is typically associated with a variety of autoimmune diseases and endocrinopathies.[222] These patients develop chronic severe *Candida* infections of the skin, nails, mucous membranes, and esophagus, and occasionally visceral dissemination occurs.[223] As in AIDS patients, in these patients the diagnosis of *Candida* esophagitis is made with endoscopic biopsy. Daily ketoconazole is the usual treatment, and long-term suppressive therapy is usually required.[224, 225] Fluconazole has been shown to be efficacious as well in these patients.[226] Visceral involvement with invasive *Candida* should be treated initially with amphotericin B.

B Cell Disorders

Selective IgA deficiency, the most common congenital immunodeficiency, has a variable clinical presentation.[227, 228] These patients typically have low levels of serum and secretory IgA.[229] Although sinopulmonary infections are more common complications, these patients may also develop intestinal symptoms.[230, 231] Up to 25% of these patients may develop chronic diarrhea, and *G. lamblia* is the most important pathogen in these individuals. Multiple stool examinations and duodenal fluid aspiration may be required for diagnosis of giardiasis. Metronidazole is effective in most patients and might be tried empirically in some patients with selective IgA deficiency and chronic diarrhea. For those

patients who do not respond to empirical therapy, the possibility of other noninfectious causes of chronic diarrhea associated with IgA deficiency must be considered, such as inflammatory bowel disease[232] or milk allergy.

Patients with X-linked agammaglobulinemia (X-LA) have extremely low serum levels of all classes of immunoglobulin as a result of a congenital defect in B cell differentiation.[233] There is an absence of plasma cells in the rectal mucosa of patients with X-LA, which may be associated with crypt abscesses and leukocyte infiltration of the lamina propria.[234] These patients typically present with recurrent pyogenic infections such as sinusitis, otitis, osteomyelitis, and pneumonia. In addition, they may present with chronic diarrhea, although less frequently than do common variable immunodeficiency (CVID) patients. The agents most commonly associated with diarrhea in these patients include *C. jejuni, Salmonella, Giardia, Cryptosporidium,* and enteric viruses, especially adenovirus, coxsackievirus, and echovirus.[234, 235] Enteroviral infections are associated with dissemination and high mortality.[236, 237] Therapy with intravenous and oral gammaglobulin may provide symptomatic relief of diarrhea in some patients without eradication of the virus. Given the frequent use of antibiotics in patients with X-LA, acute and chronic *C. difficile* colitis should be considered in patients with diarrhea. Common variable immunodeficiency is a group of disorders characterized by abnormal antibody responses and hypogammaglobulinemia that typically presents in young adults.[238] Although usually characterized by recurrent sinopulmonary infections, frequent complaints of patients with CVID include steatorrhea and chronic diarrhea.[234, 239] Again, *G. lamblia* is the most common pathogen identified as the cause of chronic diarrhea in CVID,[234] but cryptosporidiosis, strongyloidiasis, and *Campylobacter jejuni* infection have also been reported.[240–243] Diagnosis of giardiasis in this population may be difficult because patchy involvement of the small intestine is possible and has been described. Multiple biopsies and duodenal aspirations may be required. Metronidazole is effective therapy in this population and may be indicated empirically in patients with diarrhea and dysgammaglobulinemia since diagnostic measures are difficult to perform. In some CVID patients, malabsorption may also result from small bowel bacterial overgrowth. In many CVID patients, no cause can be found, and the infections are resistant to treatment. As in patients with other primary immune defects, patients occasionally develop the characteristic autoimmune syndrome of Crohn's disease but respond to sulfasalazine and corticosteroid therapy.[244] Other GI complications of CVID to be considered include nodular lymphoid hyperplasia, seen in 20 to 60% of patients, achlorhydria, identified in up to 50% of patients, and pernicious anemia.[237, 245]

Phagocytic Disorders

The most common primary defect of phagocyte function is the X-linked disorder chronic granulomatous disease (CGD). The GI complications of this disease include chronic perianal, hepatic, and splenic abscesses. As expected, the most important organisms include staphylococci, enteric gram-negative bacteria, *Candida,* and *Aspergillus.* These granulomatous abscesses can occasionally occur throughout the GI tract, leading to obstructive symptoms. If an organism can be isolated, specific antimicrobial therapy is indicated in these patients. Empirical antibiotic therapy for staphylococci may be reasonable, however, when a specific cause is unknown.

Combined Disorder

Children with SCID have both hypogammaglobulinemia and absence of T cells.[246] The GI histopathologic examination reveals an absence of lymphocytes in the lamina propria, with blunted villi and friable mucosa. Chronic diarrhea and malabsorption are common. Severe wasting due to malabsorption and chronic diarrhea are a common feature of this syndrome. Viral causes are the most important in this population and include adenovirus, coxsackievirus, and rotavirus. Although oral therapy with gamma globulin has been attempted and has met with mixed results, symptoms usually persist until definitive therapy with BMT can be initiated. These patients also frequently develop candidiasis of the oral mucosal and perirectal area, which can usually be controlled with nystatin or clotrimazole.

REFERENCES

1. Cooper AD, Gold J, Maclean P, et al. Acute AIDS retrovirus infection: Definition of a clinical illness associated with seroconversion. Lancet. 1985;2:537–540.
2. Giorgi JV, Detels R. T-cell subset alterations in HIV-infected homosexual men: NIAID multicenter AIDS cohort study. Clin Immunol Immunopathol. 1989;52:10–18.
3. Polk BF, Robin F, Brookmeyer R, et al. Predictors of the acquired immunodeficiency syndrome developing in a cohort of seropositive homosexual men. N Engl J Med. 1987;316:61–66.
4. Goedert JJ, Biggar RJ, Melbye M, et al. Effect of T4 count and cofactors on the incidence of AIDS in homosexual men infected with human immunodeficiency virus. JAMA. 1987;257:331–334.
5. Lane HC, Masur H, Edgar LC, et al. Abnormalities of B cell activation and immunoregulation in patients with the acquired immunodeficiency syndrome. N Engl J Med. 1983;309:435.
6. Crawford DH, Weller I, Iliescu V. Polyclonal activation of B cells in homosexual men. Lancet. 1984;2:536.
7. Sieber G, Techihmann H, Ludwig WD. B-cell function in AIDS. Blut. 1985;51:143–144.
8. Janoff EN, Douglas JM Jr., Gabriel M, et al. Class-specific antibody response to pneumococcal capsular polysaccharides in men infected with human immunodeficiency virus type 1. J Infect Dis. 1988;158:983–989.
9. Roberts CJ. Coccidioidomycosis in acquired immune deficiency syndrome: Depressed humoral as well as cellular immunity. Am J Med. 1984;76:734–736.
10. Murray HW, Rubin BY, Masur H, et al. Impaired production of lymphokines and immune (gamma) interferon in the acquired immunodeficiency syndrome. N Engl J Med. 1984;310:883.
11. Smith PS, Ohura K, Masur H, et al. Monocyte function in the acquired immunodeficiency syndrome: Defective chemotaxis. J Clin Invest. 1984;71:2121.
12. Rodgers VD, Fassett R, Kagnoff MF. Abnormalities in intestinal mucosal T cells in homosexual populations including those with the lymphadenopathy syndrome and acquired immunodeficiency syndrome. Gastroenterology. 1986;90:552–558.
13. Ellakany S, Whiteside TL, Schade RR, et al. Analysis of intestinal lymphocyte subpopulations in patients with acquired immunodeficiency syndrome (AIDS) and AIDS-related complex. J Clin Pathol. 1987;87:356–364.
14. Kotler DP, Scholes JV, Tierney AR. Intestinal plasma cell alterations in acquired immunodeficiency syndrome. Dig Dis Sci. 1987;32:129–138.
15. Jackson S. Secretory and serum IgA are inversely altered in AIDS patients. In: MacDonald TT, Challacombe SJ, Bland PW, et al, eds. Advances in Mucosal Immunology. Lancaster: Kluwer Academic Publishers; 1990:665–668.
16. Greenspan D, Greenspan JS. Oral lesions of HIV infections: Features and therapy. In: Volberding P, Jacobson MA, eds. AIDS Clinical Review 1990. New York: Marcel Dekker; 1990:81–93.

17. Phelan JA, Saltman BR, Friedland GH, et al. Oral findings in patients with acquired immunodeficiency syndrome. Oral Surg Oral Med Oral Pathol. 1987;64:50–56.

18. Eversole LR, Jacobsen P, Stone CE, et al. Oral condyloma planus (hairy leukoplakia) among homosexual men: A clinicopathologic study of thirty-six cases. Oral Surg Oral Med Oral Pathol. 1986;61:249.

19. Greenspan D, Greenspan JS, Conant M, et al. Oral "hairy" leukoplakia in male homosexuals: Evidence of association with both papillomavirus and a herpes group virus. Lancet. 1984;2:831–834.

20. Eisner MS, Smith PD. Etiology of odynophagia and dysphagia in patients with the acquired immunodeficiency syndrome. Gastroenterology. 1990;98:446A.

21. Tavitian A, Raufman JP, Rosenthal LE. Oral candidiasis as a marker for esophageal candidiasis in the acquired immunodeficiency syndrome. Ann Intern Med. 1986;104:54–55.

22. Cone LA, Woodward DR, Potts BE, et al. An update on the acquired immunodeficiency syndrome (AIDS): Associated disorders of the alimentary tract. Dis Colon Rectum. 1986;29:60–64.

23. Furio MM, Wordell CJ. Treatment of infectious complications of acquired immunodeficiency syndrome. Clin Pharmacol. 1985;4:539–554.

24. Raufman JP. Odynophagia/dysphagia in AIDS. Gastroenterol Clin North Am. 1988;17:599–614.

25. Horowitz L, Stern JO, Segarra S. Gastrointestinal manifestations of Kaposi's sarcoma. In: Friedman-Kine AE, Laubenstein LJ, eds. AIDS: The Epidemic of Kaposi's Sarcoma and Opportunistic Infections. New York: Masson; 1984:364–371.

26. St. Onge G, Bezahler GH. Giant esophageal ulcer associated with cytomegalovirus. Gastroenterology. 1982; 83:127.

27. Wilcox CM, Diehl DL, Cello JP, et al. Cytomegalovirus esophagitis in patients with AIDS. Ann Intern Med. 1990;113:589–593.

28. Chachoua A, Dieterich D, Krasinski K, et al. 9-(1,3-dihydroxy-2-propoxymethyl)guanine (ganciclovir) in the treatment of cytomegalovirus gastrointestinal disease with the acquired immunodeficiency syndrome. Ann Intern Med. 1987;107:133–137.

29. Koretz SH. Collaborative DHPG treatment study group: Treatment of serious cytomegalovirus infections with 9-(1,3-dihydroxy-2-propoxymethyl)guanine in patients with AIDS and other immunodeficiencies. N Engl J Med. 1986;314:801–805.

30. Friedman S, Wright T, Altman D. Kaposi's sarcoma and the gastrointestinal tract: The San Francisco experience. Gastroenterology. 1983;84:1160.

31. Rose HS, Balthaar EJ, Megibow AJ, et al. Alimentary tract involvement in Kaposi's sarcoma: Radiographic and endoscopic findings in 25 homosexual men. Am J Roentgenol. 1982;139:661–666.

32. Clumek N, Sonnet J, Taelman H, et al. Acquired immune deficiency syndrome in African patients. N Engl J Med. 1984;310:492–497.

33. Malebranche R, Arnoux E, Grerin JM, et al. Acquired immunodeficiency syndrome with severe gastrointestinal manifestations in Haiti. Lancet. 1985;2:873–878.

34. Murquart KH, Muller HA, Sailer J, et al. Slim disease (AIDS). Lancet. 1985;2:1186–1187.

35. Kamradt T, Niese D, Vogel F. Slim disease (AIDS). Lancet. 1985;2:1425. Letter.

36. World Health Organization. Acquired immunodeficiency syndrome (AIDS). WHO/CDC case definition to AIDS. Wkly Epidemiol Rec. 1986;61:69–76.

37. Kotler DP, Gaetz HP, Lange M, et al. Enteropathy associated with the acquired immunodeficiency syndrome. Ann Intern Med. 1984;101:421–428.

38. Antony MA, Brandt LJ, Klein RS, et al. Infectious diarrhea in patients with AIDs. Dig Dis Sci. 1988;33:1141–1146.

39. Bartlesman JF, Sars PR, Tytgat GN. Gastrointestinal complications in patients with acquired immunodeficiency. Scand J Gastroenterol. 1989;24:112–117.

40. Chlebowski RT, Grosvenor MB, Bernhard NH, et al. Nutritional status, gastrointestinal dysfunction, and survival in patients with AIDS. Am J Gastroenterol. 1989;84:1288–1293.

41. Centers for Disease Control. Revision of the CDC surveillance case definition for acquired immunodeficiency syndrome. MMWR 1987;365:150–155.

42. Quinn TC. Gastrointestinal manifestations of human immunodeficiency virus. In: Gottlieb MS, ed. Current Topics in AIDS. New York. 1987;2:155.

43. Smith PD, Lane HC, Gill VJ, et al. Intestinal infections in patients with the acquired immunodeficiency syndrome (AIDS): Etiology and response to therapy. Ann Intern Med. 1988;108:328–333.

44. Dworkin B, Wormser GP, Rosenthal WS, et al. Gastrointestinal manifestations of the acquired immunodeficiency syndrome: A review of 22 cases. Am J Gastroenterol. 1985;80:774–778.

45. Laughon BE, Druckman DA, Vernon A, et al. Prevalence of enteric pathogens in homosexual men with and without acquired immunodeficiency syndrome. Gastroenterology. 1988;94:984–993.

46. Rene E, Marche C, Regnier B, et al. Intestinal infections in patients with acquired immunodeficiency syndrome. Dig Dis Sci. 1989;34:773–780.

47. Greenson JK, Belitsos PC, Yardley JH, et al. AIDS enteropathy: Occult enteric infections and duodenal mucosal alterations in chronic diarrhea. Ann Intern Med. 1991;114:366–372.

48. MacDonell KB, Glassroth J. Mycobacterium avium complex and other nontuberculous mycobacteria in patients with HIV infection. Semin Respir Infect. 1989;4:123–132.

49. Connolly GM, Shanson D, Hawkins DA, et al. Non-cryptosporidial diarrhoea in human immunodeficiency virus (HIV) infected patients. Gut. 1989;30:195–200.

50. Horsburgh RC. Mycobacterium avium complex infection in the acquired immunodeficiency syndrome. N Engl J Med. 1991;324:1332–1338.

51. Hawkins CC, Gold JWM, Whimbey E, et al. Mycobacterium avium complex infections in patients with the acquired immunodeficiency syndrome. Ann Intern Med. 1986;105:184–188.

52. Gray JR, Rabeneck L. Atypical mycobacteria infection of the gastrointestinal tract in AIDS patients. Am J Gastroenterol. 1989;84:1521–1524.

53. Damsker B, Bottone EJ. Mycobacterium avium–Mycobacterium intracellulare from the intestinal tracts of patients with acquired immunodeficiency syndrome: Concepts regarding acquisition and pathogenesis. J Infect Dis. 1985;151:179–181.

54. Kiehn TE, Edwards FF, Brannon P, et al. Infections caused by Mycobacterium avium complex in immunocompromised patients: Diagnosis by blood cultures and fecal examination, antimicrobial and seroagglutination characteristics. J Clin Microbiol. 1985;21:168–173.

55. Gillin JS, Urmacher C, West R, et al. Disseminated Mycobacterium avium–intracellulare infection in acquired immunodeficiency syndrome mimicking Whipple's disease. Gastroenterology. 1983;85:1187–1191.

56. Agins BD, Berman DS, Spicehandler D, et al. Effect of combined therapy with Ansamycin, clofazimine, ethambutol and isoniazid for Mycobacterium avium infection in patients with AIDS. J Infect Dis. 1989;159:784–787.

57. Hoy J, Mijch A, Sandland M, et al. Quadruple-drug therapy for *Mycobacterium avium-intracellulare* bacteremia in AIDS patients. J Infect Dis. 1990;161:801–805.

58. Horsburgh CR, Havlik JA, Metchock BG, et al. Oral therapy of disseminated *Mycobacterium avium* complex infection in AIDS relieves symptoms and is well tolerated. Am Rev Respir Dis. 1991;143:A115. Abstract.

59. Celem CL, Chaisson RE, Rutherford GW, et al. Incidence of salmonellosis in patients with AIDS. J Infect Dis. 1987;156:998–1001.

60. Sperber SJ, Schleuner CJ. Salmonellosis during infection with human immunodeficiency virus. Rev Infect Dis. 1987;9:925–934.

61. Bottone EJ, Wormser GP, Duncanson FP. Non-typhoidal *Salmonella* bacteremia as an early infection in acquired immunodeficiency syndrome. Diagn Microbiol Infect Dis. 1984;2:247–250.

62. Jacobs JL, Gold JW, Murray HW, et al. *Salmonella* infections in patients with acquired immunodeficiency syndrome. Ann Intern Med. 1985;102:186–188.

63. Smith PD, Macher AM, Bookman MA, et al. *Salmonella typhimurium* enteritis and bacteremia in the acquired immunodeficiency virus syndrome. Ann Intern Med. 1985;102:207–209.

64. Levine WC, Buehler JW, Bean NH, et al. Epidemiology of nontyphoidal *Salmonella* bacteremia during the human immunodeficiency virus epidemic. J Infect Dis. 1991;164:81–87.

65. Gilks CF, Brindle RJ, Otieno LS, et al. Life-threatening bacteriaemia in HIV-1 seropositive adults admitted to hospital in Nairobi, Kenya. Lancet. 1990;336:545–549.

66. Glaser JB, Morton-Kute L, Berger SR, et al. Recurrent *Salmonella typhimurium* bacteremia associated with the acquired immunodeficiency syndrome. Ann Intern Med. 1985;102:189–193.

67. Mayer KH, Hanson E. Recurrent *Salmonella* infection with a single strain in the acquired immunodeficiency syndrome. Confirmation by plasmid fingerprinting. Diagn Microbiol Infect Dis. 1986;4:71–76.

68. Connolly GM, Forbes A, Gazzard BG. Investigation of seemingly pathogen-negative diarrhoea in patients infected with HIV-1. Gut. 1990;31:886–889.

69. Baskin DH, Lax JD, Barenberg D. *Shigella* bacteremia in patients with the acquired immune deficiency syndrome. Am J Gastroenterol. 1987;82:338–341.

70. Simor AE, Poon R, Borczyk A. Chronic *Shigella flexneri* infection preceding development of acquired immunodeficiency syndrome. J Clin Microbiol. 1989;27:353–355.

71. Dworkin B, Wormser GP, Abdoo RA, et al. Persistence of multiply antibiotic-resistant *Campylobacter jejuni* in a patient with the acquired immunodeficiency syndrome. Am J Med. 1986;80:965–970.

72. Perlman DM, Ampel NM, Schifman RB, et al. Persistent *Campylobacter jejuni* infections in patients infected with the human immunodeficiency virus. Ann Intern Med. 1988;108:540–546.

73. Mintz L, Drew L, Miner RC, et al. Cytomegalovirus infections in homosexual men: An epidemiologic study. Ann Intern Med. 98:326–329.

74. Jacobson MA, Mills J. Serious cytomegalovirus disease in acquired immunodeficiency syndrome (AIDS): Clinical findings, diagnosis, and treatment. Ann Intern Med. 1988;108:585–594.

75. Dieterich DT, Rahmin M. Cytomegalovirus colitis in AIDS: Presentation in 44 patients and a review of the literature. J Acquir Immune Defic Syndr. 1991;4:S29–S35.

76. Frances ND, Boylston AW, Roberts AHG, et al. Cytomegalovirus infection in gastrointestinal tracts of patients infected with HIV-1 or AIDS. J Clin Pathol. 1989;42:1055–1064.

77. Meiselman MS, Cello JP, Margaretten W. Cytomegalovirus colitis: Report of the clinical, endoscopic, and pathologic findings in two patients with the acquired immune deficiency syndrome. Gastroenterology. 1985;88:171–175.

78. Chachoua A, Dieterich D, Krasinski K, et al. DHPG (ganciclovir) in the treatment of cytomegalovirus gastrointestinal disease with acquired immunodeficiency syndrome. Ann Intern Med. 1987;107:133–137.

79. Nelson MR, Connolly GM, Hawkins DA, et al. Foscarnet in the treatment of cytomegalovirus infection of the esophagus and colon in patients with the acquired immune deficiency syndrome. Am J Gastroenterol. 1991;86:876–881.

80. Safrin S, Crumpacker C, Chatis P, et al. A controlled trial comparing foscarnet with vidarabine for acyclovir-resistant mucocutaneous herpes simplex in the acquired immunodeficiency syndrome. N Engl J Med. 1991;325:551–555.

81. Janoff EN, Orenstein JM, Manischewitz JF, et al. Adenovirus colitis in the acquired immunodeficiency syndrome. Gastroenterology. 1991;100:976–979.

82. Levy JA, Margaretten W, Nelson J. Detection of HIV in enterochromaffin cells in the rectal mucosa of an AIDS patient. Am J Gastroenterol. 1989;84:787–789.

83. Fox CH, Kotler DP, Tierney AR, et al. Detection of HIV-1 RNA in the lamina propria of patients with AIDS and gastrointestinal disease. J Infect Dis. 1989;159:467–471.

84. Jarry A, Cartez A, Rene E, et al. Infected and immune cells in the gastrointestinal tract of AIDS patients: An immunohistochemical study of 127 cases. Histopathology. 1990;16:133–140.

85. Kotler DP, Francisco A, Clayton F, et al. Small intestinal injury and parasitic diseases in AIDS. Ann Intern Med. 1990;113:444–449.

86. Harriman GR, Smith PD, Horne MK, et al. Vitamin B_{12} malabsorption in patients with acquired immunodeficiency syndrome. Arch Intern Med. 1989;149:2039–2041.

87. Ullrich R, Zeitz M, Heise W, et al. Small intestinal structure and function in patients infected with human immunodeficiency virus (HIV): Evidence for HIV-induced enteropathy. Ann Intern Med. 1989;111:15–21.

88. Soave R, Danner RL, Honig CL, et al. Cryptosporidiosis in homosexual men. Ann Intern Med. 1984;110:504–511.

89. Madi K, Trajman A, DaSilva CF, et al. Jejunal biopsy in HIV-infected patients. J Acquir Immune Defic Syndr. 1991;4:930–937.

90. Garcia LS, Current WL. Cryptosporidiosis: Clinical features and diagnosis. Crit Rev Clin Lab Sci. 1989;27:439–460.

91. Malbranche R, Arnoux E, Guerin JM, et al. Acquired immunodeficiency syndrome with severe gastrointestinal manifestations in Haiti. Lancet. 1983;2:873–878.

92. Colebunders R, Francis H, Mann JM, et al. Persistent diarrhea strongly associated with HIV infection in Kinshasa, Zaire. Am J Gastroenterol. 1987;82:859–863.

93. Ravn P, Lundgren JD, Kjaeldgaard P, et al. Nosocomial outbreak of cryptosporidiosis in AIDS patients. Br Med J. 1991;302:277–280.

94. Current WL, Reese NC, Ernst JV, et al. Human cryptosporidiosis in immunocompetent and immunodeficient persons: Studies of an outbreak and experimental transmission. N Engl J Med. 1984;388:1252–1257.

95. Wolfson JS, Richter JM, Waldron MA, et al. Cryptosporidiosis in immunocompetent patients. N Engl J Med. 1985;312:1278–1282.

96. Soave R, Armstrong D. *Cryptosporidium* and cryptosporidiosis. Rev Infect Dis. 1986;8:1012–1023.

97. Janoff EN, Reller LB. *Cryptosporidium* species, a protean protozoan. J Clin Microbiol. 1987;25:967–975.

98. Lefkowitch JH, Krumholz S, Feng-Chen KC, et al. Cryptosporidiosis of the human small intestine: A light and electron microscopic study. Hum Pathol. 1984;15:746–752.

99. Ma P, Soave R. Three-step stool examination for cryptosporidiosis in 10 homosexual men with protracted watery diarrhea. J Infect Dis. 1983;147:824–828.

100. Sterling CR, Arrowood MJ. Detection of *Cryptosporidium* and cryptosporidiosis. Rev Infect Dis. 1986;8:1012.

101. Saez-Llorens X, Odio CM, Umana MA, et al. Spiramycin vs. placebo for the treatment of acute diarrhea caused by cryptosporidium. Pediatr Infect Dis J. 1989; 8:136–140.

102. Fafard J, Lalonde R. Long-standing symptomatic cryptosporidiosis in a normal man: Clinical response to spiramycin. J Clin Gastroenterol. 1990;12:190–191.

103. Shadduck JA. Human microsporidiosis and AIDS. Rev Infect Dis. 1989;11:203–207.

104. Cali A, Owen RL. Intracellular development of *Enterocytozoon*, a unique microsporidian found in the intestine of AIDS patients. J Protozol. 1990;37:145–155.

105. Eeftinck-Schattenkerk JK, van Gool T, van Ketel RJ, et al. Clinical significance of small-intestinal microsporidiosis in HIV-1–infected individuals. Lancet. 1991; 337:895–898.

106. Orenstein JM, Chiang J, Steinberg W, et al. Intestinal microsporidiosis as a cause of diarrhea in human immunodeficiency virus–infected patients: A report of 20 cases. Human Pathol. 1990;21:475–481.

107. Peacock CS, Blanshard C, Tovey DG, et al. Histological diagnosis of intestinal microsporidiosis in patients with AIDS. J Clin Pathol. 1991;44:558–563.

108. van Gool T, Hollister WS, Eeftinck-Schattenkerk J, et al. Diagnosis of *Enterocytozoon bieneusi* microsporidiosis in AIDS patients by recovery of spores from faeces. Lancet. 1990;336:697–698.

109. Weber R, Bryan RT, Schwartz DA, Owen RL. Human microsporidial infections. Clin Microbiol Rev. 1994;7: in press.

110. Faust EC, Giraldo LE, Caicedo G, et al. Human isosporosis in the Western hemisphere. Am J Trop Med Hyg. 1961;10:343–350.

111. Dehovitz JA, Pape JW, Boney M, et al. Clinical manifestations and therapy of *Isospora belli* infections in patients with the acquired immunodeficiency syndrome. N Engl J Med. 1986;315:87–90.

112. Soave R, Johnson WD Jr. *Cryptosporidium* and *Isospora belli* infections. J Infect Dis. 1988;157:225–229.

113. Pape JW, Johnson WD Jr. *Isospora belli* infections. Prog Clin Parasitol. 1991;2:119–127.

114. Restrep C, Macher AM, Radny EH. Disseminated extraintestinal isosporiasis in a patient with acquired immunodeficiency syndrome. Am J Clin Pathol. 1987;87:536.

115. Ng E, Markell EK, Flemming RL, et al. Demonstration of *Isospora belli* by acid fast stain in a patient with acquired immune deficiency syndrome. J Clin Microbiol. 1984;20:384–386.

116. Quinn TC, Stamm WE. Proctitis, proctocolitis, enteritis, and esophagitis in homosexual men. In: Holmes KK, Mardh PA, Sparling PF, et al., eds. Sexually Transmitted Diseases. New York: McGraw-Hill, 1990:663–683.

117. Quinn TC, Stamm WE, Goodell SE, et al. The polymicrobial origin of intestinal infections in homosexual men. N Engl J Med. 1983;309:576–582.

118. Pearce RB, Abrams DI. *Entamoeba histolytica* in homosexual men. N Engl J Med. 1987;316:960–961.

119. Allason-Jones E, Mindel A, Sargeaunt P, et al. *Enta-*

120. Hall-Crags M, Soltzberg DM. Fulminant amebic colitis in a homosexual man. Am J Gastroenterol. 1986; 81:209–212.

121. Reed SL, Wessel DW, Davis CE. *Entamoeba histolytica* infection and AIDS. Am J Med. 1991;90:269–270.

122. Senay H, MacPherson D. *Blastocystis hominis:* Epidemiology and natural history. J Infect Dis. 1990;162:987–990.

123. May RG, MacLeod CL, Whiteside ME. Intestinal colonization of *Blastocystis hominis* in a homosexual male community. In: Am Soc Trop Med and Hygiene. Proc and Abst of the 32nd Annual Meeting. Baltimore: American Society for Tropical Medicine and Hygiene. 1983.

124. Garavelli PL, Scaglione L, Bicocchi R, et al. Blastocystosis: A new disease in the acquired immunodeficiency syndrome? Int J STD AIDS. 1990;1:134–135.

125. Cello JP, Grendell JH, Basuk P, et al. Effect of octreotide on refractory AIDS-associated diarrhea. Ann Intern Med. 1991;115:705–710.

126. Johanson JF, Sonnenberg A. Efficient management of diarrhea in the acquired immunodeficiency syndrome (AIDS): A medical decision analysis. Ann Intern Med. 1990;112:942–948.

127. Connolly GM, Ellis DS, Williams JE, et al. Use of electron microscopy in examination of faeces and rectal and jejunal biopsy specimens. J Clin Pathol. 1991;44:313–316.

128. Nerurkar L, Goedert J, Wallen W, et al. Study of antiviral antibodies in sera of homosexual men. Fed Proc. 1983;42:C109.

129. Siegel FP, Lopez C, Hammer GS, et al. Severe acquired immunodeficiency in male homosexuals manifested by chronic perianal ulcerative herpes simplex lesion. N Engl J Med. 1981;305:1439–1444.

130. Samarasinghe PL, Oates JK, MacLennan IPB. Herpetic proctitis and sacral radiculomyelopathy: A hazard for homosexual men. Br Med J. 1979;2:365–366.

131. Abcarian H, Sharon N. Long term effectiveness of the immunotherapy of anal condylomata acuminata of the anus. Surg Gynecol Obstet. 1982;155:865–867.

132. Douglas JM, Rogers M, Judson FN. The effect of asymptomatic infection with HTLV-III on the response of anogenital warts to intralesional treatment with recombinant alpha 2-interferon. J Infect Dis. 1984;154:331–334.

133. Law CLH, Qassim M, Cunningham AL, et al. Nonspecific proctitis: Association with human immunodeficiency virus infection in homosexual men. J Infect Dis. 1992;165:150–154.

134. Glasgow BJ, Anders K, Layfield LJ, et al. Clinical and pathologic findings of the liver in the acquired immune deficiency syndrome. Am J Clin Pathol. 1985; 83:582–588.

135. Margulis SJ, Honig CL, Soave R, et al. Biliary tract obstruction in the acquired immunodeficiency syndrome. Ann Intern Med. 1986;105:207.

136. Blumberg RS, Kelsey P, Perrone T, et al. Cytomegalovirus and *Cryptosporidium* associated acalculous gangrenous cholecystitis. Am J Med. 1984;76:1118.

137. Kavin H, Jonas RB, Chowdhury L, et al. Acalculous cholecystitis and cytomegalovirus infection in the acquired immunodeficiency syndrome. Ann Intern Med. 1986;104:53–54.

138. Defalque D, Menu Y, Girard PM, et al. Sonographic diagnosis of cholangitis in AIDS patients. Gastrointest Radiol. 1989;14:143–147.

139. Wilkins MJ, Lindley R, Dourakis SP, et al. Surgical pathology of the liver in HIV infection. Histopathology. 1991;18:459–464.

140. Krown SE, Gold JW, Niedzwiecki D, et al. Interferon-α with zidovudine: Safety, tolerance, and clinical and virologic effects in patients with Kaposi sarcoma associated with the acquired immunodeficiency syndrome. Ann Intern Med. 1990;112:812–821.

141. Lane HC, Davey V, Kovacs JA, et al. Interferon-α in patients with asymptomatic human immunodeficiency virus infection. A randomized, placebo-controlled trial. Ann Intern Med. 1990;112:805–811.

142. Sonnerborg A, Abebe A, Strannegard O. Hepatitis C virus infection in individuals with or without human immunodeficiency virus type 1 infection. Infection. 1990;18:347–351.

143. Schneiderman DJ, Arenson DM, Cello JP, et al. Hepatic disease in patients with acquired immune deficiency syndrome (AIDS). Hepatology. 1987;7:925.

144. Armstrong D, Young LS, Meyer RD, et al. Infectious complications of neoplastic disease. Med Clin North Am. 1971;55:729–745.

145. Engleman EJ, Benike CJ, Hoppe RT, et al. Autologous mixed lymphocyte reaction in patients with Hodgkins disease. J Clin Invest. 1980;66:149–158.

146. Cline MJ. Defective mononuclear phagocytic function in myelomonocytic leukemia and some patients with lymphoma. J Clin Invest. 1973;52:2815–2819.

147. Rampling A, Warren RE, Bevan PC, et al. Clostridium difficile in haematological malignancy. J Clin Pathol. 1985;38:445–451.

148. Fekety R, Kim KH, Brown D, et al. Epidemiology of antibiotic associated colitis: Isolation of Clostridium difficile from the hospital environment. Am J Med. 1981;70:906–908.

149. Chang TW, Lauermann M, Bartlett JG. Cytotoxicity assay in antibiotic-associated colitis. J Infect Dis. 1979;140:765–770.

150. Silva J, Batts DH, Fekety R. Treatment of Clostridium difficile colitis and diarrhea with vancomycin. Am J Med. 1981;71:815–822.

151. Cherry RD, Portnoy D, Jabbari M, et al. Metronidazole: An alternative therapy for antibiotic-associated colitis. Gastroenterology. 1982;82:849–851.

152. Schimpff SC, Young VM, Green WH, et al. Origin of infection in acute nonlymphocytic leukemia: Significance of hospital acquisition of potential pathogens. Ann Intern Med. 1972;77:707–714.

153. Schimpff SC, Moody MM, Young VM. Relationship of colonization with Pseudomonas aeruginosa to development of Pseudomonas bacteremia in cancer patients. Antimicrob Agents Chemother. 1970;10:240–244.

154. Schimpff SC. Surveillance cultures. J Infect Dis. 1981;144:81–84.

155. Karp JE, Merz WG, Hendricksen C, et al. Oral norfloxacin for prevention of gram-negative bacterial infection in patients with acute leukemia and granulocytopenia: A randomized, double-blind, placebo-controlled trial. Ann Intern Med. 1987;106:1–7.

156. Decker AW, Rozenberg-Arska M, Sixma JJ, et al. Prevention of infection by trimethoprim-sulfamethoxazole plus amphotericin B in patients with acute nonlymphocytic leukemia. Ann Intern Med. 1981;95:555–559.

157. Verhoef J, Rozenberg-Arska M, Decker AW. Prevention of infection in the neutropenic patient. Rev Infect Dis. 1989;2(suppl 7):S1545–S1550.

158. Qi-nan W, Zhong-da Q. Infection in acute leukemia: An analysis of 433 episodes. Rev Infect Dis. 1989;2:S1613–S1620.

159. Mulholland MW, Delaney JP. Neutropenic colitis and aplastic anemia: A new association. Ann Surg. 1983;197:84–90.

160. Alt B, Glass NR, Sollinger H. Neutropenic enterocolitis in adults: Review of the literature and assessment of surgical intervention. Am J Surg. 1985;149:405–408.

161. Rampling A, Warren RE, Berry PJ, et al. Atypical Clostridium difficile colitis in neutropenic patients. Lancet. 1982;2:162–163.

162. Feyer P, Hoffmann FA, Standke E, et al. Acute and late effects in the course of and after total body irradiation following bone marrow transplantation in patients with different forms of leukemia. Folia Haematol. 1989;116:487–491.

163. Vogler WR, Winton EF, Heffner LT, et al. Ophthalmological and other toxicities related to cytosine arabinoside and total body irradiation as preparative regimen for bone marrow transplantation. Bone Marrow Transplant. 1990;6:405–409.

164. Meyers JD, Atkinson K. Infection in bone marrow transplantation. Clin Haematol. 1983;12:791–811.

165. Milliken ST, Powles RL. Antifungal prophylaxis in bone marrow transplantation. Rev Infect Dis. 1990; 12:S374–S379.

166. Jones RJ, Lee KS, Beschorner WE, et al. Veno-occlusive disease of the liver following bone marrow transplantation. Transplant. 1987;44:778–783.

167. Shulman HM, McDonald GB, Mathews D, et al. An analysis of hepatic veno-occlusive disease and centrilobular hepatocyte degeneration following bone marrow transplantation. Gastroenterology. 1980;79:1178–1191.

168. Wade JC, Newton B, Mclaren C, et al. Intravenous acyclovir to treat mucocutaneous herpes simplex virus infection after marrow transplantation: A double-blind trial. Ann Intern Med. 1982;96:265–269.

169. Yolken RH, Bishop CA, Townsend TR, et al. Infectious gastroenteritis in bone marrow transplant recipients. N Engl J Med. 1982;306:1009–1012.

170. Blakey JL, Barnes GL, Bishop RF, et al. Infectious diarrhea in children undergoing bone-marrow transplantation. Aust N Z J Med. 1989;19:31–36.

171. McDonald GB, Sharma P, Hackman RC, et al. Esophageal infections in the immunosuppressed patients after marrow transplantation. Gastroenterology. 1985; 88:1111–1117.

172. Spencer GD, Hackman RC, McDonald GB, et al. A prospective study of unexplained nausea and vomiting after marrow transplantation. Transplantation. 1986; 42:602–607.

173. Yolken RH, Kim HW, Clem T, et al. Enzyme-linked immunosorbent assay (ELISA) for detection of human reovirus-like agent of infantile gastroenteritis. Lancet. 1977;2:263–267.

174. Middleton PJ, Holdaway MD, Petore M, et al. Solid phase radioimmunoassay for the detection of rotavirus. Infect Immun. 1977;16:439–444.

175. Carlson JAK, Middleton PJ, Szymanski MT, et al. Fatal rotavirus gastroenteritis: An analysis of 21 cases. Am J Dis Child. 1978;132:477–479.

176. Collier AC, Miller JD, Meyers JD. Cryptosporidiosis after marrow transplant: Person-to-person transmission and treatment with spiramycin. Ann Intern Med. 1985;103:218–221.

177. Glucksberg H, Storb R, Fefer A, et al. Clinical manifestations of graft-vs-host disease in human recipients of marrow from HL-A–matched sibling donors. Transplantation. 1974;18:295–304.

178. Weisdorf DJ, Snover DC, Haake R, et al. Acute upper gastrointestinal graft-versus-host disease: Clinical significance and response to immunosuppressive therapy. Blood. 1990;76:624–629.

179. Lerner KG, Kao GF, Storb R, et al. Histopathology of graft-vs.-host reaction (GvHR) in human recipients of marrow from HL-A–matched sibling donors. Transplant Proc. 1974;6:367–371.

180. Slavin RE, Woodruff JM. The pathology of bone marrow transplantation. Pathol Annu. 1974;9:291–344.

181. Beschorner WE, Yardley JH, Tutschka PJ, et al. Deficiency of intestinal immunity with graft-vs-host disease in humans. J Infect Dis. 1981;144:38–46.

182. Ely P, Dunitiz J, Rogosheske J, et al. Use of a somatostatin analogue, octreotide acetate, in the management of acute gastrointestinal graft-versus-host disease. Am J Med. 1991;90:707–710.

183. Armitage JO, Burns CP, Kent TH. Liver disease complicating the management of acute leukemia during remission. Cancer. 1978;41:737–742.

184. Beschorner WE, Pino J, Boitnott JK, et al. Pathology of the liver with bone marrow transplantation: Effects of busulfan, carmustine, acute graft-versus-host disease, and cytomegalovirus infection. Am J Pathol. 1980; 99:369–385.

185. Zahradnik JM, Spencer MJ, Parker DD. Adenovirus infection in the immunocompromised patient. Am J Med. 1980;68:725–732.

186. Lepinski SM, Hamilton JW. Isolated cytomegalovirus ileitis detected by colonoscopy. Gastroenterology. 1990;98:1704–1706.

187. Bromiker R, Korman SH, Or R, et al. Severe giardiasis in two patients undergoing bone marrow transplantation. Bone Marrow Transplant. 1989;4:701–703.

188. Higuchi CM, Thompson JA, Petersen FB, et al. Toxicity and immunomodulatory effects of interleukin-2 after autologous bone marrow transplantation for hematologous malignancies. Blood. 1991;77:2561–2568.

189. Storb R, Prentice RL, Sullivan KM, et al. Predictive factors in chronic graft-versus-host disease in patients with aplastic anemia treated by marrow transplantation from HLA-identical siblings. Ann Intern Med. 1983;98:461–466.

190. McDonald GB, Shulman HM, Sullivan KM, et al. Intestinal and hepatic complications of human bone marrow transplantation, part II. Gastroenterology. 1986;90:770–784.

191. McDonald GB, Sullivan KM, Plumley TF. Radiographic features of esophageal involvement in chronic graft-vs.-host disease. Am J Roentgenol. 1984;142:501–506.

192. Lenssen P, Sherry ME, Chenev CL, et al. Prevalence of nutrition-related problems among long-term survivors of allogenic marrow transplantation. J Am Diet Assoc. 1990;90:835–842.

193. Gratwohl AA, Moutsopoulos HM, Chused TM, et al. Sjögren-type syndrome after allogenic bone-marrow transplantation. Ann Intern Med. 1977;87:703–706.

194. Shulman HM, Sullivan KM, Weiden PL, et al. Chronic graft-vs.-host syndrome in man: A long term clinico-pathological study of 20 Seattle patients. Am J Med. 1980;69:204–217.

195. Snover DC, Weisdorf SA, Ramsey NK, et al. Hepatic graft-versus-host disease: A study of the predictive value of liver biopsy in diagnosis. Hepatology. 1984;4:123–130.

196. Peterson PK, Anderson RC. Infection in renal transplant recipients. Am J Med. 1986;81(suppl 1A):2–10.

197. Sutherland DER, Chan F, Foucar E, et al. The bleeding cecal ulcer in transplant patients. Surgery. 1979; 86:386–398.

198. Plotkin SA, Drew WL, Felsenstein D, Hirsch MS. Sensitivity of clinical isolates of human cytomegalovirus to 9-(1,3-dihydroxy-2-propoxymethyl) guanine. J Infect Dis. 1985;152:833–834.

199. Berk MR, Meyers AM, Cassal W, et al. Non-typhoidal salmonella infections after renal transplantation: A serious clinical problem. Nephron. 1984;37:186–189.

200. Peterson PK, Ferguson R, Fryd DS, et al. Infectious diseases in hospitalized renal transplant recipients: A prospective study of a complex and evolving problem. Medicine. 1982;61:360–372.

201. Grove DI. Strongyloidiasis in allied ex-prisoners of war in Southeast Asia. Br Med J. 1980;280:598–601.

202. DeVault GA, King JW, Rohr MS, et al. Opportunistic infections with *Strongyloides stercoralis* in renal transplantation. Rev Infect Dis. 1990;12:653–671.

203. Beaver PC, Jung RC, Cupp EW. Rhabditoidea: *Strongyloides* and related forms. In: Beaver PC, Jung RC, Cupp EW, eds. Clinical Parasitology. 9th ed. Philadelphia: Lea & Febiger; 1984:253–268.

204. Igra-Siegman Y, Kapila R, Sen P, et al. Syndrome of massive hyperinfection with *Strongyloides stercoralis*. Rev Infect Dis. 1981;3:397–407.

205. Fagundes LA, Busato O, Brentano L, et al. *Strongyloides:* Fatal complication of renal transplantation. Lancet. 1971;2:439–440.

206. Powell RW, Moss JP, Nagar D, et al. Stronglyloidiasis in immunosuppressed hosts: Presentation as massive lower gastrointestinal bleeding. Arch Intern Med. 1980;140:1061–1063.

207. Boram LH, Keller KF, Justus DE, et al. *Stronglyoides* in immunosuppressed patients. Am J Clin Pathol. 1981;76:778–781.

208. Purtilo DT, Meyers WM, Connor DH. Fatal strongyloidiasis in immunosuppressed patients. Am J Med. 1974;56:488–493.

209. Dwork KG, Jaffe JR, Lieberman HD. *Strongyloides* with massive hyperinfection. N Y State J Med. 1975;75:1230–1234.

210. Purtilo DT, Meyers WM, Connor DH. Fatal strongyloidiasis in immunosuppressed patients. Am J Med. 1974;56:488–493.

211. Eveland LK, Kenney M, Yermakov V. Laboratory diagnosis of autoinfection in strongyloidiasis. Am J Pathol. 1975;63:421–425.

212. Kenney M, Webber CA. Diagnosis of strongyloidiasis in Papanicolaou-stained sputum smears. Acta Cytol. 1974;18:270–273.

213. Drugs for parasitic infections. Med Lett Drugs Ther. 1993;35:111–122.

214. Fowler CG, Lindsay I, Levin J, et al. Recurrent hyperinfestation with *Strongyloides stercoralis* in a renal allograft recipient. Br Med J. 1982;285:1394.

215. Kusne S, Dummer JS, Singh N, et al. Infections after liver transplantation: An analysis of 101 consecutive cases. Medicine 1988;67:132–143.

216. Ho M, Wajszczuk CP, Hardy JS, et al. Infections in kidney, heart and liver transplant recipients on cyclosporine. Transplant Proc. 1983;15:2768–2772.

217. Mavoral JL, Loeffler CM, Fasola CG, et al. Diagnosis and treatment of cytomegalovirus disease in transplant patients based on gastrointestinal tract manifestations. Arch Surg. 1991;126:202–206.

218. Augustine SM, Yeo CJ, Buchman TG, et al. Gastrointestinal complications in heart and in heart-lung transplant patients. J Heart Lung Transplant. 1991;10:547–555.

219. DiGeorge AM. Congenital absence of the thymus and its immunologic consequences: Concurrence with congenital hypoparathyroidism. Birth Defects. 1968;4:116.

220. Ammann AJ, Hong R. Disorders of the T-cell system. In: Stiehm ER, ed. Immunologic Disorders in Infants and Children, 3rd ed. Philadelphia: WB Saunders; 1989:257–315.

221. Hallak A, Yust I, Ratan Y, et al. Malabsorption syndrome, coccidiosis, combined immune deficiency and fulminant lymphoproliferative disease. Arch Intern Med. 1983;142:196–197.

222. Cahill LT, Ainbender E, Glade PR. Chronic mucocutaneous candidiasis: T-cell deficiency associated with B cell dysfunction in man. Cell Immunol. 1974;14:215–225.

223. Ammann AJ, Hong R. Disorders of the T-cell system.

In: Stiehm ER, ed. Immunologic Disorders in Infants and Children, 3rd ed. Philadelphia: WB Saunders; 1989:257–315.

224. Meade RH. Treatment of chronic mucocutaneous candidiasis. Ann Intern Med. 1979;86:314–315.

225. Rosenblatt HM, Byrne WJ, Ament ME, et al. Successful treatment of chronic mucocutaneous candidiasis with ketoconazole. J Pediatr. 1980;97:657–660.

226. Hay RJ, Clayton YM, Moore MK, et al. Fluconazole in the management of patients with chronic mucocutaneous candidiasis. Br J Dermatol. 1988;119:683–684.

227. Bachman R. Studies on the serum gamma A-globulin level III. The frequency of a gamma-A-globulinemia. Scand J Clin Lab Invest. 1965;17:316.

228. Ochs HD, Wedgewood RJ. Disorders of the B-cell system. In: Stiehm ER, ed. Immunologic Disorders in Infants and Children, 3rd ed. Philadelphia: WB Saunders; 1989:226–256.

229. Ammann AJ, Hong R. Selective IgA deficiency: Presentation of 30 cases and a review of the literature. Medicine. 1971;50:223.

230. Crabbe PA, Heremans JF. Selective IgA deficiency with steatorrhea: A new syndrome. Am J Med. 1967;42:319.

231. Burgio GR, Duse M, Monafo V, et al. Selective IgA deficiency: Clinical and immunological evaluation of 50 pediatric patients. Eur J Pediatr. 1980;133:101–106.

232. McCarthy DM, Katz SI, Gazze L, et al. Selective IgA deficiency associated with total villous atrophy of the small intestine and an organ-specific anti-epithelial cell antibody. J Immunol. 1978;120:932–938.

233. Gabrielson AE, Cooper MD, Peterson RDA, et al. The primary immunologic deficiency diseases. In: Miescher PA, Muller-Eberhard HJ, eds. Textbook of Immunopathology. New York: Grune & Stratton; 1969;2:385–405.

234. Ament ME, Ochs HD, Davis SD. Structure and function of the gastrointestinal tract in primary immunodeficiency syndrome: A study of 39 patients. Medicine. 1973;52:227–248.

235. Ochs HD, Ament ME, Davis SD. Giardiasis with malabsorption in X-linked agammaglobulinemia. N Engl J Med. 1972;287:341–342.

236. McKinney RE, Katz SL, Wilfert CM. Chronic enteroviral meningoencephalitis in agammaglobulinemic patients. Rev Infect Dis. 1987;9:334–356.

237. Good RA, Page AR. Fatal complications of virus hepatitis in two patients with agammaglobulinemia. Am J Med. 1960;29:804–810.

238. Hermans PE, Diaz-Buxo JA, Stobo JD. Idiopathic late onset immunoglobulin deficiency. Am J Med. 1976; 61:221–237.

239. Stiehm ER, Clin TW, Haas A, et al. Infectious complications of the primary immunodeficiencies. Clin Immunol Immunopathol. 1986;40:69–86.

240. Nime FA, Burek JD, Page DL, et al. Acute enterocolitis in a human being infected with the protozoan Cryptosporidium. Gastroenterology. 1976;70:592–598.

241. Shelhamer JH, Neva FA, Finn DR. Persistent strongyloidiasis in an immunodeficient patient. Am J Trop Med Hyg. 1982;31:746–752.

242. Ponka A, Tilvis R, Kosunen TU. Prolonged Campylobacter gastroenteritis in a patient with hypogammaglobulinemia. Act Med Scand. 1983;213:159–160.

243. Ahnen DJ, Brown WR. Campylobacter enteritis in immune-deficient patients. Ann Intern Med. 1982; 96:187–188.

244. Strauss RG, Ghisan F, Mitros F, et al. Rectosigmoid colitis in common variable immunodeficiency disease. Dig Dis Sci. 1980;25:798–801.

245. Wright PE, Sears DA. Hypogammaglobulinemia and pernicious anemia. South Med J. 1987;80:243–246.

246. Gelfand EW, Dosch HM. Diagnosis and classification of severe combined immunodeficiency disease. Birth Defects. 1983;19:65.

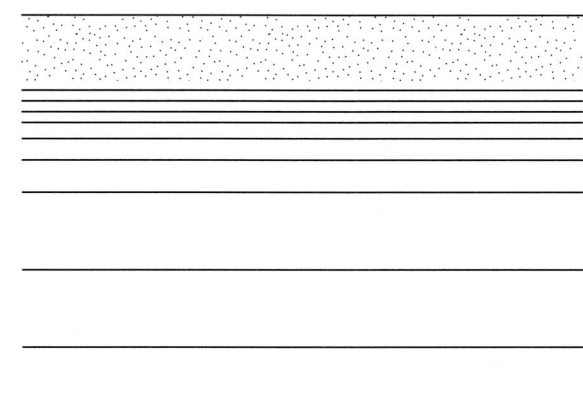

Index

Note: Page numbers in *italics* refer to illustrations; page numbers followed by t refer to tables.

C

F

ISBN 0-7216-4062-1

90038

9 780721 640624